OBSTETRICS AND THE NEWBORN

OBSTETRICS AND THE NEWBORN

An Illustrated Textbook

SECOND BRITISH EDITION

Norman A. Beischer, M.D., B.S., M.G.O., F.R.C.S. (EDIN.), F.R.A.C.S., F.R.C.O.G., F.R.A.C.O.G.
Professor of Obstetrics and Gynaecology, University of Melbourne.
Senior Obstetrician Gynaecologist, Mercy Maternity Hospital.
Chairman of the Board of Examiners for Midwifery, Victorian Nursing Council.
Editor of The Australian and New Zealand Journal of Obstetrics and Gynaecology.

Eric V. Mackay, M.B., B.S., M.G.O., F.R.C.S. (EDIN.), F.R.A.C.S., F.R.C.O.G., F.R.A.C.O.G., F.A.C.O.G. (HON.).
Professor of Obstetrics and Gynaecology, University of Queensland.
Senior Obstetrician Gynaecologist, Royal Women's and Royal Brisbane Hospitals.
Editor of The Australian and New Zealand Journal of Obstetrics and Gynaecology (1960–1982).

Baillière Tindall

LONDON PHILADELPHIA TORONTO
MEXICO CITY RIO DE JANEIRO SYDNEY TOKYO HONG KONG

Baillière Tindall   1 St Anne's Road
W. B. Saunders   Eastbourne, East Sussex BN21 3UN, England

West Washington Square
Philadelphia, PA 19105, USA

1 Goldthorne Avenue
Toronto, Ontario M8Z 5T9, Canada

Apartado 26370—Cedro 512
Mexico 4, DF Mexico

Rua Evaristo da Veiga 55, 20° andar
Rio de Janeiro—RJ, Brazil

ABP Australia Ltd, 44–50 Waterloo Road
North Ryde, NSW 2113, Australia

Ichibancho Central Building, 22–1
Ichibancho, Chiyoda-ku, Tokyo 102, Japan

10/fl, Inter-Continental Plaza, 94 Granville
Road, Tsim Sha Tsui East, Kowloon, Hong Kong

Original edition published in 1976 by Holt-Saunders Pty Ltd,
9 Waltham Street, Artarmon, NSW 2064, Australia
  Reprinted 1977, 1978, 1979, 1980, 1981, 1983, 1984
Original British edition published in 1978 by W. B. Saunders
Company Ltd
  Reprinted 1979, 1980, 1982
Second British edition 1986

Printed and bound in Great Britain by
Butler and Tanner Ltd, Frome and London

British Library Cataloguing in Publication Data

Beischer, Norman A.
   Obstetrics and the newborn: an illustrated textbook.—2nd ed.
   1. Obstetrics
   I. Title   II. Mackay, Eric V.
   618.2   RG524
   ISBN 0–7020–1163–0

Contents

This book is dedicated to
The Women in our lives
Our Mothers, Daughters, Colleagues
Our Patients and Our Wives

Preface

We have written this book because we believe that there is a need for a well-illustrated textbook of obstetrics and the neonate suitable for medical and midwifery students and primary care physicians. The textbook must be complete so that readers do not require supplementary volumes, which add to the total expense, and often cause confusion because of contradictions. There will of course be differences in learning emphasis for different members of the obstetric team. In many centres the midwife or obstetric nurse is now undertaking a significant component of the obstetric practice load, and for this reason a greater depth of knowledge is required. Many of the nursing details, deliberately omitted, can best be learned at the bedside, where the rationale for particular procedures within the institution concerned can be emphasized. In preparation of the text we have relied heavily on advice from our nursing colleagues, especially Sister Kathleen Grant (Chapter 10) and Sister Maureen Gleeson (Chapter 72).

The first chapter deals with terms and definitions; this provides a ready reference in relation to the basic language of obstetrics and facilitates understanding of the succeeding material in the text. The detailed section on questions and answers is included not only for the purposes of revision and to help the reader obtain clinical perspective, but because there should be no secrets in teaching. In the past 25 years we have spent many hours listening to coexaminers in undergraduate and postgraduate midwifery and medical examinations, and we have attempted to pass on to the reader the essence of this experience. We hope that this textbook will help students to respect the pregnant patient and to approach delivery room tuition recognizing that it is a privilege and not a right to care for a woman in labour and assist at her confinement.

A textbook of obstetrics and the neonate is only as good as its illustrations. We have avoided gruesome pictures that might upset the beginner. In writing the legends we have stressed the importance of the patient as well as the disorder, and although each illustration is referred to in the text, it has an intrinsic teaching message. We hope that the colour plates will capture the imagination of readers. We offer no apology for inclusion of rarities since they often kindle interest and provide insight. Since normality can only be stated in retrospect, it is an obligation of the obstetric attendant (midwife or doctor) to know what abnormalities may arise, enabling early detection and appropriate management. Although most of the photographs are our own, we have supplemented these from the files of the Queen Victoria Memorial Centre and Royal Women's Hospital, Melbourne.

Since the first edition was written, there have been many changes in the philosophy and practice of obstetrics and neonatal care. Perhaps the most significant has been the family-centred approach, with paternal (and sibling) roles becoming better established. Education of the parents has encouraged them to become more active in decision making, especially in relation to the many options available during labour and delivery.

One of the great strengths of obstetric care is its emphasis on prevention and early diagnosis, and this aspect has been stressed in the text. In the area of assessment of fetal well-being (both during pregnancy and labour) there have been many advances, particularly in *cardiotocography*. *Ultrasonography* has revolutionized obstetric diagnosis and management, and all relevant aspects of this modality have been included. A criticism of health care attendants, particularly doctors, is that they are now too technologically oriented. This has come about not because of the technology itself, but because its impact has not been met by sufficient empathy on the part of the attendant – the touch of a caring hand is needed as well as the ultrasonic linear array probe! An increased emphasis has been given to medical disorders; this was necessary because many patients with severe medical diseases, which are a threat to life (see Chapter 14), are aware of recent technological advances and expect to be able to reproduce with safety. The additional details included should save readers the need to purchase one of the many textbooks concerned solely with medical disorders in pregnancy.

Most chapters are introduced by an *Overview* which whets the appetite, gives perspective to the subject under discussion, and also serves as a useful revision framework. We believe that the reader will gain a bird's eye view of the subject by initially taking in the overviews and then the illustrations with the learning-orientated legends.

To help give readers perspective we have used statistics from a consecutive series of 41,000 confinements at the Mercy Maternity Hospital, to indicate the facts of clinical obstetric practice and the complications encountered – these data are summarized in Chapter 16 and are considered in more detail in the appropriate chapters.

Two new colour sections and 184 new monochrome illustrations have been included. Ultrasonographic pictures often lack the magic many patients now experience when viewing a realtime image of their fetus moving in utero – nonetheless, when studied together with the message locked in the clinical data included in the legend, the many applications of this important modality should be apparent to the reader.

A number of factors have influenced us not to continue the tradition of including references at the end of each chapter. We feel that in the present book, the current literature has been well sifted, and the student, primary care physician or obstetric nurse will have little enough time as it is to master the text provided. Adequate monographs and retrieval systems now exist to expand the reader's knowledge of the past, and current journals are more appropriate to keep abreast of newer developments.

Again, significant effort has been devoted to the index, since it is realized that text learning is often matched to clinical experience and the learner needs access to relevant material; text, illustrative and examination material have been designated separately.

No matter how often witnessed, the miracle of birth and the appeal of the newborn infant will always remain, and this, together with the modern emphasis on quality of survival, is what obstetrics and this textbook is all about. We hope that it will help others to care, in the fullest sense of the word, for the mother and her baby. We also hope that our readers will derive the enjoyment from the text that we did in attending to the many details of its preparation.

Acknowledgements

We wish to thank our colleagues at the Mercy Maternity Hospital, Queen Victoria Medical Centre, Royal Brisbane Hospital and Royal Women's Hospital for permission to reproduce photographs of patients. We also acknowledge our indebtedness to our patients who agreed to be photographed! Although we have systematically collected photographs for this Illustrated Textbook of Obstetrics and the Newborn, the acquisition of many of them could not have been planned. We are fortunate to have been granted access to the private collections of our colleagues — an acknowledgement to these is included individually in the legends. Dr Christine Acton and Dr Susan Woodward provided advice on all aspects of ultrasonography, especially the technical details in Chapter 13, and they collaborated with us in the selection and description of all the ultrasonographs. Dr Susan A. Wheildon arranged access to the photographic files of the Queen Victoria Medical Centre and Dr Denys W. Fortune to those of the Royal Women's Hospital. Mr H.G. Berkshire, medical photographer, Queen Victoria Medical Centre, provided colour plates 5, 6, 8, 12, 33, 38, 39, 46, 49, 52, 55, 56, 58 and monochromes 22.3, 39.1A, 49.7, 49.10, 59.18, 63.6, 64.12, 65.2ABDE, 65.6, 65.7, 65.12, 65.20, 65.22–65.24, 66.6, 66.8 and 67.1. Miss M.L. Johnson, medical photographer, Royal Women's Hospital, provided colour plates 4, 13, ·14, 22, 23, 34, 36, 40, 45, 78, 80, 102, 145 and monochromes 4.3, 9.1, 14.1–14.3, 17.3, 18.2, 18.6, 19.2, 19.8, 26.1, 30.7, 37.1A, 38.4, 38.6, 43.8–43.10, 49.2, 53.2A, 54.4, 57.1, 57.2, 59.17, 65.19 and 68.1. Dr Neil Roy, Director of the Newborn Emergency Transport Service of Victoria provided monochromes 62.1, 63.10, 65.13 and 71.1.

It is a pleasure to thank the following colleagues for careful review of special chapters: Dr Jill Morrison (Chapter 8), Mr David Jeffery (Chapter 11), Dr Victor Siskind (Chapter 12), Dr John Rogers (Chapters 17 and 65), Dr Richard Kemp (Chapter 27), Dr John Price (Chapter 28), Professor Mervyn Eadie (Chapter 29), Dr Robyn Mortimer (Chapter 30), Dr Jack Fidler (Chapters 30 and 32), Dr Harry Smith (Chapter 34), Professor Lawrie Powell (Chapter 35), Dr Graeme Ratten (Appendices IIIA and IIIB), Mr Maxwell Lockhart and Dr John Wilson (Appendix IV).

It is also a pleasant duty to acknowledge the secretarial assistance of Miss Adele Hallowes, Mrs Shirley Hamilton and Miss Sylvia Dupes. The preparation of the manuscript of this textbook was made possible by the facilities provided by the Mercy Maternity Hospital Research Foundation.

This second edition is larger than its predecessor, but 10 years have seen many changes in obstetric practice — and we have further developed the theme of using illustrations to facilitate the learning process. We wish to thank Miss Pat Evans, Managing Director of Holt-Saunders Pty. Limited, Australia, for her willingness to publish this expanded textbook without changing our 2 objectives of maintenance of quality, and yet keeping the volume within the financial reach of all our readers.

The adaptation of the first edition of the book for use in the United Kingdom proved a great success. Consequently the second edition has been adapted to accommodate the differences between Australia and the United Kingdom and the Republic of Ireland, in terms of definitions and statistics, social and legal aspects, product and drug names, and, when necessary, clinical practice and responsibility. The work of adaptation has been performed admirably by Dr Tony Falconer, now Consultant Obstetrician and Gynaecologist, Plymouth General Hospital, formerly Senior Registrar in Obstetrics and Gynaecology, University Hospital, Nottingham. In addition, Miss Margaret Adams, Senior Midwife Teacher,

Queen Charlotte's Hospital, London, and her colleagues have produced the section entitled *Midwifery Notes* to enhance the text for its UK midwifery readership.

We would like to thank Her Majesty's Stationery Office for their permission to use data from *Confidential Enquiries into Maternal Deaths in England and Wales (1976–1978)* (1982), and Macfarlane, A. & Mugford, M. (1984) *Birth Counts: Statistics of Pregnancy and Childbirth*, Volumes 1 and 2. These data are Crown copyright.

chapter one

Terms and Definitions

TERMS AND DEFINITIONS (THE VOCABULARY OF OBSTETRICS)

Obstetrics is learned in the wards as well as the classroom. The basic principles are, relatively speaking, few in number. Complications are interrelated, and one cannot know a part without the whole. The best way to learn obstetrics is to think it and speak it, and of course, thoughtful conversation is impossible without an adequate vocabulary. This section is at the beginning of the book because students must master the terminology of obstetrics if they are to understand the clinical conversations of nurses and doctors in the antenatal clinic, delivery suite, nursery, and postnatal ward. Most of this information appears elsewhere in each appropriate chapter of the book. It is collected here to help the beginner get away to a good start.

Abortion. The process by which the products of conception are expelled from the uterus via the birth canal before the 28th week of gestation.

Abruptio placentae (accidental haemorrhage). Bleeding from a normally situated placenta causing its complete or partial detachment after the 28th week of gestation. The diagnosis is confirmed by the demonstration of an old retroplacental clot after delivery (figure 19.3).

Acidosis. The fetus is acidotic when the blood pH is 7.20 or less in labour or at birth, or 7.25 or less if tested at induction of labour or after elective Caesarean section.

Afterpains (after-birth pains). Uterine contractions due to release of oxytocin from the posterior lobe of the pituitary gland, especially during suckling; more intense in multiparas. They promote involution of the uterus.

Amniocentesis. Aspiration of a sample of amniotic fluid through the mother's abdomen for diagnosis of fetal maturity and/or disease by assay of the constituents of the fluid (figure 21.10).

Amnion. A smooth membrane enclosing the fetus and amniotic fluid; it is loosely fused with the outer chorionic membrane.

Amnioscope. A lighted tubular instrument which is introduced through the internal os in late pregnancy; it enables an inspection of the colour and amount of amniotic fluid through the intact membranes (figure 21.7).

Amniotic fluid embolism. Entry of amniotic fluid into the maternal venous circulation. Fetal squames, hair, and vernix become impacted in the pulmonary arterioles, and thromboplastic substances cause intravascular coagulation (colour plate 62).

Amniotomy. Surgical rupture of the membranes to induce or enhance labour.

Anaemia. A maternal haemoglobin value below 11.5 g/dl in the first trimester or below 10.5 g/dl in later pregnancy.

Anencephaly. Absence of the brain and vault of the skull (figure 51.4); the cerebellum and basal ganglia are sometimes present.

Antepartum haemorrhage. Bleeding from the birth canal in excess of 15 ml in the period from the 28th week of gestation to the birth of the baby.

Apgar score. A numerical scoring system usually applied at 1 and 5 minutes after birth to evaluate the condition of the baby, based on heart rate, respiration, muscle tone, reflexes and colour.

Areola. The pigmented zone of skin around the nipple which contains sebaceous glands. The nipple and areola become further pigmented during pregnancy (colour plate 42).

Asphyxia neonatorum. Term used to describe the condition of an infant who fails to breathe within 60 seconds of birth.

Asymptomatic bacteriuria. Bacteria in a concentration of 10^5 or more per ml of urine without symptoms. This is present in about 8% of pregnant women, about half of whom will, if untreated, develop signs of urinary tract infection during pregnancy.

Asynclitism. When the sagittal suture of the fetal skull does not lie midway between the maternal sacral promontory and pubic symphysis; there is usually disproportion, and the head is rocking fore and aft to enter the pelvis.

Attitude of the fetus. Relationship of fetal head and limbs to the fetal trunk — usually flexion (colour plate 4).

Axis traction. A fitting for the obstetric forceps which enables the direction of pull to be in the axis of the pelvic canal corresponding to the station of the head.

Bandl ring. The groove between upper and lower uterine segments; it is situated at the level of the pubic symphysis at the onset of labour.

Birth palsy. Brain damage due to intrauterine hypoxia (oxygen shortage) or cerebral haemorrhage during labour or delivery.

Birth-weight. The first weight of the newborn obtained preferably within 1 hour of birth before significant postnatal weight loss has occurred.

Bradycardia. Fetal heart rate below 120 beats per minute.

Brandt-Andrews method of expressing the placenta from the uterus: controlled cord traction is applied with one hand while the contracted uterus is pushed upwards away from the placenta with the other hand on the mother's abdomen (figure 43.3).

Braxton Hicks contractions. Spontaneous painless uterine contractions described originally as a sign of pregnancy. Occur from the first trimester onward, and probably promote uterine blood flow and transfer of oxygen to the fetus.

Breech presentation. (a) Complete: the fetus is flexed and buttocks, genitalia, and the feet present. (b) Incomplete: (i) frank breech — the legs are extended and buttocks and genitalia present; (ii) footling — one or both feet present; there is a 10% risk of cord prolapse.

Bregma. The large diamond-shaped anterior fontanelle (figure 2.14).

Brow. That part of the fetal head between the root of the nose and the anterior fontanelle (figure 51.3).

Caesarean section. Surgical removal of the uterine contents by the abdominal route after fetal viability (28 weeks) (colour plate 92).

Caput succedaneum. Oedema from obstructed venous return in the fetal scalp caused by pressure of the head against the rim of the cervix or birth canal (figures 2.16–2.19).

Cardiotocography. Use of Doppler ultrasound to make an immediate assessment of fetoplacental well-being in high risk pregnancies (figure 23.3).

Cephalhaematoma. A collection of blood beneath the periosteum of a skull bone, limited to that bone by periosteal attachments (colour plate 142).

Cervical dystocia. Difficult labour due to failure of the cervix to dilate, in spite of adequate uterine contractions (figure 49.1).

Chloasma. The brown, pigmented mask of pregnancy. Usually patchy and simulates suntan (colour plate 13); it also occurs in some women who are taking oral contraceptives.

Chorion frondosum. The part of the chorion forming the placenta.

Chorion laeve. The part of the chorion forming the extraplacental membrane.

Chromosomes. Deeply-staining bodies in the nucleus of the cell which contain the hereditary material (genes); 23 are derived from each parent, making the normal complement of 46.

Colostrum. Yellowish fluid expressed from the

breasts during pregnancy and before the onset of true lactation.

Congenital dislocation of the hip. The baby has a relaxed joint capsule and shallow acetabulum which allow the head of the femur to become displaced (colour plate 136).

Constriction ring. A localized spasm of the uterine muscle.

Coombs test. Detects sensitized red blood cells (antibody attached) — e.g. in erythroblastosis.

Cord presentation. The cord is below the presenting part with the membranes intact.

Cord prolapse. As for cord presentation except that the membranes have ruptured, and pressure on the umbilical cord vessels is more likely to occur.

Corpus luteum. The yellowish body formed from the Graafian follicle after ovulation which produces oestrogen and progesterone.

Cotyledons. The lobes of the placenta (colour plate 33).

Couvelaire uterus (uterine apoplexy). Occurs with severe abruption of the placenta. The uterus is purple due to haemorrhage within its musculature (colour plate 14).

Cramps. In most women they occur in the legs 3 to 4 times during pregnancy, and usually at night.

Crede method of placental delivery: the uterus is squeezed to express the attached placenta.

Cross-infection. Infection of a person by another person or object.

Crowning of the head. Visualization of the fetal head as birth becomes imminent. The widest diameter has passed the bony pelvic outlet and emerged from under the pubic arch (figure 42.8A).

Curve of Carus. The 90° curve of the birth canal (figure 2.13).

Decidua. The exaggerated endometrial reaction to oestrogen and progesterone during pregnancy. The glands become tortuous and the stromal cells enlarge.

Decidual cast. Decidua shed from the uterus as a single piece; a sign suggestive of ectopic pregnancy (figures 18.2 and 18.3).

Delay in the second stage of labour. More than 1 hour in a nullipara or a half-hour in a multipara.

Dextrorotation of the uterus. The pregnant uterus usually is rotated towards the right side, due to the presence of the rectum and sigmoid colon on the left side. This is relevant when avoiding injury to uterine vessels during lower segment Caesarean section.

Diameters. The distance between certain important bony points in the fetus and maternal pelvis. The following 10 should be known. (i) anteroposterior of brim (true conjugate) — 11.5 cm; (ii) transverse diameter of pelvic brim — 13.5 cm; (iii) bispinous (transverse diameter of narrow pelvic plane) — 10.5 cm; (iv) anteroposterior of outlet — 11.5 cm; (v) biparietal (between the parietal eminences) — 9.5 cm; (vi) bitemporal — 8.0 cm; (vii) occipitofrontal (from occipital protuberance to above the orbital margins) — 11–12.0 cm; (viii) suboccipitobregmatic (nape of neck to middle of anterior fontanelle) — 9.5 cm; (ix) bisacromial (between tips of acromial processes) — 12.5 cm; (x) bitrochanteric (between outer aspects of greater trochanters) — 9.5 cm (figures 2.8, 2.9 and 2.15).

Diastasis of the rectus abdominis muscles. The separation which occurs when the muscles can stretch no more. The peritoneum bulges between them when the patient coughs. Postnatal exercises are required (colour plate 75).

Discharge. Physiological vaginal secretion increases in pregnancy. The vagina has a stratified squamous epithelial lining but no glands; its moisture is provided chiefly by secretion of cervical mucus (and at coitus by vaginal transudation). If there is itching or the discharge is yellow or offensive then speculum examination is required to exclude vaginitis. Copious (perhaps blood-stained) discharge may be due to cervical incompetence.

Double monster. A fetus from a single ovum with duplication of head, trunk or limbs (colour plates 45 and 50).

Down syndrome (mongolism). A congenital abnormality characterized by the presence of an extra chromosome 21 (figure 65.2).

Dublin method of placenta delivery. The uterus is used as a piston to push the separated placenta out of the cervix and vagina.

Ductus arteriosus. The channel between pulmonary artery and descending arch of aorta which allows the right ventricular output to be shunted away from the unexpanded fetal lungs.

Duration of labour. Average is 16 hours for a

nullipara and 8 hours for a multipara.

Dystocia. Difficult or abnormal labour due to cephalopelvic disproportion or a primary disorder of uterine action.

Eclampsia. 'To flash forth'. A clinical state characterized by convulsions, not attributable to cerebral conditions such as epilepsy or cerebral haemorrhage, and usually superimposed on preceding severe preeclampsia.

Ectopic pregnancy. Implantation of the fertilized ovum outside the uterine cavity. The commonest site is in the Fallopian tube (colour plate 5).

Effacement of cervix. The cervical canal becomes taken up from above down; usually occurs during the early (latent) phase of labour (figure 40.1).

Embryo. The name given to the conceptus up to the 10th week of gestation (8th week postconception); after this, the word fetus is used.

Endometrium. The mucous membrane lining the uterus which responds to ovarian hormones during the menstrual cycle.

Engagement. The fetal head is engaged when its maximum diameters (suboccipitobregmatic and biparietal when the head is well flexed) have passed the pelvic inlet (figure 6.8).

Engorgement of breasts. Full, red, hard, sore breasts due to increased blood flow before milk secretion commences (figure 60.4).

Epidural analgesia. Injection of analgesic agent outside the dura which covers the spinal canal. A sacral (caudal) epidural gives complete analgesia of all pelvic structures (figure 41.14).

Episiotomy. An incision of perineum and vagina that enlarges the introitus and lessens the curve of the birth canal (figure 45.2).

Ergometrine. The active oxytocic principle derived from ergot.

Erythroblastosis. Haemolytic disease of the newborn due usually to rhesus antibodies. Hypoxia due to fetal anaemia stimulates production of primitive red cells (erythroblasts) which are present in excessive numbers in the blood (colour plate 123).

Exchange transfusion. The blood of the baby is gradually replaced with donor blood; most commonly used in babies with erythroblastosis, to remove harmful bilirubin pigment and rhesus positive cells, as well as to treat anaemia (colour plate 124).

Face. The area of fetal head below the root of the nose and the orbital ridges (figure 51.5).

Ferning. During the proliferative phase of the menstrual cycle cervical mucus forms a palm-leaf pattern when it dries on a slide.

Fertilization. The union of one sperm and the mature ovum; usually occurs in the outer half of the Fallopian tube.

Fetal growth retardation. Birth-weight below the tenth percentile according to gestational age for infants born in the community concerned. The term is synonymous with '*small for dates*'. Many but not all growth retarded infants show evidence of malnutrition (*placental insufficiency, dysmaturity*) (figure 21.4).

Fontanelle. Space at the junction of 3 or more skull bones, covered only by a membrane and skin (figure 2.14).

Foramen ovale. An opening in the interatrial septum which allows oxygenated blood from the umbilical vein to flow from the right to the left side of the heart.

Fourchette. The fold of skin formed by merging of the labia minora and labia majora posteriorly (figure 2.1).

Funic souffle. The sound of blood passing through the umbilical cord, synchronous with the fetal heart beat.

Funnel (android) **pelvis.** A pelvis in which midpelvic and outlet diameters are more contracted than those at the pelvic brim.

Gene. The functional unit of heredity; large numbers are situated in each of the 46 chromosomes in the cell nucleus.

Generalized oedema. Excessive accumulation of fluid in the tissues demonstrated by swelling of the legs, hands, and face (colour plate 9); one of the definitive signs of preeclampsia.

Genotype. The hereditary constitution of genes of an individual.

Grand multipara. Para 4 or more; a patient likely to have powerful uterine contractions — hence the risk of uterine rupture if there is cephalopelvic disproportion.

Gravid. Means pregnant; a primigravida is a woman pregnant for the first time.

Haemorrhoids. Enlarged haemorrhoidal veins of the lower bowel. These are common during pregnancy, particularly in labour when the head distends the perineum. Push them back after delivery to prevent them becoming swollen and painful (figure 57.1).

Heartburn. A common symptom in late pregnancy due to regurgitation of acid from the compressed stomach, more usual when the patient lies down.

Hegar sign of pregnancy. Bimanual palpation of a soft uterine isthmus between the cervix below and the uterine body above. Used before modern urine tests for pregnancy became available (figure 6.3).

High forceps. Forceps application when the head is not engaged; should not be performed because of the risk of trauma to mother and fetus.

Hyaline membrane. A homogeneous eosinophilic membrane lining the alveoli, alveolar ducts, and respiratory bronchioles; an important cause of death in premature infants (colour plate 64).

Hydatidiform mole. A condition in which there is partial or complete conversion of the chorionic villi into grape-like vesicles (colour plates 36–39). The villi are avascular and there is trophoblastic proliferation. The condition may result in malignant trophoblastic disease (invasive mole or choriocarcinoma).

Hydrocephaly. Accumulation of excessive amounts of cerebrospinal fluid within the ventricles of the brain (figure 49.4).

Hydrops fetalis. Gross oedema of fetal subcutaneous tissues together with ascites, pericardial and pleural effusion; usually due to erythroblastosis (colour plate 123).

Hyperemesis gravidarum. Vomiting during pregnancy sufficient to warrant admission of the patient to hospital.

Hypertension. A blood pressure of 140/90 or above, or a rise of 15–20 systolic and 10–15 diastolic. Essential hypertension is diagnosed when hypertension is known to be present before or during early pregnancy.

Hypofibrinogenaemia. The commonest cause of blood coagulation failure in obstetrics. The blood fibrinogen level falls below the normal of 4–6 g/l. Usually secondary to severe placental abruption, prolonged retention of a dead fetus, or amniotic fluid embolism.

Hypospadias. A malformation of the male penis where the urethra opens on its under surface or on the perineum (colour plate 58).

Hysterotomy. Removal of fetus by incision of the uterus via the abdominal route before the 28th week of gestation; after this time the operation is termed a Caesarean section.

Implantation. Penetration of the endometrium by the early fertilized ovum (blastocyst) which becomes completely surrounded by decidua (colour plate 1). Occurs 6–8 days after ovulation.

Incarceration of the gravid uterus. The uterus is retroverted and with enlargement becomes imprisoned in the pelvis, impacting beneath the sacral promontory; urethral obstruction and acute retention of urine may result (figure 37.2).

Incidental antepartum haemorrhage. Bleeding after the 28th week of gestation due to local causes (cervicitis, carcinoma of cervix, vaginitis); diagnosis is made by speculum examination.

Incompetent cervix. The cervix dilates silently during the second trimester with the result that the membranes bulge and rupture and the fetus drops out (colour plate 35). A curable cause of habitual abortion and prematurity.

Incoordinate uterine action. Fundal dominance is lost, intrauterine tension between contractions is increased, the uterus is tender on palpation, and the patient complains of backache.

Infant mortality. Death in the first year of life of infants born alive (includes neonatal deaths). The rate is 10–15 per 1,000 births in developed countries.

Introitus. Entrance to the vagina.

Inversion of the uterus. Uterus turned inside-out, usually due to pulling on the cord with the uterus relaxed (figure 54.10).

Kernicterus. Yellow staining of the baby's brain due to high blood levels of bilirubin causing severe neurological damage (bilirubin encephalopathy) or death (figure 68.1).

Labour. The process by which the products of conception are expelled from the uterus via the birth canal after the 28th week of gestation.

Lactiferous sinus. A dilatation of the mammary duct just before it enters the nipple (figure 60.1).

Left lateral position. The preferred position for rest in bed in late pregnancy; when a patient turns from the supine position to her right side, cardiac output increases 10%; from supine to her left side the increase is 20%.

Leucorrhoea. Colourless (white), nonitchy, nonoffensive vaginal discharge.

Lie of the fetus. Relationship of the long axis of

fetus to the long axis of the uterus. Usually longitudinal, but can be transverse or oblique.

Lightening. Usually occurs after 36 weeks and is commoner in nulliparas; the presenting part enters the pelvis and thus reduces the pressure on the diaphragm; the mother notices that it is easier to breathe. Lightening is not synonymous with engagement; often 3–4 cm of head remain palpable abdominally.

Linea nigra. Brown or black line of pigment in the midline of the abdominal wall during pregnancy (colour plate 65).

Living ligatures. The interlacing spirally-arranged muscle fibres of the middle muscle layer in the uterine wall; contraction of these fibres closes the blood vessels and prevents postpartum haemorrhage.

Lochia. The discharge from the uterus during the puerperium; it is initially red (lochia rubra), then yellow (serosa), and finally white (alba).

Lovset manoeuvre. Rotation and traction of the fetal trunk during breech birth to facilitate delivery of the arms and shoulders (figure 50.3).

Low birth-weight. Less than 2,500 g. Includes premature infants and growth retarded infants of maturity beyond 37 weeks. *Very low birth-weight* infants are those weighing less than 1,500 g; they comprise 1% of all births and provide 50% of perinatal deaths.

Lower uterine segment. The thin expanded lower portion of the uterus which forms from the isthmus in the last trimester of pregnancy; it provides the usual method of approach to the baby in the operation of Caesarean section (colour plate 92).

Manual removal of the placenta. Removal of the placenta by means of a hand inside the uterus; it is performed when other methods fail (figure 54.3).

Manual rotation of the occiput. Performed prior to forceps application as an alternative to forceps rotation when the mechanism of anterior rotation of the head has failed (figure 46.5).

Maternal death. Death occurring during pregnancy, childbirth, or in the first year following birth or abortion, from any cause related to or aggravated by the pregnancy or its management. The maternal mortality rate ranges from 10–40 per 100,000 total births in developed countries.

Mechanism. A formal description of how the fetus is expelled during labour.

Meconium. Greenish-black, fetal faeces composed of cellular debris, bile, lanugo, and vernix caseosa (colour plate 60).

Menarche. Onset of menstruation.

Meningomyelocele. Protrusion of the meninges and spinal cord through a defect (spina bifida) in the vertebral arches of the spine.

Montgomery follicles. Hypertrophied sebaceous glands which appear as lumps scattered throughout the areola surrounding the nipple (colour plate 41).

Morula. The mulberry-like mass of cells formed by repeated divisions of the fertilized ovum.

Moulding. Alteration in shape and diameters of the fetal head during labour. The fontanelles and sutures permit the force of contractions to compress the head against the bony pelvis and adapt its shape to that of the birth canal (colour plate 103).

Mullerian duct. An embryonic tubular structure which forms the female genital tract (Fallopian tubes, uterus, vagina).

Multigravida. A woman who is pregnant for the second or subsequent time.

Naegele rule. To estimate the probable date of confinement add 9 months and 7 days to the first day of the last menstrual period. A correction is required if the patient does not have 28-day cycles.

Narrow pelvic plane or plane of least pelvic dimensions. From the lower border of the symphysis pubis, to the ischial spines laterally and to the lower border of the fourth sacral vertebra posteriorly. This is below the midpelvic plane which runs from the middle of the symphysis, above the ischial spines, to the junction of the second and third sacral vertebrae (figure 2.13).

Neonatal death. A liveborn infant who dies within 28 days of birth.

Normal labour. A labour in which the fetus presents by the vertex, the occiput rotates anteriorly, and the result is the birth of a living, mature fetus with no complications, the duration of labour ranging from 4–24 hours.

Obstructed labour. There is no descent of the presenting part in the presence of good contractions. Usually there is extensive caput and moulding, a malposition or malpresentation, and a retraction ring (figure 52.4); the fetus is often large and the pelvis small or abnormal in shape.

Occiput. The back of the fetal head behind the posterior fontanelle.

Oligohydramnios. An insufficiency of liquor amnii (0–200 ml in the third trimester). Not uncommon and usually associated with fetal growth retardation ('intrauterine malnutrition' or 'placental insufficiency') (figure 21.6).

Operculum. The plug of mucus that occludes the cervical canal during pregnancy (colour plate 83).

Ovulation. Extrusion of the ripened ovum from the Graafian follicle in the ovary to the peritoneal cavity (and then into the tube).

Oxytocic. Hastens birth of fetus and/or placenta by stimulating contractions of the uterine muscle; by definition may accelerate first, second or third stages of labour.

Parous. The woman has delivered a viable (28 weeks or more) child. A nullipara is a woman who has never reached 28 weeks in a previous pregnancy, although she may have been pregnant more than once (multigravida).

Partograph (cervicograph) is a graphic representation of cervical dilatation and descent of the presenting part; used to indicate departure from normal and the need for active management of labour, especially in nulliparas (figure 49.9).

Pawlik grip. Suprapubic palpation with the outstretched hand to identify the presenting part of the fetus, its position, flexion and its station within the mother's pelvis (figure 6.7).

Pelvic brim or inlet. The plane (flat surface) of division between the true and false pelvis. The plane passes from the upper border of the symphysis pubis, along the pubic crest to the iliopectineal eminence, then to the sacroiliac joint, along the wings of the sacrum to the centre of the sacral promontory. The shape is transversely oval with the promontory causing a projection posteriorly (figure 2.8).

Pelvic outlet. A diamond-shaped opening which runs from beneath the symphysis pubis along the ischiopubic ramus to the ischial tuberosity (on which we sit), along the sacrotuberous ligament to the fifth piece of the sacrum (the coccyx being mobile folds back in labour) (figure 2.9).

Pelvimetry. Measurement of the size of the pelvis, either clinically or by radiography.

Pendulous abdomen. Characteristic of the obese multipara with poor muscle tone and diastasis of the rectus muscles. The uterus bulges forward and malpresentations are common.

Perinatal mortality. Stillbirths plus neonatal deaths expressed per 1,000 total births. The rate is 10–15 per 1,000 births in developed countries.

Perineal body. A triangular-shaped wedge of tissue based on the perineum, separating the lower one-third of the posterior vaginal wall from the anal canal.

Period of gestation. The number of completed weeks from the first day of the last menstrual period to the date in question.

Persistent occipitoposterior or face to pubis. Birth of the fetus with the occiput directed posteriorly; anterior rotation of the occiput fails to occur (figure 52.3).

Phenylketonuria. A hereditary enzyme deficiency which can cause mental retardation; a test is taken a few days after birth to exclude this condition; incidence 1 in 10,000 births.

Phototherapy. Use of light energy (wavelength 450 nm) to convert the bilirubin molecule in the jaundiced infant's skin to a form which can be excreted without conjugation in the liver (figure 68.3).

Pica. Eating of a substance usually considered inedible.

Placenta. The organ of communication (nutrition and products of metabolism) between the fetus and the mother. Forms from the chorion frondosum with a maternal decidual contribution (colour plate 92).

Placenta accreta. Deficiency of decidua basalis, with chorionic villi attached to uterine muscle (figure 19.8). In *placenta increta* the villi are *in* the muscle wall; in *placenta percreta* the villi are *through* the muscle wall (a variety of uterine rupture).

Placenta circumvallata. Placenta with a double fold of amnion forming a ring on the fetal surface some distance in from the edge of the placenta (figure 43.8).

Placenta membranacea. A thinner, larger placenta where there is failure of atrophy of the usual proportion of the chorionic villi (figure 43.9).

Placenta praevia. Placental implantation encroaches upon the lower uterine segment; the placenta comes first and bleeding (maternal) is almost inevitable (figure 19.7).

Placenta succenturiata. Accessory lobe of the placenta (figure 43.5); may be multiple.

Placental separation mechanisms: (a) *Schultze*. Retroplacental haematoma turns the placenta inside-out and the shiny fetal surface, with umbilical cord attached, presents. (b) *Matthews Duncan*. The placenta separates edge first and slides out with the maternal surface (cotyledons) exposed (figure 43.1).

Polyhydramnios. The clinical diagnosis of an excessive amount of liquor amnii (more than 1,500 ml) (colour plate 12).

Position of the fetus. The relationship of a defined area on the presenting part (called the denominator) to the mother's pelvis.

Positive signs of pregnancy. Signs that are infallible — fetal heart sounds, palpable fetal parts or movements, X-ray, and tests for the presence of chorionic gonadotrophic hormone in the urine or blood.

Postanal palpation. A means of recognizing that delivery is imminent — when the fetal head is palpable between anus and coccyx.

Posterior fontanelle. Small triangular space in the fetal or infant skull situated at the posterior end of the sagittal suture (figure 2.15).

Posterior position of the occiput. The fetal occipital bone is directed to the posterior aspect of the maternal pelvis, either to the left (LOP) or right (ROP). It occurs in about 15–20% of labours and is commonly associated with prolonged and difficult labour (figure 52.2).

Postpartum haemorrhage. (a) *Primary*. Blood loss in excess of 500 ml from the birth canal during the third stage and for 24 hours afterwards (colour plate 91). (b) *Secondary*. Bleeding occurring in the interval from 24 hours after delivery until the end of the puerperium.

Precipitate labour. Labour of less than 4 hours' duration.

Preeclampsia. Diagnosed when any 2 of the following signs are present: hypertension (140/90 or above), generalized oedema, proteinuria not due to infection or contamination of the urine.

Premature infant. One born before 37 completed weeks' gestation i.e. 259 days (previously, one weighing less than 2,500 g). The incidence of prematurity is 8% and it accounts for 80% of all neonatal deaths.

Premature rupture of the membranes. Spontaneous rupture of the membranes before the onset of contractions; usually the membranes rupture at the end of the first stage of labour (this flushes the vagina with a sterile fluid before the fetus is born).

Presenting part. That part of the fetus felt on vaginal examination.

Proliferative phase of menstrual cycle. The interval after menstruation and up to ovulation during which growth of the endometrium is stimulated by oestrogen from the developing Graafian follicle.

Prolonged labour. Labour of more than 24 hours' duration.

Prolonged pregnancy. Pregnancy prolonged 14 days or more past the due date of confinement (full term); the incidence is approximately 6% (table 16.1).

Prostaglandins. Naturally occurring substances in decidua, semen and many tissues. The E_1, E_2 and F_2 compounds stimulate uterine muscle activity and also cause oxytocin release from the posterior lobe of the pituitary.

Pseudocyesis. A phantom pregnancy — the patient thinks she is pregnant but she is not. A royal illness (Queen Mary) seen typically in the premenopausal nullipara anxious for a child.

Pudendal nerve block. Bilateral injection of local analgesic in the region of the ischial spines which renders the vagina and perineum insensitive to pain.

Puerperal infection. An infection of the genital tract arising as a complication of childbirth.

Puerperal morbidity. All deaths due to infection and all patients in whom the temperature reaches 38°C on any 2 of the first 14 days after delivery.

Puerperium. The period during which the reproductive organs return to their prepregnant condition — usually regarded as an interval of 6 weeks after delivery.

Quickening. When the patient first becomes aware of fetal movements; add 5 calendar months (22 weeks) to calculate the due date.

Red degeneration. A common complication of large fibromyomas in pregnancy. The cause of pain is ischaemic necrosis — the fibroid has had a 'coronary occlusion'.

Respiratory distress syndrome in the newborn. Term used to describe any infant who develops a respiratory rate above 60 per minute, has difficulties in breathing as shown by retraction of the sternum and lower costal margin, has an expiratory grunt and central cyanosis. The incidence is about 3% of neonates and the mortality rate is about 20%.

Restitution. When the fetal head is born it is free to undo any twisting caused by internal rotation.

Retained placenta. Placenta still in utero 1 hour after birth of the baby.

Retraction. The quality of uterine muscle whereby permanent shortening occurs after contractions in labour. The uterine fundus thickens and pulls up the dilating cervix like a hood over the presenting part.

Retraction ring. Occurs in obstructed labour when Bandl's ring rises to about the level of the umbilicus and becomes visible and palpable (figure 52.4).

Retroversion of the uterus. The uterine fundus lies in the rectovaginal pouch of Douglas instead of anteriorly on the bladder. Occurs in 20% of women.

Rhesus factor. An antigen attached to red blood cells capable of causing production of antibodies when introduced into the circulation of a person lacking this factor (an Rh-negative person).

Rotation of the head. (a) *Internal.* The occiput rotates to the anterior position, rarely (1–2%) posterior. (b) *External.* The head rotates after it is born because the shoulders (bisacromial diameter) are turning into the anteroposterior diameter of the pelvic outlet.

Round ligament strain. Causes pain in midpregnancy that may be confused with renal infection or red degeneration of a fibroid. The hypertrophied muscular ligament is in spasm and is readily palpated.

Sclero-oedema. Cold oedema of the newborn.

Secondary powers in labour. Voluntary muscles of the abdominal wall and diaphragm, which by their contraction increase intraabdominal pressure in the second stage of labour. Intrauterine pressure rises to 110 mm of mercury with the combined effect of primary uterine action (35–60 mm) and secondary powers (50 mm).

Secretory phase of menstrual cycle. The interval between ovulation and the succeeding menstrual period during which oestrogen and progesterone from the corpus luteum stimulate growth of the endometrium and glycogen secretion of the glands.

Shoulder dystocia (impacted shoulders). Obstruction to the passage of the shoulders through the bony pelvis, the head having been delivered — the neck fails to appear and the baby's chin burrows into the mother's perineum when the occiput is anterior.

Show. A discharge of mucus and blood at the onset of labour when the cervix dilates and the operculum (cervical mucus plug) falls out.

Sinciput. That part of the fetal head in front of the anterior fontanelle — it is subdivided into the brow and the face.

Spalding sign. Overlapping of the cranial bones seen radiographically; is a sign of fetal death if moulding due to labour can be excluded (figure 23.4).

Spurious or false labour. Painful uterine contractions without cervical effacement or dilatation.

Stages of labour. (a) The *first stage* is that of dilatation of the cervix and is finished when the uterine cavity and vagina are no longer separated by a rim of cervix (figure 40.3). (b) The *second stage* is that of expulsion of the fetus. (c) The *third stage* is that of expulsion of the placenta and membranes (secundines).

Station. The level of the presenting part within the mother's pelvis. The ischial spines are the reference points on vaginal examination (figure 41.3).

Stillbirth. An infant born after 28 weeks of pregnancy who did not breathe after birth or show any signs of life.

Striae (stretch marks). Are red or purple in colour during the pregnancy in which they first appear, later become white (colour plates 66–75).

Stripping of the membranes. A method of inducing labour. Less effective than amniotomy, but also carries the risk of infection.

Supine hypotensive syndrome. In late pregnancy 10% of patients experience faintness when lying supine due to inferior vena caval obstruction causing reduced venous return and a fall in cardiac output, there being an inadequate collateral circulation via the paravertebral veins (figure 48.1).

Suture. Term applied to the membranous junction between the bones of the fetal (and infant) skull; the chief sutures are between the frontal bones (frontal), parietal bones (sagittal), parietal and frontal (coronal), parietal and occipital (lambdoid) (figure 2.14).

Symphysiotomy. Division of the pubic symphysis to enlarge the diameters of the bony pelvis.

Tachycardia. A fetal heart rate above 160 beats per minute and a maternal heart rate above 100 beats per minute; in each case is indicative of distress.

Talipes. A deformed or twisted foot (clubfoot) (figure 65.16).

Term. From 37 to 42 completed weeks' gestation (259–293 days) — neither *premature delivery* (< 37 weeks) nor *prolonged pregnancy* ($\geqslant 42$ weeks). *Full term* is 40 weeks — the due date of confinement (often mistakenly referred to as 'term' in contradistinction to the above definition).

Thalassaemia minor. A hereditary disorder of haemoglobin synthesis present in about 6% of patients who were born in Greece and 4% of those born in Italy. May cause severe pregnancy anaemia.

Third degree tear. A perineal laceration passing through the anal sphincter and laying open the anal canal.

Threatened abortion. Any bleeding from the birth canal before 28 weeks' gestation, with or without uterine pains, signifies a threat to abort (figure 18.1).

Thrush. Infection with Candida albicans; usual sites are the mother's vagina and the baby's mouth (figure 27.2).

Trial of labour. Continuous careful assessment of the progress of labour usually in a nullipara with clinical evidence of cephalopelvic disproportion insufficient to indicate elective Caesarean delivery (figure 49.8).

Trimester. A period of 3 months (13 weeks).

Trophoblast or chorion. The cells which line the blastodermic vesicle and surround the embryonic cell mass. Chorionic processes or villi develop with outer syncytial and inner cytotrophoblastic layers (colour plate 1).

Turner syndrome. A genetic abnormality where the individual has 45 chromosomes instead of 46 (XO karyotype) and is sex chromatin negative, despite being female in appearance.

Ultrasonography. Use of high frequency, short wavelength, sound wave reflections to diagnose pregnancy, assess gestational age, diagnose multiple pregnancy, malpresentations and hydatidi-form mole, identify nonviable pregnancies, locate the placental site, investigate fetal dynamics and detect fetal malformations.

Umbilical cord. The connecting lifeline between the fetus and placenta; it contains 2 umbilical arteries and 1 umbilical vein encased in Wharton jelly (figure 43.12).

Uterine inertia. (a) *Primary.* Inefficient uterine activity. (b) *Secondary (uterine exhaustion).* Occurs usually in the late first or second stage, when uterine action becomes poor or ceases. The commonest cause is obstruction due to a tight perineum in a nullipara.

Uterine souffle. Noise made by maternal blood passing through the uterine vessels.

Uterine tetany. Generalized tonic contraction of the uterus usually due to misuse of oxytocic drugs.

Vacuum extraction. Operation to deliver the fetal head by traction on a suction cup placed on the scalp (usually the occipital region).

Varicose veins. Dilatation of veins of the lower half of the body. Usually occur for the first time or get worse in pregnancy.

Vasa praevia. Fetal vessels lying in the membranes in front of the presenting part. There must be an associated velamentous insertion of cord, succenturiate lobe, or bipartite (2-lobed) placenta (colour plates 84 and 85).

Velamentous insertion of the cord. The umbilical cord inserts onto the membranes over which the vessels course to reach the fetal surface of the placenta (figure 43.6).

Vernix caseosa. Produced by sebaceous glands this 'complexion cream' prevents waterlogging and maceration of the fetal skin by the amniotic fluid (colour plate 92D).

Version. A turning of the fetus in utero whereby the presentation is changed, usually from breech to vertex.

Vertex. Top of the skull — the area between the anterior and posterior fontanelles and the parietal eminences.

Weight gain. The average weight gain in pregnancy is about 12.5 kg. A weight gain of more than 0.5 kg per week in late pregnancy often precedes generalized oedema, and thus pre-eclampsia.

Wharton jelly. The mucoid connective tissue supporting the umbilical cord vessels (figure 43.11).

ANATOMY AND PHYSIOLOGY OF REPRODUCTION

chapter two

Anatomy of the Reproductive System and Fetus

OVERVIEW

Anatomy, with physiology and biochemistry, is one of the major basic sciences. This subject is usually taught as a prelude to clinical medicine and is often regarded as dry and too factual. It is difficult, however, to practise perceptive and accurate medicine without a reasonably sound knowledge of the way structures relate to each other, the nature of their nerve and blood supply, and what happens when a certain area is cut or traumatized.

The process of labour is to some extent a matter of mechanics — the negotiation of the birth canal by the fetus, the propulsive force being the *myometrial motor*; variations in anatomy of the mother's bony pelvis (size, shape) and the fetal skull (size, shape, position, presentation) determine to a significant degree behaviour of the presenting part in labour. A critically important aspect is a detailed knowledge and 'feel' of the external *anatomical features of the fetus*. This is essential for an accurate diagnosis of the presenting part and its spatial relationship to the *maternal pelvis*, the readily palpable ischial spines being the reference point for designation of descent (station).

The placenta has its own anatomy and normal variations and these must be appreciated; sometimes a clue is provided that suggests the need for a wider search — e.g. the presence of 2 rather than 3 umbilical vessels can be associated with other congenital anomalies in the fetus or a gap in the maternal surface of the placenta can indicate a missing cotyledon (colour plate 33).

THE GENITALIA

In the female the organs of reproduction are subdivided into 2 main types — external and internal.

EXTERNAL GENITALIA

These are visible on inspection and, together with the vagina, subserve the function of coitus. The different structures are shown in figure 2.1.

Mons veneris (mount of love, or mons pubis). This is a fibrofatty cushion lying anterior and superior to the junction of the 2 pubic bones (symphysis pubis). It is covered by hair (the escutcheon or shield), the distribution of which is different in the 2 sexes — in the female, there is usually no extension upward onto the abdominal wall, whereas in the male, an extension toward the umbilicus is characteristically present, giving a different outline (male △: female ▽).

Labia majora (major lips). These are hair-covered, fibrofatty folds that extend from the mons above to the perineum below. They have both sweat and sebaceous glands, and are homologous with the scrotum in the male. The average measurements are 7.5 × 2.5 × 1.5 cm, but before and after the childbearing period are much smaller.

Labia minora (minor lips). The lesser labial folds are enclosed by the labia majora and are smaller and more delicate. They are pink in colour and devoid of hair, but contain sebaceous glands and a few sweat glands. They are richly vascular and plentifully supplied with nerve endings. Superiorly, they enclose the clitoris and, inferiorly, merge to form the fourchette, or posterior ring of the vaginal introitus. In the male, these structures form part of the penile urethra.

Clitoris. This is the homologue of the male penis. It is composed of a vascular plexus (erectile tis-

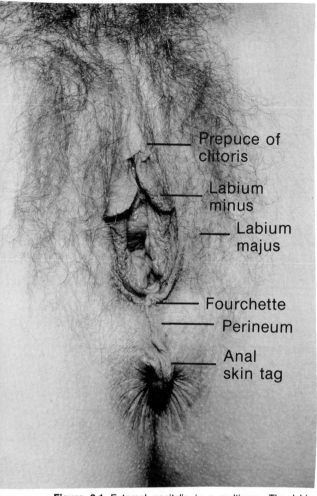

Prepuce of clitoris

Labium minus

Labium majus

Fourchette

Perineum

Anal skin tag

Figure 2.1 External genitalia in a multipara. The labia minora meet in the midline and cover the external urinary meatus and anterior part of the vestibule; superiorly they fuse to form the prepuce of the clitoris.

sue) arranged in a central corpus with 2 crura which are attached to the inferior rami of the pubis. The clitoris measures 1.5–2 cm in length, the terminal 0.5 cm being called the glans; the latter is richly supplied with nerve endings and is thus extremely sensitive. The folds of the labia minora sweep upward to enclose the clitoris, forming the prepuce above and the frenulum below.

Vestibule. This is the area enclosed by the labia minora. The urethra and vagina open into it, as do the paired Bartholin and Skene ducts. It represents the lower portion of the embryological urogenital sinus.

Urethral meatus. The external urinary orifice is situated 1– 1.5 cm below the clitoris. It is often covered by the folds of the labia minora, which must be separated to expose it, e.g. for passing a catheter. The reddish mucus membrane of the urethra often pouts onto the external surface (figure 2.2).

Paraurethral ducts (Skene ducts). These ducts come from the paraurethral glands (which have a lubricating function) and their tiny openings usually can be seen just below and beside the urethra.

Vaginal orifice. The vagina opens onto the lower part of the vestibule. Before puberty, the orifice is closed by the hymeneal membrane, which may have 1 or more small orifices in it. During reproductive life, the hymen is broken down and the interior of the lower vagina is visualized when the labia are parted. The remnants of the hymen

Figure 2.2 Technique of catheterization. **A.** The labia minora are separated to expose the urinary meatus. The vagina often has many folds (rugae) which simulate the urinary orifice. This patient has large thin labia, a relatively large clitoris and a patulous vagina. **B.** A Mediterranean-born primigravida being catheterized preparatory to Caesarean section. Note sebaceous glands on the perineum, small thick labia minora and hence easy identification of urinary meatus.

A
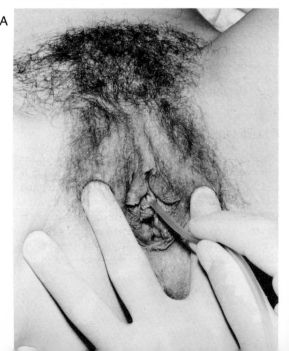

B
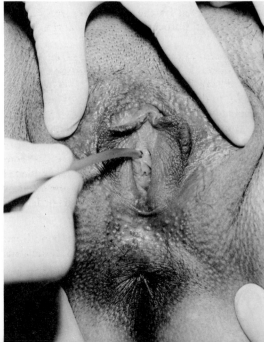

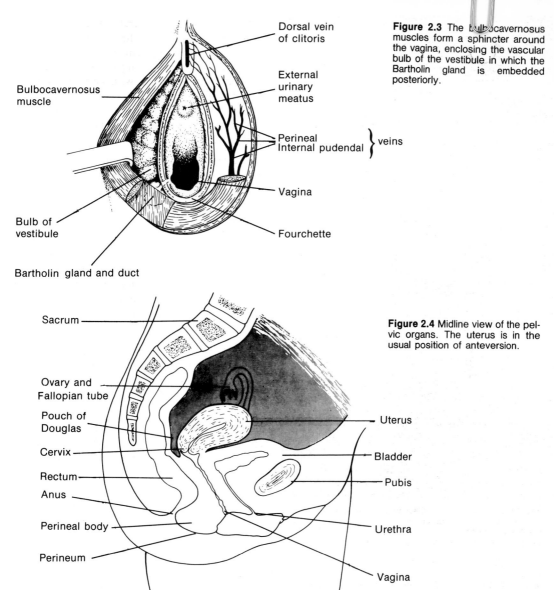

Bulbocavernosus muscle

Dorsal vein of clitoris

External urinary meatus

Perineal
Internal pudendal } veins

Vagina

Bulb of vestibule

Fourchette

Bartholin gland and duct

Figure 2.3 The bulbocavernosus muscles form a sphincter around the vagina, enclosing the vascular bulb of the vestibule in which the Bartholin gland is embedded posteriorly.

Sacrum

Ovary and Fallopian tube

Pouch of Douglas

Cervix

Rectum

Anus

Perineal body

Perineum

Uterus

Bladder

Pubis

Urethra

Vagina

Figure 2.4 Midline view of the pelvic organs. The uterus is in the usual position of anteversion.

are represented by the carunculae myrtiformes — nodules of fibrocutaneous tissue at the vaginal orifice.

Bartholin ducts open onto the vestibule at its posterolateral aspect, just outside the hymen (figure 2.3). The ducts are 1.5–2.0 cm long and run up to the paired Bartholin glands, which are situated posterolaterally (5 and 7 o'clock) above the constrictor muscles of the vagina (bulbo-cavernosus). The glands are pea-sized and are responsible for lubricating the introitus, particularly at the time of sexual arousal. Badly-placed episiotomy incisions will either sever the ducts or involve them in the subsequent repair or fibrous scarring.

Perineum. The area of the perineum is outlined by the vaginal fourchette anteriorly and the anus

posteriorly. Deep to it lies the perineal body. It is this area that is incised in the operation of episiotomy, where the introitus is enlarged to facilitate the birth of the baby (figure 45.2). The perineal body lies between the anal canal and the lower one-third of the posterior vaginal wall (figure 2.4).

INTERNAL GENITALIA

Vagina. The vagina is a musculomembranous tube which links the uterus to the vestibule. It is 8–12 cm in length and, in the resting state, the walls are opposed. Its main function is as a receptacle for the male penis during coitus. It is capable of remarkable distension during the process of childbirth. Anteriorly, the vagina is closely related to the base of the bladder and the

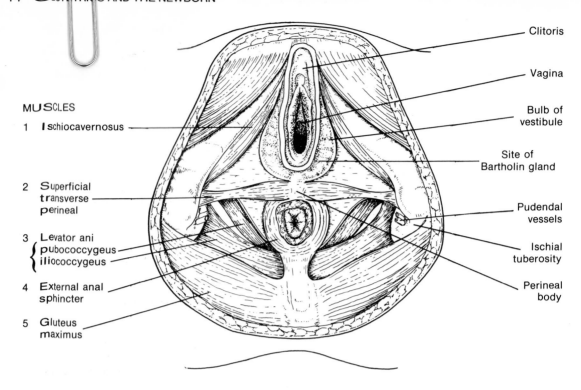

MUSCLES

1 Ischiocavernosus

2 Superficial transverse perineal

3 Levator ani
{ pubococcygeus
iliococcygeus

4 External anal sphincter

5 Gluteus maximus

Clitoris

Vagina

Bulb of vestibule

Site of Bartholin gland

Pudendal vessels

Ischial tuberosity

Perineal body

Figure 2.5 Muscles of the perineum.

urethra, and posteriorly, to the pouch of Douglas, rectum, and anal canal (figure 2.4). If overdistension of the vagina occurs during childbirth, the fascial supports (vesicovaginal and rectovaginal septa) separating the vagina from the bladder and rectum tear, usually in the midline, allowing prolapse to occur (cystocele, urethrocele, rectocele).

The vagina *passes through 2 muscular diaphragms — pelvic and perineal*. The muscles comprising the superficial perineal compartment join behind the vagina to form the strong perineal body (figure 2.5). It is these structures, with their attendant blood vessels, that are involved in perineal incisions and tears at the time of childbirth.

The *internal pudendal vessels* and *pudendal nerve* pass across the base of the ischial spine into the ischiorectal fossa and divide to supply the perineal structures (figure 2.6). The vestibular bulb, like the lateral crura of the clitoris, is highly vascular and bleeds freely if injured.

The uterine cervix projects into the upper 1–2 cm of the vagina, outlining the 4 fornices — anterior, posterior and lateral (left and right).

The *lining* of the vagina is thrown into folds like a concertina (allowance for expansion during childbirth) and these are known as rugae. The vagina has a stratified squamous epithelial lining, but no glands. Its moisture is provided chiefly by the secretion of the cervical mucus

glands and, to a variable extent, by vaginal transudation. In women who are not in the childbearing age, the vaginal walls are paler in colour, thinner, and a pale pink rather than a red or reddish-blue. This is because of the lack of ovarian hormones to which the vaginal lining is responsive. The vaginal squamous cells contain considerable glycogen, and this provides a pabulum for the *lactobacilli* (of Doderlein) which are normal inhabitants of the vagina. Since they produce lactic acid, the pH of the vagina is on the acid side (4.0–5.5) and this minimizes infection by other organisms.

The main blood supply of the vagina is from the vaginal arteries which arise from the internal iliac arteries and the descending branches of the uterine arteries, aided by the arteries to the bladder above and middle rectal and internal pudendal arteries below (figure 2.7). There is a profuse network of veins accompanying the arteries.

Uterus. The uterus is the centrepiece of the reproductive apparatus — its destiny being the nurture of the embryo and fetus until the time of parturition. It is composed of 2 functional elements — *a lower cervix*, which functions at different times as a passageway, a barrier, and a reservoir; and *an upper body*, in which the fetus develops. The cervix in the infant is twice as large as the uterine body, whereas in the adult

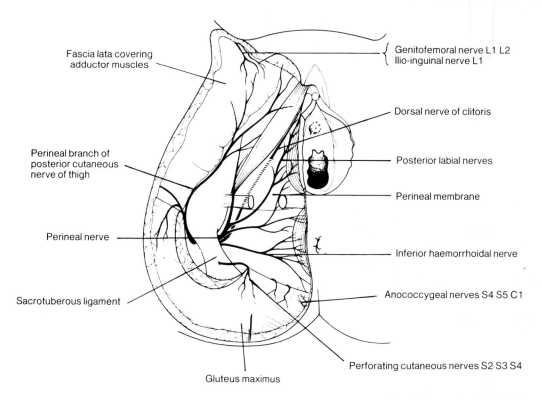

Fascia lata covering adductor muscles

Genitofemoral nerve L1 L2
Ilio-inguinal nerve L1

Dorsal nerve of clitoris

Perineal branch of posterior cutaneous nerve of thigh

Posterior labial nerves

Perineal membrane

Perineal nerve

Inferior haemorrhoidal nerve

Sacrotuberous ligament

Anococcygeal nerves S4 S5 C1

Perforating cutaneous nerves S2 S3 S4

Gluteus maximus

Figure 2.6 Nerve supply of the perineum. The pudendal nerve gives off the inferior haemorrhoidal within the pudendal canal which is formed by obturator fascia; as it emerges, the pudendal nerve divides into the perineal nerve and dorsal nerve of the clitoris. The perineal nerve gives off the labial branches and supplies the muscles in the deep and superficial perineal pouches. Note that the perforating cutaneous and posterior cutaneous nerves supply the perineum and unless a nerve block includes them as well as the pudendal nerve, the patient will experience pain when an episiotomy is sutured.

Figure 2.7 Arterial blood supply to the internal genitalia. There is free anastomosis between vaginal and uterine arteries. Coiling of vessels allows elongation as the uterus enlarges in pregnancy.

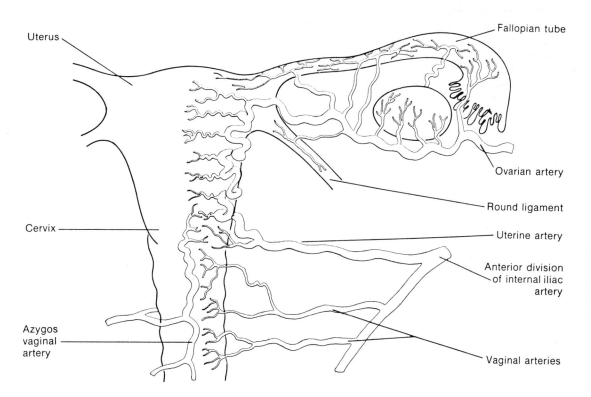

Uterus

Fallopian tube

Ovarian artery

Round ligament

Cervix

Uterine artery

Anterior division of internal iliac artery

Azygos vaginal artery

Vaginal arteries

this relationship is reversed. The uterus as a whole measures 7.5 × 5.0 × 2.5 cm and the length of the cavity is 5–6 cm in the mature woman.

(i) *Cervix.* There is a vaginal and supravaginal component to the cervix. The relations are similar to those of the upper vagina. The cervix is a strong pivotal point for uterine stability, being attached to the pelvic walls by radiating fascial condensations called ligaments — pubocervical anteriorly, uterosacral posteriorly, and transverse cervical (Mackenrodt) laterally. Premature bearing down by the patient in labour, or forceful downward pressure on the uterus after delivery, may seriously stretch and weaken these ligaments, causing uterine prolapse. The cervix is 2–3 cm in length and is delineated inferiorly by the *external os* and superiorly by the *internal os*. The shape of the external os is spherical in the nullipara, but usually transverse and more gaping in the multipara. In the latter, the reddish columnar epithelium lining the canal may be seen (perhaps exaggerated by ectropion formation), and also the small orifices of the cervical mucus glands. When the ducts of these glands are blocked by inflammation or scar tissue, small retention cysts form and these are obvious on the surface as *Nabothian follicles*.

(ii) *Uterine body.* The uterus is a hollow, muscular organ, the interior being roughly triangular in shape. The upper angles of the triangle are formed by the interstitial portions of the Fallopian tubes. The uterus is covered externally by peritoneum, except the lower part anteriorly, where the peritoneum is reflected onto the bladder. It is at this loose attachment that the incision is made in the 'lower segment' Caesarean section operation (figure 47.1). The lower segment lies at the junction of the uterus and cervix and, during pregnancy and labour, expands to some 10 cm in length.

The uterus is globular in shape, but flattened in the anteroposterior direction. Normally, it is both anteverted (rotated forward) and anteflexed (bent forward on itself). In some 20% of patients, the uterus is rotated backwards, lying more in relation to the rectum than the bladder. It is in this group that the rare complication of *incarceration of the uterus* occurs late in the first trimester of pregnancy, the enlarging uterus being caught in the hollow of the sacrum.

The Fallopian tubes are continuous with the uterus, the latter representing the fused distal portions of the Mullerian ducts, the former the unfused proximal portions. Occasionally, evidence of this process going awry can be seen in the various duplications and deletions of the uterus which occur.

The structure of the uterus is similar to that of most other hollow muscular organs in the body, although each of the 3 layers is specialized for the function of childbirth. (i) The *endometrium* or lining is composed of columnar epithelium which dips into the submucosa in the form of branched, tubular glands. Both the epithelium and the glands are responsive to the ebb and flow of the 2 ovarian hormones — oestrogen and progesterone. The thickness of the lining depends on the stage of the menstrual cycle — ranging from 0.05–0.5 cm. An additional feature of the endometrium is the typical coiled arteries, which also are under hormonal influence. During pregnancy, they greatly enlarge, especially in the region of the placenta, and they form the maternal contribution to the blood supply of this organ. (ii) The *myometrium* is the middle muscular layer and is composed of several interlacing layers of smooth muscle. During pregnancy, chiefly under the influence of oestrogen, great enlargement of the muscle fibres occurs, ready for the task of expelling the fetus in the process of parturition. The content of muscle in the cervix is quite small — about 10% although there is a recognizable sphincter in its upper part. (iii) The *serosa* is formed by the peritoneal covering and its associated blood vessels, lymphatics and nerves.

The *blood supply* of the uterus is from the uterine arteries on each side. These arise from the iliac arteries, pass down to the junction of cervix and uterus, where the cervical and vaginal branches are given off and the vessels continue upward at the side of the uterus in a tortuous manner, linking up with the ovarian arteries in the upper part of the broad ligament. Numerous branches arise from the uterine artery, passing into the muscular substance of the uterus on its front and back surfaces.

Fallopian tubes. These structures are 10–14 cm in length and their function is indicated by their alternative name — oviduct — that is, transfer of the fertilized ovum to the prepared bed in the uterus. The Fallopian tube is composed of 3 sections — *interstitial*, which runs in the outer cornu, or horn, of the uterus; *isthmus*, a narrow portion adjacent to the uterus; *ampulla*, a gradually widening trumpet-shaped outer third, which ends in a series of finger-like projections (fimbria) which wrap themselves around the ovary at the time of ovulation (figure 18.8). The inner portion of the tube is very narrow, and the epithelium is thrown up into a complex series of branching folds — hence, there is a strong tendency for blockage to occur should the tube become infected, especially as a result of gonorrhoea or following an abortal or puerperal infection. *The structure* of the tube is similar to that of the uterus, though on a miniature scale, and the responses to the ovarian hormones are less obvious. The tubes lie at the top of the broad ligaments, which are composed of peritoneum, folded over the tubes and round ligaments like sheets on a line. Since the prime function of the tubes is to facilitate transport of the ovum, the epithelium is generously supplied with hair-like processes, called *cilia*, which beat like the banks of oars in the ancient galleons, creating currents in the direction of the uterus. Partial obstruction of the lumen (whether congenital or acquired), delay of the fertilized ovum for other reasons, or untimely reflux of menstrual blood, may result in implantation of the conceptus in the tube rather than in the uterus (ectopic pregnancy, colour plate 5).

Round and ovarian ligaments. These 2 ligaments are really continuous, representing an embryonic structure called the gubernaculum, which, in the male, is responsible for pulling the gonad into the scrotum. In the female, the gubernaculum crosses the Mullerian duct and fuses with it at the point where the uterus and Fallopian tube are delineated. The round ligaments provide some anterior support for the uterus, especially during pregnancy, when they enlarge markedly. Stretching may cause discomfort or pain (*round ligament strain*) which can readily be appreciated by gentle palpation at the sides of the uterus late in pregnancy.

Broad ligaments. These are folds of peritoneum, lying between the uterus and the lateral pelvic wall. In the upper part lie the round ligaments and Fallopian tubes; at the base lie the uterine vessels and ureters, and the remainder is taken up by delicate areolar tissue, vessels, nerves, and embryonic remnants related to the defunct Wolffian (male) system of ducts and tubules. Uterine perforation or rupture may occur into the broad ligament and, similarly, tubal ectopic pregnancy may rupture downwards into it.

As the lateral pelvic wall is approached, the blood vessels supplying the ovary sweep upward out of the pelvis — carrying a process of the broad ligaments called the *infundibulopelvic ligament.*

The embryological importance of the vestigial Wolffian or mesonephric structures is that they may become cystic and enlarge. The duct (termed Gartner duct in the female, vas deferens in the male) runs down anterolateral to the cervix and vagina.

The tissue adjacent to the uterus in the broad ligament is called the *parametrium*, and is important for the reason that it represents one of the pathways in the spread of uterine infection — parametritis.

Ovaries. Otherwise known as gonads, these are paired structures which are situated on the back of the broad ligaments attached by a mesentery (mesovarium). Each ovary is almond-shaped and measures 2–4 cm in length. Its functions are the production of ova during the woman's reproductive years, and secretion of the key hormones involved in pregnancy — oestrogen and progesterone. The ovaries have a yellowish-white irregular surface, often characterized by developing Graafian follicles or active or regressing corpora lutea. The uteroovarian and infundibulopelvic ligaments have already been mentioned.

In *structure*, the ovary possesses an *outer cortex* in which are primordial and developing follicles and specialized connective tissue (theca), and an *inner medulla*, mainly composed of loose connective tissue and blood vessels.

There are probably some 400,000 primary oocytes (sex cells) in the ovary at birth. There is usually only 1 sex cell released each month; the majority of the remainder develop incompletely and regress.

The blood supply of the ovary comes mainly from the *ovarian arteries* (which arise from the aorta), aided by the anastomosis with the uterine arteries.

It is unusual for the ovary to be involved in developmental disorders, the chief disturbance being failure of development — primary ovarian dysgenesis.

SKELETOMUSCULAR SUPPORTS

Supporting the external and internal genitalia are the bony and fibromuscular structures which make up the birth canal.

The Bony Pelvis

This is made up of 4 bones joined together by ligaments. At the sides are the *paired innominate (hip) bones.* These are joined in front at the symphysis pubis and, behind, they articulate with the ala (or wings) of the *sacrum* forming the sacroiliac joints (figure 2.8). The fourth bone, the *coccyx*, is loosely articulated with the lower border of the sacrum. Both the sacrum and the iliac bones are strong and heavy, since it is through them that the weight of the head and trunk is transferred to the legs. The innominate bone is composed of 3 separate elements — pubis, ischium and ilium. These finally ossify in early adulthood. The different parts of the bone are shown in figures 2.8–2.11.

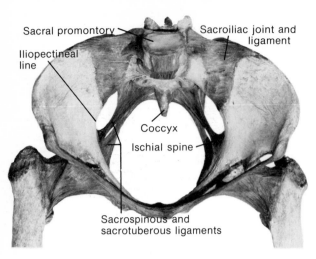

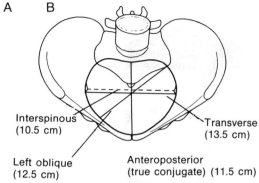

Figure 2.8 The pelvic brim. A. View from above of a large articulated pelvis. The brim is almost round — the pubic arch is generous and there is minimal projection of the sacral promontory. B. The diameters of the pelvic brim and their normal dimensions.

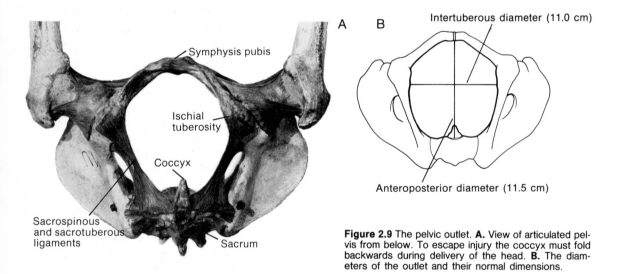

Figure 2.9 The pelvic outlet. A. View of articulated pelvis from below. To escape injury the coccyx must fold backwards during delivery of the head. B. The diameters of the outlet and their normal dimensions.

Figure 2.10 Sagittal view of the bony pelvis.

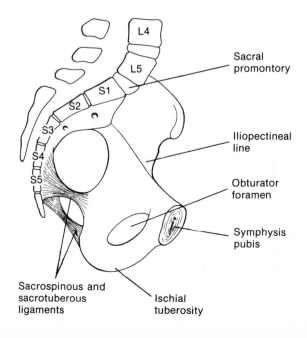

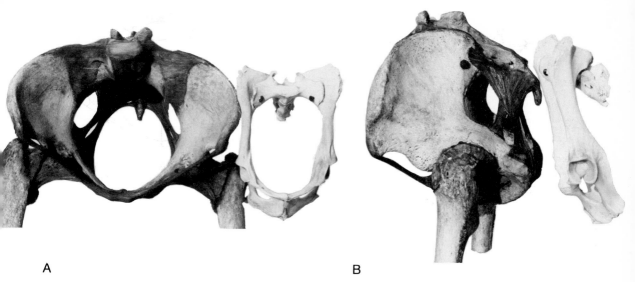

A   B

Figure 2.11 Parturition is a different proposition for human females than for quadrupeds such as ewes, whose infants have the same average birth-weight as humans. The human pelvis is a bony basin not a mere bony ring as in the ewe. In animals the sacrum is not directly opposite the pubic symphysis and during birth the fetus does not have to pass both bones simultaneously. The effect of the erect posture is to push the pubes upwards (via the femoral heads) and the sacrum downwards (effect of the weight of the trunk) — hence the mechanical difficulties of human parturition. **A.** Pelvic brim of a human (11 X 13 cm) and a sheep (12 X 9 cm). **B.** Lateral view of the pelves of a human and a sheep.

The sacrum is composed of 5 fused vertebrae, and a large intervertebral disc separates it from the fifth lumbar verebra above. The sacrum is directed backward as well as downward, and this throws its superior border into prominence as the *sacral promontory*, an important bony landmark in assessing the size of the pelvis, especially the anteroposterior diameter of the brim. The sacrum is concave on its pelvic aspect, providing in part the characteristic curve of the birth canal.

Looking into the pelvis from above, one can ascertain 2 parts — the false pelvis above and the true pelvis below. These are delineated by the iliopectineal line (figure 2.8). The true pelvis can best be appreciated by viewing the pelvis from the side (figure 2.10). It will be seen that the canal in front is made up only of the symphysis pubis and is quite short (4–5 cm). Posteriorly, there is the sweep of the sacrum and coccyx (11–13 cm) which, when added to the fibro-muscular perineal body, describes the *curve of Carus*. The dimensions of the true pelvis can be appreciated by studying 3 arbitrary planes — the brim, the midpelvis and the outlet, the shape and dimensions of which are shown in figures 2.8 and 2.9. Largely as a result of careful radiographic studies, 4 basic pelvic types have been described, and the features of these will be mentioned at each plane.

The brim is bounded by the superior aspects of the pubic bones, the iliopectineal eminences and lines, the ala and promontory of the sacrum. The basic pelvic shapes show quite characteristic brim outlines (figure 2.12). The normal *gynaecoid* (female) pelvis is almost round, apart from the intrusion of the sacral promontory posteriorly. The *anthropoid* (ape-like) pelvis is oval, with the large diameter running antero-posteriorly, in contrast to the *platypelloid* (flat) pelvis, where the largest diameter is in the transverse. The final type is the *android* (male) pelvis, which is characterized by a heart-shaped outline, with narrowing anteriorly. These differences in pelvic shape are of more than radiological interest, since they determine, in large measure, the mechanism which is adopted by the fetus in passing through the birth canal.

In general, the pelvis is considered to be mildly contracted if the diameter is reduced 1 cm, moderately contracted if reduced 1–2 cm, and markedly contracted if reduced 2 cm or more.

The anteroposterior diameter (obstetrical conjugate) (11.5 cm) is measured from the back of the symphysis to the tip of the sacral promontory. This measurement can only be made accurately by radiography, but an approximate idea is given by the diagonal conjugate, from the bottom of the symphysis pubis to the sacral promontory as measured during vaginal examination.

The transverse diameter (13.5 cm) is the largest of the brim diameters and is taken at the widest part of the brim.

The oblique diameters (right and left) (12.5 cm) run from the right and left sacroiliac joints to the opposite iliopectineal eminences, respectively.

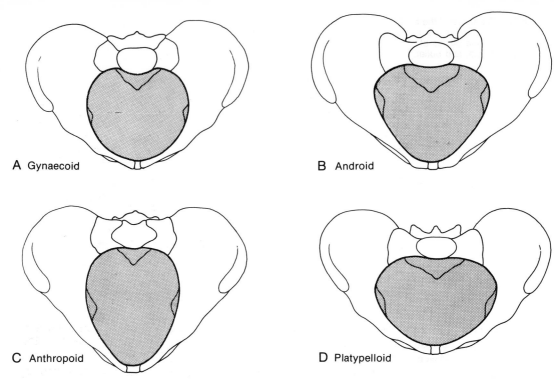

Figure 2.12 Variation in shape of the pelvic brim. **A.** Gynaecoid — almost round; 55% of women. **B.** Android — heart-shaped due to projecting sacral promontory and narrow fore-pelvis; 20% of women. **C.** Anthropoid — oval and like the android pelvis tends to have midpelvic narrowing; 20% of women. **D.** Platypelloid — transversely oval; usually a shallow pelvis with capacious outlet; 5% of women.

Pelvic cavity. This is the *area between the inlet above and the outlet below*, and is bounded by the pubic bones anteriorly, the curve of the sacrum posteriorly, and parts of all 3 components of the innominate bone laterally. The upper part of the cavity is roomier than the lower, the latter being known as the plane of least dimensions (figure 2.13). This passes from the back of the symphysis pubis to the lower part of the sacrum (disc between S4–S5) at the level of the protruding ischial spines. The latter are especially prominent in the android type of pelvis, and to a lesser extent in the anthropoid type. The *ischial spines* are very important landmarks, not only as indicators of the type of pelvis and its size, but also as reference points for designation of the station of the presenting part. Since they are approximately midway down the birth canal (about 5 cm in the central axis), the head is assumed to be engaged when it has reached this point, since the distance from the vertex of the skull to the maximum diameters of the head (biparietal and suboccipitobregmatic) is slightly less than 5 cm.

The outlet. This is outlined by the subpubic arch, the ischial tuberosities, the sacrotuberous ligaments, and the coccyx (figure 2.9). The pelvic configuration has a significant bearing on the diameters which are available to the fetus. Where the subpubic arch is narrow, as in the android pelvis, the angle may be 60–70°, compared with the normal of 90°. This means that much of the anteroposterior diameter will not be available for use by the fetus.

Pelvic inclination. The lateral view of the pelvis indicates that the pelvic brim makes an angle of 40–50° with the horizontal; this is called the angle of inclination. The inclination lessens as the birth canal is descended, being about 30° in the midpelvis and 10° at the outlet (figure 2.13).

The Pelvic Joints

The sacroiliac joints are partly cartilagenous, partly fibrous and are very strong. Despite this, pain is often experienced late in pregnancy as *joint mobility* increases with softening of the ligaments, and the weight of the pregnant uterus is added to that of the head and trunk.

The lumbosacral joint lies between the fifth lumbar vertebra and the sacrum. Because of the backward inclination of the sacrum, considerable strain also occurs here during pregnancy. In extreme cases (spondylolisthesis), the fifth lumbar vertebra projects downward and forward into the area of the pelvic brim.

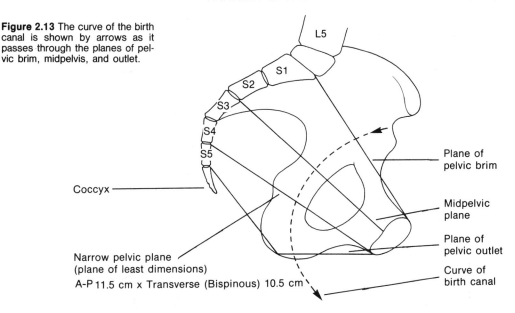

Figure 2.13 The curve of the birth canal is shown by arrows as it passes through the planes of pelvic brim, midpelvis, and outlet.

L5

S1

S2

S3

S4

S5

Coccyx

Narrow pelvic plane
(plane of least dimensions)
A-P 11.5 cm x Transverse (Bispinous) 10.5 cm

Plane of pelvic brim

Midpelvic plane

Plane of pelvic outlet

Curve of birth canal

Symphysis pubis. The 2 pubic bones are joined anteriorly by fibrous tissue, although a layer of cartilage remains between them. It is through this cartilage that the operation of *symphysiotomy* is occasionally carried out to increase pelvic diameters to allow vaginal delivery in cases of obstructed labour.

The sacrococcygeal joint is much looser than the others, allowing the coccyx to bend backwards as the fetus passes through the birth canal. Undue displacement may, however, overstretch the ligaments, giving rise to the condition of coccyodynia or pain, which is especially noticed on sitting.

Ligaments. These are well developed in the pelvis because of the stresses to which the pelvic bones are subjected. Apart from the ligaments specifically related to the above joints, there are 2 others of importance — the *sacrospinous and sacrotuberous.* These run from the sacrum to the ischial spine, and ischial tuberosity, respectively (figures 2.8 and 2.9). Together, they form, with the coccyx and lowest part of the sacrum, the posterior aspect of the pelvic outlet.

The Pelvic Soft Tissues

The bony pelvis is clothed by a number of muscles, the chief of which form the floor of the pelvis and the perineum.

The pelvic floor. This comprises the various parts of the *levator ani muscles* which run on each side from the back of the symphysis pubis around the lateral pelvic wall on the fascia over the obturator internus muscle to the ischial spine and side of the coccyx, together with the special muscular bundle, the *puborectalis,* which

decussates or joins with its opposite number around the vagina and lower rectum. The urethra, vagina and rectum all pass through this muscular diaphragm, which is completed by fascial condensations on its upper and lower surfaces. The muscles of the 2 sides slope downward and forward in the form of a gutter, and this is one of the factors aiding rotation of the fetal head, as it reaches the pelvic floor level. The puborectalis is important in helping to maintain closure of the outlet by drawing the different structures passing through it anteriorly toward the shelf of the symphysis pubis. Inability to relax this part of the levator at the time of delivery is often responsible for delay in the birth of the baby during the second stage of labour.

The urogenital diaphragm. This is a triangular-shaped diaphragm through which pass the urethra and vagina. It occupies the space between the inferior borders of the ischiopubic rami (figure 2.5) and extends posteriorly to the front wall of the rectum. On its deep aspect are 2 sets of muscles — the constrictor of the urethra and vagina, and the deep transverse perinei. Superficially, there are the *ischiocavernosus muscles* (passing from the ischiopubic ramus on each side up to the clitoris), the bulbs (erectile tissue) with the associated *bulbocavernosus muscles,* the *superficial perineal muscles,* and *Bartholin glands.* Between the vagina and rectum, the superficial and deep perineal muscles, including the anal sphincter, decussate and join, forming the strong *perineal body.* Behind the anal canal, the sphincter muscles decussate to form the *anococcygeal raphe.* It is in this region that the presenting part is felt for (by postanal palpation) as it approaches the pelvic outlet. The important internal pudendal blood vessels and the pudendal nerve pass forward from the inner aspect of the ischial tuberosity across the fat-filled ischiorectal fossa (which lies between the tuberosity and the rectum) to supply the perineal structures (figure 2.6).

THE FETUS

The size, position and attitude of the fetus influence the mechanism of birth — i.e. the movements that the fetus undergoes during negotiation of the birth canal.

THE SKULL

The shoulders normally represent the largest fetal diameter but the skull diameters are the more important since the cranium is less compressible. The bones of the cranium comprise 2 frontals, 2 parietals, 2 temporals and 1 occipital — these are separated by sutures and fontanelles and so the cranium is more compressible than the base of the skull.

The anatomical landmarks and diameters of the skull are shown in figures 2.14 and 2.15.

Landmarks. (i) Frontal suture: between the 2 frontal bones. (ii) Coronal suture: between the frontal and parietal bones. (iii) Sagittal suture: between the 2 parietal bones. (iv) Lambdoidal suture: between the occipital bone behind and the parietal and temporal bones in front. (v) Temporal suture: between the temporal and parietal bones. (vi) The anterior fontanelle or bregma is the large diamond-shaped depression at the anterior end of the cranium where frontal, coronal and sagittal sutures meet. It allows moulding in labour and growth of the skull after birth. It closes at 18 months of age. (vii) The posterior fontanelle is a smaller triangular space at the posterior end of the cranium where the sagittal suture meets the lambdoidal sutures.

Transverse diameters. (i) Bitemporal (8 cm): between the lower ends of the coronal sutures. (ii) Biparietal (9.5 cm): between the parietal eminences. The upper surface of the cranium thus narrows anteriorly.

Sagittal diameters. (i) Suboccipitobregmatic (9.5 cm): foramen magnum (nape of neck) to the centre of the bregma. It is the diameter which presents when the head is flexed; the latter then presents as a 9.5 cm × 9.5 cm sphere (biparietal × suboccipitobregmatic). (ii) Occipitofrontal (11–12 cm): occipital protuberance to the root of the nose. This diameter presents when the head is partly deflexed (military 'eyes front' attitude). *Thus deflexion has the effect of increasing the presenting diameter of the fetal head by about 20%.* (iii) Mentovertical (14.0 cm): point of the chin to the centre of the sagittal suture. This diameter is seen with a brow presentation, and if the fetal head is of normal size and shape, it cannot negotiate a normal sized pelvis. (iv) Submentobregmatic (9.5 cm): angle between neck and chin to the centre of the bregma. This diameter presents when the head is completely extended — i.e. a face presentation.

Areas of the skull. (i) *Vertex* (top of the skull): the area between the anterior and posterior fon-

Figure 2.14 Anatomy of the fetal skull. **A.** Viewed from above. Note narrowing of the cranium anteriorly from parietal to frontal eminences. **B.** Lateral view of cranium, face, and base of the skull.

A

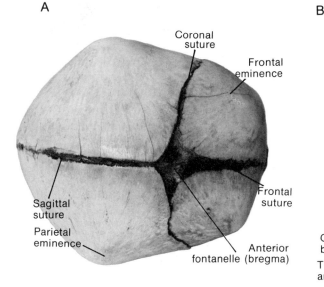

B

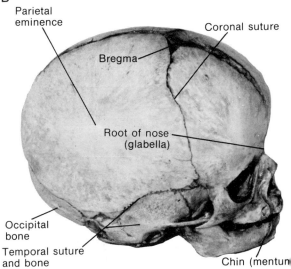

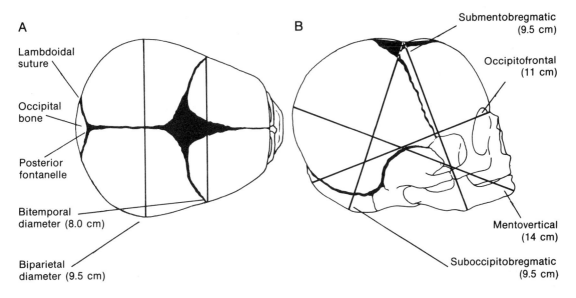

Figure 2.15 Diameters of the fetal skull. **A.** Transverse diameters seen from above. **B.** Lateral view showing sagittal diameters.

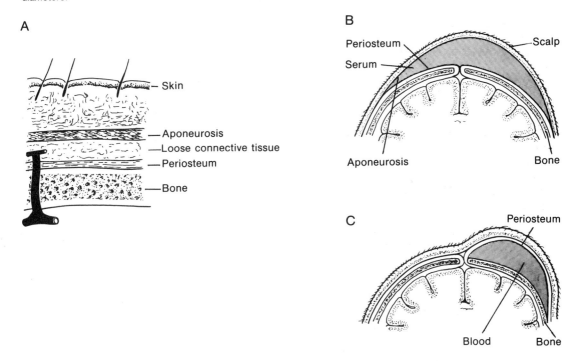

Figure 2.16 Caput succedaneum and cephalhaematoma. **A.** Anatomy of the scalp. **B.** Caput succedaneum is a swelling between aponeurosis and periosteum and can cross the sagittal suture. **C.** A cephalhaematoma is situated between bone and periosteum and cannot cross the sagittal suture.

tanelles and the 2 parietal eminences. (ii) *Sinciput*: that part of the head in front of the anterior fontanelle. It is subdivided into the *brow* (the area between root of nose and anterior fontanelle), and the *face* (the area below the root of the nose and the orbital ridges). (iii) *Occiput* (the back of the head): that part which lies behind the posterior fontanelle.

Caput Succedaneum and Cephalhaematoma

During labour, pressure of the cervix on the fetal head impedes venous and lymphatic drainage and a serous effusion collects between aponeurosis and periosteum (figure 2.16). Caput formation is most marked when there is slow dilatation of the cervix and when the patient bears down before full cervical dilatation — it is a sign of incoordinate uterine action and is accompanied by excessive moulding when labour is obstructed. Caput succedaneum disappears within a few hours of birth. It must be distinguished from a *cephalhaematoma* which is subperiosteal collection of blood. This presents some hours after birth and may enlarge for 12-24 hours; because of the attachments of periosteum to suture lines, a cephalhaematoma only overlies a single bone — usually the parietal (figure 66.1, colour plate 142).

Moulding

Moulding is due to compression which the head undergoes during its passage through the birth canal. There is diminution of those diameters most compressed and compensatory elongation of those least compressed. The degree and direction of moulding are determined by a number of factors. (i) Size, shape, elasticity and attitude of the fetal head. (ii) Size and shape of the maternal pelvis. (iii) Presentation and position of the head. (iv) Strength of uterine contractions and duration of labour. (v) Rate of cervical dilatation and position of the cervix (anterior or sacral).

In most accounts of moulding the importance of the *innate shape of the fetal head* is understated. Moulding is extreme when there is a cephalopelvic disproportion and strong uterine action (e.g. obstructed labour in a multipara). The soft head (large fontanelles) of the premature fetus moulds relatively easily, whereas the hard, inelastic fetal head characteristic of prolonged pregnancy resists alteration in shape. In face or brow presentations, moulding affects the area of the skull anterior to the bregma, whereas in vertex presentations the area behind the bregma is involved.

Moulding is common when there is posterior position of the occiput, because of its association with a larger fetal head (often there is prolonged pregnancy) and abnormal size and shape of the maternal pelvis. These points are illustrated in figures 2.17-2.19, which are paired views of infants shortly after birth and again 24-48 hours later.

THE FETAL TRUNK

Diameters. (i) *Bisacromial* (12.5 cm): the distance between the tips of the acromial processes. (ii) *Bitrochanteric* (9.5 cm): the distance between the outer surfaces of the greater trochanters.

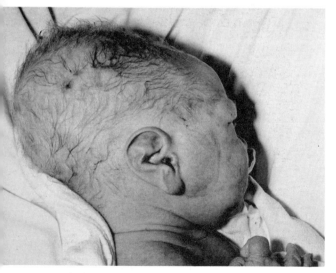
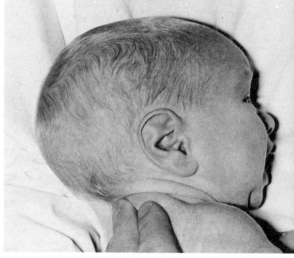

A   B

Figure 2.17 This baby was delivered from the occipitosacral position by forceps rotation and delivery. The mother was a primigravida with a contracted pelvis (transverse of brim 11.7 cm, bispinous 9.1 cm, available AP of outlet 10.2 cm) and a high fetal head at 41 weeks' gestation. After 48 hours of labour the cervix was fully dilated and the head was engaged in the persistent occipitoposterior position. There was much caput and moulding. **A.** The baby immediately after birth showing gross elongation of the head and the mark of an accurately applied forceps blade; birth-weight 3,610 g. **B.** The next day all trace of moulding has disappeared. It is seen that the baby has a long oval head.

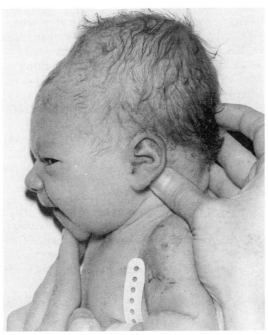
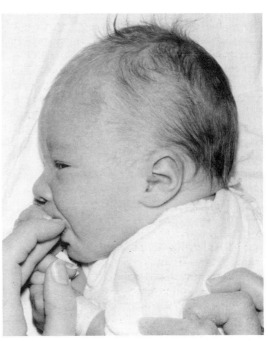

A   B

Figure 2.18 This child was born by Caesarean section performed after 21 hours of labour in a primigravida with obstructed labour and fetal distress at 40 weeks' gestation. There was gross caput and moulding. The head was deflexed and in the left occipitoposterior position. **A.** The baby immediately after birth showing moulding in a vertical direction (sugar loaf head); birth-weight 3,330 g. **B.** Two days later, moulding has gone and it is seen that the baby has a round head. Shape and attitude of the head rather than position in the pelvis has determined the direction of moulding.

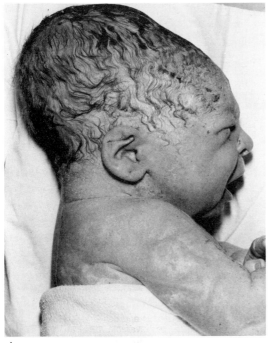
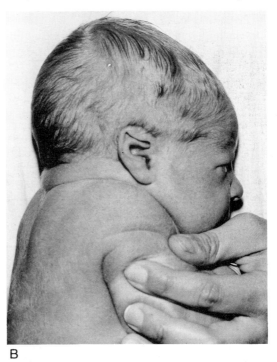

A   B

Figure 2.19 This baby weighed 3,250 g at birth and was born after a 4-hour labour, induced at 37 weeks' gestation because intrauterine death had occurred at 40 weeks in the previous pregnancy. The occiput was anterior at amniotomy and at delivery. **A.** The baby immediately after birth showing elongation of the head. **B.** Next day the moulding has gone and the natural oval shape of the head is shown. This baby had large shoulders and sustained a fractured left clavicle when shoulder dystocia occurred during delivery.

chapter three

The Physiological Basis of Reproduction

OVERVIEW

Although the reproductive period in the female extends from puberty to the climacteric, *fertility* is maximal from mid-adolescence to the end of the third decade.

For *conception* to occur, the fertilizing spermatozoon and ovum must meet, and this usually occurs in the outer end of the Fallopian tube at mid-cycle. The development of the mature sperm and ovum (spermatogenesis, oogenesis) is the result of a complex series of hormonal interactions between hypothalamus, pituitary gland and gonad. Shortly before fertilization, a special form of cell division occurs called *meiosis*; this results in a halving of the normal 46 chromosomes in each gamete (sex cell), so that the normal number will be restored when the male and female cells unite.

After fertilization, the conceptus rapidly increases in size due to repeated cell division, and after 6 days the embryo, now at the *morula* stage, implants into the endometrium of the uterus.

Preparation for *implantation* has been effected by *oestrogen* and *progesterone*, initially from the developing *Graafian follicle* of the ovary and then from the *corpus luteum*, the specialized structure which develops from the cells of the vacated Graafian follicle. Regression of the corpus luteum, which normally occurs at the end of the menstrual cycle (day 28), is prevented by a special hormone (*chorionic gonadotrophin*) released from the outer layers of the embryo (the chorion).

Errors are not uncommon in the genetic process — if major, the conceptus is usually lost, often in the initial week or so after fertilization, this being nature's mechanism for rejection of the imperfect; if less serious, the fetus may survive with anomalies, either structural or biochemical.

The Reproductive Epochs

From a reproductive viewpoint, a woman's life may be divided into 5 epochs; prepuberty, puberty, maturity, climacteric, and involution.

(i) *Prepuberty*. The structures involved in reproduction are inactive, except for a short period after birth when the high levels of placental and ovarian hormones from the mother stimulate target organs (uterus, breasts) in the baby.

(ii) *Puberty* is not a single event, but rather a *series of physiological changes* over a period of several years. The changes that occur at puberty are initiated by the hypothalamus which alters the activity of the endocrine glands; *oestrogen* from the ovaries causes growth and development of breasts and genitalia, and *androgens* from the adrenal glands are responsible for growth of pubic and axillary hair. The first changes occur in the breasts — initially enlargement of the nipples, followed by growth of the ducts and alveoli which will be responsible for provision of milk for the baby at the conclusion of pregnancy.

There is also an accumulation of fatty tissue, not only in the breasts, but also around the hips and buttocks, providing the typical feminine contour. Pigmentary changes of the nipple and surrounding areola occur a little later. After 6–12 months, pubic hair commences to grow and this continues well into the teens. Although body growth is observed to increase progressively in childhood, there is usually a spurt between the ages of 10 and 14. Finally, between the years of 11 and 14, the *menarche* (onset of menstruation) occurs. Also about this time growth of hair in the axillae commences. The onset of breast development precedes menstruation by about 2 years (range 6 months to 6 years).

(iii) *Reproductive maturity.* The early menstrual cycles are usually anovular, and the regular cyclic fertile pattern is not established for 2–3 years. As the other extreme of reproductive life is approached in the forties, ovulation and menstruation again tend to become irregular.

(iv) *Climacteric.* This is a period, similar to puberty, which heralds the end of reproductive capacity. Although the most prominent event is the menopause or cessation of menses, there are a number of other changes seen, chiefly of a physiological (neurovascular) and psychological nature.

(v) *Involution.* Regressive changes occur in the reproductive organs and in other body tissues which come under their influence, particularly those responding to oestrogen secretion from the ovary (musculoskeletal, urinary tract, skin).

The Menstrual Cycle

In essence, the menstrual cycle is a process initiated by the hypothalamus, mediated by the hormones of the anterior lobe of the pituitary gland and ovary, and directed to the production of a sex cell from the ovary (ovum) and the preparation of a bed in the uterus for its reception should fertilization occur.

For harmonious function of this delicate system, each part must know what the other is doing, and must at times be able to stimulate or inhibit one of the other parts. The basic process by which this is done is called *feedback*, similar to the information which is fed back to the brain by the nervous system, but, in this case, the messengers are usually the hormones themselves.

Events in the cycle. The first event is the secretion of *follicle stimulating hormone* releasing factor (FSH-RF) by the hypothalamus, which acts on the pituitary gland to produce *follicle stimulating hormone* (FSH). As the name implies, this causes the primordial or quiescent follicles in the ovary to grow. As the follicles develop, the granulosa and theca cells which surround the ovum secrete *oestrogen*. This hormone has a growth stimulating effect on the blood vessels and glands of the uterine endometrium, and on the myometrial muscle cells, as well as on the duct tissues of the breast. In addition, it has 2 effects on the hypothalamus — pituitary system: firstly, it progressively inhibits further FSH secretion, and secondly, at about the 10th–12th day of the cycle, a sudden oestrogen peak or surge is produced, which triggers secretion of *luteinizing hormone releasing factor* (LH-RF) from the hypothalamus, and this stimulates LH release from the pituitary gland.

The LH in turn, causes the mature Graafian follicle to release the ovum (*ovulation*); this usually occurs between the 12th–14th days of the cycle. The ovum passes into the fimbrial end of the Fallopian tube to await its rendezvous with the first and strongest of the ascending spermatozoa.

The space formerly occupied by the ovum is filled with blood and then granulation tissue, and the lining granulosa and theca cells develop under the continued secretion of luteinizing hormone to form the *corpus luteum* (yellow body). These specialized cells produce the second ovarian hormone, *progesterone*. Like oestrogen, it has effects on uterus, breasts, and the hypothalamus-pituitary system. In the uterus, whereas oestrogen is the growth hormone, progesterone is the hormone which directs the cells towards provision of nutrients — particularly glycogen. The ovum will thus have both bed and board in the important early weeks of development. In the breasts, there is a stimulation of the alveolar system and, finally, there is a feedback inhibition of the hypothalamus to shut off both FSH-RF and LH-RF.

The corpus luteum is programmed by nature to perish after some 14 days, and this sets in train the events of menstruation. As the corpus luteum regresses, the level of progesterone falls and the spiral arterioles supplying the endometrium go into spasm, causing ischaemia and then shedding. The fall in level of both oestrogen and progesterone releases the hypothalamus from feedback inhibition and a new cycle commences.

If fertilization occurs and successful embedding takes place, the *chorionic villi* which surround the embryo (colour plate 1 and figure 4.3) release a gonadotrophic (i.e. acting on the gonad) hormone (HCG) which prevents regression of the corpus luteum, and thus its secretion of oestrogen and progesterone continues, allowing the embryo to develop in peace in its endometrial bed.

Gametogenesis

This is the process whereby the gametes (mature germ cells) are formed in the female and male gonads, respectively. Although only 1 ovum is produced each month compared with millions of spermatozoa in the male, the fundamental process (oogenesis, spermatogenesis) is the same.

Essential to the understanding of the early development of the sex cells are firstly, the chromosome structure of the cells, and secondly, the 2 basic forms of cell division. In both the female and male primary sex cells (and, indeed, in all cells in the body except those gametes about to be joined in the process of fertilization) there are 46 *chromosomes* (female 44, XX; male 44, XY). It is obvious that, if this number of chromosomes is to remain constant when the ovum and sperm finally unite, each must shed half its complement. This special type of reduction division is called *meiosis*, as opposed to the process which occurs at all other times of cell division which is known as *mitosis*.

Thus, we have stem cells in the ovary and testis which have the normal number of 46 chromosomes and these divide by ordinary mitosis to produce daughter cells — the primary oocytes and spermatocytes. When these divide by the process of meiosis to form the secondary oocytes and spermatocytes, there are only 22 autosomal chromosomes and 1 sex chromosome (X or Y) to each cell. Each daughter cell has lost half of its genetic material, but this will be restored when it unites with its partner at the time of fertilization. It will be apparent that the oogonia (female sex cell) can only produce a daughter cell with a female or X chromosome, while the spermatogonia (male sex cell) can produce an X or a Y daughter cell. At conception, if the conjunction is XX, a female will result; if XY a male.

There is a further process of differentiation in the male, called spermiogenesis, whereby the spermatid cell becomes changed to the elongated, motile spermatozoa with head, mid-section, and tail.

chapter four

Fetal and Placental Development

OVERVIEW

After *conception* in the outer third of the Fallopian tube, rapid cellular division occurs in the fertilized ovum. By the time of *implantation* into the endometrium 6 days later, the *morula* (ball of cells) has changed to a *blastocyst*, with beginning of the major subdivision into embryo and future placenta. *The embryonic period commences with the formation of the embryonic disc at the start of the 2nd week after fertilization and ends at the 8th week when all the major structures have formed.* The development of the fetus is rigidly scheduled: the period of gestation is readily apparent from the progress of fetal organization. The various structures of the fetus are derived basically from 3 layers — the *outer ectoderm* supplying the skin and its appendages as well as the nervous system; the *middle mesoderm* supplying the supporting structures such as the skeleton, muscles and connective tissue, as well as the haematopoetic system, and the *inner endoderm* supplying the gut and related structures. The renal, reproductive, and respiratory systems are formed from specialized condensations — the former 2 from the intermediate cell mass on the posterior abdominal wall, and the latter from an outpouching in the pharyngeal region.

A knowledge of normal embryology assists in understanding the not infrequent anomalies of fetal development.

The *placenta* is derived from the trophoblast as a specialized development of that portion which is in closest relation to the underlying uterine decidua. Its first task is to break open maternal blood lakes and establish a means of oxygenation, nutrition and waste disposal for the fetus. The circulations are separated by the wall of the fetal capillary in the villus, a variable amount of villous connective tissue, and finally the trophoblastic epithelium which covers the villus. The 2 circulations become progressively more intimate as these tissues thin out during the pregnancy. The placenta assumes a mature form at about 14–16 weeks. Growth after this lags behind that of the fetus, the relative weights at full term being between 1:5 and 1:6.

The fetus is capable of independent life at approximately 32–34 weeks; with modern intensive care, survival may follow births as early as 24–26 weeks.

The well-being of the fetus is of vital interest to those attending the pregnant woman; this can now be assessed in a number of ways — *electronic* (fetal heart and brain patterns), *biochemical* (fetal and placental products), and *ultrasonic* (size, breathing, movement). With the current sophistication of realtime ultrasonography, much new information is becoming available in relation to organ development and function, and fetal behaviour in utero; activities such as thumb-sucking, bladder emptying, eye movements and penile erection can now be observed and quantitated. These aspects are considered in later chapters.

CONCEPTION

The process of conception, or fertilization, is initiated by sexual intercourse (coitus) at a time in the menstrual cycle related to ovulation — approximately the 11th–14th days. The male ejaculate, of 2–4 ml and containing some 200 million spermatozoa, is deposited in the upper vagina, and from there the sperms ascend through the cervical mucus and uterus and pass to the *outer third of the Fallopian tube, where the ovum is fertilized.* Although the granulosa cells surrounding the ovum are largely cast off as it enters the tube, it is probable that more than one sperm is necessary to complete this process (by enzyme action) and so allow the fertilizing sperm to penetrate the outer membrane of the ovum (*zona pellucida*) and trigger the process of cell division.

It is also probable that the ovum begins to degenerate after 36–48 hours and, allowing for the fact that the sperm are only viable in adequate numbers for a little longer time, the fertile period in each month does not normally extend much beyond 5–6 days. Very rarely, the fertilization process may occur in the abdominal cavity or even the ovary itself, to provide rare examples of primary abdominal or ovarian ectopic pregnancy. In the more usual type of *ectopic pregnancy*, the fertilized ovum embeds in the tube, having failed to reach its uterine destination (colour plate 5).

PREIMPLANTATION DEVELOPMENT

After fertilization, the body formed by the united gametes or sex cells is called the *zygote* (figure 4.1). *Rapid cell division* or cleavage now takes place by the process referred to as mitosis. Here, each of the 46 chromosomes, containing a vast number of genes (units of genetic information) duplicates itself and splits lengthwise, each daughter cell (blastomere) receiving the same material as was in the parent cell. The daughter cells so formed, although separate, adhere to each other, eventually forming a ball of cells (blastomeric ovum or *morula*). Occasionally,

complete separation does occur, and we have one of the forms of twinning (identical or monovular). At this stage, we see the beginning of integration of the cells and they are no longer totipotent (that is, able to form a complete individual) if separated away from the other cells.

At the 5th to 6th day after fertilization, the conceptus passes into the uterus and prepares to embed in the endometrium, where it will differentiate and grow over the ensuing 9 months. At this stage, a fundamental change occurs in the cell mass. A fluid space appears and a division occurs into an *inner cell mass*, which will form the embryo (embryoblast), and an outer *trophoblast*, which will form the placenta (aided in part by the underlying maternal endometrium). This is the *blastocyst* and it is in this form that embedding takes place (table 4.1 and figure 4.1).

IMPLANTATION

This occurs 6–8 days after fertilization. The primitive conceptus, after contact with the lining of the uterus, erodes through it and sinks into the deeper layers of the endometrium. The smaller blood vessels and the glands provide early nourishment as they are opened up by the digestive enzymes secreted by the trophoblastic cells (colour plate 1). The subsequent development of the 2 elements will now be considered separately.

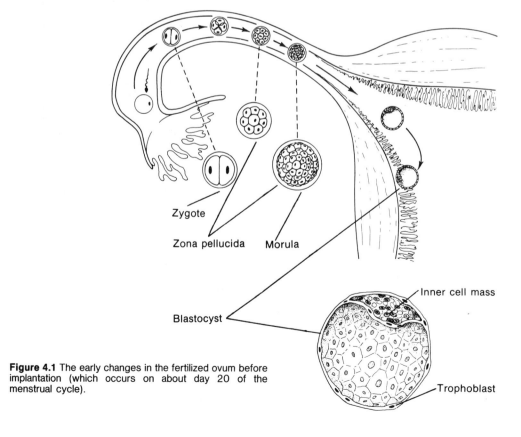

Zygote

Zona pellucida   Morula

Blastocyst

Inner cell mass

Trophoblast

Figure 4.1 The early changes in the fertilized ovum before implantation (which occurs on about day 20 of the menstrual cycle).

TABLE 4.1   DEVELOPMENT OF THE CONCEPTUS, EMBRYO AND FETUS

Stage	Age*	Size	Weight (g)	Characteristics
A. *CONCEPTUS*	1			Blastomeres form from progressive division of zygote to produce the morula (1–3 days), blastocyst (4–6 days) and trophoblast (7 + days)
		(mm)		
B. *EMBRYO* (5–10 weeks)	2			Inner cell mass differentiates into bilaminar embryonic disc. Primitive amniotic and yolk sac cavities. Trophoblast erodes maternal blood vessels and forms lacunae; primitive uteroplacental circulation
	3			Chorionic sac measures 1 cm diameter; villi around whole surface. Well-defined embryonic disc and body stalk. Somites forming. Fetal vascularization of villi; intervillous space forming. Major developmental activity in nervous system and heart
	4	4–5		Fetal sac 2–3 cm. Somites forming to provide muscles, bones and nerves of trunk. Heart and pericardium prominent. Arm and leg buds forming. Branchial arches (maxilla, mandible, hyoid); otic pit and lens placode present. Adopting C-shaped curvature
	5	10–12		Amnion enveloping fetus and body stalk. Eyes, ears, and nasal organs forming. Heart and circulation formed. Differentiation of thyroid gland and special outgrowths from the gut (liver, pancreas, gall bladder). Digital ridges indicate future fingers
	6	20–25	1	The head is large compared with the rest of the body. Digits well-formed. Intestines enter coelom. Ears and eyes developing. Genital tubercle present. Lungs separating from gullet. Fetus begins to move
	7–8	40		Head rounded; eyes and ears still forming. Neck region delineated. Abdominal protrusion less marked. Definitive kidneys starting to develop; separation of urinary and rectal passages is complete; anal membrane ruptures. Facial clefts have closed. Beginning function of special endocrine glands
		(cm)		
C. *FETUS* (11–40 weeks)	10	8	15	Ossification centres in most bones. Appearance of nails on fingers and toes. Functioning of nervous system at a primitive level (reflex responses). Teeth are beginning to form. Blood formation transferring from yolk sac and liver to bone marrow
	14	16	110	Sexual differentiation definite
	18		315	Stage of organ growth rather than differentiation
	22		620	Development occurring in the brain; progressive budding, leading to maturation and increase in size in the kidneys, lungs and gastrointestinal tract.
	26	36	1,050	
	30	42	1,700	
	34	46	2,500	
	38	50	3,400	Progressive appearance of centres of ossification, especially at ends of long bones

* Weeks after conception

EMBRYONAL AND FETAL DEVELOPMENT (table 4.1)

The inner cell mass becomes flattened to form the *embryonic disc* at the start of the second week after conception; this soon differentiates into 3 basic layers (ectoderm, mesoderm, and endoderm). The dorsally-placed *ectoderm* will provide the entire nervous system, the skin and its appendages (such as hair and glands), and the peripheral elements of the other sensory organs, such as the eyes and ears. The intermediate *mesoderm* will form the supporting structures — bones and joints, muscles, and connective tissue — together with the vascular and urogenital systems. Finally, the ventrally-placed *endoderm* is responsible for the gastrointestinal tract (including derivative organs, such as the liver, gall bladder, and pancreas), together with other outpouchings such as the thyroid and parathyroid glands, thymus, and lungs.

By the second week, the embryonic disc has become elongated and *2 cavities develop.* Dorsally, above the ectoderm, the *amniotic space* appears and this progressively enlarges over the next 10 weeks, so that it covers the entire embryo except at one point — the body stalk — where the embryo is attached to that part of the trophoblast that is to form the placenta (figure 4.2). By the 14th week of pregnancy, the amniotic sac fills the entire uterine cavity, pressing the nonplacental trophoblast against the endometrium of the opposite wall. Ventrally, another space appears — *the yolk sac.* This forms from endodermal cells, but unlike the amniotic sac, it never attains a large size and soon disappears as the fetus begins to obtain nourishment from the placenta.

The *extraembryonic coelom* is a fluid-filled cavity which arises in the extraembryonic mesoderm which surrounds the embryo. It splits the extraembryonic mesoderm into 2 layers; the *somatic* mesoderm which together with the trophoblast forms the *chorion*, and the *splanchnic* mesoderm, which with a fold of ectoderm forms the *amnion.* The chorion forms a sac inside which the embryo and its amnion are suspended by the body stalk. As indicated earlier, continued growth of the amniotic cavity eventually obliterates this sac. Originally, the extraembryonic coelom communicates with a similar but smaller space in the intraembryonic mesoderm — the intraembryonic coelom. As the embryo grows and folds, the 2 coelomic cavities become separated, that in the embryo forming the *pleural, pericardial* and *peritoneal cavities.*

The *body stalk* provides the connection between the blood vessels of the fetus and those of the trophoblast (which is specializing to become the placenta). As development progresses, great elongation occurs in the stalk, and it becomes the *umbilical cord,* containing the 2 arteries and a single vein.

From the 3rd to 8th weeks, the 3 embryonic layers progressively differentiate to provide the definitive organs of the body.

Ectodermal Layer

The ectodermal cells thicken in the midline to form the primitive streak and this is the forerunner of the *nervous system.* A depression forms in this — the neural groove and the lips of the groove convert it into a tube which becomes the future spinal canal and ventricular system of the brain. The spinal column, derived from mesoderm, develops around the neural axis. The cranial portion of the nervous system enlarges to

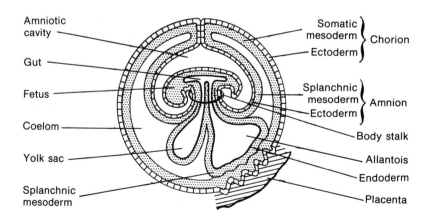

Figure 4.2 Diagram of 21-day embryo (3 weeks after fertilization is the same as 5 weeks' gestation in the language of the clinician).

form the brain. Neuroblasts differentiate to form the white and grey matter of the brain.

Primitive nervous reflex activity is seen as early as 7-8 weeks' gestation; *whole body movements* occur from 10 weeks, and the *grasp reflex* and *facial grimacing* are present at the end of the first trimester. At 16-18 weeks, fetal movements are sufficiently strong to be felt by the mother.

The brain is highly susceptible to *teratogenic agents*, the critical period being from the 10th to the 30th days of embryonic life (Chapters 11 and 17). A major spurt in brain growth occurs in midpregnancy and this continues for up to 4 years postnatally.

The *eye* develops as an outpouching of the forebrain at the side of the facial cleft; by the 6th week there is a fusing of the *optic vesicle* and overlying *lens placode*. The optic vesicle becomes cup-shaped, the narrow open end forming the pupil; the lens placode differentiates to form the lens. There are 2 layers — an inner vascularized pigment layer (retina) and an outer fibrous layer (choroid, sclera and cornea). Eyelid folds are fused until the 6th month (colour plate 119); after the 7th month the eye will respond to light. At birth, the infant fixes on patterns rather than colours; the optimum focal length is about 30 cm.

The eye is highly susceptible to insult between the 18th-30th days.

The *ear*, like the eye, is a compound development — from the *first pharyngeal pouch* and the *otocyst*. Development occurs largely over the second half of the embryonic period (4-8 weeks). The ossicles of the middle ear develop from related mesenchyme and central nervous connections are established to the cochlear and vestibular portions. Myelination of auditory fibres occurs from about the 24th-26th weeks. Sound perception develops slowly over the third trimester; it is geared especially to the type of noises heard in utero (especially vascular souffles).

Mesodermal Layer

The *mesoderm* forms a number of internal structures by processes of proliferation and sculpturing, which are often quite complex. For example, the *vascular system* is seen initially as a simple network of tubes. In the thorax, the initially straight tube undergoes folding and division, and eventually the *heart* is formed, with its intricate system of chambers and valves — subserving first the requirements of the fetus where the lungs are by-passed, and later those of the baby, when the pulmonary circulation becomes operational.

In the fetus, only 10% of the cardiac ouput

goes to the lungs; of the blood in the descending aorta, 60% goes to the umbilical arteries (and the placenta) the remaining 40% to the trunk and lower limbs.

The heart rate reaches a peak in late embryonic life (170-175 beats/minute); this slowly decreases to the normal range at term (120-160). The pressure in the right side of the heart is higher than that in the left side, but this changes rapidly after birth. Detailed data on cardiac and vascular morphology and function can now be obtained with realtime ultrasonography.

The *blood cells* are initially formed from mesoderm in the yolk sac (3rd-6th week), then the liver (6th-36th weeks), and lastly in the bone marrow (20th week onwards). Most of the early red blood cells are nucleated (*erythroblasts*) and contain a different type of haemoglobin.

The embryonic haemoglobin (Gower types 1 and 2) gives way to fetal haemoglobin (haemoglobin F which contains 2 alpha and 2 gamma chains). This is an adaptation to the relative hypoxia of intrauterine life, as is the significantly higher haemoglobin concentrations (14-22 g/dl) at birth. After delivery, adult haemoglobin (haemoglobin A which contains 2 alpha and 2 beta chains) rapidly increases from its 10-15% level to 97-98%. White blood cells and lymphocytes appear in the peripheral blood late in the first trimester; the white cell count is low early in pregnancy — $1.0 \times 10^9/l$ at the 25th week, but reaches $8.0 \times 10^9/l$ at term.

Immune globulins are produced after the first trimester, and the presence of an infection in fetal life can be inferred by the finding of disease-specific IgM in cord blood. Only IgG passes across the placenta from the mother.

The *urogenital system* is derived from swellings on the dorsal body wall. Ridges form and these invaginate to form tubes (Wolffian — male accessory duct system; Mullerian — female genital system). The gonads are populated by sex cells which have migrated from the primitive yolk sac, and these are juxtaposed to the upper part of the genital ducts. The testis can be differentiated from the ovary by about the 6th week. The LH-like activity of HCG is thought to accelerate testicular development, so that by the end of the first trimester, fetal testosterone levels are comparable to adult male levels.

The *kidneys* form from metanephric tissue which is invaded by an outpouching of the metanephric duct (the ureteric bud). As with other organs such as the lung and liver, repeated branchings occur until the final units of function are achieved (in this case the nephron — there being 1 million or more in each kidney).

At the end of the first trimester, the fetal kidney is able to filter and reabsorb urine, but concentrating ability and acidification is poorly developed until after birth.

The *bladder* forms when the urorectal septum descends and separates the bladder in front from the rectum/anal canal behind. The urethra is formed from grooves which appear on the vulva and close over; the female lacks the penile urethra, the folds remaining open to provide the labia minora. Ultrasound studies have demonstrated that the duration of the bladder cycle in the third trimester ranges from about 1–2.5 hours; hourly urine production is about 10 ml/hour at 30 weeks, rising to 25–30 ml at term. Glomerular filtration and tubular absorption rates are significantly less than in the adult on a surface area basis.

Endodermal Layer

The *endoderm* becomes enclosed as the embryonic disc folds during the 4th week, and thus the primitive *foregut*, *midgut*, and *hindgut* are outlined; the midgut leads to the yolk sac at the umbilicus (figure 4.2). Considerable elongation, folding, and outpouching occur to form the final gastrointestinal system. The abdominal bulge seen in the embryo represents the gut, which is too large to be accommodated in the abdominal cavity. Occasionally, this persists and is known as an *exomphalos* (figure 65.12).

The *foregut* comprises the pharynx, oesophagus, stomach and proximal duodenum. The stomach rotates and its mesenteries form the greater and lesser omentum.

There are a number of *derivatives from the foregut. Lung* development begins at the 3rd–4th week from a *tracheobronchial bud* which grows downward in relation to the developing heart. There is progressive budding and vascularization and by about 24 weeks air sacs are appearing in the terminal branches. These basically determine whether the immature infant will survive if born in the latter part of the second trimester. The lining cells are of 2 types — squamous and granular pneumatocytes; the latter, which appear at about the 6th month, produce *surfactant* which lowers surface tension in the alveolus. Primitive *breathing movements* can be observed by ultrasonography as early as the 12th week of fetal life; they become progressively more frequent, deep, and coordinated as gestation advances. The frequency of chest movement is 30–70 per minute and usually such activity occupies 50–90% of any sustained recording period.

The *thyroid, parathyroid,* and *thymus glands* are all derived from the pharyngeal pouches over the 3rd to 5th weeks; function usually commences late in the first trimester.

The *liver bud*, which also forms the *gall bladder*, arises from the first part of the future duodenum. The liver is a comparatively very large organ in fetal life, especially during the period of *haematopoiesis*. Gluconeogenesis is occurring from the 10th week and glycogen storage is a feature of late fetal life (providing an emergency energy store). Bile formation commences in the 4th month, but many enzyme systems are relatively undeveloped until after birth.

The *pancreas* forms from 2 buds and the acinar and islet cells develop side by side.

The *midgut* extends from the duodenum to the left one-third of the transverse colon. *Meckel's diverticulum* indicates the midpoint of the gut. Muscle tissue develops around the endodermal epithelium, and anatomical developments (formation of the appendix and caecum, rotation of the gut) occur in the embryonic period. *The fetus swallows amniotic fluid from the end of the first trimester*; the amount reaches 50 ml or more per hour in late pregnancy. Digestive enzymes can be demonstrated from the second trimester.

The *hindgut* forms the remaining portion of the large bowel. Communication with the allantois ceases at about the 7th week by the formation of the *urorectal septum*. Originally there is an occluding membrane or *proctodeum* similar to that at the entrance to the foregut (the stomodeum). The former may fail to break down, resulting in the condition of *imperforate anus* (figure 65.14).

Ultrasound examination is often helpful in the pregnant woman and this is particularly so when there is bleeding in the first trimester. The following milestones are sought: formation of the *gestation sac* (5–6 weeks), *embryonic outline* (6–7 weeks), *heart activity* (6–7 weeks), early *placenta* (8–9 weeks).

The morphology of the embryo is shown in figure 4.3, while table 4.1 gives the crown-rump (sitting) height and weight at different stages of development. The *fetal weight* increases rapidly in the last trimester of pregnancy and a rough estimate of final weight is given by the formula: maternal weight gain in the last trimester divided by 2. Factors favouring heavier birthweight include a white, tall, multiparous, high socioeconomic status, overweight, nonsmoking mother with a male infant born past term. Figure 4.4 shows the ultrasonic features at 9.5 weeks' gestation. The chief milestones are also indicated. The overall composition of the fetus changes mainly in relation to the amount of fat — 0.5% in the first half of pregnancy to 16% at term; in the placentally insufficient fetus, both

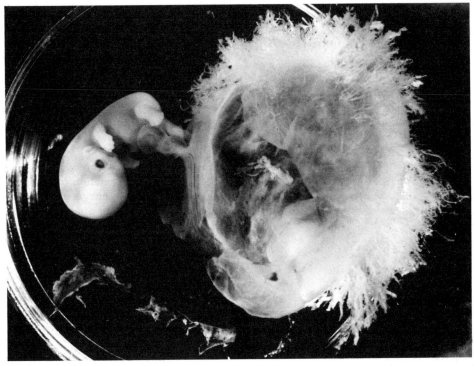

Figure 4.3 Complete abortion at 8 weeks' gestation. Villi are present over the entire surface of the chorion. The limbs, eyes and ears have formed, and the abdomen is protuberant.

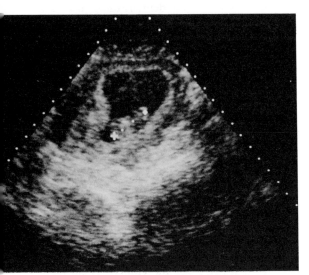 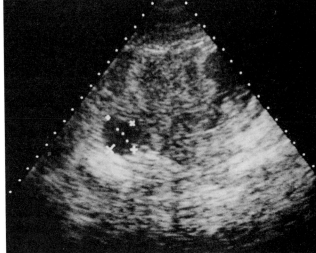

A   **Figure 4.4** Sectoscan showing fetus, a Braxton Hicks contraction and corpus luteum at 9.5 weeks' gestation — the scan was performed because of threatened abortion in a 28-year-old para 1. **A.** A single fetus is shown, crown-rump length 2.7 cm corresponding to a normal pregnancy at 9.5 weeks; fetal heart movements were present. Note irregularity of the uterine wall adjacent to the placenta caused by a Braxton Hicks contraction. **B.** A 2.5 cm diameter corpus luteum is shown to the right of the gestation sac. The pregnancy proceeded uneventfully, resulting in a normal delivery (birthweight 3,710 g) at 39.5 weeks' gestation.   B

glycogen and fat stores can be markedly depleted (figure 8.1).

PLACENTAL DEVELOPMENT

The function of the placenta is to provide a link between the fetus and the mother during the 9 months of intrauterine life. The 4 most vital functions it must carry out are *gas exchange*, *provision of nutrients*, *disposal of waste products* back to the mother, and *hormone production*.

That is, it must play the role of lungs, alimentary tract, liver and kidneys. To accomplish this effectively, it must bring the circulations of the fetus and mother into intimate contact. It has, in addition, a *barrier function*, preventing or limiting the passage of foreign material from the mother and vice versa.

(i) *Blastocyst.* As already mentioned, the mass of dividing cells becomes arranged into 2 groups — a smaller *inner cell mass*, which will develop into the embryo and later the fetus, and a larger surrounding mass, the *trophoblast*, destined to produce the placenta.

(ii) *Early trophoblast.* As embedding (or nidation) is occurring at the 6th–8th day, the rapid proliferation of cells continues. Quite early, the trophoblastic cells differentiate into 2 layers — an inner *cytotrophoblast* and an outer *syncytium*. The cells forming these layers have 2 important functions to perform at this stage; firstly, to invade and break down maternal cells and blood vessels in the decidual layer of the endometrium, so that intimate contact can be made by the trophoblastic blood vessels which will shortly develop, and secondly, to elaborate hormones which are essential to the life of the developing embryo. The most important hormone is secreted from the inner cytotrophic (Langhans) layer of cells — *human chorionic gonadotrophin* (HCG). This hormone provides the message to the corpus luteum in the ovary that conception has occurred and prevents it from degenerating as it normally does at the end of the menstrual cycle. Thus, the ovarian hormones (*oestrogen* and *progesterone*), which are indirectly essential to the growth and nutrition of the embryo by their action on the endometrium, continue to be secreted until the same hormones from the syncytium or outer trophoblast layer can take over this function about 4-6 weeks later.

(iii) *Formation of villi and the intervillous space.* At about 11-13 days after conception, that is, about 5-7 days after embedding, the trophoblastic cells have sent out processes into the endometrium, and soon, spaces or lacunae appear between them which are filled with maternal blood — the result of invasion of thin-walled vessels (colour plate 1). The outgrowths become finger-like and are termed *villi*. In the mesenchymal core of the villi, fetal blood vessels develop in parallel with those in the fetus, and they link up through the body stalk which will become the umbilical cord. By the 16th–18th day, the villi have branched several times, and both fetal and maternal blood vessels are functioning. The latter develop from the *spiral arterioles in the endometrium*, although it is not until some time later that these larger vessels open directly into the *intervillous space*. It should be emphasized that the fetal vessels, unlike the maternal vessels, are at all times separated from the intervillous blood lakes by the trophoblastic covering — *the fetal circulation is thus a closed one* and does not mix directly with the maternal blood and, if placental separation occurs it is

maternal — not fetal — blood that is lost. The heart of the embryo starts to beat on about day 22 after fertilization, so we can say that the fetal circulation, albeit primitive and sluggish, is now functional.

(iv) *Further changes in the trophoblast and decidua.* Up to this point, trophoblastic growth has occurred over the entire circumference of the embryo and, if aborted, the chorionic vesicle looks like a tiny shaggy ball (figure 4.3). With further growth, the villi in contact with the deeper part of decidua (decidua basalis) continue to proliferate to form the *chorion frondosum*, while those in contact with the superficial part (decidua capsularis) atrophy, forming the *chorion laeve* (figure 4.5). Thus, the fetal part of the placenta will be formed by the basal chorion frondosum, and the maternal part by the decidua basalis which is subjacent to it; the atrophic chorion laeve will lose its villi and become the outer layer of the membranes, expanded into the cavity of the uterus by the amniotic membrane which becomes the inner amniotic layer. Fusion of these 2 layers and obliteration of the uterine cavity occurs at the 12th–14th week.

(v) *Final form of the placenta.* By the 14th week, the placenta has attained its definitive form and, for the remainder of the pregnancy, the only changes are in the degree of branching of the villi and increase in the intervillous space. The increase in size of the placenta is less than that of the fetus, particularly in the second half of pregnancy, so that the *fetal:placental weight ratio* steadily increases, reaching a value of almost 6:1 at term. Thus the average birthweight of an infant born at 36 weeks' gestation is about 2,500 g or 75% of the average weight at 40 weeks (3,400 g), whereas the average placental weight at 36 weeks is 550 g or 90% of the average weight at 40 weeks (600 g).

The placenta encroaches upon the lower part of the uterus in about one-third of women before the 20th week, but by term this is less than 2% due to differential growth (figure 19.6).

(vi) *Gross structure and function of the placenta.* A schematic cross-section of the mature placenta is shown in figure 4.6. From the basal area, maternal blood enters the cotyledon via the spiral arterioles. There are approximately 100 such major arterioles supplying the placenta. The blood enters in the form of spurts or jets and cascades down over the villi which are floating in the intervillous space like seaweed in the ocean.

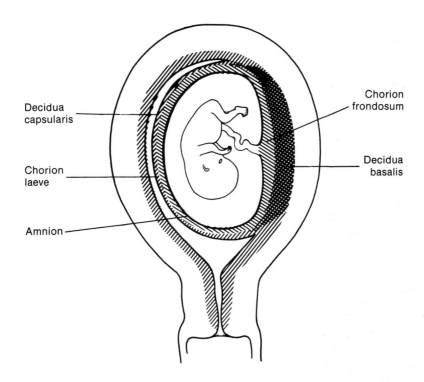

Figure 4.5 Stage of development of fetus and placenta at 8–10 weeks' gestation. The amnion lines the chorion laeve and fetal surface of the placenta, and becomes continuous with the epithelial covering of the umbilical cord.

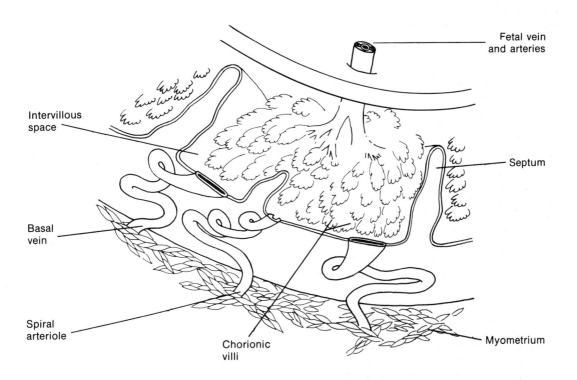

Figure 4.6 Circulation of maternal blood around the chorionic villi; the latter are pulsating in the intervillous space due to the pumping of the fetal heart.

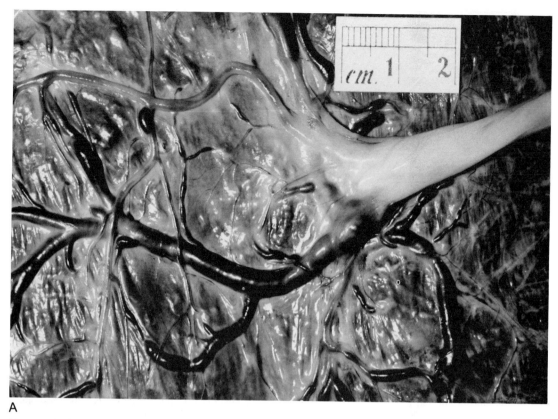

A

Figure 4.7 The placenta at term. **A.** Fetal surface: vessels ramify as they disperse from the insertion of the umbilical cord. They are covered by the glistening, transparent amnion. **B.** Maternal surface showing the usual number (20) of fleshy cotyledons (lobules) packed together. There is no retroplacental clot or macroscopic evidence of infarction or calcification.

B

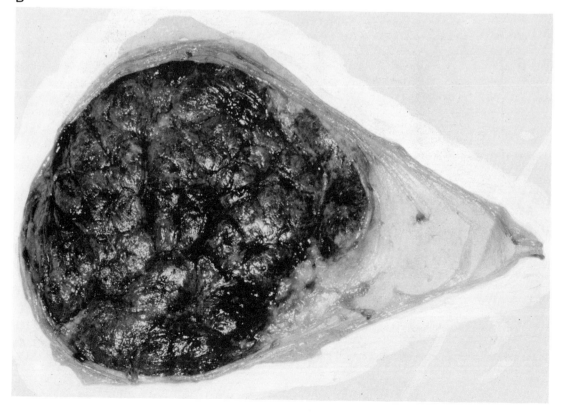

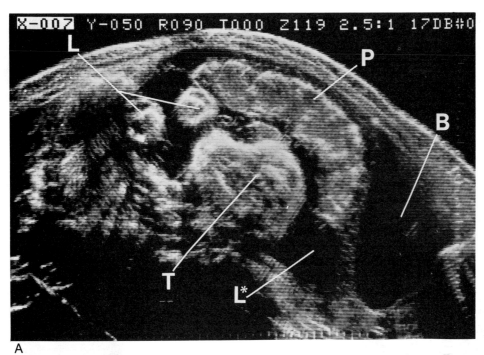

A

Figure 4.8 Placental calcification is not always associated with fetal growth retardation. **A.** This longitudinal ultrasound scan was performed at 30 weeks' gestation to exclude placenta praevia in a 24-year-old para 1 following an antepartum haemorrhage associated with a transverse fetal lie. The placenta (P) is located on the anterior uterine wall and shows an unusual degree of calcification. B = bladder, T = cross-section of fetal trunk, L = fetal limbs, L* = pool of liquor above the cervix. The patient had a forceps delivery at 38 weeks' gestation of a healthy 2,670 g infant. **B.** Following a clomiphene-induced pregnancy, labour was induced at 39.6 weeks' gestation in an obese (101 kg) 28-year-old nullipara with essential hypertension (155/110). She had a normal delivery of a healthy 3,520 g infant and this grossly calcified placenta which weighed only 460 g. It is of interest that there was no antenatal evidence of placental dysfunction (normal weight gain, liquor volume, oestriol values, cardiotocography) and the baby showed none of the features of placental insufficiency (colour plate 20).

B

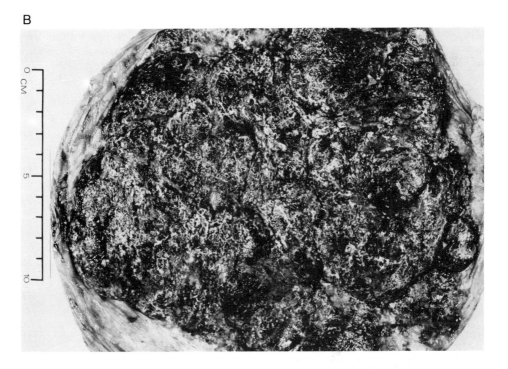

Oxygen and nutrients are provided in exchange for carbon dioxide and waste products from the villi. The deoxygenated blood is carried away by large veins, also situated at the basal area. The *cotyledons* are the units of the placenta, and are based on the arteriolar vessels supplying it. Each cotyledon is functionally independent, although there is no clear separation of one from another, except by incomplete septa. The *intervillous space* is thus potentially traversable throughout the entire placenta.

The 10–35 major and minor subdivisions of the maternal surface of the placenta seen on inspection after delivery are also termed 'cotyledons', but are more properly termed *lobules or lobes* (figure 4.7 and colour plate 92). These are anatomical rather than functional divisions, each containing a number of the latter.

The *mature placenta* measures approximately 18–20 cm in diameter and its thickness ranges from 1 cm at the edge to 4 cm at the centre (colour plates 66 and 92).

(vii) *Fine structure of the placenta.* The *histological unit* of the placenta is the *villus* (colour plate 21). The finer fetal vessels (capillaries) form loops in the connective tissue core of the villus. As pregnancy progresses, there is an increase in the size and number of capillaries and, towards term, they lie close to the intervillous space, often with no perceptible trophoblastic cover.

The tissues separating fetal and maternal blood (*placental barrier*) are trophoblast, connective tissue and endothelium of the fetal blood vessel; because of the thinning of this 'barrier' near term, there is increased efficiency in exchange of nutrients, waste products and gases between mother and fetus. Oxygen and carbon dioxide pass across the villus membrane.

Although the fetal-maternal pressure gradient for *carbon dioxide* is quite low (0.9 kPa or 7 mm Hg), this is compensated by its high diffusability. The transfer of *oxygen* to the fetus depends partly on the difference in gradient (7.3 kPa or 55 mm Hg), but also on the higher binding capacity of fetal blood. As indicated earlier, the *epithelial cells* are of 2 types. The *inner cytotrophoblast* (Langhans layer) is mainly responsible for the production of the hormone HCG, and these cells begin to disappear in the second trimester when the placenta has taken over the role of the corpus luteum as the producer of oestrogen and progesterone. The *outer syncytial layer*, so-called because the cells seem to merge with one another without cell boundaries, produces the above 2 hormones, and this layer persists until delivery, although often becoming quite thinned out or gathered into groups of cells at the periphery of the villi (syncytial knots).

By means of microscopic examination of the villi after delivery, valuable information can often be obtained as to the pathological processes involving the fetus (colour plate 17).

Calcification. Placental calcification increases towards term and is probably a normal physiological process, since it is not more evident when the infant is stillborn. It is excessive in about 5% of placentas, resulting in a gritty maternal surface (figure 4.8). Placental calcification has no well established relationship with either fetal hypoxia or growth retardation. It is probably related to maternal calcium levels (dietary intake, vitamin D intake, ultraviolet exposure) rather than to degenerative changes in the placenta.

NORMAL PREGNANCY

chapter five

Diagnosis of Pregnancy and Parity

OVERVIEW

Although the diagnosis of pregnancy is usually simple if care in history-taking and examination is exercised, there is sufficient variation in the clinical features for difficulty to arise. In addition, the picture may be blurred as a result of disturbances to the pregnancy (abortion, ectopic pregnancy, or hydatidiform mole) and the mimicking of pregnancy by conditions producing secondary amenorrhoea. In some patients, the menstrual pattern is irregular, or its reliability reduced by the patient's poor memory or the effect of the contraceptive pill. Examination difficulties may result from such conditions as obesity and uterine fibromyomas.

Over the past decade there has been a steady improvement in the accuracy of urine pregnancy tests. Today, with specific monoclonal HCG antibodies, a highly accurate test result is available in 2 minutes.

Occasional false positive results still occur, usually because of protein in the urine, occasionally because of a tumour secreting HCG.

False negative results are more common, mainly because it is too early in pregnancy or there is a lower than normal amount of HCG in the urine (blighted ovum, ectopic pregnancy). Because of this, *the patient must always be advised that a negative test does not exclude pregnancy* — it may need repetition if too early or other investigations may be needed if pregnancy pathology is suspected (sensitive serum radioassay, ultrasonography).

It is possible that factors other than HCG (e.g. early pregnancy factor) may be used for very early pregnancy detection in the future.

PREGNANCY

The diagnosis of pregnancy is based on 3 groups of findings — symptoms experienced by the patient, physical changes on examination, and finally laboratory tests.

SUBJECTIVE CHANGES

The classical symptoms are *amenorrhoea, nausea and vomiting* (especially in the morning), *breast soreness or tenderness* (more significant in primigravidas), frequency of micturition, fatigue, and constipation. All of these symptoms are individually nonspecific and not infrequent, even in the nonpregnant woman; however, taken together with the examination findings they present a fairly reliable recognition pattern.

PHYSICAL EXAMINATION

The most characteristic signs are confined to the reproductive organs. Fairly early there is a dilatation of the superficial veins of the breast. Later, there is a general fullness of the breast and changes in the nipple region — increase in pigmentation and prominence of Montgomery follicles (enlarged sebaceous glands within the areola (colour plate 41)).

On speculum examination, the vagina and cervix are a deep bluish-red colour, in contradistinction to the pink colour seen in the nonpregnant state. This is due to venous dilatation caused by the hormone progesterone.

On bimanual examination, the most characteristic change is in the size and consistency of the uterus — from being somewhat flattened and firm it becomes enlarged, globular and cystic. The pulsation of blood in the uterine arteries can sometimes be felt with the fingers in the lateral fornices, and there is a softening of the ecto-cervix (from the consistency of the nose to that of the lips).

It is only by experience that the size equivalent of gestation periods of 6, 8, 10, and 12 weeks can be confidently determined. At the 12th week, the uterus is becoming an abdominal organ and usually can just be palpated suprapubically on abdominal examination.

Diagnostic confusion arises when the above changes are mimicked. Conditions which increase the size of the uterus include new growths (almost always the benign fibromyoma), adenomyosis, retained blood (haematometra). Few other conditions cause the pronounced softening of the uterus and cervix. Hyperoestrogen states may do so — e.g. anovulation, with prolonged, unopposed oestrogen excretion from the Graafian follicle which is characteristic of the woman in later reproductive life; oestrogen from granulosa-cell tumours of the ovary may act similarly.

SPECIAL INVESTIGATIONS

Urine Tests

The majority of pregnancy tests depend on the production of chorionic gonadotrophic hormone (HCG) from the trophoblast. In the older biological tests the patient's urine (containing HCG) was injected into various animals and the stimulating effect on the reproductive organs was observed (ovulation, formation of corpora lutea, discharge of spermatozoa). Nowadays, immunological tests are used.

Most systems employ marker particles (sheep red cells, latex particles) coated with HCG. When in contact with serum containing antibodies to HCG, agglutination will occur. If the patient's urine is first mixed with serum containing antibodies and she is pregnant, the antibodies will be absorbed and none will be left to react with the marker particles — hence no agglutination (pregnancy reaction). If not pregnant, antibodies are free to react with the marker particles — hence, agglutination (nonpregnancy reaction). In some tests (DAP, Gonavislide) the HCG antibodies, not the HCG itself, are attached to the marker. In this case, the urine is directly reacted with the marker and agglutination indicates the presence of HCG in the urine, i.e. pregnancy.

Soon after implantation, HCG is secreted in amounts which can be picked up by sensitive assays on a blood sample. A peak is reached at about the 10th week and thereafter there is a slow fall to the 20th week.

Immunological tests have an accuracy of approximately 98%, provided instructions are carefully followed, the reagents have not deteriorated due to age or improper storage, the glass-ware is clean, and controls are used.

A summary of the features of commonly used pregnancy tests is given in table 5.1 and the levels of beta HCG in blood (and urine) during pregnancy in figure 5.1.

Most laboratories prefer to use slide tests since they are much faster and the sensitivity difference between them and the longer tube test is the equivalent of only a couple of days of pregnancy. Newer tests use monoclonal antibodies (beta HCG) and no longer suffer from the disadvantage of cross-reaction with LH, FSH and TSH (pituitary hormones which share a common alpha subunit with HCG).

The urine should be a morning specimen (which is more concentrated) and free of blood and debris. If a negative result is obtained and clinical suspicion remains, the test should be repeated in 1–2 weeks.

TABLE 5.1   FEATURES OF PREGNANCY TESTS

Feature	Urine immunoassay		Serum immunoassay	
	Slide test	Tube test	Radioimmunoassay (beta subunit)	Radioreceptor assay (alpha and beta subunits)
Time for test result	2 minutes	1–2 hours	1–2 hours	1 hour
Sensitivity (1U/l)	1,000–5,000	200	3–5	200
When '100%' accuracy can be expected (days after LNMP)	42	28	20	28
Cost	+	+ +	+ + + +	+ + +

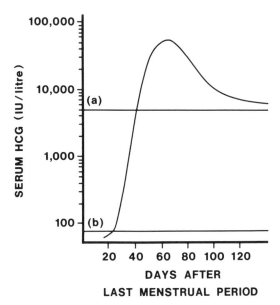

False positive results (test positive, not pregnant). Use of the specific beta-subunit HCG has eliminated many of the false positives formerly due to LH and the other hormones mentioned above.

One remaining problem is the interference by higher than normal protein levels in the urine. The protein may coat the particles carrying the immunological reagent or react immunologically with it. If proteinuria is present, the test may need repeating in 1–2 weeks when HCG levels will have increased.

If the reagents and urine are tested straight from the refrigerator, agglutination may not occur in the 2 minutes usually allowed for the slide test.

Occasionally malignant tumours (e.g. ovarian teratoma) may occur in the childbearing period and secrete significant amounts of HCG.

Figure 5.1 Curve for HCG in serum (IU/l) in early pregnancy shown on a logarithmic scale. Threshold levels are shown for a standard pregnancy test (a) and radioimmunoassay (b). The latter test is positive 10 days after ovulation at its sensitivity limit of 3–5 IU/l. Note the steep rise from days 20–60 which is characteristic of normal pregnancy. The peak occurs at about the 10th week. Thereafter the values fall from a mean of about 50,000 IU/l to plateau at about 5,000 IU/l with a slight rise near term. Urine values show the same pattern — the values in IU/l being the same as for serum. After 16 weeks' gestation a normal pregnancy may have an HCG value of below 5,000 IU/l in serum or urine which could result in a false negative standard pregnancy test.

Figure 5.2 Sector of a realtime scan at 12.5 weeks' gestation showing a fetus with a crown-rump length of 5.9 cm lying with its back on the uterine wall. Ultrasonographic assessment of fetal maturity utilizes measurement of gestational sac volume (until 6.5–7 weeks), crown-rump length (7–13 weeks) and biparietal diameter, length of femur and abdominal girth after 13 weeks' gestation.

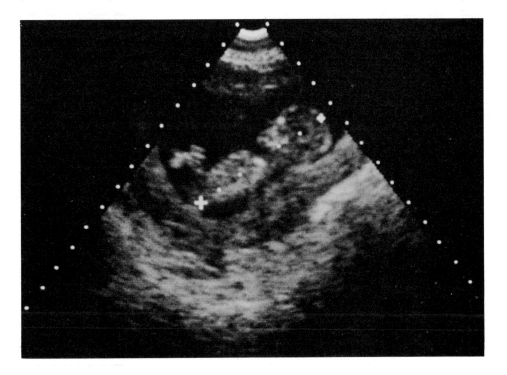

False negative results (test negative, pregnant) arise from errors in technique, test performed too early, and abnormality of the pregnancy (ectopic, abortion).

It must be emphasized that a negative test does not exclude pregnancy and this message should be clearly understood by the patient. If an ectopic pregnancy or blighted ovum is suspected, a more sensitive serum assay should be ordered. If too early, the test should be repeated in 2 weeks' time.

Sensitive Serum Assays

Two main techniques are currently in use — radioreceptor assay and the radioimmunoassay (table 5.1). These have the advantage of sensitivity, allowing diagnosis of pregnancy some 5–7 days after conception — i.e. well before the first missed period.

The principle of these assays is similar to that of the urine tests. In the radioreceptor assay, HCG is detected by measuring its competition for specific cell membrane receptor sites. It is less sensitive than the radioimmunoassay because it utilizes the whole HCG structure rather than the beta-subunit. Both assays are much more expensive than the slide test on urine and are reserved for special indications where sensitivity is necessary (embryonic failure, ectopic pregnancy).

Ultrasound (figure 5.2)

Instruments employing the Doppler principle can detect fetal heart reflection echoes at 6–7 weeks of gestation, but these only become 100% reliable at about 8–9 weeks.

With the vastly more complex compound B scanner, the fetal sac can be outlined from the fifth week of pregnancy and the embryo shortly afterwards.

Fetal Electrocardiogram

The fetal electrocardiogram can be detected at approximately 10 weeks, but only achieves 100% reliability at 18–20 weeks.

Thermometry

As early as the fourth week of pregnancy, there is a distinct elevation of skin temperature over the breast compared with that over the sternum (0.7°C). This can be detected by a sensitive infrared thermometer.

Radiography

Fetal bones become visible on radiographs at 14–16 weeks. Because of the possibility of radiation damage to the fetus and the lack of sensitivity of this technique, it is no longer used unless ultrasonography is unavailable.

Hormonal Withdrawal Test

If a relatively large dose of an oestrogen/progesterone preparation is given for 2–3 days, there will usually be withdrawal bleeding within a further 3–5 days if the patient is not pregnant. This test has now been abandoned because of possible harmful effects on the developing embryo if the patient is pregnant.

PROBLEM OF THE ABNORMAL PREGNANCY

(i) Abortion. If the abortion is only threatened, the pregnancy test will remain positive; if products of conception have been passed, the test usually becomes negative within 5 days. The same applies to missed abortion, although with more advanced pregnancies the test may be positive for a longer period. It is now realized that malformation of the embryo is relatively common (40–50% of pregnancies) and these abnormal conceptuses are usually aborted in the first 2–3 weeks after conception. Urine tests will often give a negative value, although the more sensitive radioassay on serum will be positive.

(ii) Ectopic pregnancy. The pregnancy test may be positive in the early stages, but is often negative, particularly if tubal abortion or rupture has occurred or the pregnancy is early. An important clue to this diagnosis is the finding of decidua without chorionic tissue on curettage, usually performed because a diagnosis of incomplete abortion has been made. As with early abortion, a serum test should be carried out (together with ultrasonography). The values will be below those expected for the period of gestation, and usually will fail to show the rapid rise characteristic of early normal pregnancy (figure 5.1).

(iii) Hydatidiform mole. The test is usually positive in high dilutions of urine (1/100 or more) when performed before molar evacuation has occurred. The highest urine beta HCG value in normal singleton pregnancy is about *300,000 u/24 hours* (figure 5.1) — higher values are suggestive of hydatidiform mole or *multiple pregnancy*.

LATER SIGNS

After the 12th week of pregnancy, the uterus is palpable above the symphysis pubis. Special investigations (e.g. ultrasonography) may be required to distinguish such conditions as hydatidiform mole and ovarian cyst. The 'positive clinical signs' of older obstetrical parlance (fetal heart sounds, palpable fetal parts, or movements) will usually not be demonstrated until well into the second trimester.

PARITY

Women do not always admit to a previous pregnancy, and because of the difference in clinical behaviour of parous and nonparous patients (particularly in labour) the signs of parity should be known.

Breasts. There may be pigmentation of the areolae earlier than expected (normally occurs at the 12th week). The nipple is more prominent and the breast is flabbier.

Abdomen. Striae may be present and the skin is looser. Because of the greater laxity of the abdominal muscles, the fetus is easier to palpate.

Vagina. The vagina and introitus are lax, and there may be evidence of a perineal tear or episiotomy scar.

Cervix. The external os usually provides the most revealing clue, the small circular aperture of the nullipara having become a larger transverse slit which easily admits the finger tip.

chapter six

Antenatal Care. Education of the Patient

OVERVIEW

Antenatal care has been an integral item in the management of the pregnant patient for the past 60 years. The essence of such care is a thorough assessment at the first visit (history, examination, routine and indicated investigations) followed by assessments thereafter at appropriate intervals. Major emphasis is thus placed on the preventive aspects of care — detection of preexisting abnormalities and future deviations from normal at the earliest opportunity. This allows proper action to be undertaken — be it patient education and motivation, immediate medical care, referral for investigation or expert opinion, or an increase in the tempo of surveillance.

Because of the normality of many obstetric patients, the antenatal visit is often conducted as a run of the mill exercise, and because of this, perception is often based on what is expected, rather than what is actually present. In this way, *twins* may not be detected at 26–30 weeks' gestation or *breech presentation* at 30–32 weeks, when they should be, and so on. Each antenatal visit should thus be an occasion when the attendant takes careful stock of the situation.

Proper antenatal management involves seeing the patient as *early as practicable in the pregnancy*, considerable care in obtaining all relevant information about the patient by *history, examination and special investigation* and, having this information, thinking carefully about its obstetric significance and taking appropriate corrective action.

In recent years there has been a trend toward fewer antenatal visits, particularly in the multiparous patient. With much improved patient education regarding optimum health behaviour during pregnancy, and more extensive and sophisticated investigative procedures (e.g. ultrasonography, cardiotocography), this policy is probably justified, although the decision should be made by experienced medical personnel.

An overriding consideration of antenatal care is *detection of the risk factor(s) for both mother and baby*, and reducing these to manageable and safe proportions. In the extreme case, this may involve the antenatal diagnosis of *major fetal anomaly* and termination of the pregnancy if thought to be necessary.

Financial considerations will determine the extent to which *modern special investigative procedures* (ultrasonography, cardiotocography, glucose tolerance testing) are used in addition to the established brigade of *routine tests* (haemoglobin, blood group and rhesus type and antibodies, serology for the detection of syphilis, urine dip-slide for detection of bacteriuria). The potential value of routine testing is that many conditions that affect fetal well-being have no clinical marker e.g. fetal deaths due to placental insufficiency often occur in clinically normal women. *Fewer than 50% of all perinatal deaths occur in identifiable high risk pregnancies* — hence the crusade of the modern obstetrician to investigate fetal well-being in 'normal' pregnancies. Only recently have antenatal tests been subjected to critical analysis, with an assessment of their performance in terms of sensitivity, specificity and accuracy. It is evident that fetal function tests in particular are not 100% reliable and should be interpreted together with the usual clinical considerations when decisions are made regarding the *timing of delivery*.

The antenatal period is the ideal time to provide the mother with appropriate *health education*: e.g. diet, rest, exercise, breast feeding; the potential harm to the baby of *alcohol* and *smoking* should be indicated. Salicylate abuse is often overlooked and routine enquiry should be made and the dangers to the mother and her baby pointed out (prolongation of the pregnancy, difficult delivery, bleeding tendency). The attendant should be aware of the many information, counselling, and support groups that now exist to help the pregnant and puerperal mother and should refer the patient when appropriate.

The following trends have been suggested — greater responsibility of the mother for her obstetric record, screening procedures, and care options; greater involvement of the woman's partner in antenatal care; better accessibility of clinics, continuity of care, and care of other children.

Definition

'A planned programme of observation, education, and medical management of pregnant women directed toward making pregnancy and delivery a safe and satisfying experience'
— American College of Obstetricians and Gynaecologists.

THE FIRST VISIT

The particular routine through which the patient passes depends on such variables as private or public care and the size of the institution in the latter case.

History

'The ability to communicate with patients never goes out of date'.

The history should be taken in a quiet and private atmosphere, since some of the details are of a personal nature. The information will be gathered under the headings indicated below, special enquiry being directed to factors likely to be relevant to pregnancy. Some favour self-taking histories, at least in the first instance, since this represents a significant saving of time; others feel that an important interaction with the patient is thereby lost.

Administrative details. In all cases, the patient's general particulars — name, place of abode, date of birth, occupation, next of kin, religion are documented.

Family. Conditions likely to be inherited by the patient are recorded (diabetes, hypertension, psychiatric disorder, twinning) and/or the baby (deafness, blindness, twinning, chromosomal or metabolic disorders). In some couples a detailed genetic history may be necessary.

Medical. Allergies, cardiac disease, hypertension, renal diseases, central nervous disorders (particularly epilepsy), psychoses, gastrointestinal, metabolic (particularly thyroid disorders and diabetes), blood transfusions, rubella; any medications should be recorded.

Surgical. Abdominal or pelvic operations or injuries, cardiac surgery.

Gynaecological. A history of venereal disease is important. Also previous disorders, such as abnormal cytology, infertility, and gynaecological surgery are relevant.

Social. Relevant socioeconomic data are obtained, including information on family adjustment and living conditions, and unusual stresses. Consumption of *alcohol* and *drugs of addiction* should be determined.

Obstetrical. Accurate details of all previous pregnancies (not just living babies) must be obtained, including the year, period of gestation, duration of labour, nature of delivery, and outcome, including sex and weight of the baby; also complications arising during pregnancy, labour, and the puerperium. A history of *termination of pregnancy* should be specifically enquired about in view of the possibility of cervical incompetence. Breast feeding experience and attitudes are noted together with the mother's general attitude to her childbirth experiences. In many cases, the patient is vague about the history, not having been told the details or understood the explanation provided. The need for obtaining *past records* cannot be emphasized too strongly — if any doubt exists, the previous practitioner or hospital superintendent should be requested to provide the relevant details.

The history of the present pregnancy is then obtained, which includes a careful review of all systems. Particularly important is the date of commencement of the *last normal menstrual period* and the *date of quickening* if that milestone has already passed. It is important to enquire about the regularity of the menstrual cycle, whether the last period occurred at the normal time, and whether it was itself normal in duration and amount. Because ovulation delay may follow use of the *contraceptive pill*, information about this should also be ascertained. The duration of marriage is important in patients with infertility. If the patient is unmarried, a number of details will need to be explored, preferably with the assistance of a social worker.

A list of *all drugs taken* by the patient during the first trimester should be noted, and also any infections she has suffered. The patient's diet during the pregnancy is assessed, particularly the amount of protein, vitamins and calories in relation to her activity. Since some patients improve their diet only after they become pregnant, prepregnancy habits should also be recorded.

There are other facets of history which, although not directly obstetrical in nature, are helpful in management. These include the mother's general attitude to health care, her maternal strength and degree of acceptance of the pregnancy, pain tolerance, educational level, and the degree of personal and/or environmental stress and her resources for coping with this. The attitudes/supportiveness of the husband/partner should also be ascertained.

Examination

A complete physical examination is necessary since, if abnormalities occur later in the pregnancy, a base-line will have been established. Furthermore, if a lesion such as rheumatic carditis is not detected, unexpected cardiac failure or even death of the patient may result (colour plates 4 and 94).

If the patient is in the first trimester, it is most unlikely that the uterus will be palpable in the abdomen unless the patient is thin and/or the uterus is extremely anteverted.

It is valuable, while the patient is being examined, to gain an idea of her general state of health, both mental and physical. Points to look for include degree of tension, general physique, physical fitness, posture, and weight/height ratio.

It is important for the midwife to be present at the time of this examination and to ensure that embarrassment to the patient is prevented by adequate draping and screening. A supply of the appropriate instruments and materials likely to be required should be available (various sizes of vaginal specula, gloves, lubricant, materials for Papanicolaou smear, sponge-holding forceps, cotton balls, swabs for microbiology). The bladder should be emptied prior to the examination.

The patient is assisted onto the couch, where she rests comfortably in the dorsal or supine position (figure 6.1). In the last trimester, the patient should either sit up or lie on her side, unless the doctor is to see her immediately. This is to prevent occurrence of the *supine hypotensive syndrome*, which results from the heavy uterus falling on the large vessels carrying blood to and from the heart (figure 48.1). A blood pressure cuff is placed firmly around the upper arm. This is an appropriate opportunity for the nurse to make the patient feel at ease by showing an interest in her, ascertaining how she is feeling, and whether she has any anxieties or questions.

Areas of Special Importance

Teeth. Both gums and teeth are examined, and the number of decayed and missing teeth recorded. The need for immediate and/or long-term dental care is assessed and referral arrangements, if necessary, are made.

Colour. The mucosal surfaces of the mouth and conjunctivae, and palms of the hands are observed for signs of obvious pallor, indicating anaemia. Cyanosis may be present in patients with major heart or chest disorders.

Neck. Some thyroid enlargement is normal in pregnancy, but if this is associated with warm, moist hands, tachycardia and a 'jumpy' patient, thyrotoxicosis should be considered, and appropriate tests carried out.

Breasts. General inspection and palpation is carried out, firstly to determine the regularity of the breasts and absence of any lumps which might indicate neoplastic disease, and secondly,

Figure 6.1 The blood pressure is estimated carefully at every antenatal attendance. The angle lamp is used during speculum examination of the vagina and cervix.

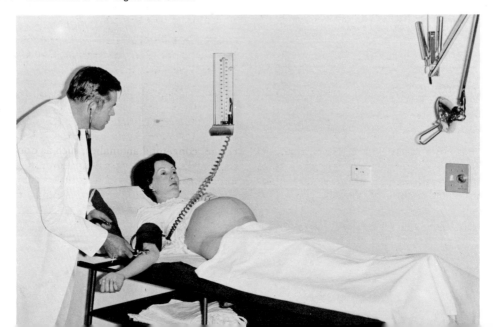

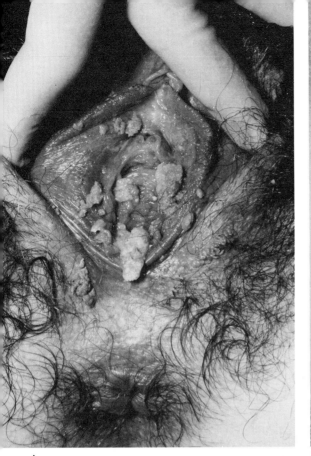
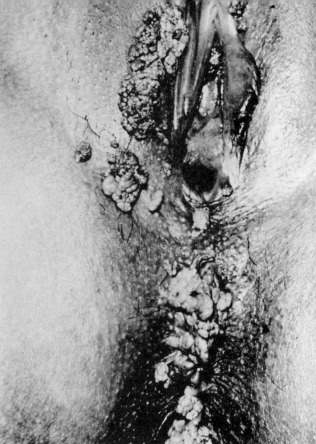

A   B

Figure 6.2 Condylomata acuminata. **A.** Involving mainly vagina and labia minora. These lesions are caused by the papilloma virus but occur in response to discharge and irritation due to infection usually with trichomonas or candida. The lesions are often smaller and more numerous and usually disappear spontaneously when the infection is treated. **B.** More extensive lesions situated mainly on the perineum. Condylomata tend to grow rapidly during pregnancy. Gonorrhoea and syphilis should always be excluded. Such large lesions usually require electrocoagulation for cure. (Courtesy of Dr Jennifer Wilson).

to assess the nipples. If the latter are flat or inverted, the patient is instructed on drawing them out, and the wearing of a special shield is considered (colour plate 44).

Heart. This is carefully checked for size, rate, and the presence of murmurs which might indicate congenital, rheumatic, or other disease. The blood pressure is measured, making sure that the cuff size is appropriate for the size of the patient's arm. Referral to a cardiologist is arranged if an abnormality is detected.

Chest. The configuration and symmetry of the chest wall is noted and the degree of expansion assessed. This gives some idea of the patient's vital capacity. More important, however, in assessing her cardiopulmonary state is to gauge her *exercise tolerance.*

Abdomen. Only rarely will any abnormality be revealed in the abdomen at the first visit. Enlargement of the liver, kidneys, or spleen may be detected. The tone of the abdominal wall

musculature should be assessed, and this is an appropriate time to bring up the subject of physiotherapy and antenatal classes.

Limbs. The limbs are tested for oedema and the lower limbs for varicosities. The latter should be done with the patient standing. The size of shoe, as well as the height of the patient, are a fairly good indirect gauge of the size of the pelvis — a small shoe and a height under 153 cm are indicative of possible contracture.

Vulva. Of relevance are varices, previous tears and episiotomies, state of the perineal body, and laxity of the introitus.

Vagina. Of relevance are infection (monilia, trichomonas, gonorrhoea, or nonspecific cervicitis); abnormalities of the cervix (laceration, erosion, tumour); laxity of the vaginal walls and cervix; congenital anomalies, such as double cervix and vagina, or vaginal septum. A Papanicolaou smear is taken and a swab for appropriate culture if infection is suspected (figure 6.2).

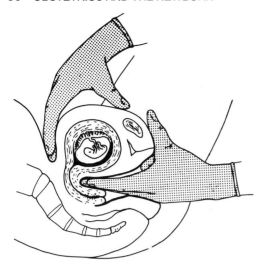

Figure 6.3 Hegar sign of pregnancy at 6–8 weeks' gestation. Because of extreme softening of the lower segment, the abdominal fingers almost meet those in the anterior fornix at bimanual examination in a thin, relaxed patient (dorsal position, bladder empty). In 80% of patients the uterus is anteverted as shown here.

Bimanual Examination

This examination is only omitted if there is active or recent bleeding or a history of repeated abortions, when it may be deferred until the second trimester. In any event, it should be handled in a systematic but gentle manner. Information is sought on the following points. (i) *Uterus.* Consistency — soft and cystic or firm, size in relation to period of amenorrhoea, regularity, anteverted or retroverted (figure 6.3). (ii) *Cervix.* Regularity, softening, size of the external os and internal os. (iii) *Fornices.* Abnormal masses, suggesting ovarian tumour, ectopic pregnancy, or bicornuate uterus. (iv) *Muscular tone.* Ability to relax muscles of the pelvic and perineal diaphragms. (v) *Bony pelvis.* Diagonal conjugate, curve of sacrum, prominence of ischial spines, width of sacrospinous ligaments, angle of subpubic arch (figure 6.4).

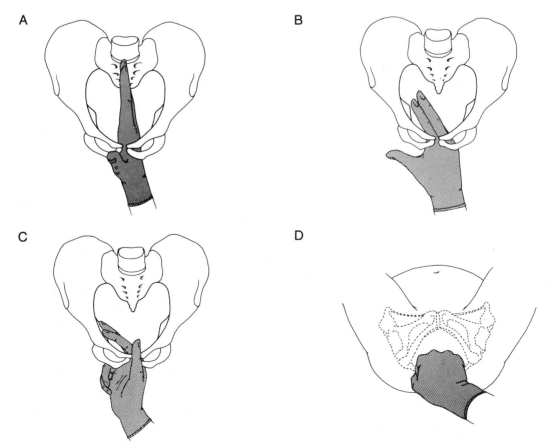

Figure 6.4 Examination of the bony pelvis. **A.** The shape of the sacrum and prominence of the coccyx is noted. If the sacral promontory can be reached (diagonal conjugate), pelvic contraction should be suspected. **B.** Breadth of the sacrosciatic notch and prominence of the ischial spine is noted. **C.** Palpation of lateral pelvic wall for convergence as occurs in an android or funnel pelvis. **D.** Assessment of the pelvic outlet — the 4 knuckles fit comfortably between ischial tuberosities (bituberous diameter) in a pelvis of normal dimensions.

TABLE 6.1   STANDARD ANTENATAL INVESTIGATIONS

Essential

(a)   First visit

    (i)   Blood grouping and rhesus typing
    (ii)   Indirect Coombs in both rhesus negative and positive women
    (iii)   Haemoglobin with full blood examination if below 10–11 g/dl
    (iv)   Haemoglobin electrophoresis if indicated
    (v)   Mid-stream urine for bacteriuria
    (vi)   Serology to exclude syphilis
    (vii)   Papanicolaou cervical smear

(b)   Subsequent visits

    (i)   Ultrasonography at 14–18 weeks if fetal maturity uncertain
    (ii)   Genetic counselling amniocentesis if indicated
    (iii)   Repeat haemoglobin at 30 weeks and postpartum
    (iv)   If rhesus negative, repeat indirect Coombs at 30, 36 and 40 weeks

Recommended

(a)   First visit

    (i)   Rubella antibodies
    (ii)   Hepatitis B antigen in high risk patients

(b)   Subsequent visits

    (i)   Glucose tolerance or diabetic elimination test at 30–32 weeks
    (ii)   Cervical swab for group B beta haemolytic streptococcus at 32 weeks
    (iii)   Test of fetoplacental function at 36–38 weeks

Additional Procedures — Investigations (table 6.1)

The height and weight of the patient will be measured and the results entered on the patient's record along with those of the urinalysis.

Before the patient sees the doctor, she will usually have had a *blood specimen* taken for *grouping, rhesus factor* and *antibodies, haemoglobin*, and screening tests for *syphilis* (one of the reagin tests) and antibodies (to *rubella* and possibly other 'TORCH' infections). In many centres, screening for the *thalassaemia trait* is undertaken if red blood cell indices are abnormal; similarly, screening for the *sickle cell disease* is carried out in populations at risk (Chapter 34). If the patient is a known or suspected *hepatitis B carrier*, special precautions should be taken: materials used for the taking of blood should be carefully disposed of; a warning note made on the specimen slip; and hypochlorite disinfectant used for spilt blood. In some centres maternal blood is examined routinely for hepatitis B status. A *urine specimen* (mid-stream) is taken for the *bacteriuria screening test* (usually by one of the 'dip-slide' methods). Sugar and protein are tested (usually by the dip-stick method). The pH and specific gravity may be recorded. If microscopy and culture of the urine specimen is to be performed, the specimen must be either refrigerated or sent to the laboratory within 10–15 minutes, since bacterial multiplication is quite rapid at room temperature. In some centres, a 'drug screen' is carried out to detect users of narcotics and other drugs of addiction.

After the conclusion of the examination, the patient should be reassured as to the findings, particularly in relation to the progress of the pregnancy, the seeming normality of the baby, and her own normality in relation to coping with the pregnancy, labour and puerperium. The *expected date of delivery is provided*; usually this is based on the first day of the last normal menstrual period, adding 7 days and 9 months (Naegele rule). If the menstrual date is vague, or the menses abnormal or irregular, *ultrasonography* is often carried out. If a problem does exist, either one already known to the patient or discovered during the visit, the significance of it should be indicated to her in words which are as simple and as reassuring as possible.

The importance of antenatal visits is stressed to the patient, as well as the need for adequate rest and sleep, and a good diet. She should be made aware of the importance of this for the baby as well as for herself. Habits which may be injurious (smoking, alcohol, drugs), are discussed. *She is requested to record the date of first fetal movements.* This is important since the date of quickening, noted *prospectively,* is as accurate as ultrasonography in assessment of fetal maturity and requires no expensive equipment — ultrasonography is employed when menstrual data, date of quickening and clinical assessment of uterine size do not correspond.

The patient is given a careful explanation of the hospital facilities, including educational and physiotherapy classes, ancillary services, and other aspects of prenatal care (maternity and other social benefits), and this is usually reinforced by giving her a booklet on the subject (which should include chapters on the hygiene of pregnancy, minor disorders, and symptoms which should be reported), and a small list of books on different aspects of pregnancy if she wishes to have more information. In many communities there is a surprising number of parent support services of value during and after the pregnancy and, when indicated, these should be brought to the patient's attention.

At the conclusion of the interview, the history and examination findings should be critically reviewed to assess their significance to the present pregnancy. That is, a compilation of *risk factors* should be made which perhaps can best be divided into major (examples being habitual abortion, previous premature deliveries, repeated pyelonephritis, diabetes, rhesus isoimmunization, Caesarean section) and minor (examples being a single miscarriage, an isolated attack of pyelonephritis, low forceps delivery). Apportionment of risk can usually be made on the basis of history (35–40%), current pregnancy (50–55%), and current labour (5–10%).

If the patient has been unduly late in seeking antenatal care, the reason should be ascertained (e.g. working, low health care interest, cultural, pregnancy unrecognized, fear etc), and the value of the early initial visit for future pregnancies emphasized.

Relevant information is sought, by letter or case notes, concerning previous pregnancies or illnesses. If further examinations are indicated, these will be arranged. A decision is made as to whether special consultation is required (e.g. physician for cardiac disease or diabetes) and how/where the patient is to be delivered. If social assistance, physiotherapy, dietetic advice, or dental treatment is required, this is also arranged.

A final consideration is that of *genetic counselling.* Whether on the basis of maternal age, family history or findings on routine antenatal testing (e.g. plasma alpha fetoprotein (AFP), haemoglobin electrophoresis), the questions of serious fetal abnormality/genetic

amniocentesis/pregnancy termination may arise (see Chapter 17).

SUBSEQUENT VISITS

Frequency of Visits

The normal routine is for the patient to be seen monthly until the 28th week, fortnightly until the 36th week, and weekly thereafter. These intervals are usually shortened if there is any condition, threatened or present, which may adversely affect the mother or baby.

Medical and Nursing Routine

The routine is similar to that of the initial visit, but the history and examination are restricted to the pregnancy itself, unless there are non-obstetrical problems present. Particular care is taken with the accurate recording of the blood pressure (figure 6.1). The patient's minor disorders, if any, are discussed, and reassurance and therapy given as indicated. The antenatal preparation of the breasts and nipples for the mother who is intending to breast-feed is

Figure 6.5 Amniography-fetography at 32 weeks' gestation. The water-soluble dye has been swallowed and 24 hours later outlines the fetal intestines, thus excluding bowel atresia as cause of the polyhydramnios. The fat-soluble dye has been absorbed by the vernix caseosa and outlines the fetal surface, showing male genitalia and excluding such defects as meningomyelocele. Note deflexed fetal attitude which is usual with polyhydramnios. Cytomegalovirus was cultured from the liquor and infant; the latter died 3 weeks after birth as a result of the infection (colour plate 126).

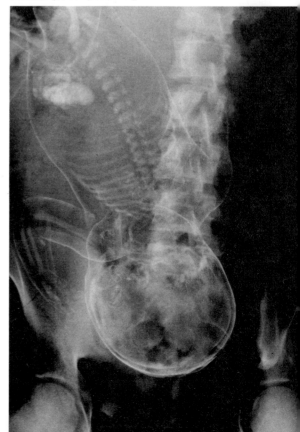

explained and supervised if necessary (Chapter 60). At the end of the first trimester the heartbeat of the fetus can be identified by the Doppler instrument. Some obstetricians routinely assess each pregnancy with a realtime ultrasound scan early in the second trimester. Routine clinical tests — weight, urinalysis for protein and sugar — are performed, and *special laboratory tests* as indicated (table 6.1): haemoglobin level at first visit and 30 weeks and perhaps near 40 weeks; rhesus antibodies; a screening test for fetal well-being (urinary oestriol or HPL assay) and/or fetal growth (ultrasonic measurement) at 34–38 weeks.

Abdominal Examination

There is usually little of significance to note on abdominal palpation of the uterus during the second trimester, apart from deviations of size. Fetal growth retardation rarely manifests itself clinically until the last trimester; a uterus larger than expected is the most likely problem to be encountered, with the need to exclude *multiple pregnancy* and *polyhydramnios* (colour plates 70 and 71). In the third trimester, accurate palpation becomes increasingly important, since preventative steps may need to be taken for abnormalities of fetal disposition.

The patient should lie comfortably in the supine position, with the arms by the sides and the head well supported by a pillow. The bladder should be empty. The drapes are arranged to give access to the whole abdomen.

Because of the occurrence of the *supine hypotensive syndrome* in some women, particularly in late pregnancy, the mother should be warned to lie on her side if she feels faint.

(a) *Inspection.* The *general contour of the abdomen* is noted — whether it is rounded, indicating a well-flexed fetus (C-shaped), or elongated, indicating a deflexion attitude (S-shape) or a breech with extended legs. A heart-shaped outline indicates the presence of a *bicornuate uterus*, and this is supported by the finding of a sideways bulge of the uterus in the mother's flank due to the fetal limbs (colour plate 72).

The normal uterine contour is oval or pear-shaped; this is obliterated if there is an abnormal amount of intrauterine contents (multiple pregnancy and/or polyhydramnios). Also, with increasing parity, the classical contour is less evident; in the extreme case, the uterus becomes floppy and pendulous due to lack of muscular and ligamentous supports. If the fetus is lying transversely, the fundus will be lower than expected, and the transverse diameter will be widened.

In late pregnancy, posterior positions of the fetal head are characterized by a prominence above the umbilicus and a depression below it. Fetal movements may be seen and, with palpation, help to fix the position of the limbs and back, which is on the side opposite to the limbs.

(b) *Palpation.* The greatest mistake of the inexperienced attendant is to palpate too vigorously with the tips of the fingers rather than with the palmar surfaces, and/or with cold hands. In such cases, the cooperation of the patient will diminish and, very often, the abdominal muscles and the uterus will be made tense and irritable (Braxton-Hicks contraction), making further palpation more difficult. A safe rule is to keep the hands flat on the abdominal wall, gliding them gently from one grip to the next.

The *fundal height* is estimated by placing the ulnar border of the straightened hand comfortably at the highest point of the uterus and comparing this with accepted levels for different periods of gestation. The xiphisternum is taken as the reference point for full term pregnancy, and the *umbilicus for 20 weeks* (figure 38.1). Each 4-week period is approximately equal to 2–3 finger-breadths or, alternatively, the area between umbilicus and xiphisternum is divided into 5 equal divisions, each representing a period of 4 weeks. The variability in position of the umbilicus and the length of the symphysis pubis-xiphisternum distance in different individuals should be remembered: for example, there is a biological variation of 15–18 cm in the abdominal length of pregnant women. In the extreme case this would produce an error of 14 weeks, assuming that the uterus grows about 2.5 cm per fortnight. The umbilicus can also vary in position by up to 12.5 cm in different women. For assessment of fetal growth in the individual patient, a reasonable estimate is obtained by successive measurements of the distance from the top of the symphysis pubis to the fundus of the uterus by tape measure. The distance in cm usually equals the gestation period in weeks up to the end of the second trimester. Because of the phenomenon of *lightening* in late pregnancy (descent of the head into the pelvis), the fundus (particularly in the nullipara) may appear to be stationary or even to drop as full term approaches (figure 38.1).

The 4 Classical Techniques of Palpation

The term, palpation, is preferred to 'grip', which does not accurately describe the procedure adopted.

(i) *Fundal palpation.* The patient should be examined from the right side, unless the examiner is left-handed. Facing the patient's head, the hands of the examiner are placed on the sides of the fundus following its contour. In 95% of patients, the *breech* will be felt, differing from the head in its less definite outline, lack of independent movement from the trunk, softer consistency, and poorer ballottement (ability to 'bounce' backwards and forwards between the examining hands).

If the head is in the fundus (i.e. the breech is presenting in the pelvis), its smooth round, hard feel is characteristic. The features may be obscured by the lower limbs if these are extended, by an anterior fundal placenta, or by the head slipping under one or other costal margin. Also, the mother often complains of greater *tenderness* in the fundal region, both spontaneously and during palpation, presumably due to a greater pressure effect of the harder skull.

If no pole can be felt, the possibilities are transverse lie or a breech presentation in an anencephalic fetus.

(ii) *Lateral palpation.* This is used to ascertain the position of the back in those cases where the lie is longitudinal. The examiner remains in the same position, but the hands are moved down to the level of the umbilicus. With gentle pressure, supplemented with dipping movements, the resistance of the back is sought and its distance from the midline noted. This procedure is made easier if alternate hands are used to steady the

trunk and push it toward the opposite examining hand. *The fetal limbs will be on the side opposite the back*; they are best felt by gliding the hands over the surface of the abdomen, seeking the mobile irregularities by which the limbs are characterized. Often, movements of the limbs will be both observed and palpated as the fetus shifts under the stimulus of the palpation.

If limbs are felt on both sides of the midline, it is indicative of a markedly *posterior position* of the fetus (occiput and back), and this position is still probable if they are clearly palpable anteriorly on one side. With lateral ('transverse') positions of the occiput and fetal back, the limbs are felt well laterally at the sides of the uterus, while, if the occiput and back are anterior in position, the limbs cannot be felt since the fetus is facing the back of the uterus and the limbs are posteriorly placed (figure 6.6).

The *anterior shoulder*, because of its prominence, is often used as a distinguishing landmark, both for assisting in the determination of *position of the fetus* and *descent of the presenting part* into the pelvis. It may be found by following the resistance of the back downward, or by palpating upward from the neck region. In anterior positions, it lies 2–4 cm on the side opposite to the back; in lateral positions, it lies in the midline, since the head is at right angles to the shoulders; and, in posterior positions, it is more than 6–8 cm from the midline on the side of the back (figure 6.6). The *fetal back*, because

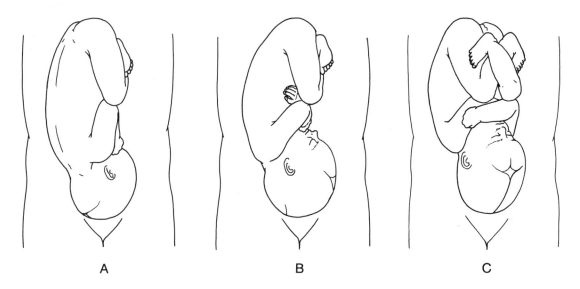

A   B   C

Figure 6.6 Right positions of the occiput. In these diagrams the head is well flexed and so the posterior fontanelle is at a lower station than the anterior fontanelle. **A.** Right occipitoanterior. The anterior shoulder is 2 cm to the left of the midline. **B.** Right occipitolateral (often incorrectly called occipitotransverse). The anterior shoulder lies in the midline and causes a firm convexity between umbilicus and symphysis pubis. **C.** Right occipitoposterior. The anterior shoulder is in the flank causing subumbilical flattening which is most noticeable during a uterine contraction (Braxton Hicks or in labour).

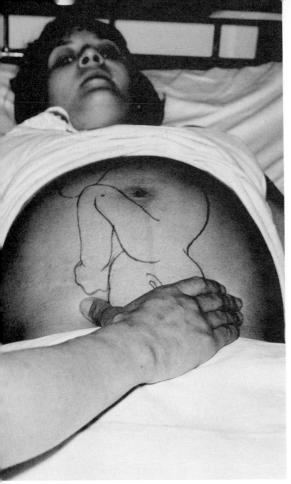

Figure 6.7 Pawlik method of palpation identifies the presenting part of the fetus and its station.

of the flexed attitude of the fetus, lies away from the midline, the respective distances being 2–3 cm, 6–8 cm, and 10 + cm, for the 3 positions discussed above.

If the lie is transverse, the characteristic features of the head and breech will be felt in each flank.

(iii) *Pawlik palpation.* Here, the right hand only is used. The fingers are well spread and are placed in the suprapubic skinfold which runs out to each iliac fossa (figure 6.7). With both this and the next palpation, gentleness must be exercised, since the lower segment is more sensitive than the upper segment. Information is mainly derived from the thumb and middle finger, which move in a coordinated scanning fashion to determine which *pole* is present, the degree of *flexion*, the *station*, and the *position*. Since the position of the back is known, the degree of flexion (*attitude*) can be determined from the relative levels of the occiput and sinciput. The station (amount of descent) is determined from the amount of the presenting part (usually the head) which is out of the pelvis. Different

notations are in use in different hospitals. For example, a numerical system may be used (5/5, 4/5, 3/5, 2/5, 1/5), indicating the amount of head entering the pelvis — 4/5 indicating that the head is just entering, — 2/5 just engaged, 0/5 deeply engaged (as in advanced labour). Alternatively, a descriptive system may be used — high, entering the pelvis, engaged, deeply engaged, and so on. The terms 'mobile' and 'fixed' indicate station in a broad sense, but fixation (immobility) depends considerably on parity (in nulliparas, the head fixes usually at 36–38 weeks; in multiparas, only at the start of labour) and, to a lesser extent, on cephalopelvic relationship (if the pelvis is large and the head is small, the head may be engaged but still mobile).

Engagement of the head has occurred when the maximum diameters have passed through the pelvic brim. When the vertex is the presenting part, the maximum diameters (biparietal and suboccipitobregmatic) are at right angles to each other. Engagement is best determined clinically by Pawlik palpation. Since passage of the suboccipitobregmatic diameter through the brim is the criterion of engagement, it follows that, if the occiput is still palpable above the brim with this technique, the head is not engaged, whereas, if it is no longer palpable, the head is engaged. Fixity of the head has no consistent relation to engagement.

Engagement is also defined by descent of the presenting part to the level of the *ischial spines*, determined by pelvic examination or radiography; this carries the proviso that the head is not unduly moulded. Accurate abdominal examination as well as pelvic examination is thus most important in difficult labour. Radiography (erect lateral) will most accurately describe the cephalopelvic relationship (figure 6.8).

Usually, Pawlik's method is modified to a combined palpation, where the left hand is placed on the fundus in a mirror image of the right hand. A simultaneous comparison is thus available between what is felt in the upper and lower poles, and the examiner is more likely to be correct as to the presentation.

(iv) *Deep pelvic palpation.* This is applied as a routine when the head is entering or has entered the pelvis, particularly in late pregnancy or during labour; if the head is not in the pelvis, it provides additional information concerning the cephalopelvic relationship. In this palpation, the examiner turns and faces the patient's feet. The hands are placed over the sides of the lower uterus in the depression which lies medial to the anterior superior iliac spine and above the inguinal ligaments (figure 6.9). Initially, the outline

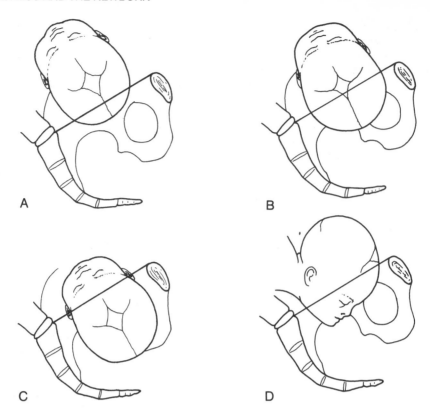

Figure 6.8 Engagement. **A.** The biparietal and suboccipitobregmatic diameters have not negotiated the pelvic inlet. **B.** Engagement has occurred — the biparietal diameter lies at the level of the true conjugate and the vertex is 1 cm above the ischial spines. **C.** Although the head is deeply engaged, about 2 cm of sinciput remains palpable abdominally — the maximum diameter has not passed the narrow pelvic plane, and cephalopelvic disproportion at the level of the midpelvis has not been excluded. **D.** In face presentation, two-thirds of the head must enter the pelvis before the maximum diameter passes the pelvic brim, whereas in vertex presentation engagement occurs when one-third of the well-flexed head has entered the pelvis.

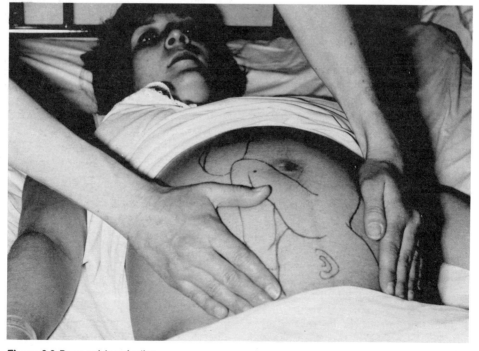

Figure 6.9 Deep pelvic palpation.

and nature of the presenting part is determined. With cephalic presentations, the 2 prominences of the head are located and an estimate is made of attitude, by comparing the relative heights of sinciput and occiput. If the head is well flexed, the sinciput (which lies on the side of the abdomen opposite the back) will be 2–4 cm higher than the occiput. Station is similarly determined by measuring the distance of the occiput and sinciput above the brim. Engagement is not determined by this palpation, since the fingers dip into the true pelvis (see above, Pawlik palpation). Position is determined by shifting the fingers around to the anterior surface of the abdomen, about 2–4cm from the midline, at a level corresponding to the greatest diameter of the fetal head. Estimation of the relative depths of sinciput and occiput below the skin surface is then made. If this is equal, the position is transverse (left or right occipitolateral); if the sinciput is more superficial, the position is posterior (LOP or ROP) and, finally, if the occiput is more superficial, the position is anterior (LOA or ROA) (figure 6.6).

Determination of attitude and position presupposes that the fetal back has been located accurately. Ultrasound studies have confirmed the clinical finding that the fetal back and occiput are directed to the left side in the majority of women in late pregnancy, especially nulliparas.

Auscultation

The fetal heart becomes audible with the clinical Doppler instrument at about 12 weeks' gestation and on stethoscope auscultation at about 18–20 weeks. It is one of the *positive signs* of pregnancy and proof that the fetus is alive. It is of indirect assistance in placing the side on which the fetal back is lying, particularly if palpation is difficult as a result of uterine irritability or obesity. Accurate detection of the fetal heart requires experience, and the beginner should not be discouraged if difficulty is encountered initially.

The point of maximal intensity is over the area of abdomen which is related to the left chest wall of the fetus, but is often only determined by trial and error. Generally, the site depends on the period of gestation, and the presentation and position of the fetus. For example, in the second trimester, it is usually heard best at the midline below the umbilicus; in breech presentations, it is located above, rather than below, the umbilicus; and in posterior positions, it is best heard well out in the flank, unless there is a significant deflexion.

The rate slowly falls from about 160/minute in the first trimester to 130–140/minute at the end of pregnancy. If an obstetrical stethoscope (Pinard type) is used, it must be kept perpendicular to the fetal back, well applied to both abdomen and ear, and not held by the hand (figure 6.10). Extraneous noises should be excluded as far as possible. There are several sounds which may be confused with the fetal heart. Firstly, a maternal pulse echo, coming from one of the major arteries in the pelvis (usually the uterine) can be quite confusing if the rate is elevated as a result of maternal exhaustion, infection, or haemorrhage. It is best to take the maternal pulse rate simultaneously at the wrist. The term *uterine souffle* has been given to the blowing sound of blood in the maternal uterine vessels. The *funic souffle* is a higher-pitched sound arising from the fetal vessels in the umbilical cord, usually when there is some compression present.

Assessment of Cephalopelvic Disproportion

An estimation of the size of the pelvis will have been gained at the first antenatal visit from *internal clinical pelvimetry*. Because of the apprehension of the patient at the first visit, particularly if she is having her first baby, this examination is repeated at approximatley 36–38 weeks, when there is greater softening of tissues and the patient is more relaxed. If suspicion is raised either by a history of difficulty in past labours or by clinical examination, an *X-ray pelvimetry* may be ordered. Late pregnancy, when the fetus is almost fully grown, is the best time for clinical estimation of the cephalopelvic relationship. The first evidence we may have of disproportion is failure of normal descent of the presenting part in the last few weeks of pregnancy (particularly in the nullipara). In addition, the head may be quite high and mobile, or obviously overlapping the symphysis nullipara pubis.

Several manoeuvres are described to improve the assessment. The simplest of these is to get the patient to stand or to sit up and determine the degree of overlap, aided by downward and backward pressure on the presenting part (i.e. in the direction of the upper part of the birth canal). This and other methods described are indicative, rather than conclusive, and indicate the need for closer and more accurate assessment by vaginal examination and radiography, and further management based on these results, usually trial of labour or elective Caesarean section.

Summary

The following important anomalies may be detected during antenatal palpation. (i) *Uterus large for dates* — error in dates, multiple preg-

A

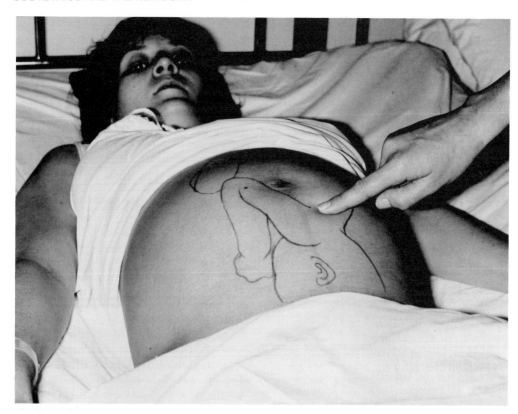

Figure 6.10 Auscultation of the fetal heart. **A.** The fetal heart sounds are best heard over the anterior shoulder where there is close contact with uterine and abdominal walls. **B.** Use of the obstetrical stethoscope: the heart sounds are best heard close to the midline in occipitolateral positions.

B

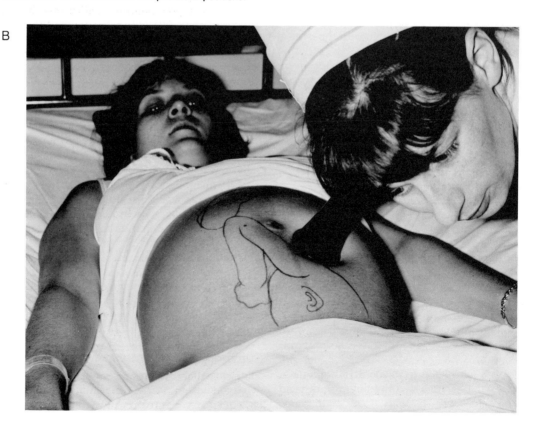

nancy, hydatidiform mole, polyhydramnios, large fetus, uterine fibroids. (ii) *Uterus small for dates* — error in dates, fetal growth retardation, small fetus. (iii) *Tumours* — either pelvic or abdominal (fibroids, ovarian tumours, nonpregnant uterine horn). (iv) *Abnormal uterus* — bicornuate, arcuate, double, pendulous. (v) *Abnormal fetus* — anencephaly, hydrocephaly. (vi) *Abnormal lie* — oblique and transverse. (vii) *Abnormal presentation* — breech, face and brow. (viii) *Fetal death in utero.* (ix) *Cephalopelvic disproportion.*

Some laboratory studies may need to be repeated later in pregnancy (e.g. syphilis screen), others are more informative if performed in the third trimester (e.g. tests for gestational diabetes) (table 6.1).

Defaulting

Patients who do not attend for their antenatal visit on the appointed day must be identified and a letter sent by the doctor or hospital administration officer, giving a further appointment and requesting further information if this appointment cannot be kept. If this is not answered, a home visit is arranged.

THE SIGNIFICANCE OF ANTENATAL TESTS

A number of deviations from normal may be detected during antenatal care. It is important to *sift the serious or potentially serious problems from the minor ones*, and to *assess the rate of deterioration*.

Excess Weight Gain

(i) *Abnormal accumulation of extracellular fluid* by the mother. It is important to recognize this, since it is usually the first sign of preeclampsia. Although many patients gain weight to excess (more than 2kg/month) without developing preeclampsia, the reverse is seldom true unless there is an underlying cardiovascular or renal disorder. The excess weight gain is followed by *generalized oedema*, which usually only occurs when fluid retention in excess of 4–6 litres has taken place (colour plate 82). Heart, kidney, or liver failure, can all cause fluid accumulation. (ii) *Increase in body fat.* This will usually be obvious, and results from excessive intake of calories in relation to body activity; it can be measured accurately by skin-fold thickness calipers. (iii) *Increase in the fetal compartment.* Polyhydramnios and/or multiple pregnancy: care should be taken to exclude these conditions before patients are put on 'reduction' diets.

Low Weight Gain

(i) *Fetal starvation* (placental insufficency): this is usually only apparent after the 28th week of gestation. (ii) *Fetal death.* (iii) *Administration of diuretic drugs* for the treatment of oedema, preeclampsia, or hypertension. (iv) *Inadequate dietary intake* (nausea, psychoneurosis) or malabsorption (chronic diarrhoea). (v) *Idiopathic.* Some mothers gain little weight and, although the fetus is smaller than normal, it is usually otherwise well and thrives satisfactorily.

Fetal Movements

Regular physical activity is a feature of fetal existence and use is made of this in assessing well-being. Although movements diminish during quiet sleep periods, there should be definable activity every day from about the 18th week of gestation. Reduction in activity should be reported to the health care attendant (see Chapter 23).

Proteinuria

This may result from preeclampsia, acute or chronic renal disease, pyelonephritis or cystitis, and in other conditions when a serious stage of the disease has been reached (hyperemesis gravidarum, cardiac disease, anaemia). Careful history, examination, and laboratory investigation will usually indicate the cause. In general, proteinuria in preeclampsia signifies that there is need for *immediate hospitalization* and that the disease will not completely reverse with conservative management; thus termination of pregnancy must be considered. In chronic renal disorders, the amount of proteinuria gives no clue to functional impairment, which must be tested for separately. In infections of the urinary tract, the degree of proteinuria is seldom very marked, but usually parallels the severity of the disease.

It should be remembered that 'proteinuria' may represent *contamination by vaginal discharge*, and a repeat specimen with proper precautions against this should be taken (cleansing of the vulva, and separation of the labia during mid-stream collection).

Glycosuria

In testing for glycosuria at each visit, *we are screening the patient for diabetes*, which may be present before the pregnancy or only revealed because of the stress effect of the latter on carbohydrate metabolism. Recent work has shown that glycosuria is very variable — its appearance following no definite pattern. To serve its object, that is, to identify diabetic mothers, it should be collected after a normal meal, not as a fasting specimen (i.e. before breakfast). The majority of patients with glycosuria during pregnancy have *renal glycosuria* and are distinguished from those with early diabetes by either a *diabetes elimination test* or full *glucose tolerance test* (see Chapter 30). Late in pregnancy and during lactation, *lactose* appears in the urine in increasing amounts. This, however, will not give a positive 'dextrostix' reading.

Haemoglobin

A test for haemoglobin level at the initial antenatal visit will indicate the presence of anaemia before the fetus makes any demands and before the major effect of haemodilution is operative; the test must be repeated at 30 weeks and postpartum. There is no universal standard for haemoglobin level in pregnancy — in general, values of 11.5 g/dl in the first half, and 10.5 g/dl in the second half may be accepted as lower limits of normal.

Rhesus Antibodies

The need for repeating this test arises because antibodies may appear at any time during the pregnancy, and, if already present, the titre may rise significantly. If no antibodies are detected at the initial visit, repeat tests are taken at 30 and 36 weeks, and at delivery. Now that anti-RH (D) gamma globulin is given in many centres at 28 and 34 weeks, as well as after delivery, it is necessary to be sure that antibodies are not present before the first injection is given.

GENERAL HEALTH EDUCATION

It is now generally accepted that health education is an integral component of medical care.

Aims

(i) Reduction or elimination of fear and anxiety in the health setting. (ii) Adoption of healthy life practices. (iii) Acceptance of preventive medicine by means of regular health care. (iv) Knowledge and prompt use of health services. (v) Adoption of a behaviour which will favourably influence environmental conditions.

Technique

The qualities required of the health educator are those of any teacher — knowledge and wisdom are acquired by learning and experience, and this is imparted to the 'pupil', in this case the patient. The message must be expressed clearly and in terms the patient can understand (low 'fog index'), and its content relevant to her experiences and attitudes (a talk on bathing the baby or family planning would best be given late in pregnancy or early in the puerperium, rather than early in pregnancy). The sequence of the message should be from general to specific, and simple to more complex. It is important to get on the patient's 'wavelength', which is determined by her basic intelligence, education, physical and mental state at the time, and interest in health matters (is she interested in, or does she know about the value of different foods? Does she give her children flouride? Does she attend the dentist for regular checkups?). This can only be done by general conversation, when her interests, motives, intentions, and ideas can be determined. Finally, by gentle questioning, it should be ascertained whether the message has 'sunk in', and, if so, whether the patient's behaviour is likely to be altered by it. Most messages need to reinforced several times before the above can be achieved.

The educational setting may be formal (class lecture or film), semiformal (small group in the clinic, ward, or nursery), or informal (usually a spontaneous, casual discussion).

Instructional aids will include apparatus that the patient may be required to use (e.g. gas and oxygen machine), models, charts, pictures, pamphlets, booklets, combined audiovisual presentations (tape-slide, movie or TV films).

Problems. The outcome of the above interaction may be summarized as follows: (i) message learnt, instructions followed (ideal patient); (ii) message not learnt, but instructions followed (dull, passive or dependent patient); (iii) message learnt, but instructions not followed (low health regard, lazy); (iv) message not learnt and instructions not followed (dull and/or don't care patient).

Patients in the latter 2 groups form a hard core who are possessed of a poor standard of health behaviour, and a reluctance to change. In the majority of cases, such characteristics are tied to levels of understanding and patterns of living which existed in their formative years. This problem is a challenge to the educators of the children of the future. It would be unduly pessimistic to believe, however, that there is more than the occasional antenatal patient whose health education and outlook will not be improved to some extent.

The Educational Programme for Pregnancy, Childbirth and Parenthood

In the United Kingdom, hospital groups including medical staff, physiotherapists and midwives have been involved in providing educational programmes for patients and their husbands. In addition, non-professional organizations such as the National Childbirth Trust are actively involved in providing appropriate courses, often in conjunction with hospital groups.

Aims. (a) A *course of instruction in the theoretical and practical aspects of reproduction.* (i) Anatomy and physiology of reproduction; conception; development of the fetus (including positive and negative influences). (ii) Anatomical, physiological, and psychological changes in the mother, and their relationship to the minor disorders of pregnancy where applicable. (iii) Antenatal care, routines, problems to watch for. (iv) Hygiene of pregnancy and nutrition. (v) Anatomical and physiological changes in labour and parturition. (vi) Methods of pain relief in labour, psychological and pharmacological. (vii) The normal puerperium; infant feeding; minor disorders. (viii) The role of the husband in pregnancy, labour, and puerperium.

(b) A *course of instruction in the theoretical and practical aspects of the physiotherapy of reproduction.* (i) The role of physiotherapy. (ii) Muscles and joints of significance in reproduction; effects of pregnancy; contraction and relaxation; coordination; posture, good and bad; physical fitness; exercises; perineal massage to relax vaginal introitus. (iii) Respiration: Patterns of breathing in pregnancy and labour; effects on fetal oxygenation and maternal venous blood return; role in psychoprophylaxis; recommended breathing patterns in the first and second stages of labour and during delivery.

More detailed information, suitable for inclusion in the above course is given in Appendix I. Criticism of some antenatal education courses is that they are too idealized — i.e. the couple are unprepared for major complications. When things do go wrong, there is a greater sense of disappointment and perhaps anger, and the latter may be projected onto the medical attendant. There should be discussions on such aspects as unplanned outcomes (what if?), and the risk-benefit of different options/interventions. At some time in the later antenatal period, a tour of the hospital is arranged to familiarize the couple with the layout and facilities, particularly of the labour ward and nursery.

chapter seven

Hygiene of Pregnancy

OVERVIEW

Although pregnancy does not require any major reorganization in the patient's life-style, definite changes occur in psychological outlook and in the body's physiology and needs. The major changes will be given in separate sections on psychology and physiology.

The present chapter describes the practical advice that should be given to the pregnant woman consequent upon the above changes.

Exercise

The amount of exercise desirable for the pregnant woman has never been defined. *If fatigue occurs, this would appear to be the desirable limit.* It is also prudent to discontinue exercise of a jolting nature, such as horseback riding, unless the person is very accomplished, or sport where physical injury may be sustained. In most centres, *special classes* are arranged where *both exercise and relaxation are taught by physiotherapists.* It is as important to *strengthen some muscles,* such as those used in expulsion of the baby, as to learn to *relax others,* such as those of the pelvic and perineal diaphragms.

Jogging is currently popular: this can usually be continued, but at a more leisurely pace (e.g. able to maintain comfortable talking capacity). This type of exercise should not be commenced for the first time in pregnancy.

Bathing

A daily shower or bath is recommended. Care should be exercised in later pregnancy when the patient becomes less well-balanced. Swimming is an excellent exercise and is recommended if the temperatures are not extreme or the conditions boisterous.

Coitus

It is probable that coitus during pregnancy may have adverse effects in some patients, particularly in the first and last trimesters. There is the possibility of *direct trauma,* and *prostaglandins in the seminal plasma may stimulate the uterus to contract,* especially in later pregnancy. Some recent studies suggest that there is an increase in *placental abruption, premature rupture of the membranes,* and *amniotic and fetal infection* if intercourse has occurred in the 4 weeks before delivery, with the risk of pneumonia/respiratory distress; other studies have shown a less significant effect. The reconciliation of such diverse views must reside in differences in methodology, population samples etc.

Restriction would only seem necessary if there has been a bad obstetric history or major complications in the present pregnancy (threatened abortion, threatened premature labour, premature rupture of the membranes, antepartum bleeding, or cramping following coitus). Coitus should not be censured without proper reason, and an explanation provided.

It is often observed that many women, and their husbands, lose interest in coitus during pregnancy, their thoughts having become focused upon the growth and development of their unborn child. This switch-over may affect one partner more than the other and is more common when there has been previous fetal loss (abortion, fetal malformation or prematurity). A patient is always anxious until her pregnancy has advanced beyond the period at which the previous interruption occurred. During the second and third trimesters, the woman may worry that the physical changes of pregnancy have reduced her attractiveness, and this, together with fatigue and awkwardness, steadily reduce her inclination for sexual activity.

The couple should be encouraged to communicate their feelings freely to each other; the husband should realize the importance of his wife's need for affection and physical contact. Love play techniques can be modified to satisfy changing circumstances. Coital techniques can be adjusted so that the uterus is not subjected to undue pressure (female above or posterior entry).

Employment

The amount of work outside the home that can be undertaken by the pregnant woman depends largely on the type of activity (sitting, standing, stooping, bending, climbing, lifting), amount of physical exertion involved, the number of children and thus the extent of the home duties she has in addition, the amount of home help she has, and the extent of her fatigue at the end of the day. Recent studies suggest that stand-up jobs are a significant hazard; fetal weight and head circumference are reduced and large (> 3 cm) placental infarcts are increased. Each patient should be advised individually since, in addition to the above, there may be obstetrical and/or medical factors in the past history or present pregnancy suggesting that employment should be given up. Most women, even if the pregnancy is proceeding normally, would prefer to cease full employment at the middle of the third trimester; some tolerate work well, however, and continue uneventfully until near to full term. Sleep patterns tend to be less regular in late pregnancy (e.g. more frequent wakenings, less deep REM sleep), and this often leads to fatigue and the need for catch-up naps during the day. It is usually recommended that air hostesses cease flying duties by the end of the second trimester. The pregnant woman should avoid chemicals, noxious fumes, temperature extremes, and working to exhaustion.

Travel

Restrictions largely apply to those women at high risk. After 28 weeks, a statement of fitness to fly is often requested by airlines, and travel after 36 weeks is usually not permitted, even for those with apparently normal pregnancies. Long car journeys are fatiguing, and stops every 1–2 hours should be made for short exercise spells. The jolting over bad roads may be harmful if the pregnancy is unstable. Patients should be counselled to wear *seat belts* when travelling by car; the mother will thereby be more likely to escape injury in the case of an accident, although occasionally a seat belt localizes injury to the uterus and the baby (figure 23.1).

Women travelling in late pregnancy should be provided with a summary of their antenatal progress in case of emergency. Problems of immunization are considered in Chapter 39.

Housework

The same rules apply as to exercise in general. It should not be done to the point of over-fatigue. It is best to divide the work into segments and separate these with a rest, a snack, or an outdoor walk.

Rest

This should not only be a cessation of activity, but there should be definite periods set aside — preferably in both the morning and afternoon — when the mother rests with her feet up. The duration of such periods are increased as pregnancy progresses. This aids return of blood to the heart, resolution of oedema fluid in the legs, reduction in the incidence and severity of pre-eclampsia, improvement in varicose veins (or their prevention), improvement in blood flow to the uterus, and probably in a reduction of prematurely terminated pregnancy.

Sleep

This is important, especially in the second half of pregnancy, when a large increase has occurred in the metabolic demands on the body — and, as so aptly put by Shakespeare, sleep 'knits up the ravelled sleeve of care'. In late pregnancy, sleep is often difficult, and a sedative may be requested. If pain or anxiety is preventing sleep, again, appropriate medication should be given.

Clothing

The basic requirements are a well-fitting brassiere and loose-fitting maternity clothes. It is probable that poor support of the breasts during and after pregnancy is a greater cause of future breast laxity than the act of breast feeding, which is often charged with this offence. A maternity belt is often of help to patients whose abdominal musculature is weak, especially after the 20th week of gestation; this, however, should not be tight or constricting. The use of constricting garters or stockings rolled and drawn in is to be discouraged — leg veins have trouble enough already in returning blood to the heart.

Generally, a shift to flat-heeled shoes early in the pregnancy is advisable. They provide a better base and are more in keeping with the posture necessary to balance the forward growth of the pregnant uterus.

Alcohol

There is evidence that even a moderate intake may be harmful to the fetus, and certainly, serious problems result in the babies of mothers who consume alcohol to excess.

Smoking

There is now clear evidence that the babies of mothers who smoke are smaller (average 200 g) than those of nonsmoking mothers. Furthermore, there is also reasonable evidence that the pregnancies in such women are complicated by an increase in the rate of premature termination and an increase in overall perinatal mortality.

There is however a slight bonus in that pre-eclampsia is less common: this may be a direct effect of the drugs contained in the tobacco, or perhaps related to different dietary habits or other unknown actions.

The medical attendant has a role in indicating to the mother the possible harm that may result to the delicate and developing tissues of the fetus (the right of the fetus to normal development). However, it is difficult to persuade heavy smokers to give up the habit during pregnancy, and the abolitionist approach can be overdone. It is all too easy to induce guilt complexes in patients admitted to hospital because of pregnancy complications when they are unable to discontinue smoking. We favour a policy encouraging our smoking patients to reduce their intake to less than 5 cigarettes per day, especially when oestriol excretion is subnormal.

The effects of smoking marihuana (pot, hashish) have not been evaluated critically, but, with their greater effect on the brain and behaviour, concern at least equal to that relating to ordinary cigarettes must be held regarding this substance.

Narcotics and other Drugs

It may be stated that very few drugs should be taken in the organ-forming period (1–14 weeks), the exceptions being well-tested antinausea preparations, hypnotics, and analgesics in limited quantities. Drugs specifically contraindicated in pregnancy are discussed in the chapter on drug therapy.

The apparent effects of *narcotic drug addiction* on the outcome of pregnancy are increased incidences of fetal growth retardation (× 4) and premature birth before 37 weeks (× 4). However, the problem is complex, because narcotic addicts often have the additional problems of an inadequate diet, unfavourable socioeconomic conditions, alcohol consumption and heavy cigarette smoking. It may be that the main hazard to these infants lies in the environment to which they return.

Dental Hygiene

The importance of using the antenatal period for conservative dental treatment and dental health education has been mentioned earlier. It is unlikely that 'a tooth is lost for every child' unless the mother uses the pregnancy as an excuse to put off seeing the dentist. However, changes do occur in the gums in pregnancy — they tend to be more swollen and to bleed more easily (figure 7.1). Continuation of cleansing, perhaps with a softer brush or flannel, should be emphasized. If extractions are required during pregnancy, local analgesia is usually employed. Antibiotic cover is given if there is a rheumatic or congenital heart disorder.

Personal Hygiene

Douching should rarely, if ever, be necessary, and should be carried out only after discussion with the doctor. The hair may be washed as frequently as desired. Pregnancy may affect the hair of some patients quite markedly, the most obvious change being loss of curl. Diet and care of the bowels are considered elsewhere.

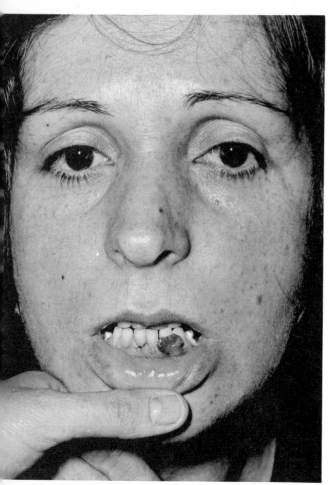

Figure 7.1 Epulis (vascular granuloma) of the gum in a 28-year-old para 2 at 28 weeks' gestation. The lesion had occurred at the same site in each of her previous pregnancies and had, as is usual, disappeared after delivery. These lesions are uncommon (1–2%) and occur in an area where the gum is irritated (tartar accumulation, caries, food pack). They are usually adjacent to the molars and cause bleeding when the teeth are brushed. Treatment is excision if the lesion, which is due to pregnancy-induced change in collagen, persists after pregnancy. Incomplete excision can result in rapid enlargement of this benign tumour.

chapter eight

Nutrition

OVERVIEW

'Let foods be your medicine, and medicines be your food' — Hippocrates.

Nutrition is concerned with the type and amount of food that is taken or administered. Throughout the world, there is a large variation in diet — from the high meat and fat diet of the Eskimo to the almost pure vegetarian diet of some tropical races. Again, some races eat entirely 'off the land' whereas others eat entirely 'off the shelf'. Studies have shown that many millions of pregnant women live in conditions of semistarvation, with almost certain ill-effects on the developing fetus. Although *calorie lack* is unusual in Western countries, *poor dietary balance* is not unusual due not only to socioeconomic considerations but food fads, drugs and voluntary malnutrition, the latter often occurring in women with privileged socioeconomic circumstances.

Those caring for the pregnant patient are in an unique position to *provide health care information, and nutritional advice* is one of the most important areas in this regard. Not only will there be a more favourable outcome to the pregnancy, but the mother's general attitude to nutrition in future years will be improved. Hopefully, she will encourage proper dietary habits in her children, particularly in the balance between proteins, vitamins, and minerals on the one hand and the obesity-producing refined carbohydrates on the other.

Initially, a broad *dietary assessment* should be made. The patient's knowledge of, and interest in nutrition should be noted, as well as the manner that this is put into practice. The often detrimental effect of food processing and cooking on food quality should be remembered when discussing nutrition with the antenatal patient. *General medical disorders* may affect nutrition (e.g. malabsorption states), as may *pregnancy complications* (e.g. hyperemesis gravidarum, hiatus hernia). In a proportion of women with hyperemesis, vomiting continues during the pregnancy and in such cases, particularly in the third trimester, assessment of both mother (liver and renal function) and baby (oestrogen excretion, cardiotocography) is necessary. Some conditions, such as *diabetes mellitus*, may be affected quite significantly by pregnancy and the diet may need modification.

Recent interest has focused on the nutritional needs of the fetus. In a normal pregnancy, most nutrients pass freely across the placenta from the mother. Of prime importance is an adequate supply of *glucose*; because of this, some dietary practices which may be relatively innocuous in the non-pregnant state (e.g. skipping breakfast) may result in a degree of *maternal hypoglycaemia* that is harmful to the fetus. If placental function is sufficiently compromised, fetal growth retardation and even death may ensue.

The mother's *dietary behaviour should be assessed several times during the antenatal period*, with appropriate praise or admonition given according to progress. In this way the patient will perceive that the medical attendant is genuinely interested in the relevance of the subject.

The importance of an optimum diet for the *lactating woman* should also be emphasized, since the baby will be needing a progressively increasing supply of milk.

GENERAL REMARKS

It is often said 'You are what you eat'; it could equally be said 'You are what you don't eat'. The idea that some foods are of good value to the body and others (even though they have a nice taste) are of less value has taken time to penetrate the general consciousness. The least useful food — refined sugar in its many guises — is often preponderent in many diets, because it is relatively cheap, it is the food of minor social gatherings, and finally it is the prized food from childhood (the reward for being good).

While it is true that the fetus is only extracting major amounts of nutrients in the third trimester of pregnancy, there is much evidence to suggest that good nutrition is important at the time of implantation and early fetal growth. It is logical to think that even before conception the state of nutrition may affect the quality of the germ cells — ovum and sperm.

The pregnant woman should be made aware of the elements of a good diet and the virtually continuous need of the fetus for nutrients. She will not be expected to remember the complexities of individual nutrients and their daily requirements, but she should have a balanced diet spread over 3-4 meals per day and have a working knowledge of the different classes of foodstuffs and the best sources of the substances that make up a satisfactory diet. The importance of the inexpensive substance called *water* (preferably without caffeine modification) should be mentioned.

Although difficult to prove, the importance of such additional factors as *adequate rest* (sleep, leisure and tranquillity of mind) during pregnancy should be remembered.

CLASSES OF FOODSTUFFS

There are a number of classifications of foods — the traditional one describes *proteins, fats, carbohydrates, minerals, and vitamins.* The lay person is more likely to think of them under their market headings; and nutrition educators now usually stress the importance of the *5 basic food groups* — bread and cereals, vegetables and fruits, meat and alternative high protein foods, milk and milk products, and fats. A balanced selection from each of these groups will ensure that daily recommended allowances of all nutrients will be obtained.

An *ideal diet should be balanced,* i.e. it should contain all the essentials listed above in adequate amounts. It is important to remember that some components (fats, vitamins, minerals) can be stored in the body for considerable periods (30–1,000 days), whereas others are rapidly depleted (amino acids, carbohydrates, folic acid, some vitamins).

The daily *caloric intake* during pregnancy depends to some extent on the woman's activity; the average intake ranges between 8,500–10,500 kJ (2,000-2,500 kcal). This total is derived from protein 50–80 g, fat 80–100 g, and carbohydrate 150–200 g.

FUNCTIONS AND SOURCES OF MAJOR NUTRIENTS

Proteins, Fats, Carbohydrates

Protein promotes growth of the fetus, placenta and accessory tissues (uterus, breast, red blood cells) and production of breast milk.

Best sources. Animal protein: meat, fish, poultry, eggs, milk, cheese; *vegetable protein*: dried beans, dried peas, lentils, nuts.

Deficiency is not uncommon in the special groups referred to above. It is reflected by low serum albumin levels and the ratio of urea nitrogen/total nitrogen in the urine is less than 60.

Fats are important sources of energy; they provide the fat soluble vitamins (A, D, E and K), and are essential components of cell membranes and the central nervous system. Phospholipids are responsible for lowering surface tension in the lung of the newborn, thus preventing respiratory collapse.

Best sources. Animal fats are widespread — all dairy products, most meats, and eggs; such fats are usually highly 'saturated' (hydrogenated, fewer double bonds between carbon atoms). They contain larger amounts of the low carbon number fatty acids (stearic and palmitic). Vegetable fats (safflower, corn, olive oil) contain more unsaturated fat (linoleic, linolenic acids). The diet should have a proper balance of the 2 types.

Deficiency . Rare; usually the most sensitive indicator is vitamin A, a fat soluble vitamin.

Carbohydrates, like fats, are important as sources of energy. Most modern diets suffer from an excess of carbohydrate, especially in the form of refined sugar (sweets) or refined flour (cakes). These provide little stimulus to mastication or intestinal motility. It is claimed that a relative excess of carbohydrate over dietary fibre (vegetables) is a factor in slow and difficult intestinal transit and a number of acquired disorders (dental caries, constipation, diverticulitis, haemorrhoids, hiatus hernia).

A summary of the important vitamins and minerals (requirement, biological function, sources and effects of deficiency) is given in tables 8.1 and 8.2. Intakes significantly above the recommended daily allowances are not only costly, but may cause metabolic upset and even fetal malformation. Although definitive figures are given in the tables, they represent a 'best estimate'; further research is needed in this still controversial area.

GROUPS AT SPECIAL RISK

(i) *Socially deprived.* Poor economic circumstances as a result of low family income. (ii) *Biologically immature.* Teenage girls, often unmarried, tend to have poor diet habits (irregular meal patterns, junk food). (iii) *Unusual demands*. Patients of high parity; those having children in rapid sequence; those with multiple pregnancy; those with intestinal parasites (round worm, hookworm). (iv) *Underweight for height*. (v) *Obesity*. Although total calories are adequate, the diet is often unbalanced. (vi) *Unusual dietetic practices or fads*. Examples are restricted vegetarian or reducing diets. (vii) *Low weight gain during pregnancy*. (viii) *Psychiatric or medical disorders* which result in inadequate ingestion or absorption of food (hyperemesis gravidarum, sprue, parasitic diseases). (ix) *Immigrants*. The chief sufferers are those newly arrived, often with language, financial, and social problems.

Defective nutrition may also result from poor methods of preparation, either domestic or commercial, where much of the natural goodness and roughage has been removed.

EFFECTS OF AN INADEQUATE DIET IN PREGNANCY

There seems little doubt from the experiments of nature (e.g. during famines and wars) and from research studies in animals that malnutrition does unfavourably effect reproduction; the following complications are more common.

Mother. Abortion, anaemia, preeclampsia/eclampsia, prematurity, infection, inadequate lactation.

Baby. Malformation, low birth-weight, perinatal death, prematurity, infections, neurological handicap.

Recent studies have emphasized the important links between nutrition and optimum growth of the individual. Apart from the direct effect of malnutrition on mental and physical development, there are other obstacles such as increased susceptibility to bacterial, viral, and parasitic diseases, probably the result of impaired immunological function.

ANTENATAL MANAGEMENT

A *dietary history* should be taken to assess the mother's general knowledge and attitudes to nutrition and the quantity and quality of the foodstuffs eaten. Questions should be directed to practices such as skipping breakfast which lead to hypoglycaemia (of the mother and fetus), food fads, and medical disorders likely to affect nutrition (e.g. malabsorption).

Examination will be directed to the patient's weight in relation to her height and general evidence of nutritional well-being. *Investigations*

that may reflect nutritional status include the haemoglobin and serum albumin levels; where intestinal parasites are prevalent these should be looked for.

Dietary progress should be assessed at subsequent antenatal visits; referral to the dietician may be indicated in some cases. If the patient belongs to a special dietary group (e.g. vegetarian who eats no butter, eggs, cheese, or milk), supplementation with vitamin B_{12} may be necessary in pregnancy. Fluoride tablets may be needed to protect the baby's deciduous teeth if the patient is living in a low fluoride area.

SPECIAL PROBLEMS

Obesity and excess weight gain. It is likely that there are *2 types* of obese patient, firstly the gross over eater and/or under exerciser; and secondly, the poor heat loser. The latter has a very efficient insulation beneath the skin, loses little heat (and thus has a lower skin temperature) and stays fat despite only a moderate intake of food. Apart from the general medical hazards of obesity (hypertension, diabetes, arthritis), pregnancy poses additional problems — preeclampsia, difficulty in diagnosis and management of malpresentations, increased anaesthetic and operative risk, prolonged labour if the fetus is large, thromboembolism, and failure of lactation. Many of the complications are interrelated; for example, hypertension leads to preeclampsia, induction of labour is more likely as is perinatal death, operative delivery and excessive postpartum blood loss.

In such patients dietary advice is important and this requires repeated encouragement, praise and admonishment. Bread, starches, confections, sugar, fruit and alcohol are the main offenders. In addition, it is important to obtain such background information as education level, economic circumstances, and previous dietary history (types, quantities, preparation of foods) before a satisfactory explanation can be given to the patient of the role of diet and the nutrients required and their sources in pregnancy.

Some patients will have had a *by-pass or stomach stapling operation* to control the obesity; the growth of the fetus should be monitored in such women, since growth retardation may occur.

Underweight. Some patients are thin by nature and tend to have small babies. An investigation is warranted, however, of the patient who has recently lost weight or when weight gain in pregnancy has been poor. If *nausea/anorexia* is excessive or prolonged, admission to hospital is advisable.

TABLE 8.1   MINERALS AND TRACE ELEMENTS

Element	Daily requirement (μg or mg*/day)	Biological function	Sources	Deficiency
Calcium†	800–1,200*	Major component of bones and teeth; breast milk; blood coagulation; neuromuscular function, muscle contractibility	Dairy products, eggs, meat, fish, grains, fruits, nuts	Osteoporosis, dental caries, neuromuscular disturbances
Iron	15–20*	Haemoglobin and myoglobin synthesis; oxidation-reduction enzymes	Kidney, lean pork, lean beef, egg yolk, raisins, cooked dried beans, peaches, apricots, and prunes, canned dried beans and green peas	Microcytic anaemia
Magnesium	300–400*	Trace element important for neuromuscular excitation; many enzyme systems; calcium mobilization from bone	Meats, cereals, vegetables	Tremors, CNS disorders
Cobalt	300–500	Vitamin B_{12} synthesis	Green leaf vegetables	Macrocytic anaemia (vitamin B_{12})
Chromium	2–4*	Insulin and glucose utilization; synthesis of fatty acid and cholesterol; stabilization of nucleic acid structures	Meats, fish, legumes, green vegetables	Animal syndromes reported (depression of glucose metabolism, growth)
Copper	4–6*	Enzyme constituents; important in absorption and utilization of iron; tissue metabolism; nervous system, connective tissue and bone development	Meats, fish, green vegetables	Impaired resistance to infection
Iodine	150–200	Component of thyroxine and triiodothyronine	Seafood, iodized salt, kelp tablets	Goitre
Manganese	3–4*	Synthesis of mucopolysaccharides of cartilage; activation of enzymes; melanin formation	Cereals, green leaf vegetables, tea, berry fruit, nuts	Defined syndromes only in animals (growth, reproduction, bone, CNS abnormalities)
Molybdenum	200–400	Flavoprotein enzymes, oxidase enzymes	Legumes, cereals, green leaf vegetables	None described
Selenium	10–20	An important antioxidant in tissues, protecting cell membranes in particular; red cell formation; metabolism of vitamin E, sulphur, and amino acids	Unrefined cereals, dairy products, meat	Cardiac and muscle dysfunction
Zinc	16–20*	Trace element, integral part of many metalloenzymes involved in synthetic pathways and thus in cell growth and healing, hormone production and reproduction	Dietary protein (wheat germ and bran, nuts, dairy products, meat and fish)	Impaired sexual development and healing; cirrhosis; acrodermatitis enteropathica

*   = mg/day

†   = other *major elements* include sodium, chlorine, potassium, phosphorus, sulphur, and silicon; these elements are widely distributed and do not normally present as deficiency syndromes unless general food intake/absorption is abnormal

TABLE 8.2 VITAMINS

Vitamin	Daily requirement (μg or mg*/day)	Biological function	Sources	Deficiency
(a) *Fat soluble*				
A	750–1,000	Bone and tooth, skin, vision, resistance to infection	Dairy products, egg yolk, organ meats; carotenes (converted to vitamin A in the body): dark green vegetables (broccoli, spinach), deep yellow vegetables (pumpkin, carrots), apricots, persimmons	Failure of dark adaptation; disorders of epithelial tissues, especially of eyes
D	10	Absorption and retention of calcium and phosphorus for the growth and formation of bones and teeth	Action of sunlight on skin; dietary sources are butter, egg yolk, fish oils, liver, fortified milk and margarine	Rickets and osteomalacia
E (tocopherol)	15–20*	Cell metabolism	Fats and oils, liver, egg, green leaf vegetables, seeds	Only seen in infant (usually premature)
K	30–40	Formation of clotting factors (especially prothrombin)	Green leaf vegetables, liver, egg, cereals, fruits	Haemorrhage in newborn infant (due to lack of production by intestinal bacteria)
(b) *Water Soluble*				
B_1 (thiamine)	0.8–1.0*	Coenzyme in intermediary metabolism	Whole grain and enriched bread and cereals, dried peas and beans, liver, kidney, lean pork, potatoes, nuts, oranges	Beri-beri (peripheral neuropathy, cardiac failure)
B_2 (riboflavin)	1.0–1.4*	,,	Dairy products, organ meats, green leaf vegetables	Growth retardation, glossitis, cheilosis, eye lesions
B_5 (niacin)	15–18*	,,	Fish, lean meat, liver, nuts, poultry, cereals	Pellagra (dermatitis), dementia, diarrhoea
B_6 (pyridoxine)	1.4–2.2*	,,	Pork, organ meats, cereals, legumes, bananas	Epithelial and CNS disturbances
B_{12} (cobolamine)	3	,,	Meat, fish, eggs, milk	Megaloblastic anaemia, CNS disorder
C (ascorbic acid)	50–60*	Intercellular matrix and collagen formation; iron absorption	Fruits (especially citrus) and vegetables	Scurvy
Folic acid	300–400	Coenzyme in intermediary metabolism, especially haeme synthesis	Green leaf vegetables, organ meats, fish, legumes, yeast and extracts	Megaloblastic anaemia, gastrointestinal disturbance, glossitis

Weight gain in pregnancy is often ill-understood. The obligatory gains are those associated with the mother (uterus, breasts, blood volume), and fetus (fetus, amniotic fluid, placenta), amounting to 10–12 kg (figure 8.1). The increase in maternal extracellular fluid is variable, but can be up to 5 litres or more (5 kg). It is now appreciated that this increase in fluid (which may produce oedema) is usually physiological, and such mothers have healthy babies of normal birth-weight. The dangers of salt in pregnancy may have been over emphasized. Although the majority of people probably use more salt than is necessary, there is little evidence that drastic curtailment in pregnancy is of any value in the normal patient. The weight gain should be assessed in relation to the patient's prepregnant weight, and the relation of this to the ideal weight for her height and bone structure. Other pathological causes of excess weight gain should always be borne in mind (*early pre-eclampsia, multiple pregnancy, and polyhydramnios*). The major fetal demand occurs in the last 8–10 weeks when growth is rapid. Some increase in protein and other dietary essentials should be taken to allow for this.

Medical and surgical disorders. There will need to be some differences in the diet for such conditions as diabetes because of the changed physiology of pregnancy. In some metabolic disorders (e.g. phenylketonuria), there is a serious risk to brain development in the fetus if the mother's diet is not strictly controlled — i.e. blood phenylalanine levels maintained between 4–10 mg/dl.

Labour. When contractions become painful, digestive processes virtually cease. It is therefore little use feeding such patients. *If the labour is likely to last for more than 12 hours, an intravenous infusion should be commenced.*

Figure 8.1 Final contributions to maternal weight gain in pregnancy. Normal weight gain is 10–12 kg (22–27 lb). There are different rates of increase for the various components. The fetus gains weight rapidly from 30–40 weeks (1,500–3,350 g) whereas placental weight (650 g), like blood volume (1,500 ml) and extracellular fluid volume (3,000 ml), increase progressively from 10 to 32–34 weeks' gestation, then plateau to 40 weeks. The amniotic fluid volume (850 ml) peaks at 35–36 weeks then decreases progressively. Enlargement of the breasts (650 g) occurs early in pregnancy whereas uterine growth (900 g) and fat deposition (1,000 g) are progressive.

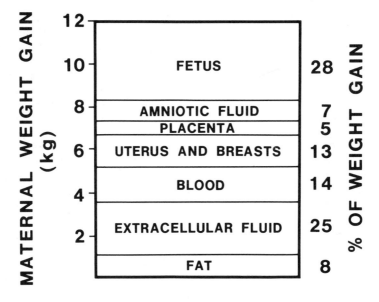

chapter nine

Minor Disorders

OVERVIEW

During pregnancy, a number of so-called 'minor disorders' may arise. Usually these are annoying rather than disabling to the patient, but merit sympathy and appropriate management since, in some cases, the disorder (e.g. oedema) may herald a more serious state, or lack of treatment may result in unnecessary aggravation of the condition (*varicose veins, heartburn*). The disorder may be due entirely to the pregnancy (*morning sickness*, heartburn) or merely be aggravated by it (*haemorrhoids*).

Since the patient will often not raise the question, specific enquiry is warranted regarding the more frequent and troublesome disorders.

Nausea and Vomiting

Although the cause of this condition is debated, it is most likely related to oestrogen production, to which the vomiting centre is initially sensitive. The majority of pregnant women experience nausea of some type at some time in the first trimester, and approximately one-half will actually vomit. The condition is usually worse when the patient gets up in the morning and is aggravated by the act of cooking or the smell of food. It is seen more frequently in those subject to motion sickness and in primigravidas and, if severe, suggests the possibility of *multiple pregnancy* or *hydatidiform mole*. In only 0.6% or less of patients is the vomiting severe enough to warrant hospitalization (table 16.1). The importance of '*psychological overlay*' is often claimed in patients in whom *vomiting is severe* without other apparent cause and when *persistence or recurrent* episodes occur. This label should not be attached to the patient unless positive signs of psychoneuroses are present and other pathology is ruled out (obstetrical, medical, or surgical causes). Symptoms usually occur only between *6–16 weeks' gestation* — patients are often reassured when informed of this fact.

Management. (i) *Frequent small meals.* Between 4 and 6 small meals are more easily tolerated and prevent a possibly harmful fall in the mother's blood sugar levels; high protein foods (Chapter 8) help to prevent low blood sugar levels. The patient will usually soon find out which foods agree or disagree with her. Fatty, greasy or highly-spiced foods are best avoided; soda water is usually well tolerated, as is tomato juice. Carbohydrates, in the form of barley sugar, maintain caloric intake. If nausea is worse late in the day, the patient is advised to prepare the main meal after breakfast and/or to concentrate on foods requiring little or no cooking. A sweetened beverage and a biscuit/toast brought by a supportive partner first thing in the morning is helpful. A temporary reorganization of household responsibilities is often needed until the end of the first trimester, when the condition usually abates. (ii) *Antiemetic drugs.* There are many agents available — e.g. pyridoxine, promethazine, meclazine, or the rectal suppository prochlorperazine. Usually 1–2 tablets taken at bedtime, when the patient is less nauseated, is the optimum form of administration, perhaps supplemented by a further tablet after breakfast. Many antiemetic drugs cause *drowsiness*, and this should be explained to the patient, particularly if she drives a car. If the condition is troublesome, initial drug therapy may need to be given as a rectal suppository or parenterally. (iii) *Psychological support.* An explanation of the self-limiting nature of the condition, together with the above measures, copes with the problem in most cases. It is reasonable to tell the mother that the basis of the condition is the production of hormones necessary for the early development of the baby. (iv) *Admission to hospital* is advisable if the patient is unable to tolerate food, if significant weight loss occurs (2–5 kg or more), or if ketone bodies are detected in the urine (see hyperemesis gravidarum, Chapter 35).

Oesophageal Reflux (Heartburn, Water-brash)

In this disorder the patient complains of discomfort, burning, or pain in the epigastrium or retrosternal region (heartburn). This condition is a feature of the second and third trimesters. It occurs in two-thirds of all patients and results from reflux of acid gastric juice and perhaps bile into the lower oesophagus or into the mouth ('water-brash'). It is caused partly by the pressure of the enlarging uterus on the stomach and partly by incompetence of the sphincters of the stomach (lower pylorus and upper cardia). Because of the helpful effect of gravity, the condition is characteristically worse when the patient lies down. Occasionally, there is a herniation of the upper part of the stomach into the chest (*hiatus hernia*) and serious vomiting may result.

Management. (i) *An antacid preparation* (aluminium hydroxide or magnesium trisilicate) should be taken night and morning and also during the day if symptoms are noted. Since *bile regurgitation* (alkaline) can cause similar symptoms, an acid preparation (e.g. dilute hydrochloric acid) may be needed in some patients. (ii) *Meals* should be light and more frequent to prevent overdistension of the stomach; milk should be included. Meals late in the day should be avoided. (iii) *The bed* should be raised at the head some 15–20 cm, and an extra pillow used if this is compatible with a good sleep. (iv) *Smoking* has been shown to reduce the competence of the sphincter, and should be ceased or considerably curtailed; other offenders include fatty foods and peppermint. (v) *X-rays*: if the condition does not respond to the above measures, a barium swallow should be ordered and a subsequent film taken with the patient in the head-down position and the uterus shielded, to diagnose hiatus hernia. Rarely, pathology in the stomach or elsewhere in the digestive system may be present.

Constipation

This may mean emptying the bowels less often than normal and/or the passage of hard faecal material. The latter usually follows the former, since the longer the time that faecal residue stays in the large bowel, the more water is reabsorbed from it. The rate of passage of material in the lower bowel is largely related to the relative *proportion of fibre and sugar* in the diet. The greater the proportion of fibre, the less resistance there will be, the faster will be the passage, and the more normal will be the motion. The higher the sugar content, the slower will be the passage, because it is more sticky and hard to propel. The latter is compounded by inadequate fluid intake; the ingestion of strong tea and coffee, which are diuretics, may aggravate the situation because of their dehydrating effect. Other factors include lack of sufficient exercise and neglecting the call to stool (or being unaware of the filling of the terminal colon).

Management. (i) *Bowel retraining.* Poor bowel habits (ignoring the call to stool) should be corrected; in some patients this may be related to a painful local condition (e.g. anal fissure) which itself will need treatment. An increase in the amount of exercise taken is suggested if the woman is very sedentary. (ii) *Dietary reform.* Increase of dietary fibre (bran, green vegetables) and a reduction in sugar will ameliorate the condition, as well as contributing to a decrease in the incidence of preeclampsia, bowel disorders in later life (diverticulitis), and venous congestive states aggravated by straining at stool (haemorrhoids and varicose veins). (iii) *Specific drugs.* These may be used until the dietary reform is established. They comprise stimulants (Senokot, Milk of Magnesia), lubricants (Agarol, paraffin) or water imbibers/bulk producers (Metamucil). Bulk-forming laxatives are as effective as irritant laxatives and cause fewer side-effects.

Epistaxis

This is often related to engorgement of the profuse network of veins lining the nasal passages. Often the bleeding follows overheating and blowing of the nose too forcefully. Usual measures, such as pressure and ice packs, will be sufficient. If it recurs, investigation may be required.

Varicose Veins

The prime *cause* of varicose veins in pregnancy is the increase in the steroid hormones, oestrogen and *progesterone*, added to later by the *increase in blood volume* and *pressure of the uterus on the pelvic veins*. Oestrogen has a growth-promoting effect, and progesterone a relaxing effect on the smooth muscle of the vein wall. When this latter effect is added to the effect of gravity (standing), incompetence of the valves in the upper leg occurs, causing further aggravation. Although there is a *strong hereditary tendency*, each pregnancy makes the condition worse. *Some 10–20% of women suffer from varicose veins of the legs*, higher figures occurring in multiparas and those over 30 years (colour plate 77). Varicosities of the *vulva* and *vagina* are less common (about 3% and 2%, respectively), are seen mainly in parous women (figure 9.1), and tend to occur later in pregnancy.

The main *complaint* is of aching, tiredness or pain in the legs, night cramps, and oedema. In

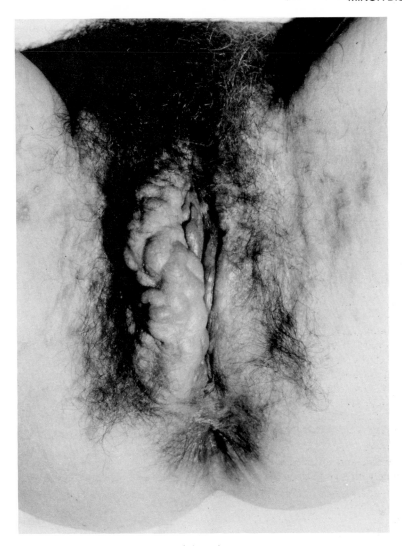

Figure 9.1 Severe varicose veins of the vulva.

the vulva, fullness, tension and warmth are complained of, especially in the posterior part.

Complications. (i) *Thrombophlebitis* (thrombosis) occurs in 5% of patients with varicose veins, usually in the puerperium (table 16.2, colour plate 76). (ii) *Haemorrhage.* If the vein is damaged, bleeding can be profuse, but being of low pressure, is readily controlled by a pressure pad. If a varix in the leg is bleeding, the patient must lie down, elevate the leg, and have pressure applied to the bleeding site. Haemorrhage from varicose veins usually occurs during delivery when an episiotomy incision or tear involves vulval or vaginal varicose veins.

Management. (i) Some authorities recommend *injection of a sclerosing solution*, but most suggest (ii) full-length *supporting hose* (2-way stretch nylon) or *elastic stockings* if the condition is troublesome. The stockings should be removed at night and applied with the feet elevated before getting out of bed next morning. Constricting clothing (e.g. garters, rolled tops of stockings) should be avoided. (iii) Proper *rest periods* (an hour twice daily) with the feet elevated, are important; conversely, long periods of standing will aggravate the condition. (iv) *Stretch panties* may be necessary if vulval varicosities are causing symptoms. (v) Care should be taken at the time of delivery to control haemorrhage from damaged vulval varices by simple pressure until medical assistance is obtained. (vi) Occasionally, *surgical excision* of incompetent veins may be necessary during pregnancy if the leg or vulval symptoms are distressing. The increased distensibility of the veins persists for 8–10 weeks after delivery and definitive treatment options are best deferred until this time to gauge persisting disability.

Haemorrhoids

This term describes varicose enlargement of the veins of the anal canal (inferior haemorrhoidal plexus). The aetiology and behaviour during pregnancy are the same as described above.

The main aggravating factors are constipation (see above) and prolonged pushing down during the second stage of labour (figure 57.1). Bleeding may occur as well as thrombosis. The former is usually associated with the passage of a hard motion, and is rarely severe. Thrombosis of a haemorrhoid is often very painful and may require surgical attention — incision and evacuation of the clot under local analgesia.

Management. (i) This is mainly preventive — avoidance of straining as far as possible. (ii) If prolapse has occurred, replacement is carried out after the patient has been rested in the head down position, and (iii) cold astringent packs placed over the haemorrhoidal mass (hypertonic saline, magnesium or zinc sulphate solution). Bleeding from haemorrhoids is so common during pregnancy and the puerperium that a *tumour*, causing the same symptom, can be overlooked; *rectal examination* should be performed when the patient reports bleeding, and if it persists after pregnancy, further investigation (*sigmoidoscopy* etc) is indicated.

Thromboembolism

Inflammation of the superficial veins, usually in the leg, may occur (thrombophlebitis) or, more seriously, a 'silent' thrombus may develop (phlebothrombosis), usually in the deeper veins. These conditions are commoner in the puerperium (see Chapters 34 and 57).

Breast Soreness

As a result of the stimulatory effects of oestrogen and progesterone on the breast parenchyma, as well as a general increase in vascularity, the patient often experiences fullness, discomfort and tenderness in the breasts. This is similar to the mastalgia many women experience late in the menstrual cycle.

The main aspects of management are reassurance regarding the cause of the symptoms and their temporary nature. Symptomatic relief is obtained by adequate breast support and local warmth.

Oedema

This is a very common finding, especially in hot weather. It is probably due to the venous engorgement (gravity plus progesterone effect) causing greater passage of fluid into the tissues of the leg; a low serum albumin level is often a contributing factor. It may be the first indication of *preeclampsia*, but here the oedema is usually *generalized* (colour plate 82). It usually subsides after resting at night and is aggravated by prolonged standing. The condition is managed largely by increasing the rest periods, with the legs well elevated; diuretics are contraindicated.

Compression Neuropathies

The most troublesome of these is the carpal tunnel syndrome, so called because the median nerve (which supplies the 'thumb half' of the hand) passes through the bony-aponeurotic tunnel at the wrist and becomes compressed if there is swelling, which often occurs in pregnancy. Numbness and tingling is experienced. Other peripheral nerves may suffer similarly (see Chapter 29).

Management is by reassurance, and perhaps diuretics; in median nerve compression, splinting of the wrist is often helpful as is the injection of a small quantity of methylprednisolone (0.5 ml) into the tunnel; an operation may rarely be needed to relieve the pressure by incising the fibrous roof of the tunnel.

Headache

This is a common complaint, and must be attributed to intracranial vascular changes related to the steroid hormones, oestrogen and progesterone. It is also complained of by patients taking the contraceptive pill. Like morning sickness, it usually passes off after the first trimester, but, in some patients, persists throughout pregnancy. Analgesics are prescribed, and rest during the attacks is advised. Investigation may be required if the attacks are frequent, severe, or persistent (Chapter 29).

Fainting

This is probably related to the general vasodilatation of pregnancy (resulting from progesterone) which occurs before the increase in blood volume which is required to fill the expanded vascular space. The effect is compounded by standing in a hot atmosphere. In *late pregnancy* the faintness may be the result of pressure on the aorta/inferior vena cava by the gravid uterus (*supine hypotensive syndrome*, Chapter 33).

Management. Reassurance and avoidance of predisposing factors is all that is necessary, the condition usually passing off after the first trimester. First aid treatment consists of either lying down or sitting with the head between the legs at the first sign of giddiness (Chapter 33). The supine hypotensive syndrome should be prevented by adequate explanation to antenatal patients of the inadvisability of lying supine for any length of time during the third trimester.

Fatigue

This is again more prominent in the first trimester. It probably reflects the major physiological readjustments that are taking place and is one of the early 'nesting' phenomena, whereby nature is ensuring that the mother plays a quieter role during the early months when the fetus is embedding and establishing lines of communication (placentation). The allied symptom of breathlessness is probably related to increased filling of the pulmonary vasculature as the blood volume expands.

Fatigue in early pregnancy is often Nature's reminder of an *accumulated sleep deficit*. The patient should be told that she will not enjoy her pregnancy as she should, or *look her best*, until she rests — many patients are surprised when they find themselves able to 'sleep for days' when they stop work in pregnancy.

The mother should be encouraged to have extra rest for 6–8 weeks, after which time the symptom is less troublesome.

Backache

Many pregnant women complain of a backache or sense of strain in the lower back, particularly as pregnancy advances. The most likely causes are altered mechanics, as the upper body is thrown back to counter-balance the forward growth of the uterus ('pride of pregnancy'), and the softening of the ligaments and muscles which support the weight-carrying joints of the pelvic girdle; occasionally, the latter may be quite marked — e.g. separation of the symphysis pubis). Rarely, an intervertebral disc may herniate, producing acute back pain, which may radiate to the leg along the distribution of one or more of the sciatic nerve roots. Sacroiliac joint strain is relatively common and is detected by elicitation of tenderness over the posterior aspect of the joint.

Management. (i) *Rest* is important in the acute phase, coupled with (ii) *heat* in the form of a hot water bottle or infrared lamp, and (iii) *analgesia* given as necessary. (iv) The support of a *maternity corset* is often helpful, and change to shoes with a lower heel is advisable. (v) *Physiotherapy* is considered if the condition does not respond quickly (posture improvement, pelvic and back exercises). (vi) *Orthopaedic consul-*

tation and investigation by radiography may become necessary to eliminate such conditions as congenital bony anomalies and prolapsed intervertebral disc.

Muscle Cramps

These are also common (33% of patients; severe in 5%); they usually occur late in pregnancy and are *worse at night*; they are often precipitated by sudden contraction of the calf muscles. The exact cause is not known, but must be related either to a temporary shunt of blood away from the muscle (ischaemic cramp) or to a change in the pH or electrolyte milieu (tetanic cramp).

Management. The muscle spasm often responds to stretching of the muscle (sitting up and pulling hard on the toes) and to massage — the husband can be helpful. If persistent, advise the patient to put a pillow at the foot of the bed to prevent her plantar flexing her ankle joints. Cramps usually are caused by the woman stretching her legs out straight (plantar flexion) when *lying on her back*. Different drug remedies have been suggested (calcium lactate, vitamin B complex, quinine sulphate), but few controlled trials have been carried out to ascertain their value other than as placebos. The patient can be reassured that cramps occur only on 3–4 occasions during pregnancy in most sufferers.

Pruritus (Itching)

This may be related to a specific condition, such as drugs, jaundice, malignant disease, infestations or bites. Often, no cause can be found and it must be assumed to be related to other metabolic products, skin stretching, or altered neurovascular sensitivity.

Management. Soothing antipruritic lotions (calamine and menthol) or creams are usually prescribed, together with a nonbarbiturate sedative at night if required. Light cotton undergarments should be worn, and overheating avoided. When persistent, *liver and fetal placental function tests* should be performed because of the possibility of *cholestasis* even in the absence of jaundice (see Chapter 35).

Pruritus vulvae. This is often related to either *candida* or *trichomonas* infections, both of which should be excluded. If general hygiene is satisfactory, a check for *diabetes mellitus* should be made. Condylomata acuminata or lata will be obvious on inspection and will require appropriate treatment. The application of a soothing lotion followed by calamine or an antipruritic dusting powder is helpful. Greasy ointments should be avoided, unless given for a specific reason.

An increase in physiological discharge is common, since this is an oestrogen effect which is related to the pregnancy. A profuse egg-white type of discharge usually heralds rupture of the membranes in patients with cervical incompetence.

Frequency of Micturition

This is one of the symptoms of *early pregnancy* and probably represents a blend of reduced bladder capacity (*pressure of the enlarging uterus*) and increased amount of urine (due to increased blood flow and glomerular filtration). The result is often nocturia, which can be alleviated by reducing fluid intake after 4 pm. Prolonged standing can aggravate the nocturia, since the tissue fluid returns to the vascular system when the patient is lying down and this excess fluid is eliminated at night. If infection is present (cystitis, pyelonephritis), there is usually an associated dysuria. Many patients experience frequency of micturition *late in pregnancy* when the head enters the pelvis and presses on the bladder. Reduction in residual urine is favoured if the woman leans well forward during the terminal act of voiding.

Insomnia

Disturbances to the sleep rhythm may result from anxiety or changes in body metabolism (e.g. increased urine production). The *sheer physical size* of the uterus later in pregnancy, especially with polyhydramnios or multiple pregnancy, often makes sleep difficult (colour plates 70 and 71). Nocturnal cramps have already been referred to.

Management. An attempt should be made to ascertain the cause and often reassurance is all that is required. Agents to allay anxiety may be given in a short course, pending resolution of the problem by other means, and late in pregnancy a sedative may again be required, although preferably *only on a 'demand'* (1–2 nights per week) *rather than on a routine basis.* A sedative should be prescribed when the patient feels exhausted but is unable to sleep. *It is often helpful to explain that rest in bed is a good second best to sleep itself.* Serenity of mind is a common quality in pregnancy and is of far greater value than a drugged sleep. Heavy meals should be avoided in the evening and a milk drink before retiring is helpful, as is lullaby music!

Striae Gravidarum

See Chapter 30 and colour plates 65–75).

chapter ten

Social Aspects of Pregnancy. Adoption

OVERVIEW

Social and preventive aspects of medicine are closely related and are of particular importance in reproduction, because of the sensitivity of the developing embryo and fetus to adverse conditions.

Approximately *20% of clinic patients will require social assistance* at some stage of their pregnancy. The actual figure will depend to a large extent on the financial health of the community in question.

Social factors tend to be overlooked in antenatal history taking — the mother's adequacy in this area being largely taken for granted.

It has been evident, however, from many studies that *social deprivation can have ill-effects on the health of both mother and baby*. As indicated above, social and economic factors are usually interrelated and affect, to a greater or lesser extent, nutrition, housing, education, sanitation, and general health.

Other factors may compound financial hardship — personality defects, ill-health, racial/cultural differences, bad luck etc.

A significant social trend over the past 2 decades has been a more liberal attitude to the *single parent* which, together with greater financial assistance from government, has allowed many women to *keep their baby, rather than give it up for adoption*. Parallel with this has been a *more liberalized approach to abortion*. In many countries there has been a movement towards equal opportunities for women. This has resulted in a movement of women into the workforce, with repercussions on child rearing in some cases.

The health care attendant should be aware of any social problems that the pregnant woman may be experiencing and seek the *assistance of the social worker when indicated*. This will enable a speedier return to social well-being.

Adoption represents a special area of social work. The mother is usually young, single, and disadvantaged. She must make a number of difficult decisions concerning whether to keep the baby or give it up for adoption, and if the latter, she must decide on the amount of contact she will have with the baby in the days after birth.

The mask of secrecy which previously surrounded many aspects of adoption practice has been removed in some countries. Rather than a precious gift for adoptive parents, the *adoptee's well-being is now viewed as paramount* and the relinquishing parents' needs receive more consideration — the child's right to have access to his/her social history is recognized, and where appropriate, communication between the adoptee, the adoptive family and the relinquishing parents is encouraged.

The availability of babies for adoption has fallen markedly over the past decade. This has resulted from the greater use of contraceptives, and if the unmarried woman does become pregnant, usually an abortion is sought or the baby is kept rather than given up for adoption. This is particularly so for the late adolescent.

SOCIAL DEPRIVATION

Definition

There is a deprivation of one or more of the essentials of existence — nutrition, housing, education, and the ability to engage in normal social interaction.

Aetiology and Effects

The reasons such disadvantages may occur in society are complex, and have to be sought at a number of levels — national, special groups, small units such as families, or individuals. The causative factors may be different at different levels. From a practical viewpoint, however, it is important to categorize those patients likely to be at greatest risk.

Personal characteristics. Mental and physical handicaps can be reasonably quantified, but personality is much more nebulous with wide normal ranges of such characteristics as coping ability, anxiety state, maturity, frustration tolerance, self-sacrifice, communication ability etc. If an individual has a poor score in one or more of these personality characteristics, *difficulties may arise during pregnancy and child rearing.* Patients with mental deficiency will need additional support while those with physical handicaps will usually fare satisfactorily with appropriate medical care. The following should alert one to future difficulties — family history of abuse, social isolation, marital instability, poor utilization of health care, pregnancy unwanted, poor impulse control, futile life style.

Economic. This is the prime basis for subdivision into social classes which range from Class 5 (unskilled labourer) to Class 1 (executive, professional). Thus, the take-home salary will be an important factor. Income will usually be low if the husband is unemployed, in poor health, or in gaol or the mother is single, deserted or widowed. Modifying factors include size of family, budgeting expertise (overcommitments to hire purchase), alcohol, gambling, and heavy or unexpected financial demands.

Accommodation. To a large extent this depends on financial resources, but again modifying factors such as number of children may cause overcrowding or change to less suitable housing. Crises may arise such as eviction orders, the dwelling itself being substandard, geographical transfer without emergency accommodation being available, and families in difficulties with the law.

Malnutrition. The diet may be inadequate generally, or more usually it is lacking in important items such as protein or vitamins. This may be related to poor food selection (pies and other pastries, prepacked foods in preference to such items as eggs, fish, cheese and fresh vegetables).

Failure to Use the Health Care System

Ambulatory care. The patient may not attend for antenatal care either sufficiently early or sufficiently regularly. After delivery, she may not attend for postnatal or infant care visits.

Hospital care. The patient may not enter hospital when necessary because of her failure to attend for primary medical care; home commitments (no husband, close friend or relative to care for children, invalid household member, fear of infidelity); fear of hospitals, doctors, or procedures (many immigrants and certain cultural primitives); fear of recognition (if single).

Social services. Many patients are unaware of the welfare benefits to which they are entitled, both financial, counselling, and service (home help).

Special Problem Groups

The unsupported mother. She may be single, divorced, or deserted; her husband may be out of work, an invalid, or in prison. Usually, pregnancy makes the woman more passive and dependent, and with inadequate support, a crisis situation may arise. *The single mother,* especially if young, may experience difficulties with her family who may overreact to the situation, or later the girl's mother may wish to take over the mothering role of the baby. There is usually a conflict as to whether to *marry precipitously* (and often injudiciously), whether *to have an abortion,* whether *to keep the child or surrender it for adoption.* Often there will be some compromise to the individual's education, career, and social well-being. Those electing to keep the child are sometimes themselves a product of a broken home. Apart from these psychological stresses, this girl is often faced with prejudiced or even punitive attitudes in the community (even from those providing for her health care). She is less likely to attend early and regularly for antenatal care, and often has financial and/or accommodation problems. A further problem is the follow-up care after the mother leaves hospital with the baby. The absence of a father figure, if the girl remains single, may result in a more dependent, less masculine child, if a male.

The immigrant. The chief problem is language difficulty. Unlike the husband, who goes out into the community in the course of employment, the wife stays more at home and such language as is developed relates more to the market place than to health care. In many groups, cultural differences exist, the patients are often ignorant of social services (counselling, home help, district nurses) and are reluctant to enter hospital and anxious to leave early. Many immigrants have financial problems, aggravated if the prevailing economy is bad. Finally, they often lack the extended family network that they had in their homeland, which provides physical, psychological, and financial support.

Precivilized. Although often possessing a high degree of social order in their own territories, problems arise when these people are separated from their kin and homeland. Modern technology is disturbing or even frightening; in such groups, attitudes and taboos exist which are often unknown to the medical attendant; and finally, a set of values which works for one culture may not work for the other. For social help to be effective, these cultural differences must be recognized; an intermediary who has multicultural experience is often necessary to bridge the gap.

Marital stress. There are a number of reasons why strains may arise — forced marriage, immaturity, personality and sexual differences, religious and cultural differences, infidelity, periodic desertion, physical or mental abuse, and conflicts over family planning and child care.

Immaturity. This may be related to age (teenage marriage), but not necessarily so. There is often an idealized view of the marriage, which crumbles in the face of the physical, psychological, sexual, and perhaps situational strains that arise. Lack of responsibility is another feature, especially concerning the broader aspects of parenthood, including the child's psychological and emotional needs. Often single mothers, lacking an adult partner, expect an adult-type of affection and response from the child, or paradoxically, expect the baby to remain a baby to fulfil maternal needs.

Inadequate coping ability. The social worker is familiar with this patient. For one or a variety of reasons, she is unable to cope with the ordinary tasks of living, and pregnancy and child care impose a further burden on her ability to manage the household, look after finances, and care for the children.

Child care. A special problem is that of the *handicapped child. Preventive aspects* include counselling by an experienced person if there is reason to suspect the patient or her husband is genetically abnormal, and possibly amniocentesis at 15–17 weeks' gestation to detect an abnormality in the fetus. If the patient has given birth to a malformed or handicapped child, a full explanation must be given to both parents concerning the cause if known, the prognosis in terms of progression, handicap, and any special care that is likely to be necessary. *Voluntary and governmental agencies* likely to be of assistance should be mentioned and help with appointments given; red tape and buck-passing should be sorted out. Other difficulties include the lack of *child care facilities* (day care for children of

working mothers, residential care when the mother requires hospitalization or a rest), lack of child recreation facilities (high rise flats during holidays, terrace-houses).

THERAPEUTIC MEASURES

The chief role of the health care attendant (student, nurse, doctor, or paramedical) is to recognize the need for social counselling and assistance, arrange for appropriate referral, and follow-through with any support necessary. Health care personnel should be fully familiar with the social services available, both in the hospital and in the community. They should be careful not to give false reassurances to patients concerning what the social workers can do for them. In the following discussion, specific items of assistance and procedures are given merely as examples; actual practice differs from country to country and even within each country.

Patient Assessment

An average figure for antenatal clinic patients needing social assistance is 20%. This need should be recognized by the members of the medical care team, preferably at the initial antenatal visit.

The social worker will need to look into the patient's life situation and assess the number of social risk factors that are present. Basic information will be recorded in relation to such factors as age, marital status, developmental history, financial support, accommodation, interpersonal relationships and support figures, personality problems, drug taking, medical handicaps, cultural and language difficulties, coping strength, maturity, employment, attitude to pregnancy, and any particular stress factors that exist, such as handicapped members of the family.

Types of Assistance

General. The social worker has a broad role in assisting patients with social stresses. Apart from direct help with assessment, education, and counselling, he or she is able to tap a variety of sources of financial and other support. The social worker will at times act as mediator, catalyst, and interventionist, in order to assist the patient to resolve these stresses as rapidly as possible. The counsellor must be available, approachable and non-judgemental, so that rapport and trust will be rapidly gained — this forming the basis of the therapeutic relationship.

Financial. Many social service entitlements are available for the pregnant woman and details of these are available at all hospital antenatal clinics or local social security offices. Alterations in the provision and amount of specific grants occur periodically and up-to-date details are available from the Department of Health and Social Security. Legislation is currently being reviewed by Parliament and alterations to the allowances as detailed below may occur in 1986.

Types of assistance:

(i) *Welfare benefits*. When the expectant mother visits her general practitioner for the first time she will be given a Certificate of Expected Confinement signed by him or a certified midwife. This entitles her to claim exemption from dental and prescription charges. Free dental treatment is also available during the 12 months after the birth of the child.

(ii) *Maternity grant*. A non-contributory grant of £25 is available for any woman resident in the United Kingdom or who has lived in the United Kingdom for at least 26 of the 52 weeks prior to delivery. The grant is also paid to those whose pregnancy results in stillbirth. In the event of a multiple pregnancy, a grant is allowed for each child that lives for more than 12 hours.

(iii) *Maternity allowance*. This is a weekly grant paid for 18 weeks commencing 11 weeks prior to the expected week of confinement. The amount paid is dependent on whether the woman has paid full rate National Insurance contributions and details are available from the local social security office.

(iv) *Child benefit*. This is payable for all children, including a first or only child, and is not means tested. It is paid monthly and the amount paid is under regular review.

Other family benefits which may be relevant to the patient are family income supplement, supplementary benefit, attendance allowance, and one parent benefit. In addition, grants are available to assist with transportation fares to and from hospital.

Payment of maternity leave. Under the terms of the Employment Protection (Consolidation) Act 1978, a woman who has been in continuous employment for 2 years with the same employer is entitled to maternity leave and payment. She is entitled to 6 weeks payment (beginning 11 weeks before the expected week of confinement) at nine-tenths of the normal week's pay, less the flat rate National Insurance maternity allowance. The woman/employee then has the right to return to her employment at any time before the end of the period of 29 weeks beginning with the week in which the child was born.

Accommodation. Help may be provided in obtaining temporary or permanent accommodation for families; however, emergency accommodation is recognized as an acute but unmet need in many centres. In the case of single mothers, special 'shelter' homes may be contacted, or private accommodation arranged.

Child care. This may be short-term, as for an antenatal visit; or long-term to cover admissions to hospital (antenatal and/or for delivery). Another problem is the care of children of a working mother, especially if she is unsupported. The most difficult situation arises when one or more of the children is handicapped, mentally or physically.

Home help. A number of home help services are available, both nursing and domestic.

Legal aid. This may be requested by the unmarried mother if she is taking an action of affiliation (proof of paternity) or alimony (maintenance allowance). Free legal services are subject to a means' test and the government may pay the benefit without requiring court action if the latter is deemed to be fruitless in view of the father's record.

Special referral. In certain circumstances, specialist referral may be required — psychiatrist, physician, venereologist, marriage guidance. This will be arranged by the patient's doctor.

ADOPTION OF CHILDREN
Definition
An adoption order is an order which vests the parental rights and duties relating to the child on the adoptees, made on their application by an authorized court. This order transfers all parental responsibilities from the biological parents to the adopting parents.

Trends
In many Western Countries there has been a change in social pattern in recent years: many unmarried mothers now choose to keep their babies. This has been facilitated by a change in community attitudes to the single parent and to improved social services to this group. Insufficient follow-up studies have been reported to assess fully the social prognosis of the children, but in some, at least, the outcome is not ideal.

Social Aspects
It is desirable that an experienced social worker interview all patients intending to have their baby adopted. A full social history is necessary as indicated earlier. Help is provided in decision making and at crisis periods in the pregnancy

(usually early in the antenatal period and then at delivery and the early puerperium). The record should be marked that the baby is to be considered for adoption; this will obviate remarks by attendants that could cause distress to the mother. The labour ward staff should be aware of the situation. The mother may need advice on seeing and holding the baby after delivery, assuring herself of its normality, and perhaps obtaining a photograph. She is likely to be upset at the loss of the baby, and psychological and social support will be helpful, not only in hospital, but also after her return home.

The adopting parents should be provided with a leaflet regarding adoption procedures and a list of relevant monographs and pamphlets for further reading if needed. Their character and suitability for adopting should be established. Important factors include their motivation, general attitudes to children and their own relatives, stability, personalities, infertility background, concordance of opinion of husband and wife regarding adoption, general health, and housing adequacy. Supervision should be continued after placement. The confidentiality of all records should be maintained. In some countries there is a move towards *open or semi-open adoption*.

Deferment of adoption may be necessary on the grounds of physical problems in the baby (malformation, immaturity, infection), mixed race, and indecision or illness of the natural mother. Eventually, the great majority of such babies will be adopted or fostered; the remainder will require institutional care.

Legal Aspects

The legal aspects of child care and adoption were studied in depth by the Houghton Committee which reported its findings in 1973. The Children Act, 1975 is based on this report. The Act has 3 main sections: (i) adoption; (ii) custody; and (iii) care.

The child care provisions of the Act protect the interests of children in care by imposing a duty on the local authority, in reaching any decision in relation to the child, to give first consideration to the need to safeguard and promote his welfare throughout his childhood and, so far as is practicable, to take into account his wishes and feelings, having regard to his age and understanding. They impose restrictions on the abrupt removal of a child who has been in care for 6 months or more and enable a local authority to assume parental rights over a child who has been left in care for 3 years. They enable the courts to order that a parent shall not represent a child in care or in related proceedings where there may be a conflict of interests between child and parent, and to

appoint a guardian *ad litem* to represent the child's interests. A special onus rests on the court to apply the provision in unopposed proceedings for the discharge of a care or supervision order.

The Children Act 1975 also requires local social services departments to establish a comprehensive adoption service in co-operation with voluntary agencies approved by the Secretary of State. Single persons of either sex may apply to adopt a child. The upper limit of age for a child for adoption is 18 years. The child's wishes and feelings must be taken into account, with regard to his age and understanding. The adoption agency will investigate the health, character and finances of the adopting parents and will make every effort to match the child to the adopters. Agreement to adoption can no longer be withheld on religious grounds. The natural parent(s) must supply written agreement to the adoption, witnessed by a Justice of the Peace or Officer of the Court. This agreement is not valid until the child is 6 weeks old. Agreement can be dispensed with in special circumstances, for example if the parents cannot be traced or in cases of persistent neglect or ill-treatment.

The court will appoint a Guardian *ad litem* who will look after the child's interests during the probationary period before the court hearing, the date of which will be set for not less than 3 months after the application. The adoptive parents must have continuous actual custody of the child for the whole of this time.

The court hearing is held in private. Evidence is given by the guardian *ad litem* and a full medical report is made on the child. It is up to the court to grant an order. Details of the order are given to the Registrar General who will record them in the Adopted Children's Register together with the details of original parentage. Certificates of birth are issued from the Adopted Children's Register in the same way as those issued from the birth register.

Confidentiality and Anonymity Between Parties

These were cornerstones of adoption practice. It was the duty of all who were involved in the process to ensure that adopting parents did not learn of the identity of the child for adoption, and the natural parent(s) did not learn the identity of the adopting parents. However, in recent years this traditional adoption practice has changed to a more honest and open approach, giving the adoptee, the relinquishing parent(s) and the adoptive parents information about each other. This goes hand in hand with recognition of the right of the adoptee to have access to information about his/her social history.

Problems

The rules concerning who can legally arrange the adoption again differ from place to place. In some countries it can be done directly by the natural parent(s), or via an intermediary who might be a medical practitioner, adoption society, or governmental authority. Occasionally, the law may require that all adoptions are controlled by a governmental department. This restriction has arisen because of the hazards that surround more private arrangements. These include overlooking of legal requirements (notifications, consents, religious upbringing restriction); change of mind of the adopting parents; and inadequate matching of the child to the adopting parents.

The remaining problems relate mainly to psychological disturbances that arise later in the parents and/or the child. It is preferable that the child is adopted as early as possible, so that a mutually satisfying relationship can be established. Also the adopted child should be the youngest in the family at the time of placement.

If the baby has a medical problem, the adoption may be delayed for a short period if the condition is not serious (interim order) and a review made at a specified time; if the condition is serious, the adoption may be deferred until the situation becomes clarified.

Foster Care

This is an arrangement made between a parent or guardian for another person to have custody of a child, but the legal relationship between the natural parent and child is maintained. Foster care often gets over the problems arising in difficult or deferred adoption.

chapter eleven

Pharmacology

OVERVIEW

'Asking not wisdom, but drugs to charm with' W. Osler

The science of pharmacology is relatively new, but has advanced dramatically in the past 2 decades. Specific and often powerful drugs have replaced the less specific remedies of former times. In addition, the growth of the pharmaceutical industry has been responsible for the multiplicity of available preparations of the same drug.

Pregnancy is associated with a considerable number of upsets and minor disorders. The temptation to use drug therapy should be balanced against by the benign nature of a great majority of these upsets and their temporary nature. In obstetric practice, a sound knowledge of drugs in common use is important, since errors of administration may have serious consequences for the mother and/or baby. The ability of drugs to pass *to the baby*, either through the *placenta* or in *breast milk*, should be appreciated, as should the altered pharmacokinetics of pregnancy (slower *gastrointestinal absorption*, increased *volume of distribution*, increased *renal clearance*, increased *metabolism*, reduced *protein binding*). In any prescribing during pregnancy, the tables listing drug safety should be consulted; if the drug is not in the safe list, its use should be looked at critically in terms of benefit to the mother versus potential harm to the fetus. Unfortunately, many of the newer drugs will remain therapeutic orphans as far as the pregnant woman is concerned because of the complexities of assessment of fetal toxicology.

Studies in many hospitals have shown that there is often an unacceptable number of prescriptions written by doctors that are illegible or contain errors in the specification of *drug dosage* or *method of administration*. Similarly, there is often a failure by the nurse to give the proper drug, at the prescribed dose, dosage interval and by the route specified. Ignorance, inattention, fatigue and lack of proper communication all play a part. The verbal ordering of potent drugs offers the greatest potential for a serious mistake to occur.

Many patients are worried by tales, often anecdotal, of the effect of drugs on the fetus. It is important that this aspect be discussed at the initial antenatal visit. In the case of patients already taking therapy for disorders such as epilepsy and asthma, preconceptual counselling is wise. As already mentioned, the physiology of the pregnant woman is altered significantly and it is not surprising that changes occur in drug metabolism (e.g. delayed absorption, decreased binding to albumin, increased renal clearance, increased liver enzyme activity, fetal-placental involvement). Therefore, it may be necessary to monitor blood or salivary levels of some drugs e.g. phenytoin. It is also understandable that there will be significant differences in the excretion of drugs by the mother and baby. One major difference relates to the immaturity of the liver and kidney in the newborn — sites of detoxification and elimination of drugs. Another important difference is the weaker *blood:brain barrier* in the baby and drugs acting on the brain, for example narcotics, will thus have a relatively greater effect. These differences are magnified in the premature infant.

The times of greatest concern are the *organogenetic* period (*risk of malformation*) and the last few weeks of intrauterine life (effect on the functional state of the newborn).

Drug Nomenclature

To illustrate the method of naming drugs we can take a compound discovered in the last century, but still in common use today — aspirin. Its *chemical name* is acetylsalicylic acid, its *generic* name is aspirin; and it has a *proprietary or trade name* according to the company making the drug. Because many drugs are quite complex, with long chemical names, the generic name or the trade name is often used.

Maternal Drug Consumption

A study of reviews of maternal drug use over the past 10–15 years reveals that significant changes have occurred as an aftermath of the thalidomide disaster. In particular, there has been a drop in the consumption of antiemetics and antihistamines, and to a lesser extent of hypnotics and sedatives. The prescribing of *diuretics* has been markedly reduced with the realization that they are harmful in the patient with preeclampsia. Ovarian steroid hormone use has also dropped after the discovery of genital tract malformations in both sexes, clear cell neoplasia in the female due to stilboestrol (DES), and abnormalities of primary sexual development from progestational agents. Antiemetics have come under a cloud from reports of occasional and possibly coincidental fetal malformations and resultant litigation publicity. *Consumption of analgesics has* largely persisted in spite of the above trend and they are still consumed at some time during the pregnancy by *at least 50% of women in most survey groups.*

Dynamics of Drug Action

A number of steps are involved in the handling of a drug by the body.

Absorption. This often depends on the route, with the rate of absorption usually increasing from oral → subcutaneous → intramuscular → intravenous administration. *If the patient is in pain from any cause or is markedly anxious,* for example in labour or after placental abruption, *absorption from the gastrointestinal system is very slow.* If the patient is in *shock,* absorption is most effective by the intravenous route, due to slowing of the blood supply to the tissues. With the oral route, there may be a question of whether the *patient has really taken the drug,* and absorption is more variable because of changes in bowel motility and pH. *Vomiting* may occur, especially in labour, and it may be very difficult to estimate how much of the drug has been retained. In the future, it is likely that the *transdermal route* (the self adhesive drug patch) will be increasingly used because of better compliance and more even blood and tissue levels.

Binding to plasma proteins or tissues. This is sometimes of practical importance. For example, some anticoagulant drugs are almost entirely bound to plasma proteins. If another drug is given which displaces the anticoagulant from the binding site, overdosage can occur. Once free within the tissues, the unbound drug will induce an effect only by *attraction to receptor sites* where it will produce stimulation or depression of specific cells e.g. oxytocin and myometrial cells.

Inactivation and excretion. The *liver and kidney* are the 2 organs largely responsible for *clearing drugs from the body.* The liver cells often *inactivate the drug* by chemical modification and the altered drug is then more easily *excreted by the kidneys or intestine.* If the liver and kidneys are functioning poorly, as in preexisting disease or significant preeclampsia, drugs may accumulate to toxic levels. The same effect may result when several drugs compete for the same excretion pathway, for example penicillin and probenecid in the renal tubules. This interaction is used in treating patients with venereal and other infections, high blood levels of penicillin being readily achieved if the drugs are given together.

Individual Variability and Side-effects of Drugs

It is now recognized that the same dose of a drug may affect people differently, either in its specific action or in its side-effects. This difference is partly due to individual variation, which is a feature of biological behaviour, and partly to specific genetic differences.

Idiosyncrasy is the term given when a person reacts abnormally to a standard dose of a drug.

There are numerous general factors which have to be considered — e.g. *those at the extremes of life are more susceptible,* as are those who are *underweight.* The general health of the person may also be important (*malnutrition* or *medical disorders*).

The intake of *alcohol and tobacco* influences many drugs, and even differences in place of living (urban, rural) are significant.

If a person is *receiving more than one drug,* the possibility of drug-drug interaction should be considered with a net diminution or enhancement of drug effect.

Obstetrical factors are important. Drug metabolism in the liver may be significantly impaired in conditions such as *preeclampsia.* The *amount of drug reaching the fetus* depends on the amount administered, the route, and the degree of placental transfer. It should be noted that *the majority of drugs cross the placenta in significant amounts.* If the concentrations of maternal plasma proteins are low (haemodilution, low protein diet) more of the drug which usually binds to these proteins will be in a free state and available for transfer to the fetus.

The problem of side-effects is also complicated by *psychological influences*. Recent work has shown that inert 'dummy' tablets (controls, placebos) may produce a wide range of side-effects e.g. fatigue, tremor, headache, nausea and other gastrointestinal upsets, insomnia, and even rashes. However, the side-effects of most drugs are now known fairly accurately and differentiation from 'placebo' reactions can be made more easily.

Toxicity is a *normal reaction to excessive levels of the drug* in the body. It may result from an overdose, or the body's failure to detoxify or excrete a drug.

Drug allergy is an *immunological reaction* and is very important since fatality may result, e.g. penicillin allergies occur in 1–10% of patients in reported series, and about 1 in 2,000 patients exhibit *anaphylaxis*. Enquiry will usually elicit a history of this, but in some a reaction may occur without prior warning. Urticaria, severe itching, angio-oedema, dyspnoea, and vascular collapse are the characteristic features. If this occurs the attendant must assist the patient into the head-down, feet-up position *and insert an airway if necessary*, call for medical aid, apply a tourniquet (or blood pressure cuff) above the injection site if this is feasible, give adrenaline 0.5 ml of a 1 in 1,000 solution subcutaneously (if in shock, 0.1 ml IV and 0.4 ml IM), and administer oxygen (by mask preferably). Thereafter, an intravenous infusion may be necessary, with further drug administration (cortisol 500 mg IV; diphenhydramine (Benadryl) 50 mg IV, 50 mg IM; metaraminol (Aramine) 100 mg).

The person who faints at the time of injection should not be confused with the one described above. An allied complication is *serum sickness*, which occurs much later — a week or so after exposure. The symptoms are malaise, fever, skin reactions and lymphadenopathy. Treatment is by antihistamines and analgesics.

One should differentiate the terms 'experience' of side-effects and 'complaint' of side-effects. Many patients will experience some change, but will not bother to report it, either because it is mild, she does not relate it to the drug, or she is not the complaining type. When a patient complains, the reverse of the above is likely. Also, however, it is often a 'signal' that the patient is anxious, unhappy, or is antagonistic to those looking after her, no rapport having been established.

Some reasons for *failure to take prescribed medication* include prolonged illnesses, absence of symptoms (hypertension) or where therapy is prophylactic (for prevention of anaemia), poor education, language difficulties, complex regimens of multiple drugs, side-effects, and failure to spend enough time explaining to the patient why the drug is necessary, how to take it, and what side-effects may occur.

If the patient has faith in her medical attendants, she is more likely to comply with her treatment regimen.

Drug Dependence and Addiction

One needs only to see the number of prescriptions written in one year in a particular country for sedatives, hypnotics, tranquillizers and analgesics, to realize the habituating tendency of such drugs. Recent surveys have indicated, for example, that 15–20% of antenatal patients regularly take aspirin (usually for 'headache'). Proper health education should enable the patient to gain insight into the habituating tendency of such drugs and promote a climate of opinion that restricts their use to emergency and short-term use, *not as a routine*. We are still far from knowing the effects of such drugs on the developing fetal brain, although the study of the babies of drug-addicted patients shows effects lasting up to 6 months in some cases. *Addictive drugs* are of many types e.g. *narcotics* (heroin, methadone), *stimulants* (amphetamines, *cocaine*), *depressants/tranquillizers* (barbiturates, belladonna, solvents, benzodiazepines, phenothiazines), *hallucinogens* (cannabis, LSD, psilocybin, mescaline), *alcohol*. It is important to realize that drug abusers may consume these agents in various combinations. Cognitive functions are often dulled by overdoses and child care is often suboptimal.

Other disease states which may be associated with narcotic abuse include *venereal diseases* (*often from prostitution*), *hepatitis*, bacterial endocarditis, and other infections. Menstrual irregularity is common in drug users, and calculations of date of delivery often unreliable.

Recent studies in opiate-dependent pregnant women have demonstrated multiple and often *serious lesions in the brains of the babies of such women* — haemorrhages, cysts, and necrosis. It is postulated that these might result from overdose and/or withdrawal of the drug, effects of the narcotic itself, *adulterant substances* and perhaps other associated drugs or alcohol. Overall neonatal mortality is about 5%. The blood:brain barrier of the fetus and newborn is much less efficient than in the older subject.

The incidence of known narcotic drug addiction in pregnancy in our experience *is about 0.06%*; the figure, however, will be related to overall drug use in the community in question.

One study reported 45 cases in 80,950 pregnancies: the main complications were *fetal growth retardation* (30%) and *premature birth before 37 weeks* (30%); there were no fetal malformations and only 1 perinatal death. Follow-up information is necessary to ascertain if the main hazard to these infants lies in the *environment to which they return*. It is probable that addicts who identify themselves and comply with the treatment programme (see below) are much more likely to have healthy infants.

It should be part of antenatal care to identify the drug addicted patient and institute appropriate management, including *detoxification, methadone maintenance*, implementation of a *proper diet*, psychotherapy, social support, and regular monitoring of fetal well-being.

The *fetal alcohol syndrome* is now well recognized. It is likely that the breakdown product, acetaldehyde, is the toxic component and those babies of women with deficiencies of the aldehyde dehydrogenase system are probably at greater risk.

Legal Requirements

Since strong analgesics are in relatively common use in obstetric practice, the nurse and doctor must be fully conversant with the legal requirements involved with such dangerous drugs, and provisions of the relevant Poisons Acts (prescriptions, supply, storage, records, checks).

Drugs and the Fetus (tables 11.1–11.3)

Experience has clearly shown that the fetus must be accorded separate consideration in relation to drug use. *Thalidomide* has shown that a drug harmless to the adult (and several experimental pregnant animals) can cause major fetal malformations. *Diethylstilboestrol* (DES) has demonstrated the latency that may occur before the real impact of a drug is seen. Unfortunately, the effect of some drugs may be both delayed and subtle, perhaps affecting CNS function, behaviour or other performances, cancer induction, or genetic change. In the first trimester there is the risk of *teratogenicity*; in later pregnancy damage to growing tissues may still occur; towards term drug effects may persist and affect neonatal behaviour as a result of immature *detoxification mechanisms*.

A point of importance is the possibility that the harmful effect of a drug may be added to by a coincident illness in the mother or fetus — genetic defect, infection, metabolic disorder, anoxia, pesticide or herbicide, food toxin etc.

The fetus and newborn differ from the adult particularly in drug penetration of the brain barrier, immaturity of detoxifying (liver) and excretory (liver/kidney/lung) pathways.

As mentioned earlier, drugs may reach the fetus by *transplacental passage* before birth or in *breast milk* after birth (table 11.4). Most lipid-soluble drugs pass the placenta as do those with a molecular weight less than 600 (heparin, with a molecular weight greater than 1,000 passes only slowly, and is thus useful as an anticoagulant to cover the baby's birth). *Clinicians now restrict prescribing in the organogenetic period to the absolute minimum* (antiemetics for troublesome vomiting, and other strictly indicated medications).

Important critical organ growth periods are as follows: *heart* 18–40 days, *brain* 18–604 days, *limbs* 25–35 days, *eye* 25–40 days, *genitalia* 35–65 days. In the growth period from the 15th week to term, the fetus is still at special risk from some drugs: androgenic and adrenal steroids (masculinization); tetracyclines (staining and abnormal growth of teeth and bones); antithyroid drugs (hypothyroidism, goitre); anticoagulants of the coumarin type (late dysmorphogenesis and bleeding); narcotic analgesics (respiratory depression, dependence); barbiturates, anaesthetics (sedation). In addition, even the mature baby is deficient in those *enzymes* responsible for metabolizing such drugs as chloramphenicol, morphine, succinylcholine, sulphonamides, isoniazid, pethidine, imipramine, phenacetin, barbiturates, tolbutamide, and in its kidneys' capacity to *excrete* the drug. These defects will be more apparent in the premature baby.

Two new drugs which are derivatives of vitamin A — *isotretinoin* used to treat *acne* and *etretinate* used to treat *psoriasis* — have a great propensity to cause severe birth defects (central nervous and cardiovascular systems). Because these drugs have a long biological half-life, adequate contraception is essential — pregnancy should be avoided for 6–12 months after the final dose.

Cigarette smoking and *analgesic consumption* deserve special mention since they are outside usual prescribing and enter the realm of *health education*. It should be remembered also that the fetus may suffer indirectly from drugs given to the mother, particularly those affecting uterine action or the blood supply to the uterus. A common example is the overactivity of the uterus resulting from excessive amounts of oxytocin or prostaglandin.

The whole range of drugs which may affect the fetus or baby is too large to be considered in detail. However, tables 11.2–11.4 provide a guide for commonly prescribed agents.

Drugs and Lactation

In recent years, the benefits of breast feeding have been realized, and the rate on discharge approaches 95% in some hospitals. Whilst knowledge of drug pharmacokinetics in lactation is still limited, this situation is being remedied with improvements in methodology of drug assay, particularly the small amounts which are in breast milk and the infants' plasma.

A number of factors influence the passage of a drug into the breast milk and maternal milk:plasma ratios vary quite widely e.g. from less than 0.01 to more than 1. The concentration of a drug in milk is usually quite small.

Drug prescribing during lactation should be regarded in a similar way to prescribing during pregnancy. i.e. (i) No drug should be taken unless considered essential; (ii) shorter-acting drugs are preferable; (iii) drugs should be chosen which have the lowest excretion in breast milk; (iv) breast feeding may need to be ceased temporarily or permanently; (v) the baby should be monitored carefully; (vi) precautions in relation to pesticides/herbicides should be encouraged e.g. stop smoking, wash foodstuffs, reduce fat consumption, reduce exposure to household/garden sprays. The list of drugs which are safe or unsafe in pregnancy provides a guide to lactation management with drugs specifically contraindicated being shown in table 11.4.

Educating the Patient

Fortunately, most patients will have been subjected to media discussion about the dangers of drugs (during pregnancy). However, this subject should be specifically discussed at the initial antenatal visit. The patient's drug history should be ascertained as well as *any* drugs currently or occasionally being taken since many women disregard 'over the counter' drugs in such discussions. The effect of drugs during the different gestational periods should be pointed out. If drugs are prescribed, the need for compliance is stressed and the intended therapeutic effect and possible side-effects are mentioned. Some patients are unaware of the secretion of drugs in breast milk.

Summary

Our knowledge of the effect of drugs on the fetus is far from complete, particularly from a long-term point of view. Prescribing for the pregnant and lactating woman should be undertaken with considerable care and health care personnel should be familiar with the correct dose of each drug, its effect and side-effects, route of administration, duration of action, method of elimination, and management of untoward effects.

TABLE 11.1   SAFE OR RELATIVELY SAFE DRUGS FOR USE DURING PREGNANCY

Acetaminophen	(analgesic)
Albuterol	(sympathomimetic)
Alphaprodine	(narcotic analgesic)
Amoxycillin	(antibiotic)
Amphotericin B	(antifungal antibiotic)
Ampicillin	(antibiotic)
Benzene hexachloride	(scabicide, pediculcide)
Betamethasone	(synthetic corticosteroid)
Butorphanol	(analgesic)
Caffeine	
Calcitonin	(calcium regulating hormone)
Carbenicillin	(antibiotic)
Cephamandole	(cephalosporin, antibiotic)
Cefotaxime	(,, ,,)
Cefoxitin	(,, ,,)
Cephalothin	(,, ,,)
Chlorpheniramine	(antihistamine, antiemetic)
Cimetidine	(histamine (H_2) receptor antagonist)
Clindamycin	(antibiotic)
Clotrimazole	(antifungal)
Cloxacillin	(antibiotic)
Cyclizine	(antihistamine/antiemetic)
Dexamethasone	(synthetic corticosteroid)
Digitalis	(cardiac glycoside)
Erythromycin	(antibiotic)
Ethambutol	(antituberculosis agent)
Fenoterol	(sympathomimetic)
Fenphenazine	(tranquillizer)
Hydralazine	(antihypertensive)
**Ibuprofen	(antiinflammatory)
Insulin	(antidiabetic)
Isoniazid	(antituberculosis agent)
Magnesium sulphate	(anticonvulsant)
Mandelic acid	(urinary antibacterial)
Meclozine	(antihistamine, antiemetic)
Meperidine	(see pethidine)
Methenamine	(urinary antibacterial)
Methicillin	(antibiotic)
Methyldopa	(antihypertensive)
Metronidazole	(antitrichomonal)
Miconazole	(antifungal)
Nalidixic acid	(urinary antibacterial)
Nitrofurantoin	(urinary antibacterial)
Nystatin	(antifungal)
Penicillin	(antibiotic)
Perphenazine	(tranquillizer)
Pethidine	(analgesic)
Phenacetin	(analgesic)
Phenobarbitone	(sedative, anticonvulsant)
Piperazine	(anthelmintic)
Prednisolone)	(corticosteroid)
Prednisone)	
Probenecid	(uricosuric/renal tubule blocker)
Promazine	(tranquillizer)
Quinidine	(antiarrythmic)
Rifampicin	(antituberculosis)
Ritodrine	(adrenergic sympathomimetic)
Spectinomycin	(antibiotic)
Sulphonamides	(antibacterial)
**Sulphasalazine	(antibacterial)
Terbutaline	(adrenergic sympathomimetic)
Trimethoprim	(antibacterial)
Vasopressin	(posterior pituitary lobe hormone)

** Use in third trimester

TABLE 11.2 POSSIBLE HARMFUL EFFECTS OF DRUGS ON THE EMBRYO, FETUS, AND NEWBORN INFANT

Drug	Adverse effect
Alcohol (ethanol)	Retarded growth; craniofacial, cardiac and limb deformities
Anaesthetics Halothane, nitrous oxide, ether Thiopentone Lignocaine	May influence fetus in theatre workers, respiratory depression CNS depression CNS depression, bradycardia
Analgesics Aspirin	Prolonged prothrombin time, leading to neonatal haemorrhage; may displace bilirubin from protein binding sites, with risk of kernicterus. Altered platelet function. Prostaglandin inhibition; premature closure of ductus arteriosus
Phenacetin	Methaemoglobin formation
Drugs of addiction — diamorphine, methadone, morphine, pethidine, pentazocine, marijuana	Withdrawal symptoms (e.g. hyperirritability, increased tone, myoclonus, shrill cry, vomiting and diarrhoea, dehydration, overventilation) usually appearing toward end of first 24 hours of life; depression of respiration if administered close to birth. Growth retardation
Antiacne Isotretinoin	Dysmorphism syndrome
Antibacterials Nitrofurantoin	Haemolytic anaemia in glucose-6-phosphate dehydrogenase (G6PD) deficient infants
Streptomycin (and dihydrostreptomycin)	Occasional 8th nerve damage (vestibular and auditory); hearing loss slight, sometimes unilateral
Sulphonamides	Haemolytic anaemia in G6PD deficient infants
Sulphonamides (long acting)	Displacement of bilirubin from protein binding sites, with risk of kernicterus. Drug very slowly excreted by infant
Tetracycline	Molecule chelates with calcium, deposited along with it in tissues undergoing mineralization, e.g. bone, tooth buds. Yellow-brown staining and deformity of primary dentition may result; certain teeth of secondary dentition are involved if drug is given in the last trimester
Chloramphenicol	Cardiovascular collapse (grey syndrome)
Hexachlorophene	Toxic absorption from abraded skin. Predisposes to Gram-negative bacterial colonization
Anticoagulants Coumarins	Fetal and neonatal haemorrhage due to prolonged prothrombin time
Heparin	Increased risk of stillbirth
Anticonvulsants Ethosuximide	Low teratogenic potential
Phenytoin	Hypoplasia distal phalanges, cleft palate and lip, haemorrhagic disease of newborn
Carbamazepine	Fetal head growth retardation
Antidepressants Monoamine oxidase inhibitors	Can interact with pethidine or anaesthetics
Antidiabetic drugs Oral hypoglycaemic agents — sulphonylureas (tolbutamide)	Insulin release from pancreatic cells; hypoglycaemia, sometimes prolonged

Antihistamine	
Promethazine	Suspected cause of hip dislocation
Antihyptertensive drugs	
Reserpine	Stuffy nose, nasal discharge, respiratory depression, hypotonia
Ganglion blockers	Paralytic ileus
Diazoxide	Alopecia if administration lengthy
Propranolol	Low birth-weight, hypoglycaemia, bradycardia, respiratory depression
Antimalarials	
Quinine	Thrombocytopenic purpura
Chloroquine	Deafness and abnormal retinal pigmentation
Primaquine	Haemorrhage
Antimitotics	
Aminopterin	Skeletal malformations, growth retardation, microcephaly
Chlorambucil	Congenital anomalies, growth retardation
Antithyroid drugs	
Carbimazole, methylthiouracil propylthiouracil, sodium iodine,	Goitre and hypothyroidism if dosage not well controlled (symptoms of neonatal thyrotoxicosis masked in first days of life)
Sodium iodide (^{131}I)	Hypothyroidism
Bronchodilator	
Aminophylline	Vomiting, jitteriness
Cholinergic drugs	
Edrophonium chloride, neostigmine, physostigmine, pyridostigmine bromide	Transient muscular weakness in some infants
Corticosteroids	
Cortisol and analogues	Theoretical risk of adrenal depression. Low oestriol values often seen
Other hormones	Androgens, synthetic progestins may masculinize the female fetus. Oestrogens may cause vaginal tumours at adolescence, and urinary anomalies in males
Diuretics	
Ethacrynic acid	Hyponatraemia
Thiodiazine group	Possible thrombocytopenic purpura. Slight salt and water depletion
Nicotine	Low birth-weight
Sedatives	
Thalidomide	Phocomelia, deafness
Phenobarbitone, phenytoin	Neonatal haemorrhage due to deficiency of vitamin K dependent factors; neonatal depression
Tranquillizers	
Chloropromazine	Respiratory problems, jaundice
Diazepam	May decrease conjugation of bilirubin because of competition, and thus predispose to neurological damage. Can cause delay in initiation of breathing
Haloperidol	Limb malformations
Lithium	Cyanosis, flaccidity and lethargy, cardiac and other anomalies
Vitamin K	Hyperbilirubinaemia

TABLE 11.3   DRUGS ASSOCIATED WITH
TERATOGENESIS

Drug	Condition
Alcohol	Fetal alcohol syndrome
Aminoglycosides	Deafness
Aminopterin	Multiple defects
Antithyroid drugs	Goitre
Anticonvulsants	CNS and skeletal anomalies, cleft lip and palate, congenital heart disease
Chloroquine	Deafness, neurological deficit
Corticosteroids	Cleft palate
Diazepam	Cleft lip and palate
Diethylstilboestrol	Genital tract abnormalities
Hormones	Feminization in males, clitoral hypertrophy in females
Isotretinoin	Dysmorphism syndrome
Lithium	Cardiovascular anomalies
Tetracycline	Stained teeth, depressed skeletal growth
Thalidomide	Phocomelia, hearing loss
Warfarin	Hypoplasia of nasal structure, skeletal anomalies

TABLE 11.4   MATERNALLY INGESTED DRUGS
WHICH CAN HARM BREAST-FED INFANTS

Drug	Potential effects in the infant
Alcohol	Vomiting and drowsiness
Anticoagulants	Bleeding
Antimetabolites	Bone marrow depression
Atropine	Tachycardia, constipation and urinary retention
Barbiturates	Drowsiness
Chlorothiazides	Thrombocytopenia
Ergot alkaloids	Vomiting, diarrhoea, weakness
Iodine	Hypothyroidism, goitre
Laxatives	Diarrhoea
Metronidazole	Blood dyscrasias, vomiting
Narcotics	Addiction
Nicotine	Reduced milk production
Radioactive preparations	Thyroid, bone marrow depression
Reserpine	Nasal congestion, lethargy, diarrhoea
Sulphonamides	Bilirubin displacement from serum albumin causing kernicterus in neonatal hyperbilirubinaemia
Tetracyclines	Teeth discoloration, interference with bone growth
Thiouracil	Hypothyroidism, goitre
Warfarin	Bleeding

THE ASSESSMENT OF ABNORMAL PREGNANCY

chapter twelve

Statistical Methods and Vital Statistics

OVERVIEW

For many people, if not most, statistics is a great turn-off. This is unfortunate, because it is basic to the scientific practice of medicine and integral to the introduction of new drugs and techniques as well as the interpretation of observed trends in different populations.

The student and practitioner should have a grasp of the fundamentals of statistical methods in order to interpret his or her own practice of medicine and to evaluate the reports and claims of others.

Such methods help us to know whether samples are true representations of the populations from which they are drawn, how one set of data is related to another, and if so what is the strength of that correlation and how likely it is to have occurred as a result of the chance fluctuations that occur in all biological material.

Experimental design of research studies abounds in traps for the unwary. Usually the help of a statistician is necessary in guidance of such matters as sample size, selection bias, randomization, response rate, type of design, appropriate method of analysis and significance of results.

Clinical trials can waste a great amount of time and money if the likelihood of finding an important difference is not large enough.

Population and Sample

It is important to distinguish between the concepts of 'population' and 'sample'. A population can be a finite number of identifiable individuals, such as all women confined at a given hospital in a given year; more often it is rather more open-ended. In our case it is usually 'all pregnant women and/or their babies'. This is often the target population, about which we wish to learn something, while the population actually sampled may be more like the first-mentioned finite one. (There are of course implicit restrictions of at least time and place in defining a population: for most purposes one would not regard Australia or the United Kingdom in the 1980's and, say, China or the USA in the 19th century as giving rise to a common population of pregnant women).

If we treat (medically, that is) one group of women differently in some way from another, we in effect create 2 subpopulations; we could then be interested in how these subpopulations differ from one another, or in medical terms, whether the treatments affect women differently (on average). To this end it is necessary to select a workable number from each population; this is called a sample. *Statistics can be regarded as the assemblage of methods for making inferences about populations from samples.*

Picking a representative sample is not as easy as it sounds: many sources of bias exist so that the chosen sample does not represent the entire population. This is especially the case if one uses a *'convenience' sample* — i.e. one that one can collect most easily. A *random sample*, picked in an orderly fashion by means of random numbers will usually get over this difficulty.

Incidence and prevalence. These terms are often confused. They are measures of the size of the abnormal sample in relation to the normal sample. *Incidence* refers to the number of patients with a certain condition presenting over a set period of time; *prevalence* refers to the total number of patients with the condition in a defined population.

Main Types of Data

(a) *Quantitative*. (i) Measured on a continuous scale (within the limits of accuracy of the measuring instrument); examples are weight of the baby or placenta. (ii) Counted in discrete units, such as number of stillbirths or neonatal deaths.

(b) *Qualitative*. Described by a quality or attribute rather than by a measurement or count e.g. blood group or sex of baby. Sometimes the categories of the attribute can be ordered with respect to one another, such as degree of pain relief — adequate, barely adequate, inadequate. This is called an ordinal variable.

Ratio is the number in one group compared with that in another, thus the *sex ratio* at birth = number of males/number of females = 105/100 = 1.05. The *proportion* of males in the population is 105/(105 + 100) = 0.51, while the *percentage* of males in the population is 100 times this: 105/(105 + 100) × 100 = 51%.

Rate represents the frequency with which an event is taking place per unit of time. Perinatal death rate = number of perinatal deaths per year/number of babies born per year (live and still) × 1,000.

Arrangement and Summarization of Data

Pie chart. The different groups in a sample are arranged as slices in a pie — the size of the slice representing the relative number in the sample.

Bar chart. Used for either measured or counted data, as long as they can be aggregated into suitable groups. As the size and number of groups become larger, we may join the midpoints of the tops of the bars and obtain a frequency polygon.

Frequency polygon. For very large samples with many groups, the frequency polygon will start to resemble a theoretical 'frequency distribution', representing the relative proportions of values in the population from which the sample was drawn. Much of statistical theory is based on the assumption that the form of the distribution is bell-shaped (and thus symmetrical and unimodal), the so-called 'normal' or Gaussian curve. For example, for the weight of the normal baby, the largest number may cluster around the value 3,400 g for a certain population, but there will be an equal number of very large and very small babies. This allows us to describe the whole group very simply with certain 'population parameters'. However, not all populations have this shape.

Measures of Location or Central Tendency

(i) *Mean*. This is given by the sum of the observations divided by the number of observations made.

(ii) *Mode*. The value (or range of grouped values) which occurs most frequently in a series.

(iii) *Median*. The middle value in a series arranged in order of size.

These 3 values are the same only in unimodal symmetrical populations. For example, if we calculated the mean period of gestation for fetal death, it might be 16 weeks — a value between the first and last trimesters; the mode would be perhaps 9 weeks, since most fetal deaths result from abortion; and finally, the median value would perhaps be 12 weeks.

Percentiles. If a large number of sample values, arranged in increasing order, are divided into 100 equal parts, each part represents 1%. The midpoint of this series occurs at the median which divides it at the 50th percentile; that is, half of the values in a distribution lie below this point and half above. If we refer to figure 23.2B, we see percentile curves — the 10th, 50th, and 90th. The 10th percentile curve indicates that 10% of the values lie below the curve and 90% above; conversely, in the 90th percentile curve, 90% of values lie below the curve and only 10% above. If we wish to define a larger 'normal' group, we may include all the values between the 5th and 95th percentiles, or even those between the 1st and 99th percentiles.

The Variation or Scatter of Data in a Sample

Range. This is the simplest form: the range of fetal weight observed during a 12-month period may be from 950–4,500 g.

Standard deviation. This gives a measure of how closely or otherwise the different values cluster about the mean; i.e. in the case of normal populations whether the bell is narrow or broad. It is very important to determine, for example, whether a small baby born at 36 weeks is outside the range of normal. The standard deviation gives us a good idea of this. If we have normal figures for babies born at 36 weeks we can derive ± 2 standard deviations (SD) (this includes about 95% of the population), or ± 3 SD (99% of the population). Thus, if the weight of the baby is more than 3 SD from the normal mean for that period of gestation, it has only 3 chances in 1,000 of being normal, and 997 chances of being either abnormally large or growth retarded (provided the dates are correct).

Correlation

In obstetrics we are frequently faced with problems of causation. For example, what causes preeclampsia? Although we have no definite answer, we may have a fairly accurate idea of the *association* which other conditions have with it. One measure of association is the *correlation coefficient*, which can be applied to pairs of variables which are jointly distributed normally, or approximately so.

The closeness of the association is given by the correlation coefficient (r), and is measured on a scale of -1 to $+1$. The nearer the coefficient comes to these extreme values the closer will be the correlation (in a negative and positive sense, respectively). The initial step is usually to construct a *scatter diagram*. The more tightly the points cluster about a straight line, the larger (in absolute value) is the correlation coefficient. After a statistical association has been found, there are the possibilities that it may be *causal* (i.e. A causes B), *indirect* (A and B are both caused by C), or *artifactual* (a rare chance event — A and B appear to be related, but a different sample would not support this finding).

Techniques to further define a statistical association include the *strength and consistency of the association*, *temporal relationship*, *dose-response effect* (e.g. the more cigarettes smoked by the mother, the smaller would be the baby's weight), and *biological plausibility* (cigarettes contain nicotine, carbon monoxide, and cyanide which may be expected to affect growth).

The Significance of Results Obtained

When we perform a certain manoeuvre or give a new drug to a patient, we like to know with a reasonable degree of certainty whether this is better than some other manoeuvre or drug, as the case may be.

'Significance' in statistical terms is really a measure of the likelihood that the change is due to chance, rather than the new procedure or drug. It is expressed as a *probability value (p)*. If we state that the administration of folic acid supplements caused a significant reduction ($p < 0.05$) in the incidence of anaemia in late pregnancy, we are saying that the improvement we noted in haemoglobin values would only have occurred by chance at most 1 in 20 times ($1/20 = 5/100 = 0.05$). This is usually accepted as the borderline of statistical security. We would be on much safer ground if our test gave us a 'p' value of < 0.01 (occurring by chance at most only 1 in 100 times).

Clinical Trials

In many hospitals, such trials as those indicated above will be carried out. In most cases, there will need to be 2 closely-matched groups — a *study group*, to whom the new therapy will be administered, and a *control group*, who will not receive the therapy. Because the well known power of suggestion affects not only patients, but also those attending them medically, the *double-blind trial* has come into favour in the case of new drug testing. In essence, this means that neither the patient nor the doctor know who is having the drug under test and who is having a standard or inert preparation (placebo) with which comparisons can later be made. If the outcome of the trial can be expressed in a qualitative form (death versus survival; improvement versus no improvement), the results are usually tested by a statistical procedure known as the *Chi-squared (χ^2) test*, which depends on an analysis of the difference between observed results and results which would be expected if there was no difference between treatment (i.e. if the 'null hypothesis' was true). The greater the difference, the larger will be the value of χ^2 and the more signficant will be the result.

Student t test. This is used when the outcome is a continuous variable, such as drop in blood pressure. Early in this century WS Gosset (under the pseudonym of 'Student') described a technique for assessment of the difference between population means on the basis of means of relatively small samples (e.g. < 30) where the population variance was unknown and had to be estimated from the samples. The t test refines the more general procedure in which the difference between sample means is divided by the standard error of the difference. By means of tables, different values are obtained, according to the sample size, for the modified multiple of the standard error (1.96 being no longer appropriate). Probability values can then be calculated.

Vital Statistics

This is the particular branch of statistics relating to events such as births, deaths, marriages, populations, and sickness. It enables an overall view to be obtained of how a given population is 'behaving' in the broadest sense. Such figures are important for all levels of planning — from governments down to ward units — and to enable comparisons to be made from one centre to another (e.g. in perinatal mortality).

Collection of data. There are 2 main groups — firstly, those which are legally required by governments, such as births and deaths, or those required by medical or nursing boards; and, secondly, those which are gathered by special groups (maternal and/or perinatal mortality committees), hospital staffs, or individuals for the purposes of planning, audit, or research. From the former, the Registrar-General's Department is able to compile a report which is published annually. In many countries, a standard form is in use for the entry of all data relevant to the mother and baby, and this is transferred to a computer for rapid analysis.

Definitions

(a) *Births.* The *crude birth rate* is the number of births (live and stillborn) from the 28th week per 1,000 total population. The *fertility rate* is the same figure related to the number of women aged 15–44 in the population.

(b) *Deaths* (see Chapters 14 and 15). (i) The *maternal death rate* is defined as the number of deaths of women during pregnancy or within one year of delivery or abortion per 100,000 total births. (ii) The *stillbirth rate* is the number of stillborn babies (babies showing no signs of life born after the 28th week of pregnancy) per 1,000 total births. This gives a measure of the wastage of fetal life during pregnancy and labour. (iii) The *neonatal mortality rate* is the number of babies dying in the 28 days after birth per 1,000 total births. (iv) The *perinatal mortality rate* is the number of stillbirths and deaths in the first week after birth per 1,000 total births. It provides a measure of the hazards of pregnancy and labour. The overall picture of pregnancy wastage is given by the number of abortions and perinatal deaths. (v) The *infant mortality rate* is the number of infants dying in the first year of life per 1,000 livebirths.

(c) *A premature baby* is one born before 37 completed weeks' gestation. Formerly, this definition was applied to a baby weighing 2,500 g or less at birth. The different categories will be discussed in more detail in separate sections.

Trends

By studying the figures for births and deaths over a period of time, graphs can be drawn which illustrate trends. The data can also help us to make predictions about future population changes, if we know the fertility rate the number in the 15–44 age group, and the net change in migration.

Trend graphs may be used to portray the overall or individual *congenital malformation rates*, this reflecting the presence of unfavourable environmental influences (drugs, ionizing radiation, air and water pollution with metals, and other chemicals such as the pesticides used in foodstuffs). An attempt can also be made to gauge the social climate by calculating the *illegitimacy rate* (= number of births per 1,000 unmarrieds aged 15–44). Such figures must be taken with a grain of salt, however, since they cannot take into account such factors as falsification, marriage after the pregnancy is discovered, and illegal abortion.

Special Note — International Reporting

At present, the definitions of stillbirth, neonatal death and maternal death used throughout the world lack uniformity. This should be taken into account when comparisons are made of mortality statistics in different countries. Different practices regarding registration of births and deaths also result in omission of a proportion of deaths in mortality statistics published in some countries. In others, deaths occurring in minority racial or socioeconomic subgroups of the population are excluded or reported separately. All this is in addition to the inevitable variation in efficiency of documentation and reporting from one centre to another. For example, careful autopsy of women killed in *motor car accidents* will reveal a number of early first trimester pregnancies. These cases might inadvertently be excluded from mortality statistics, although pregnancy complications (faintness, sleepiness due to drug therapy for nausea and vomiting) may have been responsible for the death.

The most important difficulty concerns the definition of abortion and fetal viability. This involves legal as well as statistical considerations, because legality of an abortion may be dependent upon the duration of pregnancy. In the UK, birth before 28 weeks' gestation (27 completed weeks from the first day of the last menstrual period) is defined as abortion. One objection to this definition is that a proportion of infants born before 28 weeks survive with modern paediatric intensive care, and this is statistically untidy! More importantly, use of the 28 week definition distracts attention from some of the deaths due to *cervical incompetence, premature rupture of the membranes,* and *premature labour*; unfortunately so, since many of these deaths are avoidable, and relaxation of the abortion law in many countries has resulted in an increase in the number of such cases, which therefore warrant full obstetric consideration. The fact that 1 % of women deliver between 20 and 28 weeks, yet such cases are responsible for approximately 33% of all perinatal deaths, supports this viewpoint.

Ultimately, agreement will probably be reached, and all centres will report perinatal results according to *weight* of the infant at birth. Fetuses weighing less than 500 g will be classified as cases of abortion (or 22 weeks' gestation when birth-weight is unknown); mortality and morbidity results will then be reported in the weight ranges 500–1,000 g, 1,001–1,500 g, 1,501–2,000 g, 2,001–2,500 g and 2,501 g and above. The present UK definition of neonatal death (a liveborn infant who dies within 28 days of birth) is unsatisfactory: if strictly observed, many abortuses weighing 200–300 g or even less, who move slightly after birth or have a transient heart beat recorded, would be included. Use of a birth-weight criterion does away with the need to exercise judgement in such cases.

chapter thirteen

Special Investigative Procedures

OVERVIEW

One of the fastest growing areas of health care is investigative medicine. In many cases, the advances have represented spinoffs from industrial and space technology; in others, basic and applied research in the biomedical field has led to the newer methods. Undoubtedly, the greatest leap forward has been in the field of *ultrasonography*. Because of its apparently innocuous effect on the fetus, it has, with few exceptions, replaced radiography in obstetrics. Sensitive ultrasonic scanners now permit an undreamt of resolution in both the maternal and fetal tissues and there are few areas in which some light has not been cast by this technique. Further refinements are inevitable with incorporation of more sophisticated microprocessors and other advances. A notable accuracy is achievable in the *assessment of gestational age of the fetus* in the first half of pregnancy, the weight and growth of the fetus, the presence of fetal structural abnormalities and the placental site and size, to name but a few. The safety of ultrasonography when used repetitively during pregnancy has opened up many avenues of understanding such as the behaviour of the placenta, the attitude and position of the fetus, and the frequency of *fetal breathing* and *movement*. The danger of several invasive procedures (e.g. *amniocentesis, fetoscopy, intrauterine transfusion*) has been much reduced by being performed under ultrasonic control. The introduction of realtime scanning has introduced another dimension to antenatal care.

Radiography retains its role in the provision of accurate pelvimetry (not possible by ultrasonography), largely to assist in formulating the most appropriate route of delivery in the patient with a breech presentation or the one who has had a previous Caesarean section. It is also used for its former indications (presentation uncertain, fetal abnormality suspected, multiple pregnancy suspected, fetal maturity uncertain) in centres where facilities for ultrasonography do not exist.

Radio-isotopes are now seldom, if ever, used.

The well-being of the fetus during pregnancy was formerly assessed largely by clinical and biochemical methods. *Cardiotocography* (the analysis of fetal heart patterns in response to uterine contractions) has now assumed a major role in third trimester fetal assessment as well as in labour. Cardiotocography is used antenatally to assess fetal condition (intrauterine hypoxia causes identifiable patterns of fetal bradycardia and loss of beat to beat variation in heart rate) and thereby assists decisions relating to the *timing of delivery*, i.e. to indicate when it is no longer in the interests of the fetus to attempt to prolong the pregnancy. In labour, use of the cardiotocograph to monitor the fetal heart rate pattern is of value, albeit not always decisive, in determining the *route of delivery*, by indicating when fetal distress demands immediate delivery — by Caesarean section if conditions do not allow spontaneous or safe forceps delivery. *Ultrasonography and cardiotocography are among the greatest advances introduced to obstetric practice in this generation.* Many advocate their routine use in *all* patients rather than only in high risk pregnancies for specific indications.

Inevitably there will be cost-benefit analyses that will determine the extent to which special investigative procedures are employed. Such considerations will become even more acute as technology becomes even more expensive — e.g. nuclear magnetic resonance imaging.

DIAGNOSTIC ULTRASOUND

Ultrasonic study has revolutionized investigative obstetrics, because the fine detail of soft tissues as well as bone outlines can be recorded. Ultrasound uses a pulse echo principle: a short pulse (1 microsecond) of ultrasound with a pulse repetition rate of 100 per second is transmitted and travels through tissues at a constant speed until it encounters a reflecting surface, i.e. an interface between 2 different types of tissue. At such a surface some of the sound beam is reflected back. This reflected echo is received by the scanner which converts the time of travel of the beam to distance and plots the received echo at its correct position on the screen.

In spite of extensive scrutiny provoked by expressed concern about possible harmful effects of diagnostic ultrasound to the fetus, it has been reaffirmed that *follow-up studies of infants and children have not shown developmental abnormalities or changes in chromosomes due to exposure to diagnostic ultrasound* i.e. there is no evidence available to contraindicate ultrasound investigations during pregnancy.

Modes of Display

A-mode. The echoes are displayed as vertical reflections along a baseline with the height of the deflection proportional to the amplitude of the detected echo. Originally A-mode was used in measuring the fetal head, the midline echo being obtained from the falx (figures 13.1 and 13.2).

M-mode (motion display). Timed photographic exposure records moving tissues — for example, in cardiac evaluation the heart valves are identified and excursions and velocities measured (figure 13.3).

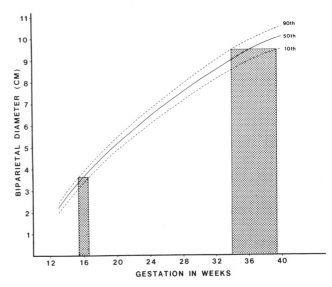

Figure 13.2 The range of the biparietal diameter according to the period of gestation is shown. The normal range is much greater in the third trimester. Estimation of the biparietal diameter early in pregnancy provides a more accurate assessment of gestational age; note that a value of 3.5 cm is in the range of 15–17 weeks, whereas the value of 9.5 cm is in the range 34–39 weeks, although most likely to be 36 weeks (the 50th percentile). Note that the rate of increase of the biparietal diameter lessens in late pregnancy.

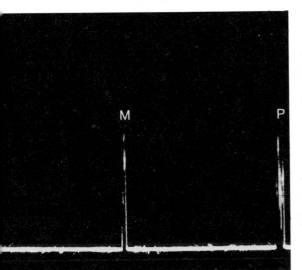

Figure 13.1 A-scan of the fetal head. The echoes from the parietal bones (P) and the midline of the brain (falx cerebri) (M) are seen.

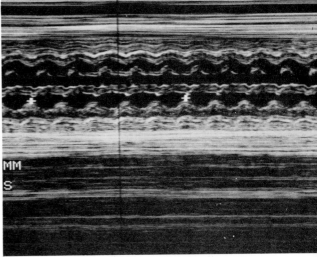

Figure 13.3 M-mode illustrating fetal heart rate. There are 5 beats within the 2 seconds between the markers — i.e. a heart rate of 150/minute.

B-mode (brightness modulation). In this mode the returning echo is demonstrated as a point of illumination with intensity related to the strength of the returning echo. The B-scan makes up a picture by the transducer moving over the skin to make a 2-dimensional image in varying shades of grey (figure 13.4A).

Realtime image. By using either multiple transducers fired in sequence or an oscillating transducer, motion can be detected by using a frame rate of more than 15 per second to show the moving B-scan image. *Dynamic views of anatomy improve the diagnostic quality.* Although resolution of these images initially was not as good as the static B-scan unit, improvements have occurred to make these of good diagnostic quality.

Doppler technique. Echoes returning from moving structures are altered in frequency. This frequency shift is detected and can be used to measure blood flow. This technique uses a continuous wave rather than a pulsed wave of ultrasound and a major application is *fetal cardiotocography*. Pulsed Doppler can separate structures at various depths and a velocity profile within blood vessels can be determined. A combined Doppler-B-scan system can present images of *blood flow pattern*, for example in the umbilical vein. This is likely to be developed as an important means of assessment of fetoplacental function.

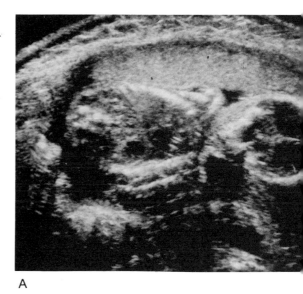

A

Figure 13.4 Assessment of fetal anatomy. **A.** Overall view of uterus at 24 weeks' gestation showing a longitudinal section of the fetus and an anterior placenta. **B.** Transverse section through the fetal head at the level of the lateral ventricles, at 14.5 weeks, showing a normal ratio of cerebral hemisphere (XX) to ventricular width (+ +). **C.** Sections of umbilical vein (V) and nearby arteries at 32 weeks' gestation. The intrahepatic umbilical vein can be cannulated within the fetus under ultrasound control after immobilization of the fetus by curare injection into the thigh. **D.** The 4 chambers of the fetal heart at 28 weeks' gestation. **E.** Penis and scrotum at 36 weeks' gestation. **F.** Wavy double line (W) indicates fetal obesity (thickened subcutaneous tissue) in a diabetic mother at 32 weeks' gestation.

B

C

D

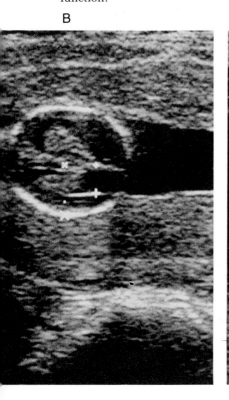

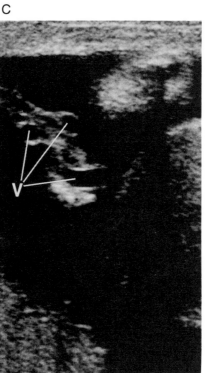

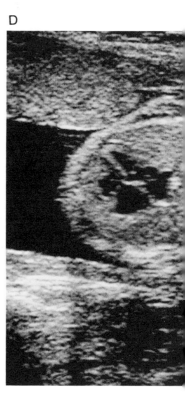

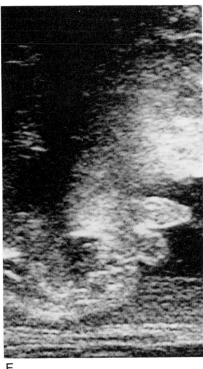

E

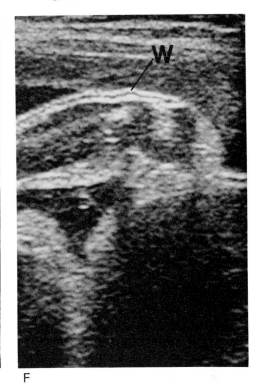

F

Apparatus and Procedure

Typical ultrasound units in operation are shown in figure 13.5. The procedure takes 5–20 minutes, depending on the amount of information required. Unlike most other investigations, the patient should present for examination with a *full bladder*. This provides an acoustic window which permits examination of structures within the pelvis. Oil or acoustic gel is smeared on the skin as a coupling medium, to allow the waves to pass in and out of the skin interface without interruption.

Clinical Applications

Early pregnancy. The *gestation sac* can be visualized from the 5th week of gestation as a 1 cm sac, and as the pregnancy progresses, fetal and placental details are seen. The *fetus* is seen within the gestation sac between 6–7 weeks and *fetal heart movement* can be detected from about 6.5 weeks and is recorded by the M-mode (figure 13.3). This is particularly valuable if there is *abnormal bleeding* or if *fetal death* is suspected (figure 13.6). Ultrasound-guided *chorion biopsy* can be used from 6–13 weeks' gestation to diagnose *genetic disorders* (DNA and karyotype analysis); the preferred gestational age for this procedure is 8–9 weeks, since at this time trophoblastic villi are more equally distributed over the periphery of the chorionic membrane (figure 13.7 and 17.1). Measurement of the gestational sac, the fetal *crown-rump length*, and the *biparietal diameter* after 13 weeks allows an accurate estimation of the period of gestation to be made (figures 13.8 A and B); other measures of *fetal (gestational) maturity* are *abdominal circumference and area*, and length of the *femur* and *humerus* (figures 13.8 C and D). An accurate fix on gestational age carries many benefits — e.g. interpretation of alpha fetoprotein levels in neural tube defect diagnosis, greater precision in the timing of genetic amniocentesis, and, later in pregnancy, in the management of many obstetric problems where the pregnancy may need to be terminated before maturity.

If *low implantation of the placenta* is detected, the chance of later placenta praevia is increased (figure 19.6). The absence of a fetus in the uterus suggests a diagnosis of *ectopic pregnancy*, especially if pain has been experienced (figure 18.10). If the *uterus is larger than expected*, the presence or absence of *twins* can be determined (figures 25.9 and 25.12), or a tumour associated with pregnancy (uterine fibromyoma, ovarian cyst) may be detected (figure 38.7). Rarely, the uterus will present a uniform echogenic appearance characteristic of *hydatidiform mole* (figure 18.12).

Realtime scanning complements antenatal fetal assessment, and is in increasing use because of its improvements in resolution, speed, simplicity, and accuracy in trained hands. The main danger of ultrasonography is that it will be

A

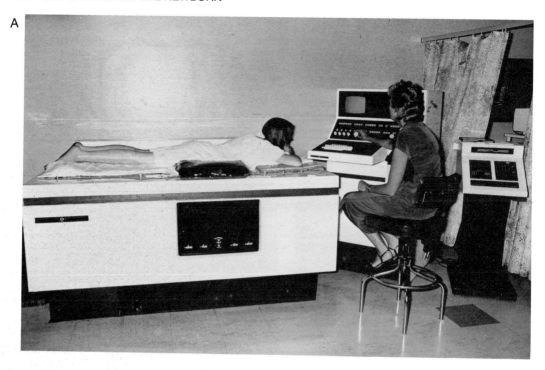

Figure 13.5 A. Octoson, an ultrasound machine designed and manufactured in Sydney, is used to obtain an overall view of uterus, placental site, fetal lie and liquor volume (figure 13.10). The patient lies on a membrane with her abdomen suspended in a water bath, from the bottom of which 8 transducers on a curved arm provide the beam. Note that the operator positions the screen so that the patient can see and 'bond' with her baby — an important byproduct of ultrasonography. Many husbands also attend ultrasound examinations for this reason. The video camera on the right of the picture is for recording the image. **B.** Realtime ultrasound scanner (Aloka Linear Array manufactured in Japan) has high resolution suitable for inspection of fetal anatomy for anomalies, measurement of biparietal diameter, abdominal circumference, and length of femur; it can also provide guidance to the operator during amniocentesis. Oil is painted onto the patient's abdomen and the operator then manipulates the ultrasound transducer. The video display unit can be moved so that the patient can see her baby — here it has been arranged to face the camera. The video camera is to the left of the picture.

B

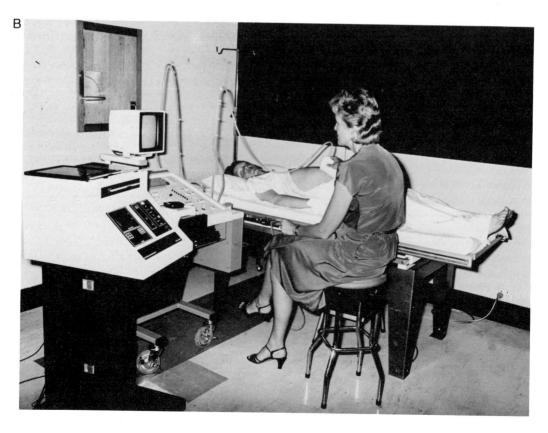

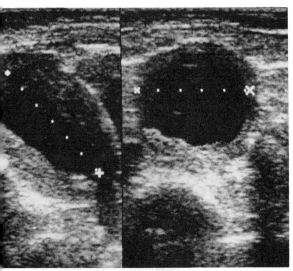

Figure 13.6 Blighted ovum 14 weeks after the last menstrual period. The longitudinal scan (left) and transverse scan (right) demonstrate a gestational sac equivalent in size to a maturity of 13 weeks but containing no fetal parts.

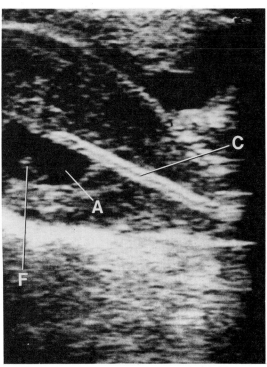

Figure 13.7 Ultrasound-guided chorion biopsy at 8 weeks' gestation. The biopsy catheter is shown with its tip in the chorionic tissue, having been introduced through the cervix. F = fetus; A = amniotic fluid; C = catheter. (Courtesy of Dr John Anderson.)

overused to the detriment of clinical skill acquisition/maintenance and the economics of the health care system.

Later pregnancy. Similar studies to those outlined above will help in the following conditions: (i) estimation of *fetal weight and rate of growth* (ultrasound can diagnose more than 50% of cases of fetal growth retardation); (ii) confirmation of *multiple pregnancy* and other causes of a *large for dates uterus* (figure 25.12); (iii) diagnosis of *fetal abnormalities* (testing indicated by high alpha fetoprotein level, polyhydramnios, low oestriol excretion, abnormal cardiotocograph — figures 13.9, 17.2, 65.4 and 65.8); (iv) diagnosis of *fetal morbidity* (oedema, ascites) or *death* (figures 21.2, 21.3 and 22.4); (v) diagnosis of the different causes of *antepartum haemorrhage* (placenta praevia, placental abruption — figures 13.10, 13.11 and 19.9); (vi) diagnosis of *cervical incompetence* and the state of *Caesarean section scars* (figures 18.4 and 13.11); (vii) estimation of *volume of liquor*; (viii) selection of the correct site for *amniocentesis* (a pocket of liquor away from the placenta, fetus and umbilical cord), and as an adjunct to *fetoscopy* and *intrauterine transfusions*; (ix) investigation of *maternal disease* (gall stones, hydronephrosis) when the cause of abdominal pain is uncertain (figures 37.1 and 38.7).

Doppler ultrasound study. Gated, pulsed, Doppler ultrasound can be used to measure blood flow velocity in deep-lying vessels such as the uterine arteries and umbilical vein. This can give an early warning of *impaired uteroplacental perfusion*. *Fetal echocardiography* has a useful place in assessing the normality of the heart chambers, septa and valves, as well as the great vessels (figure 13.4D).

In labour. If indeterminate clinically, the *lie, presentation and position* can be determined as well as cephalopelvic relationships.

Puerperium. Abnormal involution of the uterus and retained products of conception can be detected and the presence of soft tissue masses and bladder residual urine can be determined. *Intracranial haemorrhage in the newborn* may be identified (figure 64.15) together with subsequent complications such as the development of hydrocephalus (figure 65.18). Ultrasonography can also assist in the diagnosis of *abdominal masses* in the baby (hydronephrosis, adrenal haemorrhage — figure 65.21).

For the reader's perspective the following 12-year audit of ultrasonic and radiographic

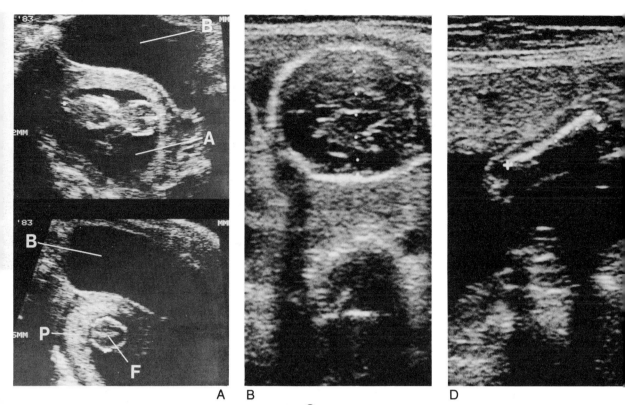

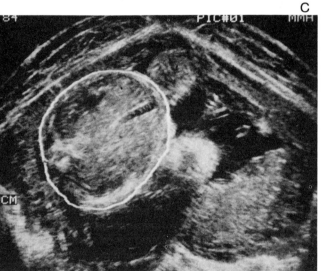

Figure 13.8 Assessment of fetal maturity. **A.** Ultrasound scan through the uterus at 13.5 weeks' gestation showing a fetus with appropriate crown-rump length (7.2 cm) and biparietal diameter (2.5 cm) (A = amniotic fluid, B = mother's distended bladder, P = anterofundal placenta, F = falx cerebri). **B.** Biparietal diameter (5.8 cm) at 23 weeks' gestation. **C.** Abdominal circumference at 32 weeks' gestation — the machine automatically calculates the fetal maturity from the area enclosed by the circle (note umbilical vein at about 2 o'clock). **D.** Length of the femur (4.2 cm) at 23 weeks' gestation. Note surrounding soft tissue of thigh.

investigations in an obstetric hospital is presented. The percentage of obstetric patients examined by *ultrasound is now 60%*. The incidence of *obstetric radiography* has fallen from *14%* of all patients delivered to *0.8%*. In contradistinction, patients having *X-ray pelvimetry* remained constant at *6%*. Table 13.1 shows the *indications for diagnostic ultrasonography* in this large series; two-thirds were scanned before 20 weeks' gestation, 75% of these because of *uncertain dates*.

TABLE 13.1   INDICATIONS FOR DIAGNOSTIC ULTRASONOGRAPHY — 12-YEAR AUDIT

Indications	Number	%
Uncertain dates	10,243	59.5
Threatened abortion	2,927	17.0
Identification of placental site/ antepartum haemorrhage	1,784	10.4
Suspected multiple pregnancy	855	4.9
Intrauterine growth retardation	430	2.5
Fetal death	216	1.2
Miscellaneous	711	4.1
Total	17,168	99.7

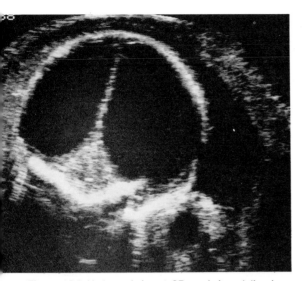

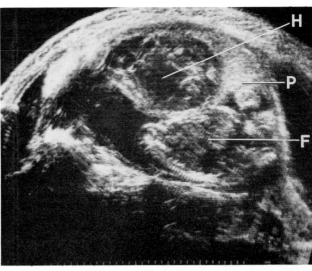

Figure 13.9 Hydrocephalus at 37 weeks' gestation in a 33-year-old para 2 scanned because of a breech presentation. There is huge bilateral enlargement of the lateral ventricles with extreme thinning of the overlying mantle of cerebral tissue; a large meningomyelocele was also demonstrated. Labour was induced by amniotomy. The fetus (birth-weight 3,180 g) died during assisted breech delivery.

Figure 13.10 Ultrasound scan performed at 24 weeks' gestation in a 32-year-old nullipara following the onset of abdominal pain and cessation of fetal movements — the diagnosis of concealed placental abruption was confirmed by demonstration of a large retroplacental haemorrhage (H) (P = placenta; F = fetal trunk). After resuscitation by blood transfusion, labour was induced by amniotomy. The infant was stillborn, birth-weight 540 g; there was a 200 ml old blood clot adherent to the placenta.

In a recent consecutive series of 40,982 patients it was estimated that if a routine ultrasound scan had been performed it would have contributed significantly to the management of the pregnancy in approximately *14.5%*, either by *assessment of gestational age*, or by detection of unsuspected *major fetal malformation, placenta praevia* or *multiple pregnancy*. Accurate knowledge of gestational age allows proper timing of induction of labour and elective Caesarean section. Use of routine ultrasonography to confirm gestational age also allows about an 80% reduction of amniocentesis for determination of fetal pulmonary maturity. The *disadvantages of routine ultrasonography* are *cost*, misdiagnosis of fetal malformations, and detection of an apparent placenta praevia that causes the parents and medical attendants unnecessary worry. Well trained ultrasonographers using appropriate equipment are required to keep false positive diagnoses at a low level to minimize the cost of needless hospitalization, intervention and patient anxiety.

ANTENATAL CARDIOTOCOGRAPHY

Cardiotocographic monitoring of the fetal heart using Doppler ultrasound enables an immediate assessment to be made of fetoplacental well-being in high risk pregnancies (figure 13.12).

When *fetoplacental function is normal*, the fetal heart has *short-term variability* greater than 7 beats per minute, and at least 4 accelerations of more than 15 beats per minute in a 20-minute time interval in response to *Braxton Hicks contractions or fetal movements* (figure 13.13). Unless an acute catastrophe supervenes (e.g. placental abruption), fetal death is highly unlikely within 7 days of such a reactive or satisfactory tracing. *This enables the clinician to defer delivery in high risk pregnancies with safety*, unless clinical indications dictate otherwise, *thereby avoiding unnecessary prematurity*.

As *fetoplacental reserve diminishes*, the fetal heart rate variability diminishes and accelerations occur less frequently (figure 13.14). As this pattern can also be the result of fetal sleep or drug-induced sedation, monitoring for more than 40 minutes is necessary to confirm that it is due to fetoplacental compromise. *If fetal maturity is more than 36 weeks, consideration should be given to delivery.* If obstetric circumstances or prematurity dictate otherwise, close daily monitoring is indicated.

The *most ominous pattern* is the appearance of *decelerations* coupled with absent accelerations and reduced variability (figures 13.15 and 13.16). The fetus with critical reserves has inadequate glycogen and brown fat stores to compensate even briefly for the hypoxaemia that occurs during Braxton Hicks contractions. The resultant acidosis directly, and indirectly through the

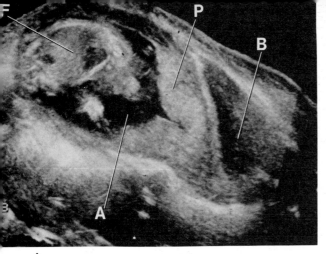

A

Figure 13.11 Placenta praevia percreta. Ultrasonography is indicated to localize the placenta in all patients with a Caesarean section scar so that the diagnosis of placenta praevia percreta can be anticipated, and preparations made for Caesarean hysterectomy. **A.** Longitudinal ultrasound scan showing bladder (B), central placenta praevia (P) covering the internal os and extending onto anterior and posterior uterine walls, amniotic fluid (A), and an oblique section through fetal thorax and abdomen (F); this scan was performed at 23 weeks' gestation because of a 1,200 ml painless antepartum haemorrhage in a 32-year-old para 2 diabetic who had had 2 previous Caesarean sections. **B.** View of anterior lower uterine segment with adherent bladder and placental blood vessels, at 29 weeks' gestation, when repeated haemorrhage and severe lower abdominal pain necessitated delivery. The infant, birth-weight 1,900 g, survived. **C.** Anterior aspect of hysterectomy specimen showing classical Caesarean incision and finger visible through lower segment, adjacent to the morbidly adherent placenta. **D.** Uterus incised posteriorly to show central placenta praevia. In such cases it is wise not to attempt to remove the placenta separately but to proceed with hysterectomy. The patient required a 3,500 ml blood transfusion and repair to her bladder which was opened to facilitate its dissection from the vagina; thereafter her recovery was uneventful.

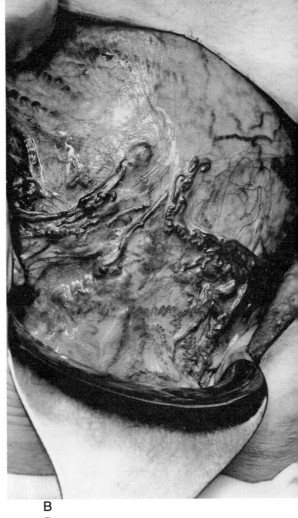

B

D

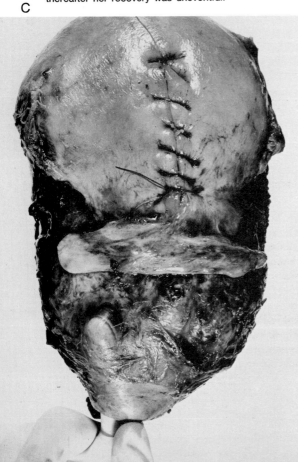

C

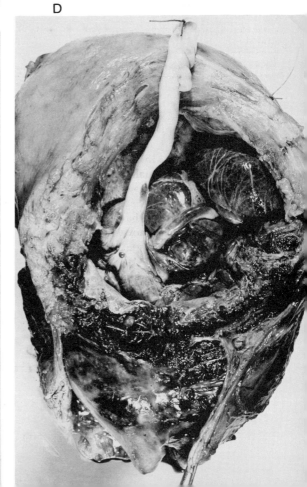

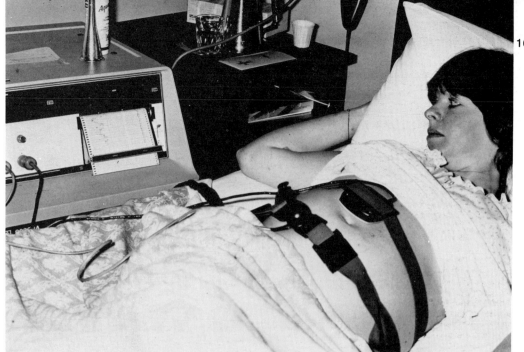

Figure 13.12 Antenatal cardiotocography at 36 weeks' gestation in a patient with clinical evidence of fetal growth retardation and low oestriol values. The tocograph above the umbilicus registers uterine contractions and fetal movements. The narrow beam Doppler transducer registers the fetal heart rate shown on the recording. The patient is in the semilateral position to avoid the possibility of supine hypotension.

TABLE 13.2   OUTCOME OF 6,438 HIGH RISK PREGNANCIES MONITORED ANTENATALLY BY CARDIOTOCOGRAPHY

Fetal reserve	Number	%	Small for dates (%)	Apgar < 6 1 min. (%)	Perinatal mortality rate (%)	Caesarean section rate (%)
Satisfactory	5,425	(84.3)	8.8	13.9	1.1	20.6
Reduced	894	(13.9)	13.8	17.3	2.8	27.7
Critical	119	(1.9)	39.5	45.4	21.8	72.3
Total	6,438		10.1	14.9	1.7	22.6

vasomotor centres, depresses myocardial activity, resulting in these late or 'type 2' decelerations. If the tracing indicates *imminent fetal demise* (e.g. figures 13.15 –13.18), delivery should be expedited, usually by Caesarean section. Despite this most unfavourable start to life, the great majority of these infants are not doomed to permanent handicap; long-term follow-up studies have shown that their *prognosis is most satisfactory* (figures 13.17 and 13.18).

The outcome of 6,438 high risk pregnancies monitored antenatally is shown in table 13.2. Noteworthy is the increasing incidences of *growth retardation, low Apgar scores, perinatal mortality* and Caesarean section as the fetal reserve diminishes. *The cardiotocograph has become the pivot upon which modern obstetric management is based in high risk pregnancies, where the timing of delivery is so important.*

RADIOGRAPHY

Formerly, textbooks of obstetrics had large chapters devoted to radiology. The realization that this investigation may occasionally be hazardous to the fetus or to the germ cells in the mother's ovaries, together with appreciation of the potential of ultrasonic echography, has tended to limit its use, and this trend will probably continue.

Since ultrasonic units are not universally available, reliance will still be placed on traditional radiographic techniques in some centres; many of the remarks regarding clinical indications are made with this consideration in mind. The International Commission on Radiographic Protection has recommended that radiation should be avoided in the first 3 months of pregnancy. The danger of radiographic studies involving multiple exposure/fluoroscopy (intravenous pyelography, barium enema) in the

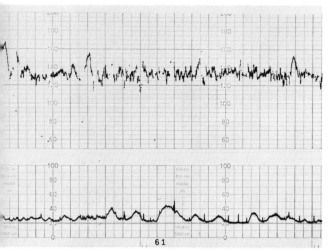

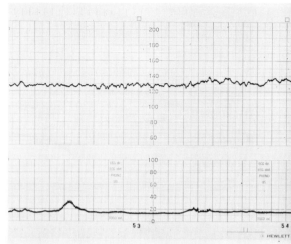

Figure 13.13 Reactive cardiotocographic tracing indicative of satisfactory fetal reserve. Note beat to beat variability of more than 7/minute and heart rate accelerations of more than 15/minute — these may occur spontaneously or in response to Braxton Hicks contractions and fetal movements (lower line).

Figure 13.14 Example of severe reduction in beat to beat variability and absence of fetal heart rate accelerations. However, there is no deceleration in response to the Braxton Hicks contraction.

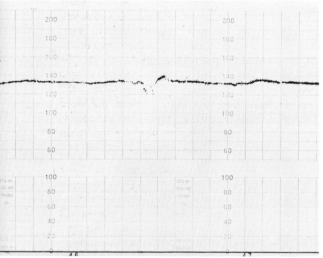

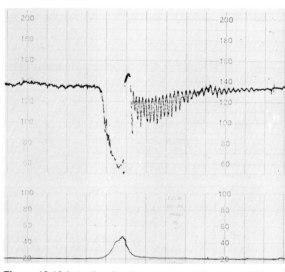

Figure 13.15 Extreme loss of beat to beat variation in association with deceleration at 31 weeks' gestation. The patient had hypertension, gestational diabetes and clinical fetal growth retardation. Caesarean section resulted in a 1,430 g infant who at 2 years of age had a cognitive score of 135 and motor development score of 96 (from Beischer NA et al Am J Obstet Gynecol 1983; 146:662–670).

Figure 13.16 Late deceleration merging with a sinusoidal pattern, then returning to severe loss of beat to beat variation at 29 weeks' gestation. Intrauterine death had occurred in the patient's 2 previous pregnancies, each at 28 weeks' gestation. Caesarean section was performed. The infant weighed 985 g at birth. Assessment at 2 years of age revealed cognitive and motor scores of 99 and 145, respectively (from Beischer NA et al Am J Obstet Gynecol 1983; 146:662–670).

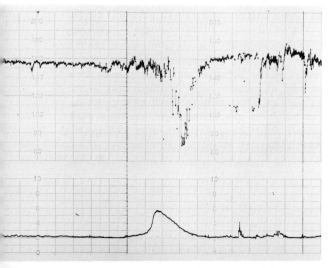

Figure 13.17 Loss of beat to beat variation followed by a late deceleration at 34 weeks' gestation. The patient was a severe diabetic with hypertension and chronic renal disease; her 3 previous pregnancies had resulted in intrauterine deaths. At Caesarean section a meconium-stained, acidotic (pH 7.12), growth retarded infant (birth-weight 1,550 g) was delivered. On assessment at 6 years of age his cognitive and motor scores were 119 and 100, respectively (from Beischer NA et al Am J Obstet Gynecol 1983; 146:662–670).

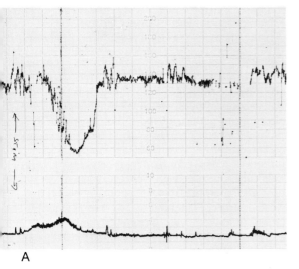

A

Figure 13.18 A. Major, late (type 2) deceleration at 37 weeks' gestation in a primigravida with clinical evidence of extreme fetal growth retardation and low oestriol values. At Caesarean section there was no amniotic fluid; although growth retarded (birth-weight 1,435 g), the infant was born in good condition. **B.** At 5 years of age the child's cognitive and motor scores are 130 and 119, respectively — within the superior range of intelligence! (from Beischer NA et al Am J Obstet Gynecol 1983; 146:662–670).

B

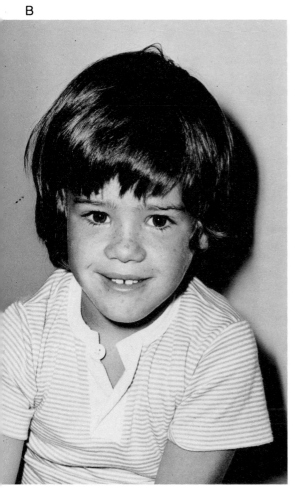

second half of the menstrual cycle, when pregnancy may have commenced, should be stressed (hysterosalpinography should be performed between day 9–13 of the cycle — i.e. prior to ovulation).

It has been calculated that 1 rad (10 mGy) carries a 1 in 1,000 chance of childhood malignancy; 2 rads has a negligible risk of fetal abnormality and *10 rads a serious risk of fetal abnormality*. If the mother has received between 2–10 rads (20–100 mGy), the fetal dose (risk) should be estimated with a view to termination, following discussion in relation to other factors such as age, parity, and desire of the patient to have the child. For perspective, a maternal chest radiograph has an absorbed fetal dose of 0.1 rad and a barium meal an absorbed fetal dose of 0.3 rad.

Clinical Indications

Early pregnancy. There are no indications as far as the uterus or fetus are concerned. Routine chest X-rays have been discontinued in many centres because pick-up rates of active *tuberculosis* have fallen markedly. X-rays may be indicated for other *maternal* reasons e.g. *cardiac disease* or *deep vein thrombosis*, in which case the abdomen can be screened. A limited *intravenous pyelogram* may be needed to demonstrate the site of obstruction to a kidney which will need surgical management, although ultrasound is used initially in investigation of abdominal pain and will identify *hydronephrosis* (figure 37.1).

Later pregnancy. (i) *Hydatidiform mole.* If the pregnancy has progressed beyond the 14th week (when the fetal skeleton normally becomes visible on X-ray), absence of fetal bony outlines will be of confirmatory value in the diagnosis. (ii) *Uterus larger than dates; suspicion of multiple pregnancy.* Since diagnosis of multiple pregnancy is important before 30 weeks to allow for rest in hospital, the diagnosis should be confirmed. If *polyhydramnios* is present, there may well be a major fetal malformation visible on X-ray — anencephaly, hydrocephaly, spina bifida. (iii) *Breech presentation.* Although the need for external cephalic version is debated, particularly under general anaesthesia, the diagnosis of this condition is important in order to plan future management. (iv) *Rhesus isoimmunization.* The procedure of intrauterine transfusion is now usually guided by ultrasonography. (v) *Fetal maturity.* Radiography for this indication is not particularly accurate (fetal growth retardation may delay the appearance of ossification centres) and better methods are now available to assess physiological maturity (phospholipids in liquor). (vi) *Fetal death.* This can now be determined quite accurately with the relatively inexpensive Doppler instrument, together with the characteristic fall in oestriol values. (vii) *Fetal position.* There is still a place for radiography in determining the fetal presentation or position. It is of particular importance in such conditions as transverse or oblique lie, and face or brow presentation. (viii) *Pelvimetry.* Radiography provides an accurate measurement of the pelvic diameters, and also a good idea of the cephalopelvic relationship (erect lateral film). The following are the major indications: (a) *Pelvic contraction* suspected on the grounds of past obstetric history (long labours, difficult deliveries), past surgical or medical history (motor vehicle or other accidents involving damage to the pelvis, poliomyelitis), or current obstetric study (small stature — less than 152 cm, clinical assessment of the pelvis, mobile head at term in a nullipara), or failure of satisfactory progress in labour. (b) *Breech presentation* or *previous Caesarean section*, where vaginal delivery is proposed and evidence of a satisfactory pelvic size has not been revealed by the previous vaginal delivery of a normal-sized baby. *Technique.* For the best results, the procedure should be carried out in the radiology department. The following standard views are usually taken: erect lateral, anteroposterior (tube shift method), and outlet. In this way, all the important diameters can be measured, and the position of the fetus can be determined, as well as its relationship to the maternal pelvis. (It should be stressed that pelvimetric study is only one element in a multifactorial problem.) *CT-scan pelvimetry,* if available, can be used to measure pelvic diameters (AP and transverse diameters of the pelvic brim, bispinous and AP of the midpelvis), and delivers only about 5% of the radiation of conventional X-ray. (ix) *Placental localization.* This should now be performed only by ultrasound — i.e. radioisotopes are no longer used. (x) *Fetal abnormality.* Major skeletal deformities are usually diagnosed, except when a single film does not show the fetus in the correct plane — e.g. an anteroposterior view of the fetal spine is needed to show a spina bifida.

NUCLEAR MAGNETIC RESONANCE (NMR) SPECTROSCOPY

This technique, discovered in 1945, is undergoing progressive development and has major potential in both morphological and functional studies.

Physiological Basis and Clinical Application

Imaging. Nonionizing radiation is beamed through a magnetic field to produce detailed cross-sectional images based on the distribution and motion of hydrogen nuclei in the body. By altering the pattern of the radiofrequency (RF) pulses, the contrast between different tissues can be enhanced. X-ray computer tomography (CT) images are dependent on a single image variable, whereas those with NMR are dependent on proton density flow effects; bone is penetrated without marked attenuation. By signal manipulation (e.g. removal of signal from fluids in motion) blood vessels will be made to appear dark; blood flow can be assessed noninvasively. This has major potential in studies of the placenta, since areas of infarction and low perfusion can be identified.

Spectroscopy. This enables components of the body to be studied at the molecular level.

One of the most interesting applications of NMR spectroscopy is estimation of fetal cerebral energy metabolism and the detection of fetal hypoxia which may have important prognostic significance. This can be calculated from the chemical shift of inorganic phosphate with reference to phosphocreatine. Another promising noninasive technique is that used to assess certain serious inborn errors of metabolism in the fetus — e.g. the use of ^{13}C in glycogen storage diseases and galactosaemia.

MISCELLANEOUS

There are a number of other instruments which are in use, and these are discussed in relation to their specific use in the appropriate chapters — e.g. Doppler fetal heart detector and the different monitoring machines for the sick or premature baby.

Invasive procedures (amniocentesis, fetoscopy) are also discussed in other chapters.

chapter fourteen

Maternal Mortality

OVERVIEW

A *maternal death* is one occurring during pregnancy, childbirth, or in the year following delivery or abortion, irrespective of the duration and the site of the pregnancy, from any cause related to or aggravated by the pregnancy or its management.

Deaths so defined are subdivided into (i) *direct maternal deaths* due to a complication of pregnancy (e.g. *eclampsia*), and (ii) *indirect maternal deaths* due to complications not specific to pregnancy but aggravated by the physiological changes of pregnancy (e.g. cardiac or renal disease). Since comparisons of national statistics are often made in the press, it should be noted that in some countries, *associated* deaths due to accidental or incidental causes (accidents, suicide, neoplasms) are also included, as are deaths occurring more than 42 days after delivery when they have their origin in illnesses related to the pregnancy.

In the past 15 years, maternal mortality rates (number of maternal deaths per 100,000 total births) have fallen more than 50% and in developed countries now range from 10–40 per 100,000 births. This reduction has been achieved almost exclusively by the reduction in direct or true maternal deaths, whereas the death rates due to associated causes remain unchanged and now account for approximately 50% of all maternal deaths. Further improvement in maternal mortality statistics will require attention to prevention of deaths from such causes as motor vehicle accidents and suicide.

Pulmonary thromboembolism, pregnancy-induced hypertension/eclampsia, haemorrhage, anaesthesia, ectopic pregnancy and *abortion* remain the leading causes of maternal death; 20% of deaths are associated with *Caesarean section. Amniotic fluid embolism* remains an uncommon but persistent problem. These causes are basically similar in most countries of the world, but the emphasis differs significantly, according to the level of health care and other local factors.

Today, successful childbirth is no longer measured in terms of maternal and perinatal mortality. Childbirth is now expected to be a joyful experience for the mother and her partner. With reduction in mortality and morbidity, many members of the public have less respect for the safety of confinement in hospital. These trends may make it difficult to maintain mortality rates at present levels. Many patients with a severe medical disease, itself a potential threat to life, now expect to reproduce with minimal inconvenience or time spent in hospital.

It should be remembered that *advanced maternal age and parity signify a 20-fold increase in the risk of maternal death*. As a corollary of this, it will be appreciated that sociodemographic changes play a significant part in the reduction of maternal mortality — i.e. the shift of childbearing into a more favourable age group (20–34 years) and an overall reduction in parity. Many countries have ethnic minorities with mortality rates 5–10 times higher than that of the overall national figure (Australia, Canada, New Zealand, United States of America).

DEFINITIONS AND GENERAL REMARKS

A *maternal death* as defined by the World Health Organization is the death of a woman during pregnancy, childbirth or in the 42 days of the puerperium, irrespective of the duration and the site of the pregnancy, from any cause related to or aggravated by the pregnancy or its management. This definition includes deaths from abortion and ectopic pregnancy but excludes deaths from accidental or incidental causes (*associated deaths*). In the reports on maternal deaths in England and Wales, all deaths occurring during pregnancy or within one year of delivery are recorded (including accidental or incidental causes of deaths, which are classified as associated deaths).

Maternal deaths are usually subdivided into 2 groups: (i) *direct maternal deaths* due to a complication of the pregnancy itself (eclampsia,

TABLE 14.1　MAIN CAUSES OF TRUE MATERNAL DEATH* IN ENGLAND AND WALES

Cause of death	Numbers of deaths (rates per million maternities in parentheses)				
	1964–1966	1967–1969	1970–1972	1973–1975	1976–1978
Abortion	133 (51.1)	117 (47.6)	81 (35.2)	29 (15.1)	19 (10.9)
Pulmonary thromboembolism	91 (35.0)	75 (30.5)	61 (26.5)	35 (18.2)	45 (25.7)
Haemorrhage	68 (26.2)	41 (16.7)	27 (11.7)	21 (10.9)	26 (14.9)
Hypertensive diseases of pregnancy	67 (25.8)	53 (21.6)	47 (20.5)	39 (20.3)	29 (16.6)
Ectopic pregnancy	42 (16.2)	32 (13.0)	34 (14.8)	20 (10.4)	22 (12.6)
Sepsis (excluding abortion with sepsis)	57 (21.9)	26 (10.6)	32 (13.9)	22 (11.4)	17 (9.7)
Amniotic fluid embolism	30 (11.5)	27 (11.0)	22 (9.6)	14 (7.3)	11 (6.3)
Ruptured uterus	30 (11.5)	18 (7.3)	12 (5.2)	11 (5.7)	14 (8.0)
Miscellaneous causes	61 (23.5)	66 (26.9)	39 (17.0)	44 (22.9)	20 (11.4)
Deaths associated with anaesthesia (excluding operations for abortion and ectopic pregnancy)					24 (13.7)
Total	579 (227.5)	455 (185.2)	355 (154.5)	235 (122.3)	227 (129.8)

* Due directly to pregnancy or childbirth

rupture of the uterus, postpartum haemorrhage). (ii) *indirect maternal deaths* due to a complication not specific to pregnancy but aggravated by the physiological changes of pregnancy (e.g. heart disease, diabetes, renal disease).

Maternal mortality rates are expressed as the number of direct plus indirect maternal deaths per 100,000 total births. The rate is now approximately 10–40 in developed countries, but shows quite a wide range, according to the particular country's socioeconomic development, the doctor : patient ratio, and so on. In former years, when maternal deaths were more common, mortality rates were expressed as the number per 1,000 or even 100 births (maternal mortality rates in many parts of the world are still of the order of 1–2 per 100 births). Perinatal deaths being more common than maternal deaths are still expressed as the number per 1,000 births (live and still). Many countries have minority groups with relatively high maternal mortality rates. For example, in England and Wales during the 1975–1978 triennium, the maternal mortality rate was 3 times higher in women born outside the United Kingdom with origins in the New Commonwealth and Pakistan compared with those born within the United Kingdom.

Direct maternal deaths constitute approximately 2% of all female deaths in the age group 15–44 years.

In England and Wales in the triennium 1976–1978, the maternal death rate was 10.8 per 100,000 total births, there being 428 notified deaths and 1,766,169 confinements (table 14.1). Although the death rate has fallen significantly,

review of the case histories revealed that a primary avoidable factor was present in almost 60% of the direct maternal deaths.

Maternal *age* and *parity* retain an important association with risk of death. The maternal mortality rate in women over 40 in their fourth or later pregnancy is more than 20 times as great as in women aged 25–29 in their second pregnancy. Although mortality rates have steadily fallen over the triennia 1964–1966 to 1975–1978 (table 14.1) in young mothers, there has been no decrease in the mortality rates for the high risk group of older mothers of high parity — approximately 1 in every 1,000 pregnancies in grand multiparas results in a maternal death.

It should be noted that international differences in mortality rates are related not only to differences in the quality of maternal care, but also to differences in the proportion of pregnancies in each country occurring in high risk women.

It is of interest, for perspective, to note that the overall risk of death due to or associated with pregnancy is less than the risk of death for women generally in the population. Although indirect and associated maternal deaths together comprise more than 50% of all maternal deaths, the numbers of deaths due to neoplasms, suicides and accidents (table 14.2) are much lower in the maternity group than would be expected from the mortality experience of the general population.

It is noteworthy that the reduction in maternal mortality rates has been achieved almost entirely by a reduction in the number of direct maternal deaths (table 14.1).

TABLE 14.2 ASSOCIATED CAUSES OF MATERNAL DEATH IN ENGLAND AND WALES

Cause of death	Numbers of deaths (rates per million maternities in parentheses)		
	1970–1972	1973–1975	1976–1978
Blood disorders	21 (9.1)	15 (7.8)	10 (5.7)
Diabetes mellitus	6 (2.6)	5 (2.6)	3 (1.7)
Intracranial haemorrhage	24 (10.4)	9 (5.1)	24 (13.7)
Neoplastic disease	27 (11.7)	21 (10.9)	33 (18.4)
Suicide	17 (2.4)	14 (7.3)	18 (10.7)
Accidental death	—	4 (2.1)	6 (3.4)
Road traffic accident	4 (1.7)	4 (2.1)	6 (3.4)
Others	152 (66.1)	83 (43.0)	100 (57.2)
Total	251 (109.2)	155 (80.7)	200 (114.4)

Aetiology. The major causes of maternal death should be known thoroughly, since preventive action is so important. It should be remembered also that it is often a train of events that leads to the fatal outcome, each complication leading to another. For example, surgical induction may be required in the management of a patient with preeclampsia; if asepsis and antisepsis are faulty, serious infection may arise in the period before delivery. Also, if control of the preeclampsia is not adequate, the rise in blood pressure may result in cerebral haemorrhage or failure of one of the vital organs (heart, kidneys, liver).

Whether or not the death was preventable is usually assessed by a panel of experts (Confidential Enquiry into Maternal Deaths) set up in most regions. The geographical location and facilities available to the medical and nursing personnel are taken into account. The fault may be assigned to the midwife, attending doctor, specialist, hospital, patient, or any combination of these. (i) *Professional factors* including shortcomings in diagnosis, judgment, management (including technique), and include failure to assess adequately risk factors or complications. Also included are failure to use currently acceptable methods, and to consult when necessary. Treatment may be inadequate, inappropriate, or badly timed (too soon or too late). (ii) *Hospital factors* are related to inadequacies in facilities, equipment, or personnel (e.g. laboratory, radiographic, anaesthesia, blood bank services). (iii) Patient factors are usually concerned with failure to attend for initial or subsequent antenatal care, disregard of evident symptoms or advice, and the patient wishing not to be confined in hospital.

In England and Wales, the causes of maternal deaths in the 5 triennia 1964–1966 to 1975–1978 are shown in table 14.1. It is seen that pulmonary thromboembolism, hypertensive diseases of pregnancy and haemorrhage, were the main causes of maternal deaths. As death rates have fallen, the 'top 10' causes have retained their place on the table but their positions have fluctuated. The main change over the 15 years has been the reduction in the number of deaths from complications of abortion. Liberalization of abortion laws has been associated with the fall in the number of deaths from septic abortion. However, maternal mortality rates could rise unless intense clinical vigilance is maintained. There are many 'near misses' for every death and many patients survive because of resuscitative efforts of heroic proportions.

The safety of childbirth in a well equipped hospital has resulted in some disregard by the general public, and even members of the medical and nursing professions, of the possibility of death. Patients with severe medical diseases, themselves a threat to life (congenital heart disease, unstable diabetes mellitus), now expect to reproduce with minimal inconvenience or time spent in hospital.

DIRECT OR TRUE MATERNAL DEATHS

Haemorrhage

The majority of deaths in this group result from *postpartum haemorrhage* (90–95% primary, 5–10% secondary). The amount of blood lost at delivery has been reduced dramatically by the prophylactic use of oxytocic drugs such as ergometrine and syntometrine. Major haemorrhage is usually caused by trauma to the upper birth canal or retained placenta (perhaps accreta — figure 14.1). Complicating factors that frequently tip the balance are preexisting anaemia, prolonged or difficult labour, dehydration, difficult delivery, and inadequate replacement of postpartum blood loss. The tendency to underestimate blood loss by almost 100% should be remembered. Uterine rupture represents a special type of trauma; with this complication, there is usually a breakdown in the standard of care — particularly the misuse of oxytocic drugs, failure to recognize obstructed labour promptly, and performance of dangerous manoeuvres (internal version).

The heroic measures ultimately employed in vain in many patients would have been unnecessary if appropriate, simple routine methods had been applied at the proper time.

Defective blood coagulation, usually the result of a lack of fibrinogen and other clotting factors due to disseminated intravascular coagulation, classically follows severe abruptio placentae, prolonged fetal death in utero, and amniotic fluid embolism; it is also seen with major sepsis and trauma and in severe preeclampsia, especially if induction of labour is delayed.

The combined deaths from the 2 main causes of antepartum haemorrhage (*placenta praevia* and *abruptio placentae*) are approximately half those from postpartum haemorrhage. Maintenance of adequate antenatal haemoglobin levels and rapid intravenous transfusion to replace the blood loss are the principles of management in both conditions, coupled with early delivery by the most appropriate route. Underestimation of the amount of blood lost is again common, particularly in abruptio, where much of the loss may be concealed.

Ectopic pregnancy is always a potential source of disaster — usually because of misdiagnosis or because operation is undertaken before adequate resuscitation has been achieved. In some cases, the patient has not called for medical assistance until it is too late. It is noteworthy that in recent years ectopic pregnancy has claimed more lives than placenta praevia, abruptio placentae, or postpartum haemorrhage.

Abortion. The majority of deaths from this condition are caused by sepsis, but major haemorrhage may occur, particularly if the pregnancy has progressed beyond 12 weeks. It is important that bleeding is controlled by the administration of ergometrine and the removal (manually or with sponge forceps) of placental tissue caught in the dilated cervix. Adequate blood must be transfused and available before curettage is undertaken.

Hypertensive Diseases of Pregnancy

Under this heading are included preeclampsia and eclampsia and other conditions of a similar but less specific nature, including liver necrosis.

The number of deaths from preeclampsia/ eclampsia provides a yardstick to the standard of obstetric care in the region, since deaths from this cause are almost entirely preventable if ordinary standards of care prevail. As indicated earlier, the disturbed physiology or therapeutic measures required (e.g. surgical induction of labour, Caesarean section), may involve additional complications (sepsis, haemorrhage, anaesthesia, thromboembolism) which are responsible for the death.

The first signs of preeclampsia may appear in the second trimester. If these are not observed or acted upon, the disease may be well advanced at the time of the patient's next visit. The importance of cerebral haemorrhage as a cause of death emphasizes the need for hypotensive drug therapy if the condition has progressed. Because ergometrine may cause a further sharp rise in blood pressure in addition to that of the labour itself, oxytocin is the preferred oxytocic drug for patients with preeclampsia/eclampsia. Failure to induce labour early enough in this type of patient is another error. The patient may not present early enough for antenatal care, and may not

Figure 14.1 Caesarean hysterectomy for placenta praevia-accreta. Placental tissue protrudes from the unsutured lower segment incision through which the fetus was extracted.

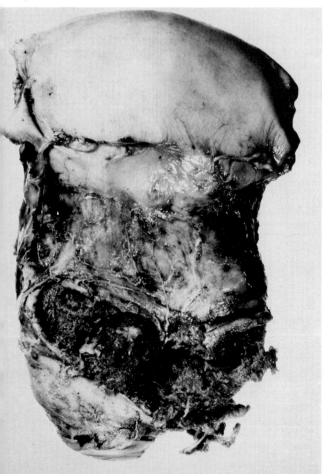

accept advice on the need for hospitalization in the early phases of the disease, or on the need for more frequent antenatal visits.

Embolism

Pulmonary thromboembolism has retained its relative importance as the main cause of maternal death, claiming the lives of 1 in 9 mothers who die as a result of pregnancy and childbirth (figure 14.2) (table 14.1). As the number of deaths from this complication has fallen, the proportion occurring during pregnancy is now about 50% of those occurring following delivery.

The patient at special risk is the elderly, obese multipara, particularly if delivered by Caesarean section.

In the majority of cases, the death is sudden and unexpected. This emphasizes the importance of prevention — reduction of predisposing factors (anaemia, infection, and trauma), wider use of physiotherapy (exercises, deep breathing, early ambulation), and specific prophylactic measures when indicated (intermittent compression of leg veins during surgery by electrical calf stimulation, anticoagulant drugs).

The use of oestrogens to suppress lactation is recognized as a possible cause of venous thrombosis, and other measures should therefore be adopted.

A special type of embolism is that from *amniotic fluid*. Collapse occurs for no apparent reason, and always when the patient is in labour or just delivered. The membranes are always ruptured, and the amniotic fluid enters the uterine veins through a tear (which can be small and difficult to find at autopsy) in the lower uterine segment. Precipitating factors are overactivity of the uterus, multiparity, and misuse of oxytocic drugs. If the patient survives, an incoagulable state of the blood follows, due to the thromboplastic activity of the liquor which has entered the mother's circulation. The administration of heparin, blood, fibrinogen, and drugs to relax the pulmonary vessels and airways (aminophylline, salbutamol) will save some of these patients.

Infection

The important association of infection and abortion has been mentioned already (see table 14.3). Another major group consists of patients with *puerperal infection*. The latter often follows *premature rupture of the membranes* and/or *prolonged labour*. Other risk factors are *cervical cerclage* and when 3 or more *vaginal examinations* have been performed in labour. In each case, organisms gain entrance to the amniotic cavity (amnionitis), after which infection of the fetus and mother is likely. Prophylactic measures include vaginal swabs for bacteriological investigation, together with antibiotics. If delivery has been by Caesarean section, the risk of infection spreading to the cellular tissues and peritoneum is increased, and so routine antibiotic therapy during Caesarean section has many advocates.

The other classical puerperal infections (*pyelonephritis* and *mastitis*) may occasionally be virulent enough to threaten the mother's life. It should be stressed that infection is far more likely to be serious if there is an upset to the mother's

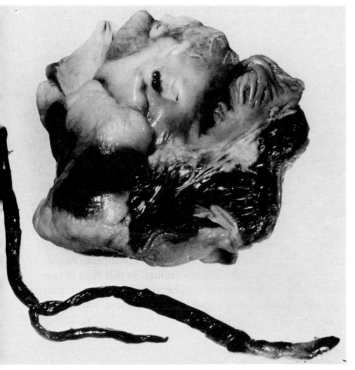

Figure 14.2 This thrombus, dislodged from the inferior vena cava and iliac veins, impacted at the bifurcation of the pulmonary trunk and caused sudden death in the puerperium.

TABLE 14.3 CAUSES OF MATERNAL DEATH IN PATIENTS WITH INFECTION IN ENGLAND AND WALES

Cause of death	Numbers of deaths		
	1970–1972	1973–1975	1976–1978
Septic abortion	38 (23)	6 (5)	7 (3)
Pulmonary infection	—	6	12
Puerperal sepsis (vaginal delivery)	15	11	8
Sepsis following Caesarean section	16	8	8
Cerebral abscess/meningitis	—	2	1
Septicaemia	—	1	2
Sepsis associated with ectopic pregnancies	—	1	1
Sepsis associated with sterilization	1	2	—
Renal tract infection	8	2	2
Total	78	39	41

Figures in parentheses indicate those abortions performed on a criminal basis.

TABLE 14.4 CAUSES OF MATERNAL DEATH IN PATIENTS HAVING CAESAREAN SECTION IN ENGLAND AND WALES

Cause of death	Numbers of deaths		
	1970–1972	1973–1975	1976–1978
Haemorrhage	8	8	10
Pulmonary thromboembolism	17	6	9
Anaesthesia	19	17	20
Sepsis	16	8	8
Hypertensive diseases of pregnancy	15	12	12
Other true causes	9	10	6
Associated diseases	27	20	25
Total	111	81	90

physiology (poor nutrition, anaemia, trauma, dehydration). It is recognized that certain types of patient are at greater risk from these complications (low socioeconomic status).

The provision of a 24-hour bacteriological service is important for maternity hospitals because of the virulent nature of some of the infections, particularly those complicating abortion and childbirth.

Caesarean Section

A considerable number of maternal deaths are associated with Caesarean section, but in many the operation has been carried out as a 'rescue' procedure, and the death is attributable more to the underlying disorder (table 14.4). In others, complications may result from the anaesthetic (inhalation of gastric contents, cardiac arrest) or the operation (haemorrhage, sepsis, pulmonary thromboembolism). Thus, Caesarean section is never undertaken without a definite indication, and patients who regard it as a less troublesome

and preferred method should be advised of its increased maternal hazards (the mortality rate is increased to about 8 per 10,000 in such operations).

Of the causes of death associated with Caesarean section, anaesthesia is the most common (table 10.4). In the 1976–1978 triannual report on confidential enquiries into maternal death in England and Wales, 38 of the 40 deaths associated with anaesthesia had avoidable factors. Most were attributable to combinations of lack of knowledge, inexperience, low general standards of care in labour and poor administrative practice. The report recommends reviewing anaesthetic services in maternity units with the aim of providing better trained anaesthetists and ensuring that administrative arrangements are inherently safe for patients.

Anaesthesia

The important causes of death from anaesthesia are cardiac arrest, inhalation of gastric contents, pulmonary oedema/infection, and failure to resuscitate adequately. A number of complex interrelationships may exist between the previous state of the patient (anaemia, sepsis, dehydration) and the blood loss during the operation on the one hand, and problems with the anaesthetic agent(s) and/or technique on the other. In other words, there may be good or bad conditions pertaining on the part of the patient, the obstetric team, and the anaesthetic team, and it is sometimes difficult to sort out where the blame should be placed if the death is considered preventable.

Cardiac arrest may be due to one or a combination of drug overdose, inadequate oxygen in the gas mixture, or operative bleeding/shock.

Inhalation of gastric contents is more common in obstetrics because of the emergency nature of many of the anaesthetics and the slowing effect of pregnancy or labour on gastric emptying. It is now accepted that anaesthesia in such patients calls for special measures (gastric emptying or administration of an alkali mixture, plus cricoid compression during intubation to occlude the oesophagus and prevent reflux of gastric contents) and special training.

Abortion

In approximately half of the deaths related to abortion, there is evidence of illegal procedures (figure 14.3). In the majority of the patients in this group, sepsis is the chief factor in the death; in a number of others, embolism results from the injection into the uterus under pressure of an abortificient solution. Continued syringing may result in the additional embolism of air. It is important for the public to be aware of the grave risks of self-interference. The most common infecting organisms are those of the clostridial (gas gangrene) and coliform groups. In some cases, the patient delays seeking medical advice until septic shock has occurred; in others, the potential seriousness of the infection is not recognized. In Clostridium welchii infections, early diagnosis is important, as is correction of anaemia due to haemorrhage.

As mentioned already, the enormous increase in the number of therapeutic abortions performed in many countries (20–40% of all conceptions) has been associated with a dramatic fall in the number of deaths from abortion. The death rate from therapeutic abortion is therefore very low, especially when performed before the end of the first trimester of pregnancy,.

It is noteworthy that, in spite of the ready availability of contraceptive measures, there is still a large segment of the population who do not seek advice. Also, all too common in those who have sought advice is the story of the discontinuance of the method because of some side-effect, without the provision of an adequate alternative.

Figure 14.3 Infection due to Clostridium welchii complicating abortion and resulting in gangrene of the uterus, ovary and tube. The uterus has been cut open and shows necrosis of the muscle wall.

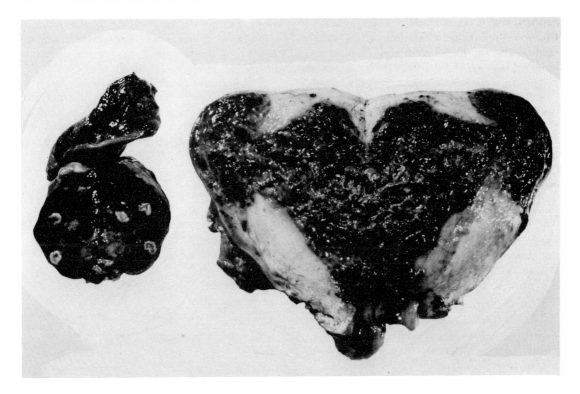

INDIRECT AND ASSOCIATED MATERNAL DEATHS

Cardiac Disease

In England and Wales during the triennium 1976–1978, 21 women died from cardiac diseases associated with pregnancy. As the number of deaths from acquired heart disease due to rheumatic carditis has fallen, as a result of better standards of health and nutrition coupled with a lower incidence of serious streptococcal infections in the community, so the numbers of deaths from coronary artery disease has risen in importance. It is apparent that the greatest danger for women with acquired disease is after the 36th week of pregnancy and for those aged 35 years or more. Congenital heart disease has not altered in incidence, but, again, advances in surgical technique have made pregnancy safe for the majority of these patients. Eisenmenger disorder, where there is a complex series of malformations, is difficult to treat and patients with this disorder remain at very high risk.

Avoidable factors are similar for most of the medical disorders which are considered in this section: (i) failure to seek consultative advice when a serious condition is diagnosed, (ii) lack of close antenatal care (including more frequent visits) to detect early deviations from normal, (iii) failure to hospitalize the patient when early deviations are observed, (iv) failure to prevent conditions known to cause deterioration. In the case of cardiac disorders, these include pre-eclampsia, anaemia, obesity, and respiratory infection. *Antibiotics* are required to cover mild respiratory infections and the early puerperium.

Hypertension

This condition is very common in the general community, but is less often seen in patients of childbearing age. If untreated, preeclampsia and eclampsia are more common. Usually, investigation for an underlying cause (renal disease) is desirable. The reasons why maternal death may occur are similar to those outlined for pre-eclampsia. Intense vasospasm causes tissue anoxia, and there is damage to the cells of such vital organs as the heart, liver, and kidney. As the pressure continues to rise, either the heart will fail or a blowout will occur in one of the vessels, with disastrous results if it happens to be in the brain. Preventive measures have already been outlined.

Renal Disease

Pregnancy represents an added strain on the kidneys as on other organs. Renal failure may be precipitated because of the limited amount of normal functioning tissue remaining (chronic glomerulonephritis), infection (chronic pyelonephritis) or hypertension (nephrosclerosis).

Subarachnoid Haemorrhage

Although the relationship of bleeding to hypertension is less clear than in the case of intracerebral haemorrhage, the grouping of episodes at the time of maximum blood volume increase in the third trimester and at the time of blood pressure peaks in labour is suggestive. The bleeding usually represents the rupture of a congenital aneurysm and requires urgent neurosurgical consultation. The potential danger of the blood pressure rise at the time of pushing during the second stage should be remembered, particularly if hypertension already exists.

Miscellaneous

Malignant neoplasms, suicide, and accidents are the main conditions in this group (table 14.2). Although considered to be independent of pregnancy, it cannot be denied that the altered anatomy and physiology may sometimes have contributed to the death. Wearing of a seat belt of appropriate design would reduce the alarming number of deaths due to motor car accidents during pregnancy (table 14.2).

Although suicide is rare in pregnancy, when it occurs in the first trimester or in the puerperium, one suspects a depressive episode related to events and circumstances that surround the pregnancy. Depression during the puerperium should always be taken seriously.

chapter fifteen

Perinatal Mortality

OVERVIEW

Perinatal mortality (Greek — peri, around; natal, connected with birth) is the combination of stillbirths and neonatal deaths occurring in the first week of life. The rate is expressed per 1,000 births, live and still, and is a measure of the standard of obstetric care and of the socioeconomic situation in the community concerned.

A *stillbirth* defines any child born after 28 weeks' gestation which did not, at any time after being born, breathe or show any other signs of life.

A *neonatal death* defines any child born alive who dies within 28 days of birth.

Different definitions are used in different countries so that for international comparisons those recommended by the World Health Organization should be used.

There are a number of uses of perinatal mortality data — improvement in the care of mothers and babies by better organization and delivery of health services; provision of information for monitoring disease trends; epidemiological studies to define high risk groups.

Prematurity, congenital anomalies and *fetal growth retardation* are the 3 leading causes of perinatal deaths. In any particular community the mortality rate is related to maternal age, parity and sex of infant, as well as to the overriding importance of fetal maturity at birth. *Social factors*, such as poor economic circumstances and poor attitudes to preventive health, are often important determinants of perinatal outcome.

The perinatal mortality rates range from 10–15 per 1,000 births in developed countries to more than 100 per 1,000 when socioeconomic conditions are less favourable.

Infant mortality (death in the first year of life of infants born alive) is another measure of the standards of medical care, nutrition and living conditions in the community concerned. Local customs can profoundly affect mortality rates, an extreme example being the high incidence of neonatal *tetanus* in primitive communities where the newborn infant's umbilicus is packed with earth and/ or cow-dung! (In Haiti and New Guinea the neonatal mortality rates from tetanus alone are 145 and 60 per 1,000 livebirths, respectively). Infant mortality rates range from 10–15 per 1,000 births in developed countries to 300–450 per 1,000 births in underdeveloped countries. It is in the former group in which cot deaths comprise the largest single group of *postneonatal deaths* (from 4–52 weeks of age).

Stillbirths comprise somewhat more than 50% of all perinatal deaths. Introduction of *ventilatory support* and intensive care for low birth-weight infants, and the introduction of *neonatal transport services* to convey sick and/or premature infants safely to major hospitals, have resulted in dramatic improvement of results in recent years. Further improvement in perinatal mortality rates will depend upon obstetrical (and *social*) rather than paediatric considerations, since major *avoidable factors* are present in approximately 25% of stillbirths and 15% of neonatal deaths. In most cases there is usually a failure of diagnosis, due to either a weak clinical appraisal or lack of appropriate investigation, or failure to act when the diagnosis has been made (appropriate therapy or referral). After delivery, there is usually inadequate resuscitation and/or ventilatory management.

The area most needing further study is the perinatal loss between 22 and 28 weeks' gestation. Genetic problems (chromosome and single gene defects), maternal-fetal infection, and disorders of the uterus (premature activity, malformation) and placenta (premature separation or bleeding) should be considered. Cytogenetic, microbiological, biochemical, and radiographic/ultrasound studies now have an established role in perinatal necropsy.

Currently, there is much debate on how far abdominal delivery (with its increased risks to the mother) should be pursued to achieve an ever-diminishing return in terms of perinatal survival.

DEFINITIONS

At present the definitions of stillbirth and neonatal death used throughout the world lack uniformity — similar to the situation with maternal death referred to in Chapter 14.

The following are the current definitions used in England and Wales.

Livebirth is the complete expulsion or extraction from its mother of a child, who after such separation, breathes or shows any other evidence of life such as beating of the heart, pulsation of the umbilical cord or definite movement of voluntary muscles, whether or not the umbilical cord has been cut or the placenta is attached.

Stillbirth (or fetal death). Any child born after 28 weeks' gestation which did not, at any time after being born, breathe or show any other sign of life.

Neonatal death. Any child born alive who dies within the first 28 days of life.

Perinatal mortality rate is the number of perinatal deaths (stillbirths and deaths in the first week of life) per 1,000 live and stillbirths.

Period of gestation is measured from the first day of the last normal menstrual period to the date of birth and is expressed in completed weeks.

For *international comparison* the World Health Organization recommends that perinatal deaths at weights under 1,000 g or neonatal deaths at ages over 7 days be excluded. Thus a *stillbirth* is a deadborn infant weighing at least 1,000 g or, if the weight is not known, born after at least 28 weeks' gestation. A *neonatal death* is death of an infant whose birth-weight was at least 1,000 g or, if the weight is not known, born after at least 28 weeks' gestation, and who dies within *7 days* of birth.

As discussed in Chapter 12, perinatal results are best defined according to *weight* of the infant at birth since this, unlike the period of gestation, is readily measured and is therefore the most appropriate criterion for statistical purposes.

Infant mortality is defined as death in the first year of life of infants born alive. It is the combination of neonatal and postneonatal deaths (tables 15.1 and 15.2, figure 15.1). For perspective, it should be noted that more than 60% of infant mortality occurs during the first month of life (table 15.1), and perinatal problems account for few deaths after this time (table 15.2). 'Cot-deaths'

TABLE 15.1 LIVE BIRTHS, STILLBIRTHS AND INFANT MORTALITY IN ENGLAND AND WALES 1979–1980

	Year	
	1979	1980
Total livebirths*	638,028	656,234
Stillbirth rate*	8.0	7.2
Perinatal mortality rate*	14.7	13.3
Neonatal death rate†		
Early	6.8	6.2
Late	1.5	1.5
Postneonatal death rate†	4.6	4.4
Infant death rate†	12.8	12.0

*Rate per 1,000 total births
†Rate per 1,000 livebirths

TABLE 15.2 CAUSES OF POSTNEONATAL DEATH IN ENGLAND AND WALES 1980

Cause of death	Rate per 1,000 livebirths
Diseases of the respiratory system	1.03
Congenital anomalies	0.77
Accidents and poisoning	0.22
Infections	0.16
Perinatal problems	0.17
Symptoms, signs and ill-defined conditions ('cot deaths')	1.43
Other	0.49
Total	4.27

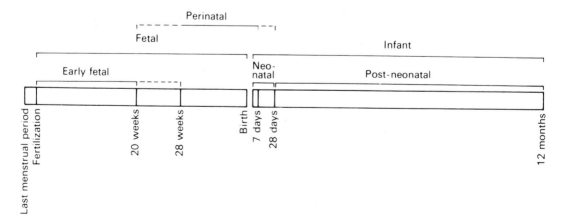

Figure 15.1 The antenatal and postnatal components of the perinatal period. The dotted lines indicate the alternative definition of perinatal — beginning at 20 rather than 28 weeks of gestation and continuing to 28 days after birth.

comprise the largest single group of postneonatal infant deaths, and often masquerade as respiratory infections.

INCIDENCE

There is a wide range throughout the world, depending chiefly on physique and health of the people, together with the density of medical services, and standards of care. The range is from 10–15 per 1,000 births in highly developed countries to 100 or more per 1,000 births where development is poor.

Its incidence reflects the general standard of obstetrical care, and the analysis of causative factors provides a more accurate idea of areas for potential improvement. Early fetal deaths (figure 15.1) are defined as *abortions* and are discussed further in Chapter 18. Although deaths in the later neonatal period (8–28 days) and the infancy period (up to 12 months) are sometimes related to disorders of pregnancy and labour, they are regarded as a reflection of the quality of paediatric care as well as the prevailing standards of social and preventive medicine in the particular community (general health standards, child welfare clinics, immunization programmes).

The perinatal death rate in England and Wales over the 6-year period 1975–1980 fell from 19.21 to 13.31 per 1,000 live and stillbirths.

INFLUENCING FACTORS

Maternal age. The perinatal mortality rate is lowest in the 25–29 year age group (12 per 1,000 total births) and highest when the mother is 35 years or more (17.7 per 1,000 total births) (table 15.3). Since 1976 there has been a decrease in perinatal mortality rates in all age groups.

TABLE 15.3 PERINATAL MORTALITY RATES BY MATERNAL AGE IN ENGLAND AND WALES 1980

Maternal age	Perinatal mortality rate
Under 20	17.0
20 – 24	13.3
25 – 29	12.1
30 – 34	12.6
35 and over	18.4
Total	13.4

Social class. The perinatal mortality rate is lowest in the professional social classes (social classes 1 and 2), where it is 10.7 per 1,000 total births and highest for the semi- and unskilled social classes (social classes 4 and 5), where it is 15.5 per 1,000 total births (figures given are for England and Wales, 1980).

Country of origin of mother. Stillbirth and neonatal mortality figures may be influenced by the country of origin of the mother, as illustrated in figure 15.2, the highest rates for both stillbirths and

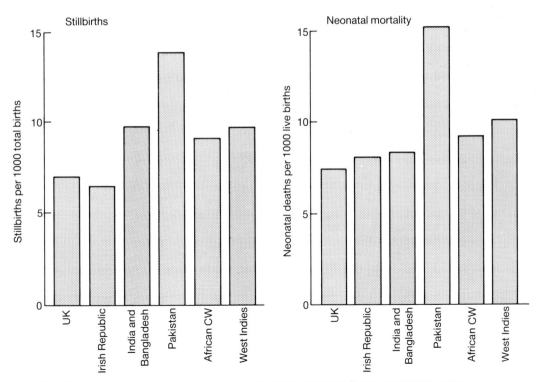

Figure 15.2 Outcome of pregnancy by selected mother's country of birth in England and Wales 1980.

neonatal mortality being recorded for mothers born in Pakistan.

Birth-weight. In England and Wales in 1980, 39% of all perinatal deaths occurred in infants weighing less than 1,500 g (table 15.4). The percentage of all deaths in this category has increased as perinatal mortality rates have fallen. Many of these deaths are due to cervical incompetence, premature rupture of the membranes and premature labour, and may be avoidable.

TABLE 15.4 PERINATAL MORTALITY RATE BY BIRTH-WEIGHT IN ENGLAND AND WALES 1980

Birth-weight	No. of stillbirths	No. of perinatal deaths	Perinatal mortality rate
Under 1500 g	1543	3239	481.4
1501 – 2000 g	783	1309	139.6
2001 – 2500 g	714	1132	34.5
2501 – 3000 g	661	1116	8.4
3001 – 3500 g	488	875	3.4
3501 – 4000 g	240	447	2.6
4000 g and over	113	199	4.0
All birth-weights	4542	8317	12.6

Time of death. In England and Wales in 1980, stillbirths comprised 54% of all perinatal deaths. Of all the neonatal deaths, 75–80% occurred within the first 7 days of life (table 15.1). These figures stress the importance of survival in the first week of neonatal life.

Sex. In England and Wales in 1980, the livebirth ratio was 105 males born to every 100 females. The ratio of perinatal deaths was 120:100; for stillbirths the ratio was 103:101, while for early neonatal deaths it was 130:100. There is no simple explanation for this extraordinary imbalance, although the higher average birth-weight of male infants for any particular gestational period explains the higher neonatal death rate in the up-to-1,500 g group, the males tending to be less mature in comparison with female infants of similar birth-weights. However, the male preponderance in perinatal deaths is present in *all* birth-weight ranges.

TABLE 15.5 MAJOR CONGENITAL ANOMALIES CONTRIBUTING TO PERINATAL DEATH IN ENGLAND AND WALES 1980

Nature of anomaly	Total	Rate (per 1,000 livebirths)
Anencephaly and similar anomalies	410	0.62
Spina bifida	256	0.39
Other congenital anomalies of central nervous system	220	0.33
Congenital anomalies of heart and circulation	298	0.45
Other	756	1.14
Total	1940	2.93

Major congenital anomalies. These were present in 22% of perinatal deaths (table 15.5). This group contained more females than males due to the greater incidence of anencephaly and spina bifida in female fetuses.

AETIOLOGY

More than 70% of perinatal deaths are due to the combination of *hypoxia* and *prematurity* (table 15.6). Another way to obtain an overall view of the

TABLE 15.6 PERINATAL DEATHS BY CAUSE IN ENGLAND AND WALES 1980

Cause of death	Number	Rate per 1,000 total births
Infection and parasitic disease	11	0.02
Disease of respiratory system	46	0.07
Congenital anomalies	1940	2.93
Conditions of perinatal period	6634	10.04
Maternal conditions	792	1.20
Multiple pregnancy	191	0.29
Conditions of cord, placenta and membrane	2062	3.12
Other complications of labour/ delivery	143	0.22
Slow fetal growth, malnutrition and immaturity	562	0.85
Birth trauma	150	0.23
Hypoxia, birth asphyxia and respiratory conditions	1774	2.68
Perinatal infections	73	0.11
Haemolytic disease of fetus/ newborn	84	0.13
Symptoms, signs and ill-defined conditions ('cot deaths')	15	0.02
External causes of injury and poisoning	26	0.04

problem is to see how many perinatal deaths occur in infants who are mature enough to survive if born alive in good condition. Table 15.7 shows that 46% of perinatal deaths occur in fetuses or infants weighing more than 2 kg, although many of these deaths are unavoidable as they are caused by major congenital abnormalities. In 20% of stillbirths, the fetus weighs more than 3,000 g. Any infant weighing 2,000 g or more at birth or of 34 or more weeks' maturity has, with modern paediatric care, more than a 98% chance of survival (figure 64.17). A major avoidable factor is present in approximately 25% of stillbirths and 15% of neonatal deaths. It is apparent that further improvement in perinatal mortality depends upon obstetrical rather than paediatric considerations.

It should be remembered that fetal growth retardation and intrauterine hypoxia can cause intellectual impairment in surviving infants.

Although the great majority of deaths are ultimately caused by hypoxia, this does not tell us much about the antecedent problems and it does

TABLE 15.7 PERINATAL MORTALITY BY BIRTH-WEIGHT AND CAUSE IN ENGLAND AND WALES 1980

Cause of death	Birth-weight (g)							
	Up to 1500	1501– 2000	2001– 2500	2501– 3000	3001– 3500	3501– 4000	Over 4000	Total
Congenital anomalies	497	319	298	319	231	111	43	1818
Conditions of perinatal period	2703	964	799	763	600	320	146	6295
Maternal conditions	432	124	94	58	32	14	9	763
Complication of cord, placenta or membranes	587	365	338	324	236	106	31	1987
Complications of delivery	12	16	19	16	29	19	26	137
Disorders of short gestation/low birth-weight	434	25	6	4	4	2	3	478
Birth trauma	34	18	17	27	23	18	4	141
Respiratory distress syndrome	439	133	49	23	18	7	4	673
Intrauterine hypoxia/birth asphyxia	140	55	82	116	111	67	30	606
All causes	3239	1309	1132	1116	875	447	199	8317

not help in our efforts to reduce wastage. In order to illustrate the problem more clearly, the 1980 figures for England and Wales are summarized in table 15.6, according to main conditions in the infant and mother. Most stillborn infants show evidence of intrauterine hypoxia at autopsy, but this finding does not explain the cause of death. Likewise, the respiratory distress syndrome in premature infants is the most common cause of neonatal death, but this does not explain the cause of the premature onset of labour. There is considerable overlap of antenatal complications — e.g. multiple pregnancy may be associated with polyhydramnios, malpresentations, pre-eclampsia and premature rupture of the membranes. It should be noted that no maternal condition was reported in 38% of perinatal deaths (table 15.6).

Multiple pregnancy ranks as an important cause of perinatal mortality. In England and Wales in 1980 the perinatal mortality rate was 59.1, a rate 4-fold higher than that for singleton pregnancies. Multiple pregnancy should be considered as a complication of pregnancy rather than a normal variant.

Errors of Fetal Development (table 15.5)
Although in many cases there are multiple deformities present, errors in the central nervous system comprise the greatest number (anencephaly, hydrocephaly, spina bifida). Then follow malformations of the heart, musculoskeletal system, chromosomes, genitourinary tract, respiratory tract and digestive tract.

Conditions Specific to Pregnancy
The major problem in this group is *immaturity*, whether idiopathic or secondary to one of the many conditions leading to it — abruptio placentae, placenta praevia, premature rupture of the membranes, preeclampsia/eclampsia, multiple pregnancy, and rhesus isoimmunization all being important. In some of the above conditions, *hypoxia* is present as an additional stress, either because of degeneration or spasm of the placental blood vessels (preeclampsia, abruptio placentae) or anaemia of the fetus (maternal isoimmunization).

Associated Conditions
Predominant in this group are diseases of the renal tract (chronic pyelonephritis and glomerulonephritis), cardiovascular system (hypertension), and endocrine system (diabetes mellitus). With some exceptions, the associated diseases are more significant as far as the health of the mother is concerned, in comparison with the other groups.

Labour Conditions
Cephalopelvic disproportion is more serious than *disturbances of uterine action*. The fetus usually suffers from progressive hypoxia because of head compression and prolonged uterine activity. The *coup de grace* may be an intrauterine infection or a traumatic delivery. Accidents to the cord (presentation and prolapse, knotting and entanglement) are relatively frequent and may be the end result of placental insufficiency. *Impacted shoulders* is also a condition of some importance.

Postnatal Conditions
These often follow from antecedent problems or insults — prematurity, intraamniotic infection, and asphyxia of diverse aetiology.

PREVENTIVE ASPECTS
Perinatal deaths can only be reduced to a minimum by continual application of the highest standards of obstetrical and neonatal care. This must take place at a number of levels — individual, hospital and government. If there is a breakdown in

any one level, efforts at the other levels will be nullified. Other skills, such as those of communication and interpersonal relationships are important if the patient is to appreciate properly her role in pregnancy, labour and the puerperium, and if we are to persuade her to cooperate fully with her medical attendants and follow the advice which she is given.

It is generally accepted that 15–20% of perinatal deaths are preventable. In the chapter on fetal well-being and in the chapters which follow, a concept of the risk factors in pregnancy and the puerperium is developed, and appropriate therapeutic measures are indicated.

As perinatal mortality rates have fallen, major congenital anomalies have emerged as a relatively more important cause of death: in 1968 in England and Wales the perinatal mortality rate was 24.7 per 1,000 total births and major anomalies were present in 17% of perinatal deaths; in 1975 the perinatal mortality rate was 19.2 per 1,000 total births and anomalies were present in 21%; in 1980 the perinatal mortality rate was 13.3 per 1,000 total births and anomalies were present in 22%. *Genetic counselling*, with induced midtrimester abortion of fetuses with identified malformations (neural tube defects, chromosomal abnormalities), will modify this trend in the future. Already in some countries nearly 20% of Down syndrome fetuses are identified and aborted and this figure would increase if all women aged 35 and older were cytogenetically monitored.

chapter sixteen

The Significance of Pregnancy and Neonatal Complications

OVERVIEW

The purpose of this chapter is to help the reader gain perspective about the main complications which occur during pregnancy and the puerperium. The significance of a complication in obstetrics depends upon its *incidence* and the *maternal* and *perinatal mortality rates* associated with it. *Placental abruption* occurs in 1% of pregnancies and has a perinatal mortality rate of 1 in 4 — this stark statistic indelibly imprints the significance of this complication, even without consideration of the maternal hazards of *hypovolaemic shock*, *renal failure*, *blood coagulation failure* and the risk of *postpartum haemorrhage*. There are relatively few major obstetric complications, but they are like birds of a feather and flock together — *multiple pregnancy* is associated with preeclampsia, anaemia, malpresentations, premature labour, postpartum haemorrhage etc; *posterior position of the occiput* results in cephalopelvic disproportion and abnormal uterine action which prolong labour and result in fetal and maternal distress and the need for manipulative delivery.

The tables in this chapter were compiled from a consecutive series of 41,000 deliveries at a large teaching hospital. They list the important complications that occur in obstetrics and show the incidence of the problem and the perinatal mortality rate associated with it. The incidences of neonatal complications are also shown.

As discussed in Chapter 14, mortality rates in developed countries may be approaching the irreducible minimum, although genetic counselling has not yet had its full impact on the prevention of malformations. With these changes, the *quality of life*, intellectual and physical, of surviving infants becomes a major consideration. Follow-up studies of high risk groups of infants (e.g. birth-weight below 1,000 g, small for dates) may provide information which will modify present obstetric methods of practice.

INTRODUCTION

About 50% of patients have a normal pregnancy — i.e. one without antenatal complication, and where there is a normal delivery after a spontaneous onset of labour. The percentage is much lower if minor disorders of pregnancy are considered (such as morning sickness, heartburn, cramps, varicose veins, haemorrhoids), or the need for episiotomy, or the occurrence of vaginal and perineal lacerations. Understandably, the incidence of conditions or procedures which render a pregnancy 'not normal' differs considerably according to the obstetric population concerned and the practices of individual obstetricians. The concentration of high risk patients in teaching hospitals is generally considered to explain why incidences of induction of labour, forceps delivery, and Caesarean section are higher in these institutions. Also, it is undeniable, although confusing for the student, that fashion influences the practice of obstetrics. For example at the Royal Maternity Hospital, Belfast, 1970–1972, the incidence of *induction of labour* was 57.2%, whereas at the Royal Women's Hospital, Melbourne, at the same time, it was 15%. At St Georges Hospital, London, the incidence of *epidural analgesia* in labour in 1982 was 35%, or more than double that at the Mercy Maternity Hospital, Melbourne. In any hospital it is essential that the doctor or nurse should record in the case notes the reason why a procedure was performed. Interference is never without some risk, and procedures such as amniotomy and Caesarean section should never be performed without a proper indication.

The significance of a complication in obstetrics depends upon its *incidence* and the *maternal and fetal mortality rates* associated with it. *Morbidity rates* are also important, but are less tangible, especially in the case of the infant, who requires follow-up for 5 to 7 years before the neurological sequelae of pregnancy or labour complications can be assessed fully. The purpose of this chapter is to help the student gain perspective by reviewing the incidences and results of treatment of the more important complications and diseases associated with pregnancy.

In developed countries, *stillbirth* and *neonatal death rates* each range from approximately 5–10 per 1,000 births, giving a range for the *perinatal mortality rate* of 10–20 per 1,000; the *maternal mortality rate* ranges from 10–40 per 100,000 total births.

Both maternal and perinatal mortality rates have fallen 50% since the first edition of this textbook was published 10 years ago. The statistics to be presented serve as a yardstick against which the hazards of any particular complication may be judged. The data in the following 4 tables were compiled from 41,000 consecutive deliveries at a large teaching hospital. These statistics include emergency as well as clinic patients, which largely explains why the hospital perinatal mortality rates (stillbirths 14.1 per 1,000 births, neonatal deaths 13.7 per 1,000 births) were double those in the community as a whole. In national studies approximately 55% of perinatal deaths are stillbirths, but in hospital practice there are relatively more neonatal deaths. This is explained by referral of nonbooked patients likely to deliver infants requiring special paediatric care (premature labour, premature rupture of the membranes, multiple pregnancy, polyhydramnios).

TABLE 16.1 STATISTICAL AUDIT AND INCIDENCES OF IMPORTANT OBSTETRIC COMPLICATIONS IN A RECENT SURVEY OF 40,982 CONSECUTIVE PATIENTS* IN A MAJOR TEACHING HOSPITAL (see note at end of chapter)

Complication	Number	Incidence %	Perinatal mortality rate per 1,000 births
Epidural analgesia			
— in labour	5,955	14.5	—
— for Caesarean section	561	1.4	—
Preeclampsia	3,978	9.7	27
Threatened abortion continuing to viability	3,237	7.9	49
Prolonged pregnancy (⩾ 42 weeks)	2,463	6.0	7
Puerperal infection (genital tract)	2,356	5.7	—
Postpartum haemorrhage (> 600 ml)**	2,150	5.2	—
Maternal obesity (> 90 kg)	1,277	3.1	20
Prolonged labour (> 24 hours)	1,136	2.8	33
Contracted pelvis	806	2.0	6
APH cause undetermined	713	1.7	107
Multiple pregnancy	571	1.4	129
Incompetent cervix	532	1.3	210
Premature rupture of membranes	442	1.0	238
Deliveries between 20–28 weeks' gestation	426	1.0	920
Abruptio placentae	419	1.0	270
Placenta praevia	375	0.9	43
Polyhydramnios	329	0.8	286
Hyperemesis gravidarum ***	263	0.6	34
Haemolytic disease (erythroblastosis)	218	0.5	74
Hepatosis or jaundice	84	0.2	60
Eclampsia****	24	0.05	167
Rupture of the uterus	18	0.04	389
Death rates and associated conditions			
Neonatal death 500 g and above — see table 16.4	516	1.25	—
Stillbirth*****	581	1.41	—
— 500 g and above	462	1.12	—
— 500–999 g	152	0.37	—
— 1,000 g and above	310	0.75	—
Maternal death	8	0.01	—
Abortion (before 20 weeks' gestation)	3,719	9.8	—
Ectopic pregnancy	144	0.4	—
Hydatidiform mole and choriocarcinoma	57	0.1	—

* Emergency (nonbooked) admissions are included
** Excluding patients delivered by Caesarean section
*** Requiring admission to hospital
**** 2 of the 24 mothers died
***** 400 g and above

SPECIFIC COMPLICATIONS

Table 16.1 lists the more important complications of pregnancy together with the incidence and perinatal mortality rate associated with each. The overall perinatal and maternal mortality rates are shown for perspective as are the numbers of patients with *abortion, ectopic pregnancy* and *hydatidiform mole* who presented to the same hospital during the 10 years that the 41,000 patients were confined. Note that the incidence of *preeclampsia* was almost 10% (included were patients in whom hypertension and proteinuria were observed for the first time during labour or within 2 hours of delivery).

A glance at table 16.1 quickly shows the importance of a condition such as *abruptio placentae (accidental haemorrhage)*, which occurred in 1% of pregnancies and was associated with a perinatal mortality rate of 27%. Note that the perinatal mortality rate of *placenta praevia* has fallen below 5%. The incidence of *prolonged pregnancy* (6%) has halved in this community in the past decade; this reflects the reluctance of obstetricians to allow pregnancy to proceed beyond 42 weeks. *Eclampsia* unfortunately is still with us and accounted for 2 of the 8 maternal deaths. *Pregnancies ending prematurely between 20 and 28 weeks' gestation* have an importance out of all proportion to their incidence; although occurring in only 1% of the obstetric population, they accounted for 35% of all perinatal deaths.

Table 16.2 shows the incidence of the important *medical* and *surgical conditions* which occur in association with pregnancy. It is noteworthy that only one had an incidence greater than 1%; it is a paradox that many of the leading causes of maternal death are uncommon conditions (eclampsia, Mendelson syndrome, blood coagulation failure, rupture of the uterus). Disorders such as *hypertension* and *chronic renal disease* have a profound influence upon pregnancy, which in turn may affect the natural history of these diseases. *Diabetes* is important because of the risk of intrauterine death near term. *Psychiatric disease* may occur for the first time during pregnancy, especially in the puerperium, and requires prompt recognition and appropriate management. *Asthma* and *epilepsy* are important diseases because they are relatively common and often require admission to hospital during pregnancy for restabilization of drug therapy. *Surgical complications* are uncommon during pregnancy. *Appendicitis* and complications of *ovarian cysts* (torsion, haemorrhage) account for the majority of laparotomies required during pregnancy (apart from ectopic pregnancy). Spontaneous *rupture of the spleen* is a rare complication that can occur without warning during pregnancy or the puerperium.

Table 16.3 shows that *surgical induction of labour* and *forceps delivery* are each performed in approximately 1 in 4 patients. The increased incidence of forceps delivery is due to the mod-

TABLE 16.2   THE INCIDENCE OF ASSOCIATED MEDICAL AND SURGICAL COMPLICATIONS IN 40,982 CONSECUTIVE PREGNANCIES

Complication	Number	Incidence %	Perinatal mortality rate per 1,000 births
Renal disease	492	1.20	42
Diabetes mellitus	358	0.87	25
Psychiatric disorder	321	0.78	—
Asthma	260	0.63	27
Essential hypertension	253	0.61	59
Venous thrombosis	160	0.39	—
— antenatal	71	0.17	—
— postnatal	89	0.21	—
Epilepsy	138	0.33	28
Cardiac disease	110	0.26	9
Tumours			
— fibromyoma	162	0.39	—
— ovarian cyst	59	0.14	—
— breast lump	11	0.02	—
— malignant neoplasm	8	0.01	—
Acute appendicitis	28	0.06	—
Acute cholecystitis	8	0.01	—
Splenectomy	2	0.004	—

TABLE 16.3   THE INCIDENCE OF ABNORMAL FETAL LIE, PRESENTATION, AND POSITION AND MANIPULATIVE PROCEDURES IN 40,982 CONSECUTIVE PREGNANCIES

Condition or procedure	Number	Incidence %	Perinatal mortality rate per 1,000 births
Forceps delivery	10,714	26.1	17
— low	6,322	15.4	—
— mid	4,392	10.7	—
— posterior position	2,059	5.0	—
— deep transverse arrest	1,029	2.5	—
— epidural analgesia	3,867	9.4	—
Surgical induction of labour	9,938	24.2	18
— Caesarean section*	753	1.8	—
Caesarean section	4,633	11.3	24
Posterior position of occiput			
— in labour**	4,363	10.6	6
— spontaneous delivery			
•occipitoanterior	1,121	2.7	
•occipitoposterior	274	0.7	
— forceps delivery	2,263	5.5	
— Caesarean section	705	1.7	
Previous Caesarean section	2,298	5.6	
— elective repeat Caesarean	1,520	3.7	—
— trial of scar	778	1.9	66
•vaginal delivery	595	1.5	
•Caesarean section	183	0.4	
Breech presentation	1,645	4.0	172
— Caesarean section	488	1.2	
Manual removal of placenta	1,766	4.3	—
— blood transfusion	190	0.5	
Transverse, oblique or unstable lie	343	0.8	78
Cord presentation or prolapse	118	0.3	237
Failed forceps	75	0.2	53
Face presentation (9 anencephaly)	55	0.1	254
Brow presentation	60	0.1	0
Caesarean hysterectomy	36	0.1	138

* 7.5% of patients having surgical induction of labour ultimately required Caesarean section
** Confirmed by vaginal examination

ern philosophy that it is best to deliver the baby once the head is on view and safely accessible. It is held that the *quality of survival* (especially intellectual) is likely to be improved by minimizing the risks of fetal hypoxia during the second stage of labour; 41% of forceps deliveries were from the midpelvis and in 29% the head had arrested in the occipitoposterior or occipitolateral positions. The *Caesarean section rate* was 11%, and since the main indication was a previous Caesarean, the pregnancy outcome in the 5% of patients who had had a previous Caesarean is shown; the operation was repeated in 66% of patients; vaginal delivery was achieved in 76% of those in whom it was considered safe for labour to occur.

Breech presentation had a perinatal mortality rate of 11% and a Caesarean section rate of almost 30%. *Posterior position of the occiput* in labour and its outcomes are shown, since this is the commonest cause of problems during labour and accounts for many of the more difficult mid-

forceps deliveries and cases of cephalopelvic disproportion; 52% of patients with an occipitoposterior position required forceps delivery, and 6% (0.7% of the population) delivered spontaneously face to pubis. Table 16.3 also shows the incidences of *abnormal fetal lie, malpresentations*, and different manipulative procedures, together with the results obtained. It is noteworthy that the incidences of *face and brow presentation* were almost identical at 0.1%.

In recent years, community studies have aimed at establishing the incidences of diseases such as hypertension, anaemia, abnormal glucose tolerance and cardiac insufficiency in the population as a whole. Such an audit allows appraisal of the disease in all stages, rather than limiting consideration to patients who already have symptoms. Such information has been available for the pregnant population since the advent of antenatal clinics and proper documentation of disease in teaching hospitals. Indeed, insight into the natural history of many diseases

TABLE 16.4   THE INCIDENCES OF IMPORTANT NEONATAL COMPLICATIONS IN 41,057 CONSECUTIVE LIVEBORN INFANTS (see note at end of chapter)

Complication	Number	%	Neonatal death	
			Number	%
Neonatal infection	5,679	13.8	102	1.8
Congenital malformation	4,865	11.8	182	3.7
— major	1,694	4.1	—	—
— minor	3,171	7.7	—	—
Hyperbilirubinaemia				
($> 154\ \mu$mol/l (9 mg/dl))	4,406	10.7	63	1.4
Birth asphyxia	3,706	9.0	427	11.5
Infants small for dates*	2,566	6.2	59	2.3
Hypoglycaemia				
($< 1.7\ \mu$mol/l (30 mg/dl))	1,517	3.6	37	2.4
Respiratory distress	1,361	3.3	261	19.2
Birth trauma	1,058	2.5	14	1.3
Cephalhaematoma	1,031	2.5	4	0.4
Infant requiring assisted ventilation	518	1.26	177	34.2
Convulsions	235	0.57	47	20.0
Necrotizing enterocolitis	24	0.05	6	25.0
Neonatal death **	563	1.37	—	—
— 500 g and above	516	1.25	—	—
— 500–999 g	116	0.28	—	—
— 1,000 g and above	400	0.97	—	—

* Incidence should by definition be 10% if percentile charts derived from the same population are used
** 400 g and above

has been achieved by detection of signs in symptomatically normal women when examined during pregnancy.

The obstetric attendant has a unique opportunity to detect many disorders such as hypertension, chronic renal disease, rheumatic carditis, diabetes mellitus and syphilis, at a very early stage. In this day of diminishing emphasis upon the manipulative aspects of obstetrics (e.g. difficult forceps and internal version and breech extraction) there is a corresponding increase in the attention devoted to the detection and treatment of medical disease during pregnancy.

Table 16.4 shows the incidences and mortality rates associated with the various neonatal complications discussed in the paediatric chapters. These complications tend to coexist; this is especially so for *birth asphyxia* which can proceed to *respiratory distress* and the need for *assisted ventilation* — infants with these problems are often *premature* and develop *hyperbilirubinaemia* and *infections*.

Note

The figures quoted in Tables 16.1 and 16.4 are from a statistical audit undertaken at a major teaching hospital in Australia. In this study legal definitions concerning the use of the terms abortion, stillbirth and neonatal death were those pertaining to Australia and are different from those in current use in the United Kingdom. As indicated in the tables, neonatal deaths and stillbirths are defined on a weight basis rather than a gestational age basis. In addition, abortion is defined as termination of pregnancy before the 20th completed week of pregnancy.

SPECIFIC DISORDERS OF PREGNANCY

chapter seventeen

Errors of Development

OVERVIEW

With improvements in the management of many other obstetric disorders, fetal errors of development have assumed a major role in perinatal morbidity and mortality; for surviving individuals, there are often major related psychological and social costs.

The obstetric attendant should be aware of the need for a careful genetic history in the antenatal patient and a review of factors predisposing to fetal developmental error (e.g. *advanced maternal age*). Additional requirements are a knowledge of the frequency of inherited and spontaneous errors; their causation (chromosomal disorder, gene defect, multifactorial); mechanisms of transmission; accuracy and risks of diagnostic methods; clinical expressions of individual disorders; treatment possibilities and long-term prognosis. The best way of getting a family history is by drawing a simple 3-generation pedigree.

Often a team approach is required at consultant level (obstetrician, geneticist, neonatologist).

Chromosomal disorders arise largely in the stages of gamete formation or early in embryonic cleavage; they are associated with 40–50% of spontaneous abortions and a lesser number of perinatal deaths, malformed or small for dates infants. Disorders of the autosomes and sex chromosomes occur with equal frequency, but the former are more damaging.

Intrauterine diagnosis is usually made on cells obtained at amniocentesis or chorion biopsy (figure 17.1); the latter may become the method of choice in the future.

Genetic disorders may be inherited in several ways: dominant, recessive, sex-linked — each having unique features of transmission. It is in this group that major progress is being made with DNA technology — currently mainly in diagnosis. Important in the group are the defects in haemoglobin synthesis and a host of inborn errors of metabolism.

Multifactorial disorders usually arise as a result of genetic predisposition brought to light by an additional adverse factor — e.g. a dietary deficiency or environmental agent (bacterial, chemical, physical). The well known example of this is *neural tube defect* (anencephaly/spina bifida). Because there is often no family history, major interest has been directed to screening methods (maternal and amniotic fluid alpha fetoprotein; ultrasonography (figure 17.2)).

Unfortunately, there are still a number of difficulties. In the moral-ethical area some may never achieve universal resolution — e.g. the right of the mother versus that of the fetus and the dilemma of nonfatal conditions. Some diagnostic methods are imperfect, and for some conditions no satisfactory diagnostic method is yet available; many disorders are usually recognized only after birth (cleft lip, cardiac defects); other conditions are diagnosed by screening all infants after birth (hypothyroidism, phenylketonuria), because clinical features are unreliable and an accurate cost-effective test is available. In some babies, one may not be sure of why a particular defect has arisen. *Counselling after the pregnancy is equally important as that during the early antenatal period even if the family is not planning to have more children.*

Further prospects look promising, with increasing sophistication of DNA probes, better prospects of heterozygote (carrier) detection, and methods of fetal assessment (including nuclear magnetic resonance studies).

Pending these developments, it is necessary that the relevant information currently available is known by physician, nurse, and paramedical personnel, as well as by the community at large. Families can choose preventive measures when applicable.

The Basis of Inheritance

Table 17.1 lists some of the important definitions relevant to genetics.

Cell Structure

The cell is basically divided into cytoplasm and nucleus; the former is responsible for the functions of the cell, the latter for the regulation of protein synthesis and the storage of genetic information. Each of the *46 chromosomes* contains a large number of genes (an average of 5,000 per chromosome), made up of deoxyribonucleic acid (DNA).

Cell Function

Protein synthesis. Proteins are composed of building blocks called amino acids. The trick is to specify which amino acid is to be selected in the building process, in the same way as the builder selects the building sequence for a house. It is done by 3 of the 4 nitrogenous bases of the DNA molecule arranging themselves in a particular sequence (a codon) to specify one of the 20 possible amino acids required.

Division. When the cell is to divide, the 2 spiral chains of nucleotides forming the DNA molecule separate and complementary chains are synthesized. At division, one set of chromosomes goes to one daughter cell and one set to the other daughter cell. This process is called *mitosis.*

ANTENATAL DIAGNOSIS

Antenatal diagnosis of *suspected major fetal abnormalities* and therapeutic abortion is now an accepted management option.

This philosophy has arisen for a number of reasons: the rapid development of accurate diagnostic methods, the emotional and economic costs of the severely handicapped, and the perceived need of most couples to have a normal and healthy family. Recent medicolegal decisions have indicated the need for all practitioners to counsel their antenatal patients adequately in this area regardless of their own moral view.

The *responsibilities of the attendant* include the following: an *awareness of which couples are at risk* (history and clinical features); the *natural history of the disorder* in question, the *range of its clinical behaviour, treatment possibilities* and *prognosis*; the possibility of *carrier detection* where indicated; the nature, accuracy, and *risks of diagnostic methods*; and finally, the *psychological implications*. Often these can be best satisfied by consultation with or referral to a medical geneticist.

TABLE 17.1 DEFINITIONS

Chromosome	Long intranuclear DNA strands containing the coding for the different genes of that individual; they become visible as homologous pairs at the time of cell division
Karyotype	The chromosome set of an individual arranged in a standard fashion
Gene	The unit of inheritance, occupying a specific locus on the chromosome; they are characterized by a short segment of DNA coding for a particular cell function
Allele	Alternative forms of a gene
Homozygous	Possession of identical alleles at a gene locus
Heterozygous	Possession of different alleles at a gene locus
Dominant trait	Expressed in the presence of a gene in the heterozygous form
Recessive trait	Expressed in the presence of a gene in the homozygous form
X-linked trait	Determined by the presence of a gene on the X (sex) chromosome
Genetic heterogeneity	A condition which at first appears to be a single disorder but is later found to consist of a number of different disorders. This may be detected by a difference in phenotype, pattern of inheritance or biochemistry
Monosomy	Deficiency of one of the pair of chromosomes
Trisomy	Addition of a chromosome to the normal diploid set
Polyploidy	Possession of 1 or more extra sets (23) of chromosomes (figure 17.3) e.g. triploid or tetraploid
Translocation	Transfer of one chromosome or piece of a chromosome to another
Mosaicism	Presence of more than 1 chromosomal cell type in an individual (e.g. 47XX + 21/46XX)
Gene expressivity*	Degree of clinical severity of a particular genetic defect among members of a particular *family*
Penetrance*	Frequency of clinical expression of a gene in a *population*
Mutation	A permanent change in genetic material
Congenital malformation	Structural or functional defect of prenatal origin (genetic and/or environmental)

* Applied largely to dominant inheritance — e.g. only 80% in the population with the gene for brachydactylia may have short digits; of that 80%, the degree may differ significantly among members of a particular family

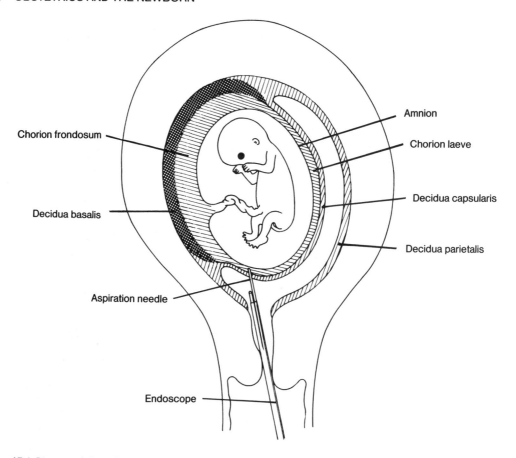

Chorion frondosum

Decidua basalis

Aspiration needle

Amnion

Chorion laeve

Decidua capsularis

Decidua parietalis

Endoscope

Figure 17.1 Diagram of 8-week pregnancy showing endoscopic needle aspiration of extraplacental chorionic villi.

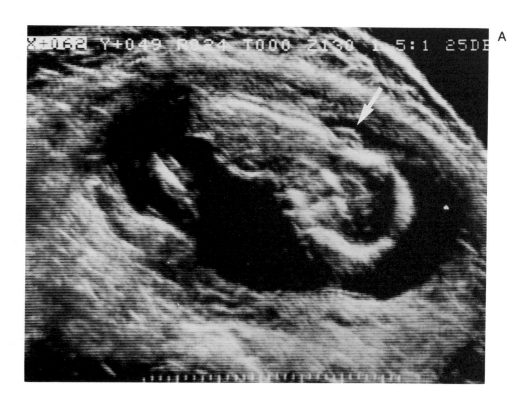

A

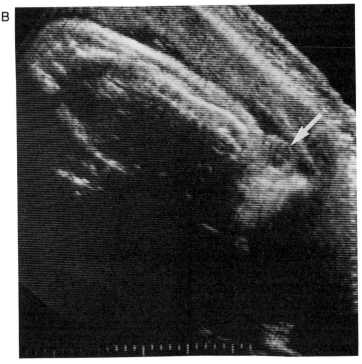

Figure 17.2 Cervical meningomyelocele. A 43-year-old para 2 had an Octoson static scan (A) performed at 16 weeks' gestation to check fetal maturity because delivery by elective repeat Caesarean section was planned. Her serum alpha fetoprotein value was 80 g/l (normal range 13–40 g/l). **A.** Oblique section through fetus showing part of the spine (cervical to lower thoracic); the meningomyelocele (arrow) was misinterpreted as a passing loop of cord. A radiograph was performed at 30 weeks' gestation because marked polyhydramnios had developed — this showed kinking of the upper thoracic spine and so ultrasonography of the fetal spine (B) was arranged. **B.** Oblique section through the fetus showing persistence of the mass (arrow) in the cervical region. Spontaneous rupture of the membranes occurred at 30.3 weeks and the patient had a normal delivery of a 1,145 g infant with multiple anomalies (including cervical meningomyelocele!) who died shortly after birth as a result of a diaphragmatic hernia. The moral is that careful screening using high quality real time equipment and expert interpretation is required to exclude neural tube defects. (Courtesy of Dr Charles Barbaro). **C.** Normal spinal cord at 16 weeks' gestation. This linear array realtime ultrasound scan shows a longitudinal section of the fetal spine (covered in 2 views) from the cervical expansion (arrow) to the sacral region. To confirm normality the spinal cord must also be screened in the transverse plane.

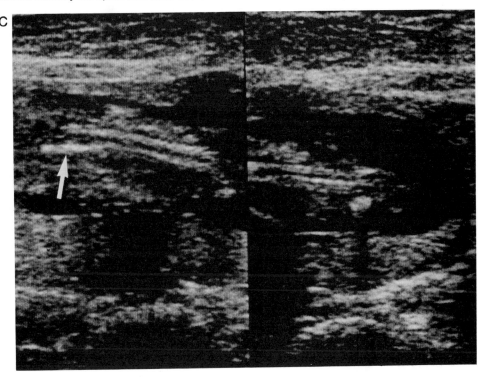

The *conditions* to be considered can be considered broadly under 3 headings — *chromosomal* anomalies, *gene* disorders, and malformations of *multifactorial* origin.

The *methods* used in diagnosis are varied and include *biochemical* analysis of amniotic fluid and its cells, fetal skin and blood, and trophoblastic tissue; *cytogenetic* analysis of fetal cells; and *physical* techniques such as ultrasound. Most of these are very sophisticated and are carried out in regional, national, or even international centres.

CHROMOSOMES AND THEIR ANOMALIES

Normal Chromosomal Complement

The 46 chromosomes in the nucleus are made up of *44 autosomes* and *2 sex chromosomes* (XX, female; XY, male). A half of the total (23) is derived from each parent at the time of fertilization. *Cytogenetics* is a recently developed branch of genetics, whereby the chromosomal makeup of the cell can be determined; it is based on the fact that each of the chromosomes differs in size, shape and staining (banding) characteristics.

Unfortunately, no method is available to study the chromosomes, except by the complex procedure of culture of lymphocytes in peripheral blood and *karyotype analysis*. Chromosomes can be studied in other body tissue cells but this is more expensive and complex. The lymphocytes must be cultured for 2–3 days, and fibroblasts from other tissue cells from 6–8 weeks and 'arrested' at the time of division (metaphase) by a chemical applied to the culture system. The chromosomes are photographed and then arranged by number (autosome pairs, 1–22; sex chromosomes, XX or XY); the complete picture is known as a karyotype (figures 17.3 and 65.3). The numbering is done according to the morphology of the chromosome — overall size and the relative lengths of the long (q) and short (p) arms and more accurately by the nature of its band structure on special staining. This enables the recognition of not only numerical differences, but the transfer of small segments of chromosomes (translocations).

Mechanism of Chromosome Anomalies

The mechanism of addition or subtraction of chromosomes from the cell can be understood from the processes of meiosis and mitosis. Before cell division, the chromosomes separate and align themselves at the centre of the cell. They then divide, and equal numbers should go to each daughter cell. Occasionally, one of the chromosomes does not separate in time (*nondis-*

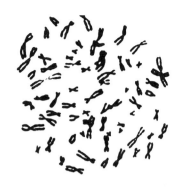

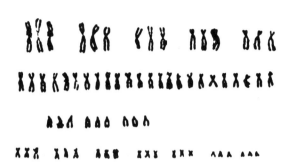

karyotype : triploid

Figure 17.3 Chromosome analysis of a malformed fetus with 69 chromosomes. The spread cell shows metaphase chromosomes. The photograph below shows the triploid karotype with XXX sex chromosome constitution.

junction), and stays with its partner in one daughter cell, leaving the other daughter cell with no chromosome of this type. Alternatively, one of the chromosomes lags as the cell is dividing and gets left out of both daughter cells (*anaphase lagging*). Thus we may have in the case of the sex chromosomes, XXX, XXY, or XYY, in one cell, and X or Y in the other. The XXX individual is known as a 'super female', and though reproductively she belies this title, she is otherwise of normal appearance, but may have learning difficulties; XXY is a eunuchoid male (Klinefelter syndrome); and XYY is a tall male (these individuals were reported to be mentally subnormal and to have criminal tendencies, but this has been disproven by further studies). The XO individual has Turner syndrome, and can be recognized at birth if the attendant is alert; the YO conceptus is nonviable. Other mechanisms which produce chromosomal anomalies include *translocation*, where part of one chromosome is added to another (this may be *balanced*, if the total complement of genetic material is normal, or *unbalanced* if this is not so), and *isochromosome* formation, where the

TABLE 17.2   APPROXIMATE INCIDENCE OF THE MORE COMMON CHROMOSOMAL ABNORMALITIES

	Per 1,000 spontaneous abortions	Per 1,000 second * trimester amniocenteses	Per 1,000 ** livebirths
Triploidy (3 × 23 chromosomes)	55	—	—
Tetraploidy (4 × 23 chromosomes)	15	—	—
Autosomal abnormalities			
Trisomy 21 (Down syndrome)	20	12.0	1.2
Trisomy 18 (Edward syndrome)	5	2.4	0.1
Trisomy 13 (Patau syndrome)	5	0.6	0.1
Trisomy 16	55	—	—
Other	80	3.5	2.0
Sex chromosome abnormalities			
47,XXX	5	2.5	1.0
47,XXY (Klinefelter)	5	3.3	1.0
47,XYY	5	0.7	1.0
45,XO (Turner syndrome)	50	1.0	0.1
Other	—	0.7	0.6
Total	300	26.7	7.1

* Figures derived from a combined series of 53,000 amniocenteses; ** figures derived from a survey of 56,000 newborn infants. The incidence and range of abnormalities is greater among abortions than livebirths — e.g. monosomy XO is about 500 times more common in abortions

separation of the chromosome pair is in the transverse rather than the longitudinal axis, producing 2 long arms or 2 short arms joined together rather than 1 short and 1 long arm in each daughter cell.

Mosaicism arises when *the abnormal chromosome formation occurs after formation of the gametes and conception* (mitotic nondisjunction); the earlier in the cleavage process that this takes place, the greater will be the clone of abnormal cells. Conversely, if later, the diluting effect of the normal cells may mask the anomaly.

Unlike Mendelian disorders, which are usually passed from the parents to their offspring, *numerical chromosomal anomalies usually arise de novo due to faulty cell division*, although translocations run within families.

Clinical Chromosomal Disorders

If there are too few or too many chromosomes, the fetus will either not develop (usually cast out as a 'blighted ovum' in the process of abortion) or will develop abnormally. Whereas development is possible with loss of one of the sex chromosomes (e.g. Turner syndrome, XO), it is not possible if there is absence of the X in the male individual (YO) or absence of one of the autosomes, since too much genetic material would be absent. The loss or addition of smaller parts of the chromosome produces less clinically obvious anomalies.

The role of chromosomal anomalies in spontaneous abortion has only been recognized in recent years. In some 40% of patients, the cause of the abortion is a chromosomal defect — the most common being a numerical abnormality

such as trisomy (e.g. for chromosome 21, table 17.2); a triple set of chromosomes (triploidy — 3 × 23 = 69, figure 17.3) instead of the normal double set (2 × 23 = 46); or monosomy (XO). The majority of conceptuses with major chromosome abnormalities (e.g. XO (Turner syndrome), trisomy 21, trisomy 18) are not viable and result in spontaneous abortion.

The *incidence* of chromosomal anomalies at birth is approximately 0.6% (table 17.2); the figure is higher if small for gestational age babies are considered (2–3%), higher again in the population of perinatal deaths (6%), and higher still in spontaneous abortions (40–50%). The chromosomal anomalies listed in table 17.2 are often associated with a characteristic clinical picture and thus the presence of a certain pattern of anomalies should suggest the need for chromosomal study. This test is expensive and time consuming and thus a consultant opinion should be sought.

One of the striking findings in relation to the incidence of chromosomal disorders is the marked increase with age, especially that of the mother. *Down syndrome* (trisomy 21) has an incidence of approximately 1 in 300 at 35, 1 in 200 at 37, 1 in 100 at 40 and 1 in 20 at 45 years (table 65.4).

The average positive diagnostic rate for patients referred for cytogenetic study is 10%; in many individuals with sex chromosome anomalies, the diagnosis is not made until after puberty, and with 'milder' anomalies (e.g. the triple X syndrome) the diagnosis is often never made because of the infrequency of structural or functional defect.

The *clinical features* of the commoner chromosomal disorders are considered in the companion gynaecological text (Illustrated Textbook of Gynaecology).

The *obstetric significance* is mainly related to *diagnosis*. This may be made *early in the second trimester by amniocentesis* if there is a known translocation carrier or advanced maternal age. The test is not usually undertaken, because of the risk to the pregnancy, if termination is not an acceptable outcome to the couple. This should be discussed before amniocentesis is performed.

The possibility of fetal anomaly should be considered in all patients with clinical evidence of fetal growth retardation, polyhydramnios or oligohydramnios. Diagnosis of the anomaly (e.g. by ultrasonography) may influence the options regarding the type of delivery.

GENES AND THEIR ANOMALIES

Genes are minute structures on the chromosomes and thus cannot be recognized. Nevertheless, their absence or malfunction can be inferred on the basis of known defects produced in the offspring or from family trees of affected individuals.

It was mentioned in the introduction that the genes regulated the sequence of amino acids (the basic building blocks) in the growth process. If a gene is damaged or is changed (i.e. undergoes a mutation) it may specify a wrong number or type of amino acid into the building process. A familiar example might be a temporarily unbalanced builder selecting cardboard sheeting for the roof of a house, rather than metal sheeting. Clinical examples are seen in the conditions

of thalassaemia (Mediterranean anaemia), and the so-called inborn errors of metabolism (phenylketonuria, galactosaemia).

In each case, there is deletion of a gene or a wrong amino acid or protein sequence in a body component (the globin molecule in the case of thalassaemia, or a vital enzyme in the inborn errors of metabolism).

Types of Gene Disorder (table 17.3)

Dominant and recessive conditions. Essentially, if a genetic defect is *clinically expressed when it comes from only one of the parents, it is dominant;* if *it is only expressed when both parents carry the gene it is recessive* (i.e. the normal gene overshadows the abnormal gene).

This is why marriage between blood relatives carries a somewhat higher risk than between unrelated individuals. The risk of the progeny receiving the same recessive gene from related parents is much greater than from unrelated parents. The more closely related the higher the risk — e.g. father–daughter 20%, first cousins 4%.

If the child has an *abnormal recessive gene from each parent, he or she will be affected clinically* and is termed *homozygous* for the particular abnormal gene; the sexes are equally affected. The parents, on the other hand, each have one abnormal recessive gene and one normal gene, and are thus *heterozygous* for the abnormal gene (carriers) and clinically normal.

Sex Linked Conditions

X-linked recessive. In some 60 disorders (e.g. *haemophilia,* and *Duchenne muscle dystrophy*)

TABLE 17.3   NATURE OF SOME IMPORTANT GENETIC DISORDERS

Nature of gene	Type of malformations
Dominant	Polycystic kidney (adult type)*
	Huntington chorea, tuberous sclerosis, neurofibromatosis
	Osteogenesis imperfecta (types 1 and 4 ± 3)*, Marfan syndrome
	Myotonic dystrophy
	Retinoblastoma, polyposis coli
Recessive	Polycystic kidney (infant type)*
	Cystic fibrosis, haemoglobinopathies, mucopolysaccharide storage disorders
	Spinal muscular atrophy (Werdnig-Hoffmann disease), hepatolenticular degeneration (Wilson disease)
	Osteogenesis imperfecta (type 2 ± 3)
	Phenylketonuria, adrenogenital syndrome, galactosaemia
	Pseudocholinesterase deficiency
Sex linked	Haemophilia A and B, Duchenne muscular dystrophy, agammaglobulinaemia, glucose-6-phosphate dehydrogenase deficiency, colour blindness
Multifactorial	Potter syndrome, cleft lip and palate, congenital heart disease, dislocation of hips, talipes

* These are examples of genetic heterogeneity

the gene mutation is *sex linked* — i.e. it is on the X chromosome. Again, the normal gene will overshadow the abnormal gene, so that females will be carriers but unaffected, whereas males will all be affected. *X-linked dominant* conditions exist, but are very rare (e.g. vitamin D-resistant rickets); in this group, females are affected since the other X chromosome is not protective as in recessive conditions. Accurate sex determination is now possible with chorion biopsy (figures 13.7 and 17.1) using a Y chromosome specific DNA probe.

Inheritance Patterns

The abnormal *dominant gene* may be transmitted from a parent or may arise in the patient's gametes or those of her husband by new mutation. Huntington chorea is typical of the former, whereas achondroplasia is typical of the latter. In contrast to the recessive gene, dominant genes produce the full clinical picture in the heterozygous state and there are no carriers. The risk for each pregnancy is 1 in 2, regardless of the sex of the fetus.

If both parents carry the same *recessive gene*, on average 1 in 4 of the children will be affected, 2 in 4 will be carriers, and 1 in 4 will be unaffected; all offspring of a person with a recessive disorder will carry the abnormal gene.

If the female is carrying a *sex linked recessive gene* (X•) there is a 1 in 2 chance that a male infant will be affected (X•Y) or normal (XY), and a 1 in 2 chance that a female infant will be a carrier (X•X) or normal (XX). An affected male can produce only normal males (XY) and carrier females (XX•).

In dominant sex linked disorders, the female (XX) can transmit to both male and female progeny, but the male (XY) can only transmit to females.

Multifactorial inheritance is when multiple genes are involved. Blood group inheritance is an all or none phenomenon, but graded characteristics such as height, eye colour, blood pressure, finger prints, and to a certain extent, intelligence, require multiple gene involvement; also, some processes of development, such as closure of the facial clefts, is determined in this way. Malfunction will give rise to such disorders as cleft lip and palate; mental deficiency, epilepsy, cardiac anomalies, and neural tube defects.

Important Gene Disorders

Haemoglobinopathies

These are of special interest because of their frequency and potential for diagnosis by modern laboratory methods. There are over 250 abnormal haemoglobins, but only a handful are of major clinical importance; these are dealt with in Chapter 34. Patients in the heterozygote state are seldom seriously affected clinically, but homozygotes may suffer fetal death, death in infancy, or major morbidity and the need for multiple transfusions throughout life. Education of groups at risk for the different types of thalassaemia and sickle cell anaemia is important as is counselling of couples before and during pregnancy. Determination of the presence of an abnormal haemoglobin gene in one or both parents facilitates decisions regarding the need for fetal diagnosis; the latter can be established by DNA studies from uncultured or cultured amniotic fluid cells (amniocentesis), or trophoblast cells (chorion biopsy — figure 17.1). Fetal blood sampling from a vein on the fetal surface of the placenta (by *fetoscopy*) or *cardiac puncture* (under ultrasound control) allows direct studies of globin chain synthesis.

Inherited Disorders of Metabolism

There are 200–300 such disorders, most being rare or very rare. Their frequency is related to the carrier state in a particular population which ranges from 1 in 50–1 in 1,000 or more; thus, the risk of 2 carriers marrying and producing an affected offspring will range from 1 in 2,500 to 1 in 1,000,000.

The defect is usually caused by reduced or absent function of an enzyme necessary for some aspect of intermediary metabolism. This results in either a build-up of toxic precursor material (e.g. absence of phenylalanine hydroxylase causes an excess of phenylalanine which normally would be converted to tyrosine), or absence of an important end product (e.g. adrenocortical hormone because of the lack of an hydroxylating enzyme). Detection of inherited disorders of metabolism involves study of enzymes in cultured amniotic fluid cells or chorion cells.

Some disorders, e.g. the relatively common cystic fibrosis, have proved to have a 'will o' the wisp' quality — each new diagnostic technique failing to stand up to critical clinical use.

Considerable progress has been made in many of the disorders — with affected and sometimes carrier individuals being accurately identified. *Phenylketonuria* is a disorder of considerable obstetrical significance. The affected baby is normal at birth because of the clearance of the toxic precursor (phenylalanine) by the mother during intrauterine life. If the disorder is not detected soon after birth, the baby will suffer from neurological toxicity (seizures, mental defect). With a low phenylalanine diet, the individual may develop normally and reproduce. A woman with phenylketonuria must have a strict diet maintained from before conception and throughout pregnancy otherwise the toxic metabolic build-up will damage the fetus. All babies are now screened for phenylketonuria by examination of a heel-prick blood sample taken before leaving hospital. This disorder can now be diagnosed in utero using DNA techniques.

The same principles of public education regarding risk groups, adequate counselling, and antenatal diagnosis apply as for the haemoglobinopathies among Mediterranean people and Tay-Sachs disease amongst Ashkenazic Jews.

NEURAL TUBE DEFECTS

Types of Anomaly
The central nervous system develops from primitive ectoderm over the cranial and dorsal part of the fetus. A neural groove develops and neural crests close over this from each side. A range of anomalies may occur as a result of malfunction of this process — from spina bifida occulta to absence of the cranium, called anencephaly (figures 49.4, 49.6 and 51.4; colour plate 110). The defect commonly allows herniation of the meninges and spinal cord, often resulting in partial or complete paralysis (usually of the lower part of the body) — called spina bifida.

Incidence
This varies from one country to another: for example, the incidence of spina bifida is 0.2% in Finland whereas it is over 0.4% in Northern Ireland. There is some evidence of a general fall over the past 5-10 years. If 1 previous child has a neural tube defect, the incidence rises to 4-5%; if 2 or more are affected, the risk is 10%.

Aetiology
It is probably partly genetic and partly environmental. Those of Celtic origin and those in lower socioeconomic classes are at greater risk; maternal nutrition is thought to be a factor.

Significance
There is a large wastage of fetuses with neural tube defects — approximately 40% will be aborted (5% of all abortions will have a neural tube defect) and 20% will be stillborn. With surgery, 50% will survive 5 years, but only 1-2% will have no residual handicap. *In the great majority of patients (90%), the anomaly will not be expected on the basis of past history.*

Diagnosis

Alpha fetoprotein (AFP). This protein is the major protein in blood in early fetal life and is normally raised in both the amniotic fluid and maternal serum when the fetus has an open neural tube defect; this is presumably due to leakage of plasma through the exposed meninges. The normal levels according to the period of gestation are shown in table 17.4.

TABLE 17.4   NORMAL RANGE OF ALPHA FETOPROTEIN LEVELS IN AMNIOTIC FLUID ACCORDING TO THE PERIOD OF GESTATION*

Gestation (weeks)	Alpha fetoprotein (mg/l)
14	7-35
15	5-34
16	2-32
17	1-28
18	< 23
20	< 21

* These values cover the time in which genetic counselling amniocentesis is performed — i.e. before it is too late for therapeutic abortion. Each reference laboratory will establish its own values — in open neural tube defects and anencephaly these are more than 2 and 5 standard deviations, respectively, above the mean

A general screening programme has been started in a number of countries where neural tube defects are relatively common. This involves taking a blood sample from the mother, usually at the 16th-17th week of gestation and analysing it for AFP level. If it is above a previously selected limit (e.g. 2.5 or 3 standard deviations above the normal mean), the patient undergoes further study — firstly by ultrasound (to verify the period of gestation, and to scan the head and spine) and then by amniocentesis. To reduce costs and improve efficiency, it is desirable that serum and amniotic fluid AFP analyses are done in the same centre.

The plasma AFP technique has a small *false positive rate* — even at a 3 standard deviation cut off there will be 1-2% of apparently normal fetuses. This may result from placental leaks or degeneration; trauma at the time of amniocentesis will act similarly if any fetal blood escapes into the amniotic fluid. In addition, a number of other conditions may cause an elevation of AFP in the amniotic fluid and/or maternal blood: these include error in dates, multiple pregnancy, fetal congenital nephrosis or renal agenesis, abdominal wall defects (omphalocele), sacral teratoma, impending abortion, and possibly maternal stress. The *false negative rate* depends largely on accuracy of menstrual dates, because the upper limit of normal falls with advancing gestation (table 17.4); sampling of *maternal urine* instead of amniotic fluid can also cause confusion — a fluid with very few cells and an AFP concentration less than 1 mg/l renders it suspect. The level in women with a Down syndrome fetus may be subnormal.

It should be emphasized that there is no truly 'diagnostic' level: the value chosen represents a compromise between *specificity* (excluding causes not due to neural tube defects, and *sensitivity* (picking up as many affected fetuses as possible).

For the above reasons, a decision to terminate a pregnancy should never be made on the grounds of an elevated maternal plasma AFP level alone. There are still a number of imponderables in a plasma AFP screening programme — ultimate cost:benefit, quality control of participating laboratories, ensuring accuracy of gestational age, and finally, the occasional results which are at variance with the fetal condition.

Amniocentesis. This is usually carried out after the period of gestation has been confirmed by ultrasound study of the fetus. Due to the increasing sophistication (and thus accuracy) of ultrasonography, all but the minor defects are usually detected and amniocentesis may not be necessary. In addition, multiple pregnancy and intrauterine fetal death will be demonstrated. If amniocentesis is performed the fluid is analysed for AFP level, as for maternal plasma. If there is doubt, additional studies are made on the fluid — particularly *acetylcholinesterase* levels and the presence of cells which adhere rapidly to glass; these tests are particularly useful if there has been contamination of the amniotic fluid by fetal blood at amniocentesis (thus giving a spuriously high level of AFP). In rare cases *fetoscopy* may be undertaken.

Management

Prophylaxis. Preconceptual attention to nutrition, with *folic acid* and *vitamin* supplementation has been claimed to reduce the incidence.

Treatment. The option of antenatal diagnosis and termination of pregnancy is offered in most centres. However, there are a number of problems — the availability of maternal plasma screening, expert ultrasonography and amniotic fluid sampling, high level laboratory facilities, and clinical expertise. If the diagnosis is made in the first trimester by ultrasonography, termination is relatively simple; if at 16–18 weeks, the problems are greater.

Regardless of the doctor's personal viewpoint, current medicolegal opinion suggests that there is an obligation to advise patients of the different options available. In counselling, the couple will wish to know the frequency of neural tube defects (especially if there is a positive history), the accuracy, technique, and side-effects of amniocentesis, and finally, the anticipated severity of the disorder and the effect this could have on the child's future. Parents must then be allowed to make their own decision on the basis of information provided.

Because of religious or other conviction, some couples will eschew antenatal diagnosis and accept the problems of care of the affected baby.

GENETIC COUNSELLING

Since *2–3% of all babies will have a major congenital malformation* (table 65.2), it is of importance to be able to talk to the mother in realistic terms about why the present mishap occurred and what is the likelihood of the same or a similar thing happening in the future. This sort of information is essential for her and her husband to make an intelligent decision concerning future childbearing. In other instances, the couple in question may not have had a malformed child, but the family history may be of concern to them.

Genetic counselling is the science of assessment of genetic risk, on the basis of all available information from the family in question, together with the known facts of the causes and incidence of congenital diseases, and the giving of advice on the basis of this assessment. Such advice should be accurate, nondirective, and confidential. The meaning of such terms as 'a 1 in 4 risk' (e.g. for recessive gene conditions) should be explained since people have a poor concept of probability: i.e. there could be 2, 3 or even 4 affected infants in succession if one was statistically unlucky. The patient's obligations to her near relatives should be indicated.

Assessment of Genetic Risk; Nature of the Disorder

An accurate diagnosis is available in about 50% of families. Where there is only a history of disease in a relative, the problem is greater. The first essential is the construction of a *family tree* which should be as complete as possible, and the gathering of all relevant information about the disease from those living and from the records of those deceased. The possibility of *consanguinity* between husband and wife must be checked.

Does it appear to be hereditary? That is to say, is the disease, which is apparent at birth or sometime after, related to hereditary material (chromosomes and genes) or can it be positively identified as an isolated happening, due to some unfavourable environmental influence during the development of the embryo or fetus? Obvious environmental causes include drugs (thalidomide) and amniotic bands (traumatic amputation of a digit or limb — colour plate 113). The malformation may be recognized as being in either the hereditary or environmental category. In the absence of a diagnosis or specific pedigree pattern, empiric risk data are used. A further problem is the variability in the degree to which a person is affected by a certain abnormal gene; in some, the clinical features are fully expressed, in others they may be mild and almost unnoticeable.

In table 17.5, a list is given of the approximate recurrence risks of a number of common malformations, based on a wide experience of many families.

With recessive conditions, we are helped by a knowledge of the frequency of such abnormal genes in the population under consideration, and whether inbreeding is common in that community. The carrier rate for the gene causing thalassaemia may be as high as 1 in 10 in some Mediterranean countries; for cystic fibrosis in Western countries it is 1 in 22, whereas that for phenylketonuria is 1 in 50.

Experience indicates that comprehension is often incomplete in counselled patients, especially in chromosomal and sex-linked recessive disorders. All patients should receive a letter restating the advice given and offering follow-up, and the opportunity to discuss the problem again.

Consanguinity. The chance of cousins marrying differs from one culture to another; in many Western countries the incidence ranges from 1 in 500 to 1 in 1,000. The risk of congenital anomaly rises, but not greatly, and is mainly the result of recessive conditions; the risk of malformation in liveborn children is 1 in 25 (normal 1 in 30). *Incest* is a different matter; the risk of fetal death or malformation is 1 in 5 (20%).

The nature of the handicap. Another thing that the couple should be aware of is the prognosis of the disorder in terms of handicap, progression with time, and what treatment, if any, is available for the condition. At one end of the scale, we might have a condition such as *colour blindness*, which is only a mild handicap and shows no progression; at the other end, there may be a condition which, if present, is inevitably fatal, such as anencephaly. More troublesome are the conditions which, although not lethal, severely handicap the child mentally and/or physically (e.g. Down syndrome or muscular dystrophy) and may result in death in childhood or early adulthood. These aspects are further discussed in Chapter 65.

Perspective. In genetic counselling, one must assess the personalities of the couple and their attitudes. Important considerations include their age, educational background, number of previous normal and abnormal children, and coping qualities.

Many couples imagine that the risk of an abnormal child is close to zero, rather than 1 in 30. A risk rate of 1 in 20 or 1 in 25 then seems more reasonable. Looking on the optimistic side, one could equally say that there is a 19 out of 20

TABLE 17.5 APPROXIMATE RECURRENCE RISKS FOR COMMON MALFORMATIONS

Malformation	Sex of index patient	Risk if parents normal, one child affected*	Risk if one parent and one child affected**
Spina bifida or anencephaly	—	1 in 25	—
Pyloric stenosis	M	1 in 50	1 in 8
	F	1 in 10	2 in 5
Congenital hip dislocation		1 in 25	1 in 10
Hirschsprung disease	M	1 in 50	—
	F	1 in 12	—
Cleft lip and palate		1 in 25	1 in 8
Heart malformation		1 in 30	1 in 20
Talipes		1 in 30	1 in 10
Diabetes (juvenile)		1 in 30	—
Mental retardation		1 in 25	—
Schizophrenia		1 in 10	—

* Risk similar if one parent affected

** Accurate figures not established for all conditions listed — risk usually 2–5 times greater than if 1 parent or child affected probability that the child will be normal. For the higher risk categories (dominant, recessive, and sex-linked), the very real likelihood of an affected child must be considered. In addition, the differences between risks to further children, and the risks to their children's children must be explained, since this is usually quite different in the 3 high risk groups mentioned above.

The great majority of chromosomal disorders are sporadic, due to a chance happening, and are not genetic in the true sense unless involving a translocation which can be passed from parent to child; such translocations account for 3% of cases of Down syndrome. Patients who have had *multiple miscarriages* or who have had several children with different anomalies may have a translocation; they should be offered investigation, and if a translocation is identified, amniocentesis is indicated in a subsequent pregnancy.

The *fragile X chromosome disorder* has recently been recognized as the second most common chromosomal cause of retardation (after Down syndrome). This condition behaves like a sex linked disorder and requires specific cytogenetic techniques to detect it.

chapter eighteen

Bleeding in Early Pregnancy

OVERVIEW

By far, the commonest cause of early pregnancy bleeding is some type of *abortion*, usually threatened. Recent technological advances have contributed greatly to understanding early pregnancy and its management. *Ultrasonography* has enabled delineation of the intrauterine contents and determination of the presence and well-being of the embryo/fetus from the 6th–8th week. *Biochemical tests* that depend on trophoblastic activity (beta HCG, placental lactogen (HPL), oestrogen, progesterone) provide supportive evidence of the amount of this tissue that is present and functioning. The diagnosis of the different types of abortion (*threatened, incomplete, complete, missed*) has been simplified by these investigations, as has differentiation from other causes of early pregnancy bleeding (*ectopic pregnancy* and *hydatidiform mole*).

The new technique of *in vitro fertilization and embryo transfer* to the uterus has focused attention to the early weeks or even days of postconceptional life; it is now realized that there is a *very high early pregnancy loss* — at least 40% — most of which is subclinical, the pregnancy being identified only by the very sensitive beta HCG assay mentioned above.

When a recognizable conceptus has been aborted, cytogenetic study has indicated that in almost 50% there is a *chromosome abnormality*.

With the relaxation of *therapeutic abortion* laws in many countries there has been a rapid rise in the number of pregnancy terminations. The use of *prostaglandins* and *suction curettage* has done much to reduce the immediate and late complications of this procedure.

Ectopic pregnancy has increased in incidence both absolutely (probably because of the effect on the Fallopian tubes of the increased incidence of sexually transmitted infectious disease) and also relatively (because of the use of the intrauterine contraceptive device, which, unlike the pill, has little effect in preventing pregnancies in the Fallopian tube). As with abortion, diagnosis and clinical management have been greatly helped by ultrasonography and beta HCG assay.

Hydatidiform mole is a rare degenerative change in the trophoblast, usually resulting from a chromosomal defect in the conceptus. Its dangers are both immediate (*haemorrhage*) and distant (change to the malignant *choriocarcinoma*). *Suction curettage* is now the standard method of emptying the often relatively enlarged uterus of its vesicular contents. Careful follow-up in a special centre is necessary for such patients to detect (by beta HCG assay) any tendency to malignant change.

ABORTION

Definition

Expulsion or removal of the products of conception before the 28th week of gestation. It is not necessary for there to be an embryo or fetus present (empty sac, hydatidiform mole), or for the conceptus to be in the uterus (tubal abortion).

The term '*habitual*' abortion is applied when the patient has experienced *3 successive spontaneous abortions*.

Incidence

Ten to 15%, but if very early abortions are considered (i.e. beta HCG present) *the figure is between 45%–55%*. The great majority of early spontaneous abortions are not diagnosed and masquerade as heavy, often late periods. This was established by laboratory biochemical confirmation of pregnancy (serial *beta HCG* assays) in patients having intrauterine devices removed because they wished to conceive, and in those followed carefully after in vitro fertilization and embryo transfer.

Classification

Abortion may be spontaneous or induced (table 18.1).

Three features may be used to distinguish the different forms of spontaneous abortion (figure 18.1). Firstly, whether the *cervix is closed* (threatened, missed, complete) or open (inevitable, incomplete); secondly, whether *products of conception have been passed* (incomplete or complete) or not (threatened, missed), and finally, whether the *uterus is equal in size to the period of amenorrhoea* (threatened, inevitable), or smaller (incomplete, complete, missed).

Aetiology

(i) *Maldevelopment of the conceptus.* This may range from complete absence of the fetus to major or minor abnormalities (colour plate 8). Similarly, the trophoblast may be defective and/or poorly embedded in the endometrium. Very often, fetal maldevelopment is caused by an addition, subtraction, or defect of one or more of the chromosomes, or a genetic defect in the presence of a normal chromosome number (46).

TABLE 18.1   TYPES OF ABORTION

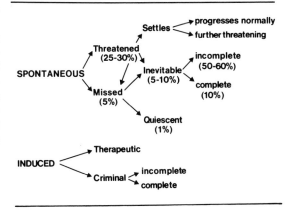

* The percentages in brackets represent the incidences of the different types of abortion when the patient is first seen.

Such abnormalities account for approximately 50% of spontaneous abortions, but mostly they are nonrecurrent. The earlier the abortion, the more likely is a chromosomal anomaly to be the cause (trisomy, especially 15, 16, 21, 22;

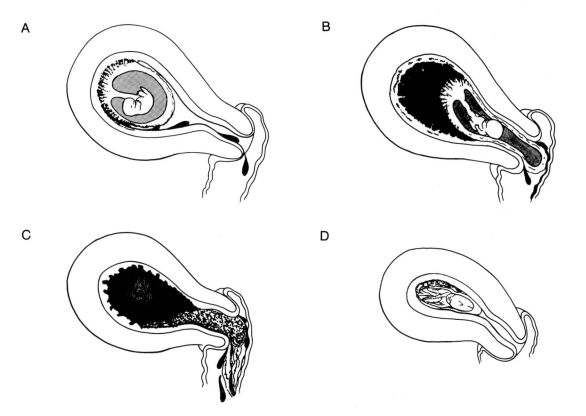

Figure 18.1 Types of abortion. **A.** Threatened: bleeding, perhaps some pain, cervix closed, uterine size commensurate with dates. **B.** Inevitable: heavier bleeding, always pain, cervix open, uterine size in keeping with dates. **C.** Incomplete: bleeding, pain, passage of placental tissue, cervix open, uterus smaller than dates. **D.** Missed: usually preceded by threatened abortion, cervix tightly closed, uterus much smaller than dates.

monosomy, especially XO; triploidy): months 1–3, 60%; month 4, 45%; month 5, 12%; month 6, 6%; term, 0.6%. *A chromosomal abnormality is present in 75–85% of blighted embryos, but only 5% or less of 'normal' embryos.*

(ii) *Endocrine.* In occasional patients, the amount of progesterone secreted from the corpus luteum of the ovary (up to 6–8 weeks) or placenta (after 8 weeks) is deficient. This may result in poor decidual development or an abnormally irritable uterus, and hence abortion. In most cases, the low level of progesterone is the result of trophoblastic/placental failure rather than the cause.

Women taking oral contraceptives are said to have twice the chance of aborting if they become pregnant; if true this could result from an effect on the endocrine system or on germ cell development, or less interest by the patient in the pregnancy. Other endocrine disorders (thyroid, adrenal) if significant, usually prevent conception, but may also cause abortion.

(iii) *Psychological.* Stress and anxiety can adversely affect the autonomic nervous system/adrenal glands, and hence blood vessels and smooth muscles. A typical example would be an unmarried mother with little family or other support.

(iv) *Mechanical.* Irritation or trauma to the uterus, either by clinical examinations, *coitus,* accidents, abdominal operations or peritonitis, may produce uterine contractions and disturbance of the implanted embryo.

(v) *Uterine abnormalities. Malformations of the uterus* (bicornuate, septate), or malpositions (marked anteflexion, retroflexion), or *fibroids* (especially submucous) may upset the normal progress of development. The presence of 2 ascending uterine arteries (rather than the normal 1) is associated with an increased tendency to abortion (and fetal growth retardation if the pregnancy continues). Diethylstilboestrol (DES) exposure in the mother's own prenatal period may produce uterine abnormalities and thus increase the incidence of abortion in later life.

An *incompetent cervix* (idiopathic, or due to previous trauma) may fail to retain the conceptus as the uterus expands in the second trimester (colour plate 3). Finally, the *decidual bed* may be relatively barren as a result of previous surgery or infection, and the embryo gains a poor foothold.

(vi) *Acquired disease.* Any disease, acute or chronic, may cause abortion if severe enough — for example, infections (pneumonia, influenza, rubella, toxoplasmosis) and hypertensive-renal disorders.

(vii) *Drugs.* Antimetabolite drugs used for treating cancer or diseases of immune origin; also anaesthetic gases (female anaesthetists and operating room nurses have an increased incidence of spontaneous abortion).

(viii) *Immunological.* There is little definite evidence, but there is a possible basis for some recurrent abortions.

(ix) *The father.* Coitus as a factor has been mentioned. Apart from creating an unfavourable psychological climate, the only other likely paternal factor is an abnormal gene or chromosome — i.e. genetic.

In *habitual abortion,* the cause is often mechanical, such as incompetent cervix or uterine abnormality. In other patients there may be a psychological, immunological, chromosomal, or infective basis. Such patients should be referred for specialist care.

Clinical Features

Pregnancy. Symptoms and signs are usually present.

Bleeding. This is most frequent and severe in incomplete abortion, less in threatened and inevitable abortion, and least in missed abortion. *In complete abortion,* the loss is variable during the abortion, but thereafter usually ceases entirely. Thus, a heavy, bright loss with clots suggests incomplete abortion; a dark brown loss suggests a missed abortion. Bright red blood indicates the process is active; brown or black loss represents a past episode of bleeding. Although in the majority of patients with threatened abortion the pregnancy continues uneventfully, the *risk of abortion is proportional to the amount of bleeding*; if the loss continues or recurs or if there is any associated *pain,* the prognosis is usually unfavourable; *if admission to hospital is necessary, 60–80% of patients will abort.* Thus, bleeding is an ominous symptom in the early months of pregnancy.

Pain. This is experienced when the cervix is dilating and products of conception are being passed. It may be barely noticed by some patients with incompetence of the cervix, but may be worse than labour in others. The pain is felt in the lower abdomen or back, is usually cramp-like, and follows the bleeding — in contrast to the sequence in ectopic pregnancy.

Passage of products of conception. The passage of definite tissue is characteristic of incomplete and complete abortion, and does not occur in threatened, inevitable, or missed abortions. A confusing picture is presented when the decidual lining of the uterus is passed in ectopic pregnancy (*decidual cast*), since this simulates trophoblastic tissue (figure 18.2). The passage of clear fluid indicates *rupture of the membranes* (chorion and amnion); whereas if the fluid is thick and albuminous it suggests that the cervix is dilating in the condition of *incompetent cervix*. In many abortions, no fetus is passed at any time, since it is either absent (blighted ovum) or rudimentary and unnoticed.

Differential Diagnosis

(i) Abnormal pregnancy (ectopic, hydatidiform mole). (ii) Normal pregnancy, *other causes of bleeding* (cancer of the cervix, erosion, vaginitis). (iii) Normal pregnancy, *other causes of pain* (appendicitis, ruptured corpus luteum cyst). (iv) Nonpregnancy conditions: amenorrhoea followed by bleeding may occur for a number of reasons (metropathia haemorrhagica, ovarian tumours or cysts) (figure 18.3).

Prognosis

Most patients are worried about both the immediate and long-term implications of bleeding in early pregnancy. No immediate assurances can be given regarding continuation of the pregnancy, but when *endocrine and ultrasound data* are added to the clinical features, a fairly reliable picture can be given of the normality or otherwise of the pregnancy and the likelihood of its progressing.

Although vaginal bleeding, no matter how minor, has a detrimental effect on the outcome of pregnancy, this should not be stressed when counselling the patient. It is equally correct, and more reassuring to state the facts in a positive manner — namely that if the pregnancy continues past 20 weeks, *95% of infants will survive* and the *incidence of major fetal malformations is*

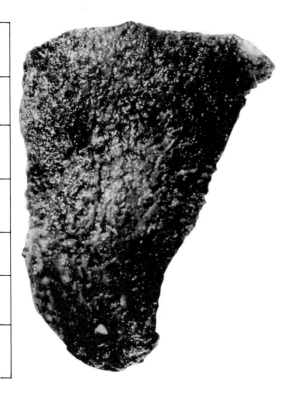

Figure 18.2 Decidual cast. After withdrawal of hormones due to death of the ectopic chorionic villi, the thickened endometrium is shed — usually in fragments as in menstruation, but sometimes as a single piece or decidual cast of the uterus, which may be mistaken for placental tissue (uterine abortion).

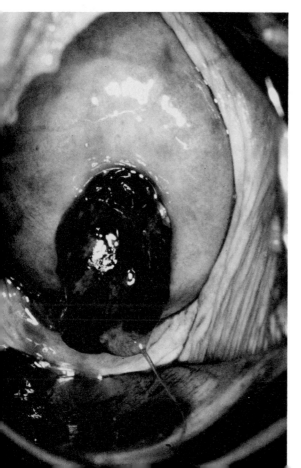

Figure 18.3 Haemorrhagic decidua and secretory endometrium protruding through the cervix and simulating an incomplete abortion. The patient was a 27-year-old para 1 who presented with 5 days' bleeding (similar to menses) after 12 weeks' amenorrhoea. The uterus was the size of a pregnancy of 10 weeks' maturity. The diagnosis of incomplete abortion was refuted by histological absence of placental villi or fetal parts. Extrauterine pregnancy could account for the amenorrhoea, uterine enlargement and extensive decidua formation. The message is that histology is required to diagnose early placental tissue.

TABLE 18.2 RESULTS IN 3,237 PATIENTS WITH THREATENED ABORTION WHOSE PREGNANCIES CONTINUED PAST 20 WEEKS' GESTATION, COMPARED WITH THE TOTAL HOSPITAL POPULATION OF 40,982 PATIENTS (TABLES 16.1 AND 16.4)

	Threatened abortion %	Total population %
Delivered between 20-28 weeks	3.0	1.0
Multiple pregnancy	2.0	1.4
Placenta praevia	2.1	0.9
Abruptio placentae	1.8	1.0
Major malformation	5.4	4.1
Minor malformation	8.6	7.1
Perinatal mortality rate	4.9	2.6

increased by only 1.3%. Table 18.2 shows the results in a series of 3,237 such patients who had vaginal bleeding before 20 weeks. *These patients comprised 7.9% of the total population.* There was a trebled incidence of *delivery before 28 weeks*, and about a doubled incidence of *multiple pregnancy, placenta praevia, abruptio placentae* and *perinatal mortality.* Most of the increase in the malformation rate was accounted for by the patients who delivered between 20–28 weeks' gestation.

Management

(i) Admission to hospital is arranged if the bleeding is causing concern. (ii) Bed rest with toilet privileges. (iii) A history of possible aetiological factors is obtained, together with details of bleeding, pain, material passed. (iv) Examination is carried out gently — speculum and bimanual palpation. (v) Vital signs must be observed and charted. (vi) Pads and aborted material are saved for inspection and possible pathological study; blood loss is charted. Vulval toilet is carried out twice a day or more often according to the amount of bleeding. (vii) Special investigations will usually include haemoglobin, blood group and Rh typing, cross-matching of blood, cervical swab for culture, blood culture if major sepsis is present, and pregnancy test. *Ultrasound study* is valuable from the 7th week to determine whether a fetus is present; realtime sonography will detect fetal movement and thus life from this time; *if fetal motion is not present, abortion is almost inevitable.* A *fetal sac* is usually identifiable between the 5th and 6th weeks, but the sac diameter may be normal up to the 9th week even if there is a blighted embryo. However, HCG levels may be normal up to the 12th week in cases of blighted ovum — i.e. the under-

lying defect (usually chromosomal) affects embryonic/fetal development more than that of the trophoblast. Tests involving placental hormones — human chorionic gonadotrophin (HCG), oestradiol, progesterone, human placental lactogen (HPL) and pregnancy specific beta$_1$ glycoprotein (SP$_1$) — are useful up to the 9th week in determining if the fetus is still alive; *if levels are low, 90–95% will abort*; the converse is less reliable — i.e. normal levels in the presence of bleeding are still associated with abortion in 20–30% of patients. (viii) An explanation is given to the patient, together with reassurance which is reasonably compatible with the presumed diagnosis; the majority of threatened abortions will settle down without incident — patients are always relieved to hear this and readily accept the explanation that abortion will occur if the fetus is not 'all right'. (ix) Tranquillizers may be helpful if the patient is anxious; diazepam settles the patient and relaxes the uterus. (x) A sedative at night is usually ordered. (xi) If pain is severe, pethidine is ordered; if less troublesome, a compound codeine preparation is given.

Further Management

This will depend on the type of abortion.

(i) *Threatened.* The conservative measures as outlined above are continued. If a fetus is shown to be present and alive, progesterone or a likeproduct may be ordered if the level is low. Ward activity is commenced when bleeding has ceased; usually the patient is allowed home in a further 2 days. Suitable advice is given concerning reasonable curtailment of activities. *Coitus should be avoided for 2–3 weeks*, longer if the abortion is recurrent. Iron and folic acid therapy is ordered; bleeding is seldom sufficient to require transfusion.

(ii) *Inevitable.* The usual picture is one of progressive cervical dilatation and cramping pain leading to rupture of the membranes, passage of products of conception, and bleeding. A special type comprises the *incompetent cervix*, with prolapse and rupture of the membranes after 'silent' dilatation of the cervix. In the last group, suture of the cervix before the membranes have ruptured may save the pregnancy. Otherwise preparations are made for anaesthesia and curettage. In the second trimester, labour may not follow membrane rupture, and stimulation by *oxytocin or prostaglandin* may be necessary. There is no place for conservative treatment if the membranes rupture before 20 weeks' gestation since serious infection may ensue. Bleeding is rarely troublesome before abortion has taken place.

(iii) *Incomplete.* This is easily the most common presentation and causes the most trouble from bleeding and shock; *blood transfusion* is required in about 3-5% of patients.

First trimester abortion is characterized by *piecemeal extrusion of placental tissue* (since the placenta has not yet developed into a discrete disc), and *continued haemorrhage* — therefore curettage is usually necessary.

Emergency treatment may be required in the form of ergometrine, 0.5 mg IV to halt haemorrhage, and elevation of the patient's legs if shock is present. Medical aid must be sought immediately. If the patient has lost a lot of blood or is shocked, *resuscitation* must be effected before transfer to hospital. An *intravenous infusion* of glucose saline, 1 litre, followed by Hartmann solution, 1 litre, or stable plasma protein solution (SPPS) or comparable plasma expander is necessary. If no medical aid is available, and the situation does not improve with ergometrine or Syntometrine, the presence of *retained products in the cervix should be sought and removed* after cleansing the vulva and applying a liberal amount of obstetric cream to the gloved hand. The abdominal hand is used to exert counter pressure on the uterine fundus. *Bimanual compression* may be useful in controlling the bleeding. Vital signs must be recorded every 5-10 minutes until the patient's condition has improved.

Usually, the bleeding is much less troublesome, and after the diagnosis has been made, the patient is prepared for curettage.

(iv) *Complete.* This type of abortion may occur after 14-16 weeks but seldom before. The diagnosis is made on the findings of minimal blood loss, a closed cervix, and passage of a complete trophoblastic sac or placenta (colour plate 3). The management is conservative.

(v) *Missed.* Although fetal death in utero has decreased in incidence, missed abortion has become somewhat more common (about 1% of pregnancies). The diagnosis is difficult to make initially, since findings are similar to threatened abortion. Usually the symptoms of pregnancy (such as nausea and breast changes) subside and the uterus becomes progressively smaller. Ultrasonic study now can readily distinguish between them because fetal heart activity can be detected very early by this method.

In early pregnancies (before 8 weeks' gestation) or when menstrual data are uncertain (and hence interpretation of ultrasound findings), estimations of plasma or urine hormone levels (*oestrogen*, *progesterone*) are useful in diagnosing the presence of an intact pregnancy

— thus avoiding prolonged hospitalization when the fetus is not viable, and incorrect management (curettage) when the fetus *is* viable.

When the diagnosis is confirmed, *dilatation and curettage* is indicated if the uterus is smaller than that of an intact pregnancy of 10-12 weeks' maturity; bleeding may be copious and the *suction curette* has advantages in these patients. At this stage a carneous mole may have formed; here the fetal sac is entombed in layers of fibrin and organizing blood from repeated haemorrhages.

(a) Dilatation and Curettage

Preliminary measures. Consent forms must be signed by the patient and husband or other relevant person. Blood is cross-matched if the patient is shocked or excessive bleeding is anticipated.

Requirements. The instruments, including the vacuum aspirator for the removal of products of conception, are shown in figure 56.5.

Anaesthetic. General, epidural, paracervical block (2.5 ml of 1% lignocaine at clock positions 2,4,8 and 10, plus a further 2.5 ml into each uterosacral ligament), or lytic cocktail (diazepam 5-10 mg, pethidine 50 mg, promethazine 25 mg serially (by slow IV injection) may be used); atropine 0.3 mg IV is also necessary.

Technique. The patient is placed in the lithotomy position and the vulva is antiseptically prepared and draped. A catheter is passed to empty the bladder so that bimanual examination can confirm the state of the cervix, the *position and size of the uterus*, and absence of adnexal masses (ectopic pregnancy, ovarian cyst). An Auvard or other type of vaginal speculum is inserted and the anterior lip of the cervix is grasped with volsellum forceps. A *sound* is passed to the uterine fundus; this confirms the uterine position and measures the depth of the cavity. If necessary, the cervix is dilated by means of *Hegar dilators* or another suitable method (vibrodilator). Polyp, sponge, or ovum forceps are used to remove large pieces of placental tissue and this is followed by systematic curettage of the whole cavity; if a *therapeutic abortion* is being done, the cervix must be dilated sufficiently to allow introduction of sponge forceps or the vacuum extractor probe. The latter is faster, safer, and requires less dilatation of the cervix.

Both curettage and vacuum aspiration are more difficult and dangerous after the 12th week of pregnancy. Uterine aspiration in particular is unlikely to be effective because of the density of fetal parts and the degree of adherence of the placenta to the uterine wall.

Oxytocin 10 units or ergometrine 0.5 mg, is usually given at the conclusion of the operation, or earlier if the uterus is large, soft, or bleeding; the injection can be given into the anterior wall of the uterus after dilatation of the cervix but prior to evacuation.

The curettings are placed in a labelled jar of formalin-saline and submitted for pathological study.

Postoperative Care

(i) *Recovery.* The patient is placed in the recovery room until fully conscious, then transferred to the ward. (ii) *Observations* of pulse rate, blood pressure, and respiratory rate are made and recorded, together with the amount of vaginal bleeding. The patient's colour and conscious state are also recorded. Instructions concerning intravenous infusion therapy are followed. (iii) Fluids are given 2–4 hours after the operation, and a light diet if the former is tolerated. (iv) *Further care.* If relevant (patient rhesus negative), *anti-D gamma globulin* IM is given to prevent rhesus isoimmunization. The patient is able to ambulate in 4–8 hours and can be discharged in 1–3 days depending on circumstances. The patient should be told to report any unusual bleeding or other symptoms, is provided with *contraceptive advice*, and given an appointment for review in 2–4 weeks.

Complications. The most serious complication of this operation is *uterine perforation* by one of the instruments (sound, sponge forceps, curette). This may result in intraperitoneal bleeding: thus the need for close postoperative surveillance; laparotomy may be necessary. Cervical dilatation beyond Hegar number 9–10 may damage the cervical sphincter and cause *cervical incompetence*: this is more likely in therapeutic abortions, where the cervical dilatation is relatively rapid. *Septic shock* may occasionally occur and requires vigorous management. Vaginal bleeding may continue, either from incomplete removal of the products of conception or from cervical or uterine trauma. Rarely, a diagnosis of *ruptured ectopic pregnancy* may have been missed, and collapse may occur because of intraperitoneal bleeding. Late complications include *infection* and *infertility*.

(b) Oxytocin Infusion

The usual indication is *premature rupture of the membranes* with failure to abort thereafter. An oxytocin infusion is set up as described under induction of labour (Chapter 44). However, because the uterus is 10–100 times less sensitive early in pregnancy, much higher concentrations may be required — up to 100 U or more of oxytocin per litre. Because of the danger of *fluid retention* (muscle irritability, headache, asthenia), the oxytocin should be added to Ringer lactate solution, a microdrip apparatus should be used, the infusion should not last longer than 12 hours, and a break of 8–12 hours should then elapse.

If the *abortion is recurrent*, a careful investigation of the factors mentioned earlier should be undertaken before the next pregnancy.

THERAPEUTIC ABORTION

Procedural Aspects and Indications

There has been a gradual relaxation in legal restrictions in many countries over the past 10–20 years. This has resulted from changing community opinion and a realization of the dangers of population pressures. Health education and advances in contraceptive technology have so far proved inadequate in many countries to control the latter. Formerly, this operation was either illegal or legal only to save the life of the mother. In the Abortion Act of 1967 in Britain, therapeutic abortion was legal if the risks to the life of the mother or to the physical/mental health of the mother or existing children was deemed greater than if the pregnancy was terminated; a further clause related to a substantial risk of handicap to the child from physical or mental abnormalities.

Regulations usually require the opinion of 2 doctors, the informed consent of both wife and husband, and that the operation be performed in a unit properly conducted for the purpose.

The *indications* may be *psychiatric ill-health* of the mother (the great majority usually); *physical ill-health* (functional impairment of one of the body systems — usually cardiac, renal, vascular, hepatic, or neurological); *diseases affecting the fetus* (viruses, especially rubella; rhesus haemolytic disease; hereditary disorders such as Down syndrome); or *sociomedical* (age extremes, rape, incest, inadequate personality).

In practical terms, unwanted pregnancies occur because there is lack of access to contraceptives, inconsistent use, or contraceptive failure; apart from bad luck, the recurrent unwanted pregnancy usually reflects a low impulse control, high libido, low realism and low capacity for integrated personal relationships. A change in life situation (e.g. desertion or imprisonment of partner) may precipitate a request for termination.

The following advantages of a more liberal

abortion programme, apart from considerations of population pressure, have been claimed: *reduction of 70% of illegal abortions* (which are dangerous, discriminatory, undignified and costly), and the provisions of *better counselling for future pregnancy prevention*.

In the history the following points should be clarified: reasons for seeking abortion; previous contraception and pregnancy experience; are there current stresses or losses — i.e. is there evidence of *emotional distress* beyond that caused by the pregnancy itself, and is the abortion expected to resolve this?; is there talk of *suicide* and does it persist after abortion is discussed?; what are the patient's plans and prospects after the abortion?; what is the degree of support by the parents and by the partner?

Examination will be directed to evaluation of physical disorders and personality characteristics (stability, maturity, intelligence, coping strength, alcohol and drug use etc).

Psychiatric referral will be necessary in all subjects with a present or suspected psychosis (schizophrenia, depression) or suicidal intention; others with significant life crisis problems or neuroses may also warrant consultation.

Methods of Termination

(a) *Very early pregnancy: menstrual regulation.* This is carried out within 2 weeks of a missed period: one technique is to use a fine suction catheter to empty the uterus (Karman catheter or Vibra aspirator); alternatively, *prostaglandin* (usually intrauterine) is used. A number of prostaglandin analogues have recently appeared and these have been effective in the *vaginal pessary* form. One successful regimen has been the use of 1 mg 15-methyl $PgF_2\alpha$ and 3 mg 3 hours later. With more experience and better compounds, termination of pregnancies up to 90 days or more after the LMP has been reported; beyond 40–45 days, however, the evacuation is seldom complete.

(b) *Mid–late first trimester.* Unfortunately, there are a number of reasons why the patient may not present early — e.g. the pregnancy was not suspected (previous sterilization, IUD or other contraceptive being used, menses irregular); patient ambivalent about pregnancy; concealed from parents if adolescent; depressed; unable to obtain medical involvement etc. These patients are usually managed by suction or classical instrumental dilatation and curettage. Failure to effect termination occurs in only about 1 in 1,000 cases, but if unrecognized may have serious medicolegal consequences.

(c) For therapeutic terminations when the uterus is larger than 12–14 weeks, the current method is administration of *prostaglandin* (Pg) E1, E2, or $F_2\alpha$ by the *intraamniotic route* ($F_2\alpha$ 30–40 mg, repeated if necessary in 12–18 hours; E_2 10 mg repeated if necessary in 12–18 hours); or *extraamniotically* via a catheter at intervals of 30–90 minutes ($F_2\alpha$ 750 μg; E_2, 200 μg) by a continuous infusion pump (1 ml = 50 μg PgE_2 per 30 minutes), or by a vaginal pessary or gel (PgE_2, 3 mg), repeated if necessary in 6 hours. *Prostaglandins are generally contraindicated* in patients with asthma, cardiovascular disease, pulmonary hypertension, and epilepsy. *Urea* (Ureaphil 80 g dissolved in 100 ml of sterile normal saline) may also be used as an intraamniotic injection. Because of the relatively high side-effects of Pg preparations when used alone, the combination of urea and Pg (e.g. 5–10 mg $PgF_2\alpha$) has been used intraamniotically. *Intraamniotic saline* (20–40 g) is also effective, but is less used because of occasional disasters if the solution is injected into the blood stream or uterine muscle. *Prophylactic antibiotics* should be given to cover both anaerobes and aerobes if the induction-abortion interval is longer than 18 hours. After expulsion of the conceptus, the cervix should be inspected for tears; curettage is usually performed to obviate delayed haemorrhage and infection from retained products of conception.

Dilatation and evacuation is quick and associated with fewer side-effects, but requires an experienced and expert operator.

Finally, *hysterotomy* (which is a miniature Caesarean section) may be necessary. This is the least desirable method, since it carries a much higher risk of immediate morbidity and mortality for the mother, and leaves a scar liable to rupture in a future pregnancy.

Follow-up

Although long-term complications are infrequent after therapeutic termination of pregnancy, follow-up is needed to assess the patient's physical and psychological health. *Psychological problems* are usually only seen in those ambivalent about having the procedure carried out, or in those in whom the termination is dictated by physical abnormalities rather than the woman's own wish; other risk factors include discord in personal relationships, adverse religious or cultural attitude to abortion, unsupportive health care personnel. Considerable effort and support may be needed when providing contraception to such patients, particularly if there are personality disorders (immaturity etc), labile life conditions, or lack of support from partner or relations. Unlike term pregnancies, there is no period of contraceptive grace after abortion.

CRIMINAL ABORTION

This is an abortion carried out in contravention of the legal requirements pertaining in the particular locality. These requirements differ quite widely not only in the statute book, but also in their interpretation by the authorities. Such abortions are carried out by the patient herself, a friend, or an abortionist, medically qualified or otherwise. A spectrum of complications may ensue if the procurer is inexperienced and proper sanitary procedure is not followed. The chief dangers are *infection*, because of failure to observe asepsis; *trauma*, because of lack of knowledge and/or skill; *embolism*, because of the syringing of air or chemical solutions into the uterus and inadvertently also into the uterine venous system.

SEPTIC ABORTION

Sepsis may complicate any of the forms of abortion, but is mostly restricted to those induced criminally and/or where retained products are neglected.

Clinical Features

In addition to the symptoms and signs of pregnancy and abortion already outlined, the patient will notice an offensive discharge, lower abdominal pain (often constant as opposed to cramping), tachycardia and fever. On examination, signs of interference may be observed on the cervix and the discharge which is present is often thick and yellowish-red in colour; uterine and perhaps forniceal tenderness is noted. In more advanced cases, pelvic or even *general peritonitis* will be evident by the marked rebound tenderness.

Bacteriology

(i) Anaerobic organisms (streptococci, bacteroides) are most commonly found, because they thrive on the pieces of dead tissue in the uterus (products of conception, blood clot). (ii) *Clostridium welchii* infections produce red cell haemolysis with resulting haemoglobinaemia (red serum), *haemoglobinuria* (port wine coloured urine), *jaundice*, as well as renal failure and muscle gangrene (figure 14.3). (iii) *Gram negative septicaemia* results from the invasion into the blood stream of organisms such as E. coli; these produce a powerful endotoxin which causes shock, damage to blood vessels, disseminated intravascular coagulation, and damage to such organs as the liver and kidney. (iv) *Gram positive septicaemia* with streptococci may also occur.

Additional features in such overwhelming infections are extreme tachycardia (> 130 minute), oliguria, shock, cyanosis, confusion passing to delirium, coma, and death.

Management

This is similar to that outlined under Shock, Chapter 54. Clostridial infections represent a special complication of abortion, largely a thing of the past, since rectal syringes are seldom used now to procure abortion. Apart from massive penicillin therapy, 10–20 million units per day, gas gangrene antiserum may be required (100,000 U: part IV, part IM, after a test dose), and *hysterectomy* if uterine gangrene (extreme local tenderness, crepitus) has resulted (figure 14.3).

INCOMPETENT CERVIX

Towards the end of the first trimester the amniotic sac fills the uterine cavity and commences to distend it; if there is a weakness in the retaining sphincteric mechanism at the junction of uterus and cervix abortion will occur.

Incidence

Approximately 1 in 1,000 deliveries, 1 in 100 abortions, 1 in 5 habitual abortions; in hospital practice the figures would be about 1 in 100, 1 in 20, and 2 in 5, respectively (table 16.1).

Aetiology

Acquired. Usually tearing of the cervical sphincter as a result of precipitate delivery or delivery through an undilated cervix; or as a result of too forceful or too rapid dilatation and curettage. *The majority of cases follow termination of pregnancy, which accounts for a recent increase in incidence* (colour plate 35, figure 18.4). *It should be noted that about 30–40% of perinatal deaths occur in pregnancies which terminate between 20–28 weeks, incompetent cervix being a major contributor.* Occasionally, the condition results from surgical procedures such as cone biopsy, cervical amputation or Manchester repair.

Congenital. In approximately 1 in 3 patients there appears to be no previous injury to account for the condition.

Clinical Features and Diagnosis

Classically there is a history of mechanical dilatation of the cervix, followed by one or more spontaneous abortions after the 14th week in which *pain has not been a feature*. The process usually commences with a feeling of fullness in the lower abdomen, followed by a *mucous dis-*

charge, sometimes urgency and frequency of micturition, and finally rupture of the membranes; significant blood loss is unusual. During the second trimester, inspection may have revealed the dilated cervix and bulging membranes (colour plate 35). Occasionally the conceptus aborts as an intact sac (colour plate 3).

Ultrasonography will usually demonstrate the effaced and dilated cervix and will be of value in excluding fetal and uterine abnormalities (figure 18.4). Ultrasonography, at 16–18 weeks and at 2-week intervals thereafter, is useful in the patient with a history of repeated second trimester abortion but without clinical evidence of cervical incompetence, to determine if ligation is indicated — by showing beaking of the internal cervical os. *Because cervical ligation has complications it is not a panacea for all patients with a past history of mid-trimester abortion.*

Between pregnancies, the presence of cervical incompetence is confirmed by the ability to pass a size 6 Hegar dilator or an equivalent-sized Foley bag, without significant discomfort to the patient. A split may be felt on digital examination of the endocervix. A premenstrual *hysterogram* also will show a characteristic funnelling or dilatation in the region of the internal os.

Treatment

(a) *Prophylaxis.* The importance of careful dilatation of the cervix (limiting it to Hegar number 10) has been mentioned. In therapeutic terminations beyond 10–12 weeks, the risk of damage is minimized by the application of local prostaglandin to the cervix 12 hours before the procedure.

(b) *Cervical repair.* The torn sphincter may be repaired in the interval between pregnancies if the cervix is badly torn or abnormal.

(c) *Cerclage during pregnancy.* This is the more usual procedure and is performed between the 14th and 20th weeks of gestation. There are a number of techniques available — purse-string suture (McDonald), buried suture, fascia or skin (Shirodkar), or right-angle mattress sutures (Wurm) (figure 18.5). In all cases, the keynote of success is placement of the suture high enough up on the cervix. The procedure is best carried out before bulging of the membranes through the internal os has occurred. The patient is usually kept at rest in hospital for several days and is instructed to report immediately if there are contractions or a vaginal loss of fluid or blood. Antenatal supervision should be more

Figure 18.4 Cervical incompetence. **A.** Longitudinal ultrasound scan at 17 weeks' gestation in a 30-year-old para 2 who, following 2 terminations of pregnancy, had lost 2 infants at 23 weeks' gestation, in spite of cervical ligation at 17 and 13 weeks, respectively. Note the beaking of the amniotic cavity into the cervical canal (C). B = bladder; V = fetal head; P = placenta. Cervical ligation was not performed because speculum examination had shown no cervical dilatation. **B.** At 19 weeks' gestation this realtime sectorscan shows amniotic fluid and membranes filling the cervical canal (C). B = bladder; V = vagina; R = rectum. Examination under anaesthesia showed membranes bulging through a 5 cm dilated cervix. A cervical suture was inserted, but the patient came into labour and delivered 2 days later. The message is that the 'beaking' sign had indicated the need for cervical ligation 2 weeks previously.

A

B

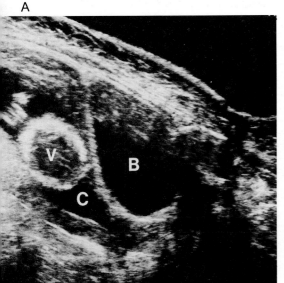
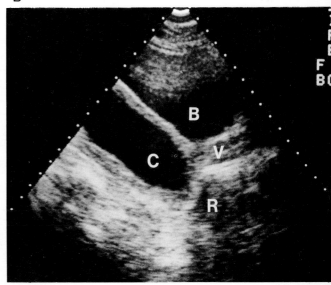

intense, with periodic inspection of the cervix being carried out. The purse-string suture can be cut towards term (37 weeks), allowing vaginal delivery; this is facilitated if the ends of the suture are drawn through a ring forceps, the latter being used to exert counter pressure against the cervix. With buried sutures it is sometimes preferable to perform Caesarean section.

These procedures are usually *contraindicated before the 12th week* (because of the 10–15% risk of spontaneous abortion in the first trimester and because the lower segment has not yet formed adequately to take the stitch), and *after the 28th week* of pregnancy, and in the presence of *ruptured membranes*, vaginal *infection*, *active bleeding* or *labour*.

After 32 weeks, conservative treatment with bed rest, sedation, mild Trendelenburg position, and perhaps progesterone is usual. Another suggested procedure is the insertion of a *Smith-Hodge pessary* as for the treatment of retroverted uterus, or alternatively a *ring pessary*.

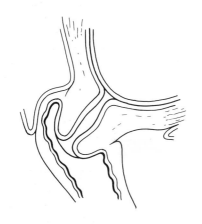

A

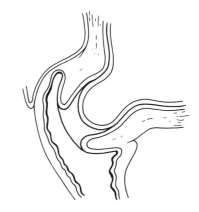

B

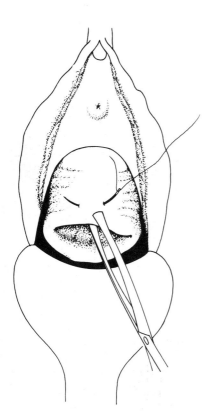

C

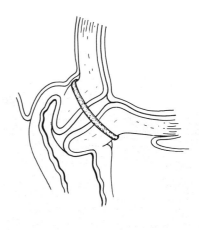

D

Figure 18.5 Incompetent cervix. **A.** Normal cervix at about 16 weeks. **B.** Incompetent internal os with bulging membranes — the operculum is shed and the patient would have copious pinkish vaginal discharge. **C.** McDonald purse-string suture (number 4 mersilk) at the level of the internal os. A simple, well-conceived operation that achieves excellent results. Sometimes 2 sutures are inserted. **D.** Buried nonabsorbable suture (mersilene tape, 5 mm wide) should be placed a little higher at the level of the internal os. Upward displacement of the bladder may be necessary if there is deep cervical laceration. Usually 3 or 4 Babcock forceps are used to hold the cervix gently.

Complications

Rupture of the membranes may occur during replacement or from careless stitch placement. Injury to the bladder base may occur during reflexion or from the suture. Subsequent dilatation of the cervix is the most common problem; damage to the cervix will occur unless the suture is removed promptly. *Infection* is rarely a problem; a low-grade chronic inflammation is often associated with non-buried sutures. *Cervical fibrosis* sufficient to cause dystocia has been reported, but this is unusual.

Success Rate

This depends on a number of factors — accuracy of diagnosis, whether the cervix has started to dilate (i.e. a therapeutic rather than a prophylactic stitch), extent of defect, stage of pregnancy, and parity. The overall rate ranges from 40–90%.

ECTOPIC PREGNANCY

Although far less common than abortion (the incidence ranges from 0.5–1% of pregnancies), ectopic pregnancy is a potentially very serious condition, because rupture usually occurs and this is accompanied by *intraabdominal bleeding which may be fatal* unless resuscitation and surgical intervention is carried out quickly (colour plates 5 and 6).

Definition

Implantation of the conceptus occurs outside the uterine cavity, usually in the Fallopian tube (figure 18.6), rarely in the ovary, abdominal cavity (figure 18.7), or cervix.

Aetiology

Kinking or narrowing of the tube will prevent the fertilized ovum making its way from the ampulla to the uterine cavity. Apart from the mechanical effect of the narrowing, damage to cells of the tubal lining (especially those with small hair-like cilia) impedes transport; there may also be malfunction of the tubal musculature. Common antecedents are gonococcal salpingitis, postabortal or postpartum salpingitis, and appendicitis. Endometriosis (ectopic functioning endometrium), congenital abnormalities, and previous tubal surgery may also impair tubal function.

Delay in transit of the fertilized ovum, perhaps coupled with an unusually receptive tubal mucosa, are additional factors.

Pathology and Clinical Features

The common sites are shown in figure 18.8.

The classical triad of symptoms is *amenorrhoea* (75%), *lower abdominal pain* (95%), and *vaginal bleeding* (75%). A similar picture may be seen with an abortion in progress, but careful examination will usually differentiate the 2 conditions. There are 3 main outcomes.

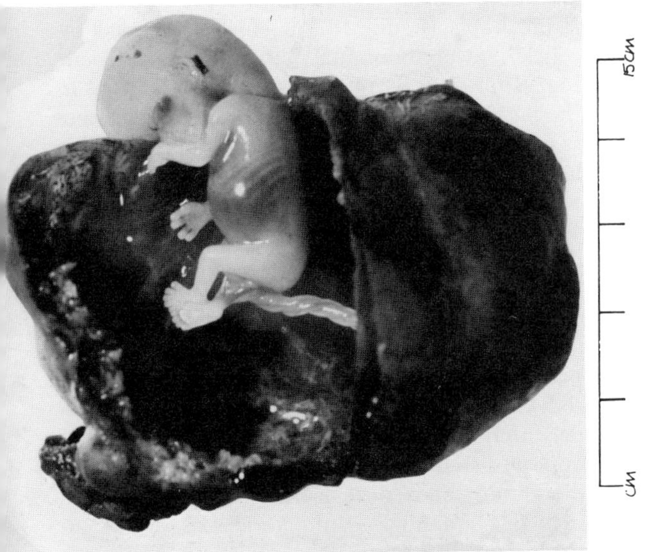

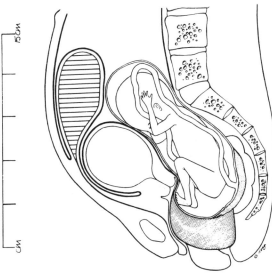

Figure 18.6 Tubal pregnancy. The tube is grossly distended and has a thickened haemorrhagic wall which accounts for the unusually advanced duration of pregnancy (9 weeks) before rupture occurred.

Figure 18.7 An unusual case of primary abdominal pregnancy in which the fetus occupied the distended rectovaginal pouch with the placenta implanted on the peritoneum posteriorly. Retroplacental haemorrhage caused a haematoma that bulged into vagina causing urinary retention at 23 weeks' gestation. (From Beischer NA. Aust NZJ Obstet Gynaecol 1967; 7: 42-46).

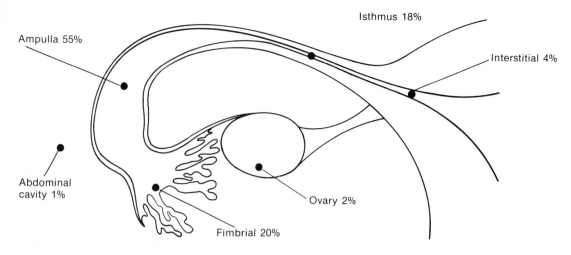

Figure 18.8 Relative frequency of sites of implantation of ectopic pregnancies.

Figure 18.9 Possible outcomes of tubal pregnancy are rupture into the tubal lumen, peritoneal cavity or broad ligament. Tubal missed abortion without rupture can occur asymptomatically and result in obliteration of the tubal lumen and later sterility.

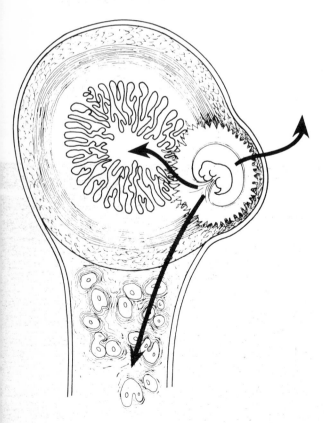

(i) *Tubal abortion.* The conceptus is extruded out the fimbrial end of the tube (figure 18.9). This is accompanied by colicky pain, followed by a more constant pain because of the presence of blood in the peritoneal cavity. This also causes pain on micturition and defaecation, and considerable pain when internal examination is carried out, particularly if the cervix is moved.

The condition may settle spontaneously, but usually bleeding continues and surgery is required.

(ii) *Tubal rupture.* If the pregnancy progresses and tubal abortion does not occur, tubal rupture is inevitable (figure 18.9). This is heralded by colicky, lower abdominal pain and vaginal bleeding. *Rupture is more likely with implantations in the narrower inner half of the tube.* The process of rupture may be gradual, with symptoms similar to those described above due to blood collecting in the pelvis. Acute rupture usually is associated with severe intraperitoneal bleeding which causes acute abdominal pain; often pain is felt also in the tips of the shoulders (due to irritation of the diaphragm by blood, the same nerve roots (5th cervical) supplying both). The patient complains of faintness and nausea and may be shocked. On examination, the abdomen is tender, both to direct and release pressure, and may appear distended because of the intraperitoneal blood and reflex distension of the bowel. Findings on bimanual examination are similar to those described under tubal abortion except that *a mass* is often palpable on one or other side of the uterus; anaesthesia may be necessary to permit adequate examination.

Rupture 'may occur downward between the leaves of the broad ligament forming a *haema-*

toma (figure 18.9). Symptoms and signs of peritonitis are absent, but pelvic pain and tenderness are marked.

(iii) *Missed tubal abortion*. The embryo dies and usually is absorbed. The clinical features are those of early pregnancy, together with a brown or red vaginal loss and perhaps mild, lower abdominal pain.

Abdominal pregnancy may occur as a primary implantation event (figure 18.7), but far more commonly, it follows a ruptured ectopic pregnancy. There is usually one or more episodes of pelvic pain and bleeding between the 6th and 10th weeks of pregnancy. This settles and the trophoblast obtains a secondary footing among the pelvic and abdominal viscera, eventually forming a diffuse type of placenta. The *diagnosis* is seldom realized before death of the fetus. The patient may complain of vague abdominal pain and discomfort and sometimes an exaggeration of fetal kicking. Often, there is a failed induction of labour. If suspected, the diagnosis can usually be confirmed by ultrasonography, which shows the empty uterus.

The *management* is strictly in the realm of the experienced consultant, because of the major bleeding that may attend the laparotomy (as a result of placental disturbance).

Diagnosis

This is usually obvious in the patient with acute rupture. If less acute, it could be confused with one of the different *types of abortion*, complication of a *cyst or tumour of the ovary*, or an inflammatory condition such as *salpingitis or appendicitis*, or *renal/ureteric colic*. A further difficulty is that the classical early features of pregnancy may not be present (amenorrhoea, morning sickness, and breast tenderness).

The most helpful laboratory test is the level of beta HCG in blood: the usual urine pregnancy test may or may not be positive. *Compound B ultrasonic scanning will demonstrate the absence of the conceptus in the uterus, and possibly its presence in the tube* (figure 18.10). Needle aspiration of the posterior vaginal fornix is sometimes carried out at the time of examination under anaesthesia to decide whether laparotomy is indicated (one is seeking the presence of old blood). *Laparoscopy is a useful investigation in the doubtful case.* Usually the history and findings clearly indicate the need for laparotomy (after *resuscitative measures* have been commenced).

Management

The initial management is similar to that for the patient with suspected abortion; essentially,

Figure 18.10 Right ruptured tubal ectopic pregnancy and right ovarian endometriotic cyst in a 31-year-old para 0, gravida 1 who presented with bleeding and abdominal pain. Her last period had occurred 10 weeks previously and beta HCG estimation was positive. **A.** Longitudinal ultrasound scan through the uterus (U) showed that it was slightly enlarged, but did not contain a gestational sac. **B.** Longitudinal scan to the right of the uterus showing bladder (B) and ovarian cyst (C) 5 X 3 cm, with a thick wall as in endometriosis, situated posteriorly in the right adnexa; also free fluid within the pouch of Douglas and a gestational sac (G), 2.5 cm in diameter, in the right adnexa, containing a fetus of 7.5 weeks' maturity. Right salpingectomy and right ovarian cystectomy were performed.

A

B

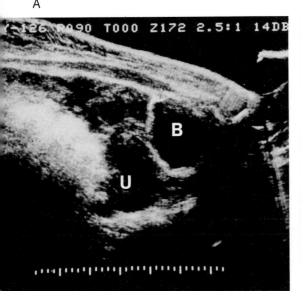
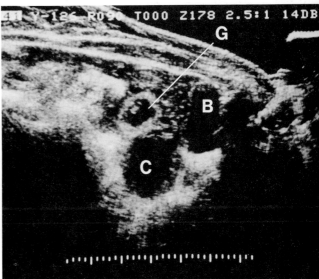

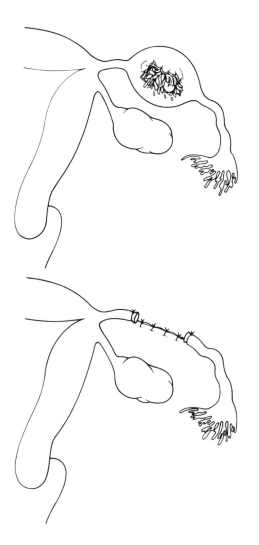

Figure 18.11 Retention of undamaged portions of Fallopian tube by resection of area of isthmus containing a ruptured ectopic pregnancy. Reanastomosis by microsurgery can be performed at a later date.

transfer to hospital (previous resuscitation if necessary). After the diagnosis has been made, surgery is indicated (salpingectomy or salpingotomy). It is important that both tubes and ovaries are inspected as soon as haemostasis has been secured. If there are serious problems on the other side, the involved tube should be conserved if possible — microsurgery may be able to restore patency at a later date (figure 18.11). In many centres *conservative surgery* is practised in 30–40% of cases of ectopic pregnancy, particularly where the tube is unruptured (now about 80%) and further pregnancies are desired.

If the patient is in shock, the measures outlined in Chapter 54 are instituted. The rare *cervical ectopic pregnancy* should be suspected if bleeding is copious and the cervix expanded. Ultrasonography is useful to confirm the diagnosis. The management is specialist in nature — usually ligation of the descending branches of the uterine arteries at the 3 and 9 o'clock positions (vaginal approach). A pack and a 30 ml Foley catheter assist control of the bleeding.

Prognosis

Ectopic pregnancy accounts for 2–5% of *maternal deaths* (from haemorrhagic shock) — due to delay in diagnosis and failure to provide resuscitation before laparotomy (table 14.1). It ranks second only to postpartum haemorrhage as a cause of maternal death from haemorrhage. *Infertility* occurs in 40%, and a *further ectopic pregnancy* in 10%.

HYDATIDIFORM MOLE

Definition

A developmental anomaly of the trophoblast or placenta in which there is a local or general vesicular change in the chorionic villi.

Incidence

The condition is commoner in Australasia (1 in 750) than in the USA, the UK and Europe (1 in 1,000–1 in 2,000), but is most frequent in South-East Asia and Mexico (1 in 150–1 in 500).

Clinical Features and Pathology (colour plates 22 and 36–39)

Typically, the mole is initially diagnosed as a case of *threatened abortion*, because of intermittent *vaginal bleeding* (95%) following a period of *amenorrhoea*.

The *diagnosis is often not made until the second trimester* (usually at about 18 weeks) when the following additional features emerge — uterus *larger than expected* (50–55%) from *retromolar haemorrhage*, and also due to cystic degeneration of the chorionic villi which form vesicles 0.5–1.0 cm in diameter; uterus feels 'doughy' rather than cystic and *no fetal heart* is heard on sonar testing; *preeclampsia* (15–20%); *hyperemesis* (25–30%); bilateral *theca-lutein* cysts in the ovaries may be palpated (10–20%) or detected on ultrasonography (30–40%); *hyperthyroidism* (5–10%) due to elevated placental production of thyroid stimulating hormone; small *vesicles* may be found in the cervix/vagina, or even passed per vaginam (20–30%), the patient suggesting the diagnosis by referring to their grape-like appearance. Symptoms from *metastatic spread* of molar tissue may occur —

e.g. *haemoptysis* and/or pleuritic pain from spread to the lung.

Occasionally the diagnosis is only made on *histological examination of curettings* from a suspected incomplete abortion. The 3 histological features are *avascularity* and *vesicular change* in the chorionic villi and *proliferation of the trophoblastic cells* (colour plate 37) — the latter explains the high levels of human chorionic gonadotrophic hormone (HCG) present in the patient's blood and urine. Usually the embryo/fetus is absent.

Great diagnostic difficulty may arise if there is a *mole with coexistent fetus* (4–6%, colour plates 22 and 36). The main differential diagnosis of hydatidiform mole is *multiple pregnancy*, which is also characterized by undue uterine enlargement, severe hyperemesis and high HCG levels in serum and urine. Other possibilities are a normal intrauterine pregnancy threatening to abort (the larger size being the result of an error in dates), or uterine fibromyomas. If the diagnosis is missed it is usually because it is not thought of. Because of the frequency of vaginal bleeding, the diagnosis should be excluded by ultrasound in all patients with a persisting threatened abortion.

Investigations

Ultrasound scanning provides the definitive diagnosis (figure 18.12); *chorionic gonadotrophin* (HCG) levels are often elevated in both serum and urine, but multiple pregnancy may cause confusion. A urinary HCG value above 300,000 U/24 hours excludes a normal singleton pregnancy, but not all cases of multiple pregnancy. In molar pregnancies the *urinary excretion of progesterone and oestrogen* is usually below the tenth percentile for normal pregnancy.

Ultrasonography has now largely superseded such other diagnostic investigations as *radiography* (absence of fetus after the 14–16th weeks), atypical vasculature on arteriography, and atypical findings on amniocentesis or amniography. Chest X-ray is needed to exclude metastatic disease.

Management

The initial treatment is similar to that outlined for the patient with suspected abortion. If the diagnosis of hydatidiform mole is established, the first procedure is to *evacuate the uterus*. Abortion may already have occurred or may be in progress, this causing the patient to seek medical attention. Since heavy bleeding may complicate this process, adequate blood must be *cross-matched*. The evacuation is similar to that described under abortion, the main difference being that *suction curettage is far superior*, the vesicles offering no resistance. After the uterus is emptied of the bulk of the mole, and reduced to a safe size, final instrumental curettage is per-

Figure 18.12 Hydatidiform mole in a 24-year-old para 1 who presented at 13 weeks' gestation with vaginal bleeding, excessive nausea and vomiting, and uterus large for dates. This longitudinal scan shows bladder (B), uterus containing a uniform echogenic mass characteristic of molar tissue (M) (and without fetus, amniotic fluid or discrete placenta), and a multilocular theca-lutein cyst (TL). Suction curettage was performed. Two weeks later the urinary HCG excretion was 47,000 U/24 hours, and the theca-lutein cysts had enlarged to the level of the umbilicus. Six weeks after molar evacuation the HCG excretion had increased to 135,000 U/24 hours, and the uterus had enlarged. Locally-invasive, nonmetastatic malignant trophoblastic disease was diagnosed (chest radiography was clear) and chemotherapy was commenced.

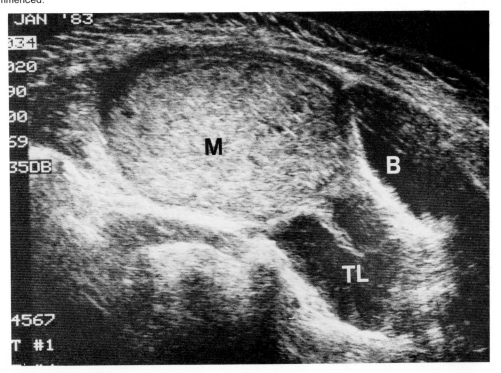

formed and the specimen is sent for pathological study.

The alternatives of *oxytocin infusion or hysterotomy for uteri larger than 12–14 weeks have been largely superseded by suction curettage; for patients older than 35, hysterectomy may be considered* if further childbearing is not desired in view of the greater risk of malignant change (invasive mole and choriocarcinoma).

Subsequent care. Since cure is not achieved initially in 10–15% of patients with hydatidiform mole, close follow-up observations are essential.

The presence of chorionic tissue is monitored by assay of beta subunit HCG in blood; a less costly alternative is to use an ordinary pregnancy HCG assay with a switch later to the more sensitive beta HCG assay after levels have fallen; check the presence/activity of chorionic tissue in the lungs by *serial radiography*; ensure that the patient understands the importance of avoiding pregnancy in the ensuing 1–2 years and provide an effective contraceptive.

Follow-up

Contraception should be commenced.

Registry. If there is a trophoblast registry in the region, the case should be notified.

Clinical examination. A careful pelvic examination should be made every 2–4 weeks if the HCG value is elevated (in 90% of patients, a negative level is reached by 42 days). *Ultrasound study may be needed to exclude pregnancy if contraceptive failure is suspected.*

Beta HCG levels. Samples are checked every 1–2 weeks until negative on 2 consecutive occasions (this usually takes 3–10 weeks). Samples are then assessed monthly for 6 months and 3-monthly for a further 6 months.

Chest radiography. This should be done every 1–2 months if the HCG value is elevated.

Persistent Disease

If the HCG levels fail to fall progressively, it is possible that all of the molar tissue may not have been removed at the previous curettage and this should be repeated. *If the levels still remain stationary or are increasing, a diagnosis of persistent disease is made on this biochemical evidence alone.* In these cases, the mole is demonstrating a more aggressive behaviour, with tissue destruction and myometrial invasion leading sometimes to perforation of the uterine wall (*invasive mole*). In some patients, metastatic spread may occur, usually to the lungs or vagina. The diagnosis may be aided by arterio-graphy (blood pooling is seen in the wall of the uterus) or laparoscopy. This type of disease is seen in *about 10–15% of patients with a classical mole*; *warning features* include age over 35, uterus large for dates, a high initial HCG titre, the presence of small vesicles and marked trophoblast proliferation on histology, and a blood group AB or B where that of the husband is O or A.

The management is similar to that described for choriocarcinoma (i.e. *chemotherapy*). If the mole has perforated the uterus, laparotomy and possibly *hysterectomy* will be needed as an emergency procedure because of haemorrhage.

CHORIOCARCINOMA

This *malignant tumour of the trophoblast* originates in a hydatidiform mole in 50%, abortion in 30–40%, and normal pregnancy in 10–20% (colour plate 40). It is a very rare condition, but important to recognize, since the chances of cure with chemotherapy are very good, whereas without this treatment, death will occur.

Characteristic features of this lesion include: *intermittent bleeding after a hydatidiform mole, abortion, or normal pregnancy*, together with the presence of a *tumour* in the vagina, uterus or lungs and a *high HCG titre*. The usual treatment is by *chemotherapy*, the primary agent being *methotrexate*. A typical course comprises 4 IM injections of 50 mg given at intervals of 48 hours followed 30 hours later by IM *folinic acid*, 6 mg. The folinic acid is an antagonist to methotrexate and mitigates toxicity to normal tissues. The course is repeated every 2–3 weeks unless there is significant impairment to bone marrow, liver or kidneys. It is ceased when the beta HCG is undetectable in the blood on 3 consecutive weeks. The side-effects of the above regimen are usually quite tolerable (gastrointestinal upset and sometimes ulceration of the mouth). The addition of additional agents (e.g. *Actinomycin D*) may be needed for high risk situations — drug resistance, disease present for 4 months or more, extensive local disease (tumour diameter > 5 cm), high HCG titre (> 100,000 U/24 hour urine), liver or brain metastases.

Long-term surveillance (5 years) is necessary for these patients. With the advent of effective chemotherapy and tumour monitoring with beta HCG, survival is now usual. Cerebral and liver metastases carry a poorer prognosis. Chemotherapy does not appear to have a detrimental effect on a subsequent pregnancy; however, it is advised that pregnancy be deferred for 12 months after ceasing chemotherapy.

chapter nineteen

Bleeding in Late Pregnancy

OVERVIEW

Antepartum haemorrhage occurs in about 5% of pregnancies: placenta praevia 1%, placental abruption 1.2%, incidental and undetermined causes 2.8%. *These causes of haemorrhage are together responsible for 20-25% of all perinatal deaths.*

A significant amount of vaginal bleeding in the second half of pregnancy is almost always associated with a placenta which is either low lying (*placenta praevia*) or prematurely separated from the uterine wall (*abruptio placentae*). Each of these conditions may cause bleeding sufficient to threaten the life of the mother; they cause about 3% of all maternal deaths (table 14.1). The baby is also at risk, from *hypoxia* due to placental separation in abruptio placentae and from the complications of *prematurity* in placenta praevia. Accordingly, the patient must be managed in a hospital able to provide appropriate high level care. Accurate diagnosis is important, since facets of management are different for the 2 conditions.

Serial ultrasonographic studies in the second and early third trimesters of pregnancy have shown that in 20-30% of patients the placenta overlies the region of the lower uterine segment, but with further development it migrates upward in 95%, so that by the 36th week it is praevia in only about 1 in 100 women. Since development of the lower uterine segment occurs progressively in the third trimester, bleeding will be inevitable if the placenta remains in this area, since its lower edge will be sheared off as the uterine muscle fibres are drawn upward. *Ultrasonography* has been a major advance in that the exact site of the placenta in relation to the lower segment can be visualized, allowing a rational decision to be made regarding route of delivery (vaginal or Caesarean section).

Placental abruption, like placenta praevia, is more common in the elderly, parous patient, particularly if suffering from hypertensive disease. Each of these characteristics is now seen less commonly in obstetric practice, explaining the decrease of the major forms of antepartum bleeding. The cardinal features on presentation are haemorrhage, premature uterine activity, uterine tenderness and fetal distress. Bleeding occurs between the base of the placenta and the adjacent uterine decidua, and depending largely on the size of the vessel involved, a variable amount of placenta is separated and thus put out of action as far as fetoplacental function is concerned. In most cases, the precise reason for the vascular blow-out is unknown. If a major separation has occurred, it represents an emergency situation for both mother and fetus, and will require energetic resuscitation and Caesarean section if the baby is still alive; in 5% of these patients *blood coagulation failure* occurs. The possibility of preventive measures should be kept in mind in the early antenatal period — reduction of smoking and aspirin intake, prevention/early detection of preeclampsia, avoidance of the supine position in late pregnancy.

Caesarean section is the method of delivery in 10-15% of patients with placental abruption and 75-85% of those with placenta praevia.

Diagnosis is not easy when the bleeding is not of great amount and is coming from the uterus: apart from lesser bleeding from the above 2 conditions, one must consider circumvallate placenta and placental edge bleeding. Finally, the bleeding may be *incidental* to the pregnancy (e.g. vaginitis, cervical neoplasia), and the cause is readily ascertained on speculum examination, which is performed gently so as not to provoke heavy bleeding if the patient has a placenta praevia.

ANTEPARTUM HAEMORRHAGE

Definition

Bleeding of 15 ml or more from the birth canal after the 28th week of pregnancy and before the birth of the baby.

Causes

(a) Placental abruption (accidental haemorrhage).

(b) Placenta praevia.

(c) Incidental and undetermined causes. These include: (i) other placental conditions (edge bleeding, circumvallate formation, vasa praevia); and (ii) local conditions.

Despite scrutiny of the placenta after delivery, no discoverable cause for the bleeding will be found in 25–35%. Since the diagnosis will often be uncertain when the patient first presents, particularly if the loss is not heavy, the general management of such a patient will now be discussed, since it differs little for each condition.

Early Management

(i) Hospitalization is essential to enable the diagnosis to be established, and to minimize the risk of further bleeding. (ii) Transport by ambulance should be made if the loss is heavy or there is any worry concerning the patient's condition. In such cases, an intravenous infusion must first be set up, and a medical attendant should accompany the patient. (iii) Sedation in the form of an analgesic such as pethidine may be necessary for restlessness and pain.

Procedures After Admission

(i) Routine admission data are obtained. (ii) A history is obtained of events before and after the onset of bleeding. An assessment is made of the amount of loss. (iii) Routine admisson procedures are carried out, including obtaining signed consent forms; the suprapubic area is shaved if operation appears likely; an enema is not given. (iv) An examination is made, including vital signs. Gentle palpation of the abdomen is performed to assess uterine tone and tenderness, contractions, fundal height, nature of the presenting part and its relation to the pelvic brim, and fetal heart rate. *A vaginal examination is not made.* (v) Most patients, even if the bleeding is not heavy, are quite apprehensive; explanation and reassurance are important, both for the patient and immediate relatives. (vi) Except when bleeding is mild, the possibility of a reduced placental blood flow exists, and thus the patient should be nursed on her side as much as possible — to avoid compression of vena cava and aorta by the uterus. (vii) Investigations will include ABO, Rh, and VDRL testing if not already performed, haemoglobin and *blood cross-matching.*

If bleeding is moderate or marked, other haematological tests will be ordered, such as haematocrit, platelet count, fibrinogen, prothrombin and thrombin times (Chapters 34 and 54). A urine specimen is tested for glucose and protein, care being taken to avoid blood contamination. (viii) Observations (intervals according to extent of blood loss): pulse rate (5–60 minutes); blood pressure (10–120 minutes); fetal heart rate (continuous monitoring — 15 minutes); fluid balance chart; amount and nature of blood loss, perineal pads to be saved for inspection; general condition of patient — abnormal symptoms or signs suggesting internal bleeding, including abdominal examination. (ix) An intravenous line should be established in case bleeding increases or a blood transfusion is indicated on test results. (x) *Further management.* If the bleeding is mild, a speculum examination is usually performed by the doctor 12–24 hours after admission to exclude local causes. If a local (incidental) lesion such as vaginitis or cervicitis appears to be the cause of the bleeding the patient is allowed home. Otherwise, she remains in hospital pending further investigations, especially *ultrasonography. Carcinoma of the cervix* is an unusual but important local cause of antepartum haemorrhage.

PLACENTAL ABRUPTION

The older name for this condition is *accidental haemorrhage,* since the placenta is normally situated in the upper segment of the uterus and, unlike placenta praevia, is not unavoidably separated as the lower segment increases in length in the last trimester of pregnancy (figure 19.1). It was postulated, therefore, that its separation must be the result of some accidental occurrence. It is *defined,* therefore, as the separation of the normally-implanted placenta (usually by haemorrhage into the decidua basalis) from the 28th week of pregnancy.

Aetiology

The causative factors are known only in a minority of cases (i) *Hypertensive disorders.* In the more serious forms of preeclampsia, hypertension, and renal disease, there are degenerative changes in the basal arteries supplying the placenta. In such cases, the complication may be looked on as a 'stroke' involving the retroplacental area rather than the brain (uterine apoplexy

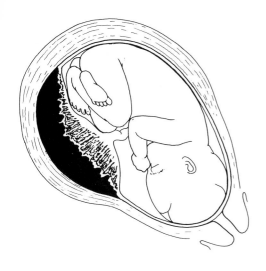

Figure 19.1 Gross degree of concealed placental abruption with complete separation of a normally situated placenta. The fetus dies of anoxia.

— colour plate 14). (ii) *Trauma.* Trauma to the abdomen may cause separation of the placenta and the commonest cause is *motor car accidents* — it can also occur during external cephalic version, particularly under anaesthesia. Shortness of the umbilical cord, absolute or relative, may contribute. (iii) *Reduction in size of the uterus.* This is seen mainly with the second twin, in the interval after the first twin has been delivered. Occasionally, the sudden loss of a large amount of liquor amnii may be responsible. (iv) *Pressure on veins draining the uterus.* Rarely, the pressure of the gravid uterus on the inferior vena cava or large pelvic veins draining the uterus (*supine hypotensive syndrome*) may sufficiently raise the venous pressure in the retroplacental veins to cause their rupture. (v) *Minor predisposing factors.* Regular aspirin ingestion, low socioeconomic status, poor nutrition, smoking and advancing parity all have some association in statistical reports. (vi) *Idiopathic.* In the majority of patients, the condition occurs without warning in the latter part of the third trimester.

Incidence

Between 0.5–1.5% of pregnancies are complicated by abruptio placentae; it accounts for 10% of emergency admissions, and 20–25% of antepartum haemorrhages. The condition is somewhat less common than formerly, perhaps the result of better management of predisposing factors, improved health of patients, and lower parity.

Pathology

Inspection of the maternal surface of the placenta after delivery reveals a depressed area of variable size at the site of separation — the result of pressure of the blood clot. The latter may or may not be adherent to the placenta. If Caesarean section is performed in the patient with major abruption, the typical features described by Couvelaire may be seen (colour plate 14) — the uterine muscle is suffused with blood, giving it a plum-coloured appearance. If the bleeding has occurred shortly before delivery there may be no obvious features on inspection. Occasionally, the condition is only diagnosed when the retroplacental clot is seen at the time of routine examination of the placenta after delivery (colour plate 16). The fetus suffers from the direct reduction in functioning intervillous space as well as the indirect effects of maternal vasoconstriction and uterine spasm. As a rule, a retroplacental haemorrhage of more than 250 ml will produce some uterine hypertonus and fetal asphyxia; if more than 500 ml, fetal death is likely; if more than 1,000 ml, serious maternal sequelae are likely (*disseminated intravascular coagulation, renal failure*). The amount of blood lost vaginally may often be in considerable excess of this due to continued loss from one or more of the spiral arterioles supplying the placenta.

Clinical Features

The clinical features may differ quite considerably from one patient to another, depending mainly on 2 factors — the extent of bleeding (and thus the amount of placenta separated), and the sites of the bleeding and placenta, respectively. The bleeding may be *revealed, concealed,* or a mixture of the two. The more extensive the haemorrhage, the more likely it is to strip the membranes from the uterine wall and pass through the cervix and vagina. Similarly, if the bleeding comes from behind the lower part of the placenta or the latter is implanted relatively low in the uterus (although not praevia), the blood will again more easily track to the exterior.

It is convenient to consider 3 grades of severity.

(i) *Mild.* Less than 1/6th of the placenta has separated; the blood loss is usually less than 250 ml. The bleeding ranges in amount from the equivalent of a light menstrual loss to heavy menstruation with free bleeding or clots. As stated above, the bleeding may be entirely concealed. The patient may experience a cramping pain in the abdomen, or perhaps only a mild ache. *Occasionally, the bleeding is painless.* There may be slight *tenderness* over the uterus, the latter being more irritable than usual. The fetal heart is normally unaffected, as are the mother's vital signs. Mostly, there is only one episode of bleeding; however, repeated small losses, or even a major haemorrhage, may follow. Therefore conservative treatment should not be continued past 37–38 weeks, and evidence of fetoplacental failure (*cardiotocography*) may suggest delivery before this time.

This type is *managed* by bed rest for the period of bleeding and for 2–3 days thereafter. Diazepam is useful initially, in that it reduces the patient's anxiety and has a relaxing effect on the uterine muscle. If the condition settles completely and placental function tests are satisfactory, the patient can be discharged home and will be followed carefully until delivery.

(ii) *Moderate*. Between 1/6th and 3/6th of the placenta has separated; the blood loss usually ranges from 250–1,000 ml, concealed and/or revealed (figure 19.2). The patient experiences pain in the abdomen — acute at first, then often becoming dull and aching. There is no periodicity to the pain, as occurs if the patient is in labour. The abdomen is tender to palpation and is firmer than usual. Fetal heart sounds are present, but there may be irregularities in rate or rhythm, particularly slowing. Although the patient is not shocked, she is often pale and anxious, and may complain of nausea or faintness. In both moderate and severe types of abruption, the compensating vasoconstriction may mask to some extent the degree of blood loss, but may imperil the fetus because of uteroplacental ischaemia. Proteinuria is usually present. *Ultrasonography* is useful in indicating the size of the retroplacental blood clot and detecting any increase in bleeding on repeat study. *Chronic abruption*. Typically this condition follows a moderate abruption which settles. A circumvallate placenta may be present. Intermittent bleeding or reddish-brown discharge occurs, perhaps with abdominal discomfort. Fetal monitoring by maternal oestriol excretion and cardiotocography is indicated, since *placental function is often reduced.*

Treatment. The general management is similar to that outlined above. Greater attention is paid to observations of vital signs in the mother and fetus. If there is a significant drop in the patient's blood pressure or the haemoglobin value is below 10–11 g/dl *blood transfusion* is given. An analgesic drug is usually necessary. A drug which relaxes the uterus (salbutamol 4–8 mg tds, ritodrine 10 mg tds) often reduces spasm and improves the fetal condition.

Labour ensues in approximately 50% of patients in this group; termination of the pregnancy may be necessary in those remaining if the fetus appears compromised. Careful fetal monitoring is essential if labour is allowed to occur.

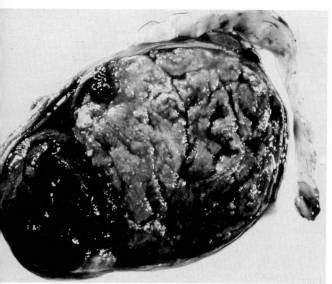

Figure 19.2 Moderate degree of placental abruption. The patient had diabetes and preeclampsia; the placenta was quite friable.

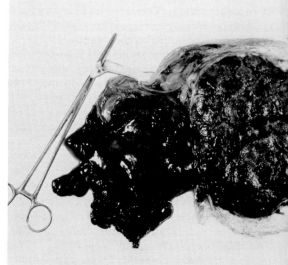

Figure 19.3 Marked placental abruption; live infant delivered by Caesarean section. Pregnancy was uneventful until the onset of vaginal bleeding and acute abdominal pain at 36 weeks. The infant was covered in meconium and was resuscitated with difficulty. The retroplacental clot weighed 900 g (equivalent to approximately 2.5 litres of whole blood).

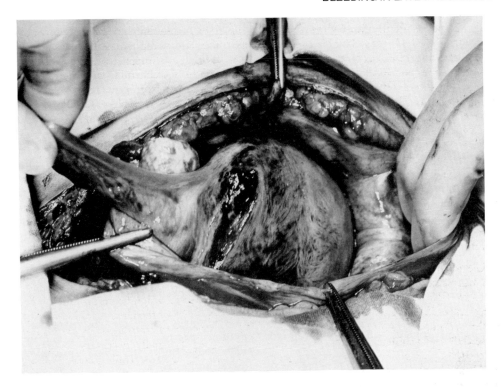

Figure 19.4 Placental abruption can mimic premature labour. This 26-year-old para 1 was admitted to hospital with abdominal pain at 35.4 weeks' gestation. There was no vaginal bleeding. Cardiotocography was normal. The pain settled and she returned to her home 3 days later. This picture shows the features of a Couvelaire uterus seen at elective repeat Caesarean section 15 days later. Blood has infiltrated the uterine wall and formed subserosal blebs at the right cornu. The infant (birth-weight 2,750 g) was born in good condition!

(iii) *Marked*. Usually more than half of the placenta is separated (figure 19.3). The symptoms are similar to those described for the moderate type, but of greater magnitude. The abdominal pain is often very severe; its location depends on the site of the placenta, whether anterior or posterior. There is usually a greater degree of *rigidity on palpation* if the placenta is anteriorly situated, and palpation of the fetus is difficult. There is also tenderness of the uterus to palpation, and the *fundus is often higher* than suggested by the dates, because of the retained blood clot (the patient's girth can increase 5–10 cm in a period of hours). The patient is often shocked; in such cases the fetal heart tones are usually absent — although auscultation may be difficult. The patient may state that fetal movements have ceased. In this group, the special complications of *disseminated intravascular coagulation* may occur, such as hypofibrinogenaemia and renal failure (Chapter 34). This results from the extensive damage to the decidual bed underlying the placenta and release of thromboplastic clotting factors, as well as the consumption of coagulation factors in the retroplacental clot itself, together with the over-stimulation of the sympathetic nervous system as a result of the shock (which slows blood flow in the smaller constricted vessels). The renal failure is caused partly by shock causing renal anoxia, and partly by blockage of small renal blood vessels by clotting; damage to other organs may occur for the same reasons.

In some cases, the extravasated blood is under high pressure as the result of rupture of a larger artery and extensively infiltrates the uterine muscle to produce a deep, reddish-blue colour (*Couvelaire uterus*; colour plate 14). Rarely, the blood may extend to the peritoneal cavity or into the amniotic cavity.

The *diagnosis* in such cases is rarely in doubt. However, if the haemorrhage is entirely concealed and extensive, there may be confusion with intraabdominal haemorrhage of other causes or *ruptured viscus*. Less severe concealed bleeding can mimic *red degeneration of a fibromyoma* or *premature labour* (figure 19.4).

The patient and her husband should be given appropriate explanation of the complication and the situation regarding the fetus, as well as the investigations and treatment which will be necessary.

If the fetal heart sounds are present, Caesarean section is undertaken urgently as a rule (figure 19.3). Otherwise, the patient is managed conservatively. The essential features in management are the accurate measurement and recording of vital signs (pulse, blood pressure, fetal heart rate, hourly urine output usually by indwelling catheter, and perhaps central venous pressure); rapid blood replacement (up to 4–5 litres may be required); analgesia; oxygen if the patient is anaemic, shocked, or cyanosed; estimation of haemoglobin, platelet count, coagulation factors; and *artificial rupture of membranes*. Fresh whole blood and/or fresh frozen plasma and platelet concentrates less than 2 days old are necessary if there is a *coagulation problem*. Intravenous administration of *fibrinogen* (4–8 g dissolved in 250 ml of normal saline) is used less than formerly because of the risk of hepatitis and the availability of fresh frozen plasma and platelet concentrates. Some patients exhibit an overactivity of the *fibrinolytic system*, but this is compensatory to the intravascular coagulation and so the use of antifibrinolytic agents such as Trasylol is not recommended. *Preeclampsia*, if present, will need appropriate therapy.

Caesarean section is indicated in 10–15% of patients with placental abruption. In one large series the incidence was 12% (52 of 419) (table 16.1).

Prognosis

Maternal death is uncommon now that the importance of early and adequate blood replacement has been appreciated, but shock (and its complications) and disseminated intravascular coagulation may be serious. The condition accounts for about 1.5% of maternal deaths (table 14.1). Postpartum haemorrhage is likely if coagulation abnormalities are not corrected (colour plate 91). The *perinatal mortality rate (table 16.1) is approximately 30%*, (stillbirth 15–20%, neonatal death 10–15%), but is considerably higher (75%) if only patients requiring transfusion are considered, and considerably lower if the fetus is alive on admission to hospital. Apart from problems related to underlying disease states (preeclampsia, hypertension), the chief risks are *prematurity* (25% of cases) and *hypoxia* (lower 1 and 5 minute Apgar scores), both of which contribute to a high incidence of *hyaline membrane disease*. Other complications include jaundice and anaemia.

The prognosis depends also on the quality of antenatal care: the placental separation is usually more severe in those patients with uncontrolled hypertension or preeclampsia, and the mortality is higher if preexisting anaemia has not been treated. *Recurrence* in succeeding pregnancies has been observed in 10–15% of patients, and in 20–25% if abruption has occurred in 2 previous pregnancies.

Occasionally, *Sheehan syndrome* may follow (pituitary necrosis from the shock and intravascular coagulation); in follow-up studies, this should be looked for.

PLACENTA PRAEVIA
Definition
The placenta is situated partly or wholly in the lower uterine segment of the uterus (figure 19.5).

Incidence
At term, 0.5–1.0% of pregnancies; it is responsible for 15–20% of antepartum haemorrhages. Ultrasonography has shown that the incidence of placenta praevia decreases progressively as gestation proceeds because of the altered relationship of placenta to lower uterine segment (figure 19.6).

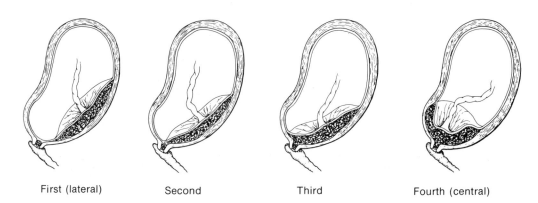

First (lateral)   Second   Third   Fourth (central)

Figure 19.5 Degrees or grades of placenta praevia. The amount of bleeding is proportional to the extent to which the placenta encroaches on the lower uterine segment.

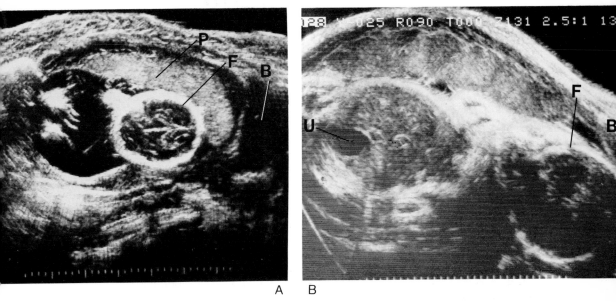

A   B

Figure 19.6 Apparent upward migration of a low-lying placenta due to growth of the lower uterine segment. **A.** Longitudinal ultrasound scan at 22 weeks' gestation showing an anterior placenta (P) between the fetal head (F) and bladder (B). **B.** At 34 weeks' gestation the placenta no longer encroaches upon the lower uterine segment. The exact position of the internal os between fetal head (F) and bladder (B) is not shown. Note urine (U) in the fetal bladder.

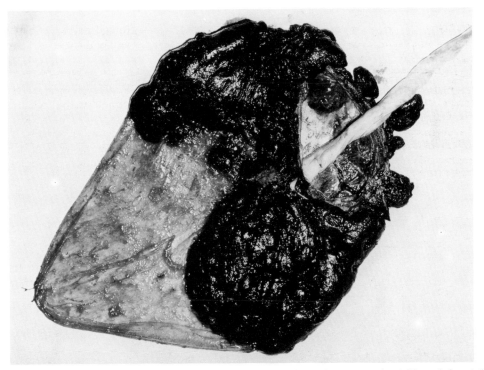

Figure 19.7 Anterior grade 3 placenta praevia. The diagnosis was made by ultrasonography at 26 weeks' gestation after the patient had experienced a 2,000 ml painless haemorrhage. Repeated haemorrhages necessitated Caesarean section at 33 weeks' gestation. The infant survived (birth-weight 2,500 g). Note that the baby was delivered through the placenta (by internal version and breech extraction). This was necessary because the lower uterine segment incision was over the middle of the placenta which was bilobed, thin and covered an unusually large area of the uterine wall.

Types (figure 19.5) and Pathophysiology

(i) *First degree.* Part of the placenta lies in the lower segment, but does not reach the internal os (lateral). (ii) *Second degree.* The lower margin of the placenta reaches the internal os, but does not cover it (marginal). (iii) *Third degree.* The placenta covers the os when closed, but not completely when it is dilated (partial) (figure 19.7). (iv) *Fourth degree.* The placenta lies centrally over the os (central).

In a series of 375 patients with placenta praevia, 46% were first degree, 26% second degree, 12% third degree and 16% fourth degree i.e. *only 1 in 4 had a major degree of praevia.*

The significance of the different types lies in the increasing morbidity and mortality to mother and fetus as the placenta becomes more centrally placed. As the lower segment of the uterus forms in the latter half of pregnancy, the placenta tends to become sheared off. Because the endometrium is less well developed in the lower uterine segment, the placenta is more likely to become attached to the underlying muscle (*placenta praevia accreta*), with consequent problems during the third stage.

Aetiology

In placenta praevia the fertilized ovum implants low in the uterine cavity. The reasons for this are not usually apparent. Higher parity is one cause, and the placenta in multiple pregnancy, because of its size, is more likely to encroach on the lower segment. *Placenta membranacea* (figure 43.9), also because of its larger size, is more likely to be praevia. There is a minor association with previous Caesarean section and early bleeding in the current pregnancy and a stronger association with previous therapeutic abortion. Smoking is another factor recently implicated.

Clinical Features

Haemorrhage without significant abdominal pain or tenderness is the outstanding feature of placenta praevia. The blood is almost invariably bright red, compared with abruption, where it is often darker. In some 20% of patients the bleeding occurs before 28 weeks, but most commonly it occurs between 34 and 38 weeks. In contradistinction to abruption, the bleeding inevitably recurs, often in a more serious degree. The initial haemorrhage may, however, be very profuse. There may be a precipitating cause, such as coitus, coughing or straining, or external ver-

Figure 19.8 Placenta praevia-accreta. Hysterectomy was required after Caesarean section because the placenta was adherent to the uterine wall and attempted removal caused torrential haemorrhage. The uterus has been opened vertically to display the retained placental tissue on the posterior lower segment.

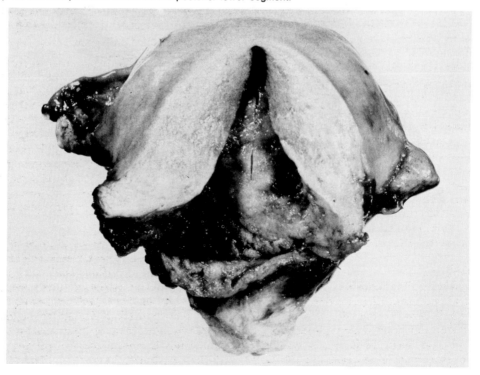

sion, but mostly the onset is spontaneous. In lesser degrees of placenta praevia, bleeding often does not occur until the cervix dilates in labour. The condition *may be suspected clinically before any bleeding has occurred* because of displacement of the presenting part from the pelvic brim, and can be confirmed by ultrasonography.

Approximately 30% of patients with placenta praevia have *no antepartum haemorrhage*, the diagnosis being made at Caesarean section (20%) or after vaginal delivery (10%). Approximately 40% of patients with placenta praevia who deliver vaginally have had no antepartum haemorrhage, the diagnosis being made when routine inspection of the secundines shows the site of fetal exit from the amniotic sac to be within 2–3 cm of the placental edge (figure III.1, Appendix IIIA).

A premature end to the pregnancy is more likely, mainly because of obstetrical interference required to control the haemorrhage; in addition, there is a somewhat greater risk of premature rupture of the membranes (displaced presenting part), and *premature labour*. The position of the baby depends on the site of implantation of the placenta: the presenting part is almost always high and placed obliquely on the opposite side of the placental attachment; if the placenta is central in position, the fetus is often placed transversely, facing the placenta. If the placenta is placed anteriorly, palpation of the presenting part is often difficult, and the breech may be mistaken for the head.

The need for *operative delivery*, particularly Caesarean section (in more than 75% of cases), has been mentioned. In a series of 375 cases at a teaching hospital (table 16.1), the *Caesarean section rate was 82%*.

After delivery, considerable difficulty may be experienced with the placenta. This results from the poor plane of separation of the placenta from its decidual bed in the lower segment. This difficulty, together with the ease of tearing the thinned-out lower segment and the considerable vascularity and poorer retraction of the lower segment muscle, contribute to a higher than normal *postpartum haemorrhage* rate. Small pieces of placenta may remain attached to the uterus and cause infection and secondary haemorrhage in the puerperium (figure 19.8).

Diagnosis

Any painless bleeding in the second half of pregnancy must be assumed to be due to placenta praevia until proved otherwise. Although the clinical features mentioned above are suggestive, a more positive diagnosis is usually sought by special investigations. One wishes to know firstly

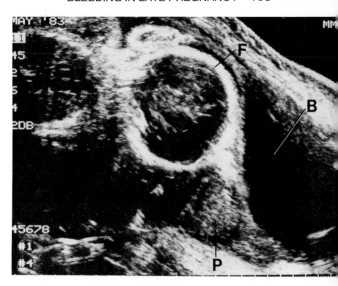

Figure 19.9 Longitudinal ultrasound scan performed at 33 weeks' gestation because of a painless antepartum haemorrhage. A posterior placenta praevia (P) completely covers the internal os and displaces the fetal head (F) 4 cm from the sacral promontory. B = maternal bladder. Lower segment Caesarean section at 37.4 weeks' gestation confirmed the diagnosis of a grade 3, posterior placenta praevia.

whether the placenta is praevia, and if so, what is the degree?

(i) *Sonicaid.* In many patients there is a characteristic auditory and ultrasonic *souffle* heard if the ear or acoustic device is placed over the region of the placenta. Although this is helpful, the greater accuracy of other methods recommends them.

(ii) *Ultrasonography.* This is the latest technique to be developed. The placenta is directly visualized on the scan, since it has slightly different properties from the uterus and amniotic fluid (figure 19.9). This technique is very accurate in experienced hands and involves no hazard to the mother and no harmful radiation to the fetus. Studies have indicated that the placenta is low-lying in 20–30% of patients studied in the second trimester, but in the vast majority (95%) of these it shifts into the upper segment (figure 19.6).

(iii) Radiographic. In the erect attitude, *the presenting part is seen to be separated more widely than usual from identifiable landmarks*, such as the sacral promontory (figure 19.10), symphysis pubis or the bladder filled with radio-opaque dye. It may be possible to visualize the placenta directly because of its greater opacity and its outline; this is more accurate if the placenta is not praevia, and thus is of limited value.

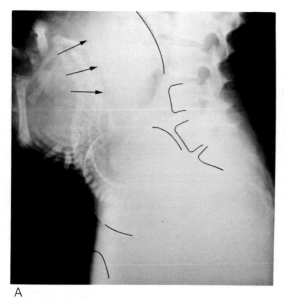
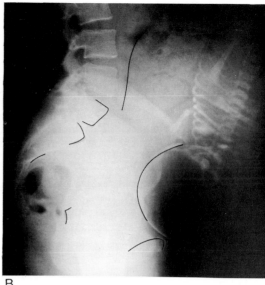

A   B

Figure 19.10 X-ray placentography. **A.** Lateral view showing placenta on the posterior upper uterine wall; the head is just engaged. **B.** Grade 3 posterior placenta praevia. Pressure on the fetal head failed to approximate it to the sacral promontory. Placentography was indicated by the head being mobile at term.

Calcification of the placenta is of some assistance, but information is usually required before 36 weeks when calcification starts to appear.

(iv) Radio-isotopes. Because of the large pool of blood contained in the placenta, short half-life isotopes (indium, technetium) injected into the maternal blood stream will be detectable by a gamma camera over the site of the placenta more easily than over nonplacental sites. Although the radiation dose to the fetus is only about 1% of that with radiographic methods, both methods have largely been superseded by ultrasonography.

Differential Diagnosis
There is usually little difficulty if the bleeding is moderate or severe in amount: bleeding of this degree is virtually always due to a placenta praevia or abruptio placentae. It is when bleeding is less serious that difficulty with diagnosis arises and further clarification must await inspection of the placenta after delivery.

Prognosis
Placenta praevia is responsible for a small but significant number (1.5%) of maternal deaths, mostly from haemorrhage and shock, and 2–3% of perinatal deaths, *mostly from prematurity* (average gestation is about 35 weeks) and intrauterine hypoxia (table 15.6). Although the conservative approach has considerably reduced this figure from the higher levels which existed previously, premature labour (20%) and intervention forced by uncontrollable haemorrhage

(35%) leave a disappointing hard core of deaths, which only partly will be overcome with the wider use of intensive care units. *The perinatal mortality rate is 5–10% (table 16.1).* The complications of Caesarean section and anaesthesia must also be taken into consideration (figure 19.7). In rare cases, the placenta is also accreta (adherent to the myometrium), a very dangerous complication (figure 19.8).

Management
Although the detection of placenta praevia before bleeding cannot be made with the same accuracy as with breech presentation or multiple pregnancy, every effort should be made in this direction by using the clues which are so often present — i.e. displacement of the presenting part by the low-lying placenta. Careful thought should be given to artificial rupture of the membranes or even vaginal examination in a patient with a high or unstable presenting part in case an unsuspected placenta praevia is present.

Diagnosis before haemorrhage is one of the advantages of *routine ultrasonography* (at about 17 weeks' gestation) which is now practised in many centres. Approximatley 50% of patients have ultrasonography performed for a clinical indication (fetal growth retardation, fetal maturity in doubt, multiple pregnancy suspected, polyhydramnios) — this has resulted in the incidental diagnosis of a high proportion of cases of placenta praevia.

The main principle of management of this condition is to treat the patient conservatively (bed rest, transfusion as indicated) until the fetus is mature (37–38 weeks). Because of the risk of sudden catastrophic bleeding, *no patient with this diagnosis should leave hospital until after delivery* unless the placenta praevia is of minor grade, the patient is within reasonable access of the hospital and can be relied on to keep the vagina inviolate. With modern techniques of investigation, the more serious grades are often diagnosed with reasonable certainty, and if the clinical features are in accord (high presenting part that does not fit into the pelvis), Caesarean section is carried out without preliminary vaginal examination. *This operation will be necessary in 75% or more of patients with clinical features.* The potential difficulties of Caesarean section for this condition should not be underestimated — large blood vessels over the lower segment, possible anterior placenta under the incision site (figure 19.7), poorly-formed

lower segment, and placenta morbidly adherent to the lower segment (figure 19.8). Caesarean section should always be performed when the patient reaches 37–38 weeks and is not in labour. If the patient is *in labour* when the diagnosis is made, vaginal delivery is favoured if bleeding is mild and the praevia is of minor degree. The use of a beta adrenergic stimulant (salbutamol, ritodrine) as a temporary measure may be indicated to relax the uterus and prevent further placental separation as well as reducing the tendency of the newborn to develop hyaline membrane disease. There is *no place for induction of labour* when the patient has placenta praevia because the poorly-fitting presenting part favours cord prolapse and delayed onset of labour.

Conservative therapy aims at prevention of prematurity and is abandoned when the fetus is mature, labour begins, or bleeding is heavy. The

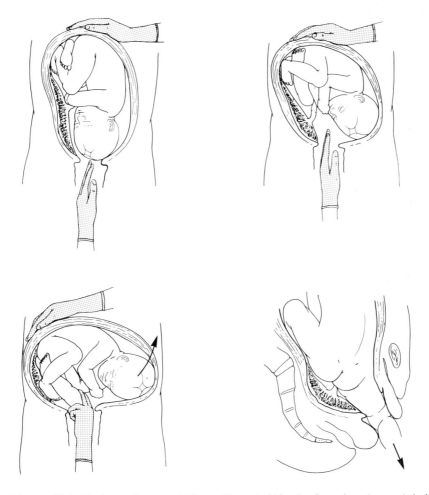

Figure 19.11 Braxton Hicks bipolar version was widely used to control bleeding from placenta praevia before Caesarean section became safe. It may still be used when the fetus is not viable, but the patient must be in labour. Because the cervix is only partly dilated, no more than the fingers can be introduced into the uterine cavity. The abdominal hand is required to bring the foot within reach of the fingers. The foot is pulled through the cervix and a weight is attached to it. Delivery is completed when the cervix reaches full dilatation.

risk of fetal anoxia from compression of the low-lying placenta or cord in labour should be remembered, and adequate monitoring techniques adopted. The paediatric staff should be alerted when labour commences or intervention is planned.

Postpartum haemorrhage should be anticipated: ligation of the vessels supplying the uterus or even hysterectomy may be required in the rare instance of placenta accreta or lower segment rupture. Anaemia should be tested for and treated in the puerperium.

OTHER PLACENTAL CONDITIONS

The following incidental and undetermined causes are responsible for 50–60% of cases of antepartum haemorrhage and as a group they have a *perinatal mortality rate of about 10%* (table 16.1). The amount of haemorrhage is often less than 100 ml and blood transfusion is seldom required. The importance of the group is the high perinatal mortality rate — approximately double that of placenta praevia, most deaths occurring as a result of prematurity.

(a) *Placental edge bleeding (marginal sinus rupture).* This is a relatively common condition where there is a rupture of the marginal sinus or vein at the edge of the placenta. The bleeding is venous in type and rarely of major degree. It is probable that in most cases the placenta is lower than normal in the uterus (although not praevia), and the edge of the placenta becomes lifted away from the uterus.

(b) *Circumvallate placenta.* This is the least common of the known causes of antepartum bleeding. Early in the development of the placenta, the trophoblast may continue to grow beyond the chorionic plate (figure 43.8). Repeated small haemorrhages (30–50%) commencing in the second trimester and hydrorrhoea (10–20%) may signal the presence of this complication. Third stage problems (retained placenta, postpartum haemorrhage) are also more common (5–10%). The perinatal mortality is between 15–25%, largely because of associated prematurity.

(c) *Vasa praevia* In this rare condition, the umbilical vessels run between chorion and amnion over the region of the internal os. The cause is *velamentous insertion* of the umbilical cord (into the membranes rather than the placenta), or a vessel passing close to the internal os when running to a *succenturiate lobe*. Usually such vessels are torn when the membranes rupture (see legends to colour plates 84 and 85 and Appendix IIIB, question 87). *In contradistinction to other types of antepartum haemorrhage, the bleeding in this condition is from the fetus,* who is placed in great jeopardy, unless speedy recognition and delivery is achieved.

It is a great thrill to diagnose a vasa praevia in labour and save a life — by immediate delivery (normal, forceps or Caesarean section if conditions are not favourable for vaginal delivery). All bleeding during labour or at amniotomy warrants testing for fetal haemoglobin.

Since fetal haemoglobin is resistant to alkali denaturation, a sample of blood from the vagina will remain pink on the addition of 10% sodium hydroxide if fetal in origin, whereas it will turn brown if maternal (*Apt test*). Diagnosis may be made by an astute observer before rupture, by noting the cord-like vessels in the membranes at the time of pelvic examination; the condition will be more evident if amnioscopy has been employed.

LOCAL CAUSES

These are revealed by speculum examination and include the following conditions.

(i) *Carcinoma of the cervix.* Usually eliminated by speculum examination at the first antenatal visit and the Papanicolaou smear test. (ii) *Cervical erosion.* This rarely bleeds to a significant degree unless marked inflammation is also present. (iii) *Cervical polyp(s).* These are seen as bright red fleshy protrusions, which usually originate in the cervical canal. (iv) *Varicose veins* are unusual causes of bleeding, and can readily be excluded by visual examination. (v) *Cervicitis and/or vaginitis.* Often due to infection with trichomonads; there is usually a profuse discharge present and the epithelium is reddened and bleeds on contact.

chapter twenty

Preeclampsia and Eclampsia

OVERVIEW

Preeclampsia and eclampsia are specific to pregnancy and together embrace a wide spectrum of clinical derangement. The disorder is responsible for a high proportion of antenatal hospital admissions, labour inductions, and morbidity/mortality to both mother and baby.

Preeclampsia, also termed *pregnancy-induced hypertension*, is characterized by the clinical syndrome of *generalized oedema*, *hypertension*, and eventually, *proteinuria*. Excess weight gain in the antenatal period usually ushers in the above features. *Vasospasm* is an important underlying abnormality, but the precise aetiology remains unclear. An *immunological basis* has been suggested because the disease is significantly more common in the nullipara or in the parous woman who has taken a different partner. The other major correlate is an excessive amount of *active trophoblast* (twins, hydatidiform mole). It is probable that the cause is multifactorial in many patients.

Much of the recent work on the subject has been concerned with *disturbed physiology and biochemistry*: important derangements include increased capillary permeability and resulting hypovolaemia, haemoconcentration, disseminated intravascular coagulation, and lowered tissue perfusion. As a result of renal tubular dysfunction, there is an increase in blood uric acid level and this occurs before there is a significant rise in nonprotein nitrogen (e.g. urea and creatinine).

Because of the great potential for serious ill-effects in both the mother and baby, the health care attendant must identify the patient at high risk for this disorder and maintain a sharp vigilance for the early signs during antenatal care. Early detection and prompt management will almost guarantee that neither mother nor baby will come to significant harm; failure to do so will expose the mother to severe *multiorgan ischaemia* and possibly to the convulsions of *eclampsia*. The ischaemia of the placenta compromises the development of the fetus and, if unchecked, is liable to cause *death in utero*.

The *essentials of treatment* in the early stage are adequate *rest*, perhaps in hospital, and a high fibre, adequate protein, and low carbohydrate *diet*. In the more advanced stages, *hypotensive and sedative drug regimens* are required to prevent intracranial and other serious haemorrhage, and eclampsia; *termination of the pregnancy* may be necessary, either by rupture of the membranes to induce labour, or by Caesarean section in the more fulminant case if induction of labour fails, there is fetal distress (cardiotocography), or the condition of the mother is causing concern.

Errors in management include lax antenatal care, failure to act on early signs of the disease, underestimation of the possible rapidity of the established disorder, delay in termination of the pregnancy, failure to use drug therapy adequately, and failure to appreciate that the preeclamptic patient is at much greater risk during anaesthesia and major operative procedures.

PREECLAMPSIA

Incidence

Although there is a wide geographical variation, an average figure would lie between 5–15%, the higher figure relating to nulliparas. In a hospital series of 40,982 patients, the incidence was 9.7% (table 16.1). The onset occurs in *labour* in 20–25% of patients.

Aetiology and Pathophysiology

Pregnancy, or more specifically, *living placental tissue* is a *sine qua non* for the appearance of the disorder. Hence strong suspicion must be levelled at the substances produced in large quantity by the placenta — particularly oestrogen and progesterone. Conditions of *hyperplacentosis* (multiple pregnancy, hydatidiform mole, rhesus isoimmunization and diabetes) are classically associated with a higher incidence of the disease. We do not know precisely how this is related to the excess water in the tissues and the subsequent vasospasm that is responsible for the rise of blood pressure.

Retention of salt (600–800 mmol of sodium) and water (6–8 litres) in pregnancy is caused by 2 mechanisms: (i) *oestrogen* and perhaps other hormones from the placenta, and (ii) a physiological response to the *upright position, whereby blood tends to pool in the progesterone-dilated veins of the lower half of the body.* This reduces the pressure on the sensory mechanisms in the great veins entering the heart, and this stimulates the release of 2 further hormones — antidiuretic/vasopressin from the pituitary gland and aldosterone from the adrenal gland, both acting on the kidney. In preeclampsia and eclampsia there is usually too little fluid in the vascular system (*hypovolaemia*) and too much in the extravascular tissues (*oedema*). This results from a rise in capillary pressure forcing fluid out of the capillaries and/or reduction of the colloid osmotic pressure which keeps the fluid in and/or a greater permeability of the vessel wall. The hypovolaemia explains why these patients show poor tolerance to blood loss, shock, and major surgical procedures. There is also an increased *viscosity* of the blood which further reduces flow through smaller vessels.

The *vasospasm* may be related to the shift of salt and water into the extravascular space or into the cell, perhaps those lining the blood vessels, rendering them more sensitive to stimulation by the *renin-angiotensin system*. Retransfusion studies suggest that vascular wall reactivity is more important than the presence of circulating pressor substances. *Prostacyclin* is now thought to be an important factor in the flow in smaller arteries.

A consistent finding in the developed condition is *disseminated intravascular coagulation* reflected by platelet consumption and fibrin split products in the blood. Since these changes can sometimes be demonstrated quite early in the disease, they may be causally involved. This would fit the theory based on animal studies that platelet activation (perhaps by immune complexes) and adhesion to endothelium is a fundamental change. Prostacyclin activity (PgI_2) is decreased in fetal umbilical vessels and amniotic fluid and this may account for the reduced inhibition of platelet aggregation and vasoconstriction. It has been observed that the incidence of preeclampsia is low if platelet inhibitors, such as aspirin, have been taken regularly in pregnancy.

Dietary fibre. Preeclampsia is less common in women whose diet contains plenty of fibre. This may be the result of changes in gut steroids or it may reflect differences in the intake of other nutrients — e.g. a high fibre diet usually has a high magnesium content.

Immunological. A number of clinical findings give support to an immunological basis for preeclampsia. There is protection by previous blood transfusion and pregnancies (less so with abortions) and this is reversed if there is a new partner. It is suggested that tolerance antibodies become effective after the initial (sensitizing) pregnancy. If there is HLA homozygosity of the partners, fewer tolerance antibodies will be produced.

Placental site. There is a relationship between preeclampsia and higher sites of placental attachment in the uterus; this may stress the ovarian venous drainage system.

Catecholamines. These are consistently lower, but the significance of this finding is still obscure.

It is likely that quite complex biochemical alterations may be involved as a result of the major homeostatic changes of pregnancy.

Clinical Features

The increase in extravascular fluid is detected *by excessive gain in weight* (more than 500 g/week, 2,000 g/month) or *oedema*, and is felt by the patient as a swelling of the feet, hands, and face (generalized oedema, colour plates 9 and 10). If pretibial oedema is still present after a night's rest, it is suspicious of early preeclampsia. Because of *vasospasm*, the next sign is *elevation of blood pressure* (at least 15–20 mm Hg systolic/ 10–15 diastolic). In addition, blood flow is reduced in the majority of the internal organs. The cells are thereby starved of oxygen and nutrients for vital processes, and dysfunction and finally death of the more susceptible cells will occur. Unless the vasospasm is relieved, small haemorrhages will occur and mark the site of the most intense hypoxia.

If the spasm is severe, very high levels of blood pressure occur (of the order 180/110 or more) and the vascular system is unable to maintain its integrity; either a blow-out occurs at the weakest point (usually the brain) or the heart itself fails. The *optic fundi* will usually reflect these changes, with arterial spasm and perhaps exudates/ haemorrhage.

The ischaemia thus produced explains the *secondary manifestations* on the brain (headache, visual upset, vomiting, fitting), kidney (proteinuria, oliguria), liver (epigastric pain which is caused by small haemorrhages in the liver or by

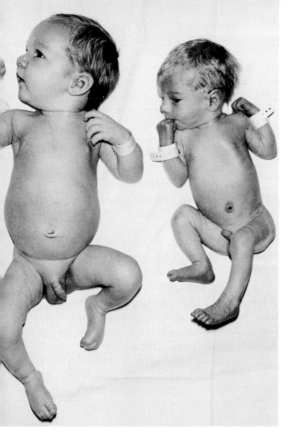

swelling of the hypoxic cells), and placenta (fetal distress, death).

The possibility of disseminated intravascular coagulation has already been mentioned.

The main *fetal risks* of preeclampsia are *intra-uterine hypoxia and malnutrition* due to *placental failure* (figures 20.1 and 20.2). Fore-warning may be obtained by special tests such as cardiotocography and oestriol values. These complications are more likely when the disease is of early onset (e.g. before the 36th week). *Neonatal death* from hyaline membrane disease is also a risk when delivery of an immature infant is necessary. The *maternal risks* of severe preeclampsia are (i) eclampsia, with the possibility of death due to cerebral haemorrhage, hepatic

Figure 20.2 Preeclampsia associated with severe placental infarction in a 33-year-old gravida 2, para 1. She had no predisposing disease (hypertension, renal disease, diabetes), but had developed hypertension in labour at 39.5 weeks in her first pregnancy. At 34.2 weeks' gestation in her second pregnancy she developed hypertension (170/100) and proteinuria (5 g/l); she had low oestriol excretion (20 μmol (5.7 mg)/24 hours), ultrasonographic evidence of fetal growth retardation, and cardiotocography showed loss of beat to beat variation. The patient was sedated and labour induced; 2 hours later a healthy, growth-retarded infant (birth-weight 1,590 g) was delivered; the placenta weighed 470 g and 75% of it was infarcted (see colour plates 18 and 19). (Courtesy of Dr Christopher Targett).

Figure 20.1 The infant on the right was small for dates (1,930 g at 36 weeks) and shows the signs of marked placental insufficiency. His mother had persistently low oestrogen excretion and developed severe preeclampsia in labour — a classical example of poor placental function for weeks before the onset of hypertension and proteinuria. The normally nourished full term baby on the left weighed 3,580 g.

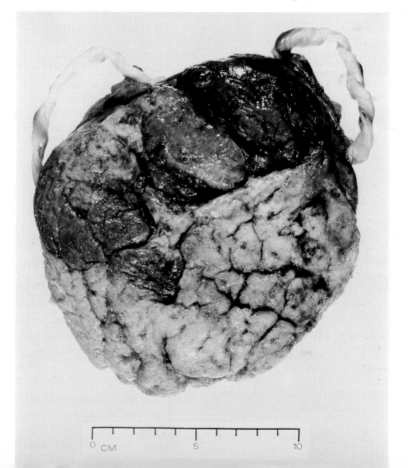

haemorrhage or failure, renal failure due to cortical or tubular necrosis, and cardiac failure, and (ii) chronic renal damage or potentiation of renal disease which is already present, as is often the case when severe preeclampsia occurs before 36 weeks' gestation.

Diagnosis

Classically, preeclampsia presents an orderly sequence of signs as above. Proteinuria, for example, does not precede hypertension except when there is chronic kidney disease. The diagnosis of preeclampsia is made when *any 2 of the 3 signs* of *generalized oedema, hypertension* (140/90 or above, or a rise in blood pressure 15-20/10-15) and *proteinuria* (more than 150 mg/24 hours and not due to contamination or infection) are present.

Many conditions produce dependent oedema (of the legs) — for example, varicose veins, standing, pressure, low blood protein levels (figure 20.3); *generalized oedema* is far less common, however, and always requires investigation. If associated with hypertension (140/90 or above) or a relative rise of blood pressure, a diagnosis of preeclampsia is made.

Probably, the commonest difficulty is in the differentiation of mild (or early) preeclampsia and essential hypertension. Often this is only evident after delivery when the elevated blood pressure fails to subside in the latter group; clinical evidence suggests that the fetal prognosis is better in these patients.

Figure 20.3 Gross pitting oedema of the feet in a short primigravida with excessive weight gain and generalized oedema. She developed hypertension and proteinuria for the first time during labour.

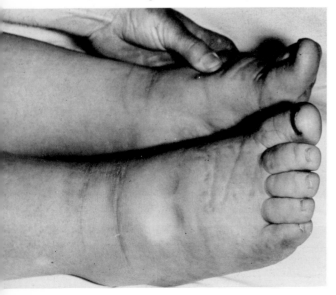

The majority of conditions mimicking the more advanced stages of preeclampsia are the different types of kidney disorder or other secondary forms of hypertension. Often, an accurate diagnosis can only be made after the pregnancy, especially if the patient is first seen in the second or third trimester.

Classification of Preeclampsia

Mild: generalized oedema, diastolic pressure less than 100
Moderate: generalized oedema, diastolic pressure 100 or more
Severe: generalized oedema, diastolic pressure 100 or more, proteinuria

Important prognostic features of disease severity are a high blood pressure, reduced urinary output, disseminated intravascular coagulation, and symptoms such as headache, visual upset, and liver tenderness.

Although preeclampsia is more common in nulliparas, it is important to remember that the disease can be severe and of sudden onset in multiparas (colour plates 9-11).

Investigations

(i) *Multichannel blood analysis.* (ii) *Urine microscopy and culture* — red blood cells and casts may mimic renal disease. (iii) *Complete blood count.* (iv) *Serum proteins* and albumin/globulin ratio — often decreased. (v) *Serum uric acid* — moderate or marked elevation. (vi) *Serum urea* — usually normal, may be a moderate elevation. (vii) *Creatinine clearance* — detects impaired renal function and may indicate underlying chronic renal disease. (viii) *Plasma or urinary oestriol excretion* — often low, especially when the disease is severe. (ix) *Coagulation studies.* Platelets and fibrogen show a progressive drop with progress of the disease; fibrin degradation products rise as does factor 8 complex. (x) *Cardiotocography.*

Management

Prophylaxis

Preeclampsia is more easily prevented or minimized than any of the other serious complications of pregnancy. Careful attention should be given to the following: (i) predisposing factors in the history — familial tendency, past history of preeclampsia, hypertension or renal disease; (ii) predisposing factors in the pregnancy — nulliparity, hyperplacentosis, excessive weight gain; (iii) high standards of antenatal care — supervision of appointments, weight, blood pressure and urine checks; and (iv) hospitalization for early deviations from normal.

Significant maternal and fetal complications usually indicate avoidable factors on the part of the mother and/or member(s) of the health team.

Therapy

The treatment required depends to a large extent on the *severity of the disease* process and the *duration of the pregnancy*. Obviously there is no place for conservative treatment if the disease is severe or moderately so, or past 40 weeks' gestation even if it is mild — conservative treatment aims at continuing pregnancy to obtain further fetal growth and maturity.

(i) *Mild preeclampsia.* The essentials are *rest* and a proper *diet* (high protein, high vitamin, high fibre, low carbohydrate). The beneficial effect of bed rest is well known clinically and is understandable in the light of the remarks made under 'aetiology'. There is an improved flow of blood to the heart and thus to the uterus and placenta, and a counteraction of the antidiuretic/aldosterone hormone release. There is a diuresis and fall in blood pressure. *Diuretic drugs are useful in essential hypertension, but are rarely if ever indicated in preeclampsia*, since they do not treat the basic disorder. *Sedation* (usually in the form of a minor tranquillizer such as diazepam) may be useful if the patient is not relaxed in hospital and is helpful also in securing a good night's sleep.

After a variable period of bed rest, usually 2–3 days, the patient is allowed up and the blood pressure is carefully assessed; if it is satisfactory, she is allowed home to continue the treatment outlined and is seen twice weekly. Later she may require readmission and finally amniotomy at 37–40 weeks according to the findings (blood pressure control, station of the head, state of the cervix), if spontaneous labour has not occurred.

(ii) *Moderate preeclampsia.* The main addition to therapy is a hypotensive drug, which is commenced if the diastolic pressure does not settle rapidly below 90 with bed rest. *Labetalol* (a combined alpha and beta blocking drug) is given orally, 100–200 mg bd as a starting dose. Other agents which have been extensively used in pregnancy include *methyldopa* and *propanolol* or one of its newer derivatives. The period of hospitalization will be longer and the likelihood of induction of labour greater in this group of patients. Corticosteroids may be given to mature the baby's lungs if indicated (Chapter 24). More intensive laboratory testing and fetal monitoring are undertaken.

(iii) *Severe preeclampsia.* When proteinuria has appeared there is usually no alternative to ter-mination *of the pregnancy*, irrespective of the period of gestation. The degree of proteinuria and the period of gestation largely determine when this will be carried out. With modern hypotensive drugs the blood pressure can usually be controlled, but despite this, very rarely does the fetus continue to grow.

Nursing Measures

Posture. The patient should be nursed on her side to maximize uterine blood flow.

Records. The type and frequency of record depends on the severity of the condition. (i) *Fluid balance.* Because of the effect of the disease process on the kidney, an accurate fluid balance is of vital importance. Oliguria or even anuria may complicate the more serious forms of the disease. (ii) *Weight.* Since the weight of the patient is a good guide to the amount of body fluid present, this measurement should be made daily before breakfast. (iii) *Blood pressure.* Twice daily measurements may be quite adequate if the process is mild and the patient is at rest in the antenatal ward. When hypotensive drugs are being used the chart should be kept 4-hourly; if the patient is in labour even more frequent estimations (every ½–2 hours) are desirable. (iv) *Urine testing.* All urine specimens should be tested for protein if the condition is moderate or marked. If mild, daily testing of the first morning specimen is adequate. (v) *Fetal heart.* Auscultation of the fetal heart should be carried out twice daily for patients in hospital and the rate recorded. In some centres monitors are used and recordings made for half an hour each day or 2–3 times each week, depending on the severity of the disease. During labour a continuous monitor should be used if available; otherwise, frequent Doppler auscultation is carried out. (vi) *Oestriol.* Urinary oestriol requires a complete 24-hour urine collection from the patient, or alternatively a blood specimen if plasma oestriol is being measured. (vii) *Temperature, pulse, and respiration rates.* These will be charted as usual. More frequent recordings will be made during labour. Special attention is given to the respiratory rate if magnesium sulphate is being given to the patient.

Drug Therapy

The following remarks apply particularly to the patient with severe preeclampsia.

Sedation. One of the main therapeutic principles is to reduce the excitation threshold of the central nervous system. (i) *Magnesium sulphate.* Magnesium sulphate 4–5 g (8–10 ml of a 50% solution) is added to an equal quantity of sterile water and given slowly IV over 5–10 minutes, followed by an infusion of 2–4 ml (1–2 g) per hour. This is equivalent to 50–100 ml per hour of a solution of 20 ml of the 50% solution (10 g) in 500 ml of infusion fluid. Alternatively, 10–20 ml of a 50% solution (5–10 g) IM statim, is followed by 5–10 ml 4–6 hourly as required; 1 ml of 2% lignocaine (lidocaine) is added to the syringe to minimize the pain of the injection. A therapeutic blood level of magnesium sulphate is in the range 3–4 mmol/l (6–8 meq/l). To check for *overdosage*, the respiratory rate should be taken half-hourly; it should be above 10/minute. The presence of the knee jerks should also be elicited half-hourly. Overdosage can be reversed with IV calcium gluconate, 10 ml of a 10% solution, which must be available. Magnesium sulphate has the virtues of rapidity of action, high efficacy, easy reversibility, minimal depression of oxygen uptake in the brain of the mother and baby, as well as a mild relaxing effect on vascular and uterine smooth muscle (resulting in increased uteroplacental perfusion). (ii) *Chlormethiazole* (Heminevrin, Hemineurine, Distaneurine). This drug is a derivative of the thiazole part of vitamin B_1. It has both anticonvulsive and sedative properties; there is also a mild hypotensive effect without effect on the pulse rate. Oral capsules and tablets are available, but the main use is by intravenous infusion in the control of severe preeclampsia and eclampsia. The solution is prepared at a strength of 0.8% and is given at 50–100 drops/minute according to the seriousness of the patient's condition, and when control is obtained the rate is lowered to 15–30 drops/minute. Side-effects are few, but may include a burning feeling in the face, phlebitis, and hypothermia. Since the solution is unstable at tropical and subtropical temperatures it must be kept cool or made up fresh from the dry pack (vial of 4 g dry powder, vial of 5 g sodium citrate buffer in 20 ml, transfer cannula for mixing). This substance passes across the placenta, but does not significantly depress the baby. It is rapidly eliminated from the body. It should be accompanied by an injection of a potent diuretic (frusemide) to produce normal levels of intracranial pressure. Combination with rapidly-acting hypotensive agents (e.g. diazoxide) may produce depression in the newborn. (iii) *Narcotics* (pethidine, omnopon, morphine) damp down painful afferent stimuli and are largely employed to cover transport, or if the patient is in labour. (iv) *Tranquillizers* (diazepam, phenergan, promazine, chlorpromazine) are used largely in conjunction with a narcotic, usually pethidine, as a

'lytic cocktail'. (v) *Sedatives* (barbiturates and compounds with a central nervous system depressive effect) are best avoided because of effects on the baby. Paraldehyde, 5–10 ml IM, is a safe and useful sedative, and for emergency use its absorption can be accelerated very effectively by adding an ampoule of hyaluronidase (Wydase) to the injection.

Hypotensive drugs. Lowering the blood pressure is essential to prevent the effects of ischaemia which result from vascular spasm, and 'blow-out' type of haemorrhage which occurs typically in the brain. (i) *Diazoxide* (Hyperstat). Given intravenously, this drug has a potent hypotensive action. It is administered in 30 mg boluses every 1 minute until satisfactory control of blood pressure is achieved. *It is unusual to require more than a total dose of 150 mg* — even less may be required if other drug therapy has already been given. There is little or no postural hypotension or cerebral ischaemia and the average duration of action is 10 hours. Because of a sodium-retaining effect, the additional use of an effective diuretic drug such as frusemide (Lasix) is recommended (40 mg IV or IM). (ii) *Hydralazine* (Apresoline). An initial 5 mg bolus intravenous dose is given, followed by an infusion of 2–20 mg per hour according to response.

Fluids. If the preeclampsia is severe, the intravascular compartment is much reduced and the extracellular space is overloaded. Expert control is usually necessary in these patients since important decisions regarding the amount of fluid replacement (and the need for a central venous pressure or even Swan-Ganz line), and its type (serum albumin, lactate) will have to be made.

Treatment in the Delivery Room

Careful monitoring and documentation of vital signs, as previously described, is continued. It is best to keep successive boiled urine specimens in test tubes in a rack so that it can be seen at a glance if the proteinuria is subsiding or getting worse (it should be remembered, however, that oliguria will cause an apparent increase in the amount of protein in the urine due to concentration).

An absolute rule is that the blood pressure and central nervous system irritability of the patient with preeclampsia should be controlled before induction of labour is performed (by rupture of the membranes). *Epidural analgesia* is useful in reducing pain stress and level of blood pressure but should be used only after confirming that the blood clotting profile is normal. Caesarean section may be needed in acute severe preeclampsia because of rapidly deteriorating biochemical indices or impending fetal death (figure 20.2).

If there is *disseminated intravascular coagulation* and *coagulation failure*, plasma concentrates and fresh frozen plasma will be needed.

The neonatal paediatrician and anaesthetist should be warned in advance, so that appropriate patient care checks and arrangements can be organized.

Remember that the signs of preeclampsia (or eclampsia) may first be observed during labour or after delivery. They always warrant sedation as the disease may be progressing rapidly. This is why blood pressure measurement and urine examination is performed regularly during labour and after delivery; sedative drugs, such as magnesium sulphate or chlormethiazole, should not be ceased abruptly after delivery. These patients are more prone to thromboembolism and simple preventive measures against this should be instituted.

Prognosis

This depends very largely on the time of onset of the disease, the speed and efficiency of medical management, and the severity of the disease process. The perinatal mortality rate is 2–4% and depends upon the proportion of cases of severe preeclampsia (table 16.1).

Maternal death may result from haemorrhage and/or shock — the chief organs involved being the brain, liver, kidney, and placenta. If the process is allowed to drift on, permanent kidney damage may result.

Fetal death occurs in 2–5% of patients. This is usually due to a combination of prematurity and intrauterine hypoxia (due to placental insufficiency).

ECLAMPSIA

Eclampsia is a very serious complication because of the high risk to the life of the mother and baby. In the great majority of cases, it represents a breakdown in the provision or acceptance of antenatal care.

Aetiology

The basic disorder is probably one of *brain hypoxia*, brought about partly by intense vasospasm and partly by oedema. In many patients there is an *underlying cerebral dysrhythmia*, and this explains why fitting occurs when the preceding preeclampsia was not particularly severe.

Incidence

Eclampsia occurs in approximately 1 in 1,000 deliveries and is 50 times less common than preeclampsia. There is, however, a wide geographical variation, due partly to differing standards of antenatal care and partly to poorly understood factors such as diet and climate. In one major teaching hospital series the incidence, including all emergency cases, was 1 in 2,000 deliveries (table 16.1).

Clinical Features

Relation to delivery. In approximately 50% of patients, eclampsia precedes the onset of labour; the remaining 50% are almost equally divided between the intrapartum and postpartum periods. With good antenatal care, it is not uncommon to find a preponderance of postpartum cases; in these patients the levels of blood pressure and proteinuria are often lower than one would expect with this complication. In the series of 24 patients shown in table 16.1, convulsions began before labour in 7, during labour in 6 and after delivery in 11.

Prodromal features. It is important to be aware of the features that often precede the actual fit: severe headache, nausea or vomiting, irritability, restlessness and twitching, epigastric pain, visual disturbance, drowsiness, oliguria and tachycardia. These really are only signs of severe vasospasm and hypoxia affecting different organs of the body.

The convulsion. Usually there is a preconvulsive stage or aura as in an epileptic fit and the patient is dissociated from her surroundings. This is followed by a *tonic stage*, lasting approximately 30 seconds, when the skeletal muscles are in a generalized spasm: because of the virtual cessation of respiration, the patient becomes cyanosed. This stage gives way to the *clonic stage* of alternate muscular spasm and relaxation, which lasts up to 2–3 minutes. In this stage, the patient is at considerable risk of self injury (tongue biting, striking herself against unyielding surroundings, or falling out of bed). Finally, there is a stage of *coma* which lasts for a variable period, sometimes hours, depending on the number of fits, degree of vasospasm, and cerebral hypoxia.

Diagnosis

There is rarely difficulty in diagnosing eclampsia because of the relation to preceding preeclampsia.

Other causes of convulsions or coma should be considered if the features are not typical — e.g.

the blood pressure is not markedly raised and/or there is little proteinuria; such conditions include epilepsy, cerebral tumour, intracranial vascular complication, inadvertent intravenous injection of a local analgesic agent, acute hypotension, amniotic fluid or air embolism, and water intoxication.

Management

Prophylaxis

If the attendant is aware of the warning signs and promptly reports their presence, emergency treatment can be given which will avert the onset of fitting. Adequate hypotensive therapy and sedation in patients with less severe preeclampsia (particularly during labour) will diminish the incidence of postpartum fitting. Preparations containing ergometrine should be avoided in third stage management when the patient is hypertensive. Patients should not be transferred from the labour ward until the blood pressure, urine output, and level of consciousness are satisfactory.

Active Treatment

The aims are to provide initial first aid, then treatment for the underlying disorder, and finally termination of the pregnancy as soon as practicable.

(a) *First aid.* (i) *Prevention of injury.* The patient should be gently but firmly restrained and a rubber airway placed in her mouth to prevent tongue biting and to aid respiration. If an airway is unavailable, a padded spoon will suffice. (ii) *Oxygenation.* If available, oxygen should be provided by means of a mask or nasal catheter. The oropharynx should be cleared of mucus and blood; if the patient is unconscious, an airway should be inserted, or alternatively, the mandible should be held forward. (iii) *Posture.* The patient should be nursed in the semiprone position to facilitate drainage and to minimize pulmonary aspiration. (iv) Because comatose patients are likely to develop bronchopneumonia, an antibiotic is given — e.g. IM penicillin, 1 million units 6-hourly. (v) *Transport.* If the patient is to be transferred to hospital it is desirable that a doctor or nurse accompany the patient in the ambulance. *Preliminary sedation* will minimize the likelihood of further fitting — e.g. magnesium sulphate 10 ml of a 50% solution (10 g) IM or pethidine 100 mg plus chlorpromazine 50 mg IM or paraldehyde 10 ml mixed with hyaluronidase IM.

(b) *Drug therapy.* This is similar to that dis-

cussed under severe preeclampsia. Metabolic acidosis may need correction with intravenous sodium bicarbonate. A diuretic (e.g. frusemide) may be necessary if there is gross fluid retention, or impending cardiac or renal failure.

(c) *Environment.* External stimuli of all kinds should be reduced to a minimum; light and noise levels should be subdued; manipulations such as blood pressure recording and catheterization should be carried out as gently as possible and preferably only when primary sedation has been effected.

(d) *Nursing care.* (i) *General.* There must be a nurse with the patient at all times. Dentures should be removed. If the patient is comatose she should be turned hourly. Immediate reporting of any abnormality is essential. An indwelling catheter and closed-drainage system is necessary for urine collection, output measurement, and testing. (ii) *Observations.* The pulse rate and blood pressure are recorded quarter-hourly initially, then half-hourly; the fetal heart rate and maternal respiratory rate are taken half-hourly. Other observations include uterine activity, fluid balance, proteinuria, level of consciousness, degree of dilatation of the pupils if the patient is comatose, and prodromal signs of fitting. (iii) *Equipment and drugs required.* Padded gag and bed rails, sucker, airway, oxygen supply with means of administration (preferably full anaesthetic set-up), routine delivery equipment, drugs as specified.

(e) *Investigations.* As outlined in the section on preeclampsia; fetal monitoring is advisable if the patient is not delivered.

(f) *Other measures.* A consultant's opinion is necessary in all cases, by telephone if necessary.

(g) *Epidural analgesia.* Lumbar or caudal epidural analgesia may be ordered (figure 41.14) since pain is relieved and there is a beneficial hypotensive effect. However, evidence of *disseminated intravascular coagulation* (low platelet count etc) is a *contraindication* to epidural analgesia because of the risk of haemorrhage causing compression of the spinal cord.

(h) *Induction of labour.* If eclampsia occurs before labour and there is no specific indication for Caesarean section, surgical induction of labour is carried out when the convulsions are fully controlled and the patient is stabilized. An oxytocin infusion is indicated if labour has not commenced in 2-4 hours.

(i) *Delivery.* Unless progress in the second stage is satisfactory, forceps or vacuum extraction should be undertaken. Caesarean section is reserved for patients in whom induction has failed, for those with specific obstetric indications, such as delay or fetal distress in the first stage of labour, or for those in whom the fits have not been controlled, which is very rare. Ergometrine preparations are contraindicated in the third stage because of their possible hypertensive effect. In these patients, oxytocin (10 units IV) is the drug of choice.

(j) *Progress.* Favourable progress is usually evident on clinical examination of the patient; symptoms such as headache and irritability will disappear, the diastolic blood pressure stabilizes below 90, the urinary output increases and proteinuria decreases. In rare cases, a serious complication may arise during the course of the disease — placental abruption, cerebrovascular accident, renal shut-down, disseminated intravascular coagulation, or liver failure; this will require additional special care. With proper management, the majority of patients rapidly return to normality after the baby is delivered. As with preeclampsia, *careful follow-up is essential* for evidence of residual hypertension or renal disease.

Prognosis

Maternal death occurs in 2–20% of patients, depending on the local facilities. The usual cause of death is cerebral haemorrhage, with renal or cardiac failure being less common. In surviving patients, there is usually complete recovery of function. *Perinatal death* occurs in 10–20% and is due mainly to hypoxia and prematurity (table 16.1).

chapter twenty-one

Amniotic Fluid

OVERVIEW

Early in developmental life, the fetus becomes enclosed by the amnion and its surrounding fluid-filled cavity. Initially, this is very similar to extracellular fluid. This buffer zone protects the fetus and umbilical cord from mechanical trauma, and allows free movement and unrestricted growth. The liquor amnii increases in parallel with fetal growth and reaches a maximum of 800–1,500 ml nearing term. Transfer studies have indicated that there is an active exchange between the liquor and the fluid compartments of the fetus and mother. The contributions of *fetal swallowing and urination* have been reasonably quantitated, but transfers between the other compartments are difficult to measure accurately.

The fluid can be sampled by the technique of *amniocentesis*, and much information obtained about the nature and condition of the fetus — e.g. *sex, congenital anomalies* (by chromosomal and biochemical analysis), extent of *haemolysis* (in the case of erythroblastosis, by the amount of bilirubin), and *maturity* (especially of the lungs, by analysis of phospholipids). Later in pregnancy, the fluid can be visualized by *amnioscopy* (carried out by passing an amnioscope through the cervix) and the condition of the fetus assessed by the amount and colour of the liquor.

Polyhydramnios (an excess of amniotic fluid — more than 1,500 ml) is often a significant pointer to problems in the fetus, particularly *congenital anomalies* which prevent the fetus from swallowing and/or absorbing the fluid (anencephaly, oesophageal atresia, duodenal atresia), and twinning. The reverse condition of *oligohydramnios* is often also disturbing, since it is usually indicative of marked *fetoplacental insufficiency*. Each of these conditions is an indication for further investigation and/or consultation.

The membranes which enclose the amniotic cavity (amnion and chorion) normally rupture at the end of the first stage of labour (at full dilatation of the cervix). In some 10% of patients, rupture occurs before this, often before labour has commenced; the earlier this occurs the more serious the outlook for the fetus because of the risk of *premature labour, infection* from vaginal microorganisms, and perhaps *prolapse of the umbilical cord.*

PHYSIOLOGY

FORMATION

The amniotic cavity develops early in fetal life. A cleft appears in the ectoderm (outer layer) of the fetus, on its dorsal aspect, and this progressively enlarges (colour plate 1). Cells lining this cavity form the amnion and, eventually, the amniotic space completely surrounds the fetus, lines the cavity of the uterus and covers the body stalk — which will become the umbilical cord. The amniotic cavity and its lining membrane are thus wholly fetal in development. The *cells of the amnion* are responsible for the formation of fluid throughout pregnancy.

The *volume of amniotic fluid* increases progressively until approximately 34–36 weeks, remains stationary until 38–40 weeks, and then decreases at a rate of about 150 ml/week. The volume is approximately 30–35 ml at 10 weeks, 125–150 ml at 15 weeks, 450–500 ml at 20 weeks, and 500–1,000 ml at 36–37 weeks. Not only the amniotic fluid, but also a large number of its constituents are exchanging constantly between the 3 main 'compartments' — the amniotic cavity, the fetus and the mother. In later pregnancy, an increasing source of removal of fluid and particulate matter is *fetal swallowing*. The amount swallowed ranges from 10–15 ml/day at 20 weeks to 400–500 ml/day at term; with conditions such as anencephaly the rate is markedly reduced (5–250 ml at term). The fetus also contributes to the liquor volume by the *passage of urine*; voiding occurs about hourly in late pregnancy; fetal *lung fluid* is a minor source. The fact that absorption of fluid still takes place after fetal death in utero suggests that there is activity of the membranes lining the uterus.

FUNCTION

The most important function of the amniotic fluid is to provide a *buffer* zone between the developing fetus and the uterus. Apart from insulation against trauma, the fluid-filled space allows equal growth of the fetus in all directions. It also enables such functions as swallowing, 'respiration', limb movement, and urination to develop normally and to be fully operative at the time of delivery. The membranes provide a *barrier to ascending infection* of the amniotic cavity, but this is less efficient after labour has commenced. Swallowed fluid provides about 25% of fetal *protein* requirements in late pregnancy — fetal malnutrition is often associated with a reduced volume of amniotic fluid.

COMPOSITION

The amniotic fluid is similar in composition to extracellular fluid. Most components (electrolytes, proteins, sugars, fats) have a lower concentration than in serum (the concentration of protein, for example, is only about 5% of that in serum). An obvious fall in *sodium* (and hence osmolarity) occurs in the second half of pregnancy, and a similar decrease is seen in the *bilirubin* level. There are a large number of substances in the fluid, especially hormones and enzymes, and the levels of some of these can be used to predict the presence of inborn errors of metabolism in the fetus or, later on, the wellbeing of the fetus. Substances excreted in the fetal urine (creatinine, urea, uric acid) rise progressively due to micturition. During labour, *prostaglandins* abruptly increase. Particulate matter exfoliated from the fetus includes hair, cells (from skin, mouth, and urinary tract) and fat from sebaceous glands (vernix); other cells are desquamated from the amnion. *Prolactin levels* are high and parallel those in the maternal circulation.

PATHOLOGY

POLYHYDRAMNIOS (colour plate 12)

In this condition, there is an excess of amniotic fluid for the particular period of gestation. *It can be temporary* and therefore not be evident at delivery. In the third trimester, this usually means a volume greater than 1,500 ml — although clinical diagnosis is often not made until the volume is in excess of 2,500 ml (the

same problems apply to estimation of the volume of amniotic fluid as to the weight of the fetus). Usually it represents an imbalance between input (or production) and output. The fetus must be regarded as being central in both activities.

Acute polyhydramnios is a rare condition (about 5% of cases of polyhydramnios), usually occurring in the second trimester. It is almost always associated with *uniovular twins*, tends to be gross, and usually is responsible for termination of the pregnancy because of premature rupture of the membranes (figure 25.12 and colour plates 12 and 71). With large accumulations of fluid, the patient experiences pressure symptoms (discomfort, dyspnoea, anorexia and perhaps vomiting).

Most of the discussion which follows refers to *chronic polyhydramnios*, a much commoner condition.

Incidence

0.5–2.0%; the higher figure is true if those patients are included who develop the clinical features of polyhydramnios between 30–34 weeks after which the excessive fluid is absorbed.

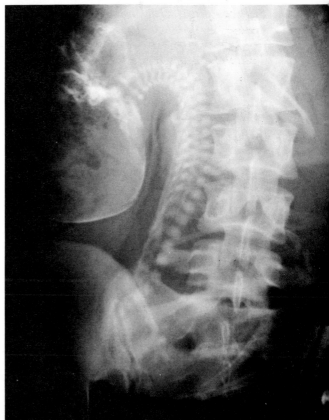

Figure 21.1 Polyhydramnios associated with extreme extension of the neck which presumably occluded the oesophagus and prevented the fetus swallowing liquor. Caesarean section is indicated in this type of breech presentation when external version fails, since difficulty would be likely with delivery of the aftercoming head.

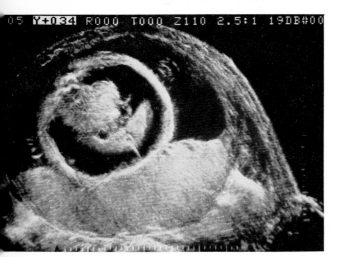
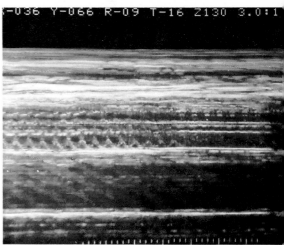

A   B

Figure 21.2 Nonimmunological hydrops fetalis and intrauterine supraventricular tachycardia identified by ultrasonography performed at 30 weeks' gestation because of polyhydramnios. Fetal congestive cardiac failure due to this cause can be treated by maternal digitalization causing reversion to sinus rhythm. **A.** Transverse scan through the fetal abdomen shows marked ascites, oedema of the abdominal wall, polyhydramnios and a thick posterior placenta. **B.** Recording of fetal heart rate of 260/minute. The large divisions in the scale at the lower margin represent 0.5 seconds. (From Acton CM et al Australas Radiol 1983; 27: 37–38).

Aetiology

(i) *Fetal malformation*. Nonclosure of cavities (anencephaly, spina bifida, umbilical hernia, ectopia vesicae). (ii) Blockage of the upper gastrointestinal tract (oesophageal or duodenal atresia). (iii) Other causes of failure to swallow (cerebral malformations, hydrops fetalis, hyperextended attitude (figure 21.1), tumours). (iv) *Obstruction of fetal venous circulation* causing nonimmunological hydrops fetalis (heart, vessels, liver). Congestive cardiac failure due to fetal supraventricular tachycardia (figure 21.2). (v) *Multiple pregnancy* (usually uniovular twins, figure 21.3). (vi) *Maternal diseases* (diabetes mellitus and preeclampsia).

In about one-third of patients there appears to be no significant aetiological factor; in some of these, there may be a *prolactin receptor* defect in the chorion which results in impaired fluid exchange across the membrane.

Diagnosis

This is fairly imprecise by clinical means. The following features are suggestive. There is a history of rapid enlargement of the abdomen (according to the patient). On examination, there is often an abnormal increase in fundal height; fetal parts are difficult to outline, and the fetal heart difficult to hear (the difficulty, or otherwise, in palpation depends on the tenseness of the uterus; in some cases, large amounts of fluid may be present at low pressure, and palpation and ballottement of the fetus is easier than

normal); the abdominal girth is larger than normal (after 32 weeks the girth size in inches approximates the number of weeks' gestation). Special investigations are helpful, and these may also diagnose associated gross fetal abnormalities. On X-ray, there is an increase in the size of the uterine cavity, the fetal parts are spread out, and there is a general haziness of the film. On

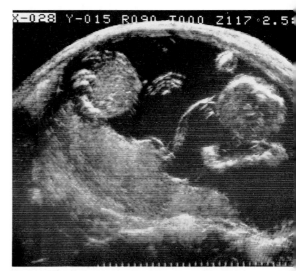

Figure 21.3 Polyhydramnios and twins at 22 weeks' gestation. The longitudinal scan shows cross-sections of 2 fetal trunks and 1 of the umbilical cords attaching to a single posterior placenta, suggestive of uniovular twins. The distended bladder is to the right. Identical, normal, twin boys were born at 38 weeks' gestation; both survived. The single placenta weighed 930 g.

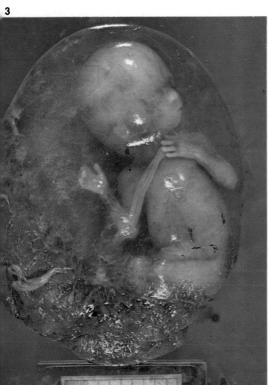

Plate 1 Recently implanted embryo (aged 10 days) obtained at premenstrual curettage for investigation of infertility. The primitive trophoblast has opened up sinusoids filled with maternal blood in the endometrium. The inner cell mass has formed. (Magnification × 100)

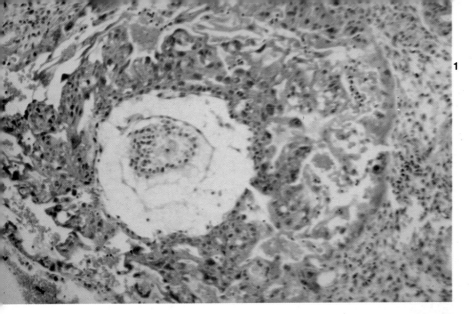

Plate 2 This embryo has a fertilization age of 48 days and a crown-rump length of 30 mm. The digits of hands and feet are clearly defined. Ribs are distinguishable. The liver occupies most of the abdomen, the intestines remaining within the umbilical cord until the 10th week.

Plate 3 Fetus at 16 weeks. Cervical incompetence is usually caused by dilatation for termination of pregnancy and is a preventable cause of prematurity and mid-trimester abortion. Usually there is serosanguineous discharge and then the membranes bulge into the vagina and burst. Abortion is not preceded by bleeding or pain.

Plate 4 The fetal attitude of universal flexion at term. The fleshy maternal surface of the placental cotyledons is shown. Note the pool of liquor between head and shoulder which is the favoured site for amniocentesis. The mother died undelivered due to cardiac disease.

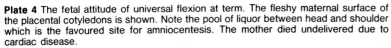

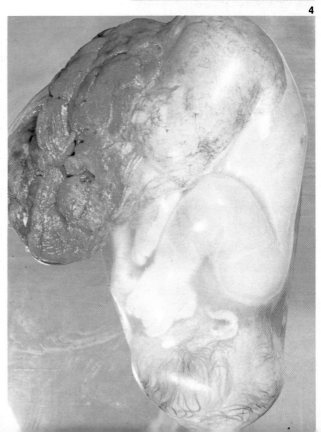

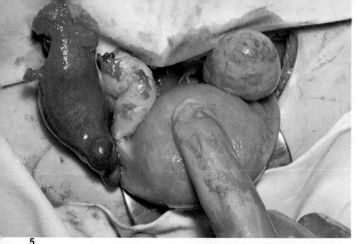

5

Plate 5 Unruptured tubal pregnancy. The patient presented with a 3-hour history of abdominal pain, 10 weeks' amenorrhoea and vaginal bleeding for 9 days. The uterus is held forwards and the distended right tube and both ovaries are shown. Right partial salpingectomy was performed.

Plate 6 Interstitial ectopic pregnancy. Fetus and placenta are shown within the distended inner end of the Fallopian tube. Rupture may not occur until the second trimester because the muscle wall is thick. Conservative treatment is sometimes possible; otherwise hysterectomy is performed as in this case.

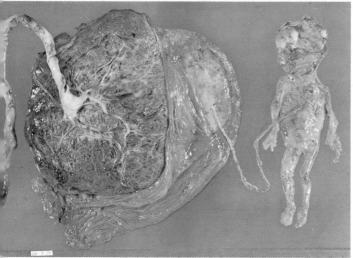

6

Plate 7 Fetus papyraceous. Any retained dead fetus who is not absorbed can become mummified (papyraceous) or calcified (lithopaedion). Fetus papyraceous usually is a complication of multiple pregnancy. The cause of fetal death may be retroplacental haemorrhage or avascularity associated with velamentous insertion of the umbilical cord. In this case the fetus was one of uniovular twins. The other survived.

Plate 8 Sirenomelus-mermaid. This fetus was aborted spontaneously at 11 weeks' gestation by a 19-year-old primigravida.

Plate 9 Comatose 39-year-old mother of 4 (aged 17, 13, 10 and 7) at 31 weeks' gestation with polyhydramnios, gross generalized oedema, oliguria and hypertensive cardiac failure. Severe preeclampsia in a multigravida may be due to fetal erythroblastosis, multiple pregnancy, diabetes mellitus, hypertension or chronic renal disease.

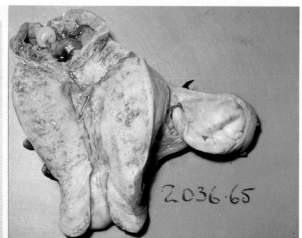

7

Plate 10 The patient made a complete recovery, this being her appearance 7 days after delivery of the conceptus shown in colour plate 11. There was no residual hypertension or intellectual impairment.

Plate 11 The fetus was grossly hydropic (birth-weight 3,160 g) and died soon after birth. The placenta weighed 1,390 g. This was an example of idiopathic (nonimmunological) hydrops which accounts for 30–40% of all cases of hydrops fetalis in Caucasian populations.

Plate 12 Acute polyhydramnios complicating a uniovular twin pregnancy at 35 weeks' gestation. This complication of twin pregnancy usually occurs late in the second trimester. Respiratory distress and preeclampsia necessitated induction of labour. Only 1 amniotic sac contained excessive liquor. The fetuses were stillborn.

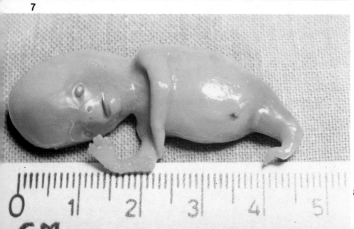

8

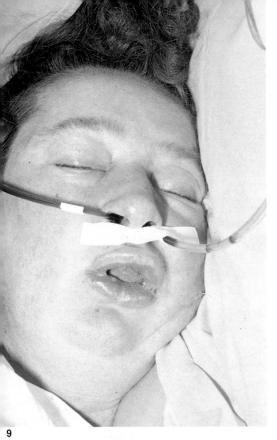

9

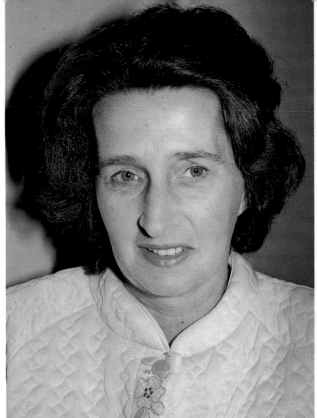

10

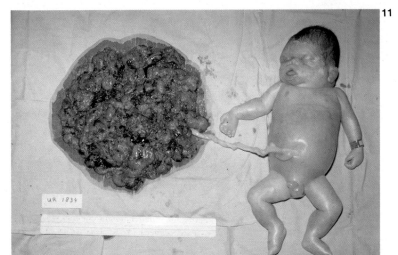

11

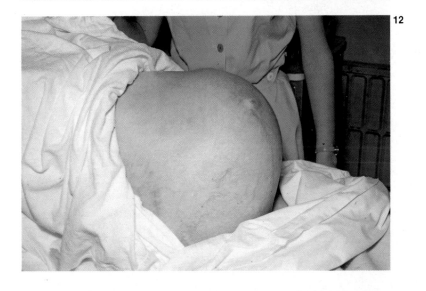

12

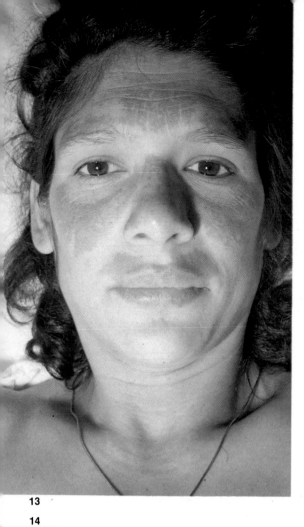

13

14

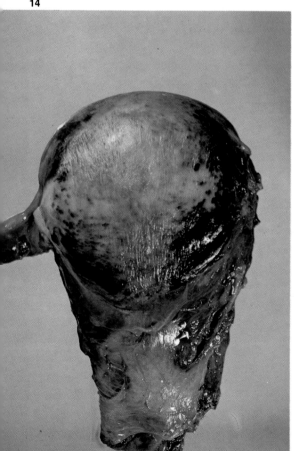

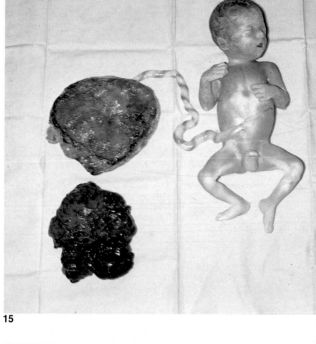

15

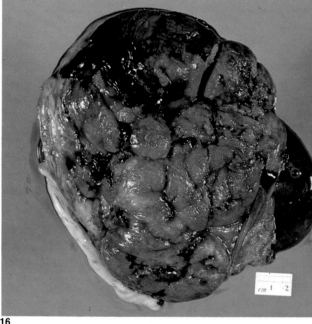

16

17

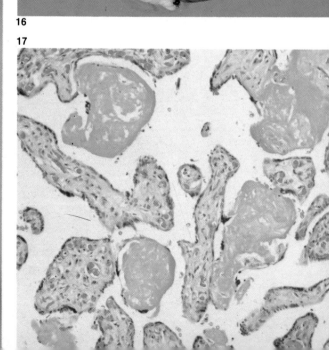

Plate 13 Chloasma or mask of pregnancy. Pigmentation is most pronounced in dark-skinned women but is seldom as marked as this. It is due to oestrogen-induced increased secretion of melanocyte-stimulating hormone by the intermediate lobe of the pituitary gland. The contraceptive pill can cause similar skin changes.

Plate 14 Couvelaire uterus. Uterine apoplexy occurs in the most severe cases (5–10%) of accidental haemorrhage. The uterus is black and appears gangrenous but complete recovery is usual. There is often associated blood coagulation failure. (From Beischer NA. Aust NZJ Surg 1966; 35: 255–258).

Plate 15 Fetal death due to massive placental abruption at 30 weeks' gestation in a 38-year-old multigravida. Blood coagulation failure was present 2 hours after the onset of abdominal pain and responded to transfusion of 2,500 ml of blood and 8 g of fibrinogen. Labour occurred spontaneously. The fetus weighed 1,710 g, the placenta 280 g and the retroplacental clot 1,020 g.

Plate 16 Chronic placental insufficiency due to clinically silent retroplacental bleeding (no abdominal pain or vaginal bleeding). Oestriol excretion was persistently low. A surviving small for dates infant (birth-weight 1,830 g at 36 weeks) was delivered by Caesarean section. Note multiple infarcts and old blood clots.

Plate 17 Section of a term placenta from a patient with preeclampsia. There is an unusual degree of fibrin deposition. The villi show reduced vascularity and there is some stromal fibrosis. (Magnification × 18)

18

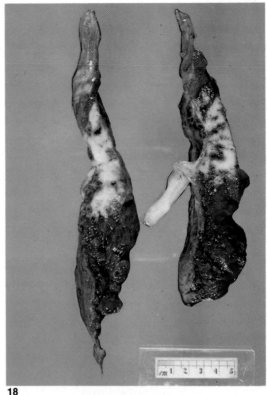

19

Plate 18 Cross-sections of a small placenta (460 g), deliverd at 39 weeks, showing a large, organized, full-thickness infarct beneath the insertion of the umbilical cord. In spite of this there was no sign of fetal distress in labour and the infant (birth-weight 3,300 g) showed no evidence of placental insufficiency.

Plate 19 Placental insufficiency due to hypertension with superimposed preeclampsia. The mother had an intrauterine death in her only previous pregnancy. Caesarean section was performed at 33 weeks when oestriol excretion fell to 11 μmol (3 mg)/24 hours. The infant, although growth retarded (1,260 g), survived. The placenta contained many infarcts and weighed 280 g.

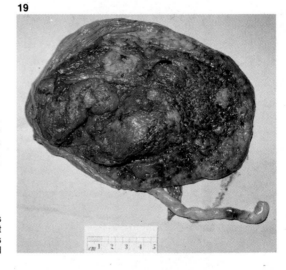

Plate 20 An extreme example of placental insufficiency. This meconium-stained, peeling infant weighed 3,440 g and was born at term. Although malnourished (absence of subcutaneous fat) he was not small for dates. Forceps delivery was performed when the fetal heart rate fell to 80/minute in the second stage of labour.

20

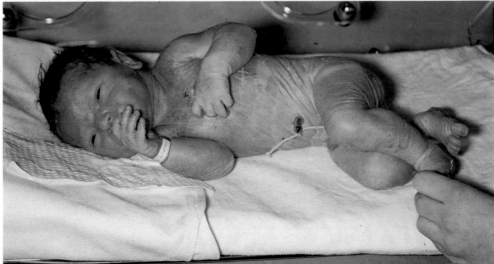

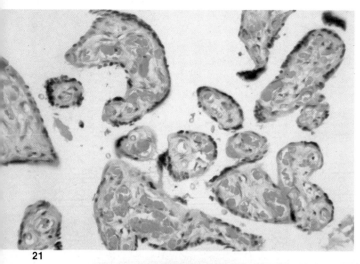

21

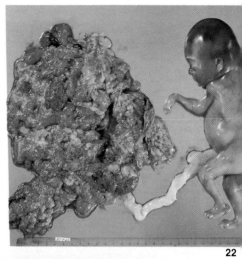

22

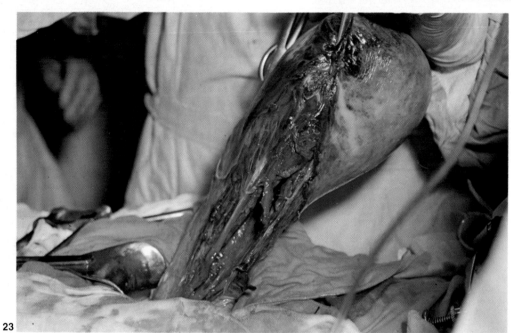

23

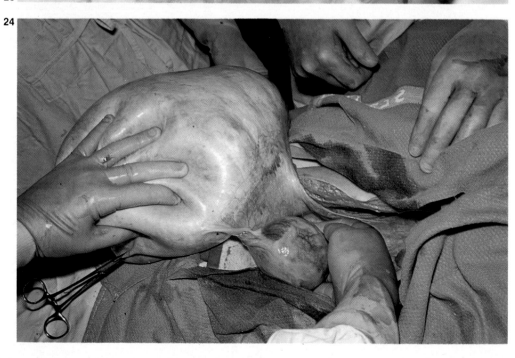

24

Plate 21 Section of a normal term placenta. Note the rich vascularity of the villi, the thinness of the trophoblastic covering of the villi, and the occasional collections (knots) of syncytial cells. (Magnification × 120)

Plate 22 Triploidy (69 chromosomes). The mother had severe preeclampsia with cardiac and renal failure and was delivered at 24 weeks. The single placenta was diffusely molar and indicates that fetal death or developmental failure is not the cause of hydatidiform mole. The chromosomally abnormal (XXX) female fetus had multiple abnormalities.

Plate 23 Uterine rupture. This uterus was weakened by severe abruptio placentae that caused fetal death. Rupture occurred during internal version and breech extraction. The huge hole in the left lower segment was seen after the broad ligament was incised during hysterectomy. The patient survived but required blood transfusion of 7,500 ml. (From Beischer NA. Aust NZJ Surg 1966; 35: 255–258).

Plate 24 Mucinous cystadenoma of the right ovary after aspiration of 1,500 ml. The patient was 6 weeks' pregnant. The uterus is discoloured due to venous congestion. The pregnancy proceeded uneventfully to term.

Plate 25 Forceps delivery. This Italian-born primigravida had outlet contraction (available AP of outlet 8.9 cm). Delay in the second stage of labour occurred with the head on view. A pudendal nerve block was inserted.

Plate 26 Using adequate lubrication the forceps blades were applied. The left blade was introduced first, the fingers preventing vaginal laceration as it was brought into position by rotation of the handle through 90°.

Plate 27 The right blade was inserted in the midline and rotated around the head so that when locked in position the blades grasped the parietal eminences with the tips overlying the fetal cheeks. A right mediolateral episiotomy is being cut commencing in the midline at the fourchette.

Plate 28 Delivery of the head by traction and extension controlled by the forceps. The sagittal suture lies in the AP diameter of the pelvic outlet and the forceps blades lie symmetrically over the fetal cheeks. Ergometrine 0.5 mg was then administered by intravenous injection.

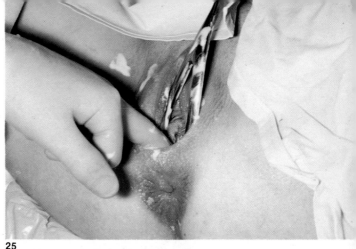

25

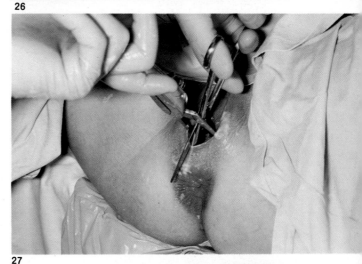

26

27

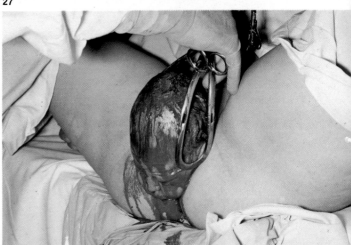

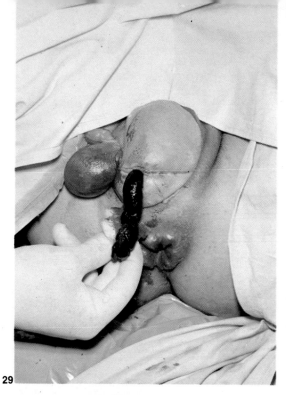

29

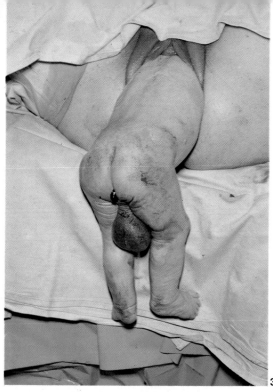

30

Plate 29 Assisted breech delivery. Birth of frank breech (also called incomplete or breech with extended legs) by lateral flexion of the trunk with bitrochanteric diameter in AP of outlet. Pudendal nerve block and episiotomy were already performed. Expulsive effort affects anal sphincters of mother and child.

Plate 30 The bisacromial diameter rotates to AP of pelvic outlet. Breech birth may be a cause of male sterility (thrombosis of testicular blood vessels). This baby weighed 3,470 g and had bilateral dislocated hips.

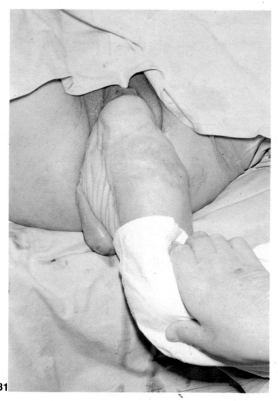

31

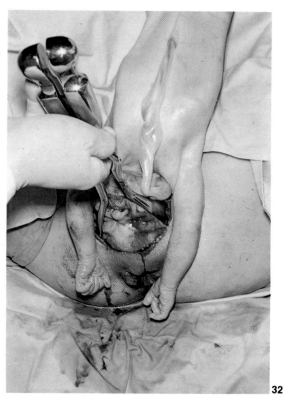

32

Plate 31 Lovset's manoeuvre for delivery of the posterior shoulder by rotation through 180° to the anterior position where it appears from beneath the symphysis pubis. The baby is grasped by the pelvic girdle to avoid injury to his abdominal organs.

Plate 32 Forceps delivery of the engaged, flexed, aftercoming head, with an assistant holding the baby up by the legs. The nasopharynx is aspirated and delivery through the pelvic outlet is slowly completed.

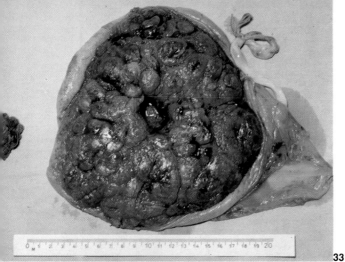

33

Plate 33 Missing placental cotyledon was noted at routine inspection of the placenta. Although there was no postpartum haemorrhage, manual exploration under general anaesthesia was performed and the missing cotyledon was found.

34

35

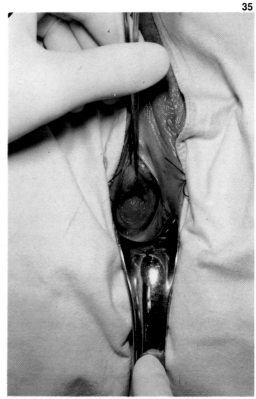

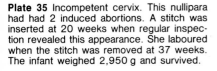

Plate 34 Vulval haematoma seen 3 hours after a normal delivery due to failure to achieve haemostasis during repair of an episiotomy. An indwelling catheter was required because of urinary retention. The haematoma was evacuated. The patient required a 2,000 ml blood transfusion.

Plate 35 Incompetent cervix. This nullipara had had 2 induced abortions. A stitch was inserted at 20 weeks when regular inspection revealed this appearance. She laboured when the stitch was removed at 37 weeks. The infant weighed 2,950 g and survived.

36

Plate 36 The patient had severe pre-eclampsia and the pregnancy was terminated at 16 weeks with an oxytocic infusion. The fetus and attached placenta containing vesicles each had male karotypes. The separate molar tissue had karotype 2AXX (female) and was thus a dizygotic twin. Was the molar disease spreading to the normal placenta?

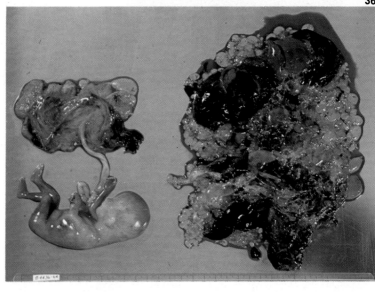

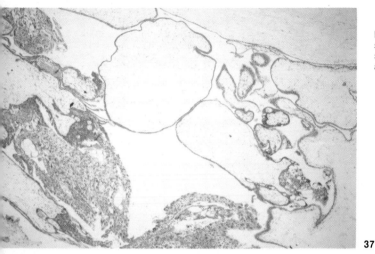

Plate 37 Section of a hydatidiform mole showing considerable trophoblastic proliferation. The chorionic villi show the typical enlargement (hydrops) and avascularity. (Magnification × 18)

37

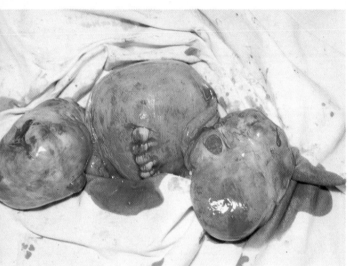

Plate 38 Uterus and bilateral ovarian theca-lutein cysts seen after hysterotomy, at 18 weeks' gestation, in a patient with a hydatidiform mole. Suction curettage with an oxytocin infusion running is the preferred method of evacuation of a hydatidiform mole.

Plate 39 Total hysterectomy specimen showing the classical macroscopic appearance of a hydatidiform mole in a patient aged 56 years. The risk of malignant change in a hydatidiform mole is 20–25% in patients over 40 years of age and so prophylactic hysterectomy is the preferred method of primary treatment.

Plate 40 Choriocarcinoma. The patient was aged 17 and presented with a haemoperitoneum. As in 50% of cases there was no preceding hydatidiform mole. Uterine perforation necessitated hysterectomy. There were multiple pulmonary metastases. Recovery was complete after treatment with methotrexate and actinomycin D.

38

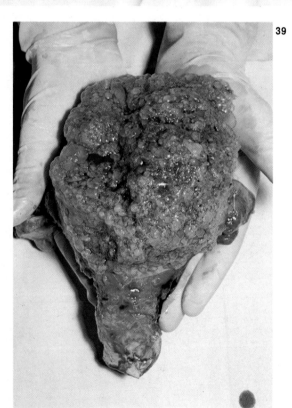

39

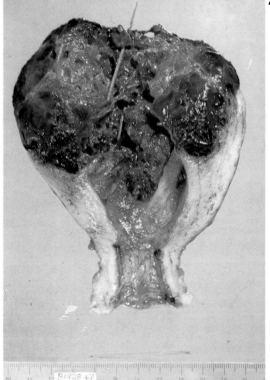

4

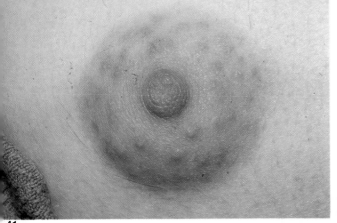

41

Plate 41 Montgomery follicles. These are enlarged sebaceous glands within the areola and are a reliable early sign of pregnancy, especially in a primigravida. This patient had her last menstrual period 6 weeks earlier.

42

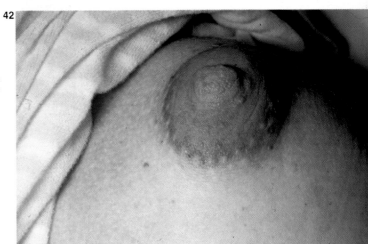

Plate 42 Pigmentation of the nipple and areola in a patient at term. The enlarged sebaceous glands are seen as nodules within the areola.

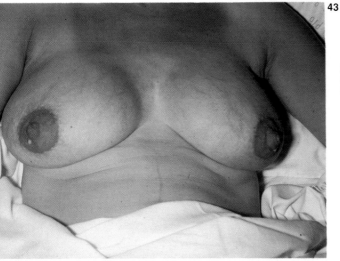

43

Plate 43 A multipara with established lactation on the 4th day of the puerperium. The vascularity of the breasts is indicated by the numerous dilated veins.

44

Plate 44 Lactation in a patient with inverted nipples. Woolwich nipple shields were used and breast feeding was persevered with for 10 days, but in vain; thereafter the baby was bottle-fed. Inverted nipples should be detected and corrected before delivery.

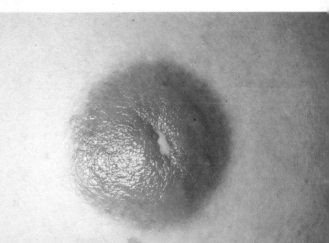

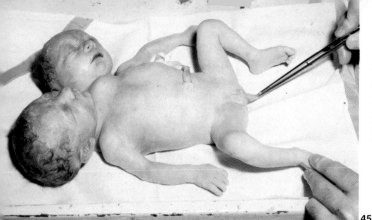

Plate 45 Double-headed monster. Incidence 1 in 40,000 births. Double monsters can be conjoined twins ('Siamese') or separated at one or other pole. In this unusual case there were also 2 anuses separated by a tail, and the double heart was in the neck due to absence of the normal attachment of pericardium to diaphragm. (From Beischer NA, Fortune DW. Obstet Gynecol 1968; 32: 158–170).

45

46

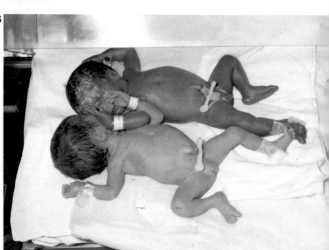

Plate 46 Twin transfusion syndrome. Born at 28 weeks the anaemic twin (haemoglobin 9.6 g/dl) weighed 1,200 g, was given a 20 ml blood transfusion (20% of her blood volume), and survived. The plethoric twin (haemoglobin 21.0 g/dl) weighed 1,490 g and died from pulmonary haemorrhage. The single placenta with arteriovenous anastomosis weighed 880 g.

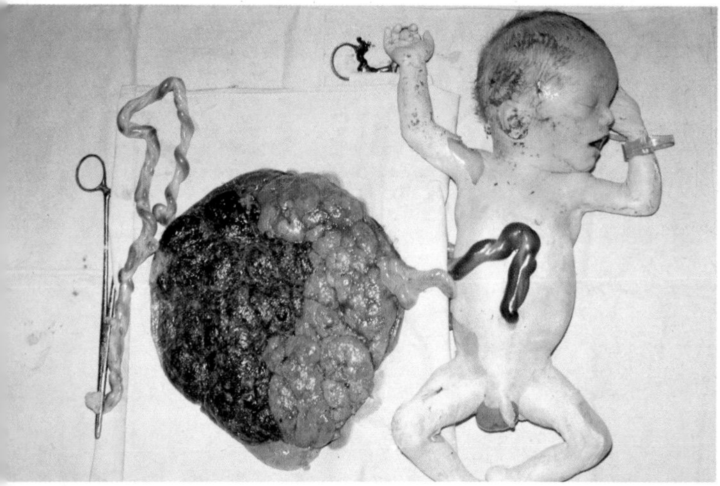

47

Plate 47 Intrauterine death of 1 of a pair of uniovular twins due to fetomaternal haemorrhage. The mother came into spontaneous labour at 38 weeks. The placenta weighed 960 g; note the pallor of the half belonging to the stillborn twin (birth-weight 1,890 g). Birth-weight of the surviving twin was 2,780 g.

48

Plate 48 This single placenta of monozygotic (identical) Korean quadruplets (see figure 25.5) weighed 1,690 g and had 4 separate amniotic sacs. Vascular communications between placental components were shown by injection of coloured gelatine into the umbilical vessels. (Courtesy of Dr Helen P. MacKenzie).

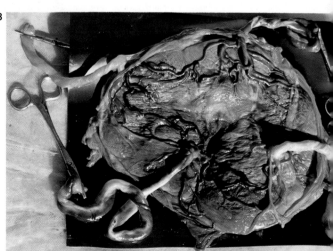

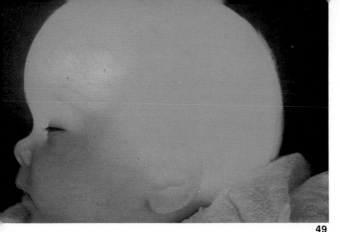

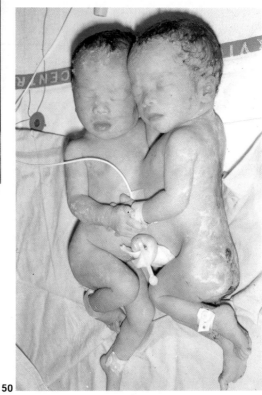

49

Plate 49 Hydranencephaly. Appearance during transillumination of the head 1 week before death in an infant aged 5 months. In hydrocephaly the cerebral tissue is thinned out but here the cerebral hemispheres are absent, there being only a fluid filled sac above the brain stem, cerebellum and choroid plexus.

Plate 50 Siamese twins. These are the first conjoined twins to be successfully separated in Australia. Diagnosis was made by X-ray studies. Delivery was by classical elective Caesarean section. They weighed 4,800 g and shared 1 umbilical cord and placenta. There was an umbilical hernia with protruding bowel. One twin has meconium on her buttocks and sacral area. (Courtesy of Dr Donald Chan).

50

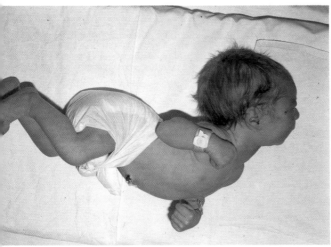

Plate 51 Face presentation due to an attitude of extension ('flying fetus') which persisted after birth illustrating that fetal muscular tone may be the primary factor responsible for the presentation.

51

52

Plate 52 Extension of the neck (face presentation) associated with thyroid enlargement. Thyroid function tests were normal and the enlargement resolved gradually without treatment. The mother had a goitre but was not taking antithyroid drugs.

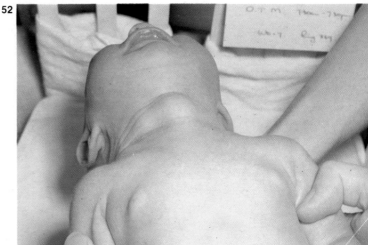

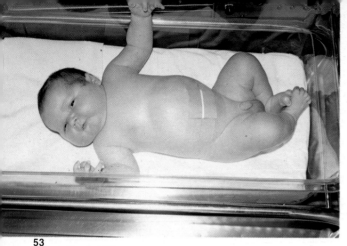

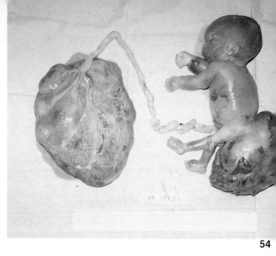

53

54

55

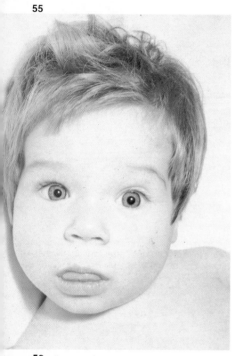

Plate 53 The 6,700 g (14 lb 14 oz) infant of a diabetic mother delivered by Caesarean section after a failed forceps. He shows the typical fat 'tomato face' and generalized adiposity. His 4 siblings all had normal births and weighed 11 lb 4 oz, 10 lb 1 oz, 12 lb and 10 lb 11 oz, respectively.

Plate 54 Sacrococcygeal teratoma associated with fetal and placental hydrops. The mother was a 23-year-old primipara. Labour was induced at 26 weeks' gestation when she developed polyhydramnios and severe preeclampsia. The fetus weighed 1,865 g and the placenta 1,250 g.

Plate 55 A 15-month-old hypothyroid infant who showed the features of cretinism: protruding tongue, lemon-coloured skin, dwarfism, hypotonia, umbilical hernia and retarded development (PBI 1.9 μg %, haemoglobin 8.3 g/dl). Administration of thyroxine (25 μg/day) resulted in intellectual and physical improvement.

Plate 56 Infant aged 4 days with gross distension of the urinary tract (hydronephrosis, megaloureters, cystomegaly) due to urethral obstruction. Difficulty with delivery of the shoulders and abdomen resulted in fracture of the right humerus. Immediately after birth the child cried, passed meconium and sucked normally.

56

Plate 57 Large pigmented naevus in an otherwise normal infant (birth-weight 3,110 g). Malignant change is very rare but these lesions have no tendency to spontaneous regression. Serial excision and grafting can be performed.

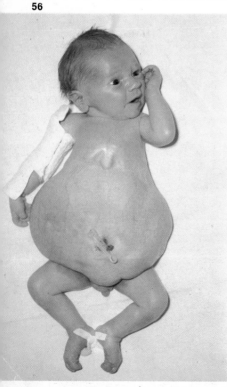

57

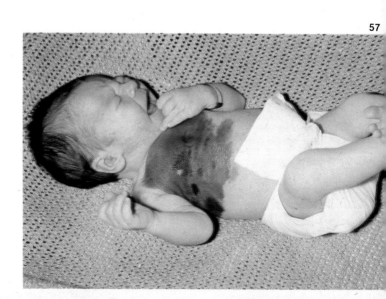

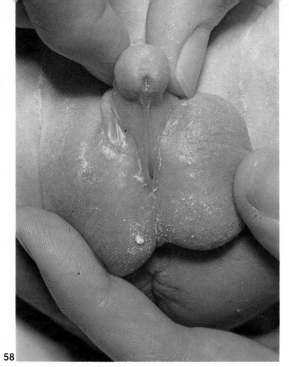

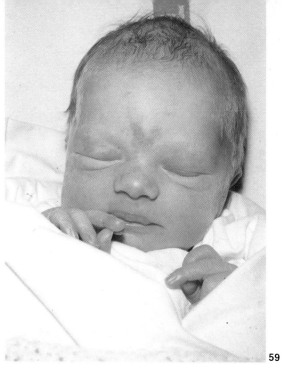

58

59

Plate 58 The rare scrotal variety of hyopospadias in a 5-week-old infant; he had 5 siblings and his father had a mild degree of hypospadias. Note the elongated urethral opening in the scrotum with a shallow groove extending to the glans. Surgery was planned for 2 years of age.

Plate 59 Naevus flammeus is the commonest of all 'birth-marks' and appears as a red area on upper eyelids, root of nose, upper lip and/or nape of neck. These mild lesions cause considerable maternal anxiety and disappointment. They are present in at least 15% of infants, and are more noticeable when the infant cries. They disappear within 18 months.

Plate 60 This plug of meconium and mucus (scale in cm) caused bowel obstruction in a premature infant. X-ray showed marked gaseous distension and multiple fluid levels at 30 hours of age. Dramatic improvement occurred when the plug was passed following a 10 ml enema.

61

Plate 61 Massive pulmonary haemorrhage which caused sudden collapse and death at 57 hours of age of a premature infant (birth-weight 2,200 g), born by mid-forceps delivery, at 35 weeks' gestation.

60

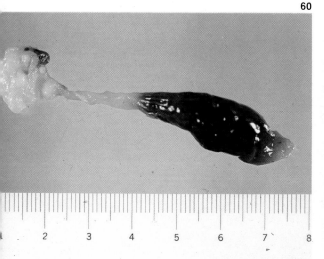

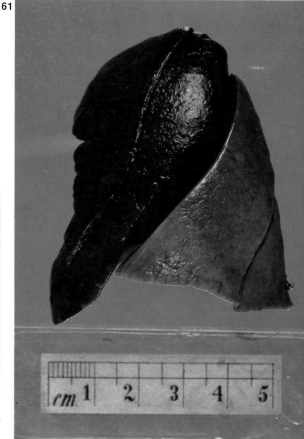

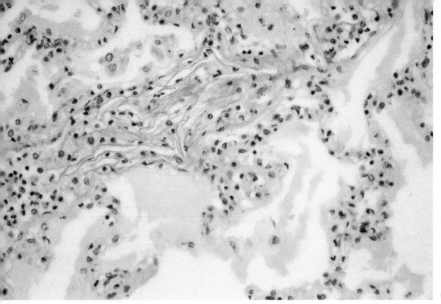

Plate 62 Amniotic fluid embolism. This section of maternal lung shows alveoli and a pulmonary arteriole containing many fetal squames and a few fibrin emboli. The patient developed blood coagulation failure and died undelivered. (Magnification × 400)

62

Plate 63 Death from hypoxia. This section of lung came from an infant who died from intrauterine hypoxia. Mauve-staining fetal squames have been inhaled with amniotic fluid and are seen within collapsed alveoli. (Magnification × 120)

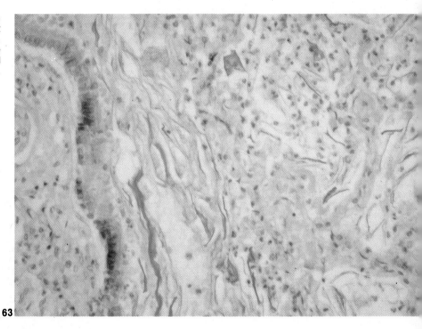

63

Plate 64 Death from the respiratory distress syndrome due to pulmonary immaturity. This section of lung came from a premature infant who died of hyaline membrane disease. Dense hyaline (red staining) membranes line the alveolar ducts and surrounding collapsed airless alveoli are shown. (Magnification × 400)

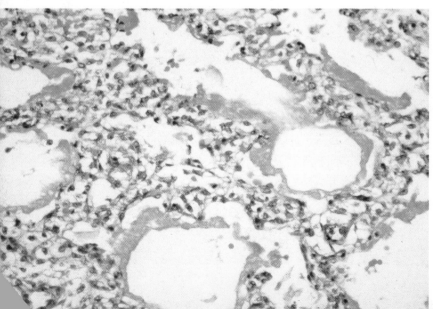

64

compound ultrasonic scanning, the relative volumes of fetus and amniotic fluid can be estimated. *Differential diagnosis* usually includes multiple pregnancy (which may, however, coexist with polyhydramnios), ovarian cyst, ascites, fetal/placental hydrops, and obesity.

Significance

It is important to recognize polyhydramnios, because of its frequent association with *fetal malformation*; this is especially important if there is a surgically correctable anomaly, such as oesophageal atresia. *Premature labour* is more common — partly because of the distension of the uterus and cervix, and partly because of the likelihood of premature rupture of the membranes. *Malpresentation* and *cord prolapse* are also more likely. Transverse or unstable lie of the fetus is present in about 10% of cases. If the condition is marked, maternal discomfort due to the distension may be considerable; herniation of abdominal contents may occur. *Diabetes* should be suspected, and so should *rhesus isoimmunization* in both Rh + ve and Rh – ve patients who have not had routine testing for antibodies. The risk of *postpartum haemorrhage* is somewhat greater, although the duration of labour is normal.

Management

Ultrasonic and/or radiographic study is always indicated, as is a *glucose tolerance test* and *indirect Coombs test*. Ultrasonography may show an absence of fluid in the fetal stomach, suggesting oesophageal atresia, or a double bubble in duodenal atresia (figure 65.4); *about 50% of fetal malformations associated with polyhydramnios can be diagnosed by ultrasonography*. If there is also evidence of growth retardation, a chromosomal abnormality may be present (e.g. trisomy 18); this can be identified by studies on the amniotic fluid obtained by amniocentesis. If the polyhydramnios is gross and the uterus is tense, or the patient is in discomfort, she should be observed in hospital. Primary causes in the mother should be treated. Diuretic drugs are sometimes prescribed, and slow release of fluid via a fine polythene catheter may be undertaken if the condition is acute and distressing. A pelvic examination should always be performed when the membranes rupture because of the likelihood of *cord prolapse*; if amniotomy is carried out, the liquor should be released slowly, and a theatre should be available for Caesarean section in case the above complication occurs.

After birth, the baby should be examined carefully for malformations, and a catheter passed into the stomach to exclude *oesophageal atresia*. Paediatric follow-up is necessary to detect other less obvious anomalies. In 40–60% of patients no cause for the polyhydramnios is apparent.

In a consecutive series of over 40,000 pregnancies the incidence of polyhydramnios was 0.8% (table 16.1). The associated conditions were *maternal diabetes* (25%), *preeclampsia* (20%), *fetal malformations* (20%), *multiple pregnancy* (10%), and *hydrops fetalis* (5%). The *perinatal mortality rate was 28%*, the important causes of death being *fetal malformations* (45%), *prematurity* (35% — largely due to cases of acute polyhydramnios) and *hydrops fetalis* (12%). Although *oesophageal and duodenal atresia* are invariably associated with polyhydramnios, they accounted for only 1.8% of cases (6 of 329) in this series.

OLIGOHYDRAMNIOS

In this condition, the volume of amniotic fluid is *less than 200 ml*. It is diagnosed less frequently than polyhydramnios, since the clinical features and effect on the mother are often unremarkable.

Aetiology

As with polyhydramnios, there is no obvious abnormality in some 40–60% of patients. In the remainder, 2 main conditions are noted. (i) *Placental failure*. This is a relatively common cause. There is a normal reduction in the volume of amniotic fluid after term. In conditions of placental failure, this is accelerated — for example, in some cases of marked fetal growth retardation, there is little liquor, even at 34–36 weeks (figure 21.4). In pregnancies prolonged beyond 42 weeks, the little liquor that is present is often mixed with meconium. (ii) *Fetal malformation* (figure 21.5). Usually, the condition responsible is absence of the fetal kidneys or obstruction to the lower urinary tract. The fetus swallows, but does not urinate. In this group, amniotic bands may form and cut into, or even amputate, parts of the growing fetus (colour plate 113); also, deformities resulting from the cramped conditions may occur (talipes (figure 65.16), wry-neck, spinal curvature).

Significance

Oligohydramnios is usually a warning that the *placental reserve is low*, especially if tests of function (e.g. oestriol values, cardiotocography) are abnormal and/or meconium staining is present. Because of absence of the protective effect of the liquor, fetal distress is often added to by compression of the umbilical cord (which has often lost its own protective cushion of Wharton's jelly). Oligohydramnios due to prolonged rupture of the membranes may be complicated by fetal *pulmonary hypoplasia*. Careful monitoring of the fetus is thus necessary during late pregnancy and labour; Caesarean section is usually carried out if other signs of distress appear (fetal heart rate abnormalities, abnormal scalp blood findings).

Renal agenesis is a lethal condition. Babies with this abnormality are usually recognized by the characteristic facial appearance with low-set, batlike ears (figure 21.6). Again, *pulmonary hypoplasia* and *amnion nodosum* may be present as a complication of the diminished amount of liquor. Ultrasonography is helpful in assessing whether the kidneys are present and whether the thoracic cage is diminished in size.

Obstructions to the lower renal tract may be corrected surgically.

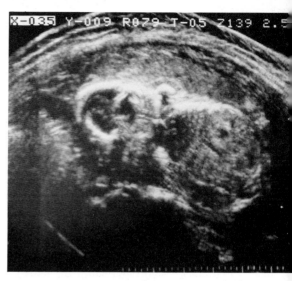

Figure 21.5 Oligohydramnios and microcephaly at 25 weeks' gestation. The longitudinal scan shows the fetus presenting by the breech, a small head, an anterior placenta and extreme oligohydramnios. The dark area to the right is the distended bladder. The infant (birth-weight 2,250 g) died 1 hour after birth at 35 weeks' gestation.

Figure 21.4 Intrauterine growth retardation due to placental insufficiency. This infant, aged 4 days when photographed, weighed 1,550 g when born at 38 weeks' gestation. The skin is wrinkled and cracked and there is loss of subcutaneous fat.

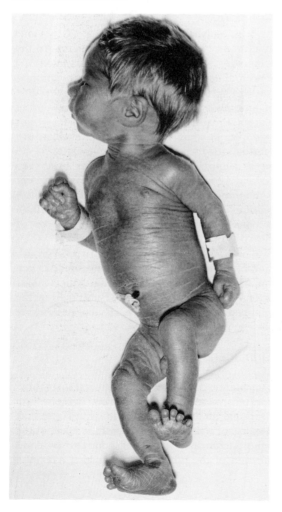

CLINICAL STUDIES OF AMNIOTIC FLUID

AMNIOSCOPY

Since a reduction in the amount of amniotic fluid and/or its contamination with meconium is usually associated with fetal distress, amnioscopy has an important screening role, especially after the 37th week.

Indications

The presence in the patient of such conditions as preeclampsia, poor reproductive history, age above 35, hypertension, chronic renal disease or other medical disorders, growth retardation of the fetus, and prolonged pregnancy.

Significance

Fetal distress may be acute, subacute or chronic. In the latter, there is a gradual resorption of liquor, and this later becomes stained with *meconium*. The latter probably occurs more commonly with acute episodes of distress. Thus, the amount of liquor present, and the freshness of the meconium (green or yellow-brown) gives an idea of the severity of fetal hypoxia and the placental reserve. Positive findings are an indication for close supervision, preferably by fetal heart and perhaps scalp monitoring (after rupture of the membranes), or even termination of

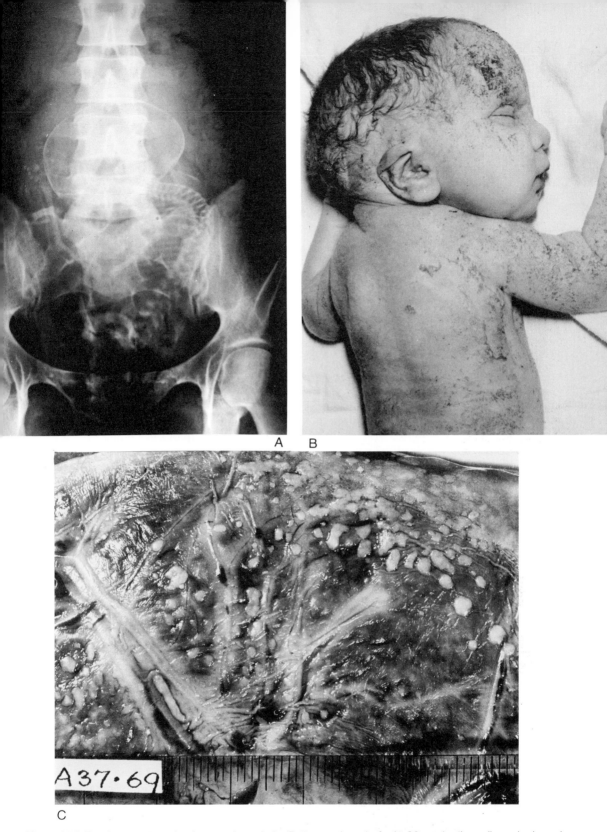

Figure 21.6 Renal agenesis and pulmonary hypoplasia (Potter syndrome). **A.** At 36 weeks the radiograph showed extreme flexion of the fetal spine due to oligohydramnios (which also accounted for failure of spontaneous cephalic version). **B.** The infant died shortly after birth and showed the typical abnormally large, low-set ears deficient in cartilage, a conspicuous crease below the lower lip with recession of the chin, and slight flattening of the tip of the nose. **C.** Nodular amnion nodosum lesions, 1–3 mm in diameter, on the fetal surface of the placenta. These lesions are related to oligo-hydramnios and represent masses of desquamated fetal epidermal cells. (From Ratten GJ et al. Am J Obstet Gynecol 1973; 115: 890-896).

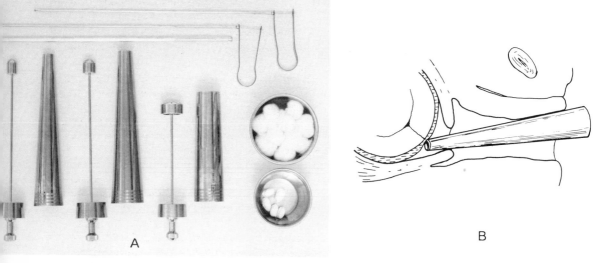

Figure 21.7 Amnioscopy. **A.** The tray as set up for amnioscopy and fetal scalp blood sampling — for the latter procedure the membranes must be ruptured. The 3 sizes of amnioscope with obturator are shown below, with pledgets (cotton wool discs) and blade carriers above. **B.** Amnioscope in position; the obturator has been removed and the light source must be attached to allow inspection of the amniotic fluid.

pregnancy by Caesarean section. Meconium staining is observed in less than 5% of so-called normal patients, and in about 10% of the high risk group mentioned above. Amnioscopy is usually repeated at intervals of 2–7 days, according to findings.

Procedure

The patient is in the lithotomy position, and sterile conditions are observed. A vaginal examination is carried out and the cervix assessed. The largest convenient size of amnioscope is chosen

and passed through the cervix (figure 21.7). The light source is connected and the forewaters are examined. Occasionally, the presenting part must be pushed up to allow liquor to pass down. The procedure is rarely carried out before the 37th week without good indication, and is contraindicated when there is an unstable lie or if there has been antepartum bleeding (unless the placenta is shown by investigation not to be praevia), or in the presence of vaginal infection. *Difficulties* include spasm of levator muscles, and a tight cervical os. The failure rate ranges from

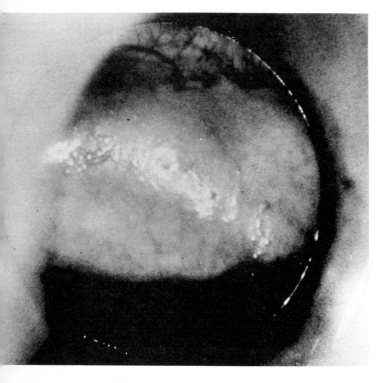

Figure 21.8 A cord presentation found coincidentally at amnioscopy is shown in the middle of this picture. Note hair on the fetal scalp above the cord. The dark crescent below the cord is amniotic fluid discoloured by meconium. Caesarean section was performed. (Courtesy of Dr Kevin Barham).

2-10% or more, depending on experience and the patient's parity and period of gestation. In experienced hands, the findings accurately reflect the intrauterine state in 95% of cases. The *chief complications* are premature labour, disturbance of a low-lying placenta, accidental rupture of the membranes, and perhaps a slightly increased incidence of puerperal pyrexia. An occasional bonus is the visualization of *cord presentation* (figure 21.8) or a *vasa praevia*, and deliberate rupture of the membranes can be effected quite conveniently through the amnioscope (*amnioscopy amniotomy*).

AMNIOCENTESIS

Indications

(i) *Rhesus isoimmunization.* In normal pregnancies, some *bilirubin pigment* is present in the liquor, but this steadily diminishes and is hardly detectable by 36 weeks. In conditions of fetal red cell destruction (especially erythroblastosis due to rhesus isoimmunization), the excess pigment enters the amniotic fluid and can be detected by the aspiration of fluid through a fine needle (amniocentesis). This test may be carried out from the 20th–36th weeks, depending on the severity of the condition, as assessed by the patient's history and level of Rh antibodies. The amount of bilirubin is measured in the laboratory and a guide is given to the nature of the treatment required (intrauterine transfusion, induction of labour prematurely, or observation only — figure 22.2). It may be necessary to repeat the test at intervals of 1–4 weeks.

(ii) *Fetal maturity.* A number of phospholipids (especially lecithin and sphingomyelin) are secreted from the fetal lung into the amniotic fluid in the second half of pregnancy. Between 34–36 weeks, there is a *surge of lecithin and this heralds fetal lung maturity.* The surface-acting properties (surfactant) of the lecithin enable the negative pressure created by the baby's chest wall after birth to expand the fine alveolar sacs in the lung and prevent them from collapsing on expiration. The test is indicated when premature induction of labour is contemplated (maternal diabetes, hypertension, preeclampsia — especially if menstrual data are uncertain). If the ratio of lecithin to sphingomyelin (*L/S ratio*) is greater than 2, lung maturity is assumed to be adequate; 1.5–2.0 is a transitional value, and if less than 1.5, the lung is likely to be immature: hyaline membrane disease and atelectasis are likely in such babies. The test may be repeated at intervals of 1–2 weeks. In recent years, much sophistication has been added to Gluck's original test, particularly in the quantitative determination of such phospholipids as phosphatidyl choline.

A reasonable idea can be obtained of the lecithin content of amniotic fluid at the bedside by shaking the tube and observing the foam on the surface (*shake or foam test*) (Chapter 24).

There are a number of other tests of fetal maturity. *Creatinine* increases steadily as a result of fetal micturition; values above 160 μmol/l (1.8 mg/dl) indicate a maturity greater than 36 weeks. *Fat cells* can be detected with 0.1% Nile blue sulphate, since they stain a bright orange; before 34 weeks, there are approximately 1% of such cells, 34–38 weeks 1–10%, and thereafter 11–60%. These cells are thought to parallel the functional maturity of the sebaceous glands in the fetal skin.

(iii) *Fetal well-being.* The presence of meconium may be detected in suspected placental insufficiency, and, thus, the test may be an alternative to amnioscopy. It should be remembered, however, that the premature or anaemic fetus, even if distressed, usually does not pass meconium. In the diabetic patient, an abnormally high insulin level (> 60 μm/l) and low glucose level indicate a less favourable fetal outlook.

(iv) *Genetic abnormalities of the fetus.* In this situation, the test is carried out at the 16–17th week of gestation.

The fluid obtained at amniocentesis may be studied in several ways.

(a) *Chromosome analysis.* The mother (or the father) may be a carrier of an abnormal chromosome — usually a translocation from one group (D) to another (G), as evidenced by the production of a previously affected baby — usually *Down syndrome* (mongolism). Down syndrome (trisomy 21) occurs most often in infants of older mothers (age less than 30 years, incidence 1 in 1,500; age more than 45 years, incidence 1 in 50 — table 65.4). Hence, if there has been a previously affected child or the mother is over 35–37 years, amniocentesis is indicated if facilities for the test are available and the patient wishes to have the investigation performed. In Australia, fewer than 50% of patients with an indication for genetic amniocentesis elect to have the test performed (religious reasons, fear of risk of amniocentesis (abortion, damage to the fetus), lack of counselling). Chromosome analysis will also provide exact information on other *autosomal anomalies* (chromosomes 5, 13 and 18), or *sex chromosome anomalies* (XO or Turner syndrome in the female, and XXY or Klinefelter syndrome in the male being common examples). (b) *Central nervous system malformation.* A

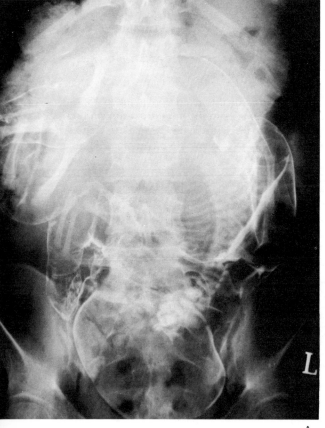
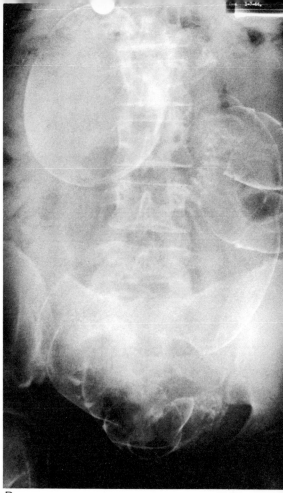

A   B

Figure 21.9 Amniography — fetography. Radio-opaque water-soluble dye introduced into the amniotic sac mixes with liquor, is swallowed, and outlines the fetal intestines. Fat-soluble dye as shown here is absorbed by the vernix caseosa and outlines the fetal exterior. **A.** A normal fetus at term presenting by the vertex and showing the usual attitude of universal flexion. **B.** An achondroplastic fetus with hydrocephaly (diagnosed after birth) and a deflexed neck presenting by the feet. (Courtesy of Dr Joan Spong).

number of congenital anomalies of the fetus, especially neural tube defect (see Chapter 17), are associated with a raised level of alpha fetoprotein (AFP) in the liquor. The normal level at 16–17 weeks' gestation is 2–30 mg/l — after this the level *falls* and the upper limit of normal at 20 weeks' gestation is 20 mg/l. The defect may be visualized by ultrasonography or radiography (amniography — figure 21.9).

(c) *Sex of the fetus.* The significance of this determination depends on the fact that, if the mother is carrying a sex-linked recessive gene, 50% of the male offspring will have the disease and 50% of the female offspring will carry and transmit it. If the fetus is a male, as shown by chromosome analysis (the presence of Y chromosome fluorescence), he will have a 1 in 2 chance of developing the disease (e.g. haemophilia, Duchenne muscular dystrophy, Hunter mucopolysaccharidosis, retinitis pigmentosa).

(d) *Metabolic disorders.* By the study of the fluid or the cells (cultured for 4–6 weeks), enzyme or other deficiencies due to a single gene mutation may be detected (mucopolysaccaride or lipid disorders; there are recent claims that cystic fibrosis can also be diagnosed).

Procedure

After the patient has emptied her bladder, she is placed in the supine position. Sterile precautions are observed. After careful palpation, usually aided by ultrasonographic localization of the placenta, a 19 to 22 gauge needle is passed into the amniotic cavity (figure 21.10). Success is most likely if the needle is directed to the region of the limbs, hollow of the neck, or below the presenting part, which is lifted out of the pelvis; 5–10 ml of fluid is aspirated and placed in clean tubes. After careful labelling, the tubes are wrapped in light-proof material if bilirubin studies are to be carried out. In most cases, the specimens should be sent to the laboratory with the minimum of delay. The most usual difficulties are those arising from *obesity*, an *anteriorly-placed placenta*, or *oligohydramnios*. Complications include *feto-maternal bleeding* (figure 22.1), bleeding from the surface of the uterus, *leakage of amniotic fluid* from the uterus (especially if the track passes through a scar in the uterus), and infection. Direct *damage to the fetus* has also been described, and *premature labour* may follow. Because of the potential risks, the procedure should only be carried out by an experienced person under ultrasonographic control. The procedure sounds formidable to the patient and adequate reassurance is necessary.

SUSPECTED PREMATURE RUPTURE OF THE MEMBRANES

The diagnosis of this condition is aided by the application of tests to the fluid draining from the vagina (fern test; study for particulate matter, such as lanugo or vernix, see Chapter 24).

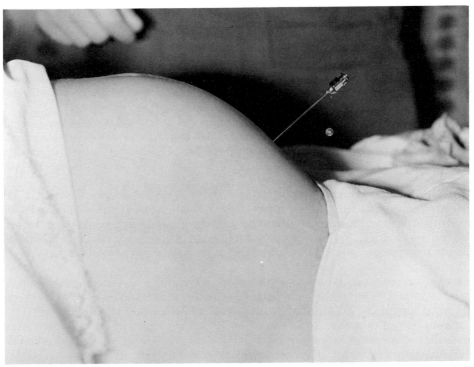

Figure 21.10 Amniocentesis. The 19 gauge needle has been inserted in the midline between the baby's head and anterior shoulder. A no-touch technique is used — some operators wear gown and gloves; 10 ml liquor has been withdrawn using a syringe. This patient has high uterine tone (due to Braxton Hicks contraction induced by the needle) and so the liquor drips out of the needle.

chapter twenty-two

Blood Group Incompatibility

OVERVIEW

Blood group incompatibility arises because the fetus inherits one or more major blood group factors from the father which are absent in the mother. When fetal *red cells leak through the placenta* into the mother's circulation, she will often react to them by *forming antibodies which will cause their agglutination and destruction.* Unfortunately, the antibodies do not remain confined to the maternal circulation, and in turn, pass to the fetus and continue their haemolytic activity.

The breakdown of fetal red cells produces an *anaemia* to which the bone marrow responds, usually liberating *immature erythrocytes* into the circulation (hence the term, *erythroblastosis fetalis*). Haemolysis also leads to another characteristic feature of the disease, *bilirubin-staining of the amniotic fluid*; amniocentesis and biochemical assessment of bilirubin level in the liquor provides an important guide to the condition of the fetus.

There are a number of reasons for the observed *variability in disease severity. Parity* is important, since the degree of maternal sensitization increases with each pregnancy; if the *husband is heterozygous* rather than homozygous for the offending antigen, the fetus will, on average, be negative for 50% of the pregnancies. The *reactivity of the immune system* varies from one individual to another and this will be compounded by differences in frequency of exposure and the number of red cells that escape into the mother's circulation.

Although *ABO blood group antigens* cause the greatest number of incompatibility reactions (65-70%), *rhesus antigens* are much more potent in terms of eliciting maternal antibody response. Other *rare blood groups* (Kell, Duffy, MNS) are involved in only 2-3%.

The frequency of rhesus incompatibility varies widely among *different races*, largely because of differences in the population of Rh-negative individuals; it is very low in Asiatic stock who are 99% Rh-positive, and relatively high in Caucasians of whom 85-90% are Rh-positive.

The *major recent advance* in management has been the *prophylactic use of anti-D gamma globulin* at the termination of pregnancy (this includes abortion and ectopic pregnancy). Such therapy subverts the normal immune response. Treatment is also necessary during pregnancy if damage to the placental barrier is suspected (e.g. abruption, amniocentesis, other trauma, fetal death); debate continues regarding the cost: benefit of routine *antenatal prophylaxis* (anti-D administration at 28 and 34 weeks to all Rh-negative women). With the introduction of an immune globulin programme, only about 1% of mothers will subsequently become immunized: failures usually result from previous incompatible blood transfusion, antepartum (rather than intrapartum) sensitization, a larger than normal fetomaternal haemorrhage, and failure to administer anti-D globulin (due to blood group error, oversight etc).

Apart from seeing that immune prophylaxis is carried out, the other *major task of the obstetric attendant is to ensure that maternal antibodies, if present, are detected by routine antenatal testing.* If no antibodies are present at the first visit, further checks are made at 28-30 weeks and 34-36 weeks. If antibodies are present at any time, the patient must be referred to a specialist or special centre dealing with this problem.

A number of complex decisions and therapeutic measures may be required if moderate or severe haemolysis is occurring in the fetus (e.g. *amniocentesis, intrauterine transfusion, induction of premature labour,* postnatal *exchange transfusion* of the baby).

ABO incompatibility, numerically 3-4 times more common than rhesus incompatibility, is very rarely if ever responsible for fetal deaths or even severe anaemia; *the usual clinical problem is early jaundice* which may require phototherapy or possibly exchange transfusion. This condition is further characterized by fetal involvement in first pregnancies, and unpredictable severity in future pregnancies.

RHESUS INCOMPATIBILITY

Incidence

The rhesus factor, present in some 85–90% of Caucasians, 95% of blacks, and 99% of Asiatics, is so named because it is present in the rhesus monkey. In the preprophylaxis era, approximately 13% of Caucasian women would be at risk of rhesus isoimmunization (Rh-negative with Rh-positive husband), but only about 0.5–1% would have an affected baby. There are a number of possible reasons for this difference. (i) The fetal cells may be of a *different ABO group* to the mother and are quickly destroyed. (ii) Some *mothers react mildly or not at all* to the fetal cells. (iii) *Red cell transfer* across the placenta is quite variable, the amount ranging from less than 0.01 ml to more than 50 ml (figure 22.1). (iv) The *husband may be heterozygous* for the rhesus factor (i.e. his children can be either Rh-positive or Rh-negative).

It is generally accepted that the first pregnancy represents a 'sensitizing' experience (IgM production) and the baby is not affected. Women previously transfused (1–2% of recipients develop antibodies) will be an exception to this; another possibility is that the mother was sensitized at the time of her own birth from an Rh-positive mother.

With an adequate prophylactic anti-D gamma globulin programme, the *incidence should be less than 1 in 500 pregnancies*.

Figure 22.1 Fetomaternal haemorrhage complicating failed amniocentesis and presumed placental damage. The baby was pale at birth (haemoglobin 8.5 g/dl). This smear of maternal blood shows that 4% of erythrocytes are of fetal origin, equivalent to a haemorrhage of about 100 ml. (Magnification X 400). This, the Kleihauer test, is based on the principle that fetal cells remain stable in an acid pH (3.2), whereas adult haemoglobin is eluted from the maternal red cells.

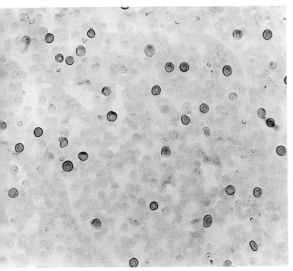

Prognosis

The overall perinatal mortality rate in rhesus isoimmunized pregnancies is 6–12% (table 16.1). The proportion of all perinatal deaths due to erythroblastosis has fallen from 5% to 0.5–1% in the past 15 years (table 15.6).

Diagnosis

In the *history*, important items include previous blood transfusion, previously affected pregnancies (number, degree of severity, nature of treatment required), whether the children have had the same or a different father. *Physical examination* will usually not reveal any unusual features unless the baby is severely affected and hydropic, in which case the mother may demonstrate signs of severe preeclampsia ('maternal syndrome' (colour plates 9–11)). Other causes of hydrops may need to be considered if rhesus antibody or liquor bilirubin levels are not high (e.g. twin to twin transfusion, infection, cardiac anomaly, alpha thalassaemia). In many patients, the diagnosis will be made by the *detection of antibodies on routine screening* using the indirect Coombs or enzyme (e.g. papain) techniques. Occasionally (1–2%), rarer Rh subgroups (C,c, E,e) or other blood groups (ABO, Kell, Duffy, Kidd, MNS) may be involved; whether an antepartum diagnosis is made in such patients depends on the depth of screening of the particular serology laboratory.

Management

In most major hospitals there is a special clinic where rhesus isoimmunized patients are managed, with close collaboration between obstetrician, biochemist, serologist and paediatrician. The major question to be answered is: *how severely affected is the fetus?* When this has been decided, a decision must be made as to the appropriate treatment option: this will be determined largely by findings at *amniocentesis* (figure 22.2) with additional help from the severity of disease in *previous pregnancies* and the current *serology results*.

General

The couple should be informed of the nature of the disorder in terms they can understand, and what tests will be necessary. They should also be reassured that in most cases the outcome will be satisfactory and the baby will develop normally.

Antibody and other serological tests. All patients will have ABO and Rh testing performed at the first antenatal visit. Tests for Rh antibodies are required as follows: no antibodies at initial test — repeat at 26–28 weeks and 34–36

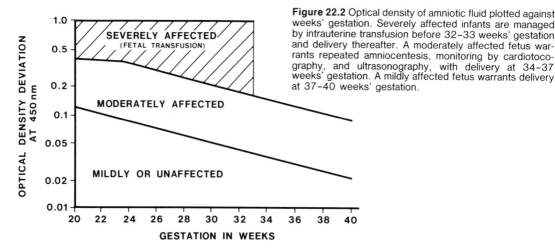

Figure 22.2 Optical density of amniotic fluid plotted against weeks' gestation. Severely affected infants are managed by intrauterine transfusion before 32–33 weeks' gestation and delivery thereafter. A moderately affected fetus warrants repeated amniocentesis, monitoring by cardiotocography, and ultrasonography, with delivery at 34–37 weeks' gestation. A mildly affected fetus warrants delivery at 37–40 weeks' gestation.

weeks; antibodies detected at initial test — further tests at intervals according to the titre and period of gestation.

There are several uses of antibody testing: (i) providing a general alert that the baby may be affected, (ii) providing a reasonably reliable indication of severity in 'first affected' pregnancies (titres greater than 40–50 IU/ml (1 in 64) are often associated with serious fetal disease), and (iii) providing reassurance if levels are low (e.g. < 5 IU/ml (1 in 16)).

In order to determine the *father's genotype* more precisely (particularly whether he is heterozygous (Dd) or homozygous (DD)), his blood and that of previous children are typed. Since no d serum exists for testing, an educated guess may be necessary, based on frequencies of the Rh gene complex in the population (e.g. CDe occurs in approximately 41%, cde in 39%, cDE in 16%, cDE in 2%, Cde in 1%, and cdE, CDE rarely).

Review of history. A careful check is made of past pregnancies, in particular the presence of antibodies, results of amniocentesis, induction of labour, state of the baby (group, Rh, haemoglobin, Coombs test, bilirubin), and any necessary treatment.

Amniocentesis. The need for this procedure is determined by the history (severity of previous disease) and results of antibody tests. Its usefulness depends on the fact that the levels of bile pigment and rhesus antibody in the fluid parallel the severity of the disease in the baby. In doubtful cases, repeated tests show whether the trend is favourable or unfavourable. The procedure may not be necessary if the antibody levels are low (< 5 IU/ml); or alternatively, it may be required as early as 20–22 weeks to determine whether intrauterine transfusion will be required. This is a specialist procedure, usually performed under ultrasound control to avoid

Figure 22.3 Intrauterine transfusion in progress at 26 weeks' gestation.

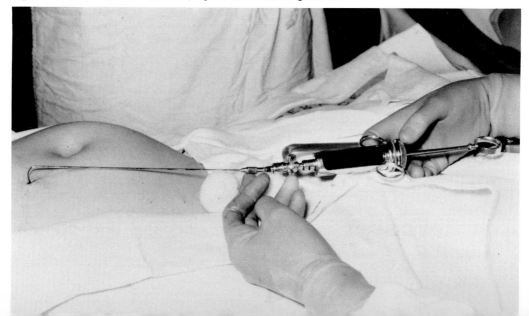

damage to the placenta or baby. The fluid is subjected to biochemical analysis (figure 22.2), particular attention being paid to the level of bilirubin (a reflection of the amount of fetal red cell destruction (figure 69.1)).

Intrauterine transfusion. In this procedure, blood is transfused into the peritoneal cavity of the fetus. This treatment option is selected when the haemolytic disease is so severe that the fetus is unlikely to survive long enough to allow delivery in the third trimester (e.g. 30–34 weeks onwards). This decision is largely based on information obtained at amniocentesis, in particular, the level of bilirubin in the amniotic fluid.

The procedure is highly specialized and usually consists of passing a needle, under ultrasound control, through the maternal abdomen and uterus into the fetal peritoneal cavity. A catheter is threaded through the needle and the latter is withdrawn. Fresh, packed, group O Rh-negative blood is transfused into the fetus at a rate of about 1 ml/minute; the amount depends largely on the gestational age of the fetus (e.g. approximately 20 ml at 20 weeks, 70 ml at 32 weeks) (figure 22.3). Initial transfusion is not practical before 20 weeks' gestation because of the small area available. Three or more transfusions at intervals of 10–20 days may be necessary. Recently, transfusions have been given *intravenously into the hepatic or umbilical vein*, again under ultrasonic guidance. Up to 50% of fetuses still die, partly because of the severity of the disease (fetal hydrops) and partly because of mishap (transfusion accidents, premature labour etc). Survival is much reduced if the procedure is necessary before 24–26 weeks.

Plasma exchange. Plasmaphoresis, using the continuous flow cell separator, has the theoretical advantage that harmful antibodies can be removed from the mother's plasma. Unfortunately, the exchanges must be started early (before the 20th week), are difficult and time-consuming, and evidence suggests that immunoregulatory factors may also be removed, allowing more rapid antibody production.

Induction of labour. A decision regarding the optimum time of delivery is made after all the necessary facts have been considered. This procedure is rarely carried out before the 32nd week of pregnancy. If the baby is considered to be only mildly affected, labour is induced at 37–40 weeks; if moderately affected, 34–37 weeks; and if severely affected, 32–34 weeks (with or without previous intrauterine transfusion).

Monitoring of fetal condition. Usual measures of fetal monitoring, such as cardiotocography and maternal oestriol values are employed, although these are less helpful than in the case of fetal growth retardation. *Serial ultrasonography* is useful in the severely isoimmunized patient to exclude signs of hydrops fetalis (subcutaneous oedema, ascites, pleural effusions) (colour plate 123 and figure 22.4). The keynote of success is skilled care after delivery.

Birth. After careful clinical assessment to detect maturity, pallor, oedema, cardiac failure, petechiae, jaundice and hepatosplenomegaly, the following routine tests are carried out. *Mother.* Antibody titre. *Baby.* Blood is preferably taken by needle from a vein near the placenta and placed in separate bottles: (i) *plain tube* for serum bilirubin (and serum proteins if required), (ii) *anticoagulant tube* for haemoglobin, blood group, Rh, and direct Coombs test. If blood is taken from the cut end of the cord it should be clear of maternal blood and the cord should not be squeezed. A sterile moist dressing should be placed over the cord, 6–8 cm of which should be left. In emergency cases, where antenatal notes are unavailable, or there has been no antenatal care, blood must be taken from the mother and umbilical cord for future study if required.

The placenta is inspected, weighed, and placed in the refrigerator pending determination whether pathology study is required. *The typical placenta, which is seen only when the disease is severe, is much enlarged*, occasionally weighing almost as much as the fetus (figure 22.4), and is more *friable* than normal.

Communication is necessary between labour ward staff and the biochemical laboratory, paediatric staff, and nursery (intensive care if necessary).

Exchange transfusion is indicated on the grounds of anaemia and/or hyperbilirubinaemia. In this procedure the blood of the baby is 'exchanged' with donor blood in *repeated aliquots of 10–20 ml* (colour plate 124). By this means, the bilirubin and harmful antibodies are removed and the haemoglobin level is raised by the transfused red cells. In general, if the haemoglobin value is 15 g/dl or more and the bilirubin less than 40 µmol/l (2.5 mg/dl), exchange transfusion will rarely be necessary; conversely if the haemoglobin value is less than 12.5 g/dl and the bilirubin more than 60 µmol/l (3.5 mg/dl), the procedure will probably be necessary. Usually 200–220 ml/kg of Rh-negative, ABO compatible blood is given and this provides an exchange of some 80% of the baby's blood. Factors such as the condition of the infant, rate of rise of bilirubin level, and degree of prematurity determine the timing of the procedure. *Repeat exchange transfusion* is usually required only because of a rising bilirubin level. *A simple transfusion* may be necessary later to restore the haemoglobin level to normal — again using Rh-ve ABO compatible blood.

Prophylaxis

As a result of generally smaller family size and *anti-D gamma globulin* administration, rhesus isoimmunization is becoming a less common disease. Immune globulin is given as an intramuscular injection of 50–300 μg within 72 hours of abortion, ectopic pregnancy, or delivery to all Rh-negative women unless the infant is shown to be Rh-negative, and provided there are not antibodies already present. In addition, any female likely to reproduce in the future is treated if Rh-incompatible blood is inadvertently given (10 μg per ml blood transfused). Failure rates with anti-

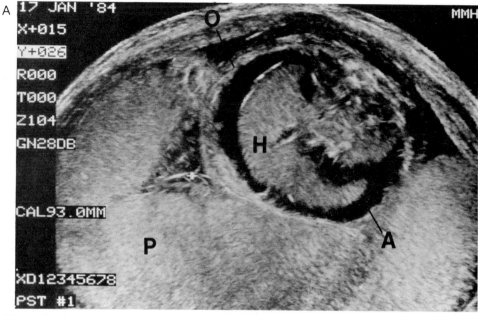

Figure 22.4 Ultrasonographic features of hydrops fetalis. **A.** Transverse scan at 31.5 weeks' gestation showing a huge placenta (P), subcutaneous oedema of the fetal trunk (O), fetal ascites (A) and hepatomegaly (H). Liquor volume was not excessive. The mother was group B, rhesus-positive with an anti-c titre of 1 in 256 (indirect Coombs). Cardiotocography showed critical fetal reserve. Immediate Caesarean section was performed. The infant (birth-weight 3,080 g) was hydropic (cord haemoglobin 4.5 g/dl) and died aged 48 hours. The placenta weighed 1,980 g. The moral is that Rh-positive mothers can be severely isoimmunized to rhesus antigens other than D. **B.** Transverse scan at 23 weeks' gestation in a patient who had had infants with nonimmunological (idiopathic) hydrops fetalis in 2 previous pregnancies. There is marked oedema of the scalp seen as a halo (H) around the fetal skull and the placenta (P) is very thick. The patient was delivered because she had preeclampsia and polyhydramnios, and the fetal prognosis was hopeless. The infant (birth-weight 450 g) died aged 5 minutes. The placental weight was 1,100 g. Nonimmunological causes account for 40% of cases of hydrops fetalis (colour plates 9–11).

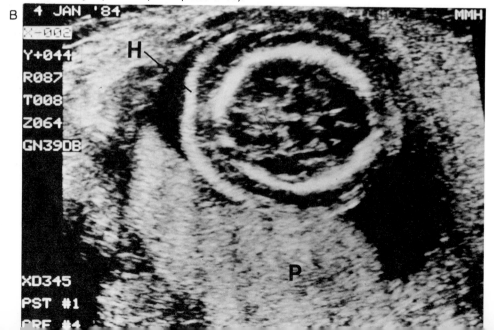

D gamma globulin are about 1%, usually because of larger than normal fetomaternal haemorrhage, unsuspected preexisting sensitization, or faulty prophylaxis. In some centres, prophylactic injections are also given at 28 and 34 weeks of pregnancy; there is evidence that this further reduces the small failure rate associated with postpartum prophylaxis, but the question of cost-benefit arises (e.g. financial, serum sickness). *Kleihauer testing* of maternal blood to detect the presence and amount of fetal erythrocytes (figure 22.1) permits a more scientific approach to prophylaxis — (20 μg of immune globulin is given for each ml of fetal red blood cells detected). In general, the dose of anti-D gamma globulin ranges from 50 μg in the first trimester to 300 μg in the third. Disturbances to placental integrity (abortion, ectopic pregnancy, chorion biopsy, abruption, 'blind' amniocentesis, external cephalic version, fetal death) all call for assessment and preventive therapy. Factors increasing fetal red cell transfer at the time of birth include Caesarean section, breech delivery, multiple pregnancy, manual removal of the placenta, and placenta praevia; if the estimated transfer exceeds 15–20 ml (about 1% of patients), extra anti-D gamma globulin must be administered in proportion to the estimated volume.

ABO INCOMPATIBILITY

The basic disorder is similar to that existing in rhesus incompatibility; i.e. the fetus possesses antigens not carried by the mother — usually blood group antigens A or B, the mother being group O. The frequency of ABO groupings in the community is approximately as follows: O 50%, A 35%, B 10%, AB 5%; group A is further subdivided into A1 70%, A2 30%.

In contrast to the rhesus system, *natural antibodies* are present to the ABO antigens lacking in the mother. That is, if she is group O (lacking A or B), she will possess 'natural' anti-A and anti-B antibodies; *some of these are of the IgG type which pass the placental barrier*. This explains why primigravidas can be affected, which is rare in rhesus isoimmunization (initial immune antibodies are of the IgM type which do not cross the placenta). In subsequent pregnancies, antibody may be produced by the sensitized mother as with rhesus isoimmunization. The disease is milder because there are fewer A and B antigenic sites on the red cell, and receptor sites for antibodies are available other than on the red cell (this is not the case with the rhesus system). Another reason why ABO is a milder form of erythroblastosis is that anti-A or anti-B antibodies are weaker haemolysins than anti-D antibody.

Incidence

Approximately 15–20% of pregnancies are ABO incompatible and it is probable that some degree of fetal red cell destruction occurs in all of these. However, clinical evidence of this is present in only 0.5–2% (table 68.3) and laboratory (serological) evidence in 2–4% (the latter is close to the calculated figure, assuming that 20% will have a significant fetal red cell transfer). In the vast majority the mother is group O and the baby is group A.

Clinical Features

It is doubtful whether the disease ever causes severe fetal anaemia or hydrops fetalis. Therefore, antenatal estimation of antibody titre, *amniocentesis and induction of labour are never indicated*. The condition is usually unsuspected until the baby becomes *jaundiced* on the first or second day of life. Hepatosplenomegaly is present in about 50%. *Kernicterus* may occur in those infants with serum bilirubin levels above 340 μmol/l (20 mg/dl) who are not adequately treated.

Laboratory Findings

(i) The mother is usually group O, the baby group A; (ii) the direct Coombs test on cord blood is negative or only weakly positive; (iii) the baby's haemoglobin level is usually within the normal range (14–22 g/dl); (iv) nucleated red blood cells, reticulocytes and spherocytes are seen in the blood film (figure 69.1); (v) the peak level of serum bilirubin exceeded 340 μmol/l (20 mg/dl) only in about 15% of infants even before the introduction of phototherapy; (vi) the enzyme, erythrocyte cholinesterase, is typically decreased; (vii) free anti-B or anti-A antibodies are usually present in fetal serum. The diagnosis is thus only suspected if there has been a previous child with the condition or there is early jaundice in the neonate, not explained by such conditions as rhesus incompatibility, prematurity, infection, drugs, or marked bruising.

During pregnancy the 'immune' antibodies can only be assessed after the 'natural' antibodies have been removed. If this is done, the significance of different titre levels is as follows: 1 in 64 or less, probably unaffected; 1 in 128–1 in 512, mild or moderate; 1 in 1,024 or greater, moderate or marked.

Management (table 68.3)

As mentioned previously, because fetal anaemia rarely if ever occurs, amniocentesis and induction of labour before 40 weeks is not indicated. *Phototherapy* is needed because of hyperbilirubinaemia in about 65% of babies; when *exchange transfusion* is required (10–12%), group O, rhesus compatible blood should be used.

chapter twenty-three

Fetoplacental Dysfunction

OVERVIEW

The fetus is at the end of a relatively unstable nutritional chain. Nutrients and oxygen are carried in the mother's blood through the uterus to the placenta, where a somewhat imperfect exchange takes place with the fetal blood which is running in the villous capillaries. From here, the enriched blood passes via the umbilical vein to the fetus.

The most vulnerable part of this supply line is the maternal component of the placenta — the decidual arterioles and intervillous lakes. These are sensitive, as are the maternal vessels elsewhere, to a number of damaging factors. These can mostly be classified into 1 of 3 groups: *specific pregnancy disorders* (e.g. preeclampsia, chronic placental abruption); *associated medical disorders* (e.g. hypertension, chronic renal disease, diabetes mellitus); and finally, *general adverse factors* (e.g. drug abuse, poor socioeconomic circumstances, malnutrition).

The nearer to the fetus that the block occurs, the more likely it is that both *nutrients and oxygen* will be affected (e.g. a knot in the umbilical cord or uteroplacental malfunction). Conversely, disorders of the lungs, heart or blood in the mother may chiefly affect oxygen availability, whereas gastrointestinal disorders will affect nutrient supply. In some cases, the placenta appears to have been imperfectly formed de novo. Where the fetus is solely or predominantly involved (e.g. chromosomal or other malformation, 'torch' infection) detection is often difficult because of the absence of an observable risk factor. The effects on the fetus depend on the acuteness of the interruption of supply.

The significance of such dysfunction is the *liability of the fetus to succumb during the third trimester, either before or during labour*; apart from fetal jeopardy, there is an additional high cost in terms of staff time and use of expensive hospital facilities.

'*Placental insufficiency*', '*intrauterine growth retardation*', and '*small for dates*' are terms used to describe the appearance of the infant and to designate when *birth-weight is less than the 10th percentile. Fetoplacental dysfunction may occur in premature, term or postterm infants.* A fetus may die in utero due to placental insufficiency without being below the 10th percentile for birth-weight. It is the chronic form of fetoplacental dysfunction rather than the acute form that is associated with fetal growth retardation. *It is the obstetrician's aim to identify the fetus at risk of death from hypoxia (fetoplacental dysfunction) whether it is growth retarded or not.*

As fetal compromise increases, there is a characteristic pattern of change. Initially there is a *depletion of energy stores* — glycogen (especially in the liver), together with subcutaneous and other fatty tissues; this is followed by a *general slowdown in growth* as bony epiphyses etc are affected; finally, there will be *deprivation of supplies to the brain* — the site most privileged (last affected) by the fetal circulatory arrangements.

The *placenta and liquor amnii* suffer the same fate as the fetus; the liquor sometimes disappears almost completely; hypoxia may also stimulate gut peristalsis and the fetus becomes covered with thick meconium.

Fetoplacental dysfunction should be *suspected* if one or more major risk factors are present and steps should then be taken to *assess fetal well-being*. The past decade or so has seen the introduction of a variety of measures for this purpose. The simplest of these is the determination by the patient of *fetal activity* over a specified time. This costs nothing and if carried out on a routine basis will usually pick up the difficult problem where the placental failure is idiopathic. Careful measurement of the *height of the uterine fundus* is also a useful indicator of suboptimal fetal growth. Confirmatory, more sophisticated tests include *cardiotocography*; *ultrasound* study of fetal size, activity, breathing pattern, and liquor volume; *biochemical analysis* of fetal/placental products; and finally, *studies of the liquor amnii.*

The key elements of the obstetric attendant's role are a high index of suspicion (allowing early diagnosis), accurate evaluation of the fetal condition, and choice of appropriate management regimen. Referral is usually indicated because of the complexity of the diagnostic tests, labour and delivery management, and care of the newborn.

It should be emphasized that without a high index of suspicion, 40–50% of cases will be missed.

The *fetal outcome* depends on several factors — the type of insult, when in pregnancy it occurs, its duration, and severity. At one end of the spectrum the fetus will die in utero, at the other the effect will hardly be noticeable. At any one point in time, the clinician needs to know the *fetal reserve* and the *rate at which this is diminishing*. Typical syndromes in the small for dates babies include brain dysfunction, coagulation disorders, and lowered immune function. In uncomplicated fetoplacental insufficiency the number of cells in the baby is usually normal and with adequate postnatal care the baby will 'catch up'. On the other hand, some disorders (genetic, infective) are associated with reduction in the cell number and the person is likely to remain small for age. Both groups should be distinguished from babies who are purely premature, since their prognosis, behaviour, and management differ in a number of respects; approximately 30% of infants weighing less than 2,500 g are small for dates.

Despite the increase in fetal hazard when intrauterine growth is retarded, the majority of these infants survive and develop normally. Evaluation of these high risk pregnancies by clinical surveillance, fetoplacental function testing, cardiotocography and ultrasonography makes possible individualized treatment and improved perinatal results. With modern obstetric and paediatric management the prognosis of the infant with intrauterine growth retardation is encouraging (see section on mortality and morbidity of the growth retarded infant in Chapter 64).

DEFINITIONS AND INCIDENCE

The most widely used definition of *intrauterine growth retardation is birth-weight below the 10th percentile according to gestational age* for infants born in the community concerned. Birth-weight below the 5th percentile or 2 standard deviations below the mean are less commonly used criteria. The terms *intrauterine growth retardation* and *small for dates* are used synonymously. *By definition, the incidence of the entity must be 10%*. However, clinically significant fetal growth retardation is present in only 2.5–5% of pregnancies; these include about 30% of babies with birth-weight below 2,500 g. *It is important to appreciate that fetoplacental dysfunction can be present when the infant is not growth retarded.*

SIGNIFICANCE

Fetal growth retardation is *1 of the 3 major causes of perinatal death*, being outranked only by *prematurity* and *congenital malformation*. *Placental insufficiency* is a term often used interchangeably with fetal growth retardation. This is a paediatric diagnosis made by inspection of the infant after birth. Its features depend upon *deprivation of calories* but the child need not be small for dates, especially when the process has been present only in the latter weeks of pregnancy. Moreover, the classical features of placental insufficiency (wrinkled and peeling skin, absence of subcutaneous fat) are often seen in infants with birth-weight appropriate for gestation, especially in those born from prolonged

pregnancies. *The signs of placental insufficiency need not correlate with those of hypoxia* (fetal distress in labour, acidosis at birth, low Apgar score). In other words placental transference of oxygen and nutriments can fail independently — significant fetal hypoxia can be present in the absence of fetal growth retardation, using the above definition. It is the obstetrician's aim, using clinical acumen combined with ultrasonographic and biochemical testing, to identify the fetus at risk of death from hypoxia whether growth retarded or not. *The ultrasonographic and biochemical methods of testing discussed in this chapter are not truly comparable (or competitive), since some aim to identify the growth retarded fetus, irrespective of its state of health, whereas others aim to detect fetoplacental dysfunction irrespective of whether or not the fetus is growth retarded.*

AETIOLOGY (table 23.1)

In spite of the numerous factors listed in table 23.1, all of which have a significant association with fetal growth retardation, the majority of cases have no known cause. However, the absence of an associated disease entity does not mean that growth retardation is benign — the infant can be born dead, die after birth, be malformed, or have neurological sequelae of hypoxia. However, the small for dates at birth are not destined to remain diminutive; in most cases smallness at birth represents intrauterine nutritional deprivation and is overcome in the first year of life with normal access to calories.

TABLE 23.1 CAUSES OF INTRAUTERINE GROWTH RETARDATION

1. *General Factors*

   Socioeconomic deprivation
   Age
   Parity
   Weight
   Race
   Personality
   Reproductive capacity — (poor past history (previous growth retardation); uterine malformations (bicornuate uterus))
   Drugs and alcohol

2. *Specific Factors*

Preeclampsia, placental abruption
Calorie and Metabolic Disturbances
   Malnutrition (poverty, persistent nausea, false pride (desire to remain thin))
   Dietary imbalance (food fads, junk food)
   Maternal hypoglycaemia
   Malabsorption states (parasites, sprue)
   Endocrinopathy (thyroid/adrenal)

Maternal Oxygen Deprivation
   High altitude
   Respiratory disease (chronic airways obstruction)
   Cardiac disease (cyanotic heart anomalies)
   Vascular disease (hypertensive — renal disease)
   Red cell disorders (anaemia, smoking effects)

Fetal Oxygen/Nutrient Deprivation
   Uterine muscle contractions
   Myodecidual arterial disease (hypertensive disorders, diabetes mellitus)
   Placental anomalies/complications
   Umbilical cord anomalies/complications

Fetal Disorders
   Malformations (anencephaly, Potter syndrome)
   Genetic disorders (metabolic, chromosomal)
   Infections (rubella, cytomegalovirus)
   Multiple pregnancy
   Fetal toxins (alcohol, heroin, antifolic agents)
   Red cell disorders (haemolysis)

General Factors

With the employment of large-scale perinatal mortality surveys and more sophisticated compilation and analysis of data, we are in a position to assess the significance of factors that might adversely affect the fetus.

Socioeconomic. Much of the pioneer work in this field was carried out in Aberdeen, Scotland. It clearly showed that social class had an important bearing on maternal and fetal outcome. *Adverse social and economic factors* are usually related characteristics, stigmata being poor and crowded living conditions, poor diet, too many to feed and clothe, poor education, and a general increase in stress.

Age. Again, there are higher complication rates at the age extremes — under 18 and over 30. The poorer outcome in the *adolescent* is largely due to the fact that usually more than 90% are nulliparas. However, this is compounded by the fact that the juvenile is not mature, and both physiological and, more particularly, psychological adaptations to pregnancy are less efficient. Antenatal care is often suboptimal due to ignorance, concealment, or not bothering: this tends to increase the rate of a number of complications such as urinary tract and sexually transmitted infection, anaemia, and preeclampsia. This will have secondary effects in increasing low birthweight and perinatal death rates.

The *elderly patient*, on the other hand, has special problems related to the natural progression of such disease processes as diabetes, hypertension, and renal disease; in addition, she is more prone to early conceptional disorders (e.g. twinning and chromosomal anomalies) and these increase the likelihood of fetal growth retardation. The effect of a long gap between children, whether due to infertility, remarriage, or mischance, has ill-effects partly due to the age increase and partly due to the reproductive apparatus 'forgetting' its role.

Parity. The second baby born has the lowest perinatal mortality rate. The first born has to be the 'trail breaker' and if there are abnormalities in the mother — either mechanical (contracted pelvis, congenital uterine malformation) or metabolic (diabetes), the baby may perish or be subject to morbidity. High parity is often associated with chronic anaemia and disorders such as rhesus isoimmunization.

Weight. As with age and parity, there is an unfavourable effect on the fetus the further deviation there is from the ideal. There may be genetic, metabolic or psychological reasons why a woman is underweight. There is a reasonable correlation between low maternal weight and low fetal weight.

Race. Classical examples of the influence of racial factors are seen in the differences in perinatal mortality rate between white and nonwhite races in developed communities (Australia, Canada, New Zealand, North America, South Africa). The rates may be up to 5 times as great in extreme cases. In some respects, there appears to be a basic inequality of reproductive performance; in other cases, there is a subtle interplay of endemic disease (infections, infestations with hookworm, anaemia), high parity, and differences in socioeconomic condition, antenatal care, diet, and education.

The problem of the *immigrant* is different. In many cases, the immigrant is going from a less favourable to a more favourable socioeconomic state. However, assimilation into the community presents problems of communication, often to the detriment of antenatal care; the reporting of complications promptly, and the confidence that the patient has in the hospital/medical/nursing complex, especially if complications do occur, are matters that can be affected adversely.

Personality. This is not a characteristic that can be coded easily like weight or height, yet we should make some attempt to assess this, since it deeply affects the patient's attitude to the pregnancy and antenatal care. *Maternal instinct* is probably a rather unique but allied phenomenon.

Reproductive capacity. This term broadly defines the overall ability of the woman to produce a normal, healthy infant. The converse is only definable in retrospect, and often defies attempts to determine why there is an undue number of abortions, infertile periods, fetal growth retardation, premature labours, and perinatal morbidity and mortality. *Fetal growth retardation tends to recur* in subsequent pregnancies (30% risk), even in the absence of predisposing conditions such as hypertension or chronic renal disease.

Uterine malformations (unicornuate, bicornuate, double uterus), minor degrees of which are quite common (5–10%), are associated with fetoplacental dysfunction.

Drug and alcohol abuse. Major abuse of tobacco, social anodynes such as analgesics, soft and hard drugs, and alcohol may have a deleterious effect on reproduction generally and on fetal growth in particular.

Narcotic drug addiction has a special association with fetal growth retardation because the patients usually have additional problems related to inadequate diet, unfavourable socioeconomic conditions, alcohol ingestion, cigarette smoking, and factors related to the drug habit such as prostitution.

The *fetal alcohol syndrome* typifies the damage that may be done to the delicate developing tissues of the embryo and fetus. The toxicity may be caused by the alcohol itself or breakdown products such as acetaldehyde.

The general incidence ranges from 0.2–0.5%, but will obviously relate to alcohol consumption patterns in the community. In some areas, mental handicap due to alcohol is exceeded only by that due to Down syndrome and neural tube defect. With heavy drinking (5–6 drinks at a time, 40–50 drinks per month), the baby is usually growth retarded, and has a typical facies due to mid-facial hypoplasia — general flattening, nose short and upturned, eyes small; there may also be microcephaly, mental disorder, abnormal palmar creases.

Specific Factors

The specific factors affecting fetal well-being are summarized in table 23.1 and will be discussed in individual chapters. The obstetric complications which are seen most commonly in cases of fetal growth retardation are *severe pre-eclampsia, threatened abortion, abnormal glucose tolerance* (*both diabetes and hypoglycaemia*), and *placental abruption.*

In some patients, the pregnancy appears to be quite normal; the cause in such cases can only be guessed at, although a disturbance at an early stage of fetal or placental development seems probable. The manner in which each complication affects the fetus often differs.

PATHOPHYSIOLOGY

In most instances of fetal growth retardation there is *deprivation of nutrients and oxygen.* With fetal starvation, there is *loss of fat and glycogen stores.* If the deprivation continues, *general body growth slows,* but there is sparing of the brain because it has preferential treatment in the distribution of oxygenated and nutrient-rich blood from the placenta. Finally, *brain development is affected* and death may occur.

The *placenta* is usually small and often infarcted and the villous surface area is reduced ($12–14 \, m^2 \rightarrow 7–9 \, m^2$). There is often atherosis and sclerosis of the placental vessels and areas of infarction. Other pathology may be evident, such as *chronic abruption* and circumvallate formation. The *amniotic fluid* shows a progressive *diminution,* and in the terminal stage is often heavily *meconium-stained.*

ASSESSMENT OF FETAL WELL-BEING AND GROWTH RETARDATION

This branch of obstetrics is a relatively new one, and, in some cases, the techniques described will be in use only at larger centres or even only in research centres. It is inevitable, however, that their use will extend in the future.

General Remarks

Although a large number of tests of fetal development and well-being are now available, there is *still a significant grey area between the normal and clearly abnormal.* This is contributed to partly because of normal biological variation (e.g. in size of the fetus, in its activities such as movement and breathing patterns, and in the levels of such products as oestriol) and partly because of variations in the 'instruments' of assessment (including the attendant).

The 2 main criteria of any test are its sensitivity (ability to detect a positive value in a population of positives) and *specificity* (ability to reject a negative value in a population of negatives). These together constitute the *accuracy* of the test. The relative values of sensitivity and specificity alter with the prevalence of the factor being studied: with low prevalence, specificity is normally at a premium over sensitivity.

When to test? Although growth retardation has been demonstrated early in the second trimester (e.g. in the diabetic patient with vascular disease), it is not cost effective to make the diagnosis unless something positive can be done to improve the fetus or remove it to the support of the intensive care nursery. This consideration, plus the fact that significant retardation is uncommon before 28–30 weeks, usually dictates a policy of waiting until the last trimester.

Who to test? How wide the investigative net is cast depends on the availability of staff and laboratory facilities. Some consider testing at 32–34 weeks should be routine, as for the earlier antenatal screening tests. Other centres will screen 'high-risk' patients only, together with those in whom current clinical findings are suspicious.

Repetition of testing. This is useful initially to *verify an abnormal finding* and then to *establish the velocity of deterioration.* The frequency will depend on the presumed or evident severity of the condition.

Number of tests. As mentioned previously, few tests of fetal well-being are 100% specific or 100% sensitive. For this reason, it is comforting to apply several tests, especially in the high-risk patient (table 23.2). In this way a *biophysical profile* can be built up which will maximize the chance of detecting the fetus in trouble. In most of the tests of fetal function, a normal result will nearly always indicate normality at that time; conversely, an abnormal result will only indicate abnormality in 20–80%, depending on the particular test.

Clinical Assessment

Maternal weight. If one allows for such factors as alterations in diet, intercurrent illness, or shifts of body fluid by diuretics, the maternal weight chart often gives a clue to chronic fetal distress. Usually, the rate of gain slows, becomes stationary, and then begins to fall. This finding must

TABLE 23.2   METHODS OF DIAGNOSIS OF INTRAUTERINE GROWTH RETARDATION

1. *Clinical*

   Maternal weight loss
   Uterine size: symphysis-fundus height measurement
   Amniotic fluid volume
   Fetal movements — kick charts

2. *Cardiotocography*

3. *Ultrasonography*

   Fetal size
   Movement
   Breathing pattern
   Muscle tone
   Amniotic fluid volume
   Doppler blood flow.

4. *Biochemical Study*

   Plasma/urinary oestrogen
   Placental lactogen
   Pregnancy-specific beta$_1$ glycoprotein
   Pregnancy-associated placental protein
   Alkaline phosphatase

5. *Amniotic Fluid Study*

   Amnioscopy
   Amniocentesis

always be assumed to indicate fetal danger until proved otherwise.

Uterine size. Obstetric experience soon tells us that a uterus which feels a certain size (and this is usually related to surface landmarks) is equivalent (or not) to a certain period of amenorrhoea — i.e. it is 'normal for dates'. For this, and indeed for most tests of fetal well-being, we need an *accurate menstrual history.* Hence the importance of this information must be emphasized in talks to mothers on educational aspects of pregnancy. The approximate height of the fundus at different stages of pregnancy is shown in figure 38.1. This assessment may be refined a little by taking tape measurements of the maximum girth (normally 70–72 cm at 34 weeks, and 96–100 cm at 40 weeks) or by measuring the distance from the top of the symphysis pubis to the uterine fundus by either tape measure or caliper. These assessments are unfortunately subject to the vagaries of observer error, position of the umbilicus, amount of fat in the abdominal wall, height of the patient (and, thus, the abdominal length), and the amount of amniotic fluid — apart from changes effected by the state of fullness of the rectum or bladder. Also, such clinical assessments are suitable only for the detection of major and chronic fetal distress in the second half of pregnancy. Despite this, if the same observer has noted a failure of the fundus to increase in size over a period of 2-4 weeks the situation must be regarded seriously, and further tests carried out.

Amniotic fluid volume. The volume of amniotic fluid increases progressively until approximately 36 weeks, remains more or less stationary for some weeks, and declines thereafter. The latter process is hastened in fetal malnutrition, so that the astute examiner may detect *oligohydramnios*, not only by the diminished uterine size, but by the absence of normal ballottability of the fetus and the feeling that the uterus is closely wrapped around the fetus.

Fetal movements. It might be expected that the well-being of the fetus would be expressed in the number and vigour of movements. Although this is true, there is a *very wide normal variation* — the range for the normal fetus is 4-100 per hour; the mean is about 25 if in hospital or 40 if ambulant. In addition, women vary considerably in their sensitivity to movements: only 25-30% are major, involving trunk activity; this is the approximate proportion detected by the average patient. An absolute standard is thus not realistic and each patient must serve as her own control. Most would accept that *3 movements per hour is a minimum*. Experience has indicated that before *fetal death* the movements are sluggish for about 2-8 days and absent for 1-5 days.

The fetus has been observed to have active periods which last about 40 minutes and passive (quiet) periods which last 20-25 minutes (in only 1% do the latter extend beyond 45 minutes). In general, the fetus is more active after the mother has eaten (glucose effect) and when she is resting (improved uterine blood flow effect). Most fetuses will also *respond to external stimuli* (palpation of the maternal abdomen, sound applied to the mother's abdomen and light via the amnioscope). A decrease is observed with maternal smoking and where the gestation is prolonged.

Despite the above problems, *maternal recording of fetal movements on a regular basis from about the 28th week is being increasingly used as a primary screening test*. There are basically 2 methods. In the first, the mother begins counting at a set time each day and records the time until a count of 10 has been reached. This is good for the mothers whose fetus is active, but tedious and often impractical if the fetus is of quieter temperament or she is not a sensitive recorder. In the other method, a set time period is used: this may be 30 minutes each morning, 20 minutes twice each day etc. If the count falls below a set limit (e.g. 10 movements per 30 minutes), a further period is used and if the count is still unsatisfactory, the medical attendant should be contacted.

It has been estimated that *maternal compliance* with this scheme runs at about 80-90%, depending largely on the enthusiasm of the attendant; the pick-up rate is 0.5-1%.

In addition, the patient should be instructed that she should report if there have been no movements for a 12-hour period.

Electronic Monitoring

Cardiotocography. The normal fetal heart rate in early pregnancy is about 160 beats/minute; the rate slowly declines during pregnancy, averaging 130-140 at term. Until recently, fetal heart rate assessment was largely confined to the patient in labour. With sophistication of electronic measuring equipment, many details of cardiac activity can now be measured not only during labour but also in the antenatal period. With improving communication links, tracings may be transmitted (usually by telephone line) from outlying centres if there is doubt regarding the significance of the pattern or its management.

The addition of uterine pressure measurement to the technique (tocography) increases the value of the test since the fetal heart response to stress (hypoxia associated with the uterine contraction) can be assessed.

The different parameters, normal and abnormal, are shown in table 23.3. As with many other tests, there is usually no 'all-or-nothing' response. Much of the test subjectivity is related to the emphasis given to the duration and amplitude of the deviation and its progression (or otherwise) with time. There is a significant maturation of the autonomic nervous system during the third trimester and this is reflected in the reactivity of the fetal heart pattern — i.e. the response to fetal movement is more pronounced after 34 weeks.

The nonstress cardiotocogram (NSCTG) (see Chapter 13). This is the simpler of the 2 CTG tests. The procedure can be done in the clinic/office or ward. The patient is in a comfortable, semirecumbent position and the recording heads for the fetal cardiac signal and uterine pressure are attached to the maternal abdomen and adjusted to give an optimal signal. An event marker is used to indicate the occurrence of fetal movements. The duration of the test is usually 30 minutes, but it may need to be run for a longer time to obtain movement/contraction responses.

Key observations: (i) normality of the baseline

TABLE 23.3   FETAL CARDIOTOCOGRAPHY

Parameter (normal features)	Abnormal features	Significance
(a) Heart rate (120–160 beats per minute (bpm))	—	Normal range after 36 weeks.
Tachycardia	Moderate to 179; marked > 179 (for 5 minutes or 2 completed contractions)	Possible fetal hypoxia if no maternal tachycardia; possible fetal cardiac anomaly
Bradycardia	Mild 119–100; moderate 99–80; marked < 80 for 5 minutes or 2 completed contractions	Severity usually parallels fetal acidosis; significance increases if other abnormal CTG features present. Exclude maternal supine hypotension and fetal cardiac anomaly
(b) Beat to beat variability (7–14 + bpm)	Beat to beat variability less than 7	Beat to beat variability reflects intact autonomic control; loss reflects fetal hypoxia. Rule out drug effect, fetal sleep state
(c) Response to fetal movement (3 accelerations of 15 or more bpm over a period of 20 minutes) lasting for 15 seconds or more	Poor response to fetal movement: acceleration less than 15	Heart unable to accelerate under the stress of fetal exertion; key observation in the nonstress test. Deceleration may occur because of cord interference
(d) Response to contraction (may be temporary acceleration)	Early or variable deceleration in relation to uterine contraction. *Severity* gauged by duration (seconds) and degree of fall (bpm) — i.e dip area	Obstruction/tension of umbilical cord; head compression by lower uterine segment or bony pelvis; 20–25% show distress in labour
	Late deceleration in relation to uterine contraction (onset after peak contraction pressure). *Severity* (see above)	Placental insufficiency usually; possibly effect of maternal hypotension (supine syndrome, epidural analgesia) or hypoxia from other causes; 50–80% fetal distress, especially if also diminished baseline beat to beat variability
(e) Sinusoidal pattern of heart trace	Minor: Major:	Occasionally hypoxia of fetus (< 5%) Usually hypoxia of fetus (> 60%); often severe

pattern (presence of normal baseline variability in rate, and absence of tachycardia or brady-cardia); (ii) reactivity of the fetal cardiovascular system to spontaneous movement (usually an acceleration of rate of 15 beats/minute); if the fetus is quiet, movements may be stimulated by external palpation and/or giving the mother a glucose drink and assessing after a delay of 30–40 minutes; (iii) the behaviour of the heart rate in relation to the stress (hypoxia) of spontaneous (Braxton Hicks) contractions.

Contraction stress cardiotocogram (CSCTG). The basis of this test is the same as that described above; i.e. one looks at heart rate behaviour in terms of baseline variability, response to fetal movement, and response to the hypoxic stress of uterine contractions. It is *reserved for patients with a suspicious nonstress test or in those where no contractions are present.* Oxytocin by infusion is used to promote contractions which should be fewer than 2 or 3 per 10 minutes and not exceeding 80–90 seconds in duration.

More attention is paid in this test to the behaviour of the fetal heart at the time of the contractions (e.g. decelerations).

It is not as popular as the nonstress test, being more cumbersome, costly and uncomfortable for the patient. More recently, the use of the oxytocin infusion has been avoided by substituting

nipple stimulation. The patient stimulates the nipple (e.g. for 2 minutes) at intervals to produce an endogenous release of oxytocin.

It should be emphasized that both tests have a low false negative rate, but a fairly high false positive rate. Even in a nonreactive test the Apgar score after delivery will be 7 or better in at least 50% of the newborns; however, if the test is nonreactive, fetal growth retardation will be present in 15–20%, and death is likely in 3–5% (table 13.2). *Late decelerations, together with loss of baseline variation, nearly always signify fetal hypoxia and acidosis* (figure 23.1).

Response to stimuli. Fetal responses to both sound and light (evoked potentials from the central nervous system and heart rate changes) are being increasingly studied.

Ultrasonography

Since the fetal sac can be visualized and measured from about the fifth week of pregnancy, and the fetus itself from about the sixth week, we have a new and powerful tool for assessing fetal growth and thus well-being. However, ultrasonography requires a skilled operator and is relatively time-consuming; it is thus not generally accepted as a routine screening procedure. Charts are available whereby the ultrasonic measurement of the *biparietal diameter*

A

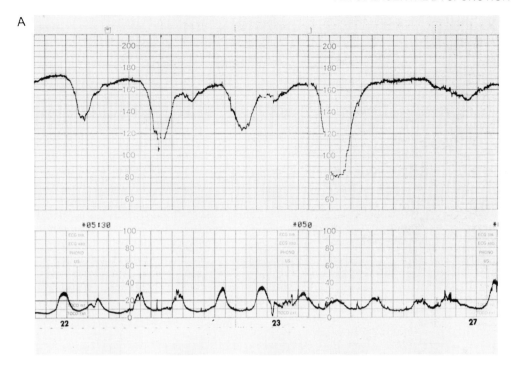

Figure 23.1 Acute fetoplacental dysfunction due to trauma — a life saved by timely cardiotocography. A 20-year-old primigravida was a passenger in a motor car accident at 36 weeks' gestation. She was wearing a combined shoulder-lap-sash seat belt, the lower band being positioned below the abdominal bulge of the uterus; the car turned over 3 times, landed on its roof and ruptured the seat belt. The patient sustained 4 fractured ribs, a pneumothorax and abdominal bruising; 2 hours after the accident she reported that fetal movements had ceased. Vaginal examination showed a closed external os and no evidence of bleeding. **A.** Cardiotocography showed a nonreactive fetal heart rate pattern, beat to beat variation of less than 5 beats/minute, and late decelerations indicative of critical fetal reserve. **B.** Caesarean section was therefore expeditiously performed, 4 hours after the accident had occurred. There was marginal placental separation; the infant weighed 2,490 g and had Apgar scores of 2 at 1 minute and 8 at 5 minutes. There was a. 300 ml haemoperitoneum due to a partial rupture on the posterior wall of the uterus which was repaired, as were smaller lacerations on the anterior wall. Recovery was uneventful. The infant thrived. The seat belt probably saved the mother's life, but localized injury to the uterus and its contents. (Courtesy of Dr Ian MacIsaac).

B

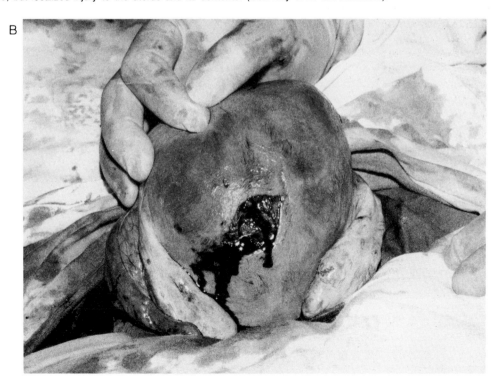

can be used to compute the maturity of the fetus (see Chapter 13). The major value of ultrasonography is in *plotting serial growth of the fetus*; in addition, comparisons of biparietal diameter (or head circumference) with abdominal circumference give an idea of growth retardation since the head region is relatively spared whereas the liver becomes depleted of glycogen stores and this reduces the abdominal measurement. The *ratio of biparietal diameter to upper abdominal diameter* in the normal fetus is less than 1 up to the 33rd–34th week; thereafter it slowly increases. In growth retardation, the ratio is less than 1; caveats include detection of hydrocephalus and fetal ascites. Various other indices have been introduced to detect the growth retarded fetus — e.g. biparietal diameter, crown-rump or femur length and trunk area will identify over 90% of cases. Abnormal biparietal values alone will identify some 60–70% of cases. Growth retar-

dation in the second trimester is usually quite ominous.

Fetal breathing activity can be studied by real-time ultrasound. Generally, breathing activity can be first detected at about 14 weeks of pregnancy and is regular and consistent from 20 weeks; the rate ranges from 30–70/minute. Some 30% of the time is occupied with breathing; it shows a circadian rhythm, with maximum activity in the evening. There is also an increase with maternal hyperglycaemia and hypercapnia, ingestion of caffeine or related compounds, and for a short time (5–10 minutes) after amniotomy. Abnormal breathing activity would be defined by inactivity for 90% or more of any 30-minute period. The rate is normally decreased before and during labour and when the fetus is hypoxic, hypoglycaemic, palpated, or the mother is suffering from the hypotensive syndrome or has ingested alcohol or sedative drugs; apnoea and

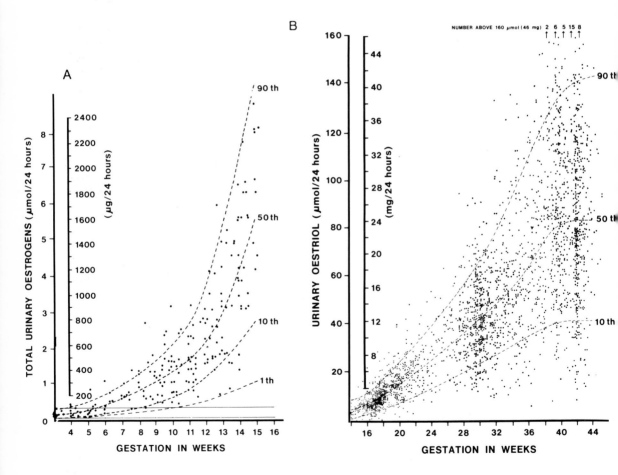

Figure 23.2 Urinary excretion of oestrogen (mainly oestriol) in pregnancy. **A.** Urinary oestrogen values in early pregnancy. The horizontal lines represent the ranges of values found in the luteal phase of the normal menstrual cycle (0.7–3.5 μmol/24 hrs or 20–100 μg/24 hrs). Abortion always occurs when values are below the 1st percentile. (From Brown JB et al. J Obstet Gynaecol Brit Cwlth 1970; 77:690–700). **B.** Oestriol values from 14 weeks' gestation showing the 10th, 50th and 90th percentiles. The lower limit of normal (from 30 μmol (8 mg) per 24 hours at 30 weeks to 40 μmol (12 mg) at 40 weeks and beyond) is similar to the 10th percentile. (From Beischer NA et al. Amer J Obstet Gynecol 1969; 103:483–495).

gasping are usually preludes to severe compromise and fetal death.

Fetal tone can be assessed by observing whether the fetus is in the normal flexed position and returns to it after back and limb extension movements. *Amniotic fluid volume* is graded according to the amount of fluid present; in the compromised fetus, there is general crowding of fetal parts and the fluid is reduced to small pockets surrounding the fetus ($<$ 1 cm vertical depth).

Doppler ultrasonography is now being used to assess blood flow in fetal and placental vessels; this promises to give earlier warning than the other tests mentioned.

Biochemical Assessment

The test most firmly established is the *measurement of oestriol in maternal plasma or 24-hour urine*. The latter requires an accurate and complete collection, otherwise the laboratory results will be unreliable, and so a careful explanation is given to the patient together with a written set of instructions. The upper and lower limits of normal oestriol values are shown in figure 23.2. Oestriol determination has retained its popularity because, unlike so many other tests of placental function, it measures what is happening in the fetus as well as the placenta, since both play an integral part in oestriol production.

The *frequency of measurement* depends on the degree of suspected or revealed distress. For example, if the mother has a condition such as chronic hypertension, the test may be carried out weekly from the 32nd–34th week, or even earlier. If normal values are obtained, weekly tests are continued; if low normal values, twice weekly; if borderline or subnormal, daily or second-daily.

Plasma and *urinary oestriol assays* have been found to be of equal clinical value in detection of fetal growth retardation and intrauterine hypoxia.

Certain conditions unrelated to fetal well-being may *depress oestriol values* and these should always be considered if the value seems out of keeping with clinical appraisal and other tests. *Placental sulphatase deficiency* (a placental enzyme responsible for oestriol production) occurs in 1 in 5,000–1 in 10,000 pregnancies; it is an X-linked recessive condition, the fetus is male, and may have ichthyosis. *Conditions affecting fetal adrenocortical activity* (anencephaly, primary adrenal hypoplasia, administration of cortisone derivatives to the mother e.g. betamethasone to enhance fetal pulmonary maturity), depress oestriol values because this organ is responsible for the initial major step in oestriol production. Other drugs which can affect the excretion of oestriol in the urine or interfere with its estimation by the methods in common use are mandelamine, ampicillin and related compounds, and certain laxatives.

There are a large number of *other placental function tests*, mainly depending on values in the mother's blood of substances which are elaborated by the placenta — *human placental lactogen* (HPL), pregnancy-specific beta$_1$ glycoprotein, pregnancy-associated placental protein (PAPP), alkaline phosphatase, oxytocinase. They are of less clinical value than the oestriol assay, for the reasons already stated. Another test, *alpha fetoprotein* (AFP) shows some promise, since it is elaborated only by fetal tissue (mainly in the liver). It is particularly useful in the detection of certain malformations where fetal serum proteins leak into the amniotic fluid and maternal serum (neural tube defects, abdominal wall defects, congenital nephrosis), but is also often elevated when there is fetoplacental dysfunction. These tests suffer mostly from the problem of high false positive rates (up to 50%), and the wide range of normal. The *dehydroepiandrosterone sulphate (DHEA-S) loading test* is a biochemical stress test (similar in principle to the contraction stress test). It tests the capacity of the fetal adrenal and liver to handle this substance which is the precursor of oestriol. Because these tests can be automated, they are useful in both screening and monitoring (perhaps using more than one test); however, their shortcomings should always be borne in mind when therapeutic decisions are being made.

Since both chorionic gonadotrophin (HCG) and chorionic growth hormone prolactin (HCGP) are produced by the trophoblast in quantity in the first trimester, they have been employed for monitoring purposes at this time.

Amniotic Fluid

Amnioscopy. In this technique, the cervix is located and steadied with the tip of the middle finger (palm upwards) and a long, illuminated metal tube of appropriate size is passed just through the cervix. The obturator is withdrawn and the amount and nature of the amniotic fluid which makes up the forewaters can be studied (figures 21.7 and 23.3). It is particularly suited to patients with suspected fetoplacental insufficiency in late and postterm pregnancy. It has been mentioned previously that fetal growth retardation is accompanied by a reduced amount of fluid. In addition, when the baby's oxygen supply is threatened, activity of the bowel is

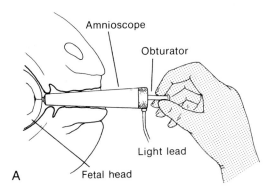

A

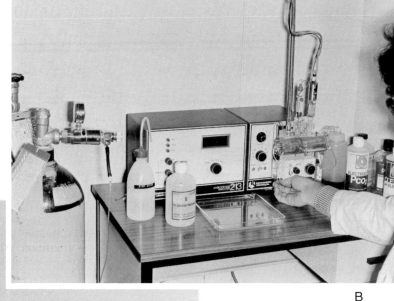

B

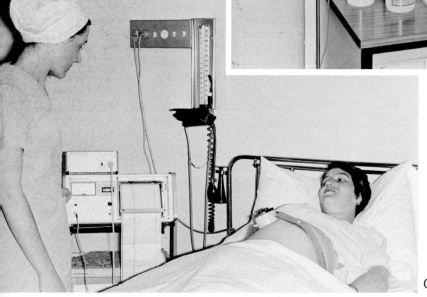

C

Figure 23.3 A. Fetal blood sampling via an amnioscope can only be done in labour since the membranes must be ruptured. The amnioscope is pressed against the scalp to keep liquor away. The scalp is incised with a guarded blade and the blood is aspirated into a polyethylene tube for pH estimation. **B.** Apparatus for measurement of fetal blood (from scalp or umbilical cord after delivery) pH and gases (oxygen and carbon dioxide). The test takes 5–10 minutes and the apparatus must be housed in or near the delivery room for ready access. **C.** Primigravida with meconium-stained liquor in the first stage of labour. The fetal scalp blood pH was normal (7.38) and the fetal cardiotocograph, obtained via a lead clipped to the fetal scalp, shows a normal heart rate pattern during and between contractions. The uterine contractions are recorded by the external pressure transducer strapped to the patient's abdomen.

TABLE 23.4 FETAL TESTS

Fetal parameter	Tests	Remarks
Structure	Ultrasonography	Standard assessment of internal/external structures
	Radiography including computer-assisted scan	Radiation hazard. Confirmatory only as a rule
	Nuclear magnetic resonance	Costly new technique; special centres only
Size/growth	Ultrasonography	Serial measurements of crown-rump length, femur length, biparietal diameter, abdominal area
Oxygenation	Cardiotocography	Nonstress and stress studies of fetal heart activity
	Ultrasonography	Realtime assessment of movement/breathing
	Fetal blood sampling	Restricted to labour; scalp or buttock sample
Maturity	Surfactant assay	Several tests of different complexity available (foam stability, lecithin/sphingomyelin ratio; other phospholipid levels and ratios)

stimulated, resulting in the passage of meconium into the fluid. A false positive result may occur because of the occasional passage of meconium as a normal event in utero; in addition, the hypoxic insult may have been transient, such as a temporary nipping or stretching of the umbilical cord, and the placental reserve will be normal.

This test scores highly on the grounds of providing an *instant result at minimal risk and cost*; there is the occasional bonus in the detection of *vasa praevia or cord presentation*. Thus, clear liquor of ample quantity indicates that the fetus is in good shape, whereas meconium-staining is a rough screening indication that all may not be well. If the distress is acute or subacute, the amount of liquor is often normal; if chronic, it is diminished or even absent. This is classically seen in prolonged pregnancies where placental failure has occurred; the familiar thick, pea-soup liquor is seen at amnioscopy or when rupture of the membranes occurs. The test has been refined by studying the fetal response to a strong light stimulus (e.g. increase in heart rate and movement).

The procedure is carried out weekly or more frequently, depending on the findings; it is not regularly used before 37 weeks because labour may occasionally be stimulated, and before this time the fetal gut is less sensitive to hypoxic stimuli.

Amniocentesis. Amniotic fluid is removed from the uterus by means of a fine bore needle and syringe (figure 21.10). This technique is mainly employed to assess *maturity of the fetus* and the degree of haemolysis (amount of bilirubin in the liquor) when the mother is *rhesus isoimmunized.* It may be used as an alternative to amnioscopy if the latter fails or is contraindicated; however, it is not popular for this purpose because of the often diminished amniotic fluid and thus danger to the fetus.

MANAGEMENT

Prevention. This implies detection at an early stage of the condition (*high index of suspicion*; *routine screening*) and institution of measures designed to minimize further damage. Adequate attention to aetiological factors (e.g. hypertension, preeclampsia, antepartum haemorrhage, renal disease, poor nutrition) is necessary. *Consultant referral* is advisable if the condition is suspected.

Treatment. *Rest in hospital* is particularly beneficial if the home environment is poor (rest difficult, nutrition suboptimal). An increase in oestriol values (a reflection of fetal well-being) occurs in many patients rested in hospital in the lateral position. Although this may partly reflect improved excretion by the mother's kidneys, evidence suggests the fetus also benefits. Attention is given to underlying medical and obstetrical problems — correction of anaemia, treatment of preeclampsia, administration of extra food to undernourished patients. Many patients are made anxious by the various tests of fetal function, and *adequate explanation and reassurance* is necessary.

Recently reported methods of improvement of fetoplacental function, apart from rest in the lateral position and attention to *maternal diet* and *drug habits*, include administration of *heparin* (to prevent intervillous thrombosis), *beta-mimetic drugs* (to relax the uterus and promote placental blood flow), and improvement of fetal nutrition by *infusion of glucose and amino acid solutions* into the mother's veins or amniotic fluid or even directly into the fetus.

When fetoplacental dysfunction is diagnosed, the important considerations are the *maternal condition* and the *maturity of the fetus.* If the patient has severe preeclampsia, uncontrollable hypertension etc she must be delivered, irrespective of the period of gestation. However, when there is no maternal contraindication, conservative treatment is instituted as outlined above, unless the fetus is mature. Fetal maturity is often difficult to establish, and when in doubt, *conservative therapy* is favoured to avoid *neonatal death* from *prematurity*. In many of these patients amniocentesis for L:S ratio estimation is not advisable because there is oligohydramnios, or fear of causing intrauterine death, especially when this has occurred without warning in previous pregnancies. The only fetal contraindication to conservative treatment, other than maturity of 37 weeks or beyond, is a *critical fetal reserve* pattern in a nonstress cardiotocograph (figure 23.1). In the presence of critical reserve, the rubicon of fetal viability meriting Caesarean section is 26–28 weeks' gestation.

The main decisions are *when and how to terminate the pregnancy*, minimizing the risk of prematurity by not terminating too early and the risk of brain damage or even death by not terminating too late. If labour is permitted, careful monitoring is necessary, and preparations should be made for intensive care of the newborn.

If *intrauterine fetal death* has occurred (figure 23.4) the approach can be conservative or active; 80–85% will deliver spontaneously within 5 weeks. Most now favour active treatment (Chapter 44) because of the emotional distress to the mother and the risk of hypofibrinogenaemia if the process extends beyond 4–5 weeks.

PROGNOSIS

The main danger to the baby is *intrauterine death*; in such cases, the diagnosis has usually been missed or not acted on promptly enough. Occasionally, the baby will die of *respiratory complications after birth*. If resuscitation is adequate, the long-term prognosis is good: although height and weight curves of such infants are a little below the 50th percentile on average, very few suffer significant mental handicap. Follow-up studies have shown that only about 2% of growth retarded infants have severe neurological handicap when assessed at the age of 7 years; this dispels previous beliefs that many infants with fetal growth retardation/fetoplacental dysfunction were doomed before birth. *Viral* or *other infection* may have caused the growth retardation and this may compromise later development.

Figure 23.4 Radiographic signs of intrauterine death. **A.** Collapse of the skull bones (Spalding sign). The fetus presents by the breech and has extended legs. **B.** Intravascular gas in the fetal heart and great vessels. A lateral radiograph is required to avoid confusion due to gas in the maternal bowel.

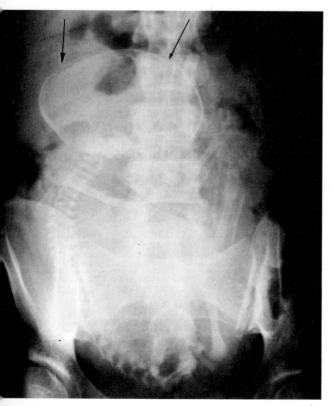
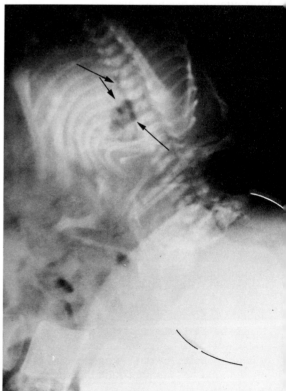

A   B

chapter twenty-four

Fetal Maturity

OVERVIEW

The following definitions are relevant: a *low birth-weight* infant is one weighing 2,500 g or less (very low birth-weight is $\leqslant 1,500$ g, extremely low birth-weight is $\leqslant 1,000$ g — see Chapter 64); a *preterm birth* is one occurring before the 37th completed week of gestation. The incidence of these complications ranges from 6–12%. A *term birth* is one occurring between 37 and 42 completed weeks of gestation; *prolonged (postterm) pregnancies* are those occurring at 42 weeks' gestation and thereafter, the incidence ranging from 6–12%, according to the rate of induction of labour (tables 16.1 and 24.1). A baby may be small at birth because of *premature birth* or *growth retardation*; the latter has many causes (table 23.1) (nutritional deprivation, malformation etc) although in the majority no predisposing cause is apparent, and the group includes infants who are small for *genetic reasons* (racial characteristic, small parents).

For centuries, the *assessment of fetal maturity* rested on such *clinical measures* as the date of the last normal menstrual period, fundal height, and the time of quickening. *Radiography* was used in an attempt to improve diagnostic accuracy, but it was not until the introduction of *ultrasonography* that the clinician had available to him an accurate means of estimation of fetal maturity when the menstrual data, clinical findings and time of quickening were contradictory. Parallel with this development has been the concept of *physiological*, as opposed to chronological maturity (or immaturity). Most attention has been directed to the fetal lungs since it is largely respiratory ability that is the arbiter of life or death in the prematurely born. It is now possible to detect the degree of *fetal lung maturity* by analysis of the fluid obtained by *amniocentesis*, particularly the ratio of *phospholipids*. This information is of major importance if premature interruption of pregnancy is being considered because of a deterioration in fetal and/or maternal condition; it is particularly important when the indication for delivery is purely in the interests of the fetus.

Spontaneous premature labour is relatively common, and is responsible for a significant amount of perinatal morbidity and mortality (80–85% of the latter, if birth defects are excluded); the causes are mainly respiratory distress and intraventricular haemorrhage. In addition, there is a very considerable financial cost in the intensive care that is required. Apart from the prematurity itself, there may be underlying obstetrical or medical problems to contend with. Unfortunately, the diagnosis of *premature labour* is not always easy, the usual definition being *the presence of uterine contractions occurring every 5–10 minutes, together with progressive cervical effacement/dilatation*.

At present, prolonged survival is exceptional before 24 weeks' gestation; between 24 and 27 weeks the survival improves from 15–20% to 55–60% with modern intensive care (figures 64.7 and 64.17).

Drugs are now available that can inhibit uterine activity; however, such *tocolytic agents* require careful thought and often fine judgement before use, since they may cause serious side-effects, and one must be reasonably certain that the fetus will be better off inside the uterus than out. Another point which is often forgotten is that only 20–25% of women whose infants are less than 2,500 g are suitable for tocolytic therapy. Failure of such therapy should prompt one to think of underlying causes — e.g. infection.

A further significant and complementary advance has been the use of *corticosteroid therapy*, which has been shown to speed up the maturation process in the fetal lungs.

Both *prevention and early diagnosis* have much to offer in terms of reducing perinatal morbidity and mortality. Prophylaxis may extend to the correction of certain problems before the pregnancy begins (e.g. uterine malformation) or reducing damage to the cervical sphincter at the time of pregnancy termination. Therapeutic time can often be gained by prompt reporting by the patient of abnormal uterine activity.

The place of Caesarean section in preventing inherent problems of the very low birth-weight baby (500–1,500 g) is still debated.

Premature rupture of the membranes is an allied problem, since labour is very prone to occur soon after. Differences of opinion regarding management exist when this complication occurs between 26 and 35 weeks' gestation: these mainly centre on whether the intensive care facilities can match those inside the uterus. The dangers to the fetus of infection and lack of protective amniotic fluid have tended to push the clinician into active management; however, these complications can be largely controlled with an intracervical multichannel balloon catheter (to prevent escape of liquor and allow instillation of antibiotics).

The reverse condition of *prolonged pregnancy* has always bedevilled the obstetric attendant. Formerly, the diagnosis was not easy to make with certainty because of the vagaries of menstrual periods, patients' memories, and their nonattendance for early antenatal care. Ultrasonography, especially in the first half of pregnancy, provides a fairly accurate estimate of the gestation period, and the problem of prolonged pregnancy can usually be approached more scientifically. It is known that there is often a decline in placental function after the 41st–42nd week, and if this is not detected and acted upon, the fetus may die, usually because of unexpected asphyxia. It should be remembered that it is not only the poorly-nourished fetus that is susceptible to this complication in women with prolongation of pregnancy. *Wholesale induction of labour at an arbitrary time limit is not recommended*; selecting the minority at risk at any one time is a more logical approach to the problem.

MATURITY ASSESSMENT

Since we can now measure fetal well-being with relative accuracy, it is important to assess the maturity of the fetus with equal accuracy, since difficult decisions will often have to be made as to when to remove the baby from an unfavourable environment. If this is done too hastily, we may defeat our object, the baby possibly succumbing to hyaline membrane disease or some other disorder associated with immaturity. On the other hand, if the baby remains too long in the uterus, placental failure may result in a critical reduction of nutrients and oxygen passing to the fetus.

Clinical

(i) *Naegele*, in 1812, formulated the rule which states that the expected date of delivery (EDD) or confinement (EDC) is given by *adding 9 months and 7 days to the first day of the last normal menstrual period.* (Most now accept that 9–10 days, rather than 7, should be added). This is quite satisfactory if the woman keeps a menstrual calendar (which is helpful) or has a good memory. Apart from this aspect, patients may have irregular periods, abnormal periods, bleeding after pregnancy starts, or unreliable menstrual data if they have conceived in the cycle after discontinuation of a contraceptive pill — because ovulation may occur more than 14 days after the period began, upsetting the assumption on which Naegele's rule is based. (ii) *Quickening*. If the patient is seen before the 18th week of pregnancy, she should be instructed to write down the date when fetal movements were first definitely felt. If 5 calendar months are added to this date, a reasonable estimate of the EDD is

obtained. (iii) *Clinical examination*. In the first trimester, *uterine palpation* is usually quite accurate (± 2 weeks) in experienced hands, provided the bladder is empty at the time of examination. *This is why it is important to perform a bimanual examination in early pregnancy.* Thereafter, a number of variables appear, such as the amount of amniotic fluid, which make it less reliable, even if such additional procedures as *measurements of symphysis pubis to fundus*, and *abdominal girth* are made.

Ultrasound

The size of the fetus and its sac can be measured accurately from early in the pregnancy, and fetal weight calculated in later pregnancy. A single ultrasound estimation of *fetal maturity* is accurate to within a few days if performed during the first trimester — using measurement of *sac volume*, crown-rump *length* and *biparietal diameter* (figure 5.2). The biparietal diameter is matched to standard tables (figure 13.2) and has greatest accuracy at 16 weeks' gestation (± 6 days) being much less reliable in the third trimester (e.g. ± 5 weeks at 36 weeks' gestation). Whenever there is a special reason to have an accurate assessment of fetal maturity (e.g. need for premature delivery (hypertension, diabetes) or elective Caesarean section), or when clinical data is confusing (menstrual data, size of uterus, time of quickening) then ultrasonography should be performed as near as possible to 16–17 weeks' gestation. When *growth retardation* is suspected, ultrasonography will need to be repeated at intervals to determine whether the fetus is small because of an error in dates (satisfactory growth rate) or because of malnutrition (slow growth rate). The biparietal diameter increases about 2.5–3.0 mm per week. In later pregnancy, fetal weight charts are now available to calculate fetal weight from ultrasound data (e.g. biparietal diameter, abdominal circumference, and femur length).

Radiography

This method is now rarely used because of the slight but definite radiation risk to maternal and fetal gonads and haemopoietic tissues, and the relatively poor precision. A general idea of fetal size can be obtained, as well as the appearance of ossification centres in certain bones (particularly at the knee, figure 24.1). As with ultrasonography, growth retardation confuses the picture because ossification is delayed.

Figure 24.1 Radiograph taken after birth of an infant weighing 2,850 g at 41 weeks' gestation, who died in labour due to placental insufficiency. Lower femoral epiphyses which appear at 36 weeks and upper tibial epiphyses which appear at 38–40 weeks are well developed and of almost equal size, indicating maturity of 40 weeks or more. Attempted resuscitation explains the partly aerated lungs.

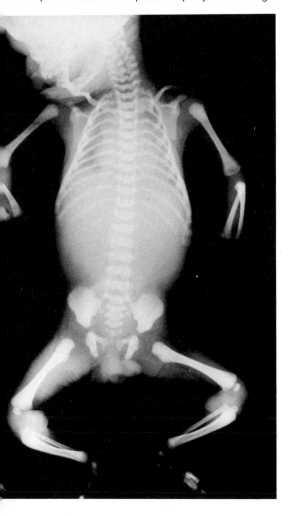

Biochemical Tests

The rapid growth of the embryo in the first 8–10 weeks of pregnancy is reflected in the steep curves of a number of biochemical indices (chorionic gonadotrophin, placental lactogen, SP_1). The serum level of these substances gives a quite accurate measure of gestational age.

In the third trimester, biochemical tests on amniotic fluid are of great value in estimating fetal physiological maturity. What is basically being measured is *fetal pulmonary surfactant* — a substance elaborated by Type 2 alveolar cells from about the 25th–26th weeks of pregnancy, although only in clinically significant amounts from the 32nd–34th week. Surfactant is composed of a number of phospholipids: *phosphatidylcholine (lecithin)* is the major constituent, with lesser contributions from phosphatidylglycerol and phosphatidylinositol. Another phospholipid, *sphingomyelin*, does not show the same progressive increase of the above compounds and it was therefore used originally by Gluck to describe the *lecithin:sphingomyelin ratio*. If this is 2 or above, the level of surfactant is considered adequate to prevent respiratory distress and hyaline membrane disease in the premature baby; a level of 1.5–1.9 is considered intermediate, and *below 1.5 the baby has a 75% risk of pulmonary problems*. It has been observed clinically that pulmonary maturity is often accelerated in the presence of hypertension, severe (vascular involvement) diabetes, narcotic use, fetal growth retardation, chronic retroplacental bleeding, hyperthyroidism; the reverse is seen in early maternal diabetes and rhesus isoimmunization.

Recently, a number of other tests have been described, all measuring surfactant activity. The *shake or foam stability test* can be done at the bedside and involves the generation of stable foam by surfactant in the presence of ethanol at a 1 in 2 dilution; there should be a complete ring of bubbles in the tube 15 minutes after a 15-minute shake. The *absorbance of light at 650 nM* is another indirect measure of surfactant: an optical density of 0.15 corresponds approximately to an L/S ratio of 2. A direct measurement of *phosphatidylglycerol* is now used in many centres: this substance is only present in surfactant and is unaffected by the presence of blood or meconium in the liquor.

The liquor is usually centrifuged at 3,000 g for 10 minutes; if there is likely to be a delay in processing it can be frozen at −20°C.

The attractiveness of the shake and optical density tests is tempered by many false negatives.

Fetal Electrocardiography

A recent test of interest is the *duration of the QRS complex* of the fetal electrocardiogram.

Retrospective Analysis

Although of no assistance in the problem of when to induce labour if there has been a doubt as to maturity, *careful paediatric examination* will assist in determining whether the baby is immature or dysmature, or a combination of both. Particular attention is paid to behaviour; reflexes; colour, opacity, and texture of the skin; development of hair, nipple and breast. If perinatal death occurs, postmortem examination, particularly of the extent of development of the renal glomeruli, provides further information.

ABNORMAL ONSET OF LABOUR

FACTORS REGULATING THE ONSET OF LABOUR

The simplest concept of the onset of labour is, by analogy with other hollow viscera, the attainment of a *critical filling pressure which overcomes the normal retentive mechanisms.*

Inhibitory Factors

(i) *Progesterone.* This hormone is secreted initially by the corpus luteum of the ovary and then in large amounts by the placenta; it serves to dampen the excitability and contractility of the smooth muscle of the uterus and to strengthen the sphincter at the internal os. (ii) *Cervix.* The action of the sphincter is aided by the strong connective tissue of the cervix. (iii) *Hypervolaemia.* The increased blood volume is thought to inhibit the hormones of the posterior lobe of the pituitary gland (oxytocin and vasopressin). (iv) *Adrenaline and sympathetic nerve fibres* act on the uterus in the same way as progesterone.

Stimulatory Factors

(i) *Oestrogen* is produced by the fetoplacental unit and causes a progressive build-up in the contractile protein (actomyosin) and hence the sensitivity of the uterine muscle. The flow of electrical current passes more easily from one smooth muscle cell to the next. (ii) *Cervix.* Probably as a result of hormonal action (oestrogen, relaxin, prostaglandin), the connective tissue of the cervix softens (ripens), and is less resistant to rises in uterine pressure. (iii) *Prostaglandin* is synthesized in the decidua and membranes in progressively increasing amounts during the last trimester of pregnancy. This may be released prematurely by mechanical, hypoxic, inflammatory and other stresses. (iv) *Oxytocin.* This hormone is released from the pituitary gland of both mother and fetus at the approach of labour. (v) *Cortisol*, an adrenal hormone, is also released in larger amounts by the fetus, and is thought to influence prostaglandin secretion. (vi) *Uterine distension* may act partly on the cervix and partly on the excitability of the uterine muscle fibres (stretch reflex). (vii) The *presenting part* normally stimulates the lower uterine segment as it enters the pelvis approaching term. (viii) *Complications* such as preeclampsia, placental abruption, and pyelonephritis often cause premature uterine activity (see aetiology).

PREMATURE LABOUR

This may be defined as labour ensuing before the 37th completed week of pregnancy. It is characterized by a progressive increase in uterine activity resulting in progressive cervical dilatation.

Incidence

As shown in table 24.1, approximately 10% of deliveries in a public hospital occur before the 37th week.

Aetiology

(i) *Idiopathic.* No obvious cause can be found; this is the largest group; in parous women there is often a history of a previous delivery of a small baby — i.e. *there is a strong tendency for premature labour to occur in subsequent pregnancies.* (ii) *Artificial induction.* The usual indications are subacute or chronic conditions in which the fetus is at increased risk of intrauterine death (preeclampsia, hypertension and other medical disorders, placental insufficiency, rhesus isoimmunization). (iii) *Spontaneous premature rupture of the membranes.* (iv) *Antepartum haemorrhage.* Abruptio placentae, if moderate or marked, usually stimulates premature uterine activity; placenta praevia may do so, but less commonly. Repeated small haemorrhages in the second trimester (e.g. from a circumvallate placenta) may cause weakening of the membranes by the action of enzyme release or secondary infection. (v) *Overdistension of the uterus* by multiple pregnancy or polyhydramnios. (vi) *Infection.* Many bacterial toxins have a stimulatory effect on the uterus. It is likely that in a significant proportion of the idiopathic (unexplained) group there is a low-grade infection, which in turn reduces lysosomal stability

TABLE 24.1   THE INCIDENCE OF PREMATURITY AND PROLONGED PREGNANCY*

Gestation at delivery (weeks)	Deliveries Number	%		Average birth-weight (g)
20–22	4	0.1		—
23–25	6	0.2		—
26–27	6	0.2		—
28–29	11	0.3		—
30–31	14	0.4		—
32	16	0.5	8.8	2,048
33	25	0.8		2,313
34	26	0.9		2,548
35	62	2.2		2,799
36	90	3.2		2,855
37	144	5.1		3,020
38	304	10.8		3,168
39	585	20.9	78.3	3,336
40	693	24.7		3,430
41	471	16.8		3,531
42	254	9.0	12.0	3,590
43 +	85	3.0		3,512
Total	2,796			3,317

* A prospective series studied from the first trimester. In this now historical series, treatment was conservative — in the group of 339 patients with prolonged pregnancy the incidence of induction of labour was 12.3%, the Caesarean section rate was 7.6%, and the perinatal mortality rate was 1.4% (Beischer NA et al Am J Obstet Gynecol 1969; 103:476–495)

and/or produces prostaglandins — e.g. the presence of *group B streptococci* in the urine is associated with an increased incidence of spontaneous premature labour and premature rupture of the membranes. (vii) *Malformations of the uterus* — unicornuate, bicornuate. (viii) *Cervical abnormality*. Trauma from previous deliveries or surgery to the cervix may weaken its sphincteric action (incompetent cervix). Abnormal biochemical responses may occur (e.g. in relation to prostaglandins, relaxin etc). (ix) *Fetal malformation*. Major malformations may be associated with premature labour. (x) *Elective induction or Caesarean section*. This may result in a premature baby if there has been a miscalculation of the gestational period. (xi) *Miscellaneous*. Socioeconomic factors, work or other stress, negative attitude to the pregnancy, poor antenatal attendance, low prepregnancy weight (< 50 kg), maladaptive cardiac responses to the pregnancy load, trauma (version, amniocentesis, vehicle accidents), coitus, burns to the body, are other observed factors.

Assessment

Clinical. The first problem to be addressed is whether the patient is in true labour. A *history* is taken of possible precipitating factors such as urinary tract infection, trauma, coitus, antepartum haemorrhage, preeclampsia.

Examination is directed to careful assessment of the nature of the uterine contractions — frequency, duration and strength — and their behaviour after the patient has been put to rest in bed. The consistency, effacement and dilatation of the cervix, the state of the membranes and the nature and station of the presenting part are checked. *It should be noted that the cervix is 2 cm dilated in 20–25% of patients at 30–34 weeks' gestation.* A tocographic record is often useful.

Special investigations may be necessary to evaluate suspected underlying factors (e.g. *urinary tract infection*). *Ultrasonography* will help in the assessment of fetal maturity, normality and well-being. It has been observed that *fetal breathing movements* show a marked reduction or cessation in the 24–48 hours preceding normal labour: this observation has been used to categorize patients with premature labour into 2 groups — those with normal fetal breathing movements in whom labour is unlikely to progress and those with reduced or absent fetal breathing movements needing tocolytic therapy.

Management

Prophylaxis. Mechanical factors (uterine malformation, *incompetent cervix*) can be managed surgically. The patient should be made aware of general risk factors (*smoking, alcohol, poor diet*) and the need for reporting promptly if there is any unusual uterine activity. Proper antenatal care will offset many of the causes listed above. Identification of risk factors (*bacteriuria,* cervical incompetence, *multiple pregnancy,* premature rupture of membranes) allows hospitalization for rest and specific therapy if indicated. If there is a *previous history* to suggest the possibility of premature labour, the patient should be instructed to report the first painful contractions which increase in frequency and intensity; immediate hospitalization is advised; regular uterine tocography has proved disappointing in predicting labour before 34 weeks. However, a 'risk assessment' (e.g. low, moderate, high) should be made late in the second trimester; if the patient falls into the high risk category, there is a 60–70% chance the baby will be immature or premature, and consultant referral or hospital transfer should be organized. Routine sterile vaginal examination may also be undertaken at intervals to assess the degree of dilatation of the internal os, and so forewarn of impending labour; this may, however, produce premature labour in some patients because of prostaglandin release or the introduction of infection.

Therapy. The decision to try and prevent the onset or progress of labour must be made individually and is usually based on the period of gestation (the dividing line is between 33–35 weeks) and any underlying complications which may be present. If labour is in progress, the patient is admitted to hospital, rested in *lateral recumbency*, and base-line observations are recorded of blood pressure, pulse rate, fetal heart, and uterine activity, the latter preferably with an external recording machine over a period of 30 minutes. A careful vaginal examination is carried out to determine *the state of the cervix and its dilatation.*

If *contractions are mild*, a sedative such as diazepam, 10 mg IM, is given, since this drug has a smooth muscle relaxing effect in addition.

If *contractions are stronger* (more frequent than 1 every 10 minutes and lasting longer than 30 seconds) and there is no indication for delivery, an intravenous infusion is commenced and a pharmacological inhibitor of uterine action is added. The success of such therapy is usually inversely related to the Bishop score.

A decision must be made at consultant level whether *transfer* to a hospital with intensive care facilities is warranted.

Beta-Adrenergic Stimulants

These drugs stimulate the beta-adrenergic receptor cells of the autonomic nervous system, and thus have a uterine relaxing effect. Before their use, 2 important questions should be answered: (i) is the *diagnosis* of premature labour correct? (ii) are there *contraindications* to the use of the drug itself (see later in chapter) or to the continuation of the pregnancy.

Ritodrine (Yutopar, Prempar), 80 mg is diluted in 500 ml of 5% dextrose in water (160 μg/ml). The initial infusion rate is 50 μg/minute, and this is increased by 50 μg/minute each 20 minutes until a satisfactory inhibition of contractions is achieved, or a level of 350 μg/minute (2 ml/minute) is reached, or a *maternal pulse rate of 130/minute* is reached. Since there is a tendency to build up the drug too quickly, some flexibility should be used in dose increment — e.g. if contractions are occurring every 10 minutes or less, the infusion can be maintained at that rate for another 20 minutes. The patient's vital signs (pulse, blood pressure, fetal heart rate) are monitored every 5 minutes initially and any unusual symptoms recorded (anxiety, dyspnoea, cardiac distress, headache, nausea). There is usually an increase in systolic pressure

and a fall in diastolic pressure. The infusion is discontinued if troublesome maternal complications arise or labour is progressive. The average infusion period is 6–12 hours (range 2–36 hours). Very close monitoring is necessary if the infusion runs beyond 24 hours. After contractions have ceased, it is continued for 1–2 hours at the same rate, then the dose is progressively tapered off over the next 10 hours. This is followed by *oral therapy*, 4–8 mg every 4–6 hours before meals, the dose usually corresponding to the amount of drug required intravenously and given to allow a period of overlap; this is continued for 4 weeks or until 37 weeks' gestation, whichever is the sooner. The patient should monitor her pulse rate, and attend at least twice weekly for assessment. Intercourse is ceased, and maximum rest obtained. If *cardiovascular side-effects* are marked, propanolol, 1 mg IV is effective. Occasionally, patients will complain of angina at high dose levels.

Salbutamol (Albuterol, Ventolin, Proventyl), 5 mg is diluted in 500 ml of 5% dextrose (10 μg/ml). The initial infusion rate is 2.5 μg (15 microdrops)/minute; this is doubled every 10–20 minutes until contractions have ceased. The infusion is maintained as described above and oral therapy 4 mg, qid, substituted when appropriate.

Contraindications to beta-adrenergic stimulants include *active bleeding* from the uterus, *fetal distress*, maternal *cardiac disease* and any contraindications to continuance of the pregnancy. Closer monitoring will be required in the patient with diabetes mellitus, since this condition may be destabilized; patients with a history of migraine headaches may experience cerebral ischaemia due to vascular effects.

Efficacy. Premature labour will be inhibited for at least 48 hours in some 65% of patients.

Observations. Careful recording of uterine contractions, maternal blood pressure and pulse, and fetal heart must be made. Side-effects are recorded.

Failure is usually conceded if the cervical dilatation is 4 cm or more, the membranes have ruptured, fetal distress unrelated to hypotension is present (or fetal death), an organic cause is revealed (abruptio placentae), or rapid resumption of activity occurs after cessation of the infusion.

Calcium Inhibitor

Verapamil, a recently-introduced drug, is given at a rate of 80–120 μg/minute. This compound blocks beta$_2$ binding sites on the smooth muscle cell. It also reduces the tachycardia and hypotension which are common side-effects of the beta-blockers.

Magnesium Sulphate

A loading dose of 4 g is given intravenously over 30 minutes and this is followed by 2 g hourly then 1 g hourly when contractions are less than 1 per 10 minutes.

Antiprostaglandins

Compounds such as *indomethacin* have been used to suppress labour, but they suffer from the major problem of *premature closure of the fetal ductus arteriosus* and in animal experiments reductions in cerebral and uteroplacental blood flow have been demonstrated. They may be tried if the situation is desperate, the other preparations have failed and use is intermittent.

Corticosteroids

Dexamethasone or *betamethasone* in a dose 6-12 mg IM bd is given for 48 hours if the period of gestation is between 26 and 34 weeks, the level of surfactant is unknown or low, there are no contraindications (infection, unstable diabetes mellitus), and labour is responding to tocolytic therapy.

Progressive labour. Apart from the usual management of labour and delivery, additional special precautions are necessary. (i) Analgesia is preferably conduction in type (epidural); if a narcotic drug such as pethidine is given there is a possibility of respiratory depression of the premature newborn infant. (ii) Preparations must be made in advance for the care of a premature baby (paediatrician in attendance, humidicrib, resuscitation facilities) (see Chapter 62). (iii) *Pelvic examination* is performed when the membranes rupture, to exclude *cord prolapse*. (iv) A close watch is kept on the patient, since delivery may be rapid and unexpected. (v) An *episiotomy* is performed when the vulval ring is just beginning to distend. A preliminary 'ironing-out' of the vulval ring helps to prevent distortion of delicate intracranial structures. (vi) Gentle forceps extraction is sometimes helpful; the vacuum extractor is contraindicated. If the baby is thought to be less than 1,500 g, especially in the nullipara, *Caesarean section* may be a treatment option to avoid damage to the delicate intracranial structures during passage down the birth canal, especially if the breech presents. This procedure is no panacea, however, since the lower uterine segment may be imperfectly formed at this time and extraction of the baby is not always as easy as might be imagined.

Because of this an upper segment (classical) incision may be required. Such patients will be managed at specialist level.

The care of the small baby is discussed in Chapter 64.

PREMATURE RUPTURE OF THE MEMBRANES

This topic is best considered in this section, since premature labour is a very common sequel.

Definition

Spontaneous rupture of the membranes before the onset of labour.

Incidence

Approximately 5-10% of labours are preceded by rupture of the membranes; in a further 25% rupture occurs before the start of the second stage. It is only in the 2-4% that occur before the 34th week that major anxiety arises because of fetal immaturity.

Aetiology

(i) *Factors causing a rise of intrauterine pressure*: multiple pregnancy, polyhydramnios, coitus, trauma. (ii) *Factors in the cervix*: incompetence (idiopathic, previous forceful or rapid dilatation, surgery). (iii) *Faulty application of the presenting part*: malpresentations of the fetus (footling, transverse and oblique lie), placenta praevia, disproportion, polyhydramnios. (iv) *Abnormal membranes*: weakening due to infection, nearby blood clot (enzyme action), acceleration of the normal loss of collagen over the last 10 weeks of pregnancy. (v) *General factors*: lower socioeconomic status (? nutrition, infection).

Diagnosis

This mainly depends on the *history of a sudden gush of fluid*, which continues to soak pads or underclothes, especially when the patient is ambulatory. *Examination by speculum* may reveal fluid escaping from the cervix (if necessary, ask the patient to cough) or the presence of a pool in the vagina with the characteristic odour of amniotic fluid. *Special study* by microscopy of the collected fluid (by sterile test tube in the vagina if necessary) may reveal ferning, fetal squames, lanugo hair, and perhaps vernix. Other investigations include the *nitrazine test* which depends on a yellow → blue colour change because of the alkaline reaction of the liquor (this may be vitiated by recent intercourse). The presence of *alphafetoprotein* can now be assessed by a rapid assay and this is a reliable test, especially if the gestation period is less than 35 weeks.

Differential diagnosis. Urine leakage is seldom continuous and has a different odour and characteristics to those outlined above. *Cervical mucus* may be profuse in patients with incompetent cervix; it is albumin-like, and has no particulate matter; the cervix will be open. *Hydrorrhoea* is usually associated with circumvallate placenta and the fluid is similar to that seen with *isolated rupture of the chorion*. No particulate matter of fetal origin is seen. Visualization of an intact membrane by the naked eye or amnioscopy is helpful but does not exclude leakage from a rupture that has 'sealed'.

Significance

The *major risks* are those of *infection* (10–30%), *premature labour* and *prematurity* (10–30%), *abnormal presentation* (10–30%), and *prolapse of the cord* (0.5–1%). *Infection* of the uterus and its contents is an everpresent menace, particularly once labour commences. Friability of soft tissues (uterine muscle) is increased, with the added dangers of rupture and haemorrhage at the time of delivery; the risk of infectious complications is also increased if Caesarean section is required some time later.

If the membranes have been ruptured for many weeks, the fetus may suffer from pressure effects (face, limbs); *pulmonary hypoplasia*; and if of considerably longer duration, short umbilical cord.

Management

(1) *Prophylaxis is related to aetiological factors.*
(ii) Therapy. Immediate admission to hospital is arranged. A careful *history* and *examination* is carried out, particular attention being paid to possible underlying factors. Fetal heart tones are checked, as well as maternal vital signs. A sterile speculum examination is usually performed (rather than a digital examination), and a sample of fluid taken for examination (microbiology, surfactant level, ferning). Other investigations which may be helpful include *ultrasound* (fetal maturity, well-being and normality, amount of liquor) and studies of fetal well-being (oestriol, cardiotocography).

A decision is made concerning induction of labour. The critical milestone of maturity lies between 33 and 36 weeks, and this represents a 'grey area' where opinion is divided as to the best approach; other factors will often swing the decision towards conservatism or radicality. Studies on the amniotic fluid will help in *assessment of the pulmonary maturity* of the fetus. If conservative treatment is decided on, bed rest with toilet privileges only is ordered. Observations are directed particularly to fetal well-being (heart monitoring, oestriol excretion); amniotic fluid leakage (soaking of pads etc); amnionitis (sterile swabs for leucocyte excretion and culture, 4-hourly temperature recording). *Chemotherapy* with a broad spectrum antibiotic is administered if subclinical or clinical infection is present. Some advocate prophylactic courses until the fetus is mature enough for labour to be induced; during labour, chemotherapy is necessary. *Corticosteroids* are indicated, with antibiotic cover, if the gestation is less than 33 weeks.

The leakage of amniotic fluid and complicating infection can both be controlled by an *intracervical multichannel balloon catheter*. Periodic sampling of the liquor can be made (to estimate maturity) and antibiotics can be infused to combat infection.

If active treatment is decided upon, an *oxytocin infusion* is commenced, provided there are no contraindications such as placenta praevia. If the pregnancy is earlier than 37 weeks, a higher incidence of breech presentation will be encountered.

Tocolytic drugs are usually only considered in *desperate situations* (e.g. late second trimester in an infertile patient, infection being controlled by adequate chemotherapy).

With either treatment, the hazard of *cord prolapse* should be kept in mind, particularly if the presenting part has not entered the pelvis.

Problems related to the labour and method of delivery are managed as for the premature baby.

Since the *baby is likely to require intensive care*, this facility should be available and ready; if not, the patient should be transferred to where it is.

PROLONGED PREGNANCY

Definition

Prolongation of the pregnancy to *42 weeks or beyond*. Postmaturity is widely used as a synonym of prolonged pregnancy, but the term is confusing as it implies the presence of placental insufficiency and the need for induction of labour.

Incidence

Approximately 6–12% of deliveries occur at 42 weeks or thereafter, and 3% at 43 weeks or thereafter (tables 16.1 and 24.1). Gestational age is uncertain in 20–50% of patients in reported series due to *uncertain menstrual data* (poor memory, lactational amenorrhoea, irregular cycles, last period related to contraceptive pill). The incidence of prolonged pregnancy is much lower in those centres where it is common practice to perform elective induction of labour when the patient has reached her expected date of confinement(table 16.1) — many obstetricians induce labour for no other reason if the patient reaches 41 weeks' gestation, especially if the head is deep in the pelvis and the cervix is favourable (soft and well effaced).

Classification

There are probably 3 subgroups (i) those whose dates are incorrect, or abnormal menstruation has occurred; (ii) those whose dates are correct, but physiological maturity is 42–43 weeks rather than 40 weeks, or fertilization has not occurred at the normal time (late ovulation); and (iii) a group (about 20–30%) whose dates are correct, the physiological maturity is 40 weeks, but labour fails to occur. In this group are included the majority of cases of placental insufficiency where the fetus is hypoxic and at risk of intra-uterine death.

Pathological Changes

The clinical features in groups (ii) and (iii) depend on *placental function* after the 40th week. If it is adequate, the fetus will continue to grow, and features suggesting simple hyper-maturity will be present — larger size, well calcified skeleton (hard skull bones and narrow sutures and fontanelles), long nails (growing over the ends of the digits), well developed ear cartilage, nipples, and genitalia etc. If it is not adequate, the characteristic changes of *growth retardation* will occur. The amniotic fluid is diminished (sometimes markedly so) and often meconium-stained, there is absence of subcutaneous fat, and the skin is dry and peeling. The typical baby with the latter condition is usually of longer than normal length (> 50 cm), but is decidedly underweight, sometimes less than 2,500 g (colour plate 20). In babies who have died, there is further evidence in the shrinkage of internal organs — e.g. the liver and heart due

Figure 24.2 Radiograph showing extreme placental calcification. The patient had prolonged pregnancy (43 weeks), oligohydramnios, and low oestriol levels. The infant was born in good condition, weighed 3,200 g and was placentally insufficient. The placenta weighed only 450 g. Placental infarction and calcification can occur before or after 40 weeks and the infant may or may not (as in this case) be small for dates.

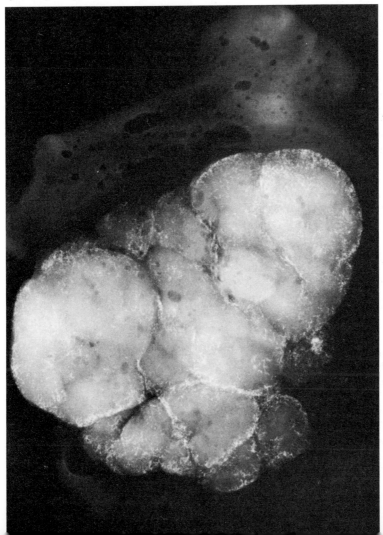

to loss of glycogen reserves. Because of the passage of meconium into the liquor, the baby is often heavily coated and stained. The umbilical cord shows loss of protective Wharton jelly — it is thus more at the mercy of entanglement and tightening, which shuts the blood vessels down much more readily. The placenta is often smaller, calcified, and is also stained (figure 24.2).

Biochemical studies of the newborn reveal that the blood sugar level is often low as are blood clotting factors.

Significance

It is apparent that such babies are at considerably greater risk — the main problems being *dystocia* (larger and less mouldable skull, incoordinate labour) and *asphyxia* (poor placental function, low glycogen stores in the baby, meconium aspiration syndrome, limp cord syndrome). The need for operative delivery is increased.

Aetiology

The most likely causes of the patient failing to come into labour are persistence of such inhibitory factors as progesterone block by the placenta, and failure of softening of the cervix and/or *lack of stimulatory factors* such as oxytocin and prostaglandin. Patients who take high doses of *aspirin* or like compounds, which are known to inhibit the synthesis of prostaglandins, have both longer pregnancies and labour. Another possibility is lack of stimulus of the cervix and lower segment by the presenting part (malpresentations, *occipitoposterior position*, short umbilical cord). The rare condition of extrauterine pregnancy should be considered if the pregnancy is grossly prolonged or resists induction.

Management

There are many approaches to this problem. Some favour inducing labour in all patients at 41 weeks; others at 42 weeks, or 43 weeks. Others only induce if evidence of fetal distress is apparent, clinically or on special investigation, or if there is an additional complication, albeit mild.

Often the state of the cervix is assessed to determine treatment — amniotomy if effaced and favourable, conservative therapy if uneffaced and unfavourable. Routine *amnioscopy* and testing of fetal function (*cardiotocography*, oestriol assay) from the end of the 41st week is probably the safest course of management. Measures to ripen the cervix before induction are recommended, since the baby's condition at birth is related to the Bishop score (itself a predictor of the work required of the uterus during labour).

Caesarean section may be performed electively if it is considered that there is insufficient reserve even for the stress of labour (meconium plus abnormal fetal function tests).

When there is meconium in the liquor, but fetal function tests are normal, the place of elective Caesarean section is less certain. A *trial of labour* may be allowed, preferably with monitoring by cardiotocography and scalp blood sampling to exclude fetal acidosis. Such patients should be under specialist care. *Routine induction of labour for prolonged pregnancy is not advocated.*

The dysmature infant often requires special care by the neonatologist because of hypoxia and meconium aspiration, and adequate preparation should be made for intensive care, at least initially.

chapter twenty-five

Multiple Pregnancy

OVERVIEW

The rate of twinning and higher orders of multiple births has remained relatively constant: although there has been some reduction due to fewer older women having babies, this has been offset by the multiple births that complicate *ovarian stimulation* or *in vitro fertilization-embryo transfer* therapy in the treatment of infertility.

Twins are basically of 2 types — monovular (identical), resulting from complete separation of the early embryo, and binovular (nonidentical) resulting from fertilization of 2 separate ova.

The general incidence of twins in *Caucasian* races is approximately *1 in 85 births*, but the rate is higher (1 in 50) if early postconceptional losses (spontaneous abortions) are included, as well as the loss (absorption) of one of the twins in the first trimester (as shown by serial ultrasound). Interestingly the incidence shows racial variation — *Asian*, 1 in 150; *Negro*, 1 in 50 viable pregnancies.

On clinical grounds it is often possible to make the *diagnosis* in the second or even first trimester if the menstrual dates are accurate and the patient presents early; the single most important clue is a *fundal height higher than expected* from the period of amenorrhoea. With the progressive introduction of routine realtime *ultrasonography* to antenatal care, the diagnosis should seldom be missed.

Knowledge that a multiple pregnancy is present should permit measures to be taken to combat the major antenatal complications — *premature labour* and *preeclampsia*. Such patients require closer supervision, more rest, and optimum nutrition. Referral for specialist opinion and/or care is necessary because of the likelihood of complications later in pregnancy and during labour. Likewise the infants are more likely to be born prematurely and require intensive neonatal care. *Multiple pregnancy has a perinatal mortality rate 3–8 times that of singleton pregnancy — twins, 80 per 1,000 births; triplets, 300 per 1,000 births — and accounts for about 10% of all perinatal deaths* (tables 16.1 and 53.1).

There is a recent trend towards more liberal use of Caesarean section when one or both twins is presenting abnormally, and also for higher orders of multiple pregnancy.

In multiple pregnancy, more than 1 fetus is present. In general, the greater the number of fetuses the higher will be their morbidity and mortality. Numbers beyond 4 rarely all survive, and beyond 5 it is exceptional for any to survive (colour plate 86). Because of the rarity of triplets and above, the main discussion will be limited to twin pregnancies.

Incidence

Hellin's law (1895) is usually quoted: this states that the frequency of twins is 1/89 births, triplets $1/(89)^2$, quadruplets $1/(89)^3$, and so on. This is roughly correct — the incidence of twin pregnancies in Caucasian races ranges from 1 in 80–1 in 90; for Negro races the incidence is higher (1 in 50), for Asiatic races it is lower (1 in 150 or less). The difference is accounted for in the number of dizygotic (twin egg) rather than monozygotic (single egg) twins. These statistics are based on clinical findings in viable pregnancies. With the increasing use of ultrasound in early pregnancy, it is now considered that in some patients one of the twins dies and is absorbed, leaving the 'stronger' to develop alone. However, when the fetuses are identifiable with beating hearts (7 weeks' gestation) it is *most unusual for one to disappear* (figure 25.1). The ultrasonic appearance of a second sac can be simulated by lack of fusion of membranes or a haemorrhage around a single sac.

One factor that has unbalanced the above figures in recent years is the use of drugs which stimulate ovulation, such as *clomiphene and*

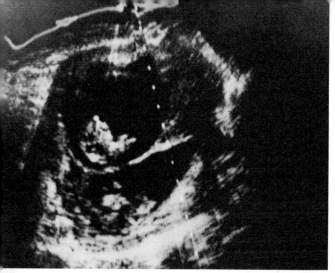

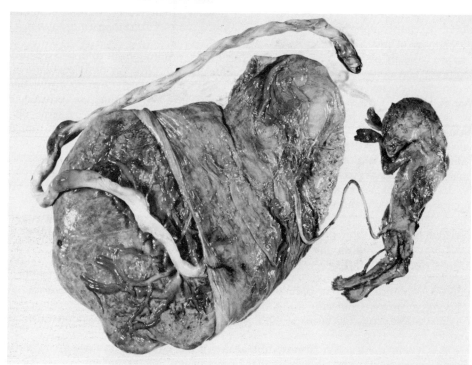

Figure 25.1 A 'disappearing' fetus. **A.** Ultrasound scan at 11 weeks' gestation showing twin gestational sacs. Both fetal hearts were identified. The crown-rump lengths were 4.3 cm and 5.3 cm. Subsequent ultrasound scans showed only a single fetus. **B.** The patient had a normal delivery at 40 weeks' gestation of a healthy male infant, birth-weight 3,350 g. The placenta (600 g) and missing twin (50 g fetus papyraceous, crown-rump length 9.0 cm) are shown.

pituitary gonadotrophins. If these are not carefully controlled, multiple pregnancies, often higher orders than twins, are produced (figures 25.2–25.4).

Types
Basically, 1 or more eggs may be fertilized as indicated above.

Monovular. If *1 ovum* only is fertilized and it separates early in development into 2 or more similar embryos — hence the term monozygous, or identical twins, triplets etc (figure 25.5). The babies are of the same sex, general appearance, eye and other colouring; finger and other prints and electroencephalographic patterns are very similar, if not identical (colour plate 107). Inherited disorders usually appear in each child

although not necessarily at the same time. The morphology of the placenta and membranes depends on when cleavage occurred to form the separate embryos — early division results in 2 separate placentas; later division results in conjoined twins (colour plates 45 and 50). With cleavage before the fifth day (33%) there will be separate amnions and chorions (and placentas); between the fifth and tenth days (64%) there will be separate amnions but a common chorion (and placenta — figure 25.6); after the tenth day (4%) both amnions and chorions will be common (as will be the placenta). An anastomosis of the 2 circulations may be seen on the fetal surface of the placenta and also on histological study of the villous structure. A rare complication (1 in 50,000) is *conjoined twins*; the degree of union can vary from as little as a skin bridge to com-

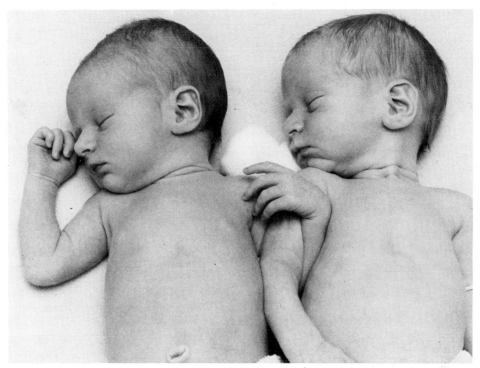

Figure 25.2 These arm-in-arm dizygotic twins were born to a 25-year-old woman who was treated with human pituitary gonadotrophins (FSH). The patient had a history of 4 years' absence of periods following oral contraceptive therapy. (Courtesy of Dr John Biggs).

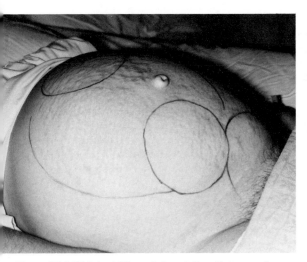

Figure 25.3 Triplets at 36 weeks' gestation. Note eversion of the mother's umbilicus.

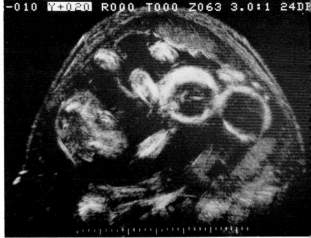

Figure 25.4 Triplets at 26 weeks' gestation. This transverse scan shows 2 heads to the right and part of the trunk of a third fetus to the left. Careful scanning is required to outline the details of each fetus. Spontaneous labour occurred at 34 weeks' gestation. All 3 infants survived. Birth-weights were 1,800 g. 1,990 g and 2,170 g.

plete fusion (usually at the thorax) with sharing of a common heart and adjacent viscera (figure 25.7).

Binovular. When *2 ova* are fertilized, the term dizygous, nonidentical, or fraternal is applied. The babies may be of the same sex; if they are not, they are certainly dizygous twins. Their similarities are limited only to those expected if they were ordinary brothers or sisters. *The pla-*

centas are usually individually identifiable, although they may fuse and give the appearance of only 1 structure. There will be 4 layers separating the fetuses and amniotic cavities — 2 amniotic layers separated by *2 chorionic layers* (figure 25.6). The overall proportion of dizygous

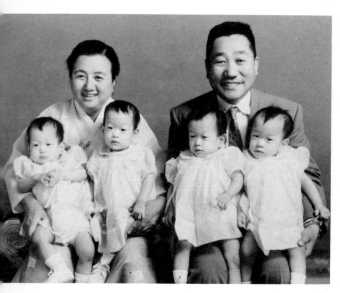

Figure 25.5 Monovular (identical) Korean quadruplets with their foster parents. Their mother died from eclampsia. (Courtesy of Dr Helen MacKenzie).

twin becomes shrunken and compressed, finally forming a *fetus papyraceous* (see colour plates 7, 36, 45–48 and 50 for illustrations of this and other complications of twin pregnancy).

Although the weights of each twin are smaller than the corresponding singleton, their combined weights are greater. The main weight deficit occurs over the last 8–10 weeks of pregnancy. It is not 'normal' for twins to be smaller than singleton infants of similar maturity. At 40 weeks' gestation, twins weigh about 400–500 g less than singletons; this is due to *fetal growth retardation* which occurs in *20–25% of twins* i.e. *more than double the incidence for singletons*. This explains why the incidence of stillbirths is 50% higher in twins than singletons. *Intrauterine growth is similar in twins and singletons until 30–32 weeks when a diminished rate of growth occurs in both uniovular and binovular twins* (figure 25.8) — the diminution is more marked in uniovular twins, especially after 37 weeks' gestation.

In ultrasound studies it is usually observed that the biparietal diameter (BPD) of twin 1 is greater than that of twin 2, and the BPDs of dizygotic twins are greater than those of monozygous twins; there are, as expected, much greater intrapair differences in the former.

to monozygous twins is approximately 60: 40. This is given by Weinberg's rule which states that the number of dizygotic twins should be twice the number of those of different sex, which is usually about 30%.

Normal and Abnormal Variations

It is unusual for twins to be the same weight at birth, especially the dizygous type, and differences of several kilogrammes may occur. Monozygous twins are usually smaller for the period of gestation and show less size variation. Occasionally, because the placental circulations may anastomose in the latter type, one twin may develop disproportionately (especially the heart) and the circulation of the weaker twin is taken over and the heart may not develop (acardiac monster). With either type, death of one twin may occur: if this is of long standing, the dead

Aetiology

Dizygous twins are distinctly more common if there is a *family history*, the patient is *over 35*, and possibly of high parity, although this factor is usually related to older age. The use of drugs to stimulate ovulation (clomiphene, pituitary

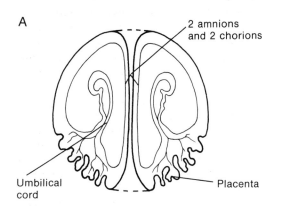

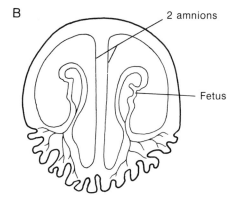

Figure 25.6 A. Binovular twins; each fetus has its own placenta, chorion and amnion — 4 layers separate them. **B.** Monovular twins usually share 1 placenta and chorion, and have individual amniotic sacs — 2 layers separate them.

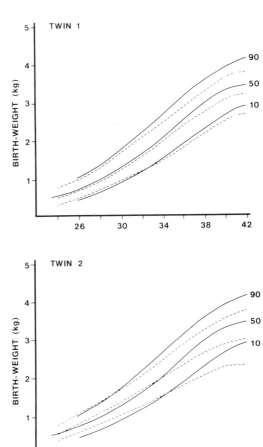

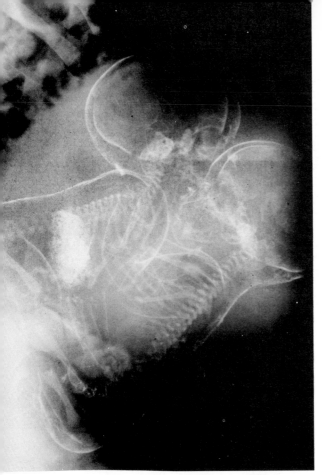

Figure 25.7 Conjoined twins diagnosed when polyhydramnios was investigated at 28 weeks' gestation. This lateral radiograph was taken after instillation of radio-opaque water-soluble and fat-soluble dyes into the amniotic sac (amniography). The vernix is outlined by the fat-soluble dye and shows the twins hugging each other in final embrace. Swallowed dye outlines the fetal gut. Ultrasonography showed extensive common tissue. They were delivered vaginally with difficulty and were stillborn. The birth-weights were 1,200 g and 1,330 g. (Courtesy of Dr Graeme Ratten).

Figure 25.8 The 10th, 50th and 90th percentile curves for birth-weight of twins (dotted lines) compared with those for singletons (solid lines). Note that intrauterine growth (birth-weight) is the same as for singleton pregnancies up to 32 weeks' gestation, but after this the fetal growth slows markedly — less so for twin 1 (A) than for twin 2 (B). (Courtesy of Dr John Fliegner).

gonadotrophins) is prone to produce multiple ova, although this is reduced when the dose is accurately controlled by daily oestrogen measurements and ultrasound monitoring of growth of ovarian follicles.

Monozygous twin incidence is unrelated to the above factors: possibly, noxious influences at the time of early cleavage may be a factor.

Clinical Features

As the result of a greater than normal amount of growing tissue inside the uterus it is to be expected that some of the *features of pregnancy will be exaggerated.* The following are more common: (i) hyperemesis, (ii) pressure symptoms: abdominal discomfort, gastrointestinal disturbances, respiratory discomfort, oedema, varices, striae (colour plates 66, 70, and 75); *separation of the symphysis pubis* can cause severe localized pain and limit mobility — like *divarication of the rectus abdominis muscles* this complication occurs more often when there are more than 2 fetuses (colour plate 75), (iii) anaemia, iron and folic acid deficiency (fetal demands), (iv) *preeclampsia/eclampsia*, (v) antepartum haemorrhage (both placenta praevia (large placenta), and placental abruption (preeclampsia), (vi) *premature labour and premature rupture of membranes* (overdistension of uterus, malpresentation), (vii) prolapsed cord (premature rupture of membranes, malpresentation), (viii) malpresentation (polyhydramnios, displacement by other fetus), (ix) obstructed labour (malpresentation), (x) manipulative delivery (malpresentation) (xi) retained placenta and postpartum haemorrhage, (xii) malformations of the infant, (xiii) feeding difficulties and other problems related to prematurity of the baby.

Diagnosis

The diagnosis of multiple pregnancy is made antenatally in 60–90% of patients, depending on the astuteness and experience of the examiner. The average time of diagnosis is 33 weeks (much earlier if the pregnancy follows ovulation induction and/or *ultrasound* is used routinely (figure 25.9)).

The first clue is given by the *history* of a similar occurrence in the patient's family or in a previous pregnancy or preconceptional use of ovulation stimulating drugs (clomiphene, gonadotrophins). The factors of higher age and parity should be borne in mind. The patient may complain of excessive vomiting. The most consistent finding on examination is a *uterus larger than expected for the period of amenorrhoea* (usually at least 4 cm more than expected after the 22nd week). This should always be regarded as indicating multiple pregnancy until proved otherwise, especially if other causes such as errors of menstrual data, hydatidiform mole, or pelvic tumour seem unlikely.

The presence of any of the complications listed above should alert the attendant to the possibility. Another consistent feature is *excess weight gain* which, although not greatly above normal,

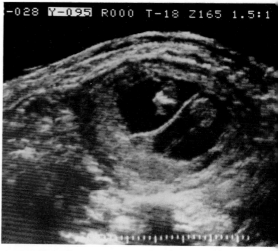

Figure 25.9 Transverse scan at 10.5 weeks' gestation showing twin sacs with an intervening membrane and placenta forming posteriorly.

is consistent each visit. The abdominal girth should be checked, since this is usually several centimetres in excess of normal. As with breech presentation, the attendant should make a positive attempt to exclude multiple pregnancy by means of careful palpation, aided by ultrasonography where necessary, early in the third trimester. In some centres, an ultrasound study is performed routinely early in the second trimester for this purpose. The mother may note

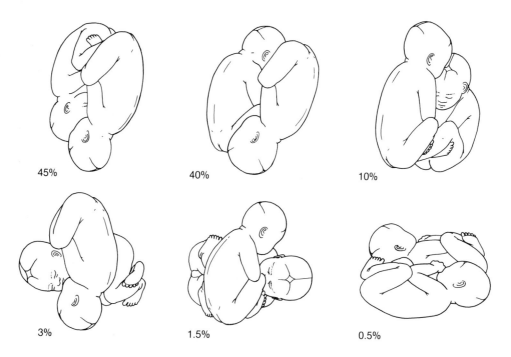

45%   40%   10%

3%   1.5%   0.5%

Figure 25.10 Varieties of presentation in twin pregnancy: vertex:vertex and vertex:breech (or breech:vertex) account for 85% of cases.

excessive fetal movements and backache may be troublesome due to a greater than normal lordosis.

The following are the characteristic features on *abdominal and pelvic examination*. The abdomen is large and globular, rather than ovoid. The division of the 2 fetuses may be felt as a sulcus or groove either at the top of the uterus or on its anterior surface. The *sine qua non* of multiple pregnancy is the presence of *more than 2 fetal poles*. The appearance of what appear to be 2 heads is less reliable since the breech may occasionally simulate the head. The degree of separation and independent mobility of the poles is highly suggestive. A multiplicity of small parts is also characteristic, although if the fetal back is directly *posterior* in a singleton pregnancy the same impression can be given. Often the *relatively small size of the presenting part on abdominal or pelvic examination can be a reliable diagnostic indicator*.

On *auscultation* by independent attendants, 2 fetal hearts will be heard: these should be independent of the maternal pulse, different from each other by more than 8 beats per minute, and reasonably separated from each other. This is only of value if both fetuses are alive. The levels of most substances used to assess fetoplacental well-being are elevated in multiple pregnancy. This may be used as a screening test: e.g. human placental lactogen (HPL) in multiple pregnancy is normally above 5 mg/dl at 30 weeks (mean 7.3 ± 2.6), but below this in singleton pregnancy (3.9 ± 2). In any case, if there is reasonable doubt or twins appear to be present with some degree of certainty, *ultrasonic* (or radiographic) study will be needed. The diagnosis may occasionally not be made until after the first twin is delivered. The abdomen will be much larger than expected unless the twin is dead, and the uterus will be cystic rather than doughy; on pelvic examination, the bag of membranes will usually be still present with the presenting part behind it. It should be a practice to palpate the abdomen before an oxytocic drug is administered in the third stage of labour.

The diagnosis of *higher orders* of multiple pregnancy is usually made early because of the large size of the abdomen. The actual number of fetuses present often requires special investigation.

The *differential diagnosis* of a uterus larger than expected early in pregnancy has been mentioned; *hydatidiform mole* is important since it mimics multiple pregnancy quite closely. Later, diagnostic difficulties may arise because of *true enlargement* of the uterus, usually due to *polyhydramnios*, rarely to large fetus, monster, fibromyomas; or to *obscuring factors* such as tense uterus, obesity, and placental abruption.

Disposition of Fetuses

The lie and presentation of fetuses in twin pregnancy are shown in figure 25.10. In 90–95% of cases, there is either Vx/Vx, Vx/Br, Br/Vx, or Br/Br. Transverse lies are uncommon (Vx/Tr, Br/Tr, Tr/Tr). That is, the fetuses are longitudinal and usually parallel to each other on either side of the maternal spine (figure 25.11). The fetus on the left hand side usually presents and is delivered first.

Management During Pregnancy

Consideration of the complications outlined above will indicate the careful attention that must be paid to the management of the patient with multiple pregnancy. Some of the problems mentioned (such as *anaemia*) can virtually be eliminated; in others (preeclampsia, antepartum haemorrhage, malpresentation, prematurity) the untoward results can be minimized by proper supervision. If the patient is not in hospital, antenatal visits should be weekly after 30–32 weeks. *Prematurity* is the greatest cause of mortality in multiple pregnancy, particularly when the pregnancy terminates before the 33rd week (15–20%, table 53.1, figure 25.12). On average, twins are born 3 weeks earlier than singleton babies. There is a progressive decrease in period of gestation at delivery and in infant size as the number of fetuses increases — for example, the mean weight of quadruplets is about 1,400 g and they are likely to be born 40–45 days early on average. *Efforts to minimize premature delivery must be instituted.* If the patient is working outside the home, consideration should be given to stopping before the 24th week of gestation. Extra help and rest at home are also important. Apart from *early diagnosis*, the patient should ideally be admitted to hospital somewhere between the 26th and 28th weeks for *bed rest*, and should remain there until 34–36 weeks. The likelihood of premature rupture of membranes and premature labour can often be gauged from the tenseness of the uterus. In some patients, the uterus appears to accommodate the fetuses easily, even if polyhydramnios is present as well, whereas in others, it will be tense and irritable. *Uterine relaxing agents* (ritodrine, salbutamol) may be used prophylactically. If premature labour does occur, preventive measure may still be undertaken. *Premature rupture of the membranes* indicates careful vaginal examination to exclude *cord prolapse*.

Because fetal growth retardation occurs in 20–25% of twins (especially monozygous), *tests of fetal well-being* are carried out routinely from the 34th week. Greater difficulty is experienced in the interpretation of many of the fetal function tests, especially those relying on fetoplacental products (oestriol, placental lactogen); trends, rather than absolute values are more useful. *Ultrasound study* is particularly useful since it enables separate studies of each twin — e.g. serial crown-rump length x trunk area, and divergence of the curve of the biparietal diameter from that of the normal singleton pregnancy. *Cardiotocography* can also assess each twin separately and assist in the timing and route of delivery if signs of severe fetal compromise are present (loss of beat to beat variation, late decelerations). Growth retardation in one twin may be caused by blood loss to the other twin through connecting placental blood vessels (*twin transfusion syndrome*).

Pressure symptoms are due not only to the twins but often to the accompanying polyhydramnios. This can only be managed symptomatically, although manifestations in the legs (oedema, varicosities) will be lessened by adherence to rest periods during the day. Frequent, smaller meals will help. Occasionally, the distress is so acute, particularly to breathing, that slow drainage of fluid from the amniotic sac must be undertaken. This is usually only required in cases of *acute polyhydramnios*, a complication of uniovular twin pregnancy that is responsible for about 15% of the perinatal deaths (from prematurity) associated with twin pregnancy (figure 25.12 and colour plates 12 and 71). This *amniocentesis* is done in a similar manner to paracentesis with a needle and fine polythene catheter.

Preeclampsia is 3–4 times more common in multiple pregnancy. The incidence was 35% in a series of 571 multiple pregnancies (including 11 triplets) in a teaching hospital (table 53.1). Although a greater weight gain is to be expected, excessive gains will have the same significance as in the patient with a singleton pregnancy. If the diastolic blood pressure rises above 90, admission to hospital is arranged. This will lessen the risk of *abruptio placentae* also.

Figure 25.11 The presence and presentations of these twins were confirmed by radiographic examination. These pictures show the 2 most common presentations of twins. **A.** vertex:vertex; **B.** vertex:breech.

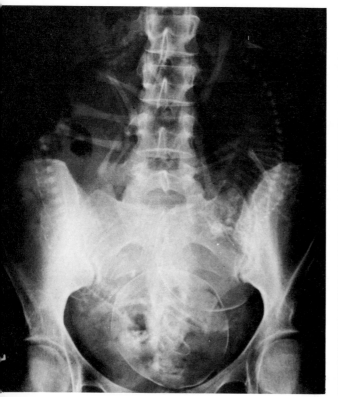

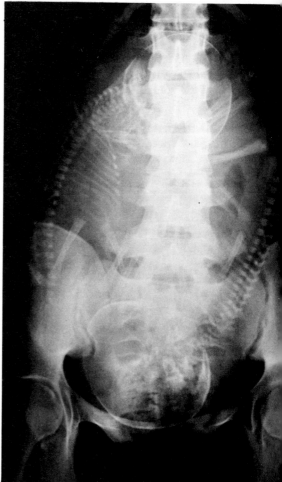

A

Bleeding from *placenta praevia* cannot be prevented, but if suspicious features exist, early investigation and perhaps hospitalization is indicated.

Anaemia is very common because of the *demands of the fetuses* for iron and folic acid; prophylactic administration of these compounds is necessary, and haemoglobin levels are checked regularly, especially in the last trimester, when the major growth of the fetuses is occurring. Because of the demand of the fetuses, women with multiple pregnancies have lower fasting values of such indices as blood sugar. Hence, a regular balanced diet with an adequate protein intake should be encouraged.

Malpresentations, particularly *breech presentation*, are common (figure 25.10). Unlike in singleton pregnancies, manipulative procedures such as external version are possible only after the first twin has been delivered. Fortunately, transverse lie (shoulder presentation) of the first twin is very rare (0.5%) and this will usually be treated by Caesarean section. Since both babies are on average 0.5 kg smaller than normal, problems of disproportion seldom arise. Occasionally, however, twins may be as large as or larger than a normal-sized singleton fetus, and if the first twin presents by the breech, and the patient is a nullipara or if the pelvis is suspect on

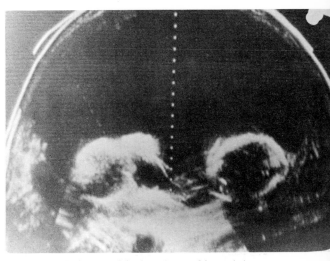

Figure 25.12 Acute polyhydramnios at 26 weeks' gestation shown in a static scan. Only 1 amniotic sac contained excessive liquor — when the patient turned from side to side only 1 twin showed free mobility. This was confirmed at delivery 10 days later after the patient came into spontaneous labour. The twins were uniovular stillborn females; birth-weights were 550 g and 730 g.

the grounds of past history or clinical examination, then pelvimetry is indicated, unless labour occurs before the 37th week.

The further aspects of multiple pregnancy (management of delivery and prognosis) are considered in Chapter 53.

chapter twenty-six

Errors of Fetal Polarity

OVERVIEW

The term polarity denotes the disposition or lie of the fetus in terms of its long axis in relationship to that of the uterus (or mother). The normal lie is longitudinal with the head down.

At term, approximately 1 in 30 fetuses will present by the breech; when labour is premature, the incidence is greater (1 in 5 at 30 weeks). Prospective *ultrasound studies* have shown that breech presentation is very common towards the end of the second trimester, but because of the relatively larger growth of the buttocks compared with the head, progressively more fetuses adopt the cephalic presentation during the third trimester. Conditions which restrict fetal turning (e.g. *extended legs, multiple pregnancy*), alter the fetal-uterine relationship (*placenta praevia, fetal or uterine malformations*) or cause *prematurity* will increase the likelihood of breech presentation in labour; occasionally *loops of cord* around the fetal neck prevent the normal cephalic presentation.

The diagnosis of *breech presentation* at 30–34 weeks is important, since *external version to a cephalic presentation* can usually be effected easily at that time. *A positive decision should be made at this time in every patient to exclude breech presentation.* This will often obviate the need for Caesarean section, which has been advocated in some centres as the appropriate treatment of all breech presentations. If obesity or firm abdominal muscles renders palpation difficult, a vaginal examination through one of the fornices will disclose the absence of the characteristic firm, rounded fetal head. If uncertainty persists, referral for consultant opinion and/or *ultrasonography* is indicated.

External cephalic version is considered to have a well-defined role by some practitioners: if carried out with care between 30 and 34 weeks it will be successful in 90% or more of patients and will often avoid a Caesarean section; others believe that it carries an unnecessary risk to the fetus.

If version does fail or is not undertaken, *expert opinion* is required to assess the risk factors involved in allowing a vaginal delivery. Such factors as the size of the mother's pelvis (*X-ray pelvimetry*), size, attitude and normality of the baby (*ultrasonography*), age, parity, period of gestation, and fetal well-being are but some of the factors which will need consideration; in some patients, the decision may wait on reassessment at the onset of labour. *We do not advocate the trial of labour finesse in breech presentation.* The delivery of the breech baby is a specialist undertaking in view of the great potential for mishap (cord compression and prolapse, difficulty with the delivery of the arms or head, i.e. the dual hazards of hypoxia and birth trauma).

Transverse and oblique lie are far less common (1 in 100) than breech presentation, but are often of much greater potential danger because of the possibility of underlying abnormalities (*placenta praevia, uterine malformation*), the greater danger of *cord prolapse* when the membranes rupture, and the virtually inevitable obstruction to labour should the latter occur. Referral for specialist care is essential in view of the probable need for Caesarean section. In some patients, the unstable lie is a transient phenomenon, and stabilization occurs as the liquor:fetal volume ratio decreases.

BREECH PRESENTATION

Definition

A breech presentation is where the caudal pole of the baby (the breech) presents in the inlet of the pelvis.

Incidence

The usual *incidence at delivery is 2–4%*, but the figure depends on the *diagnostic ability* of the antenatal attendant and policy concerning *external cephalic version* to change the presentation to cephalic; the higher figure applies to hospital practice (table 16.3) with a high incidence of complications (prematurity, multiple pregnancy, premature rupture of the membranes). Earlier in pregnancy (24–32 weeks) the breech presents much more commonly (20–30%), but spontaneous version occurs in the majority of patients.

Aetiology

Maternal. Uterine factors, such as fibroids or malformation (*bicornuate or unicornuate uterus*) may occasionally be responsible by preventing spontaneous version (figures 26.1 and 26.2); uterine malformation should be thought of if the breech recurs in successive pregnancies. Nulliparity is also a factor due to increased tone of the uterus and abdominal muscles.

Fetal. In the great majority of cases, *extended legs* are responsible; the conversion of the baby into a cylindrical rather than an ovoid form and the associated lack of movement both hinder spontaneous version. *Multiple pregnancy, prematurity,* and cornual implantation are other causes. *Fetal malformations* such as anencephaly

Figure 26.1 Note cystic teratoma containing molar teeth (arrow), which probably was the cause of this breech presentation. Both legs are extended and the breech is not engaged. Caesarean section and ovarian cystectomy were performed. Note 'moulding' due to pressure by the uterine fundus simulating Spalding's sign of intrauterine death (arrows).

and hydrocephaly are rare, but presentation by the breech occurs in about 15% and 25% of cases, respectively. Skeletal and/or muscle deformities (figure 26.3), Potter syndrome and autosomal trisomic states are occasionally present. Rarely, *cord around the fetal neck* may prevent the normal cephalic presentation. In some 20–25% of cases, no obvious cause can be found. In one large series of breech presentations (table 16.3) 308 of 1,645 cases (18.7%) were due to *multiple pregnancy.*

Varieties (figure 26.4)

(i) *Frank breech* (breech with extended legs) is the commonest variety (50–60%); the legs are extended alongside the body and the feet lie beside the head. (ii) *Complete* (flexed breech) is next in frequency; the legs are normally flexed as in the vertex position. (iii) *Knee or footling*; here one or both limbs present over the os.

Apart from the above presentations, the attitude may be one of *hyperextension* ('flying fetus') in some 5% of cases (figure 26.5). Full flexion is present in only 40% of fetuses, the remainder being in the neutral or 'military' attitude.

The *position* of the baby is given by the relation of the denominator, the sacrum, to the maternal pelvis (in the same way that the occiput is the denominator for cephalic presentations). Thus, 6 positions can be described LSA, LSL, LSP, RSA, RSL and RSP, as well as the 0° and 180° positions of SA and SP (sacrum directly anterior and directly posterior).

Figure 26.2 Transverse ultrasound scan at 24 weeks' gestation in a patient with oblique lie due to a bicornuate uterus. The placenta is anteriorly situated in the right uterine horn. A cross-section of fetal trunk is shown with one arm extending into the left horn below the septum. Liquor volume is normal. This patient had an antepartum haemorrhage and assisted breech delivery at 30 weeks' gestation in her first pregnancy, and twin breech deliveries at 32 weeks in her second pregnancy. In this pregnancy, Caesarean section was performed at 36 weeks, when she came into labour with an oblique lie and high breech presentation.

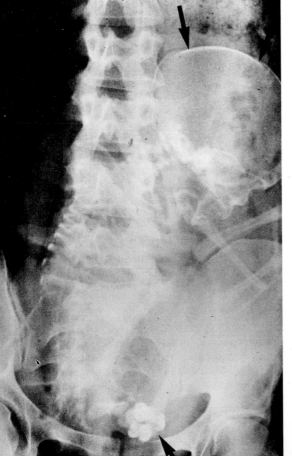

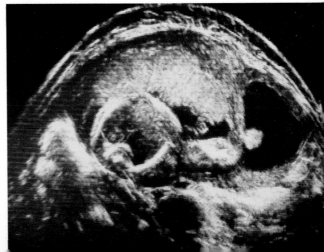

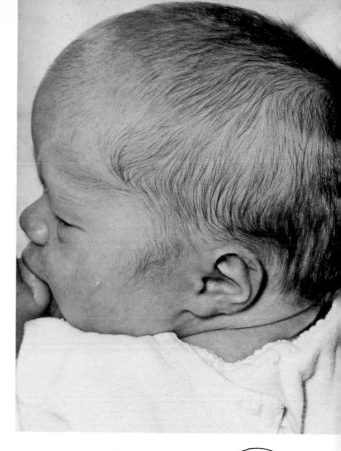

Figure 26.3 Infant aged 4 days, born at 40 weeks' gestation by elective Caesarean section because of incoordinate uterine action, in a primigravida with a breech presentation with extended legs. Birth-weight was 3,640 g. Transverse fetal lie had been corrected at 34 and 35 weeks' gestation. Note the benign postural deformity of the head ('breech head') due to force applied to the cranium by the uterine fundus. There is scaphocephaly with an increased AP diameter and protuberant occiput. This aberrant head shape is seen much less commonly in infants delivered cephalically. This condition can cause difficulty during breech delivery, but it resolves spontaneously within 1 year of birth. This infant had congenital dislocation of the right hip which is common when there is a breech with extended legs.

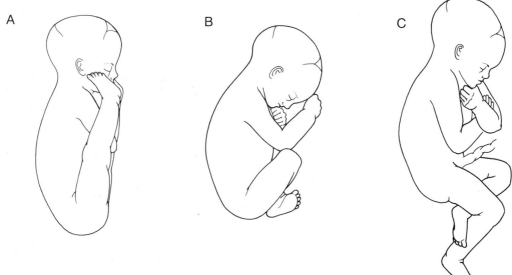

Figure 26.4 Varieties of breech presentation: **A.** Breech with extended legs. **B.** Complete (flexed) breech. **C.** Footling.

Prognosis

Perinatal mortality is approximately 5 times that of the cephalic presentation. This is largely due to increased rates of *prematurity* and *premature rupture of the membranes* (20–25%) (and the conditions leading to this, such as antepartum haemorrhage), and *congenital malformation* (5–10%). However, hypoxia (largely due to *cord* *accidents* (prolapse, pressure by the presenting part) and difficulty with delivery of the aftercoming head) and *birth trauma* (inadequate time for proper moulding; deflexion of the head) are additional problems. Follow-up statistics indicate that the breech baby has a greater likelihood of neurological disorder — e.g. they are more highly represented in a population of 'idiopathic' epileptics. It should be remembered, however,

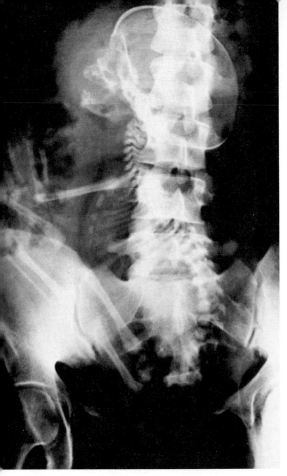

Figure 26.5 Breech with extended legs and hyperextension of the neck. Extension of the head is usually due to muscle tone, not cystic hygroma or thyroid tumour. The condition is likely to persist and cause difficulty with delivery of the head (big diameters as in brow presentation); therefore, Caesarean section is usually indicated.

that there is evidence to suggest that neurological abnormality in the fetus may cause the breech presentation rather than be the result of it (figure 26.3).

With Caesarean section rates ranging from 30–100%, the mother carries the risks of this procedure — either from the anaesthetic, or from haemorrhage, infection and thromboembolism.

Management During Pregnancy

Diagnosis

Perhaps the most important factor in breech presentation is *timely diagnosis*. The following features aid in recognition. The history may be of value — previous babies may have presented by the breech, whilst in the present pregnancy the mother may complain of tenderness under one or other costal margin as a result of pressure by the harder fetal head (figure 26.1). *On examination* the uterus will be more cylindrical than oval if a frank breech is present, although at the

time when diagnosis is most important, 32–34 weeks, the relative excess of liquor makes this sign less reliable. The most important features on antenatal examination are as follows: the rounded, hard, regular fetal head is not over the pelvis, but instead there is a softer, yielding, irregular mass which is the breech; the head in the fundus is often associated with *tenderness on palpation* and shows characteristic *ballottability*; and finally, the fetal heart is detected higher in the abdomen (usually above the umbilicus). *Failure to elicit ballottability* in spite of careful palpation may be due to extended legs, oligohydramnios, bicornuate uterus, obesity, tenderness, an anterior placenta, or the head may have slipped under the costal margin.

If the diagnosis of breech presentation is in doubt, a *pelvic examination* should be performed and the presenting part palpated through the fornices (figure 26.6). If there is still doubt, *ultrasonography or radiography* should be carried out to confirm the diagnosis and provide additional information concerning the maturity and normality of the baby, its position and attitude, and site of the placenta. It should be emphasized that if the question is asked at 32–34 weeks — 'Can I confidently exclude a breech presentation in this patient?' — the diagnosis will seldom be missed.

Further Management

If a breech presentation is found at 32–34 weeks, what is the correct treatment? There are a number of possibilities.

Figure 26.6 Sacrum, anus, genitalia and feet can be identified by vaginal palpation of a complete breech — especially in labour with the cervix dilated and the membranes ruptured. The sacrum can be mistaken for the occiput unless all fornices are palpated. An X-ray or ultrasonograph is often required.

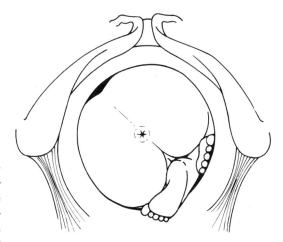

(i) *Caesarean section before maturity.* As indicated under aetiology, breech presentation is often an incidental finding between the 26th and 36th weeks of pregnancy, the primary problem being premature labour, antepartum haemorrhage, preeclampsia etc. Delivery may be called for and a decision must be made largely in the interests of the fetus. One of the major problems in vaginal breech delivery in this situation is that the small breech does not fully dilate the cervix, and the aftercoming head requires undue traction to effect delivery. Even if full cervical dilatation occurs, there is still the possibility of damage to delicate intracranial structures during passage down the birth canal as well as the greater risk of cord prolapse. Advances in neonatal intensive care have pushed survival without neurological deficit toward the 26–28 week mark, and accordingly Caesarean section has been liberalized for this group of immature fetuses.

If the emergency condition is controlled and the need for premature delivery avoided, the options discussed below will be considered.

(ii) *Caesarean section at maturity.* This will usually be the treatment if there has been a previous section or there is some other general or obstetrical indication in addition to the breech presentation. Some practitioners consider that Caesarean section should be carried out for all patients in whom the breech is still presenting in late pregnancy. The dilemma with this policy is that between 25–50 sections will be needed to save 1 infant from a nonoptimal condition at birth; i.e. morbidity is being transferred from the fetus to the mother. The possibility of a major fetal malformation should be kept in mind with this approach.

(iii) *External version.* It is obvious from the above that version is not universally accepted. It has a small risk to the fetus because of *placental separation, premature rupture of the membranes, premature labour, entanglement of the cord, fetomaternal red cell transfer* and *fetal trauma.* Such complications are, however, usually only reported if undue force has been used. The procedure is *contraindicated* if *Caesarean section is to be carried out* (the breech is easier than the head to deliver via a uterine incision), if there has been *antepartum bleeding,* or in the presence of a *multiple pregnancy, fetal death,* or *major malformation* which can be managed better as a breech (anencephaly, hydrocephaly). Considerable care should be taken if significant hypertension, preeclampsia, rhesus isoimmunization, or uterine scarring is present. As in many other obstetrical procedures, skill and experience are important. Some claim that those babies which are turned by external version would have turned anyway: this is not true for nulliparas having a breech with extended legs. Certainly the baby moves frequently and reversion after version does occur: however, it has been shown that *the incidence of breech delivery is significantly reduced when external version is practised antenatally.*

Because of the inherent risks of breech delivery and the *significantly higher incidence of Caesarean section in breech management* if morbidity and mortality are to be kept to acceptable limits, it is considered that *external version does have a place.* It is best carried out from 32 to 34 weeks. If the procedure fails, it should be repeated within the next week by a more experienced person. If failure again occurs, *X-ray pelvimetry* is carried out. If a mild–moderate pelvic contraction is present, some would then attempt version under anaesthesia which must be adequate for abdominal wall and uterine relaxation. This policy is intended to obviate the need for Caesarean section in this and in all future pregnancies, since with such contraction a trial of labour with a cephalic presentation would be reasonable (in an unscarred uterus), but not with a breech presentation. Generally, however, *elective Caesarean section is preferred to version under anaesthesia.*

Version is more difficult in nulliparas, when the legs are extended, the abdomen or uterus irritable, the uterus malformed, the liquor relatively small in amount, or the patient obese. Problems during the course of the version (fetal heart changes which persist, pain or bleeding) will indicate that the procedure should be stopped. In experienced hands, the *success rate is 90–99% in the multipara*; the problem is that the technique is becoming a lost art in many centres.

Technique of external cephalic version. Preliminary ultrasonography (or radiography) is carried out to show the normality and disposition of the fetus. *Ultrasonography* will also localize the placenta excluding placenta praevia as cause of the breech presentation. There is also a place for *cardiotocography* after attempted external cephalic version — occasionally this will reveal critical reserve requiring immediate Caesarean section. A sedative and/or analgesic may be helpful if the patient needs relaxing; some recommend a *ritodrine* or similar infusion to relax the uterus. The patient's bladder should be empty and she should be lying comfortably in the supine or dorsal position. The attendant's hands should be warm and a sprinkling of talcum powder on the abdomen is helpful in avoiding pinching of the patient's skin during the manoeuvre.

Initially, the breech is displaced upward and to one iliac fossa (assisted by pelvic examination if necessary). Then, with a simultaneous force directed to each pole, the fetus is made to perform a *forward somersault* (or backward if this fails), and a proper longitudinal alignment is secured. During the procedure the fetal head and extremities should be flexed and contact with both poles maintained until the transverse axis has been passed (figure 26.7).

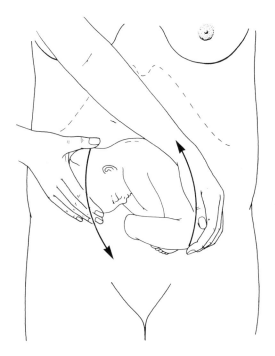

Figure 26.7 External cephalic version; at this stage of the manoeuvre wait for the uterus to relax (palpation induces contractions), then direct the head into the pelvis.

(iv) *Elective breech delivery.* In this situation, *X-ray pelvimetry* and *ultrasonography* will have been carried out and are normal, there are no particular indications for Caesarean section, and the experience and facilities for breech delivery are present. The main problem with this approach is the question of what are normal values for a breech presentation, where the head has to mould in minutes rather than hours (as in the cephalic presentation), and frequently some deflexion, rather than maximal flexion, is present? We consider that there is *no place for trial of labour with breech presentation.* Some allow labour to proceed if only a mild degree of contraction is present (not more than 1 cm reduction in diameters). In early labour the patient must

be assessed carefully. *The following factors are favourable*: period of gestation 36–41 weeks, fetus estimated not larger than 3,800 g, frank (extended) breech well in the pelvis, head not extended, cervix favourable, previous labour normal, membranes intact. A previous uncomplicated breech delivery is another favourable prognostic feature. The temperament of the patient, although difficult to quantify, is important; if clinical pelvic assessment proves difficult for attendant and patient, it does not augur well for an uncomplicated labour and delivery.

The further aspects of breech presentation (care during labour, mechanism and delivery, and prognosis) are considered in Chapter 50.

TRANSVERSE/OBLIQUE LIE: SHOULDER PRESENTATION

Transverse and oblique lie are errors in polarity of the fetus and may be *transient* or *fixed*. If labour begins when the lie is transverse, or oblique with the head in the iliac fossa, the shoulder is the part that presents — that is, the part first felt on vaginal examination. There is *no mechanism for delivery* in such cases and the lie must either be corrected (external, bipolar or internal version) or a Caesarean section performed.

Incidence

This depends upon whether transient abnormalities of lie are considered. The general figure is between 1 in 250 (multiparas) and 1 in 1,000 (nulliparas). The greater frequency in the former is explained by the greater *laxity of the uterus and abdominal muscles*. As with breech presentation, transverse and oblique lies are more common earlier in pregnancy (e.g. 25% at 16 weeks) when there is relatively more liquor and transition from breech to vertex is occurring. By 24 weeks in the nullipara and 32 weeks in the multipara the lie is longitudinal in all but 1% of patients. The incidence in a hospital series of 343 cases was 1 in 120 (0.8%, table 16.3).

Aetiology

Maternal. Any maternal condition that predisposes to *premature labour* (preeclampsia, antepartum haemorrhage) may be cited, since a transient transverse lie may be involved, also *uterine malformations* (especially bicornuate and subseptate uterus), failure of formation of the lower uterine segment, *multiparity and pendulous uterus*, tumours of the uterus or adnexa, and gross lumbar scoliosis.

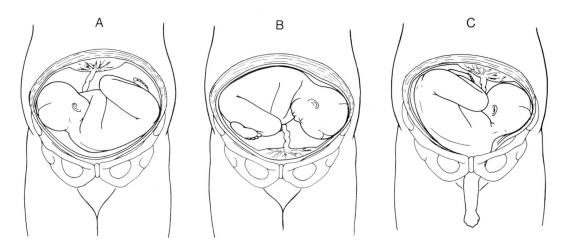

Figure 26.8 Transverse lie. **A.** Fundal placenta with fetus facing upwards. **B.** The central (type 4) placenta praevia would prevent either fetal pole entering the pelvis. **C.** Neglected transverse lie with prolapsed arm in labour. Uterine rupture would be imminent.

Fetal. *Multiple pregnancy* (more usually the second twin), extended ('flying fetus'), malformations, *polyhydramnios*, and fundal or praevial attachment of the placenta (figure 26.8).

Placenta praevia was the cause of 39 of the 343 cases (11.3%) of transverse or unstable lie in the series mentioned above. When the lie is still transverse at the onset of labour the incidence of *placenta praevia* is *20–25%*, a fact that is well worth remembering!

Varieties of Lie

Transverse lie. The main variations relate to whether the fetal head is on the right or left side of the abdomen, and whether the fetus is facing upwards or downwards. The first of these factors is a chance phenomenon, whereas the latter is related more to underlying factors, especially uterine malformations, fundal placenta (fetus facing upward), and placenta praevia (fetus facing downward) (figure 26.8).

Oblique lie. These are differentiated according to whether the head or the breech is the lower pole, and which side this pole is lying (figure 26.9). The shoulder, the torso, the elbow, and the hand may overlie the os, and thus present in labour.

Management During Pregnancy

Diagnosis. Unless obscuring features are present (such as multiple pregnancy, obesity or placental abruption), transverse and oblique lies are relatively easy to diagnose. The general contour of the abdomen often gives the first clue to transverse lie, because of *lateral expansion*. Furthermore, there is no fetal pole palpable in the fundus or lower uterus. The rounded, hard,

ballottable fetal head will then be palpated in one or other flank, with the softer breech on the opposite side. The back will usually be felt running across the abdomen — whether it is below or above the umbilicus will usually depend on the direction that the fetus is facing. The position of the back will also determine where the fetal heart is heard with greatest ease.

Vaginal examination is not employed to confirm the findings because of the possibility of placenta praevia and the possibility of rupturing the membranes accidentally. Confirmation will be by radiography and/or ultrasonography (figure 26.10).

Management. If a transverse or oblique lie is discovered on routine examination in the antenatal period between 32–35 weeks, an attempt at *external version* is made to bring the fetal head over the brim of the pelvis. If this is unsuccessful or reversion occurs, the next procedure is to review the situation in the light of the history, examination, and the special investigations in an effort to arrive at the most likely aetiological factor. *Ultrasonography* should be performed to assess the *position of the placenta* and the normality of the fetus and uterus. If placenta praevia is present, the patient is admitted to the antenatal ward and treated primarily for this condition. If placenta praevia is excluded, but the abnormal lie persists, again the safest course is for the patient to be *admitted to hospital until either the lie is corrected, definite treatment is undertaken, or labour ensues.* When transverse lie persists until 40 weeks, it is safest to perform a Caesarean section, to avoid the risk of *prolapse of the umbilical cord* should the membranes rupture.

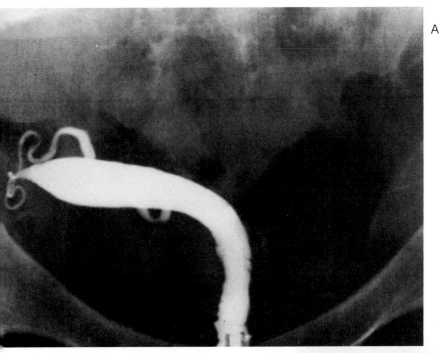

A

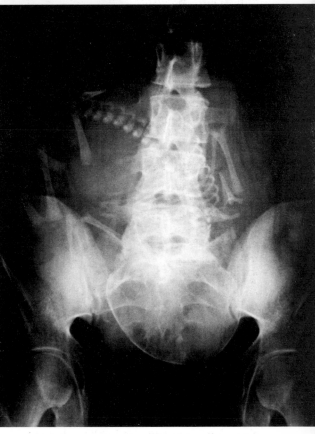

B

Figure 26.9 Oblique lie. **A.** This hysterosalpingogram, performed because of habitual abortion, reveals a single normal cervix and unicornuate uterus on the right side of the pelvis. The Fallopian tube is outlined. **B.** The same patient at 37 weeks' gestation with an oblique lie. No treatment was required because the presenting part had entered the pelvic brim and so there was no increased risk of cord prolapse. Normal delivery occurred at 40 weeks' gestation.

In some patients, premature labour may already have commenced and this situation is discussed in Chapter 50. Where there is a known cause such as uterine anomaly, fundal or praevial placenta, or pelvic tumour, it is unlikely that correction will occur. On the other hand, if the condition is due mainly to laxity of the uterus or excessive liquor, it is quite likely that as full term approaches the lie will stabilize longitudinally.

The main *complications to be anticipated* during the antenatal period are premature labour, premature rupture of the membranes (pelvic examination should be performed to exclude prolapse of the cord), and haemorrhage should the placenta be low lying. Cross-matched blood must be available if placenta praevia has been diagnosed.

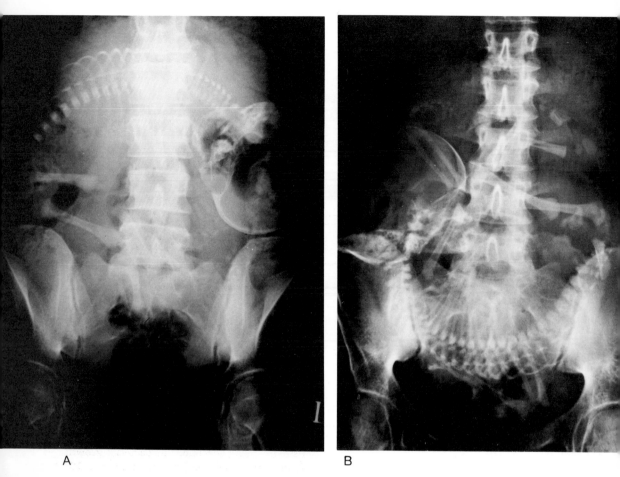

A   B

Figure 26.10 Transverse lie. **A.** Back upwards. The buttocks are in the iliac fossa with the feet dangling over the pelvic brim. If the patient was in the second stage of labour it would be relatively easy to pull down a leg and perform breech extraction. **B.** Back downwards. Internal version and breech extraction would be hazardous in this patient even if the necessary conditions were present.

chapter twenty-seven

Infections in Pregnancy

OVERVIEW

Patterns of infection in pregnancy change continually over the years; currently, *viruses* and *drug-resistant bacteria* present a major challenge. *The mother* is at risk because of certain changes induced by the pregnancy — e.g. *susceptibility to viral agents* (depression of immunity), *urinary tract infection* (changes in the urine and urinary stasis), *genital tract infection* (premature rupture of the membranes/prolonged labour; lacerations and retained products of conception), *breast infection* (stasis and cross-infection from the baby). At best, even a normal confinement leaves every woman with a *large healing placental site*, tantamount to a *surgical wound* in a potentially contaminated area, and many also have an *episiotomy* wound or sutured laceration in close proximity to bowel bacteria.

The traditional bacterial scourge of the pregnant woman, the *Group A, beta-haemolytic streptococcus*, is now rarely a problem; an important bacterial offender is a commensal organism carried in the mother's vagina, the *Group B, beta-haemolytic streptococcus*; this can cause a serious or even fatal infection in the newborn infant. Changes in the urinary tract during pregnancy encourage bacteria to grow and thus *cystitis and pyelonephritis* are more common. An effective attack on this problem has been the routine screening of a clean mid-stream urine specimen for bacterial growth (dipslide technique), and treating patients showing a *significant bacteriuria* (usually more than 10^5 organisms per ml).

Puerperal pelvic infections are usually caused by anaerobic or mixed anaerobic/aerobic flora; recently introduced antibacterial drugs usually cope effectively with such infections. *Breast infection* is nearly always due to a penicillinase-producing staphylococcus and thus a methicillin type of agent should be used. The recent increase in *methicillin resistance* by this organism has directed attention to traditional methods of infection control — accurate microbiological detection, strict hygiene measures by both patient and medical team, and isolation where necessary.

The baby is at risk from microorganisms acquired *transplacentally* (secondary to villitis and endovasculitis), or as a result of *ascending infection* from the birth canal (*chorioamnionitis*), or during passage down the birth canal. Viruses have a liking for young proliferating tissues and the fetus/newborn is thus at greater risk; infections which are often trivial in the adult (*rubella, cytomegalovirus*) can be devastating to the baby. Fetal infections in the first 4 months of pregnancy (the organogenetic period) can cause major malformations; thereafter, widespread damage to formed organs may occur — the most serious being to the central nervous system. Infections increase perinatal wastage partly because of direct fetal and neonatal damage and partly because of an unfavourable influence on the pregnancy (e.g. by causing *premature labour*). Premature and frail babies are at much greater risk. The acronym TORCH (*toxoplasmosis, rubella, cytomegalovirus, and herpes*) emphasizes a group of infections — 3 being viral in nature — which can be particularly damaging to the fetus; the first 3 of these are acquired by passage across the placenta.

Postnatally, infection may be acquired from the mother via secretions, blood, breast milk or from infected attendants or others in the immediate hospital environment.

Approximately 5% of pregnancies will be complicated by one or more viral infections (excluding the common cold). Vaccines are now being successfully developed (e.g. rubella); infections for which no vaccine is available (e.g. cytomegalovirus, herpes simplex virus) are assuming greater significance.

Bacterial infections occur mainly in the premature, hypoxic, and frail infant, with weak defence mechanisms. A variety of organisms may be involved, both aerobic and anaerobic, reflecting largely the microflora of the lower birth canal. *Anaerobic infections* have emerged as important pathogens to the mother after delivery, particularly if conditions are suitable — e.g. anaemia, and the presence of ischaemic or necrotic material. Infections due to such pathogens as *chlamydia* and *mycoplasma* are receiving increasing attention. *Prolonged labour*, particularly with ruptured membranes, is a prime cause of chorioamnionitis; to achieve therapeutic concentrations in the fetus of an antibacterial agent requires a significantly higher dose than that needed for a nonpregnant patient.

Syphilis has largely been contained as a result of the accuracy of routine antenatal testing and the continued efficacy of penicillin treatment. *Gonorrhoea* is prevalent in some communities; in pregnancy it is often present in a subclinical form being detected only when the baby develops conjunctivitis.

Infection of the mother during pregnancy usually affects the fetus directly, but such indirect manifestations as fever and endotoxin liberation (e.g. from vaginal or urinary tract infection) may precipitate premature labour.

Life-threatening infections include severe viral hepatitis, viral influenza, and malaria — also those complicating criminal abortion, prolonged rupture of membranes/prolonged labour, major childbirth trauma, and urinary tract anomaly. *Cross-infections* have decreased with acceptance of rooming-in of mother and baby.

Pregnant women living in or visiting *tropical areas* may encounter special problems, especially if hygiene/public health measures are low. *Hepatitis, malaria,* and *helminthic* infections are prevalent.

When treating infection in the pregnant/puerperal woman, the possible effects on the fetus/newborn of drugs given to the mother should be remembered. Antibiotics should never be given indiscriminately; *most of the treatable infections have relatively specific drug regimens* and these should be adhered to, unless proving ineffective.

GENERAL CONSIDERATIONS

Infecting Agents

These are usually classified as follows: bacteria, viruses, chlamydia, protozoa, fungi, spirochaetes.

Sources of Infection

Endogenous (originating in or on the body): the most important habitats are the bowel (faecal organisms), nasopharynx, skin, and vagina. *Exogenous* (originating outside the body): objects (such as linen, clothing, ward utensils) or attendants.

Factors in Infection

Changes which diminish host resistance and enhance' the capabilities of microorganisms commonly occur in obstetric practice.

(a) Host Defences

Specific factors. (i) *Epithelial barriers.* The mechanical barrier function is assisted by *bactericidal secretions* — e.g.lysozyme in the lacrimal fluid in the eye, fatty acids in the skin, acid in the stomach, and immune globulins (especially IgA, IgE) in mucous secretions. The acidity of the vagina (pH 3–3.5) is inhibitory to many pathogenic bacteria (group B streptococcus, an important pathogen in the newborn, is relatively resistant to this defence). (ii) *Immune system.* If the attacking organisms have breached the outer defences, several mechanisms are brought to bear (Chapter 39). The macrophage system of the blood and tissues consists of wandering sentinel cells which either engulf the attacker or 'memorize' its appearance and stimulate 2 types of lymphocytes (specific immune cells) to multiply: these are the *B lymphocytes* (plasma cells) which produce antibody (*humoral immunity*) and *the T lymphocytes* (killer lymphocytes) which directly attack the foreign agent (*cell-mediated immunity*). In addition, *neutrophil leucocytes* in the blood are attracted to the scene of the action because of chemical substances liberated there and they engulf the microorganisms involved.

Nonspecific factors. A large number of general factors may influence the resistance of the body — examples being race, age, nutrition, stress, alcohol, drugs, trauma, and general diseases such as diabetes. The presence of foreign bodies (such as catheters), dead tissue, or collections of blood, greatly aids the multiplication of bacteria.

(b) The Pathogens

Number of organisms. An example of this would be the contamination of the peritoneal cavity, vagina, or uterus by faecal material, which contains myriads of organisms.

Virulence. Not all microorganisms of the same species are equally 'pathogenic' or harmful to man.

Drug resistance. Many bacteria, especially the Gram-negative type (coliform, aerobacter, proteus) have genes conferring resistance to one or more antibacterial drugs.

Favourable local conditions. If epithelial barriers are injured, or there is a nidus where the organisms can multiply without fear of attack — foreign or dead tissue, blood clot — the infection will be both more serious and more difficult to treat, since neither antibiotic drugs nor defence cells will be able to penetrate into such tissue.

Cross-infection

This is the term given to the *infection of one person by another person or object*. In hospital the infection is usually passed from an already infected patient (or object used in the ward) by one of the attendants. *Staphylococcal* infection typically is transferred in such a way. The passage of *monilia* (thrush) from one baby to another is usually by an incompletely sterilized feeding bottle or teat. The prevention of cross-infection requires that all sources of infection be recognized and treated (and perhaps isolated), and every effort made to ensure that no organisms are carried either by staff or by ward articles to another patient.

THE CLASSICAL MATERNAL INFECTIONS

The mother is predisposed to infection in 3 classical sites: uterus (puerperal and post-abortal); urinary tract (pyelonephritis and cystitis); and breast (mastitis). These are also discussed in separate chapters.

Reproductive Tract

Postabortal. Predisposing factors are *blood loss* and *retained dead tissue*. In both postabortal and puerperal infections, the usual organisms are anaerobes, which thrive in such conditions. Criminal interference will often cause tissue damage and the introduction of faecal organisms or dangerous skin or throat organisms. The most serious infections result from *Clostridium welchii* — a faecal organism, which produces a powerful toxin which destroys red blood cells (jaundice, port wine urine, kidney failure), and uterine muscle (myonecrosis) (figure 14.3).

Chorioamnionitis. Infection of the fetus, secundines (placenta and membranes), and amniotic fluid is always secondary to infection (or colonization) of the mother by pathogenic microorganisms.

When the infection arises in the vagina, the membranes and amniotic fluid are primarily involved, the baby and placenta secondarily. The organisms reflect the normal vaginal flora — mixed aerobic and anaerobic bacteria, or intercurrent disease (e.g. herpes simplex). The infecting agent usually gains access to the fetus via the nasopharynx during normal 'breathing' movements in utero.

Transplacental infections occur during pregnancy, in the absence of premature rupture of the membranes or labour. There is often an unnoticed or mild illness in the mother (e.g. Listeria, or the TORCH group of organisms). The primary damage is seen in the placenta or in the fetal liver.

Early signs are maternal and/or fetal tachycardia and maternal fever. Later signs include uterine tenderness, offensive amniotic fluid, and further signs of fetal distress. Laboratory tests will usually show maternal leucocytosis and a positive culture of the amniotic fluid.

Management depends on the likely cause of the infection. The major problems are *whether to deliver the baby*, how quickly, and by what route; and what is the *most appropriate antibiotic?*

Puerperal. Predisposing factors are again *blood loss* and *retention of products of conception*. Faecal contamination can also occur if asepsis and delivery techniques are faulty, and infection from the attendant will result if scrubbing, gowning and masking are perfunctory. There is again the possibility of soft tissue trauma with instrumental deliveries and the introduction of infection during such procedures as *surgical induction of labour* and *vaginal examination*. The placental site usually becomes infected first, after which spread occurs to the surrounding tissues, resulting in parametritis and pelvic peritonitis — rarely general peritonitis or septicaemia (see Chapter 57). If the membranes are ruptured and/or labour is in progress for more than 12 hours, the risk of intrauterine infection is significantly increased. Infection complicates *Caesarean section* in 5–10% of elective and 10–30% of emergency cases.

Urinary Tract

Microorganisms grow more readily in the urine of pregnant women, due to differences in pH and the greater amounts of sugar and amino acids which escape reabsorption in the renal tubules. In addition, there is some *obstruction to urine flow* in the ureters. The risk of urinary tract infection in pregnancy is thus increased and is further aggravated by *catheterization and trauma* to the urethra and bladder during delivery.

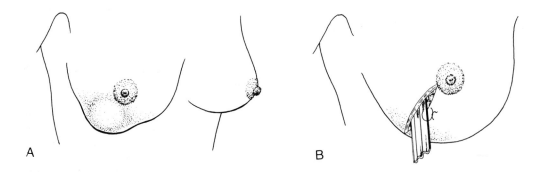

Figure 27.1 Breast abscess is an avoidable complication of breast feeding if a broad spectrum antibiotic is given at the onset of localized redness and tenderness with or without pyrexia. **A.** There is a painful fluctuant lump often deep within the breast without involvement of overlying skin. **B.** Treatment is wide incision in a radial direction from the nipple into the depth of the abscess cavity over the most dependent area with adequate drainage.

In the great majority of patients with urinary infection, a coliform or other Gram-negative organism is cultured. *In 5–10% of symptomless women*, bacteriuria will be found if a mid-stream specimen of urine is carefully examined. Urinary infections that persistently recur usually indicate an abnormality of the upper urinary tract (stone or congenital malformation) or perhaps lack of hygiene, particularly at the time of coitus.

Breast

The chief predisposing causes of puerperal mastitis are *stagnation of milk* in poorly-drained lactiferous sinuses, and trauma from suckling. It is probable that the invading bacteria (almost always Staphylococcus aureus) come from the baby rather than the mother. The baby is colonized from the hospital environment and therefore these organisms are usually *penicillin resistant*. Puerperal breast infections should be treated promptly with a broad spectrum antibiotic to prevent breast abscess (colour plate 97 and figure 27.1).

THE FETUS AND NEWBORN

Although it has been known for a long time that infection of the fetus can occur, for example syphilis or rubella, it is only recently that a true appreciation of the picture has become available.

Pathogenesis. Until late in pregnancy the fetus becomes infected almost entirely by way of the mother's blood stream and the placenta. The mother may or may not show evidence of clinical infection herself. With some infections, such as syphilis and tuberculosis, a definite placentitis precedes fetal involvement. Here the placenta is acting as a barrier, whereas with other infections such as rubella, the infecting organism can pass

more easily across the placenta from maternal blood in the intervillous space to the fetal circulation.

At the time of delivery, or during labour, if the membranes are ruptured, *ascending infection from the vagina* can occur. The amniotic fluid and membranes are first infected and finally the fetus. Primary areas of infection are the skin (including the umbilicus) and the respiratory and gastrointestinal tracts, by aspiration and swallowing, respectively. Secondary spread may occur to produce meningitis or pyelonephritis. The following factors favour amnionitis: *prolonged rupture of membranes, prolonged labour*, presence of cervicitis and vaginitis in the mother, presence of meconium in the liquor, maternal anaemia, manipulations before or during labour particularly if asepsis and antisepsis are not strictly observed. With some organisms, an ascending infection does not occur, but the *baby is infected as it passes down the birth canal*: examples are gonococcal and chlamydial *conjunctivitis, candidiasis* (thrush), and *herpes simplex infection.*

SEXUALLY TRANSMITTED (VENEREAL) DISEASES (STD)

STD now form a large group and are covered in more detail in gynaecological texts. Only those infections of particular relevance to the pregnant patient will be discussed.

Syphilis

This ancient disease is caused by the spirochaete, Treponema pallidum. It has largely been controlled in areas where antenatal care is adequate because of routine serological testing of all patients at the first antenatal visit. The *primary stage* of the disease consists of the chancre, a hard papule which breaks down into a painless indurated ulcer. The incubation period ranges from 2 –10 weeks and the chancre takes 2–4 weeks to heal. This gives way after a period of several weeks or months to the *secondary stage*, characterized by a generalized, macular, copper-coloured skin rash, ulceration of mucous surfaces, lymphadenopathy and periostitis. Characteristic flat papillary lesions may occur on the vulva (*condylomata lata*). The later stages are of considerable chronicity and the vascular and central nervous systems are particularly involved. If the *serology is positive* on screening, a more detailed study is made to confirm the presence of the disease by specific antitreponemal tests. If these are positive, the mother is treated with an adequate course of *penicillin* (benzathine penicillin 2.4 mega units IM for early syphilis; benzathine penicillin 7.2 mega units IM total in 3 divided doses at weekly intervals if duration of 12 months or more). If the patient is penicillin-sensitive, the respective doses of oral *erythromycin* are 500 mg qid × 15; 500 mg qid × 30.

The behaviour of the different serological tests during the course of the disease is shown in table 27.1. In patients with primary disease (chancre), a sample of exudate from the lesion is taken for dark field examination for spirochaetes. *Yaws* gives identical serology to syphilis (both spirochaetal) and clinical and epidemiological differences are usually relied on for diagnosis.

The major breakdown in the prevention of congenital syphilis is maternal infection during pregnancy (i.e. after initial serological testing). This has led to the suggestion that serology should be repeated at term in patients likely to be at risk (teenagers, unmarried mothers).

Fetal infection, if untreated, may result in stillbirth or generalized infection if the baby survives. The spirochaete usually does not pass the placental barrier during the first trimester, and fetal malformation is not a concern. Characteristic features in the newborn include hepatosplenomegaly, pneumonia, anaemia, jaundice, growth retardation, snuffles, skin lesions and osteochondritis. Histological study of the placenta reveals large numbers of spirochaetes.

Absence of clinical evidence of the disease at birth does not mean that the baby is free of infection.

Gonorrhoea

Gonorrhoea is caused by a *Gram-negative diplococcus*. The organism attacks mucosal surfaces and shows a preference for glandular tissue (Bartholin, urethral, cervical). The incubation period is short and the clinical features are usually characteristic (purulent discharge from the above sites (or the pharynx/rectum if sexual proclivities extended in those directions), together with associated symptoms — e.g. dysuria.

The *incidence* varies markedly throughout the world — from 0.001%–10%; higher rates are seen in the young, unmarried and sexually promiscuous.

The infection is often *chronic and subclinical*. It is in this situation that unsuspected infection of the newborn can occur. The initial manifestation is almost always a *purulent conjunctivitis* which, if untreated, may cause blindness. In some centres, prophylactic drops or ointment are used, especially if gonorrhoea is prevalent in the community. If this is not done, and the baby develops a 'sticky eye', with a purulent dis-

---

TABLE 27.1   BEHAVIOUR OF SEROLOGICAL TESTS DURING THE COURSE OF SYPHILIS

Test	Significance	Effect of disease, treatment
Reagin-type (VDRL, rapid plasma reagin etc)	Antibodies to nontreponemal lipoidal antigens. False positive in a number of disease states (leprosy, malaria, hepatitis, mononucleosis, mycoplasma infection); also positive in yaws (Treponema pertenue) and occasionally in normal women	Negative-high. (P) usually positive about 1–2 weeks after appearance of chancre. (S) high titre; variable thereafter. Disappears after treatment in 1 year (P), 1–2 years (S)
T-pallidum haemagglutination (TPHA)	Specific, quantitative; less sensitive than FTS-ABS. Usually ordered if screening test positive	Remains positive for many years, even after treatment
Fluorescent treponemal antibody (FTA-ABS)	Specific, quantitative; very few false positives. Used if TPHA negative or doubtful. Modified for detection of neonatal infection (fluorescein-labelled anti-human IgM)	IgM antibody becomes negative within 6 months of treatment; IgG antibody remains positive

P = primary; S = secondary stage of the disease

charge, a swab appropriate for isolation of the gonococcus should be taken for laboratory testing (buffered, charcoal-impregnated swabs placed in *Stuart* or similar transport medium).

If infection is recognized in the mother in the antenatal period, it is treated with *procaine penicillin*, 2.4 million units into each buttock with oral probenecid, 1 g, given at the same time (the latter blocks rapid excretion of the penicillin by the kidneys).

Chlamydial Infection

This microorganism is unusual in that, like a virus, it is an *obligatory intracellular parasite*. It is now recognized as being of equal importance with the gonococcus in the framework of sexually transmitted disease. There are a number of serotypes, producing such varied disorders as lymphogranuloma venereum, urethral and genital tract infection in both sexes, trachoma, and upper respiratory tract infection.

The clinical features are similar in many respects to those of gonorrhoea, except that the main manifestation in the lower genital tract is a cervicitis. In some centres, up to 8% of women have cervical and or urethral infection, and 30–40% of the babies of such patients will become infected. The baby's eyes are particularly susceptible to infections in the cervix and vagina. *Chlamydial inclusion conjunctivitis occurs in over 5% of babies in some centres* (colour plate 130). This may resolve without treatment, although corneal scarring may be a late result; otitis and pneumonia ('diffuse lung syndrome') are other complications in the newborn. The incubation period of conjunctival infection ranges from 5–14 days (earlier if the membranes rupture prematurely). The infection responds to *tetracycline or erythromycin*; the conjunctivitis is treated with 1% tetracycline ointment every 2–4 hours for 2–3 weeks.

If the male partner is diagnosed as having a nongonococcal urethritis, the couple should be given oral erythromycin for 7–14 days.

Mycoplasmal Infection

The female genital tract of sexually-active women is often colonized by mycoplasmal organisms — usually *ureaplasma urealyticum* and, to a lesser extent, *mycoplasma hominis*. There is evidence that chronic infection can cause abortion, chorioamnionitis, premature labour, puerperal and neonatal infection.

Like chlamydia, the organism requires special laboratory techniques for isolation, and much of our knowledge is recent and some unconfirmed.

If a mycoplasmal infection is suspected or confirmed, the mother is given a course of erythromycin (tetracycline is also effective but contraindicated during pregnancy because of the harmful effect on the developing teeth and bones of the fetus).

Common Vaginal Infections

The vagina contains a large and varied microbial flora during the woman's sexually active life and infection, although usually not of major significance to the mother, often causes considerable irritation and may subsequently affect the baby.

Candidiasis (Moniliasis, Thrush)

Some 10% of women will be infected with Candida albicans or an allied organism during pregnancy (figure 27.2). The infection may only be discovered on routine cytology, but usually there is an intense vulvovaginal irritation and on examination there is a whitish-yellow, curd-like discharge clinging to the vaginal walls and cervix. The appearance on speculum examination is usually diagnostic, but confirmation is readily obtained by culture on Nickerson or Sabouraud media.

If symptoms are acute, the discharge is removed gently with swabs soaked in dilute acetic acid (2%), and the walls are painted with 1–2% gentian violet. Follow-up treatment is given by means of one of the efficient antifungal preparations now available (*miconazole, nystatin, econazole*), in the form of intravaginal pessaries or cream.

The baby may develop oral candidiasis (which may extend to involve the gut) if the vagina is infected at the time of delivery (colour plate 131).

Trichomoniasis

This was thought to be a benign infection but recent studies suggest that it may be associated with *premature labour*. There is vulvovaginal irritation and a thin purulent, usually frothy, discharge (figure 27.3); the infection may be asymptomatic, the trichomonads being observed in the routine *Papanicolaou smear*. Clinical diagnosis can usually be quickly confirmed by mixing some of the discharge with warm, normal saline and observing under a cover slip by low power microscopy: the characteristic $20 \times 10 \, \mu$, pear-shaped, motile flagellate organism will be seen.

Treatment is by oral *metronidazole* or *tinidazole*. Although there is no convincing evidence of a teratogenic effect of these preparations, therapy is preferably deferred until the second trimester; if earlier treatment is required,

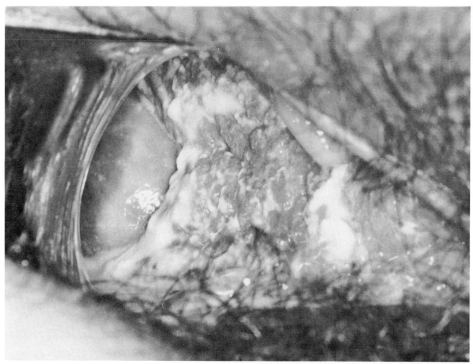

Figure 27.2 Monilial vaginitis in a 25-year-old para 1 with gestational diabetes at 31 weeks' gestation. She complained of discharge and pruritus vulvae. The patient is shown in the left lateral position with a Sims speculum exposing the cervix and oedematous anterior vaginal wall epithelium with monilial milk-like curds attached. Gentian violet (1% aqueous solution) was applied with immediate relief and Mycostatin pessaries (nystatin 100,000u), 1 at night for 2 weeks, were prescribed.

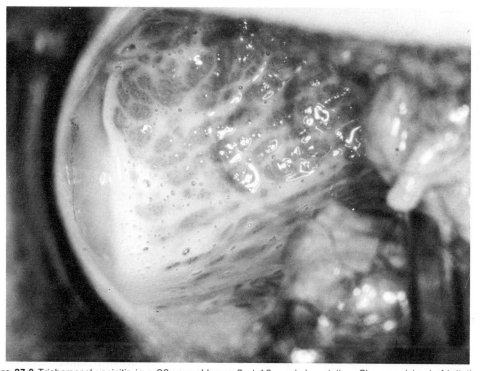

Figure 27.3 Trichomonal vaginitis in a 26-year-old para 2 at 19 weeks' gestation. She complained of irritating vaginal discharge and pruritus vulvae. This close-up view, magnification × 2, with the patient in the left lateral position, shows the typical frothy discharge and the oedematous vaginal wall. Pregnancy-induced vascularity accounts for prominence of the vaginal rugae. The husband was asymptomatic. The infection responded promptly to oral metronidazole, 200 mg 3 times daily for 7 days.

vaginal application of a less specific preparation (*natamycin*) can be used.

'Tropical' Venereal Diseases

These diseases are more common in native races in the tropics and subtropics in underdeveloped communities; *heat*, *humidity* and *poor hygiene* are predisposing factors.

Granuloma Inguinale

This chronic disease begins as a painless nodule, and like the syphilitic lesion this breaks down into an ulcer; the lesion soon extends in a destructive manner to involve the vulva and perianal areas. Lymphatic spread occurs to the inguinal glands. Often the inguinal spread represents subcutaneous infiltration rather than lymph node involvement (pseudobuboe). The usual clinical features are discharge, dyspareunia and swelling/ulceration. *Secondary infection* is usual. Granuloma inguinale is moderately contagious and autoinoculable. The causative organism is *Donovania granulomatis*, a bacterium related to the Klebsiella group; characteristic intracellular Donovan bodies are found on microscopic examination of the exudate or crushed tissue smears taken under local analgesia after antiseptic swabbing.

The differential diagnosis lies between lymphogranuloma venereum, syphilis, condylomata acuminata, carcinoma, and conditions leading to vulval lymphoedema (e.g. parasitic lymphangitis).

Treatment during pregnancy is by oral erythromycin, 1–2 g daily in divided doses for 2–3 weeks. Social and hygiene measures are also important.

Lymphogranuloma Venereum

The initial lesion is a small papule or vesicle which appears 1–2 weeks after contact; this breaks down in 1–2 weeks to produce a relatively painless ulcer. Within a further 2 –3 weeks there is inguinal adenitis. The nodes are often multiple, matted together, and adherent to the overlying skin which is also inflamed. This mass tends to break down into *multiple sinuses*.

Occasionally there is a proctocolitis and pelvic lymphadenitis; rectal stricture and intestinal obstruction may result, or perianal or rectovaginal fistulas. Elephantiasis of the vulva develops if there is lymphatic blockage.

The disease is caused by a member of the *chlamydia group of organisms* and although it responds to the usual antibiotics, extensive damage to the lymphatic system may persist.

The chief obstetric problem is the occasional severe scarring, which may necessitate Caesarean section.

The *intradermal Frei test* is positive in over 90% of patients; the complement fixation test is more easily quantitated to assess the effect of treatment. Therapy is effective with both tetracycline and erythromycin; abscesses may need surgical drainage.

Chancroid

The causative bacterium is *Haemophilus ducreyi*, a Gram-negative organism, described in 1890. It produces a soft chancre, which is quite *painful* (differentiating it from the chancre of syphilis), and there is also painful swelling of inguinal glands. Regional lymphadenitis develops in 1–2 weeks; often only 1 or 2 glands are involved, but suppuration is common. Aspiration of the pus allows laboratory confirmation of the diagnosis. The infection responds to a 10–14 day course of *sulphonamides* or to broad spectrum antibiotics.

IMPORTANT BACTERIAL INFECTIONS

Group B Beta-Haemolytic Streptococcus

This Gram-positive coccus is present in the vagina during pregnancy in approximately 10% of women; it can also be isolated from the rectum in 15–25%. Serotyping suggests a sexual mode of transmission. Unlike the Group A streptococcus, this organism is relatively resistant to the acid milieu of the vagina and grows quite well in amniotic fluid. The colonization rate ranges from 1–7% of all newborn infants. In many centres this is the most common infecting microorganism of the newborn (30% of neonatal infections) (see Chapter 67).

Clinical features. Approximately 1.5–2.0% of patients will experience puerperal infection (uterine) due to the group B beta-haemolytic streptococcus, chiefly as a complication of artificial rupture of the membranes.

In the baby there is a morbidity rate of 2–4 per 1,000 and a perinatal mortality rate of 1 in 1,000 due to this infection.

There are *2 main syndromes* — (i) An *early onset* septicaemia and pneumonia, often presenting as an idiopathic respiratory distress syndrome/cardiovascular collapse. This is seen mainly in the baby born before the 35th week of gestation; the male infant is more susceptible than the female. (ii) The *late onset* form is seen usually after the first week of life, the baby being lethargic, anorexic and jaundiced; meningitis is a common complication.

Management. Prophylaxis is mainly directed to high risk mothers — i.e. those with premature rupture of the membranes, particularly before the 36th week of pregnancy. A high vaginal swab will indicate the presence of the organism and the need for antibiotics. The mother should be treated antenatally if symptomatic; if not, she is given penicillin in labour and the baby is given penicillin after birth. In some centres, all premature babies are given penicillin prophylactically. It is considered that *routine vaginal swabs of all pregnant women (table 6.1) is not cost effective.*

Early diagnosis will enable prompt treatment. Usually, gastric, pharyngeal and ear swabs are taken and screened for Gram-positive cocci; benzathine penicillin is given if positive. A strong presumption of infection is made if the baby is unwell and has tachypnoea at birth. Immunotherapy (plasma, neutrophils) is recommended in some centres.

Maternal infections are usually nonspecific, presenting as a fever, usually on the second or third evening after delivery. There may be offensive lochia and local pelvic tenderness. The infection responds to the usual broad spectrum antibiotics; it is *resistant to the aminoglycosides.*

Tetanus

This infection is caused by a Gram-positive, anaerobic spore-forming bacterium, *Clostridium tetani.* It liberates a powerful exotoxin (tetanospasmin) which may cause death from muscle spasms leading to exhaustion and respiratory failure.

Incidence. In some developing countries (Haiti, Bangladesh, Papua New Guinea), neonatal mortality rates from this organism reach 100 or more per 1,000 livebirths (see Chapter 15).

Clinical features and diagnosis. The *incubation period* in the newborn ranges from 3–8 days. *Painful trismus* occurs due to spasm of the jaw muscles (masseters), and this prevents suckling at the breast. Soon the *spasms* spread to muscles of the neck, vertebral column and elsewhere; abdominal rigidity is usual, as is constipation. Spasms are usually set off by touching or bright light. Respiratory distress and anoxia follow. Hyperpyrexia may occur.

Death usually occurs between the 4th and 14th days after birth, depending on the severity of the infection etc.

Management. This is largely *preventive* — by institution of hygienic practices at delivery. Simple asepsis and antisepsis, the use of a sterile instrument to cut the cord, a sterile ligature for the stump, and an antiseptic or sterile dressing will largely eliminate the problem. *The use of soil and animal excreta for dressing the umbilical cord stump must be abandoned. A prior course of tetanus toxoid (2–3 doses) to the mother will protect the baby in most instances.* Because of deeply-held prejudices, an active health education effort is necessary to achieve the above objectives.

For the established condition, transfer to a special centre is necessary. The spasms are controlled by suitable anticonvulsants, positive pressure artifical respiration is applied, and repeated small doses of antitetanus serum plus betamethasone are given.

Tuberculosis

It was not uncommon, 20–30 years ago, for many obstetric hospitals to have separate wards for pregnant women with chronic tuberculosis. With improvements in hygiene and the introduction of more effective chemotherapy, a large measure of control of this once-feared infection has been obtained.

In many centres, the *once routine chest radiograph* at the initial antenatal visit has been deleted unless the clinical features are suggestive.

Ethambutol and *isoniazid* are the preferred initial drugs for treatment in pregnancy. The patient will be under the care of a specialist chest physician.

It is usually safe for the mother to handle the baby and breast-feed if the disease is not active; BCG vaccination of the latter is arranged in the puerperium.

The infection may involve the urinary tract (kidneys/bladder) and is often difficult to diagnose (pyuria and occasional haematuria, with a negative urine culture on standard media are suggestive).

Listeriosis

Although uncommon, infection of the mother with *Listeria monocytogenes* may have serious consequences for the infant (colour plate 128). Typically, the mother has a short influenza-like infection, goes into premature labour and delivers a baby with apnoea/respiratory distress; meconium-staining of the amniotic fluid is common even in the late second trimester. Unless the diagnosis is thought of and energetic treatment given, the baby has a high risk of dying as a result of disseminated infection (lung, liver, CNS). Less commonly, infection of the baby can be acquired during birth; in such cases the infection will be later in onset (several days after birth).

VIRAL INFECTIONS

Rubella

This infection is extremely important because of its frequency in the community and its very damaging effects on the fetus, especially if occurring early in pregnancy. Before the availability of an effective vaccine, rubella accounted for much of the *deafness and blindness* in the community. White races are more susceptible than black to this infection. Although 70–90% of pregnant women are immune, it is recommended that *routine testing for rubella antibodies* is carried out at the first antenatal visit (table 6.1); this enables appropriate advice to be given to the patient: i.e. if immune, they can be reassured; if not, they should avoid contact with rubella sufferers, be given immune globulin if such contact has occurred (15–20 ml IM), *and vaccinated in the puerperium if still susceptible.* On the basis of experience to date, it appears that *the vaccine rubella virus is not embyropathic* — i.e. if the vaccine is inadvertently given in early pregnancy there is no indication for induced abortion on the grounds of risks of fetal malformation or infection. However, it is still considered wisest for the patient not to be pregnant at the time of vaccination or to become pregnant within the ensuing 2 months.

Maternal infection. The infection is usually spread by droplets (pharynx, urine), and after an *incubation period of 2–3 weeks*, a fine rash appears which lasts for 1–5 days. The rash is not characteristic, but occipital lymphadenopathy, together with joint pain and swelling (particularly of the wrists and fingers) are suspicious.

The disease is usually worse in the teenager and adult. *The affected subject is highly infectious for 1 week before and 2 weeks after the appearance of the rash.* The latter is usually fine and reddish-pink in colour; it may be maculopapular.

Rubella is to be distinguished from *measles* (reddish-brown, usually coarser, rash on face, trunk and legs, Koplik spots in the mouth, cough and coryza, conjunctivitis), *roseola* (the rash lasts only 1–2 days, irritability 4–5 days, fever occurs before the rash) and *scarlet fever* (predominance of pharyngeal symptoms). Unfortunately, there is no rash in 50% of rubella patients (colour plate 125A), and 50% of rubella-like rashes are due to other conditions.

The main practical problems are firstly, is the rash due to rubella, and secondly, has the mother got a preclinical or subclinical infection?

The antibody titre is useful in assessing these problems. If the patient presents after contact with an infected subject, a *haemagglutination-inhibition (HI) test is done*; if the patient is already immune, a high titre will be present; if the titre is low or negative, a further check 2–3 weeks later is carried out (longer if immune globulin has been given, shorter if there is already a rash), *and if a 4-fold increase is observed, recent infection is suggested.* If the patient presents more than 10–14 days after exposure and the HI titre is high, the *IgM titre* is measured — a positive rubella-specific IgM result indicates a viraemia in the past 4–6 weeks (figure 27.4). IgM antibody is only present for 4–6 weeks and is *indicative of a primary infection.* The complement-fixing (CF) antibodies appear later than HI antibodies; these are seldom measured since the HI and IgM antibody

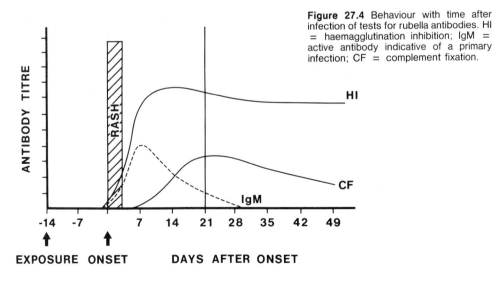

Figure 27.4 Behaviour with time after infection of tests for rubella antibodies. HI = haemagglutination inhibition; IgM = active antibody indicative of a primary infection; CF = complement fixation.

titres usually provide all the information required. Occasionally, the pregnant woman may have had a recent subclinical infection, and passed this on to one of her own or another's child. Mild or subclinical infections are not uncommon in the adult and it should be emphasized that there is no correlation between the severity of infection in the mother and fetus (colour plate 125A).

Pharyngeal swabs become positive some 5–7 days before the rash appears; although a positive diagnosis can be obtained, the procedure is not 100% successful, it is more expensive, and the result will not be available for some time.

Fetal infection.

The fetus is infected by transplacental passage of the virus during the stage of maternal viraemia; the fetal effects are largely related to gestational age (colour plate 125B). If infection occurs in the period of formation of the fetal organs (before 15 weeks), malformations are common especially of the eye, internal ear and heart. The *classical rubella syndrome* described by Dr Norman Gregg in 1941 comprises *deafness*, *cataracts*, *microphthalmia*, *cardiac defects* and *mental retardation* (colour plate 125). In 1964, additional features of congenital rubella were recognized — *the expanded rubella syndrome*: general cellular damage (*intrauterine growth retardation*), bone marrow damage (thrombocytopenia, anaemia), hepatitis (enlarged liver, jaundice), myocarditis (cardiac failure), pneumonitis and encephalitis. The risk of fetal damage from rubella is as high as *80% in the first month* of pregnancy, *30–40% in the second month* and *5–10% in the third and fourth months*. The classical malformations and the expanded rubella syndrome often occur together (colour plates 125 A and B). They are both manifestations of rubella infection in the first 14 weeks of pregnancy. Although maternal infection after this time can also result in fetal infection, it is unusual for it to cause significant damage to the fetus — i.e. *maternal rubella infection after 15 weeks' gestation is not an indication for termination of pregnancy.*

In the newborn, the general antibody titre (IgG) will be the same as that of the mother (the small IgG molecule passes the placental barrier); however IgM antibodies do not pass the placenta and their presence in cord blood is highly suggestive of infection acquired in utero (colour plate 125A).

Some 30% of babies who were infected with the rubella virus in utero will still be excreting virus at the age of 6 months and 5%–10% at 12 months (nasopharynx, urine, faeces).

Management.

(a) *Prophylaxis.* All nonimmune females should be actively immunized with rubella vaccine; this is delayed until the early puerperium in the case of the pregnant woman. In addition, all health professionals caring for the pregnant woman and her child should be tested and vaccinated if indicated. In some countries, it is recommended that *all* infants 12–15 months of age be vaccinated, usually together with vaccinations for measles and mumps; school entry is sometimes conditional on this procedure having been carried out. (b) *Therapy.* Specific measures are usually only necessary in pregnancy because of the susceptibility of the fetus. The options are *termination of pregnancy* in the first 14–15 weeks or administration of hyperimmune antirubella globulin if the former course is unacceptable. The empirical risks, related largely to the period of gestation, should be discussed with the parents.

In some centres, cord blood is routinely tested and if antibodies are present and the mother was seronegative at the initial antenatal check, paediatric referral is carried out. At the 6-week postnatal visit, it is wise to check on the success of the maternal vaccination.

If anti-D gamma globulin is required postpartum for prevention of rhesus isoimmunization, the rubella vaccination is best left to a later date, since seroconversion may not occur.

In summary, at the first antenatal visit, a check should be made as to whether the patient has noticed a recent rash or has been in contact with rubella; a rubella HI test should be done as a routine. Hyperimmune antirubella globulin or pregnancy termination are options for infection in the first 15 weeks of pregnancy, globulin alone if the infection occurs later. Serious malformations with or without evidence of systemic infection (the expanded rubella syndrome) only occur with maternal infections during the first trimester. After that time organ damage may occur but is of very low incidence and usually consists of varying degrees of deafness and mild learning difficulties that may not become apparent until school age. Nonimmune mothers are actively vaccinated in the puerperium; if anti-D gamma globulin is required, the rubella vaccine is deferred. A check of the HI titre should be carried out 6 weeks after vaccination to determine its success.

Herpes Genitalis

There are 2 main types of herpes simplex virus (HSV) infection — 1 and 2. Type 1 is responsible for most nongenital infections (lips, mouth, eyes); type 2 has a predominantly venereal (below the waist) localization. Both are double-stranded DNA viruses.

Incidence. The number of antenatal patients actively infected with HSV differs considerably according to the amount of sexually transmitted disease in the area, *but will usually be about 1%.* In some 10% of these, there will be an active infection near delivery. *Less than 1 in 5,000 liveborn infants will be affected.* Serum antibody studies indicate that 35–95% of the adult population have been infected in the past.

Pathogenesis. Infection is acquired through direct contact of abraded skin surfaces or mucous membranes with material from an infected person. After an incubation period of 3–10 days, the typical tingling, followed by blisters and then ulcers will occur. Primary attacks last for 6–12 days, secondary attacks, 3–6 days; in many the disease is subclinical and can be revealed by characteristic changes in the cervical smear. *There is no viraemia and thus no transplacental spread to the fetus:* infection is acquired after rupture of the membranes or during delivery — the mother excreting virus at the time. The virus is neurotropic and resides in the ganglia of the spinal cord between attacks.

Damage to the fetus is greater with primary attacks, partly because of the more extensive maternal infection, but also because the fetus lacks any protective IgG humoral antibody previously passed from the mother.

Like cytomegalovirus infection, and unlike rubella, the presence of antibodies in the mother may attenuate fetal infection, but not prevent it.

Fetal infection. Symptoms in the infant usually appear after an incubation period of 3–6 days. The spectrum of clinical disorder is quite wide. Severe primary infections can result in abortion, stillbirth or premature labour. The possibility of direct infection should be considered if the newborn develops skin and/or mucosal vesicles, is lethargic, feeding poorly, jaundiced, febrile or cyanotic. If the baby is *clinically affected, the mortality rate without specific antiviral therapy can be up to 90%,* usually because of viraemia and encephalitis; if the lesion appears localized to the skin etc, the mortality is low (less than 2–3%).

Diagnosis. History is very important and a question directed to past attacks involving the patient or her partner should never be omitted at the initial antenatal visit. The lesions appearing in an acute attack are so typical that diagnostic confusion seldom arises. Subclinical infection can be detected in *cytological smears* in 85% or so of involved patients. Specific diagnosis requires *viral identification in culture* from active lesions.

Management. Prophylaxis. A general awareness of the dangers of HSV, as well as the risks of infection of the patient by her partner if he has active penile herpes, should be indicated to the patient. Attendants and relatives may also constitute a source of infection.

Since the fetus is infected during passage down the birth canal, preventive measures are directed to identifying active cervical-vaginal infection and *performing Caesarean section if this is found.* Usually, weekly cultures from the 35th–36th week are taken if there has been an episode of infection earlier in the pregnancy. If there has been no viral shedding for 4 days, vaginal delivery would seem safe for the baby. Some debate exists regarding the relative risks if the maternal infection is secondary and mild.

If the membranes have ruptured for more than 4 hours, the advantage of abdominal delivery is usually lost.

Specific. Antiviral agents are becoming available clinically and will alter both the seriousness of this disease to the fetus and newborn and probably the obstetric approach.

In the *puerperium,* isolation procedures are not usually advised and breast feeding can be carried out. Careful *hand washing by the mother* is necessary and the baby should be protected from contact with infected maternal skin surfaces or secretions.

Cytomegalovirus

Cytomegalovirus (CMV) is one of the herpes group of viruses, and like herpes simplex, is probably largely sexually transmitted and widespread in most communities. Transmission is by close physical contact or by infected blood, urine or secretions (e.g. saliva, breast milk). The fetus can be infected transplacentally or during passage down the birth canal. *Unlike rubella, CMV can infect in successive pregnancies.* Nursery infections from one infant to another have been reported. Infected individuals harbour the virus for life and reactivation can occur (with or without clinical manifestations) with reexcretion of virus for a variable period.

Incidence. Approximately 50–90% of the adult population are affected serologically and *1% of seronegative women become infected in pregnancy;* in the latter case, 40–50% of the fetuses will be affected; 5–10% of fetal infections are symptomatic — *20% of these are fatal and 90% of the remainder result in major sequelae.*

Because of improving hygiene, more women are seronegative at the start of pregnancy.

Clinical features and prognosis. (a) *Maternal.* Infection in the adult is usually subclinical, but there may be pyrexia, malaise, lymphadenopathy and abnormalities in morphology of blood lymphocytes; occasionally, as with rubella and other similar viral infections, the manifestations may be more serious.

Diagnosis is made by viral culture from secretions or by demonstration of cells containing 'owls' eyes' inclusions in the urine. Serological tests are also available (complement fixation etc).

(b) *Fetal.* The clinical features are similar to those described for the rubella virus; occasionally the baby may present hydropic features (colour plate 126). Subclinical infection is common. Malformations may result from primary infection in the first trimester (colour plate 127). *CMV is the commonest cause of psychomotor retardation in children.* In contrast to rubella, a significant number of children (10–30%) are still secreting virus after the end of their first year of life. Specific CMV IgM may be detected in the serum only in a proportion of infected newborns; the virus can usually be isolated from urine and saliva.

Management. *Preventive measures* are important. General hygiene measures should be emphasized and likely chronic excretors should be avoided (congenitally infected children, immunosuppressed and debilitated subjects). If the mother has been screened for antibody at the first antenatal visit, subsequent nonspecific febrile illnesses should be regarded with suspicion. Ideally, blood for transfusion should be screened for CMV before administration to the pregnant woman or her fetus/newborn infant.

The presence of an atypical transformation zone in the cervix may be associated with viral infection. The danger of infected mothers and babies to attending health care personnel should be remembered. Virus-excreting infants should preferably be isolated.

A high index of suspicion is necessary to detect CMV infection in some infants; the likely advent of effective antiviral therapy makes such detection important.

Viral Hepatitis

Hepatitis B is one of the commonest serious infectious diseases; it has been estimated that there are 200 million carriers of the disease and some 20% of these will die of *cirrhosis* or its complication, *hepatocellular carcinoma*. The obstetric attendant is vitally concerned because of the frequency of vertical transmission of the disease (i.e. from mother to newborn) and the risk to health care workers from women (or their offspring) with clinical or subclinical disease.

Types of disease. *Type A ('infectious') hepatitis.* This is largely transmitted by the oral-faecal route, has an incubation period of 2 weeks, an illness of fairly abrupt onset and short duration, early appearance of antibodies and *absence of chronicity/carrier status. Type B ('serum') hepatitis.* In the adult, transmission is usually by infected blood or blood products or sexual contact; in the newborn, the infection is usually acquired during labour or soon after. The incubation period is 2–3 months, there is usually a prodromal 'flu-like' phase, and *chronicity (chronic hepatitis/carrier state) may occur.*

Type non-A, non-B hepatitis. Its general behaviour is similar to type B disease; the mode of spread is usually by blood transfusion (no screening test yet available), the incubation period is 1–2 months, and the disease is generally less severe; perinatal infection is not as common or as significant.

Other viral infections. Cytomegalovirus, Epstein-Barr virus, and yellow fever virus may all cause hepatitis.

Incidence. The attack and carrier rates vary very widely according to socioeconomic-cultural factors. Carrier rates range from 0.2%–20% or more. Active infection occurs in 0.01–0.2% or more of pregnancies.

Clinical features. *Mother.* There is often an initial flu-like upset (malaise, anorexia, fatigue) in hepatitis B and non-A, non-B infections and this gives way to nausea, fever, liver tenderness and jaundice; the urine is dark and the stools are pale. Symptoms due to immune complex formation (urticaria, arthralgia) may be present early in the disease. The course of hepatitis A is usually limited to 2–3 weeks. In the other 2 types, recovery may take 3–4 months or even longer; *5–10% will drift into a chronic carrier state, often with progressive chronic hepatitis.* In rare instances, the disease takes a fulminant course, with acute hepatic failure, coma and often death.

Infant. The infant rarely demonstrates the classical symptoms seen in later life; *the great majority have a subclinical infection and enter the carrier state.*

Pathogenesis and diagnosis. The virus passes from the blood stream to the hepatocyte and replicates inside the cell nucleus. The virus particles (core) leave the nucleus and are covered by a surface coat which is produced in the cytoplasm of the cell; this is the Dane particle and is the means of transmission of the disease. Damage to the liver cells is occurring *pari passu* with the above replication. An immune response occurs, with antibodies being produced to the different antigenic components of the virus. The time course of production of antigens and antibodies in relation to hepatitis B infection is shown in figure 27.5. The antigens are DNA polymerase, core(c), surface(s) and e. *If hepatitis B surface antigen (HBsAg) is present, the patient has acute or chronic hepatitis or is a chronic carrier;* if hepatitis B surface antibody (anti-HBs) is present, the virus has been eliminated *and the patient is immune* and not infectious. *HBsAg is the test of choice for antenatal screening of mothers.* Maternal carriers who also have HBeAg are a high risk group, just as in the acute disease, for perinatal transmission to their babies as well as being more infective to their medical and nursing attendants.

Diagnosis. This usually presents little difficulty because of the characteristic symptoms. Problems arise in detection of subclinical/chronic infections and carriers: it is here that *serological studies* are particularly helpful (figure 27.5). *Liver function tests* will indicate the extent of hepatocellular damage.

Figure 27.5 A. Hepatitis B acute infection resulting in self-limited disease and cure. The anti-HBs titre persists and the patient is immune. **B.** Acute infection resulting in the carrier state. There is persistence of surface antigen (HBsAg). Titres of DNA polymerase, Dane particle, e antigen and antibody have been omitted for clarity.

Perinatal hepatitis B virus (HBV) infection. Studies of the time course of HBV antigens and antibodies in the infant indicate that the vast majority of infections are acquired at the time of parturition, either during passage down the birth canal or at birth. The infant infection rate from carrier mothers ranges from 10-40%; *if the infant is infected, 85–90% will become chronic carriers (HBsAg positive) (adding to the reservoir of infection in the community) and many will experience progressive hepatic damage, with the likelihood of cirrhosis/hepatocellular carcinoma with an incubation period of 30–50 years.* The major determinant of maternal transmission (and subsequent development of the infant carrier state) is the presence of the HBeAg in her blood (a reflection of the presence of whole virus particles). There is a 70–80% chance of perinatal transmission when acute hepatitis occurs in the last trimester of pregnancy, or in the first few months after delivery.

Management

Acute hepatitis. This is managed as in the non-pregnant patient.

Prevention of newborn infection. The child is at risk in several situations. (i) The mother suffers from *acute hepatitis during the pregnancy*: the later this occurs, the greater the risk. (ii) The mother is *chronically infected.* This may be suspected for a number of reasons: previous child/family member affected, previous attack of hepatitis, drug addict/prostitute, tattooed individual, special ethnic group (Aboriginal, Asia, Africa, Pacific basin), or occupational group (exposed to blood/blood products (obstetrician,

A

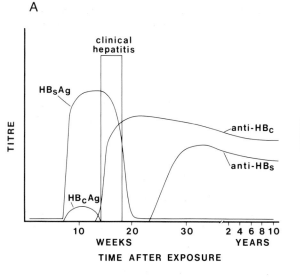

B

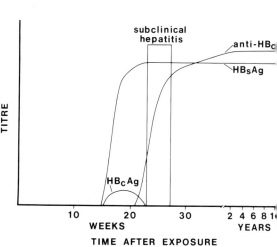

obstetric nurse, blood bank workers), care of mentally retarded). These high risk patients should be screened to identify carriers (positive HBsAg) early in pregnancy (table 6.1). *The finding of a positive anti-HBc or anti-HBs with a negative HBsAg identifies the immune individual.*

In the above groups, hepatitis B *immunoglobulin 100 IU IM is given to the newborn soon after birth, preferably together with hepatitis B vaccine 20 µg subcutaneously in a different limb and followed by similar doses of vaccine at 1 and 6 months of age.* If the vaccine is unavailable, the immunoglobulin should be repeated in 4 weeks and tests for HBsAg carried out 3-monthly during the first year of life.

Caesarean section has been suggested for delivery in mothers who are actively infectious (HBeAg positive); however, the *situation is not similar to that of mothers with herpes simplex infections* — the baby is likely to be infected from maternal blood as much as birth canal secretions.

General infection precautions. Birth attendants should exercise particular care in handling and disposing of blood-soaked articles, both at the delivery and during the puerperium. The infant, unlike the mother, is rarely a source of infection until 2 months after birth. Many hospitals have a policy requiring nonimmunized staff members to wear goggles at delivery of hepatitis B carriers.

Breast feeding. It is thought that this adds little risk to the infant if immunization has been given.

Varicella (Chickenpox)

The varicella-zoster virus is highly contagious and because of this, 90–95% of children contract varicella before reaching adolescence; infection of the pregnant woman is thus rare.

Infection in the first trimester may cause fetal anomalies (growth retardation, anomalies of limbs and eyes, skin scarring).

The incubation period is 10–20 days and infection late in the last trimester will cause disseminated neonatal chickenpox in about 25% of cases; this can be a serious problem, with a mortality approaching 20%.

New antiviral drugs (e.g. acyclovir) have shown promise and more such agents may be expected in the future. Immune globulin has a place for both the susceptible mother and infant, although the occasion rarely arises in practice. Infants need to be isolated only if the mother has contracted the disease within 20 days of delivery.

Papilloma Virus Infection

The classical disorder associated with papilloma virus infection is condylomata acuminata — genital warts. These are found chiefly on the vulva (figure 6.2), where they may become very luxuriant, but they also occur on the cervix and vagina.

There appears little concern as far as the fetus or newborn is concerned, but treatment is usually advised because of the potential of the virus to cause malignant transformation of infected cells.

In pregnancy, the safest treatment is cryotherapy, but diathermy or surgical excision are alternatives. Coexisting infections of the vagina (e.g. with trichomonas vaginalis), should be treated, since the papilloma virus appears to flourish in a moist environment.

Acquired Immune Deficiency Syndrome (AIDS)

Although 95% of sufferers are male and often homosexuals and/or drug users, this disease may be acquired by the pregnant woman. The disease is transmitted by a viral agent.

The initial symptoms comprise prolonged fever, lymphadenopathy and weight loss. Because of an induced deficiency of cell-mediated immunity (e.g. T helper lymphocytes), the subject may fall prey to rare opportunistic infections (usually fungal or parasitic), and unusual types of cancer (e.g. Kaposi skin sarcoma).

Since the infection has an epidemiological pattern of spread similar to that of hepatitis B virus, similar precautions are suggested when dealing with suspected sufferers.

At the moment there is no effective means of treatment of the underlying immunological deficiency.

Other Viral Infections

Influenza is common and can cause a troublesome maternal pneumonia requiring hospitalization; fetal anomalies have been suggested, but must be very uncommon.

Measles is rare in the adult, but major secondary bacterial infection can predispose to abortion/premature labour.

Enteroviruses. *Poliomyelitis* is rare because of vaccination. *Echo* and *Coxsackie* virus infections can cause encephalitis/myocarditis in both mother and baby; the best preventive measures are maintenance of a good standard of personal hygiene and avoidance of viral hot spots (e.g. crowded swimming pools etc).

PROTOZOAL INFECTIONS

Toxoplasmosis

Toxoplasma gondii is a protozoa, the cat being primary host and man an intermediate host. Trophozoites in the acute stage pass to the tissue to form cysts which remain viable, and oocysts are passed in the cat's faeces. The human is infected by handling the infected cat or its litter or eating vegetables etc contaminated by it; other domestic animals may have cysts in muscle tissue and so eating poorly-cooked meat is another source of infection.

Incidence. The amount of infection in the community depends largely on the latter's predilection for cats and rare meat; as assessed by positive serology it ranges from 20–40%. *Approximately 1 in 200 to 1 in 500 women are infected during pregnancy* and the fetus will be secondarily infected (by placental transfer) in nearly 50% of these.

Clinical features and diagnosis. Mother. The majority of infections in the adult are either subclinical or only mildly disturbing. Low-grade fever and lymphadenopathy are prominent, while fatigue, headache, rash, splenic enlargement, and chorioretinitis are less common. The diagnosis may be suspected on the basis of the above; a positive immunofluorescence IgM titre or a significant (4-fold) rise in complement fixing or IF-IgG titre is diagnostic.

Infant. The constellation of abnormalities is similar to that described for the other TORCH infections. However, CNS damage is usually prominent (hydrocephalus, encephalomyelitis), with calcification a late result; the infection is responsible for about a third of all cases of chorioretinitis. *It is thus a significant factor in the causation of mental retardation and blindness.* Abortion is usually the result of first trimester infection; occasionally, recurrent abortion may be caused by longstanding encysted organisms in the endometrium. Stillbirth and prematurity are other possible outcomes.

The *diagnosis* can be confirmed by a positive IF-IgM titre. Unfortunately, the majority of infections are subclinical and some 50% of these will produce serious neurological sequelae.

Prophylaxis. Pregnant women should be warned of the possible danger of handling cats and their litter, the need for hand washing before food handling and meals, and the importance of eating only well-cooked meat. If a suspected infection in the first trimester is confirmed by antibody testing, consideration may be given to therapeutic abortion, but unlike rubella and other viral diseases, therapy is available and this is the course usually advised. In some centres, antenatal women are screened for antibodies to T. gondii and if this is positive, the infant is tested with a specific IgM serum.

Therapy. The traditional treatment is pyrimethamine 25 mg and sulphadiazine 3 g, each daily for 21–28 days, together with folic acid 5 mg/day; co-trimoxazole (2 tablets daily), clindamycin (600 mg twice daily), and spiramycin (2 g daily) are alternatives. The infant is given 0.6 mg/kd/d pyrimethamine and 75 mg/kg/d triple sulpha.

Malaria

Malaria is transmitted by its vector, the anopheles mosquito. When an infected subject is bitten, the mosquito becomes parasitized; the sexual cycle occurs in the stomach of the mosquito and it is in this form that the cycle is repeated when a fresh subject is bitten, the parasites being injected into the blood stream from the mosquito's saliva. Following an initial cycle in the liver, the parasite (*Plasmodium falciparum/vivax/malariae*) attacks the subject's red blood cells, causing haemolysis and anaemia. Pregnant women have both an increased prevalence of the disease and the parasitaemia is greater, presumably due to immune depression.

Incidence. This varies very widely: the disease is endemic in many underdeveloped tropical and subtropical countries.

Clinical features and diagnosis. The *incubation period* ranges from 10–30 days. The picture depends on the immunity of the woman and the type of parasite involved — it ranges from a barely perceived chronic anaemia to a life-threatening haemolytic-type crisis. Abortion/stillbirth/low birth-weight may all complicate malaria in pregnancy. Because of the placental barrier, malaria is only rarely passed from mother to the fetus — usually during an initial attack.

The most characteristic feature of the disorder is the *fever, which recurs* every 2–4 days and is due to parasites maturing in the blood. Central nervous system symptoms often predominate — headache, irritability, even delirium, convulsions and coma. Malaise, backache, muscle and joint pain, pyrexia and sweating are common. In the chronic state, splenic enlargement and hypersplenism, as well as jaundice are often seen. Both acute and chronic forms of renal failure may occur. The anaemia is due to destruction of red cells by the malarial parasites, depression of erythroporesis, immune (complement mediated) haemolysis, and sometimes secondary folic acid deficiency. The maternal side of the placenta is often packed with parasite-containing red blood cells and macrophages.

The fetus is relatively protectd by a higher haemoglobin F level — average levels of parasitization are 3–5%, compared with maternal levels of 20–30%.

The *diagnosis* is made from microscopy of the blood film, the malarial parasites being shown by special staining techniques (Leishman, Giemsa). The placenta may be so intensely parasitized that it appears black from the malarial pigment.

Management. Prophylaxis. Chloroquine (300 mg base weekly) and proguanil (100–200 mg daily) are both satisfactory, since they are safe for the fetus. In areas where the parasite is resistant to chloroquine, one usually must resort to slightly more toxic drugs such as dapsone/pyrimethamine/(Maloprim) or sulfadoxine/pyrimethamine/(Fansidar). (A loading dose of 2 tablets is taken before entry to the malarious district, then 1 tablet weekly); a folinic acid supplement (folic acid 5 mg/day) is advisable if therapy is given in the first trimester. Pregnant women should preferably avoid such areas in early pregnancy.

When leaving a malarial district, primaquine, 15 mg/day is taken for 2 weeks to eradicate exoerthrocyte forms of the parasite (this drug is contraindicated in patients with glucose-6-phosphate dehydrogenase deficiency, since it causes haemolysis of their red cells; it is not generally advised in pregnancy).

Therapy. Many of the compounds mentioned above are administered as therapy. In acute and dangerous infections, chloroquine or quinine may need to be given intravenously, together with supporting treatment. For vivax infections and sensitive falciparum ones also, oral chloroquine is given in a dose of 600 mg, then 300 mg daily for 2–4 days. For chloroquine resistant falciparum strains, quinine is given — 600 mg tds for 7 days, combined with Fansidar, 2–3 tablets on or about treatment day 3.

Trypanosomiasis

This tropical disease is spread by the Tse-tse fly. There are several forms — *Trypanosoma brucei* (after Sir David Bruce) and *Trypanosoma cruzi* (after Carlos Chagas).

Trypanosomes can pass the placental barrier and infect the fetus, causing abortion, stillbirth, growth retardation and premature labour. The placenta is often quite large.

Helminthic Infections

Infection with the different worms that form this group (ascaris, enterobiasis, trichuriasis, strongyloidiasis, hookworm) is largely confined to tropical and subtropical areas and is contributed to by casual hygiene and/or living in close relationship to animal vectors.

Diagnosis of gastrointestinal helminthiasis is based on identification of eggs and/or worms or segments thereof in the faeces; occasionally, more specialized techniques (serology, sigmoidoscopy, radiography) may be required.

Management involves accurate diagnosis and appropriate chemotherapy. New agents are being developed rapidly, and the safest and most effective drug should be administered. Often general hygiene counselling is necessary, as well as treatment of other infected close associates.

Giardiasis

This parasitic disease is now relatively common. The upper small gut is mainly involved, causing abdominal pain/discomfort, nausea, anorexia, and diarrhoea (often bulky and malodorous). Tinidazole (4 × 500 mg tablets) is usually curative.

Amoebiasis

This, like the above, is endemic in many countries and may infect the temporary resident to such areas; it has been linked to male homosexual activity ('gay bowel syndrome'). In the usual infection, the liver is involved, often with abscess formation. Liver scan, and perhaps needle biopsy, may be needed to confirm the diagnosis. The causative organism is the Entamoeba histolytica.

Metronidazole is given in a dose of 600 mg orally per day for 7 days; if there is abscess formation, treatment may need to be continued for 3–6 weeks.

MEDICAL AND SURGICAL DISORDERS OF PREGNANCY

chapter twenty-eight

The Psyche

And such a want-wit sadness makes of me
That I have much ado to know myself.
Shakespeare

OVERVIEW

It is understandable that pregnancy — a major life event and one associated with significant physiological adaptations — is likely to engender profound psychological responses.

Many factors will determine the *success of the adaptation* of the woman (and her partner) to this event. Important among these are basic personality type, parenting strength, acceptance of the pregnancy and social support.

During the pregnancy the couple's *affiliative response to the fetus* progressively increases. This is stimulated particularly by *fetal movement*, which is the major form of communication in the antenatal period, but *visualization of the fetus* (e.g. at the time of ultrasound) often has a major effect. *The revelation comes at birth* and during the puerperium; the baby's identity is perceived and the process of bonding occurs.

In most couples, *anxiety* is heightened during pregnancy — partly from fears known and partly from fears unknown. There is above all a *concern for the well-being* and *normality of the child* and to this is added concerns regarding the *pain and difficulty of labour*.

Maladaptation may occur because of a brittle personality, poor acceptance of the pregnancy, lack of support, or an abnormal number or severity of stress factors.

The attendant should be on the lookout for early breakdown so that preventive therapy can be given.

The psychodynamics of pregnancy loss and the therapeutic measures to help the couple in this situation should be appreciated.

Psychiatric disorders. There is a significant grey area in what is regarded as a physiological response (e.g. 'postpartum blues') and psychiatric decompensation. *Approximately 1% of patients have significant psychiatric illness during pregnancy or the puerperium* (table 28.3). It is probable that personality disorder is the soil in which frank psychoneurosis grows; i.e. the obsessional or dependent personality is likely to develop anxiety with the stress of pregnancy, labour, and early child care. The *psychoses* (schizophrenia, mania, depression) are relatively rare, but because the patient often loses touch with reality, she is unable to care either for herself or for the child. Such patients must be referred immediately for specialist psychiatric opinion and appropriate care since there is a 3–6% risk of suicide.

Introduction

Emotion has been defined as a complex behavioural response with physiological and psychological components. Common examples of *positive emotions* are pleasure, elation, and love; *negative emotions* are fear, anxiety, and embarrassment: in the human, love and fear are the 2 dominant emotions. The *physiological component* is related to the autonomic nervous system and is revealed by changes in blood vessels (blushing), glands (crying), smooth or cardiac muscle (diarrhoea, palpitations). The *psychological component* is usually reflected in the patient's mood and may be positive (organizing, energizing) or negative (disorganizing, paralyzing).

In general, if the emotional experience is frightening, *sympathetic activity* predominates (heart and respiratory rates rise, sphincters tighten, and visceral activity slows); if pleasant, *parasympathetic activity* predominates and the reverse occurs. Paradoxically, things which are visually shocking (violence, brutality, blood spilling) also heighten parasympathetic tone, even to the point of causing the viewer to faint.

Emotional maturity. This is reflected by the ability to withstand frustration and pain, and to tolerate anxiety and depression. It comes partly with age and partly as a result of innate personality.

Personality

The *coping ability* of the patient is the other part of the stress equation.

A brief history will usually elicit how the patient has dealt with life's different challenges — illness, schooling, work, family discord and separations, rejections etc. To facilitate communication, it is helpful to have a general idea of school achievement and other education, and interest in health matters.

General personality factors. In very few people do we see in harmonious proportion all the attributes that make up the well adjusted personality. However, in most the accents are acceptable and compatible with satisfactory interpersonal functioning. In the remainder, a particular trait is developed to the point of caricature, and often influences the person's relationships and attitudes to pregnancy and child rearing. The terms personality or character disorder may be applied; this usually implies a deeply ingrained maladaptive pattern of behaviour; an inflexibility of mental mechanisms, inability to adapt, difficulty in assessing the environment objectively (including the needs and behaviour of others). Personality types encountered frequently in clinical practice include the following. (i) *Over-dependent*: finds it difficult to stand alone or make major decisions; depends heavily on her immediate social environment and, in the context of obstetrics, this includes the doctor, nurse, and social worker. (ii) *Obsessional*: undue importance is attached to a particular facet of daily life and inordinate trouble is taken over it. If the obsession is related to body image or tidiness in the home, pregnancy and its aftermath will cause untoward stresses in adaptation. (iii) *Rigid*: there are fixed ideas about how things should be done and, like the obsessional person, finds it difficult to make adaptive changes. (iv) *Cold, withdrawn*: unable to demonstrate warmth or affection; the maternal instinct is poorly developed and the patient finds interpersonal relationships difficult. (v) *Narcissistic*: in love with their own body image, frequently admiring themselves in the mirror. Pregnancy, with its alterations to contour and ectodermal textures, is often seen as an ugliness, and subconsciously rejected. (vi) *Aggressive*: sullenness of manner or abusiveness of speech. In some cases, this may be more a reactive change — for example, to an unwanted pregnancy or a serious problem in the baby, rather than a matter of personality or disposition.

Other factors that may influence childbearing and rearing include caring strength (in a caring occupation, keeps pets), maternal strength (desire for pregnancy, early attachment to the baby, natural birth, breast feeding), anxiety level, upset level, prevailing mood, depressive episodes, comfort in sexual role, and ease of communication.

Support figures are important adjuncts to personal coping ability and include partner, family, and friends. When enquiring about such factors a suitable phraseology is adopted: e.g. 'In times of difficulty, who are you able to turn to and rely upon for help?'

Cultural 'separation' should be assessed. A history should be taken to include past and present drug abuse. *Drug addiction* is defined as a periodic or chronic addiction that is detrimental to the individual and often to society. In addition to the compulsion to take the drug is the tendency to obtain it by any available means. The fetus often suffers directly from the agent, and also from the neglect by the active addict.

PSYCHOLOGICAL ADAPTATIONS TO PREGNANCY

Significance of the Pregnancy

There is a wide spectrum — from the greatest imaginable joy (following prolonged infertility) to darkest despair (pregnancy totally unwanted). With relatively efficient contraception now available, negative reactions are far fewer in number. In most women, pregnancy is welcomed. In some the motive for the pregnancy may not be directly related to maternal instincts and is used as a means to another end, sometimes subconsciously — e.g. to get away from the family, to trap a mate, to enchance self image etc.

Those negative feelings which are experienced, are usually related to inconveniences resulting from the pregnancy (affecting career, home accommodation, finances, social activity) and normally dissipate during the second trimester.

Also at this time, in normal couples, there is a deepening of affection and concern of each partner as romantic love receives an added dimension as the couple join in concern for the development and well-being of the fetus.

Rejection of the pregnancy may be total. This may be due to a basic nonmaternal attitude or because a seemingly impossible situation has arisen in terms of other life goals. The woman may seek a solution in abortion, or adoption after completion of the pregnancy.

Affiliative Response to the Fetus

Progressively, over the second and third trimesters of pregnancy, the mother comes to identify with her baby. Often the stimulus for this is the beginning of *fetal movements*, but it may occur earlier if she is able to *visualize the fetus* at the time of ultrasonography (e.g. for early pregnancy bleeding), hear the heartbeat on the Doppler instrument, or see pictures of early fetal life in a pregnancy atlas.

The personalization of the baby may involve a variety of aspects — appearance (relation to one or other parent, previous children), normality, sex, place in life, names etc. Subconscious anxieties may be revealed in disturbing dreams and fantasies.

Associate Responses

As the mother takes more and more interest in the developing baby, she tends to narrow other interests. This probably parallels the nesting phenomenon, the mother's activities being devoted to the preparation for birth and future care of the baby. She often becomes more passive, and depends to a greater degree on such supporting figures as her partner, parent(s), and medical attendants.

In some 50% of patients there is an increased lability of mood: this may be related to fatigue or one of the many other metabolic/physiological changes taking place.

Sexual response gradually diminishes in most pregnant women: usually there is a decrease in libido, and this is often added to by concerns for fetal well-being.

Reactions to Labour

Labour and delivery are the major hurdles in the eye of most pregnant women. Problems of pain, trauma, and coping with the physical effort all loom increasingly large as term approaches. Immediately beyond is the new individual — the baby — who will be largely her responsibility; subconsciously at least, there will be anxieties regarding normality — of appearance and behaviour.

Antenatal education has achieved much in allaying fears, and strengthening coping ability; many women experience a feeling of great pleasure, perhaps exhiliaration, even during the labour. The obstetrician is now sharing many of the fears that were formerly largely shouldered by the mother; in 15% or more of mothers the labour will end in Caesarean section or this procedure will be carried out electively.

Reality-Based Identity of the Newborn

With delivery, the 9 months of gestation reach a climax and fantasy becomes fact — the baby's appearance, behaviour, and sex are revealed. The astute observer will look for such favourable reactions as eye contact, smiles of joy and acceptance, love, and commencement of breast feeding. In some patients, as with the pregnancy itself, acceptance is not immediate, and, in rare cases, will never occur (parental instinct (maternal/paternal) may be low, the child unattractive, of the wrong sex, fretful and crying, ill-formed or suffering from some other disorder). Usually, however, parental solicitude takes over and the totally dependent baby becomes accepted. In some parents oversolicitousness results — this may be to counteract repressed feelings that the child should be rejected.

THE STRESSES AND ANXIETIES OF PREGNANCY

Although stress and anxiety form an inevitable component of living, some individuals, by virtue of their personal make-up, attract trouble and/or are less able to cope when trouble occurs. Again, others are unfortunate to encounter more than their fair share.

The *father's response* usually mirrors that of the mother, the couple achieving a new level of relatedness to each other, sharing feelings, fantasies, anxieties, and hopes. The partner may experience significant emotional changes; couvade symptoms (anorexia, nausea, vomiting, indigestion, aches and pains, faintness, headache) may occur in 20% or more. Modifying factors will be his relationship with his own parents, previous children and parenting knowledge, relationship with his wife, and basic personality (including psychosexual aspects). After the child is born, there may be ambivalent feelings engendered particularly by the strong affectional bond between the mother and baby and the focusing of her emotional and physical resources onto the latter.

It is helpful to ascertain the stress load in each patient attending for antenatal care, since helpful therapeutic assistance can usually be provided.

Many 'stress tables' have been published, with weighting being given for a variable number of stresses likely to be encountered. Although such detail is probably not helpful, a general check list is given (table 28.1) that can quickly be run through.

TABLE 28.1 STRESS AND ANXIETIES IN PREGNANCY

Past Medical History
   Infertility
   Termination of pregnancy
   Obstetrical problems in pregnancy
   Significant family history
   Genetic/inherited problems

Social
   Feelings of inadequacy
   Single parent. Present partner not the father of the child
   Dependent or sick relatives
   Poor supporting family network
   Marital dysfunction (e.g. infidelity)
   Interpersonal conflicts
   Problems related to finance, housing, career
   Drug addiction

Current Medical
   Pregnancy unplanned/not wanted
   Obstetrical complication (minor/major disorders)
   Medical/surgical complication(s)
   Separations from family (e.g. in hospital)

Rational/Irrational Fears
   Normality of reproductive organs
   Normality of baby (malformed, too large, dead)
   Loss of figure, attractiveness
   Labour, delivery (pain)
   Haemorrhage, dying
   General ability to cope

Maladaptation

The problems arising from psychological maladaptation to pregnancy are less well researched and recognized than those related to their physical counterpart. Obtaining basic stress and personality profiles will point to patients at risk and closer supervision should be given to these.

Manifestations include anxiety, fear, nervousness, guilt, rejection, irritability, interpersonal difficulties, abnormal down-turn of libido, abnormal increase in dependence, and morbid introspection.

The maladaptation may occur at one or more of the pregnancy maturational steps previously outlined; it may only appear after the mother has left hospital with her baby.

The Unsuccessful Pregnancy

An unfortunate truth of reproduction is that there is an *appreciable wastage*: of each 1,000 pregnancies, 100–150 will end in a clinically recognizable abortion and a further 10–50 in perinatal death. In a minority of these the pregnancy may not have been wanted, but in the remainder the loss is strongly felt by the couple, particularly the mother, since it is a part of herself that has died.

With abortions, at least those in the first trimester, there is often no recognizable fetus; later in pregnancy, the couple may be faced with the unsettling appearance of maceration or malformation. The woman suffering a stillbirth faces the paradox of coexisting birth and death; when there is a major malformation in addition, there is the added conflict of horror and perhaps revulsion combined with natural love and attachment. The depth of the upset will depend on such factors as the 'value' of the pregnancy, normality of the fetus/baby, number of other children and so on.

There are other disappointments not directly related to the baby — e.g. loss of a partner, failure of labour (resulting in an operative delivery), baby the wrong sex, failure to breast-feed etc.

In the *acute grief reaction* that usually follows pregnancy loss, there are a number of typical symptoms: shock, disbelief, emptiness, depression, sense of failure, frustration, anger, guilt; there may be accompanying psychosomatic dysfunctions such as insomnia and anorexia. There may be reemergence of long forgotten loss reactions experienced in childhood.

In the *management* of such patients there are a number of basic principles. (i) The *couple should be together when told of the problem* and this should be done promptly after diagnosis. Although some malformations are visually very upsetting (e.g. cleft lip and palate), the couple should be reassured where possible regarding surgical possibilities, and shown results of treatment of other children (colour plates 111 and 112). (ii) The attendant should appreciate the need for the *grieving process* to occur and should coordinate the efforts of those caring for the pregnancy to facilitate this. (iii) Full explanations should be given, since this shortens the grief period. (iv) It is usually preferable for the couple to have as *tangible a memory of the fetus/ baby as possible* and thus should be allowed to see, handle (and photograph if this is desired) stillborn babies, and be present at the terminal phase of life of the neonate; it is beneficial for a *name* to be given to the baby. (v) *Assistance* will be needed to facilitate documentation, funeral, and other arrangements. (vi) The psychological state of the couple can be helped by simple planning measures such as area of hospital domicile, early discharge, handling enquiries (often a spokesperson is helpful until the couple have sufficiently recovered), handling siblings (nature of explanation, attendance at the funeral etc). (vii) Discussion of autopsy and other investigative findings and prognosis for the future. (viii) Lactation suppression. (ix) Monitoring of progress over the next 6–9 months and provision of adequate contraception during this time. Thereafter, it is likely that grief will have run its course and a healthy perspective will have returned. Persisting negative feelings (guilt, shame, anger, depression, fear) are a danger signal indicating the need for psychiatric help. In the case of malformed or retarded children, the attendant should try and ascertain the couple's attitudes to the child — whether loving and supportive, inadequate, unhappy, or even wishing it dead. (x) In the pregnancy that follows a perinatal death, a greater than normal sensitivity, counselling, and care is needed; this will need to extend well into the puerperium.

THE PSYCHONEUROSES

There is no unanimity as to whether the neuroses stand alone as a psychopathological group or form a continuum with personality and behavioural disorders on the one hand and mild psychotic states on the other. Conditions usually grouped under this heading include anxiety states, situational depression, obsessional/manic behaviour, and hysterical states. *Drug and alcohol abuse* are usually special facets of personality disorder.

Neurotic disorders occur in *8–16% of pregnancies* and are usually manifest in the first trimester and in the puerperium.

In contradistinction to the frank psychoses, the patient is *in touch with reality* and usually realizes that the behaviour is bizarre and/or irrelevant.

The psychoneurotic patient may have problems in pregnancy because of the extra stress and anxiety involved and the intrusion of the baby may conflict with such obsessions as slimness of figure, tidiness of the home etc. Depression is usually reactive in nature; it may be related to the pregnancy (abortion, stillbirth, malformation) or to something outside. Manic tendencies tend to settle in pregnancy, but may surface after delivery. Hysterical reactions are uncommon. *The incidence of psychoneurotic disturbance in pregnancy ranges from 3–6%*, depending on criteria, population group etc. Vulnerable periods are the first trimester (difficulties of pregnancy acceptance) and the puerperium (major psychobiological adaptation).

Therapeutic Measures

Education. A typical syllabus for antenatal education is given in Appendix I. This will cover general aspects of pregnancy, labour, and the puerperium and will do much to dispel misconceptions and relieve anxieties. The couple will be greatly helped by such preparation, sharing in the labour, birth, and child rearing. The mother should be careful to avoid letting the infant *totally intrude into her life and endanger the marital relationship.*

Although major attention is directed to the mother, it should be remembered that the father may become psychologically dysfunctional and require therapy.

Identification. Specific enquiry should be made as to appropriateness of the mother's adaptational responses — i.e. is the pregnancy accepted, is the personalization process normal, is the baby accepted after birth etc. The mother's initial anxieties should settle in the second trimester, and with stabilization, her drive should increase in order to organize for the birth and beyond.

Insight therapy. A reluctance to discuss pregnancy and labour may be a clue to the existence of false beliefs: the patient is unwilling to talk because she is afraid that the doctor may confirm her worst fears. Some patients need reorientation in relation to such false or exaggerated beliefs — not only regarding the pregnancy, but also other areas of concern that may have become magnified out of all proportion. Problems that remain can then be tackled realistically, and immediate, intermediate and long-term goals suggested.

Behaviour therapy. Some patients maintain a high anxiety state, despite education and insight therapy.

There are a number of techniques of *relaxation therapy* which can be offered. Most depend on the patient settling into a comfortable position and relaxing maximally with each expiration ('letting the tension flow out of the body'). This may be preceded by sequential contraction of individual muscle groups for 5 seconds to heighten the relaxation effect. The patient should imagine that she is in the most relaxing environment — in a bubble bath, on a billowing cloud, a warm, soft, sandy beach etc. *Practical coping techniques.* Simple measures to improve efficiency may make the difference between staying on top, in psychological terms, or going under. The patient should be encouraged to make simple priority lists, delete/defer/delegate when appropriate, and halt unnecessary demands; the husband may need reorientation in relation to assistance with home activities.

Assistance. The network of family and friends should be invited to help where appropriate, and beyond this, formal social or other services may need to be tapped. This will complement the reassurance and support of the medical team.

Drug therapy. The temporary use of a sedative drug such as a benzodiazepine (e.g. diazepam) may be helpful; if sympathetic overactivity is predominant a beta-adrenergic blocker is indicated.

Expert opinion. If signs of early psychological breakdown are evident, referral for specialist opinion is indicated.

PSYCHIATRIC DISORDERS

Although there is undoubtedly a continuum in some people from personality aberration to frank psychosis, it is convenient to discuss psychiatric disorders in major subgroups. One must accept the empiric approach to diagnosis and treatment until the true biological basis of the different mental illnesses is unravelled.

Terms and Definitions

Obsession: a thought or urge that intensely and persistently intrudes into consciousness even though the patient, when it occurs, realizes that it is senseless or at least that it is dominating and persisting without cause.

Compulsion: an irresistible need to perform a certain act.

Delusion: a false unshakeable belief, out of keeping with the social and cultural background.

Hallucination: a sensory perception for which there is no appropriate external source (e.g. hearing voices).

Fantasy: a product of an unrestrained imagination (e.g. a daydream, a vivid mental image, a personally constructed set of concepts).

Illusion: a misperception of some real object or situation (e.g. optical illusion).

THE PSYCHOSES

Types of Disorder

Schizophrenia. It is probable that schizophrenia ('split mind') is a syndrome, rather than an entity, comprising several related disorders. It is more easily described by the frequency of features which may be observed. *Dominant features*

are thought disorder and lack of insight, hallucinations and delusions, flatness of affect (mood response to a situation), and catatonic motor behaviour. *Paranoid features* may predominate and will be evidenced by suspiciousness, feelings of persecution etc; if *affective features* predominate, major mood changes will be present i.e. elation or depression.

Mania. This is basically an expression of uncontrolled mental and psychological overactivity — i.e. the accelerator has jammed. It is seen more often in the cyclothymic type of personality. With progress of the disorder, the observed features become progressively more aberrant.

The early stages are characterized by mood elation, together with increased speech and physical activity (restlessness, insomnia). There may be expansory behaviour or ideas (e.g. overspending) or increased activity (e.g. of a sexual or religious nature). With progress, there are mood swings to irritability/hostility and depression, from the former prevailing euphoria. As anger increases, judgement decreases, and delusions and disordered thinking may enter the picture; overactivity is still a feature, however.

Depression. This is the other major morbid mood change. It may exist alone (unipolar) or as a partial feature of manic-depressive illness (bipolar). Manic-depressive illness tends to develop more rapidly than schizophrenia. The major features of psychotic depression are summarized in table 28.2, and are compared with those in neurotic depression. Vegetative features referred to in table 28.2 include anorexia, weight loss, decreased libido, palpitation, constipation and insomnia in the last one-third of sleep.

Depression may sometimes be masked in a cloak of hypochondriasis, other anxiety or

TABLE 28.2   DIFFERENTIATING FEATURES OF NEUROTIC AND PSYCHOTIC DEPRESSION

Feature	Neurotic	Psychotic
Age	Peaks at 25 years	Middle age
Precipitating stress	+	+ / –
Vegetative symptoms	–	+
Guilt feelings	–	+
Diurnal pattern	–	+
Sleep disturbance	First 1/3	Last 1/3
Delusional ideas, hallucinations	–	+
Anxiety	+	+
Agitation	+ / –	+
Retardation	–	+
Mood	Unhappy	Despair
Anergy	–	+
Suicidal thought	–	+
Illness duration > 1 month	+ / –	+

behaviour aberration (e.g. alcoholism). *Suicidal risk is highest in this group.*

Organic disease. Intracranial disorders (primary and secondary neoplasm, infection, trauma, vascular abnormality) may present as an acute or chronic psychosis. Prominent features include confusion, defects in intellect, and personality change. *Focal signs* should be looked for: amnesia (memory loss), asphasia (language disturbance), agnosia (perceptual defect), apraxia (disordered higher motor function) and epilepsy.

Toxic and confusional states. The patient is disorientated in time and/or space, and is often restless, not fully alert to her surroundings, sleepless and disinterested in the child. The disturbance may occur as a complication of such conditions as severe preeclampsia/eclampsia, infection, metabolic disease, prolonged and poorly managed labour, and injudicious use of drugs.

Aetiology

The basic disorder in psychotic mental illness is still not clearly understood. Its predilection for the puerperium suggests that the major endocrine/metabolic changes occurring at this time may be superadded to a genetic predisposition; there are, in addition, significant psychological stresses at this time in adapting to the baby and its demands. It is simpler to talk of risk factors for the pregnant woman. These are family and/or personal history of mental disorder, poor parental relationship, previous pregnancy breakdown, unresolved conflicts (oedipal, pregnancy acceptance, marital), poor personality integration, major childbearing disappointment, major obstetrical complication, difficult baby (fretful, feed-refusing). Less important, but additional problems include poor family/social/cultural support, career conflict, economic problems, heavy smoking, and drug addiction.

Incidence

The range is 0.2–0.8% of pregnancies. In 35–45% of patients the breakdown occurs predominantly or solely in the puerperium: in approximately 50% of these, the disorder appears after the patient has left hospital. Previously psychotic patients are less likely to marry, and if they do, the break-up rate is higher.

Nature of disorder

Most breakdowns are schizophrenic in type, usually with a major affective component (depression); catatonic and paranoid features may predominate. The mother will display disturbance of thinking and emotional reaction; she will complain of intrusion of abnormal thoughts and it will be apparent that she has lost the ability to concentrate and organize. This leads to lack of concern and later neglect of both herself and the baby.

Depression is often a component of a basic schizophrenic illness, but may represent major mood morbidity — as part of a unipolar or bipolar (manic depressive) illness. The appearance is often later — initial symptoms 2–3 weeks after the birth and the full-blown picture at about 4–6 weeks. Differentiation should be made from depression due to drugs and organic change. The picture of the mother is one of major depression, exhaustion, self-accusation, insomnia, food refusal, and feelings of futility. The mother is unable to discuss the future; she will express feelings of failure as a mother and perhaps suicidal thought. She may misperceive her child as abnormal. There is again a picture of neglect and noncoping.

Manic features may be expressed in hyperactive behaviour, which usually commences in the first puerperal week and peaks a week or so later. The patient is often agitated and exhibits excessive motor activity, confusion, and flight of ideas which may often be accompanied by delusions and hallucinations. The picture can be usually differentiated from that of the schizophrenic — stilted, colder, and perseverative.

Suicide. This accounts for 1–2% of all female deaths and approximately 4% of maternal deaths (18 out of 427 maternal deaths in the most recent national survey; table 14.2). The risk is higher if the patient has received poor mothering, there has been a previous suicide attempt by the patient or close relation/friend, there is poor social support or hostility to important life figures, age <20, drug addiction, and poor impulse control. Unsuccessful attempts are far more common, chiefly in teenagers; these usually represent an impulsive act following a dispute with, or rejection by one with whom they are emotionally involved. The method employed in these cases is usually an overdose of a hypnotic drug, in contrast to the often more violent measures adopted by psychotic patients. Accomplished suicide is usually felt to be the only answer to an uncontrollable situation. The risk is much lower if there are other children. *The overall risk is about 3–6% of patients with psychotic illness in pregnancy.*

Management

Early recognition and prevention. An adequate antenatal psychiatric history should be taken and risk factors noted. Patients who are at higher risk should then be monitored carefully. Early warning signs (tired, unable to sleep, irritable, unable to do her work and cope, deteriorating relationship with husband) should prompt an immediate evaluation and referral for consultant opinion if progressing beyond reasonable reaction to pregnancy and other experiences.

Therapy. If a psychosis is present, management will usually be at specialist level, at least initially.

Drug treatment. There is now a wide range of antipsychotic preparations. *Chlorpromazine*, up to 500 mg/day, then decreasing to 250–350 mg/day is effective in the schizophrenic patient. For maintenance therapy (especially the non-complier), depot preparations are now available (e.g. fluphenazine enanthate). In depressed patients, a tricyclic preparation is commonly used (e.g. *amitriptyline* (Tryptanol)); it should be remembered that such preparations may take 2–3 weeks to be fully effective. Low dose *phenothiazines* are useful for the tension and anxiety which often occurs in the psychotically depressed patient. If manic features are present, drugs such as phenothiazines or haloperidol are useful in the acute phase. *Lithium carbonate* is of particular value as maintenance therapy in recurrent manic illness.

Care of the baby. The baby is usually in separate care in the initial stages; the degree of supervision required when the mother and baby are together will depend on the nature of the illness and its therapeutic control.

Social therapy and milieu manipulation will be required at a later stage.

Psychotherapy. This may take a number of forms — supportive, analytical, behavioural, conjoint family and group therapy.

Medical and *general supportive treatment* will be needed for toxic confusional states; antipsychotic drugs may be needed in some patients.

Prognosis

This will largely depend on the premorbid personality and past psychiatric history. Patients whose illness began before the age of 18, those with poor social integration, illness in a first degree relative, poor personality, low social class, and low IQ fare less well.

These features provide higher recurrence rates in subsequent pregnancies (30–40% versus 5–10%).

Infanticide is rare; the patient is usually subnormal or frankly psychotic and will often attempt or accomplish their own death. Infant rejection occurs in about 5% of patients.

FATIGUE

Fatigue deserves special mention, since it has a tendency to potentiate psychiatric or emotional disturbance. Many women are physically and mentally exhausted after labour and delivery. Often they have missed one or more nights of sleep, and usually they face the challenge of motherhood with anxiety and a painful perineum, particularly if they are primiparous. *This is why it is important for every patient to receive adequate analgesia and sedation in the early puerperium.*

TABLE 28.3   METHODS OF TREATMENT ACCORDING TO DIAGNOSES IN 321 PATIENTS WITH PSYCHIATRIC ILLNESS IN PREGNANCY

	Number	Treatment				
		Drugs	Psychiatrist	Electroconvulsive therapy	Admitted to mental institution	Other*
Depression	102 (39)	94	54	5	12	23
Schizophrenia	40 (29)	38	34	3	16	4
Anxiety/depression	38 (14)	33	17	2	2	11
Puerperal depression	38 (14)	31	27	3	11	7
Puerperal psychosis	36 (16)	34	29	5	16	8
Personality disorders	22 (15)	18	19	1	6	10
Anxiety	14 (6)	12	6	—	1	4
Hysteria	13 (6)	13	10	1	2	1
Manic depression	12 (7)	11	11	—	1	1
Drug addiction	6 (4)	2	2	1	2	3
Total	321 (150)	286	209	21	69	72

Figures in parentheses indicate the numbers of patients with a known past history of psychiatric illness

* Domiciliary sister, social worker, group therapy or infant welfare worker

PSYCHIATRIC ILLNESS IN A TEACHING HOSPITAL

For perspective, table 28.3 is included to show the diagnoses in 321 patients with psychiatric disorders seen in a series of 40,982 pregnancies, *an incidence of 0.8%*. In clinic patients the incidence was 1.8%, similar to that in the general population, and 3 times higher than that recorded in private patients (0.6%), who comprised 80% of this series. It is likely that the true incidence is much higher since details of a patient's psychiatric history are not always recorded in the hospital clinical notes.

In this series of 40,982 pregnancies there were 8 maternal deaths — one was a primipara found at home, drowned in a bath, 10 days after delivery of an infant who had died from multiple malformations. This case highlights the possible dangers of discharging patients who have been delivered of dead or deformed infants without careful assessment. Emotional disturbances are common enough during the puerperium even in mothers with normal living children and stable families. Ideally all patients who have suffered the disappointment of a perinatal death or malformed infant should be interviewed by a trained counsellor or consultant psychiatrist, especially if feelings of guilt or suicidal tendencies are suspected.

Of the 321 patients shown in table 28.3, there were *150 (46%) who had preexisting disease* which continued during pregnancy, 76 (23%) in whom symptoms *began during pregnancy*, and 95 (30%) who developed symptoms for the first time *after delivery*; 48 of these patients (15%) were considered to have *suicidal tendencies*. The onset of *puerperal psychiatric disease* was often insidious with the diagnosis not being made until the patient had returned home — the condition then being recognized by the domiciliary sister or general practitioner.

The *recurrence rate in subsequent pregnancies* was 26% (13 of 49) in patients who developed symptoms for the first time during pregnancy, and 41% (27 of 65) in those with the onset in the puerperium.

In this series almost all patients received *drug therapy* and 209 (65%) were seen by a *psychiatrist*; 69 patients were referred to a *psychiatric institution* and 21 received *electroconvulsive therapy* (table 28.3).

chapter twenty-nine

Nervous Disorders

OVERVIEW

Neurological disorders form a very diverse group in pregnancy and range from conditions which are largely of a nuisance to the patient (headache, compression neuropathy) to those which are immediately life-threatening (intracranial haemorrhage).

Seizure disorders (*epilepsy*) are relatively common (0.5% of pregnancies). They are important because of difficulties in drug management; this is partly due to the narrow therapeutic range of the common anticonvulsant, phenytoin, and partly due to alterations in blood levels resulting from the metabolic changes of pregnancy.

Intracranial haemorrhage is a major emergency. The bleeding may occur into the subarachnoid space from either a berry aneurysm or an arteriovenous malformation. Early neurological consultation is required in both conditions. *Intracerebral bleeding* is usually the penalty of uncontrolled hypertension and does not have the same prospects of cure as the former group.

Headache is a common symptom and in many patients will be migrainous in nature. Oral ergotamine preparations are not first line drugs in pregnancy, but can be prescribed for the more troublesome attack.

Pregnancy imposes problems in several other conditions. In *myasthenia gravis*, care must be taken with analgesia and anaesthesia to avoid serious respiratory depression; autoantibodies to the receptors for acetylcholine pass to the newborn in 10–20% of patients and careful supervision of the baby is necessary and possible neostigmine treatment also. *Paraplegics* are prone to urinary tract infection in pregnancy and during labour uncontrolled autonomic reflex activity may occur. Labour may be premature and, depending on the level of the lesion, painless; this creates problems in diagnosis, and such patients should be supervised closely during the last trimester with these problems in mind.

Pregnancy often has a deleterious effect on Von Recklinghausen disease. This condition is transmitted by a dominant gene and is characterized by multiple neurofibromas which may swell in pregnancy and cause pressure on vital structures.

Seizure Disorders (Epilepsy)

Seizures may be either *generalized or partial*. In the former group are the common tonic-clonic (grand mal) and the less common clonic (myoclonic) seizures, as well as the non-convulsive condition of brief absence (petit mal). Focal seizures may be motor, sensory or autonomic.

Diagnosis. Most patients with a seizure disorder will have been diagnosed before the pregnancy and may be receiving appropriate medication.

When the condition first develops during pregnancy, a careful general and neurological work-up is necessary to establish the diagnosis. Non-neurological conditions which may cause confusion include eclampsia, hypoxic attack, hyponatraemia, hypoglycaemia, tetany, and drug withdrawal.

Consultant opinion is usually desirable.

Behaviour in pregnancy. In the majority of patients there is no change or a decrease in the number of seizures. Those showing an increase (30–40%), usually have suboptimal levels of drug in the blood stream which is largely due to increased hepatic drug metabolism and increased blood volume in pregnancy.

Effect on pregnancy. There is a mild increase in a number of pregnancy complications, but this depends largely on the degree of control of the disease; if this is good, the pregnancy is virtually normal.

One of the major concerns is the *teratogenic effect of anticonvulsive drugs*. An increase of 2–3 times the normal rate is seen. With diphenylhydantoin, *craniofacial anomalies*, mental retardation, cardiac and limb defects have been described. Trimethadione and related drugs have been linked to a number of central nervous system and somatic anomalies. Less information is available on newer agents such as valproic acid (spinal deformity), carbamazepine (decreased fetal head growth with no catch up after birth), and clonazepam; reports to date indicate a cautious approach to prescribing.

Management. If the patient has been clinically clear for several years and wishes to become pregnant, medication should be withdrawn. During the *first trimester*, relatively safe drugs such as barbiturates or benzodiazepines should be used. *If specific anticonvulsive therapy is needed, control of drug dosage by means of blood levels is advisable.* Because such drugs have a low therapeutic index (i.e. a low toxicity ceiling) and are difficult to use, collaboration with a physician experienced with such therapy is indicated. Blood levels are usually checked every month.

Phenytoin is usually the drug of choice for intermittent seizures, the dose range usually being 300–400 mg/day. This should produce a blood level in the therapeutic range of 40–80 μmol/l (10–20 μg/ml): side-effects are mainly due to cerebellar dysfunction (ataxia, giddiness, nystagmus). If greater seizure control is needed, phenobarbitone is added to give a blood level 65–130 μmol/l (15–30 μg/ml). Parenteral therapy may be required if absorption is poor (e.g. vomiting, prolonged labour). Sodium valproate is effective in generalized epilepsy. The dose is 400–1,200 mg/day.

In the puerperium, plasma levels of anticonvulsant drugs tend to rise and overdosage may occur unless an adjustment is made.

For *petit mal*, ethosuximide, 250–500 mg tds or diazepam, 5–10 mg tds is given.

Status epilepticus is a medical emergency requiring immediate hospitalization and intravenous anticonvulsive therapy (10–20 mg of diazepam over 3–5 minutes or clonazepam 1 mg every 1–2 minutes until fitting is controlled or vital functions begin to be compromised. General measures described for eclampsia (Chapter 20) should be instituted.

Anticonvulsants may cause a depressed folate level in the mother and this should be checked; there may also be a depression of vitamin K-dependent clotting factors in the baby and this vitamin should be given soon after birth.

Breast feeding is usually permissible if the disease is satisfactorily controlled.

The *hereditary risk* of epilepsy in the offspring is increased 8–12 times normal.

Cerebrovascular Disease

(a) Subarachnoid Haemorrhage

This is a rare (0.2–0.5 in 1,000) but serious complication of pregnancy. *Arteriovenous malformations* are more likely to bleed in pregnancy because of the increase in size of the lesion. The patient is often less than 25 years of age. Bleeding may occur in the first half of pregnancy. *Aneurysms* related to the circle of Willis tend to present in patients over 30 years of age and bleeding usually occurs in late pregnancy. Hypertension and/or preeclampsia is a precipitating factor in both conditions.

The *diagnosis* is usually obvious (vomiting, severe headache and confusion leading to coma; meningism is usually marked and localizing signs are usually absent as are convulsions). CT scanning can be used to show blood in the cerebrospinal fluid and ventricles; alternatively, evenly blood-stained fluid will be revealed on lumbar puncture. Confusion may arise from meningitis, viral encephalitis, severe migraine, benign intracranial hypertension and intracranial tumour.

Management. Urgent neurological consultation is necessary to decide on the need for surgery (craniotomy and clipping etc under hypotension).

If the patient with haemorrhage from an intracranial aneurysm is undelivered and recovers, vaginal delivery under epidural analgesia and elective forceps is usually advised, unless other conditions indicate the need for Caesarean section. Oxytocics should be given only if necessary and oxytocin is preferable to ergometrine. The risk of recurrent bleeding is greater with vascular malformations and the Caesarean approach is usually preferred; sterilization was formerly advised, but many such lesions can now be handled by neurosurgery.

(b) Intracerebral Haemorrhage

This may complicate any condition where the blood pressure is significantly elevated — e.g. a diastolic pressure greater than 100. It usually occurs late in labour or in the early puerperium.

Since ergometrine preparations may cause a sudden rise in blood pressure, their use in the third stage is contraindicated in the hypertensive patient. Otherwise *prevention* is largely a matter of *control of preeclampsia and other hypertensive disorders* of pregnancy.

Neurosurgery has less to offer in this condition, and maternal death is more likely than with subarachnoid haemorrhage. *High dose steroids* and/or intravenous *mannitol* or glycerol may be lifesaving in some patients by reducing intracranial pressure.

The *clinical features* depend on the site and severity of the haemorrhage and will vary from a mild focal disturbance to rapid collapse and death. The patient requires specialist care.

(c) Cerebral Thrombosis

Thrombosis of one of the major *cortical sinuses* (usually the superior sagittal) is a very rare complication which usually occurs after delivery. Headache, major seizure, mono- or hemiparesis, paraplegia, and papilloedema are features that would suggest this condition.

Thrombosis of one of the *cerebral arteries or veins* is again uncommon. The picture is typical of the stroke which is more common in the postmenopausal age group. Occasionally, the thrombosis may complicate a coexisting medical condition such as thrombotic thrombocytopenic purpura.

Hemiplegia of various degrees of severity is almost universal in this group; there may be preceding paraesthesia, seizure or headache.

Headache

This is a relatively common symptom and may have an endocrine basis in some patients, since it may occur in relation to the menstrual cycle and oral contraceptive therapy.

Vascular. The classical vascular headache is migraine, the pain phase being due to vasodilatation which follows a period of vasoconstriction. Other causes of vascular headache include histamine release (cluster headache), toxins (alcohol, drugs, infections), hypoglycaemia, and hypertension.

The classical migraine attack is one which is preceded by an aura, usually visual. It is typically unilateral, often triggered by a known stress, and is often associated with irritability, nausea, and avoidance of bright light.

Treatment of migraine involves (i) *avoidance of trigger factors*, and a commonsense approach to diet (avoidance of hypoglycaemia and vasoactive foods); (ii) *prophylactic use* of propranolol (40–120 mg/day), cyproheptadine (4–12 mg/day); (iii) *early treatment of the attack* with an aspirin/codeine preparation and oral ergotamine tartrate (1–3 mg) or suppository (2 mg alone or with pentobarbitone and belladonna); (iv) if the attack is severe, parenteral therapy may be required — e.g. intramuscular dihydroergotamine, 0.5–1.0 mg and chlorpromazine, 25–50 mg.

Muscle contraction. This may be associated with arthritic changes in the cervical vertebrae, myostitis, and tension states.

Treatment is directed to the basic cause.

Miscellaneous. There are a large number of causes of headache not involving the above 2 major groups. Neurological consultation is advisable if the headache is persistent.

Paraplegia

This condition is becoming more frequent as a result of motor vehicle trauma. The spinal cord may be damaged in the cervical, thoracic, or lumbar regions, producing a range of paralysis and disability. The chief obstetrical problems are troublesome *urinary tract infection* (an indwelling catheter is usual), and *pressure damage during labour* (particularly at the base of the bladder) because of loss of sensation. Careful nursing will avoid both of these complications. *Disturbed autonomic reflex activity* due to sudden catecholamine release may occur when the lesion is in the upper thoracic or lower cervical regions. It is triggered by stimuli from the pelvic structures (full bladder, catheterization, contractions, examinations), and this may be associated with marked blood pressure fluctuations, cardiac irregularity, headache, flushes, sweating and nasal congestion. Labour is usually painless, and the patient must be taught to recognize its onset. It is likely to be premature when the lesion is above the level of T11. Since catgut sutures are poorly absorbed by paraplegics, nylon or fine delayed absorbable sutures (e.g. Vicryl 00) are preferred. Breast feeding is not contraindicated; the main problem is lack of mobility on the mother's part.

Multiple Sclerosis

In this disease there is loss of myelin on the central white matter of the nervous system. The disorder is characterized by a slow downhill course with exacerbations. It may present for the first time in pregnancy, and suspicious features include weakness, incoordination, visual disturbances and paraesthesias; dysuria may be present.

Pregnancy appears to unmask the disease in some women, but does not significantly aggravate it if preexisting; relapse is more common in the puerperium.

The main problem is coping with the patient's functional and psychological disturbances, as with paraplegia.

Myasthenia Gravis

In this rare disease the patient suffers from *weakness* and *fatiguability* of voluntary muscles (a curare-like disturbance of the neuromuscular junction). The disease is occasionally congenital, but more usually arises from the third decade on. It is due, at least in part, to the formation of autoantibodies to the receptors of the neurotransmitter, acetylcholine. There is no particular trend of the disease in pregnancy — almost equal numbers exacerbate, remain unchanged, and remit. There is an increased incidence of prematurity and fetal growth retardation.

Treatment consists of pyridostigmine or a similar drug, the usual dose being 15 mg 3–4 times per day. Prednisone may be required in some patients, usually as a high dose bolus every second day. From a practical viewpoint, these patients are more *susceptible to sedatives and narcotics* which must be given first as a test dose (about 25% of the normal dose) and if there is no undue reaction, a 50% dose may be given at desired intervals. A close watch must be kept for deterioration in labour; the second stage should be assisted with forceps or vacuum extraction. Inhalational anaesthesia (ether, halothane), magnesium salts, aminoglycoside antibiotics (e.g. gentamicin) and beta blockers (propranolol) are contraindicated as all may exacerbate the myasthenia; epidural analgesia, however, may be used with safety. Breast feeding may be attempted, but the patient often finds this tiring; anticholinesterase drugs taken by the mother are secreted into breast milk.

In 10–20% of patients, the baby has *neonatal myasthenia* in the first few weeks after birth due to transplacental transfer of maternal IgG autoantibodies and this may require temporary treatment to offset lethargy and difficulties with feeding and respiration.

Peripheral Nerve Disorders

(i) *Compression neuropathies.* The fluid retention and oedema of pregnancy may cause symptoms of peripheral neuritis (tingling and paraesthesia). The median nerve at the wrist and the lateral cutaneous nerve of the thigh are chiefly affected, since they both pass through fibrous tunnels. The *carpal tunnel syndrome (median nerve)* affects the radial half of the hand and is more common and troublesome; it is treated by a diuretic or vasodilator drug, together with splinting; hydrocortisone injected into the retinaculum, is often effective. The patient should refrain from sleeping on the affected side, if the condition is unilateral. Improvement is usually dramatic after delivery, but if symptoms persist, operation to free the nerve may be required. The *lateral cutaneous nerve of the thigh* is compressed as it passes under the inguinal ligament or through the fascia lata of the thigh. It has only a sensory distribution, and the effects are limited to paraesthesias and pain in the nerve distribution. Less common neuropathies are those of the obturator and peroneal nerves. The *lumbosacral* nerve trunk may be affected by stretching, or compression (either by the baby's head or a forceps blade) as it lies in front of the wing of the sacrum. *Sciatic* pain is usually due to posture change, swelling in the nerve root tunnel, or prolapse of an intervertebral disc. The latter is usually managed conservatively during pregnancy by bed rest, perhaps traction and physiotherapy.

(ii) *Bell palsy* involves the *facial nerve* and symptoms vary according to the level of involvement. Apart from facial paralysis, there may be hyperacusis (sensitivity to noise) and loss of taste in the anterior tongue. The condition is more common in pregnancy. *Management* is conservative; prednisone 40–60 mg/day is commonly used from the outset if facial palsy is complete.

chapter thirty

The Endocrine System

OVERVIEW

The endocrine system is basically involved in the regulation of cellular processes by means of hormonal messengers which are carried in the blood stream. It thus complements the nervous system, but usually on a slower time scale.

The classical endocrine system functions in a multilevel fashion; the *hypothalamus* directs the activity of the *pituitary gland* (synthesis, storage and release of trophic hormones), which in turn directs *target endocrine organs* (eg. thyroid, parathyroid, adrenal, ovary) or peripheral tissues. By means of a delicate control mechanism, the various processes required for body function are carried out at an optimal level. Many other hormones which lie outside the above system have now been isolated — many of these being produced in the gastrointestinal system (e.g. insulin, glucagon).

In early pregnancy, there is an increase in secretion of *oestrogen* and *progesterone* from the *corpus luteum*, the latter being stimulated by human chorionic gonadotrophin (HCG) from the trophoblast. These hormones depress the release of follicle stimulating and luteinizing hormones at the hypothalamic-pituitary level. There is probably some increase in the other trophic hormones of the anterior lobe of the pituitary gland (which stimulate the thyroid gland and adrenal cortex), also a rise in the output of melanocyte-stimulating hormone (MSH), which is responsible for the chloasma ('mask') of pregnancy and the linea nigra in the midline of the abdomen (figure 30.1 and colour plate 13). The major change in the *anterior lobe* is an increase in cells which secrete the hormone *prolactin*, responsible for lactation. *The posterior lobe* of the pituitary gland secretes *oxytocin* and *vasopressin* (antidiuretic hormone). The former hormone increases during labour, probably reflexly as a result of cervical and vaginal dilatation and stimulation by the prostaglandins which are released at this time.

If the patient has loss of pituitary gonadotrophin function, and ovulation is induced artificially, progress during pregnancy is usually uneventful. The same applies in patients with diabetes insipidus, where there is malfunction of antidiuretic hormone production by the posterior lobe. Considerable interest has focussed on the fetal pituitary gland, since it has been credited with an important role in the onset of labour; if it is absent or poorly developed (as in anencephaly), there is no trophic hormone release, especially to the adrenal cortex. The adrenal cortical hormones appear to be intimately involved in the complex train of events that starts labour. It has been further shown that oxytocin is released in spurts from the fetal pituitary after labour has commenced.

The *ovary* is essential to the pregnancy until the placenta takes over the secretion of oestrogen and progesterone at about 8–10 weeks.

A knowledge of the influence of the various physiological changes of pregnancy on the endocrine system is necessary in order to interpret changes in hormone levels and organ function which take place at this time.

One of the major endocrine disorders in obstetrics is *diabetes mellitus*; it is relatively common and, if not diagnosed and managed skilfully, has the potential for serious complications to both mother and baby. Problems in the major endocrine organs are mainly related to hyper- or hypofunction; all are fairly unusual apart from *thyrotoxicosis*. Conditions in this group which have the potential for disaster include *pituitary adenoma* (rapid enlargement), *phaeochromocytoma* (hypertensive vascular blowout), and *Addison disease* (adrenal crisis).

The newborn may be secondarily involved in the mother's disorder. For example, the thyroid antibody responsible for the maternal disease may cross the placenta and cause fetal thyrotoxicosis; antithyroid drugs on the other hand may cause hypothyroidism and goitre. Because of the importance of the thyroid in neurological development, screening tests of thyroid function in the neonate are undertaken in many centres.

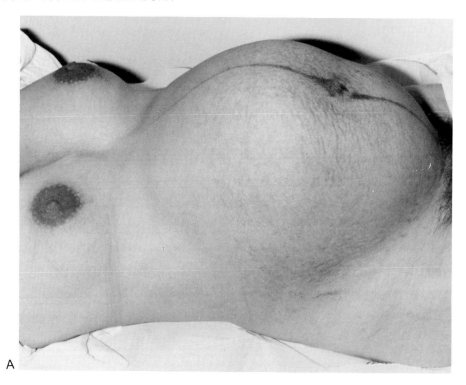

A

Figure 30.1 A. Dark-haired, brown-skinned women are more prone to pregnancy pigmentation. This Italian-born primigravida shows a full term fundus and unusually pronounced pigmentation of nipples and abdominal midline (linea nigra). Striae gravidarum are also evident. **B.** Marked chloasma of pregnancy in a beautiful 24-year-old para 2, quarter-caste Australian aborigine. She was photographed 4 days after a normal delivery of a 3,465 g male infant. The patient's skin tone is light and so accentuates the patchy pigmentation.

B

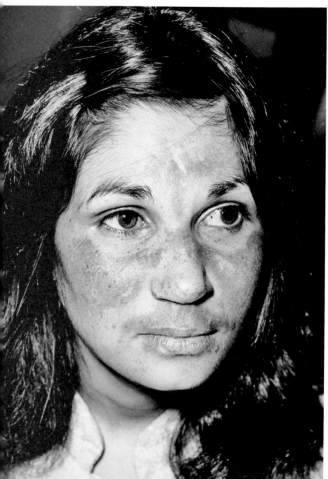

THE PITUITARY GLAND

Physiological Changes

The 2 pituitary gonadotrophins — follicle stimulating hormone (FSH) and luteinizing hormone (LH) are essential only for conception and early embryonic development; levels are low for the remainder of the pregnancy. The level of prolactin, on the other hand, increases markedly throughout pregnancy in preparation for its role in lactation, reaching a value 10–15 times the nonpregnant level (nonpregnant to 25 ng/ml; trimester 1 to 30/35 ng/ml; trimester 2 to 100 ng/ml; trimester 3 to 200 ng/ml; postpartum day 7 breast feeding, 150 ng/ml, not breast feeding to 25 ng/ml).

The posterior lobe of the gland produces oxytocin and vasopressin; there is a physiological increase in both hormones, particularly in late pregnancy, labour and suckling at the breast. *Vasopressin* (antidiuretic hormone) is mainly involved in osmolar and plasma volume regulation and responding to stress. *Oxytocin* has important actions in uterine activity and in milk 'let-down' (contraction of myoepithelial cells which surround the ducts leading to the nipple).

Pituitary Tumours

The great majority of tumours in the child-bearing age group are *prolactinomas*, mostly less than 10 mm in size (microadenomas). Usually, the patient has suffered from infertility due to the suppression of ovulation by the excess prolactin, and pregnancy has resulted from bromocriptine therapy. Such patients will be under specialist care. The major worry with larger tumours is the occasional rapid increase in size because of the stimulus of oestrogen; careful monthly monitoring is necessary of possible effects related to this (headache, visual symptoms or field changes etc). Bromocriptine, which is usually stopped when pregnancy is diagnosed, should be recommenced. In some centres, patients are advised to have surgical or irradiation therapy before embarking on the pregnancy. Breast feeding is not usually contraindicated in the patient with a microadenoma.

Acromegaly

Pregnancy occasionally occurs in such women if the disease is not advanced. Pregnancy is largely unaffected, although nerve entrapment (e.g. carpal tunnel syndrome) is common because of the increase in soft tissue.

Diabetes Insipidus

Almost invariably, the diagnosis has been made before the pregnancy on the basis of polyuria and polydipsia. In many patients the condition is idiopathic (1–2% of these are hereditary), in others it is the aftermath of a tumour or infection, resulting in lack of antidiuretic hormone.

Treatment is by a vasopressin analogue, 1-diamino-arginine vasopressin, given intranasally.

THE THYROID GLAND

Physiology

Iodine in the food is trapped by the thyroid gland and synthesized to one or other of the 2 circulating thyroid hormones, tri-iodothyronine (T_3) or thyroxine (T_4). The blood level of these hormones reflects the overall function of the gland, while the unbound or free hormone (less than 1%) reflects the amount of active hormone present in the blood. The actual production and turnover of T_3 and T_4 is increased in proportion to the mother's increase in surface area. The secretory activity of the hypothalamus (thyroid releasing factor) and the pituitary gland (thyroid stimulating hormone) is kept in check by the active thyroid hormones in the blood (negative feedback).

Common tests of thyroid function. (i) *Basal metabolic rate* (BMR). Overall activity of the thyroid is increased in pregnancy because of the added fetal and placental metabolism. (ii) *Protein-bound iodine* (PBI). The amount of iodine bound to serum protein is increased because oestrogens significantly raise the level of binding proteins (this mainly measures T_4 since this comprises 95% of PBI). (iii) T_3 *resin uptake*. Radio-active[131] Iodine labelled T_3 is added to serum in vitro — the excess is absorbed into a resin and measured. (iv) *Free thyroxine index*. This is obtained by PBI multiplied by T_3 resin uptake divided by 100 and is useful in pregnancy or if the patient is using oral contraceptives, since the increase in the globulin binding protein effect is allowed for. (v) *Urine 24-hour T_3 excretion* in pregnancy is no different from the nonpregnant value — (160–320 μmol (2–4 μg)), and is a new and useful test.

Changes in Pregnancy

(a) Mother

Normal pregnancy mimics the features of a *mild hyperthyroid state* — there is an increase in BMR, cardiac output, and pulse rate, vasodilatation, heat intolerance, and emotional lability. There are characteristic changes in some of the laboratory tests (e.g. PBI) as indicated above.

There is an increase in size of the thyroid gland (*physiological goitre*) in the majority of women. The combined effect of the 'mopping up' of free hormones (T_3, T_4) by the increased binding proteins and loss of iodine in the urine (due to the increased glomerular filtration in pregnancy) causes an increase of the trophic hormone TSH from the pituitary gland, since the latter is partly released from feedback inhibition. This stimulates activity of the thyroid gland which therefore enlarges. By 6 weeks postpartum, the gland has returned to normal size.

(b) Fetus

The *fetal thyroid* begins to accumulate iodine at the start of the second trimester and produces T_3 and T_4 under independent hypothalamic-pituitary control. Radio-iodine which is sometimes used to treat hyperthyroidism, is contraindicated in pregnancy because of damage to the developing fetal thyroid gland which has an avidity for iodine about 40 times that of the maternal gland.

Since the trophic stimulating hormones from the pituitary gland (e.g. TSH) do *not* cross the placenta, the regulating systems of the mother and fetus are independent. There is, however, a slow transfer of the free thyroid hormones (mainly T_3) and a rapid transfer of free iodine. This explains why the fetus with no thyroid may still develop normally *in utero*.

DISORDERS OF FUNCTION

Although thyroid disorders are relatively uncommon in pregnancy, their recognition is important because of the potential for harm to the fetus.

There is a 15-20% increase in thyroid gland activity in pregnancy due to the metabolic demands of the products of conception. In addition, there is a shift in normal values of a number of tests of thyroid function, largely because of the increase in thyroid binding globulin (an oestrogen effect).

Hyperthyroidism in the reproductive age group is usually the result of autoimmune disease, the thyroid antibodies being directed to TSH receptors on the thyroid cell, causing overactivity. Hypothyroidism may also be the result of autoimmune disease, but in this case the antibodies attack cell components resulting in permanent damage (Hashimoto disease).

Hyperthyroidism

Untreated hyperthyroidism lowers fertility and increases abortion, prematurity, and perinatal death rates, but severe disease is very rare nowadays.

Incidence

1 in 1,000-1 in 2,000 pregnancies.

Aetiology

The usual cause of hyperthyroidism in pregnancy is overstimulation of the gland by immune globulins (e.g. antibody to thyrotrophin receptor) (Graves disease, diffuse toxic goitre). These globulins being of the 7S variety can cross the placenta and can similarly affect the fetus, producing a temporary thyrotoxic state after birth. A preexisting nodular goitre may also produce thyrotoxicosis (Plummer disease), but usually the mother in such cases is late in the childbearing period. It is now known that trophoblastic tissue secretes a thyroid stimulating hormone; where there is an overgrowth of this tissue, as in hydatidiform mole, the thyroid gland is stimulated, sometimes markedly, with resultant thyrotoxicosis which can be severe enough to cause cardiac failure.

Diagnosis

Usually the disease has been diagnosed before the pregnancy. If not, sharp observation and

intuition may be needed, since there is considerable overlap in symptoms and signs with the changes of normal pregnancy. Goitre and tachycardia (particularly if persisting during rest or the Valsalva manoeuvre) are very suspicious; weight loss (this may be obscured by the normal increase in pregnancy), exophthalmos, pretibial oedema, diarrhoea, and hand tremor are other signs which should lead to laboratory investigation. A diffuse euthyroid goitre may occur in conditions of iodine deficiency. A thyroxine (T_4) value above 0.19 μmol/l (15 μg/dl) is fairly suggestive.

In the baby, hyperthyroidism is rare and usually acquired from the hyperthyroid mother by increased transfer of LATS (long-acting thyroid stimulator), an immunoglobulin against the receptors to TSH in the gland, which is produced in the mother's lymphoid tissues.

Treatment

For moderate or severe hyperthyroidism during pregnancy, good results are obtained with subtotal thyroidectomy preceded by iodine therapy, but most patients are now treated with drugs such as propylthiouracil or carbimazole (figure 30.2), which block the uptake of iodine by the gland and hence the formation of the thyroid hormone. Another action of propylthiouracil is to block the peripheral conversion of T_4 to T_3 (the more active tissue hormone). The usual commencing dose of propylthiouracil is 50-100 mg 8-hourly. It is the preferred drug because it is less readily transferred across the placenta.

Side-effects (rash, pruritus, nausea, fever, leukopenia) are unusual if the dose is kept low (propylthiouracil 25 mg/day, carbimazole 5-10 mg/day). It is usually possible to reduce the dose progressively during the second half of pregnancy, the free thyroxine index being kept near the upper limit of normal. If the level of thyroid-stimulating antibody globulin is high in the mother's blood, larger doses are given in order to prevent fetal/neonatal thyrotoxicosis. During the course of pregnancy the free T_4 should be checked every 1-2 months.

Concurrent thyroxine therapy, 0.1-0.2 mg/day, is sometimes used to prevent fetal hypothyroidism and goitre which may otherwise occur. A selective beta 1 adrenergic blocking drug may be useful early in treatment to control quickly the sympathetic effects of the disease. An exacerbation is often observed postpartum and an increase in drug dose will often be necessary. Although only a small amount of drug passes into the breast milk (<0.1%), some authorities

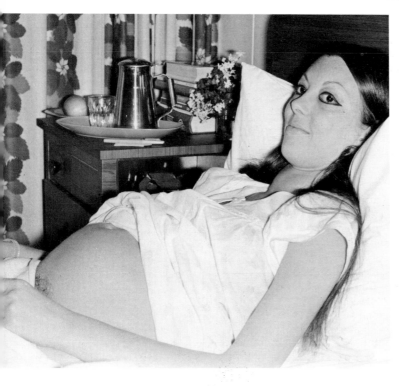

Figure 30.2 Thyrotoxicosis in a primigravida at 24 weeks' gestation. Note exophthalmos and diffuse thyroid enlargement. Palpitations, tachycardia, hypertension and tremor responded to carbimazole (an antithyroid drug) and propanolol (an adrenergic blocking drug). The patient was euthyroid 2 weeks later and was then given iodine therapy and subtotal thyroidectomy was performed.

advise artificial feeding because of the small chance of serious side-effects such as agranulocytosis.

Hypothyroidism

Unless this condition is mild, pregnancy is unlikely to occur; if it does, abortion is common. The incidence ranges from 1 in 500–1 in 1,500 pregnancies; it is more common in white than black races. Hypothyroidism may result from *lack of iodine in the diet* (endemic goitre), *disease of the thyroid gland* (aplasia, enzyme defect, autoimmune disease), or the aftermath of treatment of hyperthyroidism or thyroid carcinoma (radiation, surgical ablation or drug treatment).

Paradoxically, excessive iodine (or lithium) ingestion by the mother (e.g. in some cough mixtures) may produce hypothyroidism, the excess iodine being taken up by the thyroid and blocking the production of T_3 and T_4. The classical features are a general slowing of body functions (tiredness, constipation, bradycardia, puffy/dry skin, cold sensitivity, decreased mental alertness).

On investigation, T_4 levels are low and TSH is elevated.

Iodized salt, containing 200 μg of iodine daily, will prevent hypothyroidism in both mother and infant in geographic low iodine areas. Recent work in New Guinea has shown that iodine, apart from that incorporated in the thyroid hormones, is necessary in the first trimester, and deficiency adversely affects the developing fetal brain and is reflected by severe mental disorder in the infant (retardation, deafness, gait disturbance). Hence it has been recommended that such mothers receive iodized oil injections, the iodine from which is released slowly over a long period.

If the *mother* has established hypothyroidism, replacement with 1-thyroxine sodium will be necessary, the usual dose ranging from 0.1 to 0.2 mg/day. A small increase in dose is sometimes required in pregnancy. Maternal levels should be checked regularly (every 1–2 months) during the pregnancy.

If the *baby* is hypothyroid, 1-thyroxine sodium is again given in a dose of 0.025–0.1 mg/day. Unfortunately, the classical signs often only develop some weeks or months after birth (enlarged protruding tongue, protuberant abdomen, lemon-yellow skin discoloration, marked constipation, lethargy, poor feeding, hyptonia, noisy or distressed respiration, hypothermia — colour plate 55). For this reason, routine screening is carried out in many centres to detect the 1 in 3,000–1 in 4,000 with serious hypothyroidism.

The Thyroid Nodule

This usually represents nontoxic nodular goitre, but it may be a true adenoma or very rarely a carcinoma. Specialist referral is indicated.

THE PARATHYROID GLANDS

The parathyroid glands, as the name suggests, are in close relationship to the thyroid gland. Their major function is in the regulation of calcium and phosphorus metabolism in the body, in conjunction with *calcitonin* (a hormone derived from the parafollicular C cells of the thyroid gland).

Major functions of calcium include bone structure (85% of content), muscle and nerve excitation, coagulation, and hormone release.

The normal level of calcium in the blood is (2.3–2.7 mmol/l (9–10.5 mg/dl)); some 45% of this is protein bound, the remainder being in the ionized, active form. *Parathormone* is responsible for maintaining normal levels of calcium in the blood, chiefly by mobilizing calcium from the bones, enhancing its absorption from the upper bowel (via vitamin D) and renal tubule. Its major action in phosphorus metabolism is to limit its reabsorption in the renal tubule.

Calcitonin is the functional antagonist of parathormone, reducing calcium levels if these are too high by decreasing osteoclastic activity in bone (i.e. prevents bone breakdown). It also has a regulatory function over a number of digestive hormones (gastrin, cholecystokinin, glucagon).

Normal Pregnancy

Calcium balance is usually normal in pregnancy if the diet is adequate in dairy products. Total blood calcium levels fall as a result of the dilution of binding protein, but the ionized level remains the same. Both parathormone and calcitonin levels rise in pregnancy, although the latter returns towards normality in the third trimester. The rise in parathormone causes an increase in 1,25 dihydroxycholecalciferol (active vitamin D), which is responsible for enhanced calcium absorption from the gut.

The fetus requires significant amounts of calcium and phosphorus in the last trimester and this is achieved by enhanced maternal absorption and placental transfer. There are higher blood levels of *both of the above substances in the fetus*; the parathyroids are thus relatively suppressed, and this facilitates the growth of dental and skeletal tissue in late pregnancy. After birth, calcium levels fall, the parathyroids become more active and, as with the mother in pregnancy, vitamin D production is increased and extra calcium is absorbed from the plentiful supply in the gut.

Hyperparathyroidism

This condition is rare before the age of 35 and is mostly caused by an adenoma of the gland.

Clinical features are not very specific, but pronounced nausea and vomiting is suggestive, as is lassitude and bone tenderness. If the condition is of long standing, there is an excess of both phosphate (decreased reabsorption) and calcium (raised blood levels) in the urine and thus the risk of calcium deposition in the urinary tract or elsewhere.

Confirmation of the diagnosis is usually based on a *high level of serum calcium* and a *low level of phosphate*.

The *effect on the pregnancy* is an increased risk of abortion, premature labour, and perinatal death. The elevated calcium level causes depression of the fetal parathyroids and this may result in tetany and collapse after birth.

Treatment ideally is resection of the parathyroid adenoma.

Hypoparathyroidism

This condition is the reverse of the above, the major feature being a lowered calcium level in the blood, with ensuing *tetany*, *weakness*, and sometimes *psychiatric disturbance*. (Other causes of lowered blood calcium include sprue and renal disease). It is almost always the result of surgical ablation of the glands in the course of thyroidectomy.

Treatment will usually have been commenced before the patient becomes pregnant and consists of daily supplementation with calcium (e.g. 5–8 g of calcium lactate) and vitamin D (100,000 U). Acute insufficiency may cause stridor/laryngeal spasm and requires intravenous calcium gluconate (10 ml of 10% solution). Breast feeding is not usually recommended in view of the calcium drain on the mother.

THE ADRENAL GLANDS

There are 2 adrenal glands, each shaped like a cocked hat, situated on the posterior abdominal wall just above the corresponding kidney. The adult adrenal gland measures 3 × 1 cm and weighs 6–8 g. Each gland represents 2 fused elements — an outer cortex and an inner medulla.

(a) *Adrenal cortex.* There are 3 groups of hormones secreted from the 3 functional zones. (i) *Zona glomerulosa: mineralocorticoids* (mainly aldosterone) which promote sodium retention by the kidney, (ii) *zona fasciculata: glucocorticoids* (mainly cortisol) which influence the metabolism of carbohydrate, protein and fat, chiefly by converting protein and fat into sugar; glycogen deposition is increased in the liver, (iii) *zona reticularis: sex steroids* (mainly androgens).

Normally, about 90% of cortisol is reversibly

bound to plasma proteins (albumin and transcortin).

(b) Adrenal medulla. This is part of the sympathetic nervous system and produces adrenaline (epinephrine) and noradrenaline (norepinephrine) in times of stress. These hormones affect almost all organs in the body, enabling the individual to better deal with the emergency. Vital activities are enhanced (metabolism is speeded up, the heart and lungs are stimulated) while unessential activities are shut down (digestion, emptying of the bowel, bladder, or uterus).

Changes in Pregnancy

There is some increase in the size and function of the gland (cortex chiefly); this is reflected in a significant increase in blood cortisol; the reason for this is the same as for the thyroid gland, namely, the increase in binding protein (transcortin in this case) in the blood in response to oestrogen. More of the *cortisol* becomes protein bound, there is less free cortisol to suppress the hypothalamus and pituitary gland and more of the adrenal stimulating hormone (ACTH) is released with consequent increase in total corticosteroids. Nature thus ensures that there is a reserve for the stresses of pregnancy and parturition. The pigmentation of pregnancy is due to an increase in melanocyte stimulating hormone (MSH), which is secreted along with ACTH.

In the *mineralocorticoid* system there is a considerable increase in *aldosterone secretion*. This counteracts the sodium-losing effect of progesterone by enhancing reabsorption of sodium in the distal renal tubule. The increased secretion is probably caused partly by the high oestrogen levels and partly by greater pooling of blood in the legs, with reduced return to the heart.

There is little change in *sex hormone* secretion, the output of oestrogens and progesterone being dwarfed by that of the fetus and placenta.

The *adrenal medulla* is little changed in pregnancy, levels of adrenaline and noradrenaline in the urine being the same as in the nonpregnant woman.

The *fetal adrenal* gland weighs 3–4 g at term and has a special zone (which forms 80% of the cortex) and this produces large amounts of a precursor material (dehydroepiandrosterone) which is processed by the placenta to produce oestriol. At mid-pregnancy, the fetal adrenal gland is quite large, overshadowing even the kidney; relatively, it is 100 times larger than the adult adrenal. If the fetal pituitary gland is absent or poorly developed (as is classically the case in *anencephaly*) there is little or no stimulating hormone (ACTH) reaching the adrenal gland, hence the above system does not function, and maternal oestriol levels are very low (figures 30.3 and 30.4). It has long been known that pregnancy in the patient with an anencephalic fetus tends to be prolonged. It is thought that the fetal adrenal gland plays a role in the events leading to labour, possibly by prostaglandin effect. Another effect of cortical hormones is to hasten maturation of the fetal lung in late pregnancy (see Chapter 63).

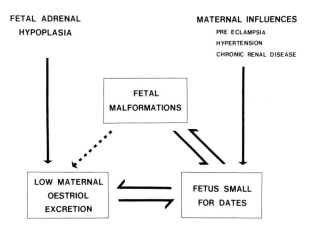

Figure 30.3 The interrelation between the various conditions that influence maternal oestriol excretion. In anencephaly there is always adrenal hypoplasia (gland weight less than 1 g) and very low oestriol excretion. Other fetal malformations have an increased incidence of low oestriol excretion (20%), mainly because the fetus is small for dates.

Striae Gravidarum

Most women develop at least a few striae, especially during the third trimester of their first pregnancy. Such marks usually occur when skin stretching is maximal. The sites involved are breasts, abdomen, thighs and buttocks. Striae are generally more numerous in nulliparas and in patients with excessive abdominal enlargement, especially when due to multiple pregnancy (colour plates 66 and 70). However, many women develop none at all, even when weight gain is excessive (colour plate 68). Others develop them early in pregnancy before weight gain or change in body shape have begun (figure 30.5). The aetiology is probably related to changes in the collagen and elastic fibres of the dermis, induced by adrenocortical hormones. They are indistinguishable from the striae which occur in Cushing syndrome. Their importance, although mainly cosmetic, can be monumental (figure 30.6).

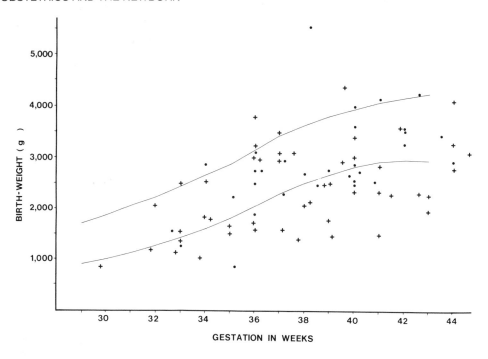

Figure 30.4 Maturity and weight at birth in 79 fetuses with major malformations. The 10th and 90th percentiles for birth-weight according to gestational age are shown. Note the high incidence of small for dates infants (37 of 79). * = normal oestriol excretion; + = low oestriol excretion. (From Macafee CAJ et al. Aust NZJ Obstet Gynaecol 1972; 12:71-85).

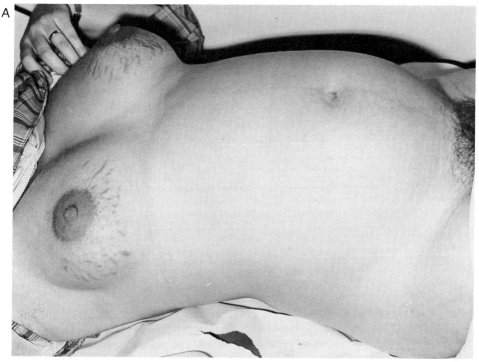

Figure 30.5 Striae gravidarum. **A.** A 19-year-old primigravida at 29 weeks' gestation. She had gained 9 kg in weight during pregnancy (57 to 66 kg). The striae had appeared on her breasts by 20 weeks and remained unchanged thereafter. She had no striae on abdomen or thighs. **B.** A 17-year-old primigravida at 12 weeks' gestation. She had nausea and had lost 4 kg in weight (76–72 kg) since becoming pregnant; i.e. she developed marked abdominal striae without weight gain or change in shape. There is more to striae than stretching!

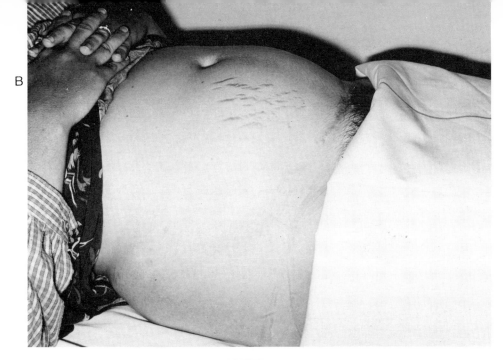

B

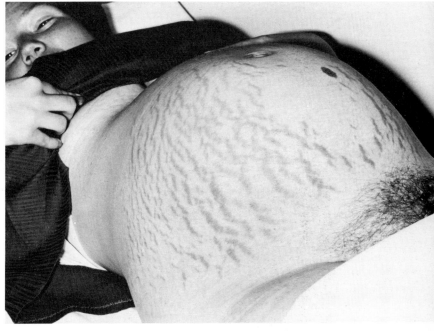

Figure 30.6 Marked striae gravidarum such as this may warn of impending preeclampsia. They are mainly subumbilical in position but also occur on the thighs and lower quadrants of the breasts. They are not simply due to stretching, but to changes in the skin perhaps induced by adrenocortical hormones. Pregnancy and Cushing syndrome (adrenocortical overactivity) have features in common — tendency to striae, acne, hypertension, diabetes and weight gain.

DISORDERS OF FUNCTION

Patients who suffer from serious glandular underactivity (Addison disease) or overactivity (Cushing disease) rarely become pregnant. With adequate treatment, however, pregnancy can occur and progress normally.

Adrenocortical Excess: Cushing Syndrome

This is a rare condition in pregnancy and may result from an adrenal adenoma or carcinoma, non-ACTH-dependent hyperplasia, or hyperfunction of the pituitary gland (usually a pituitary adenoma) causing a secondary hyperplasia in the adrenal cortex.

The classic features of Cushing syndrome are rounded, florid face, obesity, weakness, glucose intolerance, ready bruising (capillary fragility), hypertension, and psychological upsets. Pregnancy complications include diabetes and hypertensive disorders in the mother and hypoadrenalism in the baby.

The diagnosis rests on the demonstration of elevated cortisol levels and loss in the diurnal variation of this hormone; there is not the expected depression of cortisol with the dexamethasone test.

The work-up and treatment of such patients lies in the specialist field.

Adrenocortical Insufficiency: Addison Disease

This condition is again rare and has usually been diagnosed before the pregnancy.

The *aetiology* may be congenital absence or subsequent damage, usually as a result of surgical removal, tuberculosis etc. In the undiagnosed patient, there is usually an *adrenal crisis* at times of major stress, particularly after labour or operative delivery. Acute insufficiency can also result from infarction or haemorrhage into the gland (e.g. during a severe infection); these patients have acute lumbar pain and persistent shock, but no localizing abdominal features.

The *clinical features* include weakness, pigmentation, weight loss, anorexia, nausea and vomiting. The blood pressure, blood sugar and blood sodium are characteristically low. *Secondary adrenal insufficiency* occurs as a result of prolonged adrenal drug therapy for conditions such as autoimmune disease or major damage to the hypothalamic-pituitary axis.

The *diagnosis* is based on the finding of low levels of plasma and urinary free cortisol and failure of response to ACTH stimulation.

The *treatment* of the established condition involves replacement of the hormones which are lacking: e.g. cortisone acetate orally, 25 mg in the morning, 12.5 mg in the afternoon together with 0.05–0.15 mg of 9 alpha-fluorohydrocortisone daily orally. In labour, 25 mg of hydrocortisone sodium succinate (Solu-cortef) is given IV every 4–6 hours. In the early puerperium, intravenous fluids and hydrocortisone are continued. In an *adrenal crisis*, the dose of hydrocortisone is increased so that over 12–24 hours, 5–6 litres of fluid and 500–600 mg of hydrocortisone are administered; potassium levels should be monitored twice daily.

Adrenal Medulla

Phaeochromocytoma is a tumour of the adrenal medulla which by excess adrenaline secretion produces intermittent hypertension, severe headaches, tachycardia, pallor, and sweating. The condition is usually aggravated in pregnancy and the mortality is high from cerebrovascular accident. Confirmation is obtained by examining the urine for excretion products (catecholamines; vanillyl mandelic acid). Elective Caesarean section is usually indicated, followed by exploration of the adrenal and removal of the tumour.

Adrenocorticosteroid Drugs

There are a number of conditions for which adrenal cortical hormone is given (asthma, autoimmune disease, collagen and skin diseases). It is preferable to maintain as low a dose as practicable in the first trimester because of the small risk of fetal malformation. Such treatment affects not only the mother's pituitary gland, but also that of the fetus, suppressing ACTH release. This is of clinical importance because the fetal adrenal gland in turn does not produce oestriol precursors, and maternal oestriol values are low, giving the false impression that the fetus is in danger. Because of the depressed state of the maternal adrenal cortex, hydrocortisone cover is needed for stress episodes (labour, anaesthesia).

The Infant

The remarkable hyperplasia of the cortical zone (fetal cortex) has been mentioned. This regresses slowly after birth. The most important adrenal abnormality as far as the infant is concerned is *congenital adrenal hyperplasia*. Here, there is a lack of one or more of the enzymes responsible for the production of cortisol; this results firstly in an overstimulation of the gland because the normal restraint by cortisol on the release of the pituitary ACTH is diminished, and secondly, in a build-up and release of precursor hormones, some of which are androgenic. The lack of mineral and sugar regulating hormones may produce a severe and perhaps fatal outcome in the newborn if the condition is not recognized and treated. If a female baby is masculinized (clitoral hypertrophy), the above condition must be considered in the differential diagnosis (see figure 65.22).

THE PANCREAS

The endocrine function of the pancreas is carried out by the islets of Langerhans, the cells of which secrete insulin. The physiology of this hormone and alterations in pregnancy are discussed in Chapter 36.

Diabetes Mellitus

Introduction/overview

In this disease there is an inadequate amount of insulin produced by the islet cells of the pancreas in response to a carbohydrate load. This results in hyperglycaemia and glycosuria, and in the more severe forms, ketosis and protein wasting. After a number of years, deleterious changes occur in the vascular system, particularly the small vessels (microangiopathy); there are, in addition, disturbances to the microcirculation because of such changes as decreased erythrocyte deformability and increased blood viscosity: these combine to produce retinopathy, nephropathy, neuropathy and accelerated atherosclerosis. A form of the latter is seen in the blood vessels supplying the placenta during pregnancy, and this often results in fetal growth retardation.

Two major types of diabetes are recognized. Type 1 (insulin-dependent) is the one usually seen in the childbearing age group, and Type 2 (insulin-independent) which is characterized by a later onset and obesity.

Pregnancy represents a stress on islet-cell function because of the effect of pregnancy hormones on carbohydrate metabolism, and the disorder may be manifest only at this time (*gestational diabetes*).

Diagnosis is often suggested by unusual events in a previous pregnancy (e.g. macrosomic infant, unexplained stillbirth, congenital malformation), together with the presence of glycosuria, abnormal glucose tolerance on routine testing early in the third trimester, or typical clinical features (large fetus, polyhydramnios, early onset preeclampsia especially in a multipara).

Diabetes is characterized by an increased risk of *intrauterine death* in late pregnancy — hence the rationale for delivery at about 38 weeks' gestation and the need for close monitoring of fetal well-being. There is a 2-fold increase in the risk of *major malformation*, especially of the central nervous system, and *hyaline membrane disease* is more common, even in large infants born near full term — hence the need for assessment of pulmonary maturity (LS ratio > 2:1) before elective delivery.

Recent trends emphasize the need for early diagnosis, team management, close blood sugar monitoring, precise insulin dose regimen, careful fetal monitoring, and good neonatal intensive care facilities.

Improvements in perinatal mortality related to the above have highlighted the residual problem of severe fetal malformation. Improvement in this area can only come from preconceptional counselling and better diabetic control in the first 6-8 weeks of pregnancy.

Diabetes mellitus is important because of the high perinatal mortality (5-15%) and because of the deterioration which may occur in the mother if careful supervision is not given.

General Classification of Diabetes

Spontaneous diabetes. There are 2 basic types of diabetes which are now recognized.

Type 1. This is characterized by insulin dependence, the presence of circulating islet cell antibodies, an onset usually before the age of 35-40 years, and a tendency to ketoacidosis.

Type 2. Here there is usually insulin-independence, absence of islet cell antibodies, an onset after the age of 35-40 years, obesity and little tendency to ketoacidosis.

Secondary diabetes. This may complicate pancreatic disease, contra-insulin hormonal disturbances (acromegaly, Cushing syndrome), drugs, and some rare genetic syndromes.

In both types, deterioration is caused by such conditions as stress, infection, and pregnancy. The action of insulin is to restrain the excessive breakdown of glycogen, fat, and protein to glucose, and if its secretion is subnormal, blood glucose levels will rise. Another hormone from the pancreas is *glucagon* which has an effect opposite to that of insulin. In stress conditions, glucagon output is increased to mobilize sugar rapidly, whereas insulin output is depressed. In diabetic patients, therefore, the glucagon effect may at times aggravate an already high blood sugar level (e.g. in the presence of infection).

Gestational diabetes. Here the chemical or clinical upset only appears with the *stress of pregnancy*. Usually the glucose tolerance test reverts to normal after delivery. The diabetic condition is then said to be latent.

There is an additional condition termed *prediabetes*. Before clinical abnormalities appear, the underlying metabolic defect may manifest itself during pregnancy in one or more of the following ways: (i) a baby overweight for the period of gestation, (ii) unexplained perinatal death, (iii) polyhydramnios, (iv) congenital malformation, (v) preeclampsia. These effects may be due to increased levels of growth hormone and/or insulin in the fetus, together with as yet unexplained metabolic disturbances.

Classification of Diabetes Severity in Pregnancy

The special classification (Classes A to E) proposed by White and co-workers is based on the severity of the diabetes — e.g. from gestational diabetes to late stage disease with organ damage resulting from vascular pathology.

Incidence

The incidence is approximately 2-3%; the majority of these are gestational diabetics, the remainder being those known to be diabetic before pregnancy began.

Diagnosis

Where the diagnosis has not already been established before the pregnancy commenced, the features described above under 'Prediabetes' should sound a warning. Other alerting features include *maternal age over 30*, a positive family history, maternal weight over 90 kg, and heavy or persistent glycosuria.

The diagnosis is confirmed by means of a *glucose tolerance test*, where a sugar load (50–100 g) is given orally or intravenously and blood sugar samples are tested half-hourly for 2–3 hours. The latter is usually chosen because of the delayed peak in pregnancy. If the condition is clinically florid (polyuria, polydipsia, weight loss, ketonuria), a significantly elevated random blood sugar estimation (11 mmol/l; 198 mg/dl) is sufficient to diagnose diabetes. There should be an adequate amount of carbohydrate in the diet in the 2–3 days preceding the test, otherwise there may be a spuriously high result. Since glycosuria is relatively common (30% of pregnant patients), the above test is frequently preceded by a *diabetes elimination test* whereby a similar sugar load is given but only a 2-hour or 3-hour sugar level is tested. If the 2-hour level is above 6.6 mmol/l (120 mg/dl) a complete glucose tolerance test is performed. The frequency of *benign (renal) glycosuria* is explained by the higher glomerular filtration rate in pregnancy, with inability of the renal tubules to reabsorb the greater sugar load. This continues until a week after delivery when there is a return to normal values. In centres where glucose tolerance tests are carried out routinely in the last trimester, it is found that 1–2% of pregnant women will have gestational diabetes.

There is no uniform standard for glucose tolerance measurements and thus the values for the individual centre where one is practising should be known. *An acceptable definition of gestational diabetes is a 1-hour plasma glucose level of 9 mmol/l (162 mg/dl) or above AND a 2-hour level of 7 mmol/l (128 mg/dl) or above after a 50 g oral glucose load (table 30.1). Amniotic fluid insulin levels* are significantly raised in patients with gestational diabetes and can be used to identify the endangered fetus.

The Effect of Diabetes on Childbearing

The effect of diabetes on pregnancy depends largely on its severity. For example, early diabetes is characterized by effects of the elevated maternal blood sugar on the baby (secondary hyperinsulinaemia producing macrosomia in relation to insulin-sensitive tissues such as body fat and the viscera (figure 30.7), polyhydramnios etc). With increasing instability, ketoacidosis occurs with the greater likelihood of fetal malformation and/or fetal death *in utero*. Finally, at the stage of maternal vascular disease, the predominant effect on the fetus is one of growth retardation and possibly fetal death due to uteroplacental insufficiency.

Other effects include the following: (i) infertility and abortion are more common if the condition is severe. (ii) preeclampsia; (iii) bacteriuria, chronic pyelonephritis and vaginal moniliasis; (iv) the large fetus (colour plate 53, figures 30.7 and 30.8) may result in cephalopelvic disproportion, prolonged or obstructed labour (colour plate 92), and impacted shoulders during delivery — operative delivery, especially Caesarean section, is more often necessary; (v) there is a tendency for the newborn to suffer from hypoglycaemia and respiratory distress (colour plate 92).

Thus *intrauterine or neonatal death* may be the result of poor control of the diabetes, complications of longstanding diabetes (nephropathy, hypertension), specific complications of pregnancy (preeclampsia), difficulties in labour, major malformation, immaturity and/or respiratory distress.

The Effect of Childbearing on Diabetes

In the first 14–20 weeks of pregnancy there is a fall in blood glucose, partly as a result of fetal demands and partly because of diminished appetite; insulin levels also tend to be lower. In the second half of pregnancy, the above tendency is counteracted by the anti-insulin effect of placental hormones (lactogen (HPL), oestrogen, progesterone) and other hormones (cortisol), and thus the insulin requirements will be greater. After delivery the situation is reversed and the insulin requirement is rapidly reduced, often to less than that existing before the pregnancy began. If diabetic control is poor, the effect of pregnancy on the diabetes may be disastrous — e.g. on retinopathy and nephropathy.

Management

The general principles of *management of the high risk patient* are followed (e.g. consultation, more frequent visits etc). The danger of *smoking* should be emphasized, since there is a compounding ill-effect on blood flow in smaller blood vessels; this is particularly important if there is retinopathy or nephropathy. Other risk factors include previous perinatal death or serious morbidity, previous macrosomic infant, vascular disease/hypertension, polyhydramnios.

Unless the condition is mild, hospital admission is arranged at the first visit for *stabilization*, which may be by diet or insulin and further admissions for stabilization are made as indicated.

Usually the pregnant diabetic is managed jointly by a team with a special interest in this problem — usually obstetrician and internist/

TABLE 30.1   DEFINITIONS OF ABNORMAL GLUCOSE TOLERANCE

*NONPREGNANT**
    (a)   A fasting plasma glucose value of 8.0 mmol/l or above = *DIABETES*
    (b)   If fasting plasma glucose value is 6.0–8.0 mmol/l perform a 75 g oral glucose tolerance test:
        (i)   A 2-hour plasma glucose value above 11.0 mmol/l = *DIABETES*
        (ii)   A 2-hour plasma glucose between 8.0–11.0 mmol/l = *IMPAIRED GLUCOSE TOLERANCE***

*GESTATIONAL DIABETES****: a 1-hour plasma glucose value of 9.0 mmol/l or above *AND* a 2-hour level of 7.0 mmol/l or above after a 50 g oral glucose tolerance test

*GESTATIONAL HYPOGLYCAEMIA*****: a fasting plasma value of 4.0 mmol/l or less *AND* a 3-hour level of 3.0 mmol/l or less after a 50 g oral glucose tolerance test

  * WHO criteria
  ** Note that a patient with impaired glucose tolerance is likely to have gestational diabetes when pregnant unless glucose tolerance improves
 *** The 98th percentile in a series of 40,000 consecutive patients tested at 32–34 weeks' gestation
**** The 2nd percentile in the same series of 40,000 patients

Figure 30.7 This baby died during delivery by Caesarean section at 35 weeks' gestation. He weighed 6,420 g (14 pounds 2 ounces) and was 55 cm in length in a squatting position. The mother had diabetes and hypertension (200/105). The extreme obesity mimics the generalized oedema of hydrops fetalis. He had a huge liver and spleen. This classical baby of a diabetic is seldom seen — the baby is big for dates (above the 90th percentile) in 40% of diabetics.

Figure 30.8 Fetal macrosomia — birth-weight 4,400 g at 37 weeks' gestation. The mother was a 28-year-old para 1, diabetic since the age of 11 years. Her insulin requirements had fluctuated widely throughout pregnancy. When the baby's 'buffalo hump' was palpated at Caesarean section before the head was born, it was thought to be an occipital encephalocele! The copious vernix caseosa is also typical of the large for dates fetus.

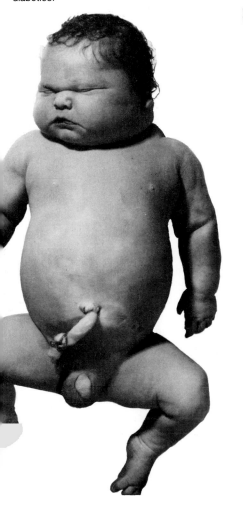

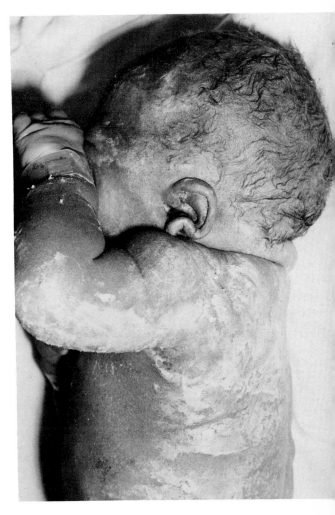

endocrinologist, consulting with nurse, dietitian, and later the paediatrician. Opthalmological examination should be carried out to assess retinal vascular changes.

Diet is an important part of management whether insulin is being taken or not.

In *Type 1 diabetes*, the patient is usually not overweight and quality rather than quantity of food is important.

In *Type 2 diabetes*, an attempt should be made to achieve ideal weight for height (by calorie reduction); with the decrease in obesity, insulin sensitivity usually returns.

The following are suggested daily intakes: protein 100 g, carbohydrate 200 + g, and fat 60–80 g; this should make up 6,700–8,400 kJ (1,500–2,000 kcal) per day. Complex carbohydrates or starches (grains and legumes) are much preferable to concentrated sucrose-type sweets.

Insulin therapy is considerably simplified if the patient understands its basis of action and the need for regular, more frequent, and sensible meals; in this way hypoglycaemia (skipping meals) and hyperglycaemia/ketosis (binges) will be avoided.

A total weight gain of around 10 kg for the pregnancy is ideal.

The particular insulin regimens differ from centre to centre; a common example would be a mixture of intermediate and regular (soluble) insulin, 2:1, in the morning and 1:1 in the late afternoon. Usually, the overall requirements will be lower in the first half of pregnancy and higher in the second half.

The vigour with which *control of blood sugar* level is pursued also differs from centre to centre. Prevention of congenital malformation, which is emerging as one of the major challenges in these patients probably requires patient education (preconceptual counselling and stabilization) as much as tight control, since many patients will have passed the organogenetic period for the heart, skeleton, and nervous system before they first seek antenatal care.

Home monitoring is now taught to many patients and unquestionably will increase in the future; with proper motivation, very good control can be obtained. Blood sugar levels 1–2 hours postprandial should be maintained in the range 4–7 mmol/l (72–128 mg/dl). A 4-point test regimen (0700, 1100, 1500, and 2100 hours) is carried out 2–7 days per week depending on disease severity. A sudden drop in insulin requirement should raise the suspicion of fetal difficulty and should be reported promptly.

A general idea of the type of blood sugar control over the preceding weeks is obtained by measurement of *glycosylated haemoglobin (Alc)*. This is checked at the first antenatal visit and at intervals of 6–8 weeks thereafter; a satisfactory value is < 8%, optimally near 6%.

Although opinion is divided on the management of the gestational diabetic, evidence suggests that insulin treatment in the last trimester (e.g. 20 U intermediate: 10 regular in the morning) will prevent fetal hyperinsulinaemia and its attendant problems (e.g. macrosomia, dystocia). The proportion of gestational diabetics who require insulin therapy as well as dietary regulation to control their blood sugar levels ranges from 10–40% in large reported series.

An important distinction, particularly in the first 14–16 weeks, is that between *starvation ketosis* (normoglycaemia) and *diabetic ketosis* (hyperglycaemia); the former requires glucose, the latter insulin.

Monitoring. The control of maternal blood sugar and ketoacidosis has already been mentioned. *Fetal monitoring* is important also in order to detect placental insufficiency. The frequency of testing (e.g. cardiotocography, oestriol) depends on the period of gestation, severity of the disease, and the presence of other factors likely to influence fetal well-being (e.g. preeclampsia). If available, *ultrasonography* should be carried out at the initial visit and serially in the last trimester to assess fetal growth and well-being (movement, breathing). This technique is also helpful in diagnosing fetal malformation and macrosomia; in the latter condition, the biparietal diameter is normal, whereas the fetal trunk and the placenta are enlarged. Growth retardation is much more likely in patients with severer forms of the disease where vascular damage has occurred and where hypertension is present. Apart from glucose control and fetal monitoring, a close watch is kept on the urinary tract (bacteriuria) and the optic fundus.

Timing of delivery. With improvements in the control of diabetes, most patients are now allowed to go at least to the 38th week, provided fetal function tests are satisfactory and there are no other obstetric complications. The management of the unripe cervix is by temporary deferment of delivery or local prostaglandin use etc, depending on the urgency of the situation. Premature delivery may be necessitated by the maternal or fetal condition. Amniotic fluid analysis will indicate lung maturity and the insulin level in the liquor is a good index of diabetic control (normal range 5–15 mu/ml).

Management during labour and delivery. Factors favouring *surgical induction and vaginal delivery* include mild diabetes, multiparity with previous normal delivery and normal-sized baby, and a good obstetrical history. In favour of *Caesarean section* is a previous section, unstable presentation or cephalopelvic disproportion, and evidence of fetal distress (cardiotocography, low oestriol values). The incidence of Caesarean section ranges from 40–70% in large reported series.

If induction of labour is planned, an IV infusion is set up and no food or subcutaneous insulin are given that morning. Plasma glucose levels are kept between 3.3–5.5 mmol/l (60–100 mg/dl) by continuous infusion. The usual insulin requirement lies between 1 and 20 U/hour given in the 5% dextrose infusion flask.

For the patient in spontaneous labour, an IV infusion is set up and insulin requirements are determined by frequent blood glucose estimations.

For elective Caesarean section, the initial procedure is similar to that for induction of labour. Glucose is usually withheld until after delivery. It is important in such cases to demonstrate *fetal lung maturity* (L:S ratio > 2:1), unless the indications for the section are pressing.

Early puerperium. There is usually a' temporary but marked drop in insulin requirement after the baby is born, and dose is guided by regular monitoring. Most patients with *gestational diabetes* no longer require insulin after delivery; they should have a glucose tolerance test 4–6 weeks after delivery to determine future management.

The Baby

In patients with nonvascular insulin-dependent disease, the baby is often overweight (excess fat and fluid), flabby, sleepy, and difficult to feed. Because of *immature behaviour*, the baby is usually treated in a similar manner to the premature baby. In addition, a close watch is kept on *blood sugar levels* (tendency to hypoglycaemia) and *respiratory function* (atelectasis, hyaline membrane disease). A careful check for *congenital malformation* should be made (figure 30.9) as well as for birth *trauma*. With more advanced

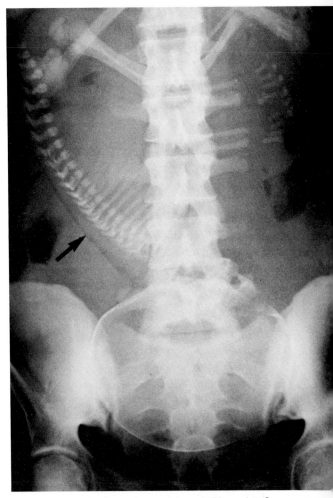

Figure 30.9 This radiograph was taken at 38 weeks, 2 days before spontaneous normal delivery. The infant weighed only 2,715 g, but had thick subcutaneous tissues as indicated by the translucent zone arrowed. The baby had hydrocephaly (ventriculomegaly), cleft palate and micrognathia and died 15 minutes after birth.

disease, the baby often shows the features of intrauterine *growth retardation*, with attendant complications of wasting, asphyxia, and meconium aspiration.

There is no specific contraindication to breast feeding, although this may be more difficult initially. The parents should be counselled regarding the inheritance risks of diabetes.

chapter thirty-one

Respiratory System

OVERVIEW

In the process of *pulmonary respiration*, the blood which is pumped to the lungs by the right ventricle and pulmonary arteries is relieved of its carbon dioxide and takes up oxygen, the carriage of these gases being effected by the haemoglobin of the red blood cell. The oxygen is then carried in the circulation to the individual cells of the body where the further process of *tissue respiration* occurs, chiefly mediated by subcellular components called mitochondria. Here, oxygen is used for the various activities of the cell and carbon dioxide is released as an end product of the metabolic processes.

In the great majority of patients, the pulmonary system copes very adequately with the added demands of pregnancy. One of the major changes is the *reduction in expiratory reserve volume* and *residual volume* (figure 31.1). This is caused by engorgement of the pulmonary vessels (increased blood volume) and, later in pregnancy, by the upward pressure of the diaphragm. Patients living at high altitudes may have smaller infants due to the oxygen deficit.

The major adaptation is an *increase* in *tidal volume* (an effect of progesterone — centrally on the respiratory centre, and peripherally on the bronchial musculature) and a corresponding increase in oxygen uptake. There is an *increase in the oxygen tension* and a *decrease in carbon dioxide tension* in the blood, both changes helping the fetus. The heightened pulmonary stretch reflex (due to engorged vessels) is reflected in a feeling of dyspnoea in some antenatal patients.

Asthma (1%) is a distressing complaint and may require hospital admission if simple measures fail (e.g. bronchodilators). Occasionally, anoxaemia may be sufficient to compromise the fetus. Intravenous therapy, including adrenal steroids, may be required. Asthma ranks third (after cardiac disease and intracranial haemorrhage) among fatal medical conditions in pregnancy.

Respiratory infections are common, especially of the upper airways. Most are of viral origin and respond to bed rest and simple measures. Bronchopulmonary involvement may require hospitalization and antibiotic therapy. Classical *lobar pneumonia* is now relatively rare and *tuberculosis* has largely been eradicated.

The traditional 'vital signs' such as temperature, pulse, respiration, and blood pressure are important in monitoring the progress of a sick patient, but it should be appreciated that, in some situations, the oxygen, carbon dioxide, and acid-base levels (pH) have altered before the clinical vital signs have indicated that there is a serious problem.

The 2 respiratory tract conditions most likely to cause major maternal morbidity or death are *pulmonary embolism* (Chapter 34) and the *aspiration of gastric acid content* during anaesthesia (Mendelson syndrome, Chapter 41).

CHANGES IN PREGNANCY

There is an *increase in tidal volume* (air breathed in and out with each normal respiration) in pregnancy, due to the effect of progesterone on the respiratory centre (figure 31.1). The 1-minute volume is similarly increased (by 40%), but unlike the heart, this represents only a small part of the total reserve. In later pregnancy, the level of the diaphragm is raised and the *residual air in the lungs decreases*. Both these changes cause a *fall in the carbon dioxide tension*

in the maternal blood ($PaCO_2$ 4.6–5.3 → 4.0–4.2 kPa (30–40 → 30–32 mm Hg)), and this in turn helps the fetus to dispose of carbon dioxide across the placenta. The PaO_2 shows a corresponding increase (11.3 → 12.2 kPa (85–92 mm Hg)). At term, the *oxygen consumption has increased by nearly 20%*. There is no significant change in the respiratory rate.

Respiratory function tests (table 31.1) show few changes; there is less resistance in the airways, presumably again related to the effect of progesterone (and perhaps relaxin) on the

TABLE 31.1   TESTS OF RESPIRATORY FUNCTION

Function	Test
Oxygenation	Arterial oxygen pressure/content Haematocrit/haemoglobin
Ventilation	Tidal volume, frequency
Ventilatory reserve	Vital capacity (VC) Forced expiratory volume in 1 second (FEV_1) Functional residual capacity
Other tests	Chest radiography Pulmonary artery/capillary wedge pressures

bronchopulmonary smooth muscle. In the third trimester there is a considerable fall in expiratory reserve volume and residual volume, due to both the upward pressure of the uterus and the engorgement of the pulmonary capillaries. The symptom of *dyspnoea* may be experienced in mid-pregnancy: this may be due to a heightened 'stretch reflex' due to capillary engorgement.

RESPIRATORY DISORDERS

Bronchial Asthma

This is the most common disease affecting the lungs in pregancy, with an incidence of approximately 1% (table 16.2).

The *effect of pregnancy* is not constant; in patients with extrinsic asthma (onset in infancy, presence of other allergic stigmata and a seasonal incidence) the dominant change is one of improvement; with intrinsic (infective) asthma, the majority of patients will show no change or an improvement. There is little evidence of any effect of the disease on the pregnancy unless the condition is serious and hypoxia results; in such cases there is an increase in abortion, fetal growth retardation, premature labour, and stillbirth.

The *general management* is similar to that in the nonpregnant state. An accurate history of the disorder and objective measurements of airflow may be necessary to differentiate the condition from emphysema and chronic bronchitis where the airway obstruction is not reversible. *Acute episodes* are treated with the inhalation of a sympathomimetic agent such as salbutamol or terbutaline (2 puffs of metered aerosol 2-hourly); if there is no significant improvement, theophylline 250 mg in 10 ml is given IV over 5 minutes or an intravenous infusion of 500 mg in normal

saline is given over 8 hours; warmed, humidified oxygen is administered if there is continued respiratory difficulty (cyanosis, severe dyspnoea). Infection is treated by appropriate antibiotics and physiotherapy is directed to improvement in aeration and sputum production. *Corticosteroid therapy* may be required if the above measures fail to produce adequate improvement; 200–400 mg of hydrocortisone is given every 2–4 hours as required, followed by 30–60 mg prednisone orally per day, decreasing as the acute phase passes. Sedatives and tranquillizers are contraindicated.

For *maintenance therapy*, a bronchodilator aerosol (salbutamol, terbutaline), 2 puffs 2–4 times daily or oral tablet (salbutamol, 2–4 mg tds; terbutaline, 2.5–5 mg tds) is given. Sodium cromoglycate (20 mg 2–4 times daily) is useful as a prophylactic agent if taken on a regular basis. Finally, corticosteroid aerosol (beclomethasone dipropionate) or systemic corticosteroid may be required.

One problem concerns the *effect of adrenal cortical hormone* treatment on the value of *maternal oestriol excretion*. Because the fetal adrenal cortex is depressed, oestriol production is low and it may be concluded erroneously that the fetus is in jeopardy. The same applies to any patient receiving cortisone or one of its analogues. Because the maternal adrenals are also suppressed by this therapy, adrenal cortical hormone is needed to cover additional stresses (normal labour, operations, haemorrhage, infection).

In *labour*, regional analgesia (*epidural*) is preferred to narcotic analgesics which release histamine and may provoke asthma and depress respiration. If the patient has recently been taking *corticosteroids* she should be given 200 mg hydrocortisone IM or IV 4-hourly during labour. *Ergometrine* or *oxytocin* should be used in management of the third stage of labour since they do not cause bronchoconstriction.

There is a 5-fold increase in asthma within the first year of life of the offspring of asthmatic patients and a lesser increase in the incidence of major respiratory disease.

Upper Respiratory Tract Infection and Pneumonia

Adeno, rhino, and para influenza *viral infections* complicate 1–3% of pregnancies; usually the process is fairly self-limited, but some patients may experience a serious *bronchopneumonia*, with high fever, chills, prostration, and dyspnoea.

There is a low risk of congenital malformation if the infection occurs in the first trimester.

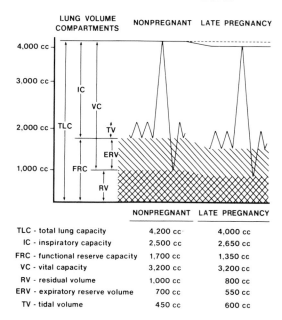

	NONPREGNANT	LATE PREGNANCY
TLC - total lung capacity	4,200 cc	4,000 cc
IC - inspiratory capacity	2,500 cc	2,650 cc
FRC - functional reserve capacity	1,700 cc	1,350 cc
VC - vital capacity	3,200 cc	3,200 cc
RV - residual volume	1,000 cc	800 cc
ERV - expiratory reserve volume	700 cc	550 cc
TV - tidal volume	450 cc	600 cc

Figure 31.1 Changes in pulmonary volumes in the non-pregnant state and late pregnancy. The appropriate mean volumes for nonpregnancy and late pregnancy are shown.

Abortion and premature labour are not uncommon and maternal mortality is possible if acute respiratory failure occurs.

Tuberculous infection (Chapter 27) and *pneumococcal pneumonia* are becoming progressively less common, together with such attendant complications such as *bronchiectasis* and *lung abscess*. Instead, we are seeing more infections related to viral agents and mycoplasmas, often in the heavy smoker. Infections acquired in hospital are likely to be due to E. coli, haemolytic streptococci, staphylococcus aureus, or Klebsiella pneumoniae rather than diplococcus pneumoniae. There may be an underlying congenital disorder (immune deficiency state, cystic fibrosis). The *aspiration pneumonitis* that accompanies inhalation of gastric content during or after general anaesthesia (Mendelson syndrome) has been mentioned earlier.

If an upper respiratory tract infection is not responding to bed rest or there is a pneumonic process present, *antibiotic therapy* is indicated. Penicillin or one of its synthetic derivatives is usually the drug of choice; erythromycin is effective against mycoplasma.

Women should be *immunized* early in pregnancy with a polyvalent influenza vaccine.

Tuberculosis. This infection is almost eradicated in some countries, but may complicate up to 2–3% of pregnancies in *developing countries*. The disease may be known and quiescent or only recognized during pregnancy because of a posi-tive chest radiograph or characteristic symptoms (malaise, fever, fatigue, weight loss, productive cough and perhaps haemoptysis).

The chest radiograph will usually suggest the diagnosis which will be confirmed by *positive sputum culture*. Tuberculosis has little effect on the course of the pregnancy, and vice versa. The main problem is prevention of cross-infection to others.

The mainstay of treatment is a prolonged, effective antituberculous drug regimen. By the time of delivery, the mother is usually not infectious, and can handle and feed her baby.

Sarcoidosis is a rather rare chronic granulomatous disease, predominantly affecting the lung and thus liable to be confused with tuberculosis. Adrenocortical therapy may be required in the acute phase.

Respiratory Failure

This may take one of several forms.

Airway obstruction may be caused by acute asthma or an exacerbation of chronic obstructive pulmonary disease. In each case, the basic problem is failure to eliminate carbon dioxide. The management is directed to improving the movement of air in and out of the lungs and so reducing the work of breathing and thus carbon dioxide production; the measures include oxygen, humidification, chest physiotherapy (including postural drainage), bronchodilators, and antibiotics if required.

Parenchymal lung damage results in a greater or lesser degree of nonoxygenation of pulmonary venous blood due to damage or collapse of lung tissue. Hypoxaemia rather than hypercarbia is the main problem. Conditions to be considered include pneumonia, chest trauma and fat embolism, severe septicaemia ('shock lung' etc). There is consolidation/infiltration evident on radiography. This type of patient usually requires treatment in an intensive care unit, possibly needing intubation, mechanical ventilation and positive end expiratory pressure.

Secondary lung failure is the term applied when the basic pathology lies outside the lungs — e.g. severe kyphoscoliosis, poliomyelitis, drug overdosage. Vital capacity is reduced, the degree and reversability depending on the underlying condition.

Conditions that are most likely to cause *acute pulmonary embarrassment in pregnancy* are acid aspiration during intubation for general anaesthesia (Mendelson syndrome), severe preeclampsia/eclampsia, severe sepsis, disseminated intravascular coagulation, amniotic fluid embolism, severe allergic reactions, and finally acute right heart failure.

chapter thirty-two

Cardiac Disorders

OVERVIEW

The *blood volume* in pregnancy increases about 40% from approximately 4.0 litres to 5.5 litres. This is necessary to accommodate the growth and metabolic needs of the fetus. The heart adapts to this load by increasing both its *stroke volume* and *rate* — i.e. *the cardiac output*. This extra load on the heart normally causes no embarrassment, but if there is an organic lesion present, cardiac failure and sometimes maternal death may follow.

The *incidence* of cardiac disease in pregnancy ranges from 0.25–1.5%, the higher figure being found in areas where control of rheumatic fever (and thus rheumatic carditis) has not been achieved. *Congenital heart disease* now provides an increasing number (25–30%) of cases in many centres, although even here, marked improvements have been made because of surgical correction in infancy and childhood. The obstetrician is tending to see relatively more of such conditions as cardiomyopathy, viral myocarditis, coronary disease, and enigmatic failure. Advances in technology (echocardiography, intracardiac catheter studies of flow and pressure) are now providing the cardiologist with precise information which can facilitate diagnosis and prognosis.

The major tasks of the primary care physician are to diagnose the disorder if this has not already been done and to seek consultant opinion as early in the pregnancy as possible. Because of the hyperdynamic circulatory state in pregnancy, certain changes occur which can mimic heart disease and even heart failure — e.g. dyspnoea, systolic ejection murmurs, accentuated heart sound, ECG changes, and exaggerated pulmonary vascular markings on chest radiography.

There are, however, certain physical signs which always denote cardiac disease: any diastolic murmur, a Grade 3 (easily heard) systolic murmur, unequivocal cardiac enlargement, and major arrhythmias (atrial fibrillation or flutter; heart block).

Conditions with a particularly bad reputation include *pulmonary hypertension, major congenital anomalies* with the potential for shunt reversal (Eisenmenger complex, tetralogy of Fallot), long-standing rheumatic carditis with weakened myocardium and atrial fibrillation, Marfan syndrome, cardiomyopathy, and aortic stenosis.

The patient with cardiac disease is traditionally placed in one of 4 functional grades according to her exercise tolerance; during pregnancy there is usually a shift down at least one grade. This grading will provide a reasonable guide as to how the patient will cope with the pregnancy, what freedom of activity she can be given, and how intensive must be her surveillance. It should be appreciated, however, that sudden and alarming deterioration can occur in some of the more serious conditions mentioned above.

With improvement in maternal mortality rates in the past decade, cardiac disease, especially congenital heart disease, has become a relatively *more common cause of maternal death* and now accounts for almost 5% of cases.

During the antenatal period, the key aim is to prevent the onset of cardiac failure, or if this cannot be achieved, to recognize it promptly and institute immediate and effective treatment. Stresses that tend to precipitate failure are *preeclampsia, hypertension, anaemia,* and *respiratory tract infection*; drugs given to stop premature labour (ritodrine, salbutamol, terbutaline) are usually contraindicated in the patient with heart disease because of their often excessive stimulation of cardiac activity.

Caesarean section is not an easy way out for the patient with cardiac disease. Vaginal delivery should be the goal in most patients. This can be made easier for the patient (especially the nullipara) in 2 ways — prelabour softening of the cervix to lessen the uterine work in the first stage, and forceps/vacuum extraction to shorten the second stage.

The early puerperium is a dangerous time: *oxytocics* (especially ergometrine) should be used with care and blood loss replaced if necessary. Special requirements may include *anticoagulants* for patients with prosthetic valves, *antibiotics* as prophylaxis for endocarditis, and carefully supervised physiotherapy postpartum.

If an operative procedure becomes necessary, local rather than general anaesthesia is better; if the latter is needed, an anaesthetist of considerable experience is advisable.

PHYSIOLOGICAL CHANGES IN PREGNANCY

The function of the heart is to pump blood to all parts of the body and to respond reflexly to changes in the circulating blood volume.

A number of adjustments are necessary in the cardiovascular system during pregnancy to provide for the demands of the growing fetus and its support systems (uterus and placenta). The primary change is probably the *increase in plasma and red cell volume*, to which the heart responds by *increase in stroke volume* (amount of blood ejected per beat) and *stroke rate*; these 2 changes are responsible for the increase in *cardiac output* (amount of blood ejected per minute). The *cardiac volume* increases by some 10-15% and the hyperdynamic circulatory state is responsible for the accentuation of cardiac sounds (closure of cardiac valves) and exaggerated ejection murmurs. The ECG shows a deviation to the left in the electrical axis; there is occasional flattening of the T wave in lead 3. The increased blood volume (1.5 litres or more) is responsible for the greater blood flow seen in several major organs — notably the uterus and kidneys (figure 8.1). The plasma volume increases about 50% (2.6 to 3.8 l) and the red cell mass 20-30% (1.4 to 1.7 l), the higher figure occurring in patients receiving iron supplements — the total blood volume, therefore, increases about 40% (4.0 to 5.5 l).

Some women with *small hearts* have difficulty coping with the cardiovascular changes of pregnancy, and at the antenatal examination they may have pulse rates of more than 90 or even 100 per minute; *premature labour* is more common in such women. During early antenatal visits, however, nervousness rather than cardiac stress is the usual cause of tachycardia.

The above changes are progressive throughout pregnancy, although a peak is usually reached at about the 8th month. This additional strain to which the heart is subjected is partially alleviated by 2 factors — firstly, the *decrease in peripheral resistance* (progesterone effect), and secondly, the *reduced viscosity of the blood* (haemodilution) which the heart has to pump through the vascular system. In the hypertensive disorders of pregnancy, where marked vasospasm may occur, there is a considerable additional burden on the heart.

CARDIAC DISORDERS

Heart disease is of special importance in view of its role in maternal mortality (table 14.1). Early diagnosis, accurate assessment and team care are the keystones of management.

Aetiology

Rheumatic heart disease accounts for approximately 60% of cases (usually with damage to the mitral valve), *congenital anomalies* for 30% (usually patent ductus arteriosus, atrial and/or ventricular septal defect, anomalous construction and/or positioning of major vessels or a combination of these — e.g. tetralogy of Fallot, Eisenmenger complex), and the remaining 10% is made up of such conditions as myocarditis, coronary disease, cardiomyopathy, endocarditis, and cor pulmonale.

Incidence

0.25-1.5% of pregnancies (table 16.2); the difference is determined largely by the higher frequency of *rheumatic heart disease* in communities with unfavourable climate and socio-economic conditions (poverty, crowding, and poor nutrition). In recent years, the number of patients with *congenital heart disease* has increased, since more defects are being corrected by surgery, whereas the number with rheumatic disease has decreased as a result of improved living standards and control of streptococcal infections.

Diagnosis

The nature of the heart lesion is usually known before pregnancy commences. The clinical features will depend on whether the left or right side of the heart is predominantly involved, the nature of the pathology, and its degree. Typically, there is a history of dyspnoea on effort, tiredness, and perhaps cyanosis. Examination reveals typical organic heart murmurs, irregularities of rhythm, heart enlargement, and changes in the electrocardiogram. If there is congestive heart failure, there will be abnormal fill-ing of neck veins, haemoptysis, tenderness and engorgement of the liver, and dependent oedema. The initial antenatal visit is an ideal time to diagnose previously unsuspected heart disease, since the physical signs are usually accentuated by the hyperdynamic state of the cardiovascular system. In some patients the diagnosis will be obscure and may require soph-isticated techniques — e.g. endomyocardial biopsy in cardiomyopathy, echocardiography in Marfan syndrome.

Assessment

There are 4 functional grades: *Grade 1*, no breathlessness on exertion; the heart lesion is detected on routine examination; *Grade 2*, breathless on moderate or heavy exertion (heavy household work); *Grade 3*, breathless on less than moderate activity (light household work); *Grade 4*, breathless without significant activity. Often the patient may slip a grade during the pregnancy: with rheumatic heart disease the deterioration is often slow and predictable; with other types of disorder (especially where shunt reversal can occur), the deterioration may be dramatic. A simple test of cardiopulmonary adequacy is the breath-holding test (maximum inspiration, expiration, inspiration and hold): normal and Grade 1 patients should manage at least 45–50 seconds.

Apart from determining the patient's func-tional grade, other important factors to consider are: (i) history of previous heart failure, (ii) behaviour in a previous pregnancy, (iii) age of the patient, (iv) socioeconomic condition of the patient (number of children, availability of home help, financial circumstances), (v) type of cardiac lesion, (vi) presence of arrhythmia, and (vii) car-diac size.

Management

Antenatal. The first essentials are exact anatom-ical diagnosis and functional classification. The patient is placed in a high risk category with an emphasis on specialist consultation, more fre-quent antenatal visits, anticipation of compli-cations, and their early treatment. If the initial assessment indicates that pregnancy may endanger the mother's life or health, *therapeutic abortion* is offered if surgical correction of the defect is not feasible.

The patient is advised of the need for additional rest and educated in relation to factors that may aggravate her cardiac status. Elastic support of the leg veins during the day is helpful in the maintenance of cardiac stability. Referral to the social worker for assessment of the need for home help may be indicated.

Patients who have undergone cardiac surgery in the past or those with mitral valve disease and atrial fibrillation may be on continuous *antico-agulant therapy*. Oral therapy will be changed to *heparin* during the first trimester and at 36 weeks, since this drug does not cross the placenta and does not carry the risk of causing haemor-rhage in the fetus or newborn. *Warfarin* does cross the placenta and may cause *embryopathy* during the first trimester (saddle nose, basophilic stippling of bones, microphthalmia and mental retardation) — the risk of these defects has been exaggerated and is less than 5%. Heparin ther-apy is ceased when the patient comes into labour and is recommenced 24 hours after delivery. Any abnormal bleeding (i.e. epistaxis) must be reported immediately. Control is obtained by monitoring heparin levels and/or partial throm-boplastin times.

Cardiac failure can be minimized if the patient is instructed about the importance of *adequate rest* and the dangers of *respiratory infections*, *preeclampsia*, *anaemia*, *overwork*, and *obesity* (colour plate 4). *Warning signs* include the appearance or increase of dyspnoea on effort, insomnia, tachycardia or irregularities of rhythm, and the finding of moist sounds in the chest or increase in fluid in the lungs on radi-ography. *Digitalis* may be ordered to offset maximal strain on the heart (30–32 weeks onward), and *hospitalization* is often recom-mended at this time and at intervals thereafter. If the patient is receiving digitalis, *overdosage* should be considered if the patient complains of fatigue, muscular weakness, anorexia and nausea, and exhibits central nervous system symptoms such as confusion, restlessness, apa-thy, insomnia, and visual disturbances; abnor-malities of heart rhythm not previously present are also suspicious.

Labour. Induction is not carried out unless there is an obstetrical indication, since spontaneous labour is less strain on the patient and *there is a tendency for the cardiac condition to improve as full term approaches*. If an oxytocin infusion is given, the overall fluid load must be carefully monitored. The patient must be observed closely in the labour ward, and reassured. The patient's head and shoulders should be kept as high as practicable during labour and delivery; the *lith-otomy position should be avoided* because of the risk of acute heart failure resulting from the sud-den increase of venous return to the heart. Usual analgesic measures are provided; *epidural anal-gesia is given only in special circumstances* because hypotension should be avoided. If nitrous oxide is given, an adequate oxygen concentration should be present (at least 30%). The cardiac and respiratory rates should be recorded every 15–30 minutes according to the patient's condition. Dyspnoea, cyanosis, undue tachycardia (above 100 per minute) or tachypnoea (above 25 per minute), or any unusual behaviour by the patient should be reported.

Forceps or vacuum extraction are used if there is delay in the second stage of labour. Caesarean section is undertaken only for obstetrical indications, with some exceptions (e.g. pulmonary hypertension, coarctation of the aorta). The use of ergometrine in the third stage should be avoided because of its action on the smooth muscle of blood vessels (coronary arteries) as well as the uterus. *These patients withstand blood loss poorly and intravenous oxytocin, 5–10 units IV, is recommended after completion of the second stage.* In a number of congenital anomalies there is a shunt between the 2 sides of the heart: reversal of this (due to a sudden drop in peripheral resistance or increase in pulmonary resistance) should be avoided, since rapid cardiac decompensation can follow. If active bleeding persists, intravenous ergometrine, 0.25 mg, may be given. If transfusion is required, packed red cells are preferable if the patient has Grade 3 or 4 disease.

Some patients with valvular lesions following rheumatic fever may be on continued penicillin prophylaxis. Otherwise, an *antibiotic cover* should be given for 5 days over the immediate perinatal period *to prevent bacterial endocarditis* in patients with organic heart lesions. Cover should also be given for dental procedures to cope with transient bacteraemia.

If *cardiac failure* occurs, the following measures must be adopted: (i) sit the patient upright, (ii) administer oxygen by mask — 8 litres per minute, (iii) rapidly digitalize the patient (intravenous digoxin) 1–1.5 mg in divided doses over 24 hours; *arrhythmias* may need correction by appropriate drug therapy or electroconversion, (iv) morphine, 15 mg, preferably intravenously, (v) aspiration of frothy mucus if present, (vi) rapid venesection of 500 ml, (vii) aminophylline, 250–500 mg, by slow intravenous injection, (viii) rapidly-acting diuretic (intravenous frusamide (Lasix), 40–80 mg), (ix) on rare occasions, emergency cardiac surgery may be necessary (usually for a tight mitral valve lesion).

Puerperium. Adequate sleep should be ensured. A careful watch should be kept on the patient, since rapid haemodynamic alterations may occur at this time, often precipitating right or left heart failure. Attention is given to the *prevention of thromboembolism* by intensive physiotherapy (deep breathing, exercises). Breast feeding is probably unwise if cardiac failure has occurred. An accurate fluid balance chart is essential. If oedema persists, an aldosterone antagonist (Aldactone A) may be added to the diuretic. Blood pressure, pulse and respiratory rates are charted and a 4-hourly temperature chart is kept to detect early infection. Immunosuppressive therapy may be dramatically effective in patients with peripartum cardiomyopathy. Commencement of ambulation can be gauged by the grade of heart disease and the patient's progress.

Postpartum sterilization is usually recommended for patients with Grade 3 or 4 lesions; with lower grades, individual circumstances will determine the course of action. Laparoscopy is contraindicated in these patients (cardiac embarrassment from pneumoperitoneum) as is general anaesthesia (risk of thromboembolism) — sterilization should therefore be performed under regional analgesia or preferably deferred until after the puerperium.

Prognosis

Maternal mortality is 0.5–1.0%. This is considerably less than formerly, due to general improvement in diagnosis and management, decrease of rheumatic carditis in the community, the lower age of childbearing and smaller families and the relief of otherwise intractible cardiac failure by emergency surgery (chiefly mitral valvotomy). Lesions carrying a particularly poor prognosis have been referred to earlier. Pregnancy does not generally accelerate deterioration in eventual cardiac status, although added complications (e.g. endocarditis) may shorten lifespan.

The *perinatal mortality rate* is 2–4%, this being largely contributed to by prematurity and hypoxia; the rate will depend upon the proportion of patients with severe disease (table 16.2). The incidence of spontaneous abortion is not increased unless there is chronic hypoxia and a significant rise in haematocrit.

chapter thirty-three

The Vascular System: Hypertension

OVERVIEW

During pregnancy there are 2 opposing influences on the cardiovascular system — on the one hand, the load on the heart and vessels increases by virtue of the *increasing blood volume*, but this is more than offset (at least until late in the second trimester) by the *relaxation of the small vessels* (and hence their resistance) by the action of the hormone *progesterone*. It is thus not until the third trimester that the full impact of the hypervolaemic load is felt by the heart and blood vessels.

If the patient is found to have hypertension before 20 weeks' gestation the presence of *primary* (essential) or *secondary hypertension* can be assumed; if first seen *later in pregnancy, it is often difficult to separate preexisting and pregnancy-specific hypertensive disorders.*

The importance of hypertension is its *potential for damage to vital organs* (brain, heart, kidney and placenta) with ensuing morbidity or even death of the mother and/or baby. The damage may be chronic and insidious as a result of atherosclerosis, or acute and dramatic as a result of a vascular blow-out and consequent haemorrhage. *Preeclampsia* is more common in the woman with hypertension and the likelihood of operative delivery is increased.

The *essentials of management* comprise accurate classification, assessment of organ damage, specialist consultation/referral, specific antihypertensive therapy, close fetal monitoring, termination of the pregnancy at the optimal time to minimize fetal risk, and appropriate paediatric care after delivery.

Physiological Changes

The *blood pressure is determined largely by the peripheral resistance* (tone in the arterioles) and the *stroke volume of the heart* (itself the resultant of the strength of each heart-beat and the blood volume). The additional blood volume in pregnancy (approximately *1,500 ml*) is largely accommodated in the blood vessels of the uterus and choriodecidual space and the peripheral veins of the mother (particularly in the limbs). The latter aids in the dissipation of heat generated by the actively-growing fetus.

The blood pressure would rise considerably as a result of the *increased blood volume* were it not for the vasodilatation caused by the *smooth muscle-relaxing effect of progesterone* from the placenta. The latter effect is dominant until about the end of the second trimester when a reversal occurs, and the blood pressure tends to rise, sometimes dangerously so.

The effects of *venous dilatation* are seen particularly in the legs, the pressure in the femoral vein rising from 8–10 mm Hg to 20–25 mm Hg. Apart from the increased blood volume and decreased venous tone, there is the growing problem of *uterine pressure on the inferior vena cava*. This explains why *oedema of the legs* is common in pregnancy and *varicosities* become worse. When patients stand too long, the blood tends to pool in the legs, venous return to the heart is reduced, and water and salt conserving mechanisms are switched on (secretion of anti-diuretic hormone and aldosterone); when the patient lies down, the reverse occurs. If the patient lies on her back too long, she may be one of the 10% who experiences the '*supine hypotensive syndrome*'. This is another effect of the uterus blocking the return of blood to the heart. Typically, the patient starts to feel faint, voices become distant, and she is noted to be pale and sweaty. The blood pressure is either low or unrecordable until she is turned on her side and the uterus no longer obstructs venal caval flow.

In the *pulmonary system* there is little change in pressures; the flow is augmented to cope with the increased blood volume and the resistance is lowered.

Definition

Hypertension is *arbitrarily defined as a blood pressure of 140/90 or more*. The diagnosis of chronic hypertension is made only before the

20th week of pregnancy, preferably on the basis of 2 separate measurements; (as a sign of pregnancy-induced hypertension a *relative rise* of pressure is an alternative definition). The blood pressure rises slowly with age (5-10 mm for each decade after the third) and this should be taken into account; in addition, as a result of genetic factors, diet, and lifestyle, it may differ significantly between racial and social groups. Apart from observer and instrument errors, additional factors that should be remembered in the measurement and assessment of blood pressure include the effects of stress (whether at home or attending the surgery/hospital), posture (lying or sitting), exertion, and obesity (tendency to false high recording), and room temperature/season of the year. Because of the somewhat imprecise predictive value of isolated blood pressure readings, some advocate admission to a day hospital in the first instance if the elevation is in the mild-moderate range.

Incidence

This depends on the age and population being studied; it ranges from 2-5% of pregnancies. This figure includes all cases of chronic hypertension (primary and secondary) but excludes cases of preeclampsia (pregnancy-induced hypertension); the latter account for 75-80% of hypertension in pregnancy (see Chapter 20).

Classification of Chronic Hypertension

(i) *Primary (essential)* (70-90%). Here, there is no cause evident, although a genetic influence is likely since hypertension is clustered in families. (ii) *Secondary* (10-30%). In the great majority of patients in this group, the underlying cause is some form of *ischaemic renal disease*, either macroarterial (hypoplasia or stenosis of the renal artery or main branches) or microarterial (chronic pyelonephritis, glomerulonephritis, or polycystic disease). Other causes include *endocrine disease* (overactivity of the adrenal cortex (Cushing syndrome) or medulla (phaeochromocytoma), or thyroid gland) or *blockage of the vascular tree* (coarctation of the aorta).

Effect of Pregnancy

(i) *Mother.* Worsening of the blood pressure often occurs, especially in late pregnancy. If the level is high (diastolic pressure above 100) a crisis can occur at any time in pregnancy, but is especially likely during labour or in the early puerperium. The most serious complication is *cerebral haemorrhage*, which may be fatal. Haemorrhage may also occur in other sites, e.g. retroplacental, leading to *placental abruption*, or hepatic, leading to rupture. There is often a preceding period of intense *vasospasm* and the consequent *ischaemia* may give rise to such warning symptoms as headaches, visual upset and pain over the liver. If sustained high pressures are not relieved, *heart failure* may result. Finally, *preeclampsia* is more common in patients with preexisting hypertension.

(ii) *Fetus.* Fetal and placental development is *often retarded* because of degenerative changes in the decidual arterioles which supply them with oxygen and nutrients; in extreme cases, abortion or *fetal death* may occur. The prematurity rate rises in parallel with the elevation of blood pressure; this is related to both spontaneous premature labour and premature termination of the pregnancy in the interests of the fetus.

Serious Omens

History. Age over 35 years; aggravation in a previous pregnancy; sustained hypertension between pregnancies (diastolic pressure over 90). *Examination.* Blood pressure already high early in pregnancy; retinal haemorrhages or exudates; evidence of enlarged heart or ECG changes in the mother; impairment of renal function. *Progress.* Poor response to treatment; development of preeclampsia.

Assessment

This will be directed to determining whether there is a *primary lesion present*, and what *secondary changes* have occurred in the heart (chest X-ray, ECG), kidneys (urine microscopy, serum uric acid and urea, creatinine clearance), and vascular system (retinoscopy).

The *family history* may point to such conditions as polycystic disease of the kidneys. The *reproductive history* may be helpful in indicating the effect of pregnancy on the hypertension and vice-versa. The patient's symptoms may relate to the hypertension itself (headaches), underlying disease (chronic pyelonephritis), or secondary organ involvement (angina).

During pregnancy the appropriate function tests will be performed to monitor both the condition of the *mother* (renal and hepatic function, coagulation screen) and *fetus* (oestriol levels, cardiotocography).

Management

An early decision which may have to be made in patients with moderate/severe hypertension is whether *therapeutic abortion* is indicated. This is usually an individual decision based on such factors as family size, height of the blood pressure, response to treatment, and involvement of vital organs such as the heart and kidneys.

Relaxation therapy. Patients' anxieties should be allayed as far as possible. Relaxation techniques should be taught since these have been shown to lower blood pressure and reduce hypotensive drug requirement and need for hospital admission.

Drug treatment. If the diastolic pressure remains elevated above 90 mm Hg, in spite of bed rest, an antihypertensive drug is indicated. The following are the hypotensive agents in common use for pregnancy hypertension; the commencing doses are given:

(i)   methyldopa   250 mg bd or tds
(ii) labetalol   100–200 mg bd
(iii) oxprenolol   40–80 mg bd
(iv) hydralazine   25–50 mg bd
(v)   prazosin   0.5–2 mg bd or tds

The mode of action and side-effects of these agents are shown in table 33.1

In the *emergency situation*, often due to superimposed preeclampsia, when the rise in blood pressure is rapid and dangerous levels are reached (diastolic > 110), a rapidly-acting drug is required by intravenous injection; the recommended intravenous drug regimens are given in Chapter 20 — note that in these circumstances both *sedation* and *hypotensive therapy* are required.

Thiazide-type diuretics may cause potassium depletion, skin rash, and a rise in blood urea, uric acid, and glucose and are now seldom used in pregnant women except for congestive cardiac failure.

Sedation. Sedative drugs are best reserved for patients who are tense, anxious and restless and preferably should be used on a temporary basis, being replaced by education and behavioural therapy directed to better coping with stress and reduction of *smoking* if relevant.

High risk categorization. Specialist referral, more frequent antenatal visits, and anticipation of complications is mandatory.

Rest. Rest periods in the morning and afternoon are advisable.

Hospitalization. The patient should be admitted initially for assessment if the *resting diastolic blood pressure is 90 or greater*, and again at any time in pregnancy if this level is reached or there is *early preeclampsia*, or *doubt about fetal wellbeing.* Confining the patient to bed carries the risk of *thromboembolism* and so the patient should be advised to move her legs regularly.

Well supervised domiciliary care has a role if the diastolic pressure is below 100 mm Hg, there is no preeclampsia, and conditions are suitable.

Prevention/early detection of preeclampsia. Attention to diet and rest, together with regular medical supervision, will minimize the occur-

TABLE 33.1   ORAL HYPOTENSIVE DRUGS COMMONLY USED FOR PREGNANCY HYPERTENSION

Agent	Mode of action	Regimen (commencing dose)	Side-effects	Remarks
Methyldopa	Acts as a false adrenergic transmitter in the brain	250 mg bd or tds	Sedation, sodium retention, fever, dry mouth, depression, constipation, postural hypotension, hepatitis	Transient effect on blood pressure of neonate
Labetalol	Combined alpha and beta receptor blocker	100–200 mg bd	Scalp tingling, rash, itch, nausea, abdominal pain, lassitude, dry eyes, vivid dreams	Can exacerbate obstructive airways disease (asthma) and impair glucose tolerance — mainly beta receptor blocker side-effects
Oxprenolol	Pure beta receptor	40–80 mg bd	Same as labetalol	Same as labetalol
Hydralazine	Peripheral vasodilator by its effect on vascular smooth muscle	25–50 mg bd	Tachycardia, palpitations, headache, nausea, fluid retention	Observe for hypotension; usually given with a beta-blocker or methyldopa to avoid reflex tachycardia
Prazosin	Peripheral vasodilator due to alpha receptor blockade	0.5–1 mg bd or tds	Same as hydralazine	Same as hydralazine

rence of preeclampsia. Predictive tests for the latter complication include the supine pressor response ('roll-over' test), angiotensin-2 infusion response, and the plasma urate level: none of these add much to careful clinical care. The emergence of preeclampsia substantially prejudices fetal outcome (see later).

Assessment of the fetus. The well-being of the fetus must be monitored (see Chapter 13), the intensity of the investigation depending on the clinical state.

Induction of labour. The usual indications for induction before term are *fetal growth retardation, poor medical control* of the blood pressure, and development of *preeclampsia.* Routine induction of labour in all patients with hypertension is not indicated, particularly if conditions are unfavourable (nullipara, head not well in the pelvis, cervix unripe) and the elevation of pressure is mild (e.g. < 95 diastolic). In general, however, *induction at 40 weeks* is practised if hypertension persists or if the patient has required hypotensive drugs.

Care during labour and puerperium. This follows similar lines to that outlined for the patient with preeclampsia. The major difference lies in the long-term management of the patient with chronic hypertension — the need for possible *further investigation* (e.g. *intravenous pyelography*), continued drug treatment and surveillance, and the probable reduction in ultimate family size.

Table 33.2 gives an overview of the clinical features in a series of 253 patients with essential hypertension. The low incidence (0.6%) is explained by inclusion only of patients with a blood pressure recording of 140/90 or above on at least 2 occasions before 20 weeks' gestation, and in whom there was no known underlying pathology (chronic renal disease). Noteworthy were the high incidences of *preeclampsia, low oestriol excretion, induction of labour,*

TABLE 33.2   CLINICAL DATA IN 253 CONSECUTIVE PATIENTS WITH ESSENTIAL HYPERTENSION IN AN OBSTETRIC TEACHING HOSPITAL

	Number	%	
Incidence	253 in 40,982	0.6	
Superimposed preeclampsia	88	34.7	(9.7)
Low oestriol excretion	60	23.7	(11.8)
Abruptio placentae	4	1.5	(1.0)
Induction of labour	134	52.9	(24.2)
Fetal distress in labour	36	30.0	
Caesarean section	66	26.0	(11.3)
Small for dates infants	32	12.2	(6.2)
Stillbirths	9	3.5	(1.4)
Neonatal deaths	6	2.3	(1.2)

Figures in parentheses denote incidences in total hospital population

Caesarean section, small for dates infants, stillbirths and *neonatal deaths* — all of which were increased by a factor of 2 or more in comparison with the total hospital population.

It was concluded that these patients should be delivered as close to 40 weeks as possible, earlier delivery being indicated by *placental insufficiency* (clinical signs, low oestriol excretion, abnormal cardiotocography), *uncontrollable hypertension* or development of *preeclampsia.* When induction is deferred because of relative contraindications (high head, uncertain dates) when the pregnancy has .reached term, the fetal condition should be closely monitored (amnioscopy, cardiotocography). During labour, a time of special risk, the fetal heart rate should be monitored continuously, and a Caesarean section performed promptly if there is evidence of fetal distress in the first stage. The second stage should generally be shortened by forceps delivery.

The risks of essential hypertension in pregnancy are principally those of *superimposed preeclampsia,* which is associated with increased incidences of low oestriol excretion, fetal distress in labour and perinatal mortality.

chapter thirty-four

The Blood: Anaemia, Coagulation, Thromboembolism

OVERVIEW

Anaemia is a common disorder, occurring in 5–20% of pregnancies. The wide incidence range is due partly to differing socioeconomic conditions and partly to specific factors such as infection (e.g. malaria) and congenital disorders of haemoglobin formation (thalassaemia, sickle cell disease).

Pregnancy imposes significant haematological demands because of the needs of the mother's red cell mass expansion plus the general demands of the fetus and placenta. The relatively greater expansion of the mother's plasma volume over the red cell mass results in a *dilution of red cells and haemoglobin*; values of the latter above 10.5 g/dl in mid–late pregnancy are acceptable.

The *major causes* of anaemia are *deficiencies of iron and/or folic acid, haemoglobinopathies*, and general medical conditions (particularly *chronic infection and renal disease*). *Anaemia is thus a symptom rather than a disease per se.* It occurs if the elements necessary for red blood cell production are not present in the diet in adequate amounts (or not absorbed), and/or the bone marrow production is defective and/or there is an abnormal loss of red cells (by haemolysis or haemorrhage).

It is important to diagnose the presence and type of anaemia, since if neglected, the morbidity and mortality of both mother and fetus are increased (*inability to withstand haemorrhage, susceptibility to infection, cardiac failure, premature labour, fetal hypoxia and growth retardation*). *Laboratory advances* in haematology have greatly facilitated diagnosis as a result of automated determination of red cell indices (e.g. mean corpuscular volume and haemoglobin), plus determinations of serum iron and ferritin, and abnormal forms of haemoglobin. Such assistance does not absolve the clinician from a relevant antenatal history and examination.

In most centres, *routine supplementation of iron and folic acid* is now given, although some concern has been expressed that this might not be necessary if the diet is adequate, and might indeed be harmful in terms of blocking the absorption of other essential trace elements, such as zinc. Early detection is important in some of the congenital anaemias because of *genetic counselling* implications.

Patients whose anaemia is not responding to standard supplementation should be referred for consultant opinion.

Coagulation disorders are much less common than the anaemias, but are potentially very serious and usually require considerable expertise in diagnosis and management.

During pregnancy there is an increase in many of the coagulation factors and although this tends to protect the mother from the inevitable bleeding which occurs at delivery, it increases the risk of *thromboembolism*, particularly in the puerperium, by 5–6 times. The latter condition is notoriously difficult to diagnose clinically, and because anticoagulant therapy carries serious risks in pregnancy, specialist referral is indicated.

Disseminated intravascular coagulation is a specific type of thrombosis with generalized involvement of small vessels. Specific pregnancy complications are usually present (*major placental abruption, prolonged fetal death, shock/sepsis, amniotic fluid embolism, severe preeclampsia*). There is a secondary consumption of clotting factors and platelets which produces a haemorrhagic diathesis; this is treated by replacement of deficient blood factors and correction of the basic disorder where indicated.

Other coagulation problems include von Willebrand disease and various platelet disorders (thrombocytopenias).

Malignant disorders of the bone marrow may present with a coagulation problem or difficulties may arise during chemotherapy of such tumours.

ANAEMIA

NORMAL CHANGES IN PREGNANCY

(a) Maternal

Although there is an *increase in both of the major components of the blood* in pregnancy, the rise in plasma (45%) is significantly greater than is the rise in red cells (25%); this results in *haemodilution* which is *physiological and beneficial* — allowing the blood to circulate more easily, and heat generated by the fetus to be lost from the dilated blood vessels in the skin. *There is an apparent fall in the level of haemoglobin, red cells and haematocrit.* The size of the red cell and its haemoglobin content remain constant except for a moderate fall in the last trimester; therefore, the mean corpuscular volume (MCV) and mean corpuscular haemoglobin (MCH) are similar to nonpregnant values. *Platelet numbers* change very little in normal pregnancy, (200–300 × 10^9/l), although they show an increased tendency to aggregate. The *serum iron* level falls, but the capacity of the serum proteins (chiefly *transferrin*) to bind iron increases by about one-third, allowing greater storage. By contrast, the *serum copper* rises quite sharply; that of the fetus remains well below the mother's nonpregnant level.

The *iron demands* of pregnancy are as follows: fetus (300 mg), placenta (75 mg), mother's increased red cell mass (400 mg); these are required particularly in the third trimester. There will be a further variable demand as a result of third stage loss (50–250 mg) and lactation (0.5–10 mg/day). This total (500–1,000 mg) will be offset by the amenorrhoea of pregnancy and lactation, and the postpartum reduction in red cell mass (together 350–550 mg). The total amount of iron in the body in pregnancy is approximately 3,500 mg, of which 60–70% is in the circulating red cells — i.e. there is about 1,200 mg in storage depots.

(b) Fetal

The level of haemoglobin in the fetus (18 ± 4 g/dl) is much higher than in the mother and it is specially adapted to receive oxygen at lower concentrations than occur after birth. Thus we find that haemoglobin A (adult) is low, whereas haemoglobin F (fetal) is high (80%); in the embryo the main haemoglobin type is Gower (figure 34.1). The fetus is able to maintain a normal haemoglobin level despite quite severe anaemia in the mother (e.g. a haemoglobin of 6 g/dl).

DEFINITION

A haemoglobin value below 11.5 g/dl in the first trimester, or below 10.5 g/dl in later pregnancy. The fall in value depends significantly on the extent of plasma volume expansion — itself a reflection of fetoplacental adequacy.

INCIDENCE

Approximately 10–20% of patients, but this figure differs according to factors such as geographical locality and the age/parity profile of the pregnant population. For example, higher figures will be experienced if socioeconomic conditions are poor, diseases such as hookworm are common, or there is a high proportion of patients of Mediterranean origin (*beta thalassaemia minor* is present in 6% of patients born in Greece and 4% born in Italy).

Figure 34.1 Patterns of globin chain synthesis during embryonic, fetal, and postnatal life; the percentages of nonalpha chains are expressed relative to alpha chain production. Two alpha chains are initially associated with 2 epsilon chains (Hb Gower) in the embryo, then with 2 gamma chains (HbF) in the fetus, and finally with 2 beta chains (HbA) in postnatal life. Prenatal haemoglobin forms persist into adult life in low concentration; HbF, 1–2%; HbA_2, 2–4%.

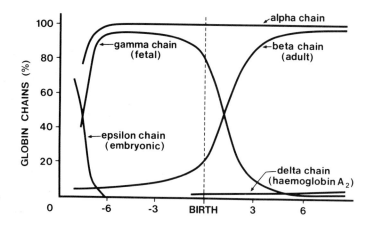

SIGNIFICANCE

The important *maternal hazards* of anaemia are the *inability to withstand haemorrhage*, an increased susceptibility to *infection*, and the risk of *cardiac failure* when anaemia is severe.

The chief *fetal risk* is that of *hypoxia*, reduction of the oxygen carrying capacity of the mother's blood aggravating placental insufficiency from any cause. *Premature labour* is more common when anaemia is severe.

When apportioning risks of anaemia in pregnancy the effects of *malnutrition* and *chronic infection* should be remembered.

CLASSIFICATION AND CAUSES

Iron Deficiency

Iron is an essential component of the haem part of haemoglobin. Normally, very little iron is lost from the body; the requirements are met by iron in the diet, 5–10% of the 10–20 mg in the food being absorbed per day. *This type of anaemia is approximately 10 times more frequent than the other types.* The patient may have depleted blood and tissue iron from: (i) poor intake (inadequate diet, anorexia); (ii) poor absorption (gastrointestinal disturbances such as vomiting and diarrhoea); or (iii) excessive loss (grand multiparity, menorrhagia, haemorrhage associated with pregnancy complications, or other causes such as epistaxis, haemorrhoids, hookworm and malarial infection). Patients with *thalassaemia* have a microcytic, hypochromic anaemia, but can be distinguished by having normal serum iron levels and *elevated haemoglobin A$_2$*.

As the serum iron progressively falls, the saturation of iron-binding proteins falls and bone marrow stores decrease.

Folic Acid and Vitamin B$_{12}$ Deficiency

Folic acid is a necessary intermediary in the metabolism of amino acids and is required for *cells undergoing division* — hence, relatively large amounts are needed in pregnancy. Up to 1,000 μg are required per day, and the fetus has top priority for what is available. Hence, anaemia from this cause is rare before 24 weeks, but increases thereafter, often insidiously, with the rise in fetal requirements. The causes of deficiency are broadly the same as for iron, although greater spoiling occurs with overcooking; it is more common in lower socioeconomic groups. Unlike iron deficiency, it may occur in the late puerperium if the patient is breast feeding and the diet is poor. In patients with haemoglobinopathies and *multiple pregnancies*, the demands are accentuated, and

deficiency is almost the rule unless the mother receives a folic acid supplement. The antiepileptic drug, phenytoin (Dilantin), may be associated with lowered levels because of decreased absorption by the mother. *Pernicious anaemia* is very rare in pregnancy: deficiencies of vitamin B$_{12}$ as well as folic acid may occur, however.

Congenital Disorders

In order to understand these disorders, brief reference must be made to the types of haemoglobin that are normally present. Figure 34.1 shows the relative amounts of the different haemoglobins present in fetal and adult life. Differences are based on the composition of the 4 basic globin chains: haemoglobin A (alpha$_2$ beta$_2$); haemoglobin A$_2$ (alpha$_2$, delta$_2$); haemoglobin F (alpha$_2$ gamma$_2$); in embryonic life there are several transient forms of haemoglobin (Portland, Gower).

These different chain types are necessary to produce the particular form of haemoglobin required at specific developmental periods.

Congenital anomalies arise (i) because not enough adult haemoglobin is being produced — either the alpha chains (alpha thalassaemia, South-East Asian type) or the beta chains (beta thalassaemia, Mediterranean type), or (ii) an abnormal form of haemoglobin is being produced — e.g. HbS (sickle cell disease) and HbC where the amino acids valine and lysine, respectively, replace glutamic acid in the beta chain. These are recessively inherited conditions (Chapter 17).

(i) *Beta thalassaemia minor* (thalassaemia trait). Commonly seen (5–8%) in Italian and Greek immigrants from the Mediterranean area (thalassa = sea) and to a lesser degree in those from South-East Asian countries. Fewer red cells are produced and the red cell has a reduced life in the blood (40 days instead of 120 days) because of a greater susceptibility to wear and tear as it circulates. Pregnancy seems to induce *haemolytic episodes* in some of these patients. In beta thalassaemia minor, the haemoglobin value usually fluctuates in the 8–11 g/dl range in the third trimester. In the major (homozygous) form of beta thalassaemia, severe anaemia necessitates repeated blood transfusion and often causes death in childhood. In homozygous *alpha thalassaemia*, the fetus is hydropic and stillborn, this being a special form of *erythroblastosis* due to inability of the abnormal haemoglobin (gamma$_4$; Hb Barts) to release its oxygen.

(ii) *Congenital haemolytic anaemia* results from increased fragility of the red cell due to its abnormal shape (spherocyte, elliptocyte). In anaemias with shortened red cell lifespan there is necessarily a hyperplastic bone marrow and greater amounts of folic acid are required. In *paroxysmal nocturnal haemoglobinuria*, there is a susceptibility of red cells to spontaneous haemolysis, particularly when there is stasis and a fall in pH in the blood, as during sleep. The morning urine is often discoloured as a result of the haemoglobinuria.

(iii) *The sickle cell gene* occurs in 5–10% of Negroes in the USA, usually in the heterozygous form (sickle cell trait (HbAS)). In this mild form of the disease there is not enough of the abnormal haemoglobin in the red cell for the molecular stacking and thus 'sickling' to occur; it is not associated with major morbidity, but requires *genetic counselling* if carried by both parents. As with thalassaemia, the homozygous state (HbSS) is far more serious; the maternal mortality may be as high as 5–10% and the perinatal mortality much higher. There is clogging of the small blood vessels by the abnormal red cells with consequent *ischaemia*, necrosis and haemolysis. The incidence of *infection* is increased (especially *pneumonitis* and *pyelonephritis*). Other complications include abortion, preeclampsia, eclampsia, prematurity, and perinatal loss. *Haemoglobin SC disease* (containing 2 abnormal haemoglobin forms, S and C) is similar to sickle cell anaemia in terms of complications; other combinations may also occur (table 34.1).

TABLE 34.1   HAEMOGLOBINOPATHIES IN BLACK RACES

Haemoglobinopathy	Approximate incidence USA	Africa*
Sickle cell trait HbAS	1 in 12	1 in 3–1 in 5
Hb AC	1 in 60	1 in 5 (Ghana) 1 in 20 (Nigeria)
Hb SS	1 in 600	1 in 12 1 in 50 (Nigeria)
Hb SC	1 in 850	1 in 200
Hb S Thal	1 in 1,600	
Hb CC	1 in 4,500	1 in 400 (Nigeria)

* High incidence areas

Acute or Chronic Renal Disease

Renal function should be investigated (serum creatinine or urea, creatinine clearance) when anaemia is marked or persistent, since the explanation may be *clinically silent renal disease*.

Haemodilution is described above under physiology.

In summary, if anaemia is noted in late pregnancy, one or more of the following is likely: the patient is not taking the prescribed iron or she is not absorbing it; there is folic acid deficiency (if routine folic acid has not been prescribed); there is a larger than usual plasma volume increase; the patient is losing blood either by internal or external bleeding or by haemolysis; or there is a primary hypoplasia of the bone marrow. In many cases, there is more than one cause operating (e.g. iron as well as folic acid deficiency).

SYMPTOMS AND SIGNS

The clinical features of anaemia are largely nonspecific: tiredness and fatigue, progressing to shortness of breath, oedema, palpitation, and eventually to faintness. A considerable variation is seen according to the rapidity of onset; if slow, values about 8 g/dl may cause little or no distress. Soreness of the tongue (glossitis), cracking of the angles of the mouth, and anorexia are sometimes complained of and usually indicate a folic acid deficiency, perhaps aggravated by vitamin lack. *Pallor* is present, but this sign differs considerably from person to person. Assessment of haemoglobin, even when inspecting palmar creases or the conjunctivae, is rather crude, particularly if values are above 8 g/dl.

INVESTIGATIONS

Before laboratory investigations are carried out, it is important to take a *history*, with particular reference to diet and drugs, gastrointestinal disorders, previous menstrual and reproductive history, and blood loss from any cause. *Physical examination* should be thorough, noting any changes in the skin (bruising), nails (koilonychia, brittleness), abdomen (hepatosplenomegaly), lymph nodes (enlargement), mouth (pallor, atrophy, gum changes, bleeding), and nervous system (peripheral neuritis).

(i) *Haemoglobin*. This test is carried out at the first visit and repeated at approximately 28 and 36 weeks. In some centres the value is checked at every antenatal visit. The initial test will detect preexisting anaemia (usually iron deficiency or congenital disorder) and the later tests are important in the detection of both iron and folic acid deficiency. As already mentioned, there is a variable drop in haemoglobin value in pregnancy as a result of *haemodilution*; however, investigation is warranted if the level falls below 10 g/dl. If there has been an abnormal loss at delivery (episiotomy, Caesarean section), a further check will be carried out in the puerperium. In the standard haematological laboratory investigation, the red cell indices, differential white cell count and platelet count are usually also assessed. (ii) *Blood film*. This is a useful screening test to differentiate between iron deficiency (hypochromic, microcytic anaemia) and folic acid deficiency (normochromic, macrocytic anaemia). Useful indices, such as the mean corpuscular volume (MCV) and mean corpuscular haemoglobin (MCH), are now routinely available from most automated cell counters; the normal MCV range is 80–96 femtolitres and the MCH is 27–31 picogrammes. Values below these ranges suggest the possibility of thalassaemia and further testing should be carried out (HbA$_2$ (normal value < 4%), HbF). The partner of a patient with the thalassaemia trait should also be tested to assist in genetic counselling. A preliminary 'iron screen' can be run of MCV (red cell iron) and serum ferritin (iron stores) and if abnormal, serum iron and iron binding capacity are assessed. (iii) *Haematocrit*. The normal value is 45%, falling to 30– 35% in pregnancy; it indicates the proportions of red cells and plasma in the blood. (iv) *Serum iron*. Normal value 15–32 μmol/l (80–180 μg/dl). This investigation is useful if the patient is not responding to oral iron (not taking tablets, malabsorption, occult haemorrhage). (v) *Reticulocyte count*. The normal value is less than 2%. It serves as an index of the rate of red cell production, and hence is raised in blood loss or haemolysis. (vi) *Serum folate*. The normal value is 3–10 mg/l, there being a slow fall during pregnancy; values are determined if folic acid deficiency is suspected. Other indices include red cell folate, study of blood neutrophils for hypersegmentation, and bone marrow for megaloblastic change. (vii) *Serum B$_{12}$ levels* may fall a little in pregnancy, usually secondary to low folic acid levels; true B$_{12}$ deficiency is extremely rare. (viii) *Haemoglobin type*. Used for the detection of abnormal haemoglobin as in thalassaemia (elevated haemoglobin A$_2$ and F). (ix) *Bone marrow examination*. Indicated especially if the patient is not responding to treatment, if the haemoglobin level is below 8 g/dl, or the blood film appearance is nonspecific or suspicious of a disease such as leukaemia. (x) *Tests on other organs. Gastrointestinal tract*: absorption studies if sprue is suspected; *urinary tract*: urine microscopy and culture, blood urea, blood nitrogen, and renal function tests. *Chronic renal disease* is present in about 8% of antenatal patients with haemoglobin values below 9 g/dl. Folic acid deficiency can be related to chronic urinary tract infections and causes an increase in perinatal mortality.

MANAGEMENT

General Principles

Education of the mother concerning *optimum diet* is important, as is the attendance for regular antenatal care. Although practices differ from one centre to another, *iron and folic acid are usually prescribed prophylactically to pregnant patients*. A wide range of preparations is available. The usual tablet contains 200–300 mg of ferrous sulphate (55–80 mg of elemental iron, of which 10–15% is absorbed), and, if folic acid is added, its dose is of the order of 100–500 μg. Organic salts of iron (gluconate, succinate) and slow-release preparations have been recommended if gastrointestinal upsets (nausea, diarrhoea/constipation) occur, but their superiority in controlled trials has not been established. The amount of elemental iron in such preparations is 60–80 mg, of which 5–15% is absorbed. The amount of dietary iron is approximately 6 mg per 1,000 calories.

Iron tablets are best absorbed between meals and, if the haemoglobin level is normal and the diet adequate, one tablet per day is probably sufficient. Iron in multivitamin/mineral preparations is less well absorbed because of the inclusion of calcium and other minerals.

It is important for the doctor and nurse to stress to the patient that *iron tablets are poisonous to small children*; tablets should be kept in a child-proof container in a safe place.

Active Treatment

(i) *Iron deficiency*. Unless the patient is not taking, tolerating or absorbing the oral iron, the haemoglobin level should rise by approximately 1 g every 7–10 days with 600–900 mg of ferrous sulphate daily (2–3 tablets). *Intramuscular iron* is not recommended just to get a quick result: it should be reserved for patients in whom there is a genuine intolerance to oral iron, continued noncompliance, or there is poor gastrointestinal absorption. The maximum dose (Jectofer) is 1.5 mg of iron/kg/day by deep IM injection into the upper, outer quadrant of the buttock, every second day. Care is necessary, particularly in obese patients, that the injection is given intramuscularly, otherwise it is poorly absorbed; poorer absorption is also observed in patients confined to bed. *Intravenous total dose iron infusion* is now rarely prescribed in pregnancy and should never be given without expert supervision and availability of full resuscitation facilities. If anaemia is marked or delivery is imminent, *blood transfusion* (usually of packed cells) is given.

(ii) *Folic acid deficiency*. Deficiency should

rarely arise if the diet (especially green leaf vegetables, liver, kidney, peanuts) is adequate and prophylactic therapy is given, even if a high risk condition is present (chronic haemolytic anaemia, *multiple pregnancy*, chronic pyelonephritis, anticonvulsant therapy for epilepsy). If malabsorption is present or there is a proven folic acid deficiency, folic acid tablets (5 mg) are prescribed 1-3 times daily. Occasionally, the intramuscular route is necessary. If there is blood loss from any cause (e.g. antepartum haemorrhage), there will be an increased need for folic acid by the bone marrow.

(iii) *Thalassaemia minor* and other haemolytic anaemias. These patients usually must accept a lower haemoglobin level than normal, since the body iron stores are usually high as a result of chronic haemolysis. It is important, however, to ensure that adequate folic acid (at least 1,000 μg/day) is being taken; if true iron deficiency anaemia is demonstrated (serum iron and ferritin studies), then iron therapy may be required. *Transfusion* is reserved for obstetrical indications (acute blood loss). The *genetic implications* of inherited disorders such as thalassaemia should be discussed. Couples should be screened where relevant and the risk of thalassaemia major explained (e.g. 1 in 4 if both parents are carrying the gene). Material obtained at *chorion biopsy* or *fetoscopy* allows an informed decision regarding pregnancy termination. Significant lowering of the gene frequency in the population will require, in addition, reduction of progeny by carriers married to normal partners.

Paroxysmal nocturnal haemoglobinuria may require intermittent transfusion with washed packed red cells, maintenance of the haematocrit at 25-30%; anticoagulants if thrombotic episodes occur; monitoring closely for signs of infection; avoidance of iron therapy.

Sickle cell anaemia. All black women should be screened for red cell sickling and if positive, prophylactic carefully-matched *packed red cell transfusions* are given to maintain donor cells between 40-50% of the total. It is important to *prevent anoxia*, since this increases change in the red cell, and also to *prevent increases in blood viscosity* (infection, preeclampsia). A partial *exchange transfusion* may be necessary in some patients with severe anaemia. Broad spectrum antibiotics and pneumococcal vaccine should be given in the early puerperium and catheterization avoided where possible.

(iv) *Tropical disorders*. Specific treatment may be needed for *malaria, intestinal parasites,* and *chronic infections.*

(v) *Miscellaneous*. Other types of anaemia are very uncommon (leukaemia and other blood dyscrasias, pernicious anaemia) and will require special management.

Gross anaemia

A haemoglobin value under 8 g/dl is uncommon unless haemorrhage has occurred or marked folic acid deficiency is present. If present, however, the patient must be admitted to hospital for immediate investigation and treatment.

COAGULATION

A number of dynamic processes maintain the correct coagulation level of the blood. In pregnancy, important physiological and potentially pathological changes occur in the system, so that *the woman treads a tightrope between thromboembolism on one hand and haemorrhage on the other*. To understand the disorders that might arise, one must understand the processes underlying haemostasis.

THE CONTROL OF HAEMORRHAGE

Basic Considerations

(i) *Blood vessels*. Injury causes a spasm of the smooth muscle fibres in the vessel wall and a liberation of *thromboplastins* which activates the coagulation process.

(ii) *Blood flow*. There is a sharp reduction in blood flow in vessels which are *constricted* as a result of damage, compression, or shock, and this slowing favours coagulation.

(iii) *Coagulation system*. Coagulation occurs when *thrombin* is formed from the inert precursor *prothrombin* (Factor 2) by the action of clotting factors and *thromboplastin* (present in platelets and tissues), and the thrombin then acts as a proteolytic enzyme on *fibrinogen* to produce *fibrin* and this by polymerization becomes insoluble, forming a network of fibres in which the formed elements of the blood become enmeshed. There are 2 systems. *Intrinsic* — changes in the blood itself, mainly platelets, set in motion the reaction which forms thromboplastin. Clotting of blood in a test tube is an example of this. *Extrinsic* — tissue injury outside the vascular system liberates the thromboplastin which then reacts directly with blood factors. Thrombus is dissolved after a varying period by the plasminogen-plasmin system, with the release of a number of 'split-products' of fibrinogen and fibrin. Figure 34.2 shows the sequence of events in the 2 systems.

The classical *clotting factors* are as follows:

1. Fibrinogen
2. Prothrombin
3. Platelet factor
4. Calcium ions
5. Labile factor
6. Accelerin
7. Stable factor
8. Antihaemophilic factor
9. Christmas factor
10. Stuart-Prower factor
11. Plasma thromboplastin antecedent
12. Hageman factor
13. Fibrin stabilizing factor

There are now more than 50 factors isolated which are considered to be involved in the coagulation process.

PREVENTION OF COAGULATION

Basic Considerations

(i) *Blood vessels.* The smooth intact endothelial lining prevents the initiation of coagulation. An additional mechanism involving the vessel wall is the production of *prostacyclin*, a potent vaso-dilator and inhibitor of platelet aggregation. It counterbalances the action of thromboxane A_2, a vasoconstrictor produced by platelets.

(ii) *Blood flow.* An adequate flow of blood in relation to the size of the vessel inhibits coagulation.

(iii) *Intrinsic fibrinolytic system.* To prevent unwanted fibrin deposition in the blood vessels and consequent blockage, there are 2 main checks — substances which limit the activity of thrombin (*antithrombins*) and substances which break down fibrin (*fibrinolysins*). In the latter system, there is an inactive precursor enzyme, plasminogen which, on activation by tissue or blood activators (chiefly kinins and clotting Factors 11 and 12) is changed to the active *plasmin* (a proteolytic enzyme) which splits the fibrin clot into 'split products' or 'fibrin degradation products' (FDP) of different size, and also attacks the precursor fibrinogen (figure 34.2). The degradation products inhibit the activator to serve as a regulating mechanism of overproduction, and as a limiting factor in fibrin formation. This system is essential also in clearing clots which have already formed in response to vessel injury (see above).

Figure 34.2 Interrelationships of blood coagulation and fibrinolytic systems.

NORMAL CHANGES IN PREGNANCY

Change in the blood coagulation system in pregnancy should be viewed in the light of life as lived thousands of years ago — before blood transfusions, oxytocic drugs, and hospitals were thought of. In those distant times, haemorrhage was one of the chief complications of pregnancy. It is understandable that nature has tended to make the blood '*hypercoagulable*' — i.e. there is an increase in major coagulation components (chiefly fibrinogen, increasing from 200 (non-pregnant) to 400–600 mg/dl and Factors 7, 8, 9 and 10), and a decrease in the anticoagulation components (the fibrinolytic system).

In the *fetus and newborn*, the fibrinolytic system acts as a protective mechanism for the removal of clots without the risk of haemorrhage, and the blood shows a decrease in clotting and platelet activity.

THROMBOEMBOLISM

Venous thrombosis and pulmonary thromboembolism combine to form a serious and often fatal complication of pregnancy and the puerperium. The nurse and doctor have vital roles to play in the prevention of these complications and in the first aid treatment of the patient with a serious embolic episode.

Incidence

Approximately 1–2% of patients develop *superficial thrombophlebitis* in association with pregnancy (colour plate 76). For *deep vein thrombosis* the figures range from 0.05–0.3% and approximately 50% are asymptomatic and the great majority occur after delivery. *Pulmonary thromboembolism* occurs in 10–15% of

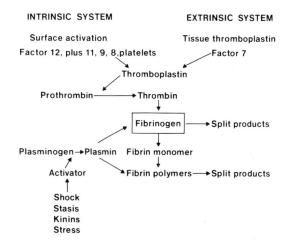

INTRINSIC SYSTEM	EXTRINSIC SYSTEM
Surface activation	Tissue thromboplastin
Factor 12, plus 11, 9, 8, platelets	Factor 7

Thromboplastin

Prothrombin → Thrombin

Fibrinogen → Split products

Plasminogen → Plasmin   Fibrin monomer

Activator → Fibrin polymers → Split products

Shock
Stasis
Kinins
Stress

patients with deep vein thrombosis and 1 in 15,000–1 in 60,000 pregnant women die as a result of this complication (approximately 10% of all maternal deaths, table 14.1). The likelihood of *recurrence of deep vein thrombosis* in subsequent pregnancies is 15–25%, the risk being significantly reduced by prophylactic anticoagulant therapy.

Mechanism of Thrombosis

When the smooth intimal lining of the vein is damaged, platelets adhere to the bare underlying connective tissue fibres. The damaged tissue and the platelets themselves release a platelet aggregating factor — adenosine diphosphate (ADP) and *thromboplastins. Thrombin* forms from *prothrombin* in the circulating plasma and is added to the platelet plug and this converts fibrinogen to *fibrin* which stabilizes the clot with interlacing strands.

It was mentioned earlier that nature is more concerned with haemorrhage than clotting. In pregnancy, especially, there is a *built-in clotting tendency* (greater concentration of factors in the blood). If we add to this a *slowing of the blood* (bed rest, anaesthesia, cardiac disease, prolonged labour) and *tissue damage*, the stage is set for the initial small thrombus to extend. This occurs as a result of further incorporation of platelets and fibrin, then red and white blood cells. If the clot spreads too far or the fibrin network is not strong enough, the clot breaks and is carried inevitably to the pulmonary arteries, and blockage of the blood supply to a part of the lung occurs.

The high risk profile. Clinical conditions predisposing to deep vein thrombosis include the following: *past history of thrombosis, cardiac disease, age over 30, para 3 or more, recently delivered by mid-forceps or Caesarean section, anaemia, obesity, varicose veins, and longer bed rest than normal.*

Lupus anticoagulant. The pregnant woman seems specially vulnerable to the effects of the *lupus anticoagulant factor.* There is a paradoxical situation of a major thrombotic tendency (arterial and venous, including the placental bed) despite an inhibitory effect on the generation of the prothrombin activator complex. The latter laboratory finding is due to the anticoagulant factor (an autoimmune 1gG antibody) reacting with phospholipid in the wall of the platelets; its more important clinical thrombotic effect may be mediated by platelet damage causing aggregation aided by an inhibition of prostacyclin in the wall of blood vessels.

Clinical Features and Diagnosis

The most serious form of thrombosis, from the viewpoint of fatal pulmonary thromboembolism, is that which forms in the deep veins of the legs or pelvis.

(i) *Superficial thrombophlebitis.* The clinical diagnosis is usually simple — there is a tender, linear, reddened area over one of the superficial leg veins (colour plate 76).

(ii) *Deep vein thrombosis.* The picture here is usually much less obvious. The patient often complains to the nurse that one or other leg feels heavy or painful. The affected leg is noted to be *tender* in the calf or thigh, slightly or obviously *swollen*, and the superficial veins are often distended. When the foot is dorsiflexed, there is pain in the calf (*Homans sign*). There are 4 main confirmatory tests. (i) *Venography* is the most accurate since it defines the precise site and extent of the thrombus; however, it requires pelvic shielding in pregnancy, skilled personnel, and is expensive, time-consuming and invasive. (ii) *Doppler ultrasound* is reasonably reliable (60–70%) (if the thrombosis is occlusive and above the calf) and is safe and easy to use. (iii) *Impedence plethysmography* is also safe, noninvasive and easy to perform and has a similiar usefulness as Doppler ultrasound. (iv) [131]*Iodine fibrinogen uptake test* can be used if the patient is not breast feeding. The latter methods are rarely sufficiently conclusive to act as a basis for long-term anticoagulant therapy. With the wider use of these techniques in some clinics, it is obvious that only a minority of deep vein thromboses were previously detected clinically. The majority of deaths from thromboembolism after vaginal delivery occurs after the first postpartum week and thus a *high index of suspicion should be maintained.* Any unusual leg symptom, unexplained tachycardia/fever should be investigated.

(iii) *Pulmonary episode.* In 10–15% of patients the deep venous thrombosis will lead to pulmonary thromboembolism and infarction; this is far more likely to occur if the thrombus detaches from a femoroiliac location. The classical features vary considerably according to the size of the embolus. At one extreme there may be complete occlusion of the major arteries to the lung with rapid death, while at the other there is no suspicion on the part of the patient or staff, the diagnosis being made on routine chest X-ray. In between these extremes, 2 syndromes are recognized. In *pulmonary infarction* there is obstruction to a small or medium-sized vessel; symptoms appear hours later — there may be tightness in the chest or pain, cough with frothy, blood-stained sputum, tachycardia, tachypnoea, cyanosis, and fever. The X-ray appearance is usually characteristic: initial radiolucency followed by single or multiple pulmonary opacities, pulmonary artery prominence, pleural effusion. More recently, *isotope lung scanning* and *pulmonary arteriography* have been used. With a *major embolism* there is occlusion of one of the large vessels. There is great oppression in the chest, severe dyspnoea and cyanosis; collapse may occur within seconds, often after the patient has called for a bedpan or started for the toilet. Examination reveals normal air entry, but usually a gallop rhythm is present over the heart. *Differential diagnosis* includes coronary thrombosis, amniotic fluid embolism and other acute pulmonary/cardiac episodes.

Management

Prophylaxis. Attention should be paid to the predisposing factors already outlined. (i) *Stasis.* Avoidance of the supine position, use of elastic stockings, adequate mobility and physiotherapy to maintain return of blood from legs and pelvic veins; also use of *calf muscle stimulators* during Caesarean section when performed under general anaesthesia. Prevention of hypovolaemia (avoidance of preeclampsia, long labour). *Immediate restoration of circulating blood volume in the case of significant haemorrhage.* Avoidance of pressure on veins (proper positioning, padding of calves when the legs are held in stirrups). (ii) *Thromboplastin release.* Avoidance where possible by minimizing tissue damage, hypoxia, sepsis. (iii) *Prophylactic anticoagulant therapy.* Because of a 10–15% risk of thromboembolism in patients with a past history of this condition, prophylaxis during pregnancy is often recommended. Usually this takes the form of twice daily subcutaneous sodium heparin injections. An adequate educational programme must be provided for the patient (often in hospital initially) and follow-up with home visits by a community nurse is helpful. Patients with *cardiac valve replacement* will already be receiving warfarin and this will need to be continued throughout the pregnancy — perhaps with heparin replacement during the organogenetic and the prelabour/labour periods. *Heparin* or *Dextran 70* have been used to *cover major surgery* (e.g. Caesarean section) in the high risk patient, but elastic stockings and/or calf compression are safer and cheaper alternatives. In patients with phospholipid autoantibody (lupus anticoagulant), treatment with immunosuppressive drugs (Chapter 39) and/or anticoagulants is necessary. (iv) *Family limitation* in high risk patients.

Superficial vein thrombophlebitis. Local treatment may consist of ichthyol and glycerine, Hirudoid ointment, together with an elastic compression bandage. *Ambulation is encouraged.* An anti-inflammatory drug, such as *aspirin* is useful (colour plate 76). If the length of vein involved is more than 10 cm, anticoagulant drugs may be ordered.

Deep vein thrombosis and pulmonary thromboembolism. Anticoagulant therapy, usually in the form of *heparin*, is necessary. The initial dose is 10,000–15,000 u and this is followed by 30,000–40,000 u per 24 hours preferably as an infusion, or in divided doses each 4–8 hours. Subsequent doses are calculated according to blood levels of heparin (0.1–0.3 u/ml) or coagulation indices (e.g. ATT 1.5–2 times normal). Self-administered subcutaneous heparin (5,000–7,500 12-hourly) may be introduced after a week or so. If the heparin is continued throughout the pregnancy (often the case if iliofemoral in location), it is discontinued temporarily early in labour and continued after delivery for a further 6 weeks, usually at a reduced dose. With long-term heparin therapy, regular heparin assays must be carried out. Side-effects of long-term heparin treatment include *haemorrhage* (colour plate 94), *thrombocytopenia*, and *osteopenia*; premature delivery and fetal loss are common to both heparin and *warfarin*. The latter, unlike heparin, *passes across the placenta*, and may produce *chondrodystrophy*, *optic atrophy* and *mental retardation in the fetus* as well as haemorrhage; it is also more difficult to adjust the degree of anticoagulation. If labour commences in a patient receiving warfarin, vitamin K should be given. Haemorrhagic complications occur in 5–10% of patients, but can be minimized by correct administration and careful monitoring; reversal of the heparin effect is obtained with 1% *protamine sulphate* — 1 mg per 1,000 u of heparin given over the previous 15–30 minutes (maximum of 5 ml, by slow IV injection). If the thrombosis occurs after delivery, an oral anticoagulant such as warfarin can be used after the initial heparinization.

Ancrod, a drug prepared from the venom of the Malaysian pit snake is useful for recent venous thrombosis in the *puerperium*.

Oral warfarin is an alternative to heparin, but suffers from the disadvantage of causing dysmorphogenesis in some fetuses. The loading dose is 20 mg and this is followed by 10 mg in 24 hours; as with heparin, further doses must be guided by coagulation studies. Reversal requires 5–15 mg vitamin K, by slow IV injection; check prothrombin time 3 hours later. Warfarin, unlike phenindione (Dindevan), *does not pass into breast milk* and can be given to lactating mothers.

Newer agents such as nafazatrom (400 mg tds), which stimulate prostacyclin synthesis, may be useful in special situations.

All patients on anticoagulant therapy should have an identifying bracelet and should be advised to avoid salicylates; any unusual symptom (e.g. indigestion) or any bleeding should be reported immediately. Procedures such as *amniocentesis* and *epidural* analgesia are contraindicated. Appropriate agents to reverse the anticoagulant effect of heparin or warfarin should be immediately available.

Inferior vena cava plication is reserved for those patients with repeated emboli or those with contraindications to long-term anticoagulant therapy.

With confirmed *pulmonary embolism*, the loading dose of heparin should be 10,000–15,000 u, and 40,000–60,000 u are given per day. *Bilateral phlebography* to determine the exact site and extent of the thrombosis is important. Treatment may be needed for right heart failure, shock, pain, and cyanosis.

If there has been a major *pulmonary embolism* (blockage of more than 60% of the pulmonary vasculature, right ventricular failure, persistent systemic hypotension), *surgical thrombectomy* (preceded by pulmonary angiography) or medical dissolution of the clot by streptokinase (600,000 u loading dose over 1 hour, 100,000 u hourly) may be undertaken — embolectomy if the block is proximal, thrombolysis if distal. Preliminary *emergency measures* may be necessary (external cardiac massage, admission to an intensive care unit).

COAGULATION FAILURE AND HAEMORRHAGIC DISORDERS

General Remarks

In obstetrics, *the great majority of patients with coagulation failure will have disseminated intravascular coagulation with secondary hypofibrinogenaemia.* However, there are a number of other disorders of the coagulation process which may occasionally be encountered. These can be classified as defects of the coagulation process itself or of platelet function.

Most of the congenital disorders will have declared themselves as a result of a positive history in the patient and her family of haemorrhagic problems, either spontaneous or related to trauma, surgery, menstruation etc. *Coagulation factor disorders* are usually characterized by ecchymoses and haematomas, whereas *platelet disorders* produce petechiae of the skin.

Basic Pathology

In most of the conditions to be considered there is *release of thromboplastins* into the blood stream; these then initiate clotting over a wide area of the vascular system, largely in the small vessels. These thromboplastins or 'procoagulants' may arise from *tissue destruction* or fetal death (trauma, hypoxia), acidosis, *amniotic fluid* (embolism), *red blood cells* (incompatible transfusion), or *bacteria* (bacteraemic shock). Enhancing factors are vascular stasis, overactivity of the sympathetic nervous system (usually as a reaction to shock), and damage to vascular endothelium.

As a result of *vascular blockage*, there may be secondary failure of the kidneys (oliguria/anuria), liver (jaundice), lung (dyspnoea, cyanosis), brain (convulsions, coma), retina (blindness), and pituitary gland (Sheehan syndrome).

Consumption of clotting factors, especially fibrinogen, Factors 5,7,8 and platelets can be demonstrated. A further complication arises when red blood cells encounter fibrin strands in the small blood vessels and become fragmented (*microangiopathic haemolytic anaemia*). Finally, the fibrinolytic system of the vascular wall is activated to dissolve the fibrin strands; this produces fibrin degradation products which can be readily detected in the laboratory.

Aetiology

The disorder is usually acute in onset (except as a late complication of fetal death) and can be caused by a variety of disease processes.

(a) *Maternal.* (i) *Abruptio placentae* (accidental haemorrhage). This is easily the most common cause (60% of cases; 5% of all abruptions), the thromboplastins being released from the damaged endometrium, placenta, and platelets. The syndrome is rare unless the abruption is severe enough to kill the baby. (ii) *Fetal death.* Usually, the fetus must have reached a certain size (at least 20 weeks) and the period of death is rarely less than 4 weeks before defibrination occurs. (iii) *Shock and severe sepsis.* Usually, the cause here is secondary sympathetic nervous system overactivity, plus the effect of bacterial toxins on the vascular endothelium and coagulation system. Also, *infections that cause haemolysis of red blood cells* (Cl. welchii, E. coli) release thromboplastin. Important infections are those complicating abortion and premature rupture of the membranes and those involving the urinary tract. (iv) *Amniotic fluid embolism.* Amniotic fluid is rich in thromboplastins and occasionally it may enter uterine veins, especially if there has been a tear in the uterus. Typically, the patient has had strong contractions (often oxytocin induced) and collapse occurs around the time of delivery, with cyanosis and severe dyspnoea (colour plate 62). If the patient survives, an incoagulable state usually supervenes. (v) *Severe preeclampsia and eclampsia.* Ischaemic tissue damage resulting from intensive vasospasm causes release of thromboplastins.

(b) *Fetal.* (i) *Hypoxia.* If the fetus suffers from major intrauterine hypoxia, the resulting ischaemia, especially in the brain, liberates thromboplastins. (ii) *Intrauterine growth retardation.* (iii) *Prematurity.* In both (ii) and (iii) the mild coagulation deficiency normally present in the unborn is exaggerated. (iv) *Severe sepsis.* (v) *Erythroblastosis.*

Clinical Features
It is noted that wounds continue to bleed, or spontaneous haemorrhage or bruising occurs. Blood collected for testing fails to clot in the tube within the normal 6–8 minutes.

Investigations
(a) *Bedside.* Take 5 ml of blood into a plain tube and observe. If, after 10 minutes, there is a stable clot, fibrinogen is > 1.5 g/l; partial clot dissolution, 1.0–1.5 g/l; rapid clot dissolution, 0.6–1.0 g/l; no clot, < 0.6 g/l. (b) *Laboratory studies* are based on the detection of the consumption of clotting factors (platelets, fibrinogen, Factors 5 and 8) and the special type of anaemia (microangiopathic) due to breaking up of the red blood cells by the fibrin strands in the small vessels. The normal values are shown in brackets. (i) *Bleeding time.* Ear lobe prick, blot every 30 seconds (5 minutes). (ii) *Clotting time.* Blood is collected into a plain glass tube held in the hand and gently tilted each 30 seconds (6 minutes). The formed clot should resist gentle shaking. (iii) *Blood film (EDTA tube).* Number and shape of red cells, number of platelets. (iv) *Fibrinogen (EDTA tube) (4–6 g/l).* (v) *Activated partial thromboplastin test* (APTT). A useful screening test (35–45 seconds), but does not detect deficiencies in platelets or Factor 7 (prothrombin time). (vi) *Prothrombin time.* If normal, defibrination/fibrinolysis is not the cause (12–14 seconds). (vii) Thrombin time (15 seconds). (viii) *Platelet count* (200–950 $\times$ 10^9/l). (ix) Tests for *fibrinolysis* (fibrin split products (FSP)) (normal value < 10 mg/l).

Treatment
The basic principles are removal of the precipitating cause if possible, correction of aggravating factors (shock, acidosis, hypoxaemia), and replacement of missing coagulation factors.

General measures as outlined for shock may be required.

Transfusion. The most effective treatment for the prevention of hypofibrinogenaemia is early and adequate transfusion, which prevents shock and the consequent overactivity of the sympathetic nervous system–adrenal response. Although solutions such as glucose-saline and plasma are valuable in replacing effective blood volume, *fresh blood or fresh frozen plasma* has the added value of replacing coagulation factors and platelets.

Fibrinogen. If serious depletion has occurred, i.e. the blood level has fallen below 1.0 g/l, intravenous fibrinogen (5–10 g) is necessary and often life-saving. This substance must be made up from the powder (usually 5 g amounts) by continued gentle shaking with added sterile normal saline.

Underlying conditions. The treatment of such underlying conditions as abruptio placentae, fetal death etc may need to be carried out.

Heparin. This drug was formerly used quite widely to prevent further coagulation and consumption of clotting factors. Its use has largely been replaced by active management of the causative process and replacement of coagulation factors.

Streptokinase. This substance may be ordered on rare occasions to dissolve established thrombi. In most obstetric patients with defibrination, the body's natural fibrinolytic activity soon clears the smaller vessels. Dose range (intravenous infusion) 250,000 u over 30 minutes and 100,000 u hourly.

Epsilon-aminocaproic acid (EACA) and Trasylol. These drugs are usually not indicated in the therapy of DIC.

INHERITED ANOMALIES OF COAGULATION FACTORS
Von Willebrand Disease
There is typically a history of epistaxis, heavy menstrual loss, easy bruising and operative/postoperative haemorrhage. The basic defect is in the Factor 8 complex, with a secondary effect on platelet function (this explains the prolonged bleeding time — a characteristic of platelet deficiency).

The main effect in pregnancy is a tendency to

postpartum haemorrhage. The likelihood of this is best gauged by the patient's past history and estimation of Factor 8 level in late pregnancy. If lower than 30-40% of normal, fresh frozen plasma or cryoprecipitate is indicated: management should have been passed into the hands of an experienced physician/haematologist. Since this is an autosomal dominant inherited disorder, there is a possibility of a haemorrhagic diathesis in the neonate.

Other Coagulation Factor Disorders

The commonest congenital disorder, haemophilia, is expressed clinically (with rare exceptions) only in the male. Any of the other classical coagulation factors may be deficient, but their occurrence is rare and will be handled at specialist level.

Platelet Disorders

The normal platelet count ranges from 150-400 $\times$ 10^9/l, and remains relatively constant during pregnancy. There is, however, an *increased aggregatory tendency*. Spontaneous bleeding is not usual until the count has fallen to 20-30 $\times$ 10^9/l.

The classical features of thrombocytopenia are petechial haemorrhages, a positive tourniquet test, a prolonged bleeding time and decreased clot retraction.

Automated platelet counting is now available in most large laboratories; bone marrow examination may be indicated if platelet production is thought to be subnormal.

Immune Thrombocytopenic Purpura

In this rare condition (0.1-0.2 per 1,000 pregnancies) there is a normal or even increased production of platelets, but these are subject to attack by the immune system and destroyed prematurely (platelet-associated IgG). A special variety of this condition is that induced by a heparin-dependent platelet-aggregating factor.

In pregnancy, there may be troublesome bleeding and treatment may be required if petechiae appear or the platelet count falls below 20-30 $\times$ 10^9/l. Prednisone, 60-80 mg/day, is given until a response occurs (usually in 7-14 days) and the dose is then tapered off to a maintenance of 5-15 mg/day. *Splenectomy* is reserved for patients failing to respond to adrenal steroid therapy.

Since the immune factors cross the placenta, the newborn may also display thrombocytopenia. Beta- or dexamethasone should be given to the mother late in pregnancy since these drugs cross the placenta more readily than prednisone and so are more effective in protecting the fetus from intracranial and other haemorrhage. In some centres a check of the fetal platelet count is made early in labour via a scalp sample and a decision made then regarding the need for prophylactic Caesarean section (e.g. if the count is less than 45-50 $\times$ 10^9/l).

Other Platelet Disorders

Thrombocytopenia may result from an idiosyncratic reaction to a number of drugs — either central (bone marrow effect) or peripheral, or from bacterial or viral infection. Serious thrombocytopenia from these causes is very uncommon in pregnancy. *Thrombotic thrombocytopenic purpura* is characterized by microthrombi in vessels and may be a manifestation of a number of disorders; the microthrombi cause dysfunction in the central nervous system, liver, kidney etc. It is often very difficult to distinguish from severe preeclampsia.

Therapy includes drugs preventing platelet aggregation, exchange transfusion, and fresh frozen plasma. As opposed to preeclampsia, the course of the disease is not dramatically improved by delivery.

Bone Marrow Neoplasia

Rarely, such conditions as *leukaemia* or other *bone marrow destroying diseases* may coexist with pregnancy. *Polycythaemia vera* has a deleterious effect on pregnancy (hypertensive disorders, abortion, preterm delivery and stillbirth). Repeated phlebotomy is the treatment of choice.

chapter thirty-five

The Digestive System

OVERVIEW

The digestive system shows many *changes during pregnancy*. The majority of these are of little importance and go unnoticed. Some have been considered in the chapter on *minor disorders of pregnancy* (Chapter 9). On occasions, medical or surgical disorders may arise in the gastrointestinal tract which pose a *serious threat to the mother's health or life*.

Incompetency of the lower oesophageal sphincter accounts for the relatively common conditions of reflux and regurgitation of stomach content. If persistent or severe, oesophagitis may result. Reflux may be associated also with *hiatus hernia*, a poorly diagnosed condition in which heartburn, dyspepsia and vomiting persist into the second and third trimesters of pregnancy.

There is an increase in mucin secretion in the *stomach* and this may account for the improvement in gastroduodenal ulcers in pregnancy. Nausea and vomiting are common disorders in the first trimester and are probably endocrine related. *Hyperemesis* is the term applied when the vomiting is excessive; weight loss and ketonuria suggest the need for hospital admission and intravenous therapy.

The *small intestine* is responsible for the digestion and absorption of nutrients. Lack of digestive enzymes or damage to this part of the bowel may result in *malabsorption* and perhaps *diarrhoea*, due to undigested/unabsorbed food. Because of the marked displacement of the small bowel by the enlarging uterus, *mechanical obstruction* may occur in late pregnancy if there are preexisting adhesions. *Ileus* may complicate Caesarean section if there is electrolyte imbalance or oral fluids are given too early.

Appendicitis in pregnancy is rare, but is potentially serious, particularly in later pregnancy, because of the greater tendency to intraabdominal spread of the infection. As with the small bowel, there is a marked upward displacement of the appendix as pregnancy progresses; this requires diagnostic and surgical reorientation.

The *colon* tends to absorb more fluid to meet the demands of pregnancy, and *constipation* is not an uncommon result. *Inflammatory bowel disease* (*ulcerative colitis, Crohn disease*) affects females of the reproductive age group. Abdominal discomfort and pain, diarrhoea, anorexia, weight loss and fever are common symptoms. Conservative treatment is the rule.

The *liver* has a significantly increased workload in pregnancy due to *increased metabolic demands* as well as the detoxification and excretion of products from the mother and fetus. *Jaundice* may need investigation. *Cholestasis of pregnancy* is a genetic condition characterized by mild jaundice, pruritus and biochemical evidence of intrahepatic cholestasis. *Acute fatty liver* of pregnancy is a rare but serious condition usually appearing in the last trimester; liver failure occurs rapidly and this must be treated energetically in a specialist unit and the pregnancy terminated. *Severe preeclampsia* and *septicaemia* are other obstetric causes of jaundice. *Viral hepatitis* is common in some countries and its course is not usually different from that in the nonpregnant person. Serological markers will identify the type and provide a basis for estimation of the risk to the newborn and thus whether protective immune globulin/immunization is needed. Patients with *chronic hepatitis* may become pregnant and complications include bleeding from engorged oesophageal varices (portal hypertension) and liver failure.

Biliary colic and *cholecystitis* are associated with gall stones; treatment is usually conservative. *Pancreatitis* in the pregnant woman is commonly the result of impaction of a small stone at the ampulla of Vater. The patient usually presents with acute upper abdominal pain and raised levels of pancreatic enzymes (amylase, lipase) in the blood.

PHYSIOLOGY

Appetite is often capricious, perhaps taking bizarre forms (e.g. pica). Usually the nausea of early pregnancy gives way to an increase in appetite which lasts until late pregnancy. The *taste threshold* is raised — that is, foods seem less flavoursome.

ORAL CAVITY

Salivary glands. There is an increase in salivary secretion (ptyalism), most obvious in the second half of the first trimester. *Teeth and gums.* There is no significant change in dental caries during pregnancy. The main change is in the gums, which become swollen as a result of gingival oedema; this explains why the *gums often bleed* after the teeth are brushed during pregnancy.

STOMACH

In late pregnancy and the puerperium there is an increase in acid and pepsin production; secretion is also high in the newborn. Gastric tone and motility are generally increased, whereas the reverse occurs in the oesophagus. Incompetence of the lower oesophageal sphincter explains the tendency to reflux, felt by the patient as *heartburn*. In late pregnancy, the enlarging uterus displaces the stomach upward under the left dome of the diaphragm and aggravates any tendency to *hiatus hernia*.

SMALL INTESTINE

There is little change in physiology with the exception of an improvement in iron absorption (due to increased demands) and a decrease in motility, with an associated slowing of the transit of food. Delayed absorption may explain the 'lag curve' often seen with oral glucose tolerance tests in pregnancy.

LARGE INTESTINE

The main function of the colon is to absorb salt and water from the succus entericus which is passed on from the small intestine. Relaxation of the smooth muscle produces a tendency to *constipation* which is aggravated if fluid intake is not optimal. With the enlargement of the uterus, the caecum and appendix shift upwards into the right flank.

LIVER AND GALL BLADDER

There is a selective, albeit mild, decrease in some aspects of function, mainly in relation to bile metabolism and excretion; there is an increase in bile viscosity and residual gall bladder content after a meal (the latter is demonstrable on ultrasonography); this is associated with a greater tendency to gall stone formation. There is little change in blood flow, in contrast to the kidneys.

PATHOLOGY
ORAL CAVITY

The only abnormality is an increase in periodontal disease.

STOMACH
Gastric and Duodenal Ulcers

Peptic ulceration is very rare in pregnancy; if already present, it tends to improve because of the increase in mucus production. The classical picture is one of epigastric pain and tenderness relieved by meals. Haematemesis and perforation occasionally occur and the symptoms of the latter are dangerously muted if the condition occurs in the puerperium. Treatment consists of avoidance of aspirin-type drugs, alcohol, and cigarettes; antacids (e.g. Mylanta, Gelusil) and after the first trimester an hydrogen receptor blocker (e.g. cimetidine) is indicated.

Dyspepsia

This condition is more common in heavy smokers and drinkers; this has been shown to be due, in part at least, to pyloric incompetence and reflux of duodenal contents.

The classical picture is one of epigastric pain and tenderness relieved by meals.

Oesophageal Reflux

Reflux of acid gastric content into the oesophagus causes the familiar symptoms of heartburn and water-brash (*reflux* or regurgitation). Oesophagitis may result, the changes ranging from mild inflammation to severe ulceration. If persistent, this may point to an associated *hiatus hernia*, a condition which is more frequent in the older, obese, multiparous patient (5–10% of pregnancies). Other suspicious features of this condition are indigestion, nausea and vomiting which persist after the first trimester, and an aggravation of symptoms when bending forward; *haematemesis* may also occur. Occasionally, most commonly in labour, the patient may experience an acute attack, with severe retrosternal pain and shock; cyanosis and dyspnoea may also be present. Other conditions to be considered in *vomiting of late pregnancy* include urinary tract infection, liver and gall bladder disease, intestinal obstruction, acute gastroenteritis and appendicitis.

Oesophageal reflux is managed by weight reduction if obese, avoidance of large meals, avoidance of food or drink for 2–3 hours before bedtime or any aggravating substances (alcohol, fats, chocolate) or drugs (e.g. anticholinergics), appropriate postural measures both during the day (avoidance of bending forward) and night (sleeping with the head of the bed raised 10–15 cm), reduction of heavy straining, and wearing of loose abdominal garments; sucralfate protects the oesophageal mucosa and metoclopramide is useful for symptomatic relief. If reflux oesophagitis has occurred, further measures are needed — antacids and antisecretory agents (cimetidine etc).

The treatment of hiatus hernia is basically that outlined for reflux and oesophagitis; the need for surgery (especially in the rolling type (paraoesophageal hernia)) may arise in the puerperium in the unlikely event that symptoms persist.

Hyperemesis Gravidarum

The usual sickness of early pregnancy becomes persistent and severe.

It is characterized by dehydration (a weight loss of 5% or more, reduced urine output, loss of skin tissue turgor), electrolyte disturbance and ketosis. If unchecked, symptoms of serious damage to body organs may occur: CNS (polyneuritis), liver (jaundice), renal damage (oliguria), and finally death.

The condition is now less common, occurring in 1 in 100–1 in 200 pregnancies. This is due mainly to improved management of the early stage of the disorder with antiemetic drugs.

In the *aetiology*, it is noted that primigravidas are more often affected, as are patients with *multiple* or *molar* pregnancies; a history of previous hyperemesis and/or unsuccessful pregnancy is more common. There appears to be some relation to *psychological stress*. Undoubtedly, the vomiting centre in some patients is in a more delicate balance than in others, as is the case for motion sickness. The agent which stimulates the vomiting centre has not been defined, but oestrogen must be regarded as the prime suspect in view of its known effects on the nonpregnant patient. Certain personality types seem more prone to the disorder. The possibility of an underlying *renal tract infection* must always be kept in mind.

It is of interest that if the reverse situation is present, i.e. if nausea and vomiting are absent, the patient is at higher risk of abortion and premature labour, presumably due to lower levels of pregnancy-supporting hormones (oestrogen and progesterone).

Management. (i) Admission to hospital is advised if ambulatory care measures have failed (dietary advice, rest, antiemetic drugs), particularly if there is evidence of dehydration or starvation as indicated above. (ii) The room should be quiet and darkened, to reduce stimuli; visitors should be reduced to a minimum. (iii) *Intravenous therapy* is given in the form of 2 litres of 10% dextrose together with 1 litre of normal saline and 1 litre of Hartmann solution per day; potassium chloride 25 meq (1g) is added if indicated on serum electrolyte analysis and also *vitamins* (Intravite plus pyridoxine). Usually the infusion can be discontinued after 36–72 hours, when a light diet is given. If more prolonged feeding is necessary, a hyperalimentation regimen must be substituted to provide the additional protein and caloric requirements. (iv) A drug to combat nausea is given, initially IV or IM (e.g. promethazine, pyridoxine, or metoclopramide). (v) Nursing measures include close attention to fluid balance, regular urine testing, vital signs, psychotherapy, and reassurance. (vi) Investigations include haemoglobin; serum electrolytes and urea (often as a multichannel autoanalyser check); mid-stream urine specimen for *microscopy and culture*; *HCG in urine or blood* (in case of mole or multiple pregnancy). (vii) If the condition is severe and/or prolonged, a careful diagnostic review must be made to exclude underlying pathology (acute appendicitis, bowel obstruction, hepatic, biliary and pancreatic disease, hiatus hernia, urinary tract infection and intracranial lesions). If nothing is revealed, deeper psychotherapy, perhaps including *hypnotherapy*, is often helpful. Only exceptionally is termination of the pregnancy necessary, usually on the basis of progressive deterioration, with evidence of parenchymal damage (CNS, liver, kidneys).

In a series of more than 40,000 consecutive antenatal patients in a teaching hospital, approximately 1% had hyperemesis of sufficient severity to warrant admission to hospital (table 16.1); 60% of these patients were admitted during the *first 14 weeks* of pregnancy; 70% had *ketonuria* and required *intravenous therapy*; 80% required only a *single admission*, and spent less than 7 days in hospital. Contrary to expectations, in this series of 263 patients there was no association with multiple pregnancy (6 cases), urinary tract infection (3 cases) or hydatidiform mole (0 case) although these possibilities must be considered. In this series there were 24 patients (9%) with a history of *past psychiatric illness*, and it was felt that many of the remaining patients had some underlying problem of anxiety, depression or psychosocial disturbance. It is probably this high incidence of psychiatric disorders in the 1% of patients with severe hyperemesis that gives rise to the belief that the aetiology of the nausea and vomiting which occur in 30–60% of antenatal patients has a psychological component!

Gastric Carcinoma

This is rare in women of the childbearing age group, but must be excluded if gastric symptoms persist despite treatment.

SMALL INTESTINE

Obstruction

This is often related to a displacement of the small bowel by the enlarging uterus causing tightening of preexisting adhesions. The characteristic symptoms are severe, colicky, abdominal pain and persistent vomiting.

Ileus

This is a paralysis of bowel function: it is usually seen after abdominal operations (Caesarean section) if feeding is commenced too early; it may also be the result of peritonitis, pelvic haematoma etc.

Malabsorption

This may have a variety of causes: *luminal* (pancreatic or bile salt dysfunction), *mucosal* (lactose deficiency, coeliac disease, sprue), *whole segment* (resection, radiation, Crohn disease, parasites, cathartics). *Investigations* include absorption tests (faecal fat, D-xylose, vitamin B_{12}); nutritional indices (blood film, serum folate, plasma albumin), and postpartum small bowel biopsy and/or barium radiography. *Treatment* is directed towards the cause — dietary modification, replacement of digestive substances, correction of nutritional deficiencies, antibiotic therapy etc.

LARGE INTESTINE

Appendicitis

This is a rare (1 in 500–1 in 1,500 pregnancies (table 16.2)) but potentially very serious complication of pregnancy, since diagnosis is more difficult and the infection is less efficiently walled-off because of the presence of the uterus. Consequently, rupture and general peritonitis may ensue; the morbidity is greatest in patients presenting in later pregnancy. The appendix is carried upward from its normal position in the

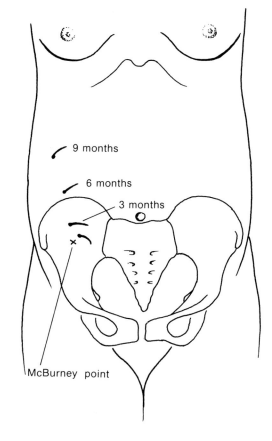

Figure 35.1 The position of the appendix alters during pregnancy, and so must the site of an incision to gain access to it.

right iliac fossa by the enlarging uterus, and pain and tenderness are thus experienced more in the flank than in the iliac fossa (figure 35.1). The characteristic features are fetid breath, abdominal pain, nausea and vomiting, together with fever, tachycardia and tenderness. The presence of diarrhoea should make one suspicious of *gastroenteritis*. The main hazard to the fetus is abortion or premature labour, precipitated by the intraperitoneal infection.

The *treatment* is appendicectomy. In the first 8–10 weeks of pregnancy, a paramedian incision is advisable in view of other possible causes of the right iliac fossa pain (complication of ovarian tumour, ectopic pregnancy, salpingitis); thereafter a high McBurney incision is needed. If the appendix is acutely inflamed, wound drainage and chemotherapy will usually be indicated in addition to the surgery to minimize the risk of abortion. If the operation has been performed in association with Caesarean section, particular attention should be paid to the appendiceal stump, since the caecum often distends markedly in the early postoperative period. Intravenous fluids are continued until there is no further danger of ileus. Drugs to relax the uterine muscle (salbutamol, ritodrine) may be given if premature labour threatens.

Constipation

This is the most common disorder of the large bowel. Appropriate management of this complication is by a high fibre diet, coupled with an adequate, nondiuretic type of fluid intake (i.e. not tea, coffee etc). The patient should be educated in the simple physiology of the bowel and defaecation. The strong gastrocolic reflex, which usually occurs after breakfast (particularly if the latter is preceded by oral fluids) results in a mass peristaltic movement of faeces into the rectum (this is postulated to be a prostaglandin effect). Ignoring this results in a decreased sensitivity to the presence of faecal material, progressive absorption of water, and hardening of the bowel contents. If a change in dietary habit is not fully successful, a vegetable bulking agent (Granacol or Normacol) will ensure the passage of a soft motion. Senokot (standardized senna) is a useful mild peristaltic stimulant.

Diarrhoea/Malabsorption

Chronic diarrhoea, if otherwise unexplained, should always raise the suspicion of intestinal dysfunction. Malabsorption may be the result of a digestive disorder (especially a pancreatic or bile salt deficiency) or absorptive disorder (decrease of absorptive surface by loss or damage — surgery, inflammation, metabolic and endocrine disorders). Modern techniques of radiology, small bowel biopsy and biochemical analysis have greatly facilitated the assessment of such patients.

If the diarrhoea is bloody, the important conditions to think of are bacillary dysentery, Crohn disease, and *ulcerative colitis*. Frank bleeding is more suggestive of polyp(s) or carcinoma of the colon or an anorectal problem such as *haemorrhoids*.

The *ileostomy patient* usually manages pregnancy satisfactorily: in some patients there may be enlargement/protrusion of the stoma and the appliance opening may need enlarging.

Inflammatory Bowel Disease

(a) *Ulcerative colitis* is an uncommon disease, but females in the reproductive age group form a significant proportion of sufferers. The symptoms are abdominal cramp, diarrhoea (often bloody), anorexia, fever and weight loss, these occurring characteristically in attacks with variable periods of remission. If the disease exacerbates it is usually early in the pregnancy or in the

puerperium. Abortion and other pregnancy complications are not significantly more common. Occasionally, a colectomy may have been performed previous to the pregnancy, and some of these patients may have an ileostomy. Treatment of the active disease includes a high protein, high calorie diet, *corticosteroids* (prednisone 60 mg/day, reducing with control of symptoms, perhaps with steroid enemas), *sulphasalazine* (0.5-2 g tds), antispasmodics, sedatives and antidiarrhoeal drugs; surgery (colectomy) may occasionally be necessary for life-threatening disease.

Total colectomy for this or other conditions of the large bowel (carcinoma) leaves a scarred area in the perineum, but this does not usually interfere with the passage of the baby's head or contraindicate episiotomy.

(b) *Crohn disease (regional enteritis)*. This is a chronic inflammatory disease affecting predominantly the terminal ileum and the colon. Symptoms are mainly intermittent lower abdominal pain, diarrhoea, weight loss, general ill health and fistulas. On examination, a tender mass may be felt, usually in the right iliac fossa. Pregnancy does not significantly affect the course of the disease, although there is a relapse rate of 20-30% in the puerperium. Treatment is usually conservative — bed rest, low residue diet, sulphasalazine, metronidazole (200 mg/day), and corticosteroids for active phases of the disease; surgery may occasionally be required for structural/inflammatory complications.

LIVER

Jaundice

This occurs in approximately 1 in 1,500 pregnancies (table 16.1); it may or may not be related to the pregnancy.

(a) *Related to the pregnancy*. (i) *Cholestasis.* There is a delay in the flow of bile and this may be due to a defect of any site from the canaliculus to the ampulla of Vater. Cholestasis of pregnancy (obstetric cholestasis) is due to an oestrogen sensitivity effect which is genetically determined and thus usually recurrent in successive pregnancies. It is more common in Scandinavia (up to 1-2% of pregnancies), South America and Mediterranean countries. The symptoms are mainly mild jaundice (the serum bilirubin is rarely more than 85 μmol/l), malaise, and itching of the skin. Liver function tests (alkaline phosphatase, urine urobilinogen) indicate biliary obstruction, and cholic acid levels are typically elevated. The condition clears up rapidly after pregnancy, and often recurs if the patient is prescribed oral contraceptives. There is some extra hazard to the mother as a result of postpartum haemorrhage (reduced vitamin K absorption). Premature labour is relatively common (30%) and the *stillbirth rate is approximately doubled. Induction of labour* is indicated at 40 weeks or earlier if oestriol excretion is subnormal or if cardiotocography indicates reduced fetal reserve. Cholestyramine resin (4–8 g per day) is usually effective (this lowers serum bile salt levels by chelating intestinal bile salts). (ii) *Acute fatty liver of pregnancy.* This rare condition occasionally follows intravenous tetracycline administration, or hepatic toxins, especially in poorly-nourished patients or those suffering from acute pyelonephritis. The condition is usually seen in the third trimester. Epigastric discomfort and vomiting lead to liver failure; the mortality may be 50% or more without energetic treatment. The patient should be placed in an intensive care unit: adequate intravenous fluids are administered, together with albumin, dextrose, and vitamin K; coagulation defects may need correction with fresh frozen plasma. The pregnancy should be terminated. Tests indicating recent liver cell damage (SGOT, SGPT) are elevated. (iii) *Severe preeclampsia or eclampsia* may occasionally result in liver necrosis, either because of the intense vasospasm producing anoxic damage or disseminated intravascular coagulation. (iv) *Severe vomiting.* Prolonged vomiting from hyperemesis gravidarum or other conditions such as hiatus hernia may cause liver damage and failure. (v) *Septicaemia* from such conditions as infected abortion and chorioamnionitis may result in jaundice and red cell haemolysis; the mechanism of the jaundice is unclear.

(b) *Unrelated to the pregnancy.* (i) *Viral hepatitis.* This is relatively rare in pregnancy (about 1 in 4,000 pregnancies), but is the most common cause of jaundice in pregnancy (50% of cases); there is considerable variation in incidence and severity according to the level of hygiene and nutrition in the community. Hepatitis types A, B and non-A, non-B all occur in pregnancy. *Hepatitis B* and *non-A, non-B* occur especially after blood transfusion or parenteral injection, and also from contaminated needles used for taking or giving serum, ear piercing, acupuncture, drug taking, and tattooing; *hepatitis A* infections usually result from contact with excretions of infected persons or carriers. Whatever the specific viral cause, the symptoms include a prodromal period of anorexia and nausea which is often marked, together with lassitude, pain in the right upper abdomen and fever; this is followed by jaundice, dark urine and pale stools.

The liver is tender and enlarged, blood levels of liver enzymes (e.g. serum transaminase) are markedly elevated, and in *hepatitis B* the specific hepatitis B serological markers will be positive (see Chapter 27). Treatment is along the usual lines. Termination of the pregnancy is not indicated. The fetus does not become infected but may die *in utero*, perhaps due to associated maternal pyrexia and toxaemia; the incidence of neonatal death is also increased because premature labour is more common. (ii) *Drugs.* Chlorpromazine, a drug sometimes given for pregnancy vomiting, may occasionally cause a cholestatic (stasis) type of jaundice which may last for many months or years. Tetracyclines have already been mentioned. The volatile anaesthetic, *halothane,* has recently been mentioned as a cause of liver failure, although usually only after repeated administration. (iii) *Chronic liver disease.* Patients with chronic hepatitis become pregnant infrequently, but increasingly so with modern immunosuppression therapy. The collaboration of a physician will be necessary if they do. The serum albumin level and the prothrombin time are good indicators of the severity of hepatocellular failure. Such patients may have *portal hypertension,* a serious and unpredictable condition in pregnancy; bleeding from portal-systemic (e.g. oesophageal) varices is the major concern. Fat soluble vitamins (A, D, K) may need to be given intramuscularly each month. Bleeding from the oesophageal varices is treated with an intravenous vasopressin infusion or a Sengstaken-Blakemore inflatable balloon tube; emergency surgery may occasionally be necessary. *Chronic active hepatitis* (CAH) usually has an autoimmune basis and if so, antibodies can be demonstrated to different normal tissues (cell nuclei, smooth muscle etc). A minority of patients may have unresolved hepatitis B and the associated hepatitis antigens will usually be present in serum. Both conditions tend to pursue a relapsing course. Autoimmune CAH is treated with antilymphocyte drugs such as prednisone and azathioprine. Premature labour and prematurity may occur, but with modern immunosuppressive therapy pregnancy and vaginal delivery can be anticipated, especially if the disease is well controlled. (iv) *Gall stones.* Repeated pregnancy predisposes to gall stone formation, and if a small stone blocks the cystic duct, jaundice may occur. The incidence of gall stones in the female is roughly 3 times that in the male. (v) *Chronic haemolysis,* e.g. from one of the varieties of haemolytic anaemic, incompatible blood transfusions, Cl. welchii infection.

GALL BLADDER

Acute Cholecystitis

Acute inflammation of the gall bladder is rare in pregnancy. The classical symptoms are right upper quadrant pain which often radiates to the back and keeps the patient immobilized, anorexia, nausea and perhaps vomiting, and fever; there is marked tenderness over the gall bladder area. The condition is treated conservatively (intravenous fluids, antibiotics, pain relief with pethidine and atropine, nasogastric suction) unless obvious progression occurs; surgery is necessary in approximately 1 in 5,000–1 in 10,000 pregnancies (drainage or cholecystectomy) (table 16.2). After delivery, a full investigation is carried out. Usually there is a coexisting cholelithiasis.

Biliary Colic

This is caused by a stone in the cystic duct or common bile duct. The pain is severe and tends to be constant; it often lasts for 12–15 hours. Treatment is conservative — i.e. pain relief.

PANCREAS

Acute Pancreatitis

The usual cause of this rare complication is a temporary impaction of a gall stone at the entrance of the pancreatic duct into the duodenum. It is characterized by severe abdominal pain (usually central upper abdomen radiating to the back), nausea, vomiting, anorexia, and flatulence; shock often ensues. Abdominal distension, tenderness, and rigidity are often present; there may be a vague mass palpable. The diagnosis usually hinges on the finding of raised levels of pancreatic enzymes in the blood (amylase, lipase); ultrasonography can be of confirmatory value. Treatment is usually conservative — supportive intravenous therapy, gastroduodenal suction, pain relief, atropine to reduce pancreatic secretion; broad spectrum antibiotics (e.g. cefoxitin) are indicated for cholangitis or pancreatic abscess.

The *endocrine function of the pancreas* (islet cells) and the subject of diabetes in pregnancy is discussed in Chapter 30.

chapter thirty-six

Intermediary Metabolism

OVERVIEW

Throughout pregnancy, the fetus is entirely dependent on the mother for the supply of raw materials for growth and energy needs. These materials are largely in the form of glucose, amino acids, and fatty acids. Synthetic mechanisms are well developed in the fetus, allowing rapid growth, and, in later pregnancy, the laying down of metabolic stores for use in the early neonatal period: both glycogen and subcutaneous fat can be used at this time, or before birth if there is deprivation of supply (e.g. placental failure). Enzyme systems for the breakdown of such stores, as well as those needed for dealing with metabolic breakdown products (e.g. those involving the ammonia-urea cycle in the liver), of necessity develop rapidly in the perinatal period.

The fetal demands, as well as the increased loss of metabolites in the urine are responsible for the relatively low levels of some biochemical values in the mother (e.g. glucose, creatinine, urea, albumin); this is added to by the haemodilution effect of pregnancy.

There are many applications of knowledge of the metabolic changes in pregnancy. It helps in the appreciation of fetal growth and its disorders, congenital disorders of metabolism (e.g. phenylketonuria and galactosaemia), and diseases such as diabetes mellitus which can profoundly affect both mother and baby. Periods of maternal fasting are less well tolerated and ketosis occurs more easily.

There are 3 primary nutrient materials — *carbohydrates*, *proteins*, and *fats*. These have both individual and interrelated metabolic pathways (figure 36.1).

CARBOHYDRATES

These substances are so called because they are primarily composed of carbon, together with hydrogen and oxygen (which form water); they provide the main source of fuel for the cells of the body.

The simplest sugars contain 6 carbon atoms — hence, are called hexoses, the most familiar example being glucose. When 2 such units are joined, we have sucrose (table sugar) and lactose (milk sugar). More complex units occur (polysaccharides) and these are used as building blocks (intercellular cement) as well as energy sources (starches).

Metabolism

A simple scheme of carbohydrate metabolism is shown in figure 36.1 Glucose may directly enter the cycle or may be derived from glycogen (a storage compound found chiefly in muscles and liver). As the breakdown of these 2 substances takes place, energy is released. Smaller molecules, particularly pyruvate, are produced which may enter one of 3 reactions: (i) Interchange with similar elements from protein and fat metabolism, (ii) breakdown to *lactate* if there is little oxygen (*anaerobic path*), (iii) breakdown in the *citric acid cycle* if there is adequate oxygen (*aerobic path*).

The level of sugar (glucose) in the blood is regulated by a number of hormones: *insulin* lowers blood sugar, whereas *glucagon* (alpha cells of pancreas), *growth hormone* (pituitary gland), and hormones from the adrenal cortex and medulla raise it. *Placental lactogen* is similar to growth hormone — it decreases glucose utilization by the mother and increases fatty acid breakdown; both of these actions provide an increased supply of glucose for the fetus. Although insulin levels rise significantly in pregnancy, hypoglycaemia is countered by the rise in antagonists, especially glucagon, which converts glycogen to glucose and favours gluconeogenesis (sugar from amino acids and fatty acids). The above hormonal actions render the mother more prone to both *hypoglycaemia* and *ketosis*, particularly if fasted.

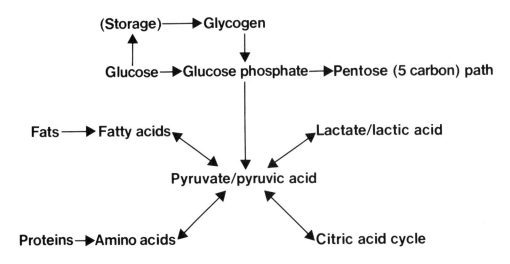

Figure 36.1 Important metabolic pathways.

Fetus and placenta. The dependence of the early embryo on *glycogen* stored in the Fallopian tube and in the lining of the uterus (progesterone effect) has been mentioned. Throughout pregnancy, the fetus depends on a constant transfer of glucose across the placenta from the mother by a process of facilitated diffusion — the difference in blood levels being 1.1–1.7 mmol/l (20–30 mg/dl); in late pregnancy, the fetus requires about 30 g of glucose per day. The fetus uses both of the energy pathways shown in figure 36.1, the *pentose path* mainly early in pregnancy when growth is very rapid (pentose sugars are needed for nucleic acid synthesis), and the *pyruvate path* mainly in later pregnancy.

After birth, levels of 2.8–3.3 mmol/l (50–60 mg/dl) are common. Only levels below 1.4 mmol/l (25 mg/dl) are considered to be significant in neonates.

At full term, the concentration of *glycogen* in the liver and heart muscle of the normal fetus exceeds that of the adult by up to 10 times; this is in preparation for the first days of independent life. Premature and growth retarded infants lack this important reserve.

Diabetes. The relation to diabetes is discussed in Chapter 30. If increased blood sugar levels are present in the mother, passage of additional sugar across the placenta to the fetus occurs; this causes the fetal islet cells in the pancreas to increase in size and produce more *insulin*. This produces more glycogen deposition, more adipose tissue and thus *fetal macrosomia*. After birth, when there is no longer a sugar transfer

from the mother, the high insulin secretion persists for a time in the baby, aggravating the low blood sugar levels — sometimes to the extent of causing brain damage, since the liver at this stage is relatively immature, and the brain requires large amounts of glucose for proper functioning and development.

Acidosis. When the muscles are contracting *strongly* for sustained periods (e.g. labour), larger than normal amounts of the breakdown products (pyruvate/pyruvic acid, lactate/lactic acid) are produced in the mother, with a tendency towards acidosis. In conditions of *fetal distress*, depending on whether it is chronic (chiefly glycogen stores depleted) or acute (oxygen lack), the acidosis is aggravated since, in the former situation, fat is used for energy, which is inefficient and produces more acidosis (fatty acids), while in the latter, more lactic acid is produced (anaerobic path). This acidosis aggravates the effects of oxygen lack in the cell. When the pH falls below 6.9, glycolytic activity ceases, and the fetus will die even if some glycogen is still remaining. Hence, during labour, the technique of *fetal scalp blood sampling* is used. If the pH (a measure of acidosis) of the scalp blood is less than 7.20 (normal above 7.30), the fetus is often in serious trouble.

PROTEINS

The proteins have the widest range of use in the body. The basic unit is the *amino acid*, of which there are 20 of importance. Most of these can be synthesized in the body, but for 8 of them (*essential amino acids*) this does not apply — they must be taken in the diet in the form of protein (meat, dairy products, eggs, legumes). Besides forming the bulk of the structural elements of the body, they have functions such as carrying the hereditary material (genes and chromosomes in the cell nucleus), providing the material for cell division, speeding up most of the chemical reactions in the body (*enzymes*) and forming the globin part of haemoglobin in the red cell.

Metabolism

Protein is absorbed from the gut after breakdown of dietary protein in the form of amino acids. These are then built up into progressively more complex compounds (peptides, polypeptides) and, finally, 'structural' or 'operational' proteins. The genetic material DNA (deoxyribonucleic acid) and RNA (ribonucleic acid) determines how, where, and when the amino acids will be built up in the body. If a 'decision' is made in the cell nucleus, or by a hormone arriving at the cell, for a particular protein to be synthesized, messengers are sent into the cytoplasm from the nucleus which have 'stamped' on them the amino acid sequence which is required (messenger RNA). Then, one of the cytoplasmic components, called the ribosome, is activated and this runs along the messenger RNA. The free amino acids are brought up to the messenger RNA in the required sequence by couriers (transfer RNA), and these await the arrival of the ribosome to pick up and build them correctly. Then, another ribosome comes up to the messenger RNA and the process is repeated until a feed-back message is received by the cell that enough new units have been produced.

Protein synthesis or build-up is influenced generally by *growth hormone* (from the pituitary gland) and *insulin* (from the islet cells of the pancreas). Many other hormones have specific actions — for example, the other hormones of the pituitary gland (thyroid, adrenal, gonads). These probably act by stimulating the ribosomes in the cell.

The *intermediary metabolism* of proteins is rather complex. Like carbohydrates, they can be broken down when not required, or used as a reserve form of energy. The main process is by *deamination* which produces ammonia from the nitrogen-containing amino group and this is then metabolized to urea by the liver and excreted by the kidney. The nonnitrogen residue can join the carbohydrate final energy path.

Fetus and placenta. The importance of an adequate protein supply can be imagined from the rapidity of fetal growth. This building material must be supplied to the fetus as amino acids or smaller residues from the mother for transfer across the placenta; these are supplied against a 1:2 gradient. If the placenta is not functioning properly (placental insufficiency) as a result of poor development or the effect of maternal disease (preeclampsia, hypertension, renal disease), the supply of materials for growth will be inadequate and *fetal growth retardation or death* will result.

It is now appreciated that some drugs, chiefly of the antibiotic group (streptomycin, chloramphenicol, tetracyclines) are bound to the ribosomes and prevent them from carrying out their work — i.e. building up new polypeptides on the messenger RNA model. This explains why the teeth and bones of fetuses are poorly formed if the mother has been given *tetracycline*.

There are a large number of *disorders of protein intermediary metabolism* (Chapter 17), the most serious being *phenylketonuria*. This occurs because a crucial enzyme is missing which is necessary to convert the amino acid phenylalanine to tyrosine. The phenylalanine banks up in the blood, becomes toxic to the brain of the growing child, and causes idiocy unless picked up by a routine blood sample after birth (Guthrie test). Such patients must remain on a low phenylalamine diet, both for their own well-being, and particularly for that of the fetus should they become pregnant.

FATS

There is a wide variety of compounds in the body which are included in this group. These provide *insulation* (subcutaneous fat), an economical store of *energy* (fatty acids), and *building components* (cell membranes, sheaths of nerve fibres). The fat distribution is characteristically different in the female and male.

Fats have the characteristic features of being soluble in chloroform and other nonaqueous solvents. The chief compounds are fatty acids, which may be saturated (palmitic, stearic) or unsaturated (linolenic, linoleic), triglycerides, or more complex compounds, such as phospholipids (lecithin and sphingomyelin), glycolipids, or steriods (cholesterol, adrenal and sex hormones, bile acids).

Metabolism

Like carbohydrates and proteins, fats in the diet are broken down into smaller units in the stomach and upper part of the small intestine and, with the help of bile acids, are absorbed into the lymphatics. Also like the other 2 compounds, breakdown and reformation is constantly taking place. The *breakdown of fatty acids* is a fairly simple process — there is a progressive splitting off of 2 carbon units which are oxidized to carbon dioxide and water by cell enzymes which are housed in special compartments of the cell cytoplasm called mitochondria. Thus, fats can directly provide energy as can carbohydrate. *In starvation or in severe exercise, when the carbohydrate stores are used up, most of the energy comes from fat.* Because the end products (ketone bodies) cannot be handled as easily as carbohydrate end products, they build up in the body, sometimes to toxic levels (ketoacidosis); this can be seen in *hyperemesis gravidarum, prolonged labour,* and *diabetes mellitus.*

Many hormones stimulate fatty acid release, including the hormone placental chorionic somatomammotrophin (HCS) (also called human placental lactogen (HPL)).

The building up process is a reverse of the above, the basic units mainly being fatty acids absorbed from the bowel, but also glucose can be converted to fatty acids as can the storage compound triglyceride under the action of insulin.

Fetus and placenta. Some fatty acids pass to the fetus from the mother via the placenta, and the fetus builds up its own complex lipids (e.g. phospholipids for lung maturity and myelin sheaths for the nerves of the brain and spinal cord). The fetus uses carbohydrate predominantly for energy, but can metabolize ketones faster than the adult, especially in the brain. After birth, with the addition of a fat-rich milk diet, there is a greater utilization of fatty acids.

Some 10–15% of the baby at birth is in the form of fat, most of which is laid down in the last weeks of pregnancy. *The premature baby* thus has little fat, and so has poor insulation (gets cold more easily) and poor energy stores to mobilize. The same applies to the baby who is growth retarded or *placentally insufficient* from any

cause. A special type of fat is also laid down in the fetus — *brown fat.* This is important in the provision of energy and prevention of cooling. It is present also in hibernating animals which, like the fetus, are often faced with the need to have a quick warming system. Brown fat, unlike the more usual white fat, can be metabolized completely in the cell itself, usually under the stimulus of the autonomic nervous system. This process needs oxygen and thus a premature baby, or one without fat insulation, particularly if hypoxic, will lose heat very rapidly and must be dried and quickly wrapped in warm covers, or placed in an incubator.

The reverse situation is seen in the *babies of diabetic mothers* — they are often oversized and fat. An excess of both glucose and insulin tends to cause deposition of fat, and both these are present in such babies (excess sugar from the mother, and excess insulin from the baby's pancreas trying to cope with it).

The change in the ratio of lung stabilizing *phospholipids* (lecithin and sphingomyelin) in the liquor as the baby matures is now used as an important test for fetal pulmonary maturity.

Mother. In the blood of the pregnant woman, there is a rise in most of the types of fat. The changes are the opposite of those described above for the baby of the diabetic mother — there is an antagonist to insulin, and fats are mobilized from the mother's stores. This antagonist is probably the placental hormone, HCS (HPL). The greatest increases are seen in the triglycerides and cholesterol (mainly low density lipoprotein type). By using these lipids for energy, more glucose can be spared for the fetus, which uses this to a much larger extent.

Although the fat contents of human and animal milk are similar, the nature of the fats themselves is different. Human milk contains more of the essential fatty acids as well as more unsaturated ('atheroma preventing') fatty acids.

chapter thirty-seven

The Urinary System

OVERVIEW

The kidneys are paired retroperitoneal organs situated in the upper part of the posterior abdominal wall. The million or so functional units (nephrons) of the kidney lie in the cortical zone; from these units the filtered plasma passes to the collecting tubules in the renal medulla, thence to the minor and major calyces which empty into the pelvis of the kidney. This in turn narrows to form the ureter, which empties into the bladder. The kidneys, renal pelvis and ureters form the upper urinary tract, while the bladder and urethra form the lower urinary tract.

The essential measures of *kidney function* are the renal blood flow (900 ml/minute), glomerular filtration rate (120 ml/minute), and tubular reabsorption; *bladder function* is usually considered in terms of capacity (over 500 ml), together with rate and completeness of emptying.

The kidneys, together with the cardiovascular system, bear a large part of the burden of the woman's adaptation to pregnancy. *There is a 40–50% increase in renal plasma flow and glomerular filtration rate*; the tubules are unable to reabsorb all of the filtered material, and so there is a waste of substances normally retained (e.g. sugar, amino acids, vitamins, minerals). There is also a significant *dilatation of the renal pelvis and ureter* (due to progesterone) which simulates obstruction on radiographic films.

The major disorder in pregnancy is *infection* — either in the kidney or the bladder. Since this infection is often silent — i.e. producing no symptoms, it is *routinely tested for by the dip-slide method on a clean mid-stream urine specimen collected at the first antenatal visit*. If there are 10^5 organisms/ml, 'significant' bacteriuria is said to be present; this occurs in 5–8% of antenatal women. Since such patients are at risk for a number of complications (anaemia, acute pyelonephritis, premature labour, increased perinatal loss), the infection is treated according to the laboratory sensitivity tests.

Overt infection may occur in the kidney (pyelonephritis), bladder (cystitis) or both of these sites. Renal infection is far more serious, since permanent damage may occur. The clinical picture usually allows the differentiation to be made. If the infection is recurrent, full investigation (including radiographic studies) must be carried out in the puerperium. Conditions tending to cause chronicity of infection in the younger adult include *congenital malformations* of the urinary tract, medical disorders which are associated with renal damage (*diabetes mellitus*), *calculus*, or unusual organisms (tubercle bacillus).

A number of other acute and chronic renal disorders may complicate pregnancy — glomerulonephritis, polycystic kidney, lupus erythematosus. In many patients, particularly if there is hypertension and depressed renal function, there is a major risk to the patient's life because of the added strain on the kidneys, and pregnancy termination will be considered. The added complication of *preeclampsia* also occurs more often in the patient with preexisting renal damage.

Acute retention of urine may occur towards the end of the first trimester because of urethral obstruction from a retroverted uterus trapped in the hollow of the sacrum; the same effect may result from pressure of the presenting part in labour. In the puerperium, the retention is more likely to be reflex in nature — micturition being inhibited by the pain of nearby tears and incisions, together with the physical effects of swelling and bruising close to the bladder neck and urethra.

CHANGES IN PREGNANCY

There are a number of changes affecting the urinary tract during pregnancy. (i) Under the influence of progesterone there is a *dilatation* of the renal pelvis and ureters (average capacity increases from 10 to 40 ml) (figure 37.1) and this, plus the increase in vascularity, increases the renal length by 1 cm or so. (ii) With the growth of the uterus, the *bladder is carried up* and becomes more an abdominal organ; the bladder neck however, does not rise appreciably, although it is displaced forwards against the symphysis pubis. (iii) In late pregnancy *the enlarged uterus compresses the ureters* at the pelvic brim, causing a further slowing of urine flow. The effect is greater on the right side, partly because of the dextrorotation of the uterus and partly because of the cushioning effect of the pelvic colon on the left side. Another factor causing ureteric compression is the great hypertrophy of the ovarian and uterine plexuses of veins through which the ureter passes. (iv) With the increase in blood volume there is a 40–50% *increase in renal blood flow and glomerular filtration rate*. As a result, the capacity of the tubular cells to reabsorb certain substances is exceeded (particularly sugar, amino acids, folic acid, water soluble vitamins, and iodine), and this explains the frequency of *glycosuria* (lowered renal threshold). Protein in the urine increases from the nonpregnant level of 35–100 mg per 24 hours up to 300 mg per 24 hours. Waste products such as *creatinine* and *urea* are also cleared more readily and this explains the lower plasma levels observed in pregnancy (normal range 0.3–0.11 mmol/l; 1.7–6.7 mmol/l, respectively). (v) There is an increase in urine produced which, together with the pressure exerted by the enlarging uterus on the bladder, *increases the frequency of micturition*. In pregnancy, and especially in the puerperium, the bladder becomes twice as full before there is a desire to micturate. (vi) There is an *increase in aldosterone, renin and its substrate*; the patient is more resistant to an angiotensin infusion.

INFECTION

(a) Bacteriuria

Incidence. Bacteria can be cultured from the urine in 5–10% of pregnant patients; of those negative at the initial test, 5% will become positive later in pregnancy if retested.

Significant bacteriuria in pregnancy is important for a number of reasons. (i) Thirty per cent

A

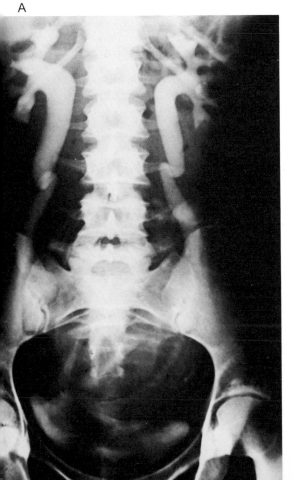

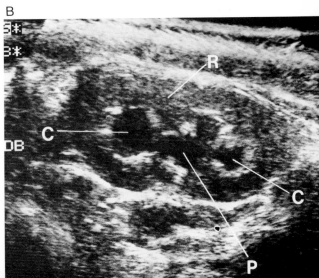

Figure 37.1 Pregnancy hydronephrosis and hydroureters. **A.** Pyelogram at 18 weeks showing a fetal skeleton in the pelvis and marked dilatation, elongation, and kinking of the ureters. This is an extreme example of the effects of pregnancy upon the urinary tract. The patient had recurrent pyelonephritis during pregnancy. **B.** This longitudinal ultrasound scan was performed at 30 weeks' gestation in a 19-year-old nullipara with left-sided loin pain thought to be renal colic. There is moderate dilatation of the renal pelvis (P) and calyces (C) without loss of renal cortical substance (R). This degree of hydronephrosis is outside the normal physiological range of pregnancy, especially for the left side. Ultrasonography can often detect a calculus in the pelvicalyceal system but not as readily in the lower ureter. If the clinical situation warrants further investigation to exclude a calculus, a limited intravenous pyelogram is performed.

B

or more of such patients develop clinical infection, which is rare (2–3%) in nonbacteriuric patients. (ii) Other complications are more prevalent — abortion, hypertension, pre-eclampsia, anaemia, prematurity and perinatal loss. (iii) Established chronic pyelonephritis will be seen in approximately one-third of these patients in 10–15 years; hence such patients should be investigated postpartum (by intravenous pyelography) for underlying abnormalities of the urinary tract.

Aetiology. The presence of significant numbers of bacteria in a properly collected mid-stream specimen indicates the presence of infection in some part of the urinary tract. Subclinical ('silent') infections are most likely to be in the kidney (chronic pyelonephritis), but may also be in the bladder (chronic cystitis). The former is more likely if there is some previous damage to the kidney (congenital hydronephrosis, stone), and the latter is more common if hygiene is poor, intercourse frequent (honeymoon cystitis) or *catheterization* has been employed. Statistically, bacteriuria is more common also in multiparas, and in those with such conditions as diabetes, hypertension, sickle cell anaemia.

Upper and lower urinary tract infection can be distinguished by careful catheterization, collection of bladder urine, running a urinary antiseptic into the bladder (aqueous Hibitane, 1 in 10,000, or a weak neomycin solution), washing it out with sterile saline, and finally collecting the urine coming into the clean bladder from the kidneys. Newer techniques such as the detection of antibody coating of bacteria, have helped to localize upper tract infections.

Diagnosis. Often there is a history of recurrent attacks of pyelonephritis, particularly in childhood, early married life, and pregnancy. Excessive analgesic intake may be noted. A *mid-stream urine test* is now routine in most antenatal clinics (table 6.1). Although each hospital has its own particular method for this investigation, the basic principles are the same: (i) proper cleansing of the vulva with a liquid soap or other nonantiseptic solution and drying; (ii) the labia may need to be separated when voiding; (iii) the patient micturates in the normal way and the mid-stream urine is collected into a sterile container; (iv) the urine container, properly labelled, is either sent immediately to the pathology laboratory or refrigerated until it can be sent or collected. Since the number of bacteria doubles in 30 minutes at room temperature, dip-slide or dip-spoon cultures should be used if the above conditions cannot be met. A tampon may be inserted in the lower vagina if contamination by discharge is likely.

In some centres, specimens are obtained by *suprapubic puncture* of the distended bladder. This is a simple and safe procedure, but is probably only indicated in the early puerperal patient if a routine clean mid-stream specimen is difficult to obtain.

Significant bacteriuria means 100,000 (10^5) organisms or more per ml of urine; a value between 10,000 (10^4) and 100,000 (10^5) is equivocal and indicates that the test should be repeated. A poorly collected specimen (contaminated) usually contains less than 10^5 organisms per ml, and the types of bacteria are often different.

Coitus will produce a transient bacteriuria in about 30% of females, and this should be appreciated when assessing positive cultures.

Treatment. If significant bacteriuria is present in a mid-stream (or catheter) specimen, a course of the appropriate antibacterial drug (determined by laboratory testing) is given. A single dose of *co-trimoxazole* is almost as effective as a 5-day course and can be used initially, with a longer course reserved for failures/recurrences. Further specimens should be tested after completion of the course and at intervals of 2–3 months during the pregnancy. If bacteriuria persists or recurs, or prophylaxis is required, a longer course — perhaps with a different drug — should be administered. Since coitus may precipitate attacks, the drug can be given soon after this activity, perhaps coupled with the use of an antiseptic cream (0.5% cetrimide) to the periurethral area. Double micturition is of benefit if there is vesicoureteric reflux of urine.

(b) Overt Infection

Incidence. The overall incidence of pyelonephritis in pregnancy is 2–4% (table 16.2).

Aetiology. (i) *Urine slowing* (stasis) resulting partly from loss of tone in the ureters and bladder and partly from pressure of the enlarging uterus and ovarian veins; (ii) *trauma* to the bladder and urethra, especially in labour; (iii) introduction of organisms by *catheterization* (now much less common than formerly); (iv) *weakness of the sphincter between the ureter and bladder* allowing reflux of infected urine upwards; (v) increase in glucose, amino acids and other bacterial growth promoting substances in the urine; (vi) *general factors* such as poor hygiene, high parity, and certain medical disorders (e.g. sickle cell anaemia and diabetes mellitus).

Organisms. The predominant organisms in urinary tract infection whether subclinical or clinical, are bowel inhabitants: E. coli, Streptococcus faecalis, Aerobacter aerogenes, Klebsiella, and Proteus species. The presence of less common pathogens and pyuria suggests that there may be underlying renal pathology.

Diagnosis. If overt infection is present, the diagnosis is usually simple. The patient complains of dysuria and frequency of micturition, pain in the flank radiating to the groin, fever and chills; anorexia and vomiting are often associated. Findings on urine microscopy usually allow an immediate diagnosis (pus cells, red cells, and organisms). Proteinuria is often present, but is seldom more than a heavy cloud on boiling or + to + + on Albustix testing. Generalized oedema is not present unless there is an associated preeclampsia or nephrotic condition. Other disorders which can be mimicked are acute appendicitis, labour, and other causes of an acute abdomen. In the puerperium, it may be difficult to distinguish from uterine and parametrial infection until laboratory tests are available.

Full blood examination, serum creatinine, and perhaps a creatinine clearance test should be carried out to assess if there is renal impairment. A plasma or urine oestriol test is often helpful in the last trimester to determine fetal well-being. After delivery, an *intravenous pyelogram* should be ordered when the physiological dilatation of the upper urinary tract has subsided (2–4 months).

Treatment. (a) *Acute pyelonephritis.* There is a wide spectrum of disease severity, ranging from the patient who is virtually asymptomatic to one who is desperately ill with septicaemia and shock. (i) *Specific measures. Chemotherapy.* This will be given according to laboratory testing, although a drug will usually be ordered pending the result. The main agents include the synthetic penicillins, a cephalosporin derivative, an aminoglycoside, trimethoprim/sulphamethoxazole. Special organisms (e.g. Mycobacterium tuberculosis) may require specific drugs. The possible effect of such agents on the fetus should be remembered (Chapter 11). (ii) *Nursing measures.* Important *observations* include pulse and respiration rates, blood pressure, temperature, fluid balance, urinalysis, and fetal heart rate. Because of the sensitivity of the uterus to coliform endotoxin, a watch should be kept for the onset of premature labour. *Symptomatic relief* is given in the form of analgesics and tepid sponging if fever is significant. An adequate fluid intake is essential. If the patient is nauseated or vomiting, an intravenous infusion is necessary, and initial chemotherapy must also be given parenterally (ampicillin, cephaman-dole, cefoxitin, gentamicin).

(b) *Chronic pyelonephritis.* Conditions likely to produce recurrent infection and renal damage include congenital abnormalities of the renal tract, calculi, diabetes, analgesic abuse, and any condition causing chronic obstruction/stasis. Management is largely directed to initial detection (significant bacteriuria), prevention of flare-ups during pregnancy by intermittent courses of chemotherapy, and full investigation in the puerperium.

GLOMERULAR DISEASES

Acute Glomerulonephritis

This is an extremely rare condition in pregnancy, and in later pregnancy may mimic severe preeclampsia, except for the presence of haematuria which is not a feature of the latter condition.

Chronic Glomerulonephritis

This is now less common, because of the reduced incidence of streptococcal infections. It may be revealed, if previously unsuspected, by the detection of proteinuria on routine urine testing in the antenatal period. It predisposes to *preeclampsia, fetal growth retardation, and stillbirth.* Diagnosis is made by renal function tests, and possibly renal biopsy. If renal function is poor and/or blood pressure is high, termination of the pregnancy may be indicated.

Nephrosis is a particular form of chronic glomerulonephritis where there is gross proteinuria; because of the subsequent lowering of albumin levels in the blood, the patients may become markedly oedematous. Often, the blood pressure is less elevated and renal function less impaired than in other forms of nephritis and the fetal prognosis is better.

Polycystic Disease

This condition is usually inherited, but often does not become manifest (hypertension, renal failure) until the patient is in her third or fourth decade or even later. In pregnancy, hypertension and preeclampsia are common and, if a family history of kidney trouble is present, one should suspect this condition. It can be demonstrated usually on ultrasonography.

General Medical Disorders

Conditions such as diabetes mellitus and lupus erythematosus may also cause extensive renal impairment (colour plate 78).

Patients with any form of chronic renal tract pathology are at *high risk*, as are their babies, and *specialist care* is advisable.

OTHER DISORDERS

Oliguria/Anuria

There are 2 main groups of patients — those with retention of urine, and those with renal failure.

(a) *Retention of urine*. (i) *Incarceration of the retroverted uterus* occurs late in the first trimester and pressure is exerted on the bladder neck and proximal urethra as the uterus expands forwards (figure 37.2). The retention may be masked by incontinence which is due to overflow. The condition is usually cured by catheterization, with the catheter indwelling for 24–48 hours, sometimes aided by the prone position and manual anteversion of the uterus. (ii) *Late pregnancy and labour.* The same obstructive effect may be caused by pressure of the fetal presenting part. The resulting bladder fullness is discomforting to the patient, encourages infection, and inhibits uterine contractions. If neglected, serious damage to the base of the bladder may result, even to the extent of fistula formation. (iii) *Puerperium.* Retention may result from *oedema of the urethra or bladder base*; also, the pain of an episiotomy, nearby lacerations, or Caesarean section wound often *reflexly* inhibits bladder function, making micturition difficult. It should be remembered that after delivery the bladder has a poor tone and considerable distension may occur without the usual discomfort or urgent desire to micturate. Voiding is encouraged by allowing the patient to get out of bed, and by other accepted nursing measures. If voiding has not occurred by 12–15 hours, the patient should be catheterized. A full

Figure 37.2 Incarceration of the retroverted gravid uterus occurs at about 12–14 weeks when it fills the pelvis. The cervix is displaced upwards and anteriorly, causing the urethra to become elongated and often occluded.

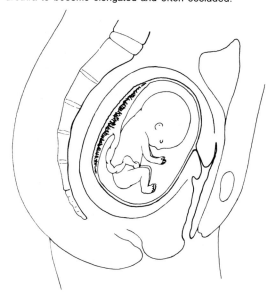

bladder will give a false idea of the height of the uterine fundus.

(b) *Renal failure.* There are 3 recognized groups. (i) *Prerenal.* Here, the kidneys are capable of functioning normally, but are not being supplied with enough blood. Thus, in major haemorrhage or shock, if the blood pressure falls below 80 mm Hg systolic, little or no urine will be produced. (ii) *Renal.* Typical causes of renal failure in pregnancy include septic abortion, severe preeclampsia or eclampsia, placental abruption and other causes of disseminated intravascular coagulation. There may be disease of the kidney antedating the pregnancy, such as chronic glomerulonephritis. In addition, conditions not specific to pregnancy, such as incompatible blood transfusion, may be at fault. (iii) *Postrenal.* Here, there is a blockage to the flow of urine. The condition is very rare in obstetrical practice.

Haematuria

The usual causes of haematuria are: (i) infection (haemorrhagic cystitis), (ii) trauma — catheters; pressure of the fetal head; damage at forceps delivery or Caesarean section, (iii) miscellaneous — stone, neoplasm, varices, idiopathic.

Distinction should be made from haemolysis of red blood cells due to such complications as C1. welchii abortion and incompatible blood transfusion where the urine is usually reddish-brown in colour (haemoglobinuria).

Postnephrectomy

If the remaining kidney is healthy, there is little disturbance to the pregnancy. If the kidney is diseased, serious consideration should be given to termination because of the seriousness of further deterioration in function.

Renal Transplant

More patients will be seen in the future who have received transplanted kidneys. Pregnancy is not contraindicated, but the patient's condition should be stable, without significant hypertension or proteinuria, or evidence of graft rejection, and care must be exercised in the use of immunosuppressant drugs in the first trimester. Such patients will be under consultant care because of the close and expert supervision necessary. The incidence of abortion, premature labour, hypertensive disorders and infection are all increased. *Ectopic pregnancy* is often more difficult to diagnose and treat in such patients: ultrasonography is helpful, as is estimation of beta HCG levels. A paramedian or midline rather than Pfannenstiel incision is advisable for Caesarean section to minimize danger to the pelvically-located kidney.

chapter thirty-eight

The Reproductive System

OVERVIEW

The centre piece of pregnancy, the reproductive system, may itself have anomalies and disorders that require recognition and treatment.

In pregnancy, the uterine body and cervix have inverse and paradoxical functions: the uterus must first relax to accommodate the conceptus and then at term expel it, whereas the cervix must first retain the conceptus and then at term relax to allow its egress. These functions are achieved as a result of some clever biochemical work evolved by nature.

The *development of the reproductive tract* takes place by a rather unusual coming together of 2 ducts (Mullerian): these fuse at their lower end and hollow out to produce the uterus and vagina. Unfortunately, this does not always go to plan, and a range of *anomalies* of nonfusion and nonhollowing may occur. The changes are sometimes subtle and diagnosis requires careful clinical appraisal. Very often there is a history of *infertility* or *recurrent pregnancy mishap* (abortion, stillbirth, prematurity, malpresentation, dystocia, third stage problems); these should always raise one's index of suspicion.

The *mechanical disorders* — incarceration of the uterus, pendulous abdomen, prolapse — are uncommon, but each requires appropriate recognition and management.

Neoplastic disorders are relatively frequent in the reproductive age group, albeit with a heavy preponderance of *benign lesions*. *Fibromyomas* can give rise to a variety of complications during pregnancy, usually related to their size (large), location (cervical), or change in blood supply (infarction). *Ovarian cysts* and benign tumours (figure 26.1) are important because of their tendency to undergo complication (torsion, rupture, infection, haemorrhage), especially after delivery. Since it is often difficult to exclude malignancy, these tumours are operated on at any time from the beginning of the second trimester, when the risk of abortion caused by laparotomy becomes minimal.

Malignant neoplasms may arise in the cervix, ovary, or breast: the first is usually detected by cytology or clinical inspection; the latter, by careful palpation. Management is highly specialized.

CHANGES IN PREGNANCY

Uterus

The most striking change is seen in the uterus. In the nonpregnant state the uterus weighs about 60 g and its cavity holds about 6 ml; at term, the weight has increased to 1,000 g and the volume to 5,000 ml. There is an increase in the number of muscle fibres (*hyperplasia*) and an increase in size (*hypertrophy*). The bulk of the increase in the muscle fibre is due to the contractile protein *actomyosin*. In later pregnancy, the fibres also become considerably stretched, so that there is an overall thinning of the uterine wall; this particularly affects the lower portion of the uterus (*lower uterine segment*).

Until the 12th week of pregnancy, the uterus is a pelvic organ, but thereafter can be palpated abdominally. At 20–22 weeks the fundus is at the level of the umbilicus; between 36 and 40 weeks it has reached the xiphisternum (figure 38.1).

Concomitantly, there is an increase in the vascular supply of the uterus (figure 38.2), as well as an increase in the lymphatic and nervous networks. The *uterine blood flow* at term ranges between 500–700 ml/minute.

Contractions occur throughout pregnancy (Braxton Hicks type — figure 38.3), but are relatively much stronger and more frequent as term approaches, due to the progressive release of prostaglandin from the uterine lining (decidua). They are painless and are instrumental in the formation of the lower uterine segment. There is a progressive increase (almost 100-fold) in the *sensitivity of the uterus to oxytocin* during pregnancy.

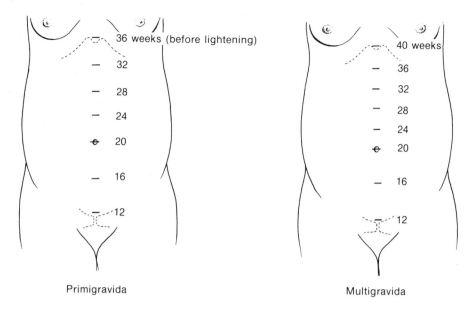

Primigravida   Multigravida

Figure 38.1 Height of the uterus fundus is a guide to the period of gestation. Nulliparas experience lightening at 36–38 weeks when the fundal height reverts to the 34–36 weeks level.

The *cervix* enlarges, sometimes markedly (figure 38.6), due to increased vascularity, and quite early its colour changes from pink to violet (progesterone effect) and it is much softened, largely due to the effects of oestrogen and progesterone. The cervical canal tends to become everted, giving the appearance of an erosion; there is an increase in the mucus secretion from the glands lining the endocervix. The *softening* (*ripening*) is accentuated as labour approaches; both *relaxin* and *prostaglandin* are thought to play a role in this by altering such tissue components as collagen and glycosaminoglycans.

Vagina

The vagina shows similar colour and consistency changes to those described in the cervix. There is a thickening of the mucosa, loosening of the connective tissue, and hypertrophy of muscle in preparation for the distension required at the time of parturition. Because of the increase in glycogen in the squamous lining cells and increased desquamation, *monilial infections* are seen more frequently (figure 27.2).

Ovaries and Tubes

The *ovaries* and *oviducts* show little change. The most characteristic feature is the *corpus luteum of pregnancy* which is maintained by the chorionic gonadotrophin (HCG) secreted by the developing trophoblast. The corpus luteum of pregnancy (figure 4.4) is responsible in turn for

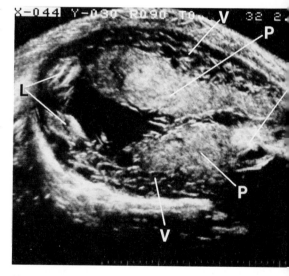

Figure 38.2 Decidual veins. Longitudinal scan at 28 weeks' gestation in a 38-year-old para 1 with an incompetent cervix. The right lateral fundal placenta (P) is shown on both uterine walls and the numerous subjacent maternal veins (V) are well demonstrated. Fetal limbs (L) and face (F) are also shown. A healthy infant (birth-weight 3,150 g) was born by Caesarean section at 36.3 weeks' gestation.

the secretion of the high levels of *oestrogen* and *progesterone* necessary for embedding of the fertilized ovum in the uterus and the early development of the ovum; by about 8 weeks the placenta takes over this function.

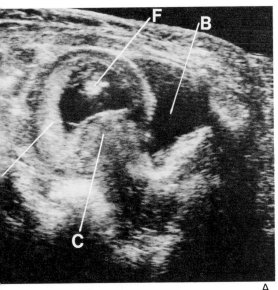

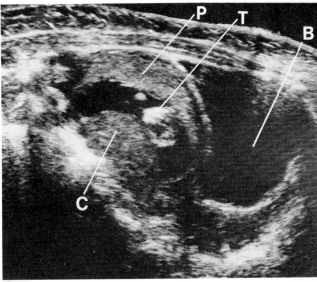

A   B

Figure 38.3 Braxton Hicks contractions, first described as a sign of pregnancy when the uterus was palpated bimanually at the end of the first trimester, are identifiable by ultrasound as early as 8 weeks' gestation. First recognized as uterine contraction waves by Dr. Beresford Buttery, these ultrasonic appearances were previously misdiagnosed as fibro-myomas. **A.** Longitudinal scan at 9 weeks' gestation showing contraction wave (C), fetus (F), bladder (B) and placenta (P) reaching almost to the site of the uterine contraction. **B.** Longitudinal scan at 13 weeks' gestation showing Braxton Hicks contraction (C), fetal trunk (T), bladder (B), and placenta (P) on the anterior uterine wall.

CONGENITAL DISORDERS

Embryology

The genital tract forms in the embryo from the paired Mullerian ducts. These form at about the 6th week from the dorsal aspect of the coelomic cavity, lateral to the genital ridge and Wolffian system. The lower ends of the ducts fuse at about 14 weeks. The suspensory ligaments of each ovary (gubernacula) cross the ducts and delineate the fused portion below (the uterus, cervix and vagina) and the unfused portions above (Fallopian tubes). The ligaments become the uteroovarian and round ligaments, respectively. The septum between the 2 ducts normally breaks down and differential sculpturing produces the anatomically distinct uterus, cervix, and vagina.

Types of Anomaly

The following 3 anomalies may occur either singly or in combination. (i) *Faulty midline fusion.* This group contains the great majority of cases. The anomaly may involve the uterus, cervix, vagina, or a combination of these. The extreme form is represented as a completely separate system on each side (uterus didelphys — figure 38.4) similar to that seen in some animals. (ii) *Faulty development of one duct* gives rise to incomplete or absent structures on that side — e.g. unicornuate uterus (figure 26.9). There are often anomalies of the renal tract on the same side, since the tissues of origin of genital and

urinary tracts lie side by side in the embryo. (iii) *Faulty canalization* of one or both ducts results in blockages or apparent absences of the corresponding structures. An extreme form of this is seen in absence of the vagina.

An unusual type of anomaly may follow the administration of *diethylstilboestrol* (DES) to the patient's mother during early pregnancy. The hysterogram often shows an abnormal uterine shape and the rates for ectopic pregnancy, abortion, and premature labour are increased. The cervix and vagina are often covered with columnar rather than the normal squamous epithelium (adenosis); this is more susceptible to neoplastic transformation.

Incidence. Approximately 0.2–4%, although if minor forms of duplication are included (arcuate and subseptate uterus) the figure may be closer to 6–8% or even higher.

Clinical features. There is a wide spectrum of clinical disorder, according to the type of anomaly and the level affected. (i) *Infertility.* Absolute if the tract is blocked, relative if there are septa or narrowings. (ii) *Abortion* and stillbirth are more common with uterine anomalies (implantation on poorly vascularized septa, distortion of cavity). (iii) *Premature labour* and (iv) *premature rupture of the membranes* occur for the same reasons. (v) *Malpresentation* is much more common as a result of the altered shape of the uterus (oblique and transverse lies;

322

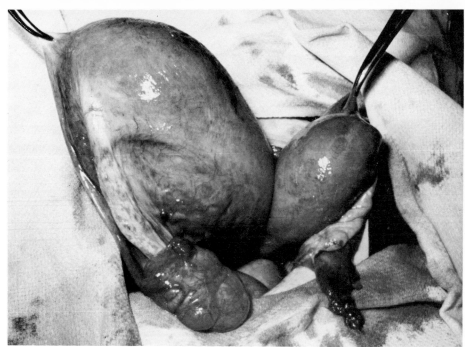

Figure 38.4 View at Caesarean section at 38 weeks. The nonpregnant half of a double uterus (uterus didelphys) was jammed in the pelvis and labour was obstructed. Ovaries and tubes are shown. Note enlargement of nonpregnant uterus due to the growth stimulus of the hormones oestrogen and progesterone.

breech presentations) and cord prolapse is a further complication. (vi) *Dystocia* from incoordinate uterine action, malpresentation, blockage by a nonpregnant uterine horn in the pelvis (figure 38.4), or obstruction by septa in the cervix or vagina. (vii) *Third stage anomalies*, due to abnormal placental attachment and incoordinate uterine action (*retained placenta and postpartum haemorrhage*).

Diagnosis. Any of the above features in the patient's obstetrical history should arouse suspicion if no other cause can be found. At the initial antenatal visit, major duplications in the uterus, and/or cervix, and/or vagina should be diagnosed if speculum and bimanual examination is thorough. An accessory uterine horn may be confused with a fibromyoma or ovarian tumour. The anomaly may only be apparent later in pregnancy, when changes in the uterine contour are accentuated, particularly when the uterus is contracting (fundal broadening, breech or limb flanking, axial deviation — colour plate 72). The fetus will often be lying transversely or obliquely, with the upper pole in one or other flank (figure 26.2). A septum may be palpated at the time of manual removal of the placenta. Finally, ultrasonography soon after delivery and/ or hysterography performed later will delineate the shape of the cavity (figure 38.5).

Management. Specialist referral is recommended because of the many complications that may arise. Obstetrical management is usually expectant, but Caesarean section may be

Figure 38.5 Hysterosalpingogram showing a bicornuate uterus. The Fallopian tubes are outlined with dye which is spilling into the peritoneal cavity, thus confirming their patency.

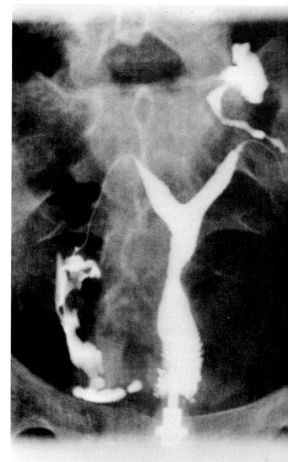

required for persistently unstable lie or cephalo-pelvic disproportion. Septa in the cervix and vagina are stretched markedly during labour and can be incised between clamps and ligated. Interval surgery may be required to excise a septum or unite a double uterus, particularly if infertility, abortion, or premature labour have occurred.

Intravenous pyelography is warranted after delivery to check for associated renal anomalies.

MECHANICAL DISORDERS

Incarceration of the Uterus

Clinical features. The uterus lies in a retroverted position in 15–20% of women. Although spontaneous correction occurs late in the first trimester in the great majority, the growing uterus occasionally becomes incarcerated in the hollow of the sacrum. With continued growth, there is pressure on the bladder neck and the patient experiences increasing difficulty in voiding, leading to complete retention (figure 37.2). Placentation is often disturbed and abortion threatens. Rarely, growth continues by an outpouching of the anterior wall of the uterus (*sacculation*). On examination, the distended bladder is palpable suprapubically, and on bimanual examination the uterus is felt posteriorly.

Treatment. The condition is relieved by the insertion of a Foley catheter which is left to drain. The uterus can then be pushed gently out of the pelvis with the patient in the knee/chest position if spontaneous correction does not occur.

Pendulous Abdomen

Clinical features. This condition is rare and is predisposed to by multiparity and gross laxity of the anterior abdominal muscles. It occurs in the latter half of pregnancy and consists of a gross anteflexion of the uterus. The patient experiences discomfort or pain when in the erect attitude. The main problem arises from the associated abnormality in the fetal lie.

Treatment. Conservative correction in the form of a well-fitting maternity corset suffices during pregnancy, and this can be replaced with a binder in labour.

Uterovaginal Prolapse

Clinical features. This also is far more common in the multipara with lax tissues. It is seen less often now that the Brandt-Andrews technique for placental delivery has replaced 'fundal pressure' methods. Usually the laxity of supports

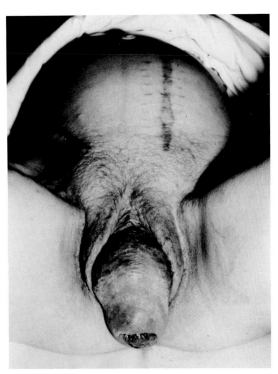

Figure 38.6 A marked degree of cervical hypertrophy and prolapse at 39 weeks' gestation. The cervix was pulled up spontaneously in labour and the patient had a normal delivery.

allows the uterus to descend so that the cervix appears at or beyond the introitus. The condition improves after the 4th month as the uterus becomes abdominal in position, but may recur late in pregnancy because of the weight of the uterus (figure 38.6).

Treatment. This consists of the insertion of a suitably-sized *plastic pessary*, antiseptic dressings for the cervix if it is infected, and appropriate periods of recumbency. Vaginal wall prolapse also responds satisfactorily to pessary treatment.

If a patient has had a *previous operation for prolapse*, some consider that vaginal delivery may be allowed usually with a generous episiotomy; however, although pregnancy itself considerably stretches the uterine supports (paracervical and round ligaments), *it is delivery through the vagina that damages the vaginal supports.* Caesarean section is the better option if it is this area that has been operated on (cystocele, rectocele, stress incontinence).

Trauma

Uterine rupture is considered in Chapter 54. *The patient may suffer uterine rupture, placental abruption, pelvic fracture etc as a result of motor vehicle injury*; although a seat belt minimizes the risk of fatal injury, it may localize trauma to the uterus and its contents (figure 23.1). A particularly difficult condition to manage is avulsion of the uterine or internal iliac artery from its origin; this may occur because of the inertia of the gravid uterus. Severe retroperitoneal haemorrhage usually ensues. Motor vehicle accidents account for a high proportion of maternal deaths (table 14.2).

NEOPLASIA — BENIGN

Uterine Fibromyomas

Incidence. 0.5-1% of pregnancies. Usually the tumours are multiple and are seen in older childbearing women (figure 38.7).

Clinical features. Usually, the tumours are symptomless, but may give rise to some of the complications outlined in the section on uterine malformations (malpresentation (breech, transverse lie), premature labour, dystocia, third stage problems). A unique feature is their tendency to undergo *degenerative change*; in pregnancy this usually takes the form of *red degeneration* (infarction), since the blood supply is endangered by the differential growth of the uterine muscle and the fibromyoma. This complication is considered in the differential diagnosis of the *acute abdomen* in pregnancy,

because of the associated pain and tenderness. Since pregnancy often causes an increase in the size of the tumour, pressure symptoms occur. Torsion and bleeding from a surface vein are rarer complications.

Management. Conservatism is the keynote — myomectomy is rarely, if ever, required except for torsion. Caesarean section may be indicated for obstruction (cervical fibroid) or malpresentation of the fetus. After delivery, *hysterectomy* may be necessary on rare occasions if there is a submucous or subserous fibroid which continues to bleed.

Ovarian Cysts and Tumours

A variety of tumours may coexist with pregnancy, and even though benign in their course, they are potentially serious because of their liability to complications (colour plate 24).

Incidence. Tumours of significant size (5 cm or more) are present in about 0.2-1% of pregnancies (table 16.2); like fibroids, they are more common in the older age group. In 5%, the tumours are bilateral.

Pathology. Two-thirds of the tumours are cystic — originating in the *corpus luteum* (luteal cyst), the covering epithelium (serous or mucinous cystadenoma), or the germinal elements (cystic

Figure 38.7 Fibromyomas. **A.** Longitudinal scan in a 43-year-old primigravida at 13 weeks' gestation showing 3 fibromyomas (FM), placenta (P), fetus (F) and bladder (B). The fibroid posterior to the placenta was the largest and measured 7.5 cm in diameter. Caesarean section was performed at 38 weeks' gestation because cardiotocography showed critical fetal reserve; the infant was born in good condition, birth-weight 2,350 g, but died from laryngeal atresia. **B.** Fibromyomas at myomectomy: the round ligaments are held by forceps. Pregnancy after 8 years of infertility had been complicated by red degeneration of the largest fibromyoma and breech presentation.

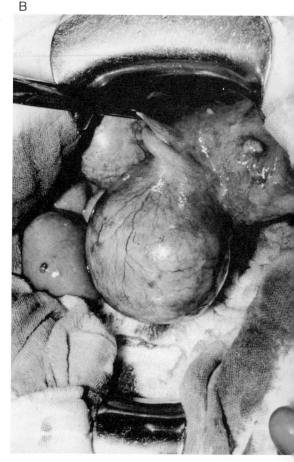

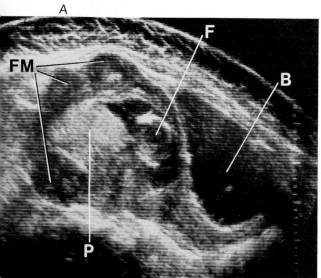

teratoma — dermoid (figure 26.1)). The solid tumours are usually fibromas.

Clinical features. Unless a *complication* occurs, such as torsion, haemorrhage, rupture, or infection, the presence of the tumour is usually unsuspected by the patient. It may be palpable in one or other parametrium at the first antenatal visit or may be revealed after delivery when the stretched and relaxed abdominal wall facilitates examination. Ultrasonic study is useful if there is doubt clinically. If the tumour is incarcerated in the pelvis, *labour may become obstructed.* The complications mentioned above are more likely in the puerperium following the trauma of labour.

Management. The patient with an ovarian neoplasm is usually managed conservatively until the beginning of the second trimester, when excision (usually cystectomy) is recommended. Earlier interference is much more likely to cause an interruption to the pregnancy, and is reserved for patients with complications such as *torsion.* Cysts smaller than 5 cm in diameter are likely to be functional in nature (corpus luteum cyst) and

can usually be observed. Caesarean section may be required if labour is *obstructed* and, in such cases, the tumour is removed at the same time. If it is discovered late in pregnancy and is not in the pelvis, normal delivery is anticipated and removal deferred until early in the puerperium.

Breast Hypertrophy

Enlargement of the breasts during pregnancy and lactation varies enormously and is quite unpredictable, as is the degree of involution that occurs when lactation ceases (colour plate 65). Diffuse hypertrophy of the breasts during pregnancy causing gigantomastia is an exceedingly uncommon condition (1 in 30,000–50,000 pregnancies) of unknown aetiology (figure 38.8). Surprisingly it can occur in patients whose breasts behaved normally in previous pregnancies. The condition, in our experience of only 4 cases, does not resolve after pregnancy, nor does it respond to bromocriptine therapy, either during the pregnancy or after delivery. Therefore reduction mammoplasty is likely to be required. In the past this condition has been mistaken for malignancy and treated by irradiation!

Figure 38.8 Pregnancy-induced gigantomastia (diffuse hypertrophy) in a 27-year-old para 1 at 16 weeks' gestation. The breasts had *not* enlarged excessively in the previous pregnancy. The patient was tall and slender (weight 67 kg). The breasts were red and oedematous; their frightening growth had commenced *before* the first missed period. By 20 weeks, continued growth and embarrassment imprisoned her at home. The plan is to suppress lactation and perform reduction mammoplasty about 6 months after delivery.

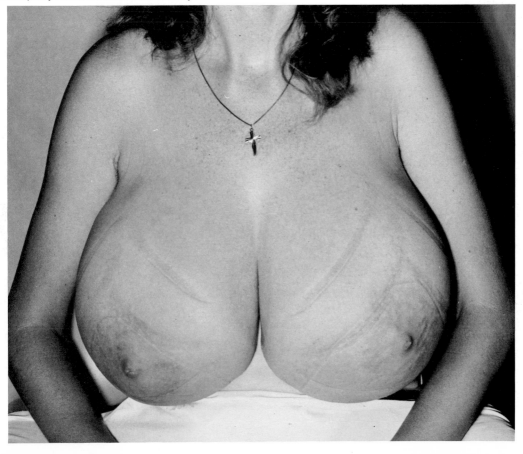

NEOPLASIA — MALIGNANT

Vulval and Vaginal Cancer

These tumours are very rare in the reproductive age group and if present are usually intraepithelial in type. Treatment is by superficial local eradication (as for the cervical lesion). Invasive lesions are treated as in the nonpregnant patient.

Cervical Carcinoma

If the lesion is early, usually no symptoms will have been noted.

Incidence. With routine Papanicolaou smear testing, preinvasive (intraepithelial) forms of the disease are not uncommon (0.2–0.5%); an invasive lesion, on the other hand, is quite rare in the pregnancy age group (1 in 5,000).

Clinical features. With invasive lesions, there is usually a watery or blood-stained discharge or frank bleeding. The patient is usually parous and over the age of 30 years.

Diagnosis. If the smear test proves positive and a target lesion is obvious, a punch biopsy is taken; if there is no evident lesion, the cervix should be subjected to *colposcopy and directed biopsy.*

Treatment. Providing an expert has seen the patient, further management of cervical intraepithelial neoplasia (CIN) is conservative until after the pregnancy, when the lesion can be eradicated by cryotherapy, diathermy, laser, or occasionally cone biopsy. In 20–50% of patients the lesion is no longer demonstrable at the postnatal visit; this may be the result of loss of the epithelium at the time of parturition or regression due to altered host:tumour relationships. If *invasive cancer* is present, radical treatment by surgery, radiotherapy, or a combination of both is necessary if the patient's life is to be saved. This is strictly a procedure for consultants experienced in the management of such conditions, to whom the patient should be referred. The major factors influencing treatment are the stage, the period of gestation, and the parity/desire for children (if the cancer is microinvasive). Most difficulties arise where colposcopy is either unsatisfactory or at marked discrepancy with the cytology, where a microinvasive lesion has been shown on punch biopsy, or where there is a possible endocervical adenocarcinoma. With *microinvasive cancers* (Stage 1A) in the third trimester, vaginal delivery is usually awaited and a cone biopsy is performed postpartum; before this, it is necessary to perform conization without delay. A properly performed cone biopsy has little effect on future pregnancies.

Ovarian Carcinoma

This type of carcinoma is uncommon in the childbearing period (approximately 1–2% of ovarian tumours, 1 in 10,000 pregnancies). The types of ovarian cancer seen in the second and third decades are the dysgerminoma, teratoma, and granulosa cell tumour; cystadenocarcinomas become increasingly more common in the fourth and fifth decades. Accurate diagnosis is difficult, and about 1 in 1,000 pregnant patients will require exploration because of an adnexal mass: 90% of these will be benign.

Ovarian cancers present great problems in management, since optimum treatment is removal of all of the internal genitalia (uterus, tubes, and ovaries). This is very radical treatment in a young person, and may be modified to oophorectomy in localized, less malignant growths.

Breast Carcinoma

Incidence. About 15% of breast cancers occur in women aged 40 years or younger and 1% occurs in association with pregnancy. Unlike cancers of the cervix, vagina and vulva, only invasive lesions are seen clinically; such lesions occur in 1 in 3,000 pregnancies.

Diagnosis. The condition is usually diagnosed by the patient at the time of breast self-examination; less often by the physician at the time of office consultation. There may be symptoms of itch, pain, nipple discharge or bleeding. If the lump is highly suspicious of malignancy a biopsy is taken; if there is significant doubt, needle aspiration is carried out, perhaps assisted by mammography and/or ultrasonography.

Treatment. This is usually by modified radical mastectomy, with removal of the axillary nodes. If the axillary nodes are involved, serious consideration will be given to termination of the pregnancy because of the need for radiotherapy and/or chemotherapy.

If the patient has been treated successfully for breast carcinoma (e.g. 2 or more years), further pregnancies do not appear to be contraindicated, as the prognosis does not appear to be altered thereby; breast feeding is not contraindicated.

chapter thirty-nine

The Immune System

OVERVIEW

The immune system is responsible for the rejection of any foreign matter that gains entrance to the body and disturbs its normal function. This not only applies to various microorganisms such as protozoa, bacteria, and viruses, but almost any protein or particulate matter.

At the centre of the immune system are the 2 major defence arms — the *humoral* (antibodies) and the *cellular*. These are distributed widely and encompass the thymus, spleen, and lymphatic tissue. This lymphocyte (immunocyte) system is assisted by other leucocytes (e.g. polymorpho-nuclear cells) and phagocytes (macrophages).

Why such an effective system allows a partly foreign intruder (the conceptus) to embed and grow is still conjectural, although the main theories suggest that the foreignness of the trophoblast (antigenicity) is masked by a protective coating, or one of the hormones secreted by the trophoblast may be immunosuppressive locally, or the presentation of the foreign antigens may be so gradual that the system fails to react.

The fetus depends for its safety largely on its protected site within the amniotic sac, together with the free passage of antibodies from the mother. Its own immune system has formed, however, in the first trimester, and slowly becomes functional as the pregnancy advances.

The major practical problem arising from a such close relationship is maternal immunization against fetal red blood cells which escape into her circulation (*blood group isoimmunization*). This also can occur, albeit to a much lesser extent, with fetal *platelets* and *leucocytes*.

The fetus may also be involved, indirectly, by the transfer of harmful maternal *autoantibodies*. These can affect all tissues; the condition (autoimmune disease) represents a breakdown of the protection normally enjoyed by the body.

Congenital defects of the immune system do occur, but are very rare; either one or both of the immune divisions (humoral, cellular) may be affected. Serious problems then arise because of inability to control infections.

Immunization during pregnancy is recommended against poliomyelitis and influenza, and increasing attention is being given to its use against such diseases as tetanus which may be prevalent in particular localities. Vaccines employing live organisms (e.g. rubella, smallpox) are contraindicated.

ANATOMY AND FUNCTION

The organs primarily involved in production of the specialized cells of the immune system (lymphocytes or immunocytes) are the *thymus gland*, *spleen*, and *lymphatic system*. The cells arise in the embryo in one of 2 sites — T cells are derived from the thymus and B cells are derived from the bone marrow. The T cells are responsible for *cell-mediated immunity*; that is, they attack the foreign material 'in person'. The B cells secrete antibody which attaches itself to the material, and so mark it for destruction (*humoral immunity*).

The immune system can be looked at as one of the *surveillance-protective systems* of the body, similar in principle to the nervous system. The information concerning the presence of foreign material is obtained by one or more of the many millions of surveillance cells patrolling the body. The latter then enter the lymph and are carried to one of the depots, where the information is transferred to cells residing there. These in turn multiply in large numbers, some producing antibody, others passing out of the depots (usually lymph nodes or spleen) to seek the foreign material. These cells elaborate a number of substances (*lymphokines*) which assist in their tasks: (i) stimulate other lymphocytes to divide (*mitogenic factor*); (ii) slow down other passing white blood cells, such as macrophages (*macrophage inhibiting factor*); (iii) transfer

TABLE 39.1   CHARACTERISTICS OF THE MAIN TYPES OF ANTIBODY

	IgG	IgM	IgA
Molecular weight	160,000	900,000	160,000*
Levels (mg/dl)			
— mother	1,100–1,150	100–150	180–250
— cord	1,000–1,050	0–12	1–3
Placental transfer	Yes	No	No
Distribution in the body	Intra- and extravascular	Intra-vascular	Secretions, colostrum, milk
Half-life in the body	25–30 days	5 days	5–7 days

* As 'secretory IgA' (molecular weight 375,000) it consists of 2 units, plus a component making it more resistant to enzymatic digestion

information to other cells (*transfer factor*); (iv) cause an inflammatory reaction (*inflammatory factor*).

The *foreign material* is usually a protein and is called an *antigen*. The *antibodies* which are produced in response to its presence are specific. Antibodies are in 4 main groups — *immunoglobulins* A, G, M, and E (IgA, IgG, IgM, and IgE, for short). Their main features are shown in table 39.1. It can be seen that *only the IgG antibodies cross the placenta*. This is quite useful in deciding whether a baby has been infected in utero since, *if there are IgM antibodies present soon after birth, they must have been produced by the baby since they do not cross the placenta*. In general, IgM antibodies are the first to be produced, whilst IgG antibodies appear later. The presence of IgA in the chorioamniotic membrane and decidua serves as a first line of defence against local infection.

In addition to the classical immune system, there are other helper systems in combating infection — the *phagocytes* (polymorphonuclear white cells and macrophages) and *humoral mediators* (the *plasma-derived* complement, kinin, and clotting systems) and the *tissue-derived* prostaglandins, histamines, lysosomes etc.

DEVELOPMENT IN THE FETUS

The thymus, spleen, and lymphatic system are present at the second month of intrauterine life, but do not become functional until the second trimester. All the important IgG antibodies of the mother are passed across to the fetus, especially in the last 6–8 weeks of pregnancy.

These protect the baby until antibody production in the newborn reaches satisfactory levels in the months after birth. In the premature baby, lower levels of IgG are present, since sufficient amounts will not have been obtained from the mother before birth. In both term and premature infants, levels often remain low for up to 6 months after birth. This explains the susceptibility of the newborn to bacterial infections, since this is largely a B cell responsibility. Some antibody production takes place in the fetus from the end of the first trimester (IgA, IgM, IgE, and small amounts of IgG); lower levels are found in fetuses suffering from growth retardation.

Lymphocytes are present in the immune organs (thymus, spleen, lymphatic tissue) from the end of the first trimester and become functional early in the second trimester (i.e. can attack viruses etc and produce antibody). The *thymus gland* reaches its maximum size early in the third trimester.

Apart from the transfer of IgG across the placenta, the colostrum and milk represent a further source of immune protection; some antibodies pass, especially in the colostrum, but the main protection appears to be derived from immune cells which help to protect the bowel. Milk contains 2,000–4,000 white blood cells per cmm. This explains the relative immunity of breast-fed infants to gastroenteritis. The immunoglobulin IgA is produced from most mucus-secreting glands and is thought to provide local protection from infection. It may also play a role in preventing the absorption of antigenic material from the gut, since antibodies to cows' milk are high in those children deficient in IgA. Levels of IgA are higher in the blood of mothers who are breast feeding.

CONGENITAL ANOMALIES

A number of rare *congenital disorders* exist where one or both types of immunity are deficient. Agammaglobulinaemia of the *Bruton type* is a sex-linked defect (males affected, females carriers) primarily of the B cell (humoral) system. The *Di George syndrome* is a primary defect of the T cell (thymus) system. In the *Swiss type* there is a combined deficiency of B and T cells. Such infants have serious problems throughout life with various types of infections.

CHANGES IN THE MOTHER

There is some general *depression of maternal immunity* during pregnancy because of the production of a special protein which may partly block lymphocytes (lymphocyte depressing factor, LDF) and also because of an increase in adrenal cortical activity. However, these factors alone are not sufficient to explain why the fetus is not rejected. Other possible mechanisms include the coating of the trophoblast by an antigenically inert material (sialomucin); blocking of maternal cellular rejection by harmless antibodies which attach to the trophoblast; and finally the *barrier function* of the placenta preventing cellular traffic until the pregnancy is well established. The main factor seems to be the inertness of the trophoblast cover, since the mother can react quite vigorously to red blood cells which escape from the fetus (rhesus isoimmunization, Chapter 22), but tolerates trophoblastic cells which break off and enter her circulation in large numbers. It is not known for certain why administration of anti-D globulin to the nonimmunized mother prevents her from making antibodies; it may be the antigenic sites on the fetal red cells are blocked, or the fetal cells so marked are more readily destroyed, or possibly the antibody-producing lymphocytes are inhibited in some way.

In rare patients (e.g. renal transplant) the *immune depression* of pregnancy may be accentuated by drugs used to suppress the rejection of the transplanted organ; these patients are particularly susceptible to infection.

Leucocytes and platelets as well as red blood cells pass the placenta, and the mother may make antibodies against them also. This explains some cases of neonatal purpura or wasting. *Strangely enough, cellular traffic in the reverse direction is rare.* When it does occur, however, it may produce a 'graft versus host' reaction — the lymphocytes attacking the baby. The same thing may happen with intrauterine transfusions if the white blood cells are not removed beforehand. Another example of mother to fetus passage of cells involves the Rh-negative female fetus whose mother is Rh-positive; in later life these women fail to produce antibodies despite the presence of an Rh-positive fetus, presumably due to *immune tolerance* induced by receipt of maternal Rh-positive cells when in utero. Some *spontaneous abortions* may be caused by incompatibility between mother and fetus.

It has been claimed also that *preeclampsia* may have an immunological basis, because it is more common in unrelated matings than in consanguineous matings. Its predilection for primigravidas and its recurrence when the pregnancy is the result of a different father supports this view. Others consider that abortion, premature labour, and even fetal death or malformation may occasionally have a basis of immunological rejection.

AUTOIMMUNE DISEASE

Early in fetal life when the immune system is immature, it accepts as normal all the developing tissues around it; they are recognized as 'self'. As the system matures, it is able to differentiate between self and nonself (i.e. 'strangers'), much the same as a guard dog differentiates between owners and visitors. Occasionally, there is a breakdown in the system, perhaps because of damage to tissues by bacteria or viruses, and the immune system starts to attack its own tissues. We thus speak of autoantibody production and autoimmune disease. All of the important organs can be affected — e.g. thyroid gland, thymus, liver, blood, kidneys, heart, and the skin (*herpes gestationis*, figure 39.1)). These harmful antibodies may pass to the fetus and cause symptoms during the month or so that they are active.

The major features of these disorders in the mother and baby are discussed elsewhere (*thymus gland*, Chapter 29; *thyroid gland*, Chapter 30; *blood*, Chapter 34; *liver*, Chapter 35). Table 39.2 summarizes the features of some other autoimmune diseases which may complicate pregnancy.

The following facts should be remembered. (i) The antibodies are of the IgG type and thus pass freely across the placenta and affect the fetus. (ii) The fetal disorder is usually self-limited (2–3 months), but permanent damage may occur — e.g. *cretinism* in the case of antithyroid antibodies; *heart block* in the case of antibodies to the cardiac conducting system in systemic lupus erythematosus. (iii) The fetus (and newborn) may be affected in the absence of maternal features (the fetal tissues are more susceptible to the antibodies), or after the mother has been treated (e.g. by thyroidectomy in the case of Graves disease or splenectomy in the case of immune thrombocytopenic purpura). (iv) The fetus is often growth retarded.

IMMUNIZATION IN PREGNANCY

An adequate level of immunity is necessary to protect the mother and fetus during pregnancy and the baby for some months afterwards. Immunization is the procedure adopted to achieve this if tests show that the level is inadequate. A distinction should be made between vaccines containing live and killed organisms, since the former may be dangerous to the fetus — for example, *rubella or smallpox*. Thus, rubella vaccination should be given to women of the child-bearing era between pregnancies, and protection against pregnancy ensured for the

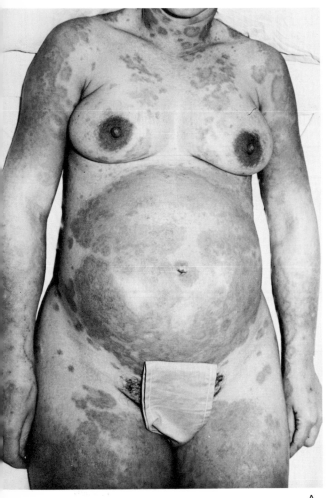 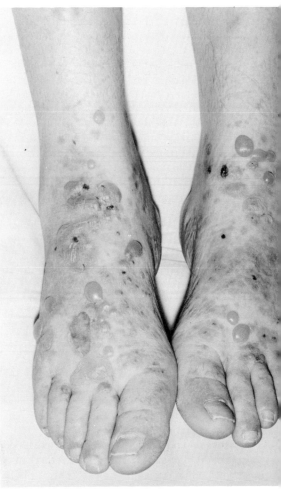

A   B

Figure 39.1 Herpes gestationis in a 27-year-old para 1. **A.** Appearance at 32.5 weeks' gestation when referred because of an itchy generalized, papular rash. The rash had commenced on the soles of her feet at 26 weeks, and progressed in spite of sedation and application of 1% phenol in calamine lotion. **B.** The legs became oedematous and vesicles developed. Oral betamethasone, 2.5 mg/day, was commenced and the rash subsided; she was maintained on a dose of 0.5 mg/day. She had a normal delivery at 39 weeks' gestation of a healthy infant, birth-weight 3,520 g. The betamethasone was ceased 10 days after delivery; 14 years later the patient reported no recurrence of the rash, although she had not had any further pregnancies.

next 2–3 months. Smallpox vaccination may cause fatal vaccinia in the fetus; this is far more likely if the vaccination is primary rather than secondary (revaccination). The safer alternative is initial vaccination with killed organisms.

Poliomyelitis and influenza vaccinations are advisable in pregnancy and provoke little reaction. *Tetanus* vaccination is often given routinely in countries such as India where the risks are higher. There is likely to be an increased use of such vaccines given early in the third trimester, since high levels of antibody (IgG) will be available to the fetus by passage across the placenta. *Diphtheria* vaccination is

not advisable unless in an emergency, because of systemic reactions; the same applies to *pertussis* and *typhoid*, since chemotherapy is available.

Before any immunization is undertaken in pregnancy, a careful history should be elicited of *past infections* or *immunizations*, and the type of reaction experienced.

The administration of immune serum globulin is often advocated to prevent or minimize the effects of rubella, mumps, hepatitis A and B, chickenpox, influenza, or tetanus, should the mother or close household contact have the disease, or there is evidence of infection in the newborn.

TABLE 39.2 AUTOIMMUNE DISEASES AND PREGNANCY

Disorder (incidence)	Major clinical features	Effect on pregnancy	Course of disease	Management	Remarks
Systemic lupus erythematosus (1 in 1,500–1 in 2,000, colour plate 78)	Renal damage, Raynaud disease; pleuritis/ pericarditis, arthritis, skin lupus; multisystem disorder	Increase in abortion, growth retardation, death in utero, prematurity, preeclampsia. Transmission of LE factor to newborn; occasional clinical involvement	Some tendency to exacerbate in pregnancy; significant risk postpartum	Preconceptional advice; collaboration with physician/ internist; pharmacother- apy — aspirin/ corticosteroids/ rarely azathioprine. Therapeutic abortion seldom indicated	Pregnancy less well tolerated if disease active, especially if cardiac or renal involvement
Obstetric lupus syndrome	Abnormal laboratory findings (coagulation and immuno- logical) systems	Thrombosis in intervillous space. High incidence of abortion and fetal death	Cortisone, platelet inhibitors	Clinical variant of SLE	
Rheumatoid arthritis (1 in 300–1 in 600)	Chronic relapsing disorder. Symmetrical inflammation of peripheral joints (swelling, pain, stiffness), fatigue and weakness; other systems may be affected	Insignificant	Improvement is usual, but most relapse within 3 months postpartum	Physical therapy: appropriate balance of rest, exercise and heat; aspirin. Other drugs under specialist supervision	Presence of rheumatoid factor in serum (anti-IgG)
Herpes gestationis (1 in 5–10,000, colour plate 80 and figure 39.1)	Generalized rash with subepidermal vesicles. Toxaemia can result in coma and simulate septicaemia	Increased perinatal loss	Usually presents late in pregnancy or in labour and resolves completely after delivery	Corticosteroids, for severe skin and toxic manifestations	Diagnosis confirmed by immunofluore- scent studies on skin biopsy
Periarteritis nodosa (very rare)	Inflammation of medium-sized arteries. Arterial thrombosis and distal organ infarction. Malaise, weakness, fever, myalgia, arthralgia	Abortion/ premature labour common	Significant risk to mother	Exclude predisposing factors (drugs, microorgan- isms). Corticosteroids	Unlike other disorders described; males and older age groups are more commonly affected. Diagnosis often missed
Systemic sclerosis (uncommon)	Skin thickened and tight; other connective tissues also injointed (joint, muscle, gastrointestinal tract); can mimic SLE	Similar to SLE if disease generalized. Renal involvement indicates poor prognosis	Variable, largely unrelated	Symptomatic relief	Disease more common in 4th and 5th decades

Anatomical and Physiological Basis of Labour

OVERVIEW

As full term approaches, the *uterus will have increased its bulk* by 1,200% — largely due to hypertrophy of the many billion smooth muscle cells which make up the bulk of the organ. Most of the individual cell enlargement is due to the accumulation of the *contractile proteins, actin and myosin*. From early in the third trimester the uterus progressively delineates into a *thick upper segment* and a *thin lower segment*; use is made of the latter in the performance of the usual type of Caesarean section. Experience suggests that poor formation of the lower segment leads to poor dilatation of the cervix during labour. Concomitantly with the growth of the uterus is an increase in vascular supply: damage to the uterus and/or its vessels is responsible for the sometimes massive bleeding which may complicate childbirth.

By the time labour commences, there has been a general *softening of the connective tissues* of the pelvis — joint ligaments, pelvic cellular tissue, and cervical connective tissue; this facilitates the passage of the baby during the process of parturition.

Throughout pregnancy the output of *progesterone*, initially from the corpus luteum and later from the placenta, serves to block stimulatory influences which would otherwise cause expulsion of the fetus (myometrial stretching, oestrogen sensitization, oxytocin, prostaglandin). At full term, the progesterone effect is overcome as stretching and the other factors achieve a critical value, and the wave of excitation is able to travel quickly across the myometrium, stimulating actomyosin into functional activity via a flux of calcium ions into the cell. Once started, the uterine contractions become stronger and more frequent, due to progressively increasing release of *prostaglandin from stressed decidual lysosomes* and release of *oxytocin from the posterior lobe of the pituitary gland* in response to cervical and vaginal stretching.

Labour is traditionally subdivided into 3 stages — the relative end points being full dilatation of the cervix and delivery of the baby. The *first stage* comprises the slower *latent phase* when the cervix is effacing and beginning to dilate, and the *more rapid dilatation phase*. The work required and the time taken is significantly greater in the nullipara.

The *physiological changes in the mother* during normal labour are relatively minor — a modest hyperventilation and respiratory alkalosis, tachycardia, blood pressure elevation, and a more significant reduction in gastrointestinal motility and absorption (especially during the painful active phase and after narcotic analgesia).

The baby shows a mild acidosis, particularly in the second stage. Breathing movements are markedly curtailed. Significant decelerations in fetal heart rate and flattening of the baseline pattern usually indicate transient or permanent hypoxia.

Labour (or parturition) is *defined* as the process in which the fetus, placenta, and secundines are expelled from the birth canal after a minimum period of 28 weeks. Before this, the term *abortion* is applied.

THE MOTHER

ANATOMY

The anatomy of the pelvis and the earlier changes in pregnancy have been described in Chapters 2 and 5.

At the end of pregnancy the uterus fills most of the abdominal cavity. Its length has increased from 7–8 cm to 30–40 cm and its weight from 60–80 g to 850–950 g. The predominant change in the third trimester, apart from increase in size, is the development of the *lower uterine segment* which at full term measures 5–7.5 cm; in the nullipara, there is usually a parallel descent of the presenting part. This part of the uterus is much thinner than the upper segment, and is recognized at Caesarean section by the fact that the peritoneum is only loosely attached to it.

Bandl described the line of demarcation between upper and lower uterine segments where the peritoneum becomes adherent to the uterus (colour plate 92B, figures 47.1A and B). In every labour there is a *physiological retraction ring* at this site, which is at the level of the pubic symphysis at the onset of labour. A *pathological retraction ring* occurs in obstructed labour when the ring is palpable and visible, often reaching to the level of the umbilicus (figure 52.4). With the increasing volume of the fetus, placenta, and liquor, the uterine muscle becomes thinner. There is almost always some *rotation of the uterus to the right side*, so that at Caesarean section the left round ligament is seen much more readily than the right (colour plate 93A). There is general thickening of the ligaments supporting the uterus and this is most obvious in the round ligaments, which may measure 1–2 cm in diameter. The blood vessels are greatly enlarged, especially the veins, explaining the severity of the bleeding if they rupture during labour.

The *ovaries and tubes* are carried higher into the abdomen, as is the appendix; the surgical approach to these organs is thus different from that in the nonpregnant patient.

The *cervix* is approximately at the level of the ischial spines. Softening, together with some dilatation and effacement, usually occurs in the last 4–6 weeks of pregnancy. This ripening process represents an alteration in the composition of glycosaminoglycans and glycoproteins in the ground substance of the cervix, with separation of the collagen bundles. When labour commences, the 'taking up' process that led to the formation of the lower uterine segment continues, the involvement of the cervix in this process causes it to become *effaced*: the cervical canal widens from above down, until only the external os remains as a thin rim (figure 40.1). This heralds the end of the *latent phase of labour*, dilatation of the cervix begins, and the *accelerated phase of labour* commences. The above sequence is classically seen in the nullipara; *in the multipara, effacement and dilatation may occur simultaneously*.

The fused amniotic and chorionic membranes line the cavity of the uterus and are attached to the endometrium except over the internal os. The amniotic fluid is usually separated into 2 compartments during labour by the ball-valve effect of the presenting part: these compartments are known as the *forewater* below, and the much larger *hindwater* above. The membranes do not usually rupture until the end of the first stage of labour provided the forewater is protected by a well-fitting presenting part. Rarely, the baby may be born with the membranes still intact (born in a caul). Occasionally, only the outer chorion may rupture, leaving the amnion intact,

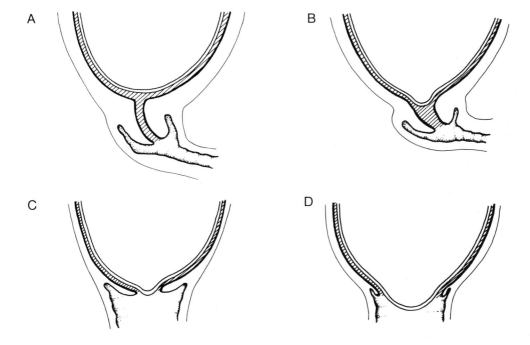

Figure 40.1 Changes in the cervix during the first stage of labour. **A.** Cervix at term — no dilatation or effacement. **B.** Cervical effacement ('taking up' to become part of the lower uterine segment) has commenced. **C.** The endocervical canal has disappeared as effacement of the cervix is complete. The external os is 2–3 cm dilated. **D.** The cervix is almost fully dilated and the intact bag of forewaters bulges into the vagina.

or fluid may accumulate between the 2 layers.

The process of cervical dilatation is greatly facilitated by a well-fitting presenting part.

The vagina shares with the uterus a general increase in size and vascularity. As a result of this, and an increase in elastic fibres, it becomes very distensible and so is able to accommodate the passage of the baby.

The other most obvious change is a general 'softening' of the pelvic tissues, probably due in part to a general increase in extracellular fluid and in part to the hormone *relaxin*. This softening extends to the ligaments of the joints — the resulting relaxation providing some increase in pelvic capacity.

PHYSIOLOGY

A. The Uterus

Like other hollow muscular structures in the body, the uterus displays several important properties.

(i) *Tone.* This is the pressure that is measured in the uterus *between contractions*; it is the basal activity that distinguishes living muscle from dead and it ranges from 2–10 mm Hg.

(ii) *Contractility.* This is the ability of the muscle fibres of the uterus to contract — usually in response to a wave of excitation (change in electrical activity). If all fibres contract in unison, the contraction is said to be coordinate or synchronous; if not, the contraction is incoordinate or asynchronous. As in the case of other smooth muscle, the contractions are *involuntary*.

The *effectiveness of the uterus* in doing its work, i.e. delivering the baby, depends on the *strength* of the contractions, their *frequency* per unit of time, their *coordination* as regards synchrony (working together) and *polarity* (fundal dominance). A general measure of the normally-acting uterus is the *Montevideo unit*, which is the intensity of the contraction (in mm Hg) multiplied by the number of contractions in a 10-minute interval; that is, 2 contractions of average intensity 40 mm Hg = 80 Montevideo units. This does not accurately express *uterine wall tension*, which is a measure of both intrauterine pressure and radius of curvature of the uterus (La Place law). The cumulative *work load* for the whole labour can be assessed. There is usually a progressive decrease in the work required for each centimetre of dilatation.

(iii) *Fundal or proximal dominance.* This means that the wave of excitation normally passes downward, the resulting contraction or peristaltic wave forcing the contents out of the organ. In the uterus, the contractions begin in areas called *pacemakers* which are situated in the region of one or other uterine horn (near the attachment of the Fallopian tubes).

A further characteristic is that the duration of the contraction is longer in the fundus than in the lower part of the uterus and it is more powerful. This provides for coordination of the contraction, with the maximum expulsive force being exerted at the one time, by different parts of the uterus.

(iv) *Rhythmicity.* Each muscular organ has an inherent rhythm of contractility depending upon its physiological function and the conditions pertaining at a particular time — e.g. for the uterus — whether it is pregnant or not, period of gestation, presence of pharmacological agents etc.

The combined effect of *Braxton Hicks painless contractions* and *relaxation of the pelvic joints* which occur late in pregnancy causes the head to descend into the pelvic brim. This phenomenon, which is termed *lightening*, is much more common in the nullipara because of the firmer abdominal musculature. As a result of the decrease in pressure on the upper abdomen, breathing, heart action, and digestion are all easier.

The labour process is probably a largely autonomous one, depending on cervical resistance on the one hand and uterine contractibility on the other; separate labours may occur where there is complete uterine duplication, with 1 fetus in each uterus.

The Onset and Continuation of Labour

There has been much debate as to the cause of labour, but in a similar manner to ripe fruit falling from the tree, there is almost certainly a balance of forces involved. Labour ensues when the forces of retention are overcome by the forces of release.

The *myometrial cell* is the basic unit in the contractile process. Under the influence of oestrogen, the contractile proteins, actin and myosin, increase in preparation for the work of labour. Their combination to the active form (actomyosin) is caused by the influx of *calcium ions* after depolarization of the cell membrane and this is regulated by the 2 proteins, *tropomyosin* and *troponin*. Adenosine triphosphate (*ATP*) is the energy source used by the actomyosin.

For efficient uterine activity, the many billions of myometrial cells must act in concert. Correct polarity, which is the basis of peristalsis, is achieved by electrical activity originating in fundal pacemaker sites; the spread of the contraction is achieved by the development of low-resistance cell:cell contacts. As full term approaches, the stage is set for the development of the long trains of action potentials of high spike activity that characterize labour. The latter is the culmination of a number of positive factors — e.g. the cell has enough contractile protein (actomyosin) to do the job and stimulatory factors have peaked (*prostaglandins* in the uterus, *oxytocin* and receptors for this hormone, *oestradiol, uterine stretch*). This is sufficient to *overcome the synergistic effects of progesterone and relaxin* (on membrane binding of calcium ions, inhibition of spread of the wave of excitation, and cervical resistance). Cervical factors play only a secondary role — i.e. labour is made difficult if the cervix is unripe, but its onset is not prevented.

The criteria used for the onset of true labour are firstly, *rhythmic, regular contractions* that show a progressive increase in amplitude and frequency, and are discomforting to the patient (unlike Braxton Hicks contractions); and secondly, a '*show*' of *blood and mucus*, which indicates that the cervical canal is opening (colour plate 83 and figure 40.2).

The Stages of Labour

Three stages of labour are traditionally described; *first*, from the onset of regular contractions to full dilatation of the cervix (figure 40.3); *second*, from full dilatation to delivery of the baby; and *third*, from birth of the baby until delivery of the placenta.

Clinical Correlations

During each uterine contraction there are 3 phases: *increment*, when the pressure is rising in

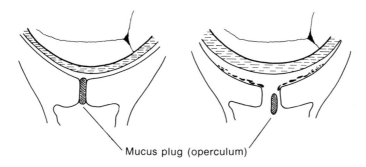

Figure 40.2 At the onset of labour, dilatation of the cervix begins and the mucus plug (operculum) which occluded the endocervical canal is shed. The show of blood at this time is due to the membranes being stripped off the uterine wall.

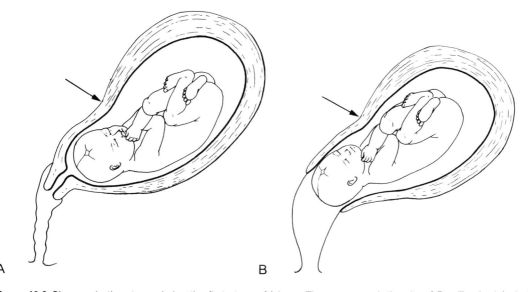

A   B

Figure 40.3 Changes in the uterus during the first stage of labour. The arrows mark the site of Bandl's physiological ring between the upper and lower uterine segments. In obstructed labour this ring rises and becomes visible as a pathological retraction ring. **A.** At the onset of labour there is neither taking up nor dilatation of the cervix. **B.** On completion of the first stage the vagina, cervix, and lower uterine segment form a continuous surface — the cervix no longer acts as a ledge preventing descent of the presenting part.

the uterus; *acme*, a brief plateau of maximum pressure; and *decrement*, when the pressure falls away.

Since *pain* is only perceived when the contraction pressure reaches 20–25 mm Hg, inhalation methods of pain relief must be used intelligently to be effective. There is considerable evidence that the pain of labour is related to dilatation of the cervix and other birth canal structures rather than the contraction itself, since Braxton Hicks contractions in late pregnancy are painless, as are those in the third stage of labour, despite reasonably high pressures being present. *Cervical dilatation* does not occur unless rhythmical contractions of at least 20 mm Hg are occurring. Clinical estimates of the duration of contractions are usually shorter than the real duration, since the beginning and end of the contraction are not perceived by the patient.

The Effects of Uterine Contractions

(i) *The first stage of labour.* Before the membranes rupture, the pressure exerted by the uterine contractions is transmitted to the centre of the cavity of the uterus and is equal throughout the amniotic fluid. However, because of fundal dominance, the lower segment becomes progressively thinner and drawn out, and in the period denoted as the *latent stage* of labour the cervix becomes effaced and continuous with the lower segment; this occupies approximately half of the duration of labour. Factors slowing the latent phase include a high presenting part, incomplete maturation of the excitatory mechanisms, an unfavourable (unripe) cervix, and sedative drugs given prematurely. When the cervix starts to dilate actively, the process is quite rapid (figure 40.4); this *acceleration phase* is similar in the nulliparous and parous patient. In general, a cervical dilatation rate of more than 1 cm/hour will result in spontaneous delivery; less than 0.5 cm/hour usually means Caesarean section unless improved by oxytocin. The *characteristic progression* is largely the result of 2 mechanisms — firstly, the increasing release of *prostaglandin* from the decidua as disruption of cell lysosomes occurs, and secondly, the increasing release of *oxytocin* with dilatation of the cervix and birth canal. The process of cervical dilatation will con-

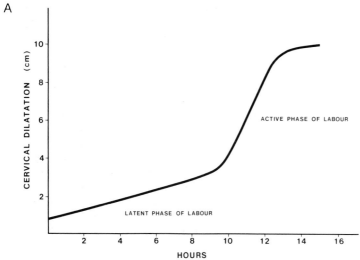

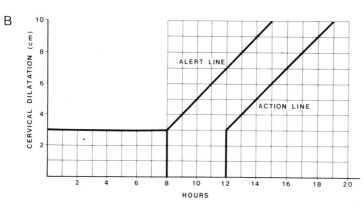

Figure 40.4 A. The duration of normal (spontaneous, nonaugmented) labour in nulliparas, as shown here, is about 16 hours, or twice as long as for multiparas. Little cervical dilatation occurs in the first half of the first stage (latent phase) but is rapid in the second half (active phase). In multiparas the 2 to 10 cm dilatation of the active phase may sometimes be achieved in 1 or 2 strong contractions. **B.** Partograph (cervicograph) as originally developed by Philpott for use by midwives in peripheral Rhodesia (Zimbabwe). The active phase of labour is designated from the time of 3 cm cervical dilatation. Subsequent rate of cervical dilatation should follow a rapid course as described by Friedman (figure 40.4 A) and exceed 1 cm per hour. Vaginal examination is performed at intervals of 2–4 hours and if the rate of cervical dilatation crosses the alert line special care is indicated. When the action line is crossed, consideration is given to amniotomy, epidural analgesia, oxytocin stimulation (enhancement or augmentation of labour) and fetal heart rate monitoring by cardiotocography. Caesarean section is indicated in the presence of fetal distress, failure of the head to descend, failure of efficient cervical dilatation within 6 hours of crossing the action line, or for other obstetric indications which would preclude active management of labour. This graph is designed specifically for use in nulliparas.

tinue whether it is the forewater membranes or the presenting part that the lower uterus and cervix are being drawn over. Hence rupture of the membranes prematurely will not impede labour — the *clinical impression is that the reverse occurs*, provided that the presenting part is fitting well into the lower segment. The force of the uterine contraction is now directed downward, rather than into the centre of the cavity. A further advantage of membrane rupture is that the liquor can be seen and this is a barometer of sorts to the well-being of the fetus (display of meconium when present). Possible disadvantages of membrane rupture are that if the labour continues to be slow, usually as a result of incoordinate uterine action and/or posterior position of the occiput, the chances of *infection* of the fetus are increased. Also, studies have shown that very high pressures exist at the level of the presenting part and the lower segment of the uterus; intact membranes may serve to lessen the pressure on the fetal skull by distributing it more equally, and furthermore, there is a lesser chance of direct pressure on the placenta or cord by the baby.

The uterus causes the cervix to dilate basically because of fundal dominance. For the explusion of the baby it is important that the uterine fundus has a *pied-a-terre*, or foot on the ground, and this is provided by the *supports* which are attached in the region of the cervix — the cardinal ligaments laterally, the uterosacral ligaments posteriorly, and the pubocervical ligaments anteriorly. It is with these ligaments to pull against that the uterus can push the baby through the soft tissues (pelvic and perineal floors) and hard structures (bony pelvis) that constitute the birth canal.

Descent occurs in an oscillatory fashion, as anyone familiar with the terminal phases of labour has observed. With each contraction the baby descends, but because of the resistance of the birth canal structures it loses some of this ground during the relaxation phase. However, with each contraction some descent occurs, albeit small, and this gain is secured by *retraction* of the uterine muscle. *In this process, the muscle does not relax to its original length, but stays at a new shorter length.* The *position of the patient* is of some relevance: if on her side, the strength of the contraction is greater, but the frequency is less; the overall activity is greater. The *duration* of the first stage of labour varies rather widely, especially in the nullipara. *The average is about 12 hours* although the median and modal values are less than this (8–10 hours); the major problem is knowing when labour actually commences. Some centres take this to be when the

patient is admitted to hospital; this is a practical though somewhat quaint idea. *In a multipara the average duration of the first stage is about 6 hours* (half that of the nullipara).

(ii) *The second stage.* When the cervix is fully dilated, the second stage of labour is entered. The contractions are usually stronger, but occur less frequently. The head descends and becomes palpable postanally. At some point in the second stage, a strong *bearing-down reflex* comes into play, similar to that which occurs when the bowels are stimulated to open. After an inspiration, the patient pushes down with the aid of the diaphragm and abdominal wall muscles (*secondary powers*). The main *stimulus to bearing down* is the reflex elicited by distension of the pelvic floor and upper vagina, and is evinced only with contractions (figure 40.5). Usually, 2–3 bearing-down efforts are made with each contraction. Such efforts made prematurely during the first stage cause an undue rise in intrauterine pressure, with detrimental effect on fetal oxygenation, and also cause overstretching of the central uterine supports, leading to later prolapse. *The patient is therefore encouraged not to bear down until the cervix is fully dilated* — if in doubt this is verified by vaginal examination. Some patients do not feel like bearing down until later in the second stage, when the presenting part is at the introitus.

The contraction/retraction sequence continues in a progressively stronger fashion, since the membranes have now usually ruptured and the uterine fundus acts directly on the long axis of the baby (*fetal axis pressure*) to force it through the lower birth canal with the aid of the secondary powers. The descent of the presenting part causes pressure on the other pelvic organs. The fundus of the bladder is displaced upward, whilst compression of the rectum often causes faecal material to escape. Final dilatation of the cervix, or distension of the vagina may cause small lacerations, and this may be accompanied by a *show of blood*.

The *normal duration of this stage ranges from 10–30 minutes in the multipara to 20–60 minutes in the nullipara.* Factors influencing the duration include the strength and coordination of uterine contractions, the strength of the mother's secondary powers (ability to push), the resistance of the lower birth canal (high in the nullipara because it has not been distended previously, and there is greater likelihood of associated spasm of pelvic diaphragm musculature), and finally, the size, presentation and position of the presenting part.

These factors must be taken into account

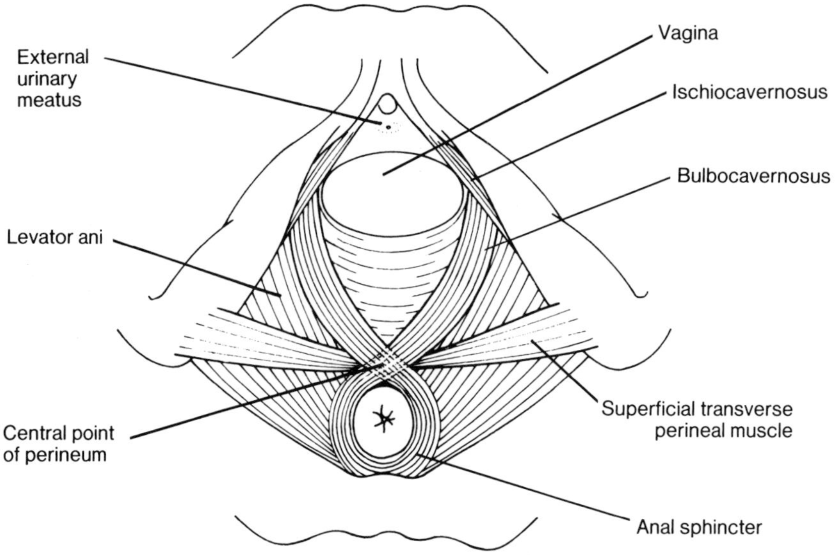

Figure 40.5 During delivery, the muscles of the pelvic diaphragm are pushed downwards and the aperture between the origins of the levatores ani muscles (from the back of the pubic bones) is greatly increased. The perineum bulges downwards 6–8 cm and its initial anteroposterior length of 5 cm in increased to 10 cm — thus forming the soft tissue component of the curve of the birth canal.

when assessing whether the second stage is prolonged in a particular patient.

When the head is on the perineum the contractions may become weak and infrequent (*uterine exhaustion*); if an episiotomy is considered necessary, it should be properly timed to make use of a commencing contraction. This prevents unnecessary delay in delivery and minimizes the risk of fetal hypoxia (the most dangerous period (risk of death) of a person's life is that preceding and following the process of birth).

During delivery, stretching and some damage is inevitable in the musculofascial structures of the pelvis; this, together with damage to nerves supplying the pelvic floor, often leaves a legacy of prolapse and varying degrees of urinary and faecal incontinence.

(iii) *The third stage.* Strong, largely painless contractions continue during the third stage, although their frequency may be reduced to 1 per 5 minutes. With the routine use of oxytocic preparations, the picture is blurred, since the ergometrine causes sustained tonic activity.

B. Other Maternal Changes

(i) *Respiratory system.* There is a *modest hyperventilation* during pregnancy, mainly due to a greater depth of respiration (tidal volume) rather than an increase in frequency. This results in a *steady fall in arterial CO_2 pressure* (P_aCO_2) from the normal of 40 mm Hg because more CO_2 is exhaled with each breath. In labour, this tendency is accentuated; during strong contractions, both rate and depth of respiration are increased. The mean level of P_aCO_2 falls from 32mm Hg at the start of labour to 22 mm Hg at the end of the first stage. In the second stage, because of breath-holding associated with pushing, less CO_2 is expired and the level rises to 26 mm Hg. Occasionally, *hyperventilation is overdone*, either spontaneously or in mistaken application of the 'psychoprophylactic' method; the P_aCO_2 levels fall below 16–18 mm Hg, clinical symptoms such as dizziness occur, and fetal asphyxia may result. The opposite effect may occur if *shallow respiration is overdone*, since the tidal volume (air in and out each breath) will be low, and too little oxygen will be delivered to the fetus. Similarly, second stage pushing can be harmful if too prolonged, either overall or during contractions, because of the drop in oxygen during breath-holding.

(ii) *Cardiovascular system.* The main change is seen in the *blood pressure*. In the first stage there is an average rise of 10 mm Hg systolic/5–10 mm Hg diastolic during contractions, but little change between contractions; in the second stage there is a rise of 30/25 mm Hg during contractions and 10/5–10 between contractions. The rise during the second stage places the patient with hypertension from any cause in jeopardy, because of the *risk of cerebral haemorrhage*. Although compression of the inferior vena cava in the supine patient lessens as the presenting part descends, aortic compression continues until birth.

If the patient is pushing strongly, there is a

compensatory and often marked fall in blood pressure as bearing-down stops at the end of the contraction; this may place the fetus in jeopardy from hypoxia, particularly if the placental circulation is not robust. Other changes in labour include a slow, but progressive *rise in pulse rate* which will be accentuated by dehydration, haemorrhage, anxiety, unrelieved pain, infection, and certain drugs (such as those inhibiting labour); a rise in cardiac output; and a fall in plasma volume. These changes will vary considerably according to the duration and strength of the labour, the amount of panting by the patient (water loss), room temperature, and fluid replacement.

(iii) *Gastrointestinal system.* During active, painful labour (particularly after narcotic administration), gastrointestinal *motility and absorption are reduced*, so there is little point in expecting to feed patients successfully at this time. Similarly, drugs given orally will be poorly absorbed. Later in labour, nausea and vomiting may occur, particularly at the time of transition from first to second stage.

(iv) *Acid-base balance.* The main factor lowering the pH of the blood is starvation (if there has not been intravenous replacement) plus the work performed by the uterus; *metabolic acidosis* may thus result. This is usually offset by a lowering of the CO_2 (respiratory alkalosis) as discussed above. The slightly raised pH of late pregnancy, 7.42 (versus the nonpregnant 7.40) falls to 7.35. This is reflected in the figures for base excess, the respective values being $\pm$ 2, 0 and -8.

(v) *Fluids and electrolytes.* As a result of reduced gut absorption, panting and sweat loss, there is a degree of haemoconcentration (reflected in the haematocrit) and a fall in plasma levels of sodium and chloride.

(vi) *Temperature.* There is usually a small drop (0.5° C) in body temperature a day or so before the onset of labour.

THE FETUS
ANATOMY

The major change to the fetus during labour is the *compression* (*moulding*) of the presenting part (figures 2.17– 2.19). In the usual situation, the head is presenting and moulding is accomplished by the table bones of the skull (occipital, parietal, frontal) approaching one another and if necessary overlapping. The flexed attitude of the fetus is usually accentuated after rupture of the membranes and drainage of liquor from the uterus.

PHYSIOLOGY

(i) *Cardiovascular system.* The most readily observable parameters are *heart rate and rhythm*. The rate usually stays within the normal range of 120–160 beats/minute. The rhythm is fairly constant, the base-line showing a characteristic fluctuation of $\pm$ 5–10 beats/minute over a selected time interval. During a contraction, there is no significant change in rate if placental function is adequate; *blood flow velocity in the umbilical arteries* (Doppler measurement) is also unaffected by normal contractions. The *rate may drop during the contraction* (*type 1 dip*) as a result of cord compression or stretching, or pressure on the fetal head (causing reduced cerebral blood flow or vagal reflex activity). If the placenta is not functioning normally, a characteristic *fall in rate may occur after the finish of the contraction* (*type 2 dip*) (figure 41.7).

(ii) *Acid-base balance.* This is of importance because of the introduction of the technique of *fetal scalp blood sampling* as a measure of fetal well-being. During labour, there is a slow fall in scalp pH from a mean of 7.30 to 7.20, largely because uterine contractions inhibit placental exchange, but partly because the pH of the mother also falls at this time. This change is more evident in the second stage, when the hypoxia consequent on pushing is added, this increasing the metabolic acidosis (Chapter 48).

(iii) *Breathing and movement.* During labour there is a sharp decrease in the time spent by the fetus in breathing activity (30–40% to about 1%); there may be hiccup-like activity. Trunk movements are largely unchanged except after artificial membrane rupture, when a decrease occurs.

Chapter forty-one

The Management of Normal Labour. Analgesia and Anaesthesia

OVERVIEW

'It is much easier to make a hospital birth homely
than to make a home birth safe'

In no area of obstetrics has the debate been keener or opinion more divided than in the philosophical approach, place of conduct, and management of labour. On the one hand, it is seen as a natural, emotionally-fulfilling event; on the other, it is seen as potentially the most dangerous period of existence, whether one is the mother or the baby (but particularly the latter). Home birth at all cost or hospital birth at all cost are practical expressions of these philosophical stances.

Community pressure has forced maternity institutions to review traditional practices and to accept consumer demand for the more family-centred, gentle, and natural approach to childbirth, and the needs of parents to have a greater input into decision-making. Initially, it was thought that this could be accomplished only by separate ('low risk', 'alternate') birth centres.

It is now realized that the main change needed was in the attitude of the health care attendant and health administrator. The low risk birth centre is still seen as having an important role, but much can be done in traditional hospital labour wards to enable the parents to experience childbirth in a fulfilling but safe manner.

The problem with low risk centres is that sometimes too much is asked of them in terms of obstetric abnormality. *The problem with home births is that the potentially fatal obstetric complication can never be anticipated with certainty.*

Confidence of the mother is particularly important to the successful outcome of the labour and this is engendered by antenatal education, psychological support, physiotherapy, and the secure knowledge that adequate skills and facilities are available should trouble arise. *The information given to the parents should be realistic*, otherwise there may be a deep sense of disappointment and failure should things not go smoothly in terms of pain control, labour progress, and type of delivery.

Other trends in labour care include freedom of the mother to adopt *positions of comfort* and accept analgesia, discretion in the use of *shaving and enema* and in the use of the more scientific approaches to *fetal monitoring*.

Many of the measures of the new wave (including relaxing in the salt water tub or pool) do result in a more contented and relaxed mother and, in general, the lower the anxiety state, the smoother the labour. A significant contributor to this in recent years is the caring and *attentive husband/partner*: the burden of the labour is shared, appreciation of the travail deepened, and the ground prepared for bonding of the new family unit.

Partographic documentation has led to the concept of *acceleration of the tardy labour* (almost exclusively in the nullipara). An *oxytocin infusion* is commenced if cervical dilatation is non-progressive in the absence of significant disproportion.

There is little unanimity in relation to *relief of pain* in labour. Many mothers do not wish there to be any attenuation of the peak emotional experience and reality of labour, birth, and *early bonding* and seek to control pain by psychoprophylactic and physiological means. Others, less tolerant, still seek relief in analgesics and increasingly, *epidural nerve block* (which has the advantages of leaving the sensorium undulled and pain eliminated).

It is evident that the modern obstetric attendant must exercise a delicate balance in labour care between imposition of a sick role on the mother on the one hand and failing to monitor adequately on the other. There will always be some degree of compromise required; good faith, based on adequate understanding of each position, should minimize potential conflict.

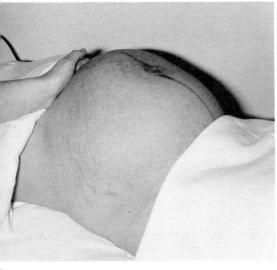

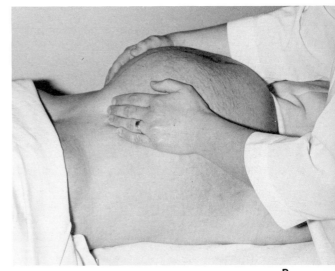

B

Figure 41.1 Examination of the abdomen. **A.** The height of the fundus is noted. **B.** The fetal pole occupying the fundus (usually the breech) is palpated. **C.** Lateral palpation ('umbilical grip') detects the fetal back on one side and flexed limbs on the other. **D.** The presenting part is identified and its station noted. This fetus is large and there is a retraction ring visible below the umbilicus and above the distended lower uterine segment. **E.** Pelvic palpation is useful in labour to follow descent of the presenting part.

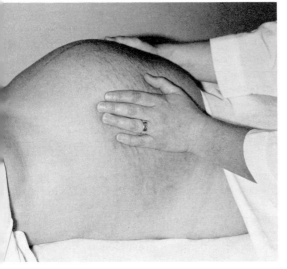

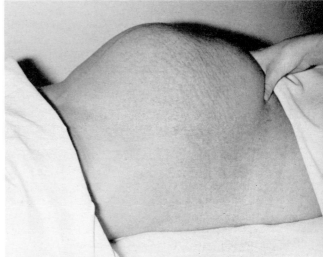

D

E

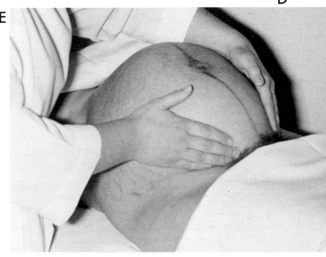

ADMISSION TO LABOUR WARD

Usually, the patient will come to hospital early in labour; table 41.1 provides a check list of the usual requisites (attire, toiletries etc) that she will have ready packed to accompany her. Her antenatal record is obtained and any abnormalities noted, since these may well have a bearing on the progress of labour or on the well-being of the mother and baby.

The patient will be asked about the following: the time when contractions started, their frequency, approximate duration, and nature; presence of a show; state of the membranes; and nature of fetal movements.

TABLE 41.1 CHECK LIST OF REQUISITES —
BIRTHING AND PUERPERIUM

Attire

Nightdresses (3–4)	Slippers
Cardigan/bed jacket	Sanitary belt (1–2)
Nursing bras (2–3)	Panties
Dressing gown	

Toiletries

Face washer(s)	Make-up
Soap	Hair kit (shampoo etc)
Brush/comb	Sewing kit
Deodorant	Hand mirror
Toothbrush/paste	Tissues
Powder	Nipple cream
Shower cap	Hand cream

Usefuls

Torch	Camera
Notebook, pen, letter pad	Grocery bags
Laundry powder	Knitting/book/magazines
Watch/small clock	

Documents

Admission forms

The precise admission procedure differs from hospital to hospital. *The traditional enema and vulval shave is now often waived.* The *enema tends to cause soiling* of the perineum with liquid faeces at delivery; it should not be given if the membranes are ruptured and the presenting part is high. *Shaving predisposes to infection* and is uncomfortable for the patient subsequently; the hair can be cut short with scissors. A shower is taken by the patient and she is dressed in a clean gown.

If the patient is in significant discomfort from strong contractions, the admission procedures should be expedited, and finalized when she has become settled.

Examination

A *general examination* is carried out, with particular attention being paid to the breasts and nipples, heart, chest and abdomen. It is important to ascertain whether the patient has an *infection* of any sort. The blood pressure is recorded, as are the temperature, pulse rate, and respiratory rate. *The abdomen* should be examined systematically (Chapter 6). The following points should be noted: the general contour of the abdomen and its size; the height of the fundus; the lie, presentation, flexion, station and position of the baby (figure 41.1). Particular attention should be paid to the 2 latter observations, since the assessment of the progress of labour depends on their accurate initial determination. The *strength, duration and frequency of contractions* are ascertained.

Provided there are no contraindications, such as antepartum haemorrhage or unstable lie, *a vaginal examination* is then performed. Again, this should be systematic. The introitus is first examined and the following points ascertained: presence of varices, discharge, size of the introitus and length of the perineal body (is an episiotomy likely to be required?). The labia are separated and vaginal examination is carried out. The tone of the levator muscles and perineal floor is noted and an assessment made of the patient's ability to let these muscles relax, if necessary, by pushing down; poor relaxation indicates the probability of a slow second stage and the possible need for forceps delivery. The *cervix* is next examined and a note made of its consistency and *dilatation*, degree of effacement, position in the pelvis (e.g. anterior, axial, sacral), and how well it is applied to the presenting part (figure 41.2); these observations should be combined to provide a Bishop score (see Chapter 44). The *membranes* are palpated and, if ruptured, the *nature of the liquor* is noted. Attention is now turned to the presenting part and confirmation of abdominal findings sought — the *presentation, position, station and degree of flexion* are determined, and also the amount of descent with a contraction (figure 41.3).

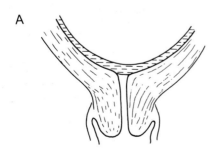 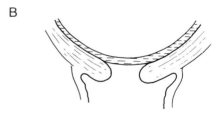

Figure 41.2 Assessment of the cervix. **A.** Primigravida in early labour; the cervix is long, undilated and not effaced; in many primigravidas the cervix is well effaced before labour commences. **B.** Multipara in labour with partly effaced cervix and 2 cm dilatation of the internal os.

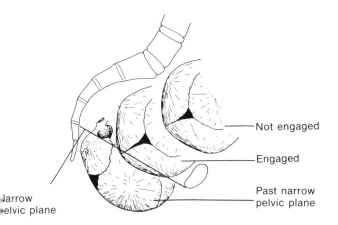

Figure 41.3 Station of the head. The fetal scalp is on view when the maximum diameters of the head (biparietal and suboccipitobregmatic) reach the narrow pelvic plane and this is the level of a low forceps delivery.

Not engaged

Engaged

Past narrow pelvic plane

Narrow pelvic plane

Finally, a check is made of the size of the pelvis — attention being directed to the sacral promontory, the hollow of the sacrum, the ischial spines, sacrospinous ligament, the subpubic angle (figure 41.4). Probably the most rewarding observation is the general degree of fit between the presenting part and the pelvis — does it feel free or is there very little room between it and the walls of the pelvis? If the labour has been in progress for some hours, the degree of *caput and moulding* are determined: the latter can be scored from 0 (nil) to + + + depending on the degree of apposition/overlap of the fetal skull bones. After the vaginal examination is concluded, a *sterile perineal pad* is applied and the patient is allowed to adopt whichever position gives her most comfort — walking, sitting, squatting on all fours, resting in bed etc.

Since patients usually admit themselves, one of the main decisions to be made is whether labour has truly started. *False* (spurious) *labour* can usually be distinguished by a failure of the contractions to increase progressively in strength and duration, and by the absence of a show.

Observations

The following observations are routinely carried out.

(i) *Temperature* is recorded 4-hourly, unless it is elevated, then every 1–2 hours. An elevation in temperature usually signifies infection, but, in cases of prolonged labour and dehydration, a rise in temperature is common.

(ii) *Pulse rate* is taken every ½–1 hour if the labour is normal, but more frequently (every ¼ hour) if an abnormality is present, or if an infusion of oxytocin is in progress. Again, prolonged labour — particularly if intravenous fluids are not given — causes an elevation in rate, as does haemorrhage, infection, cardiac or pulmonary disease, pain, apprehension, and tocolytic agents (beta adrenergic type). There is a surprising range in pulse rates even in normal patients in late pregnancy and labour.

(iii) *Respiratory rate* is observed 4-hourly, in the interval between contractions. An elevated rate usually indicates cardiac or pulmonary disease. A slower rate is usually observed in patients receiving magnesium sulphate therapy.

(iv) *Blood pressure* is normally recorded every 1 hour, but every ¼–½ hour if it is abnormally high (hypertension, preeclampsia) or low (haemorrhage or shock).

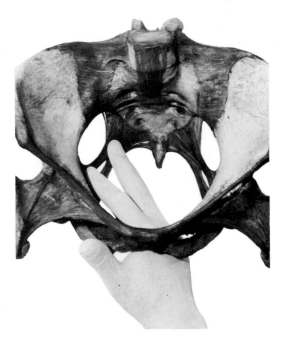

Figure 41.4 Palpation of the sacrospinous ligament, ischial spine, and subpubic angle.

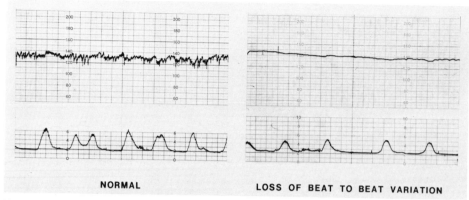

Figure 41.5 In the normal tracing, the basal heart rate (i.e. between contractions) is between 120–160 per minute. Normally, the beat to beat variation exceeds 5 per minute. Loss of beat to beat variation, if gross, as shown here, is indicative of impending fetal death.

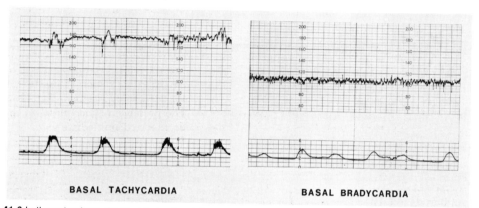

Figure 41.6 In these tracings, the beat to beat variation is maintained although the basal heart rates are abnormal. These signs warrant fetal blood pH measurement, as would the passage of meconium.

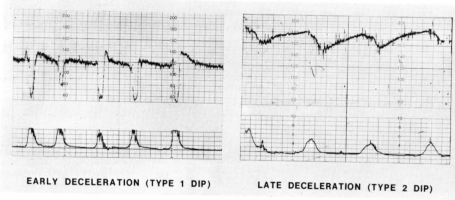

Figure 41.7 The tracing on the left shows strong contractions (top of scale) every 2–3 minutes (distance between thick vertical lines signifies 1 minute). Slowing of the fetal heart rate does not persist after a contraction has ceased, but does so in the tracing on the right which is the more ominous pattern in terms of fetal welfare. Both patterns indicate the need for fetal blood sampling or delivery.

(v) *Fetal heart rate* is counted every 15–30 minutes during the first stage of labour and every 5–10 minutes during the second stage. If there is any irregularity, or if suspicion of impaired placental function exists, the heart rate is checked more frequently (e.g. after each contraction) or *monitored electronically* (figures 41.5–41.7).

(vi) *Contractions.* The duration, strength, and interval are recorded every 30 minutes in the early first stage, (every 15 minutes if there is an oxytocic infusion), every 15 minutes in the late first stage, and every 10 minutes in the second stage. The effect of the contractions on the fetal heart provides a useful indicator of fetoplacental reserve.

With experience, a fairly accurate guide to the *strength of the contractions* can be obtained by abdominal palpation of the uterus, for example, with weak contractions, the uterus can readily be indented even at the acme, whereas with strong contractions, the uterus feels rigid, even boardlike. The duration of the contractions and intervals between them provide supportive evidence. A more precise measurement is afforded by *intrauterine catheter.* Unfortunately, these parameters do not always equate with labour progress: other factors that may confound the observer include the efficiency of the contraction (particularly fundal dominance) and ease of dilatation of the cervix and lower uterine segment. In some centres, the amount of work performed by the uterus (in kiloPascals) is calculated. Table 41.2 summarizes the characteristics of contractions during the first and second stages of labour.

(vii) *Fluid balance.* All fluids and food taken by, or administered to, the patient are recorded, as well as the loss of fluids by voiding or vomiting. A balance should be made at the end of 12 hours.

(viii) *Urine testing* should be carried out for protein and ketones.

(ix) *Bowel actions* are recorded.

(x) *Progress of labour.* A formal assessment of the progress of the presenting part by abdominal examination should be made every 1–2 hours, according to circumstances. If labour does not appear to be progressing normally, vaginal examination is performed and repeated in 1–4 hours. In many centres, a *partograph* is prepared (figures 40.4 and 49.9), based on the degree of cervical dilatation at successive vaginal examinations and descent of the presenting part. The rate of cervical dilatation provides a good guide to the ease or otherwise of the labour and delivery: a dilatation of 1.5 cm or more per hour is satisfactory, whereas a rate below 1 cm per hour usually indicates that difficulty is to be expected. The extent of caput and moulding, and position and flexion of the head are noted if the presentation is cephalic. The partograph is an important record of labour events, and facilitates continuity of care and management.

(xi) *State of membranes* and *nature of liquor* are recorded; the time of membrane rupture is noted. The presence of *meconium* in the liquor should be reported immediately.

(xii) *Blood loss.* Any bleeding greater than a show must be measured and recorded.

(xiii) *Other observations.* Any other untoward event must be recorded — e.g. headache, irritability, fitting, visual upset, unusual pain, dyspneoa, change in conscious state, or cyanosis.

Any of the above routine observations, if outside the normal range, must be reported to the sister or doctor.

TABLE 41.2   CHARACTERISTICS OF CONTRACTIONS DURING THE FIRST AND SECOND STAGES OF LABOUR*

		First stage			
	Onset of labour	*Early acceleration*	*Mid-acceleration*	*Late acceleration*	*Second stage**
Contraction					
Duration (sec)	15–20	30–40	60–80	80–100 +	80–110 +
Interval (min)	10–15	5–8	4–6	3–4	2–4
Intensity	Mild	Mild–Mod	Moderate	Strong	Strong
Pressure (mmHg)	15–30	30–40	40–60	50–80 +	50–80 +
Palpation of uterus	Indents readily	Indents	Firm	Rigid	Rigid

* Often the contractions become less frequent and of shorter duration and intensity when the head is on the perineum (impending uterine exhaustion) — these patients often require an episiotomy to facilitate delivery

PATIENT CARE

Psychological Aspects

The following information should be ascertained: whether the patient has attended antenatal classes, and how many; her attitude to the pregnancy and labour, and that of her husband; whether the patient wishes her husband, relative, or close friend to be with her during labour; her intentions concerning breast feeding; whether she has had any psychiatric upsets in the past — especially in relation to childbearing; and what emotional support she has received during the pregnancy. If the patient is unmarried, any problems still outstanding should be discussed. An assessment of the patient's emotional state and psychic stability can be made after discussion along the above lines.

Frequently, the patient has a number of questions to ask concerning the labour, pain relief, and the baby. The patient may be too shy or reserved to mention these matters, and the nurse can make it easier by asking the patient whether she has any such questions. Fear, loneliness, anxiety and uncertainty all have a deleterious effect on the patient's pain threshold and on the smooth progress of labour. Most patients wish to maintain their identity, and a request to wear their own apparel, if clean, should be respected. The partner will often assist by his presence, giving psychological support, and can help with relaxation, psychoprophylactic techniques, and timing of contractions. His presence will usually facilitate the bonding process, and he will appreciate better the efforts and difficulties inherent in the labour process. *However, it should be appreciated that not all fathers can cope with the labour scene*: some feel helpless, uncomfortable or even frightened. Some studies suggest that the memory of labour and delivery remains with the male partner longer and more vividly than with the female.

The attendant should assess the patient's anxiety level and effect of contractions; if she responds with muscle stiffening and holding her breath, efforts at relaxation should be encouraged and reinforced. Imagery is often helpful to the patient — riding over the wave of the contraction; visualization of the cervix opening and stretching over the baby's head etc.

Each centre will have guide-lines concerning the *attendance of children during labour and delivery*. Relevant factors include their age and emotional maturity, the attitude of the family to life events, the child's prenatal education, and the anticipated ease or difficulty of the labour. If children do attend, they should have been given a realistic picture, otherwise they might be disturbed by the sights and sounds of the labour.

They should preferably be in the care of a support person other than their father. Positive reactions include increased personal maturation and facilitation of the acceptance of their new sibling into the family.

There will be many opportunities during labour, delivery, and the postnatal period to build on the parent-infant bonding that has already begun during the antenatal period (table 41.3).

TABLE 41.3   FACTORS FACILITATING PARENT-INFANT BONDING

Antenatal	Pictures of the developing fetus Picture (e.g. ultrasonograph) of own fetus Hearing fetal heart beat Feeling fetal movements Good relationship with care providers
Labour	Supportive family-centred atmosphere Optimal, patient-accepted pain relief
Delivery	Presence of husband/partner Early contact/nursing of baby Early suckling of baby
Postnatal	Baby close to mother Access to special care nursery Breast feeding on demand Adequate parenting knowledge Confidence in caring for baby

Physical Care

(i) *Ambulation.* The mother ideally should be free to walk about, sit, or take up whatever position of comfort she desires during the labour. Contractions are usually more efficient, the labour shorter and labour augmentation and fetal distress less common in such cases. If the patient lies on her back she usually experiences more pain, the contractions are less effective, obstruction to major vessels is likely, there is less satisfactory pelvic opening, fetal distress and operative delivery are both more common. In some centres, the mother sits in a warm bath or pool — this aiding relaxation and reducing catecholamine release.

(ii) *General hygiene.* In early labour, the patient is able to manage her own toilet, but later the nurse can provide much comfort to the patient with washing, oral hygiene, facial sponging, and hair toilet. A perineal wash-down should be given after the bowels have opened.

(iii) *Bladder.* The bladder should be emptied every 2 hours and, if necessary, the patient is *catheterized.* Each specimen of urine should be tested for protein and ketones.

(iv) *Bowels*. Enemas are usually now restricted to those whose bowels have not opened for 24 hours or where the rectum is obviously loaded.

(v) *Nutrition*. It is now accepted that, *once painful contractions are established, little food is absorbed by the patient*. If meals are given, they will either be vomited or will provide a hazard should anaesthesia be required. In early labour, fluids and puree-type foods may be tolerated, but thereafter oral intake should be restricted to sips of fluid to keep the mouth moist. For high risk patients in whom operative delivery is likely, an intravenous infusion of Hartmann solution should be set up. *An intravenous infusion should also be set up if the end of labour is not in sight by 12 hours.*

(vi) *Pain relief*. The subject of pain relief is a large one and is considered separately in the section on pain and its management. If the patient has attended antenatal classes and wishes to manage the labour with psychoprophylactic techniques, she should be encouraged in this. *Hyperventilation* should be watched for since the baby may suffer temporary asphyxia from vasoconstriction and reduced oxygen transfer (a result of reduced carbon dioxide level in the blood). Maternal symptoms include paraesthesiae, lightheadedness, and perhaps muscle spasm.

(vii) *Sleep.* The best sleep will be provided by an opiate drug such as omnopon or pethidine if painful contractions are present; a sedative such as diazepam (Valium) 5–10 mg orally or intramuscularly or nitrazepam (Mogadon) 5 mg orally, is also helpful. If labour is prolonged because of dysfunctional uterine action, epidural analgesia is helpful in permitting a restful night's sleep. Surroundings should be as conducive as possible — darkened room and quietness of attendants.

(viii) *Monitoring of the fetus.* The extent of electronic fetal monitoring in labour varies greatly, depending on staff, facilities, and philosophy. Preferably all high risk patients should be monitored: the trace may be obtained via an abdominal electrode or a vaginal scalp electrode if the former is unsatisfactory. Intermittent Doppler monitoring is usually adequate, but is labour intensive. If the patient is not being monitored continuously and facilities are available, periods of monitoring (e.g. 20 minutes) should be carried out 2-hourly. The subject of fetal monitoring is further discussed in Chapter 13, and fetal distress in Chapter 48.

(ix) *Stimulation of contractions.* Artificial rupture of the membranes during labour stimulates contractions in 50–60% of nulliparas and 80%

of multiparas. It has the further advantage of allowing visualization of the liquor. The main disadvantage is that the head and umbilical cord have lost an important cushioning mechanism. An *oxytocin infusion* is helpful in accelerating the labour, especially in the nullipara. The resulting shorter labour is more enjoyable to the patient, the baby is less likely to be distressed, there is less amnionitis, and fewer operative deliveries (propulsion replacing traction).

(x) *Pyrexia*. If the temperature is over 38°C, a cause must be sought — uterus (especially if the membranes have ruptured prematurely or the labour is prolonged), urinary tract, or upper respiratory tract. Routine high vaginal smears and a clean urine specimen should be sent to the laboratory; appropriate treatment should then be commenced (Chapter 27).

Further Management — Second Stage

It is essential that the patient receives constant attention during the second stage to detect signs of fetal or maternal distress, and to assess the progress of descent.

Often, by the end of the first stage, the nullipara may exhibit one or more of the following: shivering, hiccups, vomiting, flushing, and a small amount of vaginal bleeding; she may be a little fed-up and irritable.

The most significant activity undertaken by the mother at this time is bearing down, although 10–15% of women do not experience this feeling. If progress is satisfactory, it is probably unnecessary to exhort the patient to 'push', otherwise she may become prematurely exhausted. This is particularly so if she has had an epidural anaesthetic. It is probably safer for the patient to push naturally, not close her glottis, and not push continuously for more than 6–8 seconds. If the patient is receiving nitrous oxide analgesia, it is necessary for the nurse to help the patient to coordinate this with the bearing down efforts. If pushing down is to be maximally efficient, the patient must relax the pelvic floor, rather than tighten it. The actual pushing is best effected by the patient partially sitting and grasping the backs of the thighs, the legs being well separated (figure 41.8). After pushing, the patient is encouraged to exhale fully and take another deep breath to take advantage of the contraction.

If contractions become weak or infrequent, and the fetal heart is satisfactory, an *oxytocin infusion* may be commenced — this *enhancement of labour* is relatively safe in nulliparas, but only after a vaginal examination has been performed to assess progress, and to exclude cephalopelvic disproportion. When an oxytocin

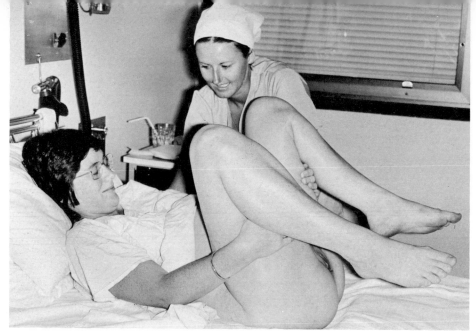

Figure 41.8 Encouraged by the attending midwife a patient bears down with contractions in the second stage of labour; she grasps her thighs to increase the expulsive force applied by her abdominal muscles.

infusion is used to enhance labour, continuous *fetal heart rate monitoring* is indicated to exclude hypoxia. We consider that an oxytocin infusion should rarely be used to enhance labour in multiparas, because of the risk of *uterine rupture*.

Progress of the presenting part during the second stage is best followed by *postanal palpation*. In this technique, the *palmar aspect of the middle finger* palpates the region between the coccyx and anal margin, the patient being in the left lateral position. If the presenting part is felt, it is good evidence that the maximum diameter is at or beyond the level of the ischial spines, and thus at the level of the cervix, which can be assumed to be fully dilated. Contributory signs are pouting and then gaping of the anus, and expulsion of faeces by the descending presenting part. Not infrequently, the pressure on the rectum causes the patient to call for a bedpan. Gaping of the vulva usually only occurs when the presenting part is very low and can be seen by parting the labia; the same applies to bulging of the perineum.

Confusion as to the true amount of progress may arise in breech presentations if a limb (or limbs) presents — it may have slipped through the not fully dilated cervix. In multiparas, strong pushing can sometimes cause the presenting part to descend to the level of the outlet, even though the cervix is not fully dilated. Finally, gross moulding and caput formation resulting from cephalopelvic disproportion can simulate deep descent of the head.

The patient is much helped by sympathetic handling and encouragement, and wiping the face and neck with a cool wet sponge is soothing.

If pressure of the presenting part on the rectum causes the expulsion of faecal material, this should be removed with a pad and the perineum swabbed. Towards the end of the second stage, the presenting part will reach the perineum and begin to distend it. The patient is now ready for delivery.

Ideally, the fetal heart should be monitored continuously, but this facility is often unavailable. As a compromise, auscultations should be carried out after each contraction. As the head descends, the point of maximum intensity of the fetal heart tones moves downwards and towards the midline of the abdomen.

BIRTH BEFORE ARRIVAL IN HOSPITAL (BBA)

A large proportion of, if not all, mothers to be (and their husbands) show much anxiety about the possibility of delivery before reaching hospital. These fears may arise because of the distance from home to hospital, lack of transport, previous precipitate labour, or well meant advice not to come into hospital until labour is established.

In one reported series of BBAs in a large teaching hospital, the *incidence was 1 in 500 births* (83 in 40,982); *parity* distribution was: para 0, 18%; para 1, 34%; para 2, 24% and para 3 or more, 24%. *Precipitate labour* (less than 4 hours' duration) occurred in 70% of patients, of whom more than 50% were having their first or second child. *Most BBAs were avoidable (65%) had the patients attempted to reach hospital at the onset of labour.*

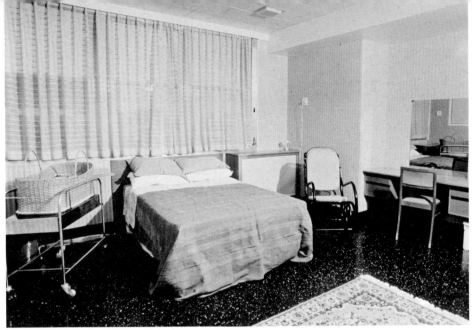

Figure 41.9 Birth centre in a major teaching hospital. Note absence of the usual hospital atmosphere. The partner remains during labour and for 24 hours thereafter — i.e. until they go home with their baby. (Courtesy of Dr Michael Kloss).

The above study showed that *a patient need not be concerned about the possibility of BBA if she presents for assessment when she believes that labour has begun* (show of blood, onset of contractions, rupture of membranes) — this applies to nulliparas as well as multiparas!

Obstetric problems mostly relate to the rapidity of the birth (birth canal trauma and haemorrhage, fetal trauma and hypoxia) and absence of third stage control (*retained placenta*, atonic haemorrhage). In the series quoted above, the perinatal mortality rate was 8.4%, 5 of the 7 deaths being due to extreme prematurity; there was no case of fetal trauma due to precipitate birth, and the only maternal complication was retained placenta (2 cases) requiring manual removal.

LOW RISK BIRTHING CENTRE

Philosophy. The low risk (or 'alternate') birthing centre concept has arisen because of the concerns of some couples about confinement in traditional hospital labour wards. The family-centred nature of a home birth is maintained — the mother can be with her husband, children and close personal figures, she is usually more comfortable and relaxed, and has greater freedom combined with adequate support (figure 41.9). Because of proximity of the centre to a traditional hospital labour ward, the critical problem that may arise suddenly in a home birth can be dealt with expeditiously and safely (resuscitation, monitoring, skilled staff, anaesthetic and operating room facilities).

The other consideration that has been advanced in favour of both home birth and birthing centre is the ability of the couple to be involved more in decision making — e.g. participation or otherwise in the many and varied hospital routines (enema, shave, labour induction, membrane rupture, analgesia, monitoring, restriction on mobility).

The impetus for such centres has slowed in recent times because the above needs (family-centred care, greater role in decision-making) have been increasingly addressed by maternity hospitals.

Procedures. The major problem concerns the screening of mothers to provide an acceptably low risk population. Each centre has its own system where factors in the history, plus current and future assessments, are graded and perhaps scored. Examples of high risk factors obtained from the patient's medical and past obstetric history are: cardiovascular and renal disease, diabetes, asthma, maternal age 37 or more, para 4 or more, previous Caesarean, difficult forceps delivery. Different centres adopt different criteria regarding intervention; the most conservative approach is to take out any woman in whom any intervention is likely.

A major medical review is undertaken at the first antenatal visit and again at 36 weeks. Intermediate care is undertaken by the midwife/obstetric nurse or medical practitioner.

The mother and baby are usually discharged during the first 24 hours, subject to satisfactory medical and paediatric review. Daily visits are made by a health care nurse for 4–5 days and further medical reviews at 1 and 6 weeks.

Outcome. In conservative centres, the transfer out rate is 40–50%. The following are the commonest indications: *antenatal* — premature labour/membrane rupture, hypertension, antepartum haemorrhage, multiple pregnancy, fetal growth retardation, prolonged pregnancy; *intrapartum* — fetal distress, hypertension, dystocia, pain requiring epidural analgesia; *postpartum* — retained placenta/postpartum haemorrhage, neonatal complication (respiratory distress, congenital abnormality). The incidence of episiotomy (especially nulliparas) and perineal tearing (especially multiparas) is usually quite significant; results in one large series were: perineum intact, 40%; tears, 40%; episiotomy, 20%.

The use of drugs for pain relief during labour in birth centres is minimal; in one large series the results were: no analgesia, 80%; pethidine (average dose 100 mg), 12%; nitrous oxide and oxygen, 8%.

Return to hospital after discharge is usually related to maternal infection (often mastitis) or bleeding, or neonatal jaundice or other complication.

HOME BIRTH

The enthusiasm for home birth varies from country to country. The great stumbling block to this seemingly attractive alternative is the unpredictability of the life-threatening obstetrical problem. The really dangerous complication is the one that is unexpected. The 4 conditions that bedevil the home attendant are *sudden fetal distress in labour*, *impacted shoulders*, *neonatal apnoea*, and *primary postpartum haemorrhage*. These are often difficult enough to deal with at specialist level in hospital. In England and Wales, the Obstetric and Paediatric Flying Squad are usually available from most major centres. They attend the patient at home on request, stabilize the problem, and transfer the patient back to a major centre.

ANALGESIA AND ANAESTHESIA

An understanding of pain, particularly its mechanism and relief, is important in obstetrics, since few labours are painless; furthermore, obstetrical procedures of a surgical nature are not infrequently required (forceps delivery, Caesarean section, and manual removal of the placenta).

There are a number of *important principles* involved which should be understood. Anxiety is very common in labouring patients and expla-

nation, sympathy and reassurance are important components in management. There is a wide range of measures available for pain relief: the choice will depend on an equally wide set of variables which will include the severity of the pain, the stage of labour, patient preference, the setting and facilities, complications in the mother and baby, and experience of the attendant. Complex techniques should not be attempted without proper training, and preexisting complications in the mother (e.g. preeclampsia, hypertension, haemorrhage) or fetus (e.g. growth retardation, prematurity, asphyxia) usually call for expert consultation. Aortocaval compression by the uterus (figure 48.1), with harmful effects on both mother and fetus, should be avoided, since it will aggravate the side-effects of analgesic and anaesthetic procedures.

Patients vary very widely in their tolerance to pain and to analgesic and anaesthetic drugs.

Definitions

Pain is the feeling which results from the noxious stimulation of special sensory receptors and nerves. *Pain threshold*: the level of stimulation at which pain first appears. *Pain relief*: (i) *amnesia* is loss of memory of pain or other experiences; (ii) *analgesia* is loss of sensation to pain; (iii) *anaesthesia* is total loss of sensation, pain included.

Classes of drug employed. (i) *A sedative/ hypnotic* causes general depression of the central nervous system: smaller doses will sedate, moderate doses will put to sleep, larger doses will produce unconsciousness; these compounds have anticonvulsant, and respiratory depressing properties. (ii) A *tranquillizer* will sedate (but in contrast to the above there is easier arousal of the patient after higher doses) and has an antipsychotic, anticholinergic, and anti-alpha-adrenergic effect. (iii) *Narcotics* have a sedative action, but also have a specific action on the pain receptors in the central nervous system.

Pain Mechanisms

The nervous system is basically quite simple — the sensations perceived in the internal and external environments are transmitted along nerve fibres to the brain, where they are decoded and a decision is made as to whether any action is required. The viscera (body cavities) are served by *autonomic nerves* (sympathetic and parasympathetic), while the musculoskeletal system and skin are served by *somatic nerves*. In the somatic system, a variety of stimuli, if sufficiently intense, will cause pain (pressure, heat, noise). It is also now appreciated that injury causes the release of a number of pain-producing substances such a H^+ and K^+ ions, substance P, serotonin, histamine, kinins and prostaglandins.

Many of the principles can be appreciated by considering what happens in labour. Early in the first stage of labour, the intrauterine pressure is less than 20–25 mm Hg and no pain is felt. As the contractions become stronger, the pressure increases (up to 100 mm Hg) and the pain threshold is exceeded. There is a latent period or delay after the contraction has started before pain is experienced, but then the rate of increase of pressure is very rapid, so that moderate and marked pain zones are reached quickly. This carries important implications when inhalational analgesics such as nitrous oxide are being used late in labour.

Pain Threshold

The *appreciation* of pain is an individual matter and varies rather widely, as does one's *reaction* to it. The components which determine our reaction to pain are not fully understood, although both physical and psychological factors are involved. Apart from such basic constitutional factors in each person, there are a number of other factors that temporarily alter pain perception or reaction.

Competing sensory stimuli. If a person is concentrating on some other activity, even marked pain may not be noticed — i.e. the brain is so preoccupied with other inputs that the messages from the pain fibres are 'jammed'. This is thought to underlie the mechanism of action of psychoprophylaxis, transcutaneous nerve stimulation and perhaps acupuncture.

Unfortunately, many women approach labour with an adverse conditioning regarding pain. Improved education by parents and school teachers is countering this and fear and anxiety are being replaced by understanding and confidence.

Factors which act in the reverse manner and *lower the pain threshold* are ignorance and fear, insecurity, starvation, dehydration, fatigue, and infection.

PAIN RELIEF IN LABOUR

General Comments

Pain relief should be administered only after *adequate discussion with the patient* and *full assessment of the progress of labour*. It often requires fine judgement in avoiding giving analgesia too soon (and prolonging labour) and avoiding giving it too late (causing the patient unnecessary distress).

Most agents will have some effect on the mother and/or her uterus and/or the baby, and a balance must be struck between maternal relief and these unwanted and/or untoward effects. It should not be forgotten that a mother suffering from *pain stress* will increase her output of catecholamines, and these may adversely affect uteroplacental circulation and uterine activity.

Physiological

This is largely preventive in nature; for example, dystocia can be minimized by the early detection of abnormalities in the antenatal period and labour. If labour is prolonged, adequate physiological support is necessary in the form of *intravenous fluid* and calories. Attention should also be given to provision of *adequate sleep* and *prevention of infection*.

Inhibition of painful sensations can be effected at *spinal cord level* by the use of nonpainful stimuli (massage, heat, pressure, counterirritation, acupuncture).

Psychological

In 1933 Grantly Dick-Read introduced the concept that ignorance of the labour and delivery process will engender fear and anxiety, and this in turn causes tension, heightened sympathetic activity, and spasm of the cervix and lower uterine segment, as well as the voluntary muscles of the pelvic outlet. Education will remove fear of the unknown and improve the patient's cooperation during labour. As mentioned earlier, pain can be blocked by selective attention and mental dissociation (*psychoprophylaxis*). The diversionary activity may consist of special breathing or visual/auditory attention. Psychoprophylactic methods aim to increase body awareness, the interaction of physical and emotional states, the achievement of physical and mental calm and relaxation, tension release, and mental imagery.

The health care attendant can reinforce such efforts by the following approaches — acceptance of the mother (regardless of sociocultural or other factors), reassurance, warmth, information transfer, and encouragement of her efforts during the labour.

Hypnosis is another form of psychological pain relief. This is usually induced by the attending doctor during labour after antenatal conditioning sessions. This is quite time-consuming, many patients are unable to cooperate properly, and disruption of the trance may occur during late labour. A rare patient may have the ability to induce an autohypnotic state.

Pharmacological

Although there are many agents and procedures

used for the relief of pain in labour, the principle is similar in each, namely, blocking the transmission of the painful stimulus. This may be done by the use of analgesic drugs which act on the pain centre in the brain, by local or regional nerve block, or by the use of anaesthetics which cause loss of consciousness.

Sedatives and Hypnotics

Drugs in this group will produce relaxation, drowsiness, and finally sleep as the dose is increased. Hence, these drugs are useful in early labour to settle the patient, and at night they will enable her to sleep. The drugs have no analgesic properties *per se*, and if pain is present, may produce a restless and uninhibited patient unless an analgesic drug is administered in addition. Hypnotics depress the central nervous system; therefore a mild lowering of the blood pressure will occur (vasomotor centre) and a depression of respiration (respiratory centre). Because of the effects on the fetus, large doses should be avoided, even where there is hypertension or preeclampsia, since better and more specific drugs are available.

(i) *Short-acting barbiturates* pentobarbitone (Pentone); quinalbarbitone; butobarbitone; the dose range is 50–200 mg, orally. Hypnotic effect is seen within 30 minutes; there is a delayed and lessened effect after a large meal or if the patient is in established labour. (ii) *Long-acting barbiturate* phenobarbitone; the dose is 50–100 mg, orally; 100–200 mg, intramuscularly. Hypnotic effect is seen within 30–60 minutes and lasts for 12–16 hours. These compounds are used to produce overnight sleep, or in the treatment of epilepsy and preeclampsia subsequent to delivery. (iii) *Chloral hydrate.* Given as a flavoured elixir (1 g in 10 ml) or in capsule form (500–650 mg); a higher dose (2–4 g) is occasionally used per rectum. This sedative is safe, but has an unpleasant, burning taste and tends to produce gastric irritation (nausea and vomiting) which is not a good start to labour.

Tranquillizers

Drugs in this group tend to have the following specific actions — tranquillizing, antiemetic, antihistamine, and sedative. (i) *Major tranquillizers* include the *phenothiazines* (promazine, chlorpromazine, promethazine, hydroxyzine), rauwolfia derivatives (rauwolfia serpentina, Serpasil); and *neuroleptics* (droperidol, haloperidol). (ii) *Minor tranquillizers* include diazepam and related compounds and meprobamate.

These drugs are useful during labour because of their calming effect and because they counteract the emetic effects of labour itself or of the narcotic drugs administered for pain relief. The total dose of diazepam should not exceed 20 mg, otherwise undesirable effects may occur in the newborn (apnoea, anorexia, lethargy, and hypothermia).

The use of sedatives, hypnotics and tranquillizers varies considerably in obstetric practice in different communities. Many practitioners rely on a single injection of a narcotic drug, together with an antiemetic agent (pethidine, 100 mg plus promethazine 25 mg IM) ± epidural analgesia for pain relief in labour. The increasing use of Caesarean section to terminate difficult or prolonged labours has also lessened the need for complicated drug regimens to control pain.

Analgesics

Nonnarcotic analgesics. Compounds in common use are codeine (3–30 mg), aspirin (250–500 mg), and paracetamol (250–500 mg).

These drugs are usually in tablet form, but are used as a mixture in some centres. Frequently they are combined and provide a fairly wide spectrum of analgesia, ranging from simpler preparations such as aspirin, 300 mg to compound codeine formulas (aspirin 225 mg, paracetamol 150 mg, codeine phosphate 30 mg, caffeine 30 mg). Since aspirin irritates the stomach, buffered compounds may be preferable. The use of drugs in this group is restricted to early labour.

Narcotic analgesics. These agents are popular because of their ease of administration, reasonable efficacy, low incidence of major complications and availability of antagonists if necessary. Troublesome side-effects may occur, however, and these include respiratory depression, nausea and vomiting, tachycardia, postural hypotension, and delayed gastric emptying. Drugs in use include pentazocine (30–60 mg); pethidine hydrochloride (50–100 mg); morphine sulphate (10–15 mg); and papaveretum (10–20 mg). The above doses are for intramuscular use. *Pethidine has largely taken the place of the other drugs*; it is given by the intravenous route in some centres either intermittently in small doses (25 mg over 1–2 minutes every 1–3 hours) or self-administered if the patient passes a reaction time test (to avoid overdosage). Newer drugs include nalbuphine (10–15 mg) and butorphanol (2–3 mg).

Narcotics depress the sensation of pain, and also the emotional response to it by allaying anxiety and fear. They are usually administered intramuscularly when the pain associated with the contractions begins to distress the patient.

Narcotic drugs depress the respiratory centre of both the mother and fetus and the premature fetus is specially vulnerable; depression of the fetal heart trace may occur (e.g. loss of beat to beat variation). To offset the respiratory depressive effect after birth, naloxone (10 μg/kg) can be given to the baby intramuscularly or into the umbilical vein; this drug has no depressant actions and can also antagonize pentazocine (Fortral).

The usual duration of action of the narcotic drugs is 2-4 hours, according to dose and conditions. Preferably, such a drug should not be administered within 1 hour of delivery — and if it is, the baby should be given *naloxone* (0.02 mg) IM immediately after birth. During this period, inhalation or regional block techniques are preferable; rapidly-acting drugs such as fentanyl may also be useful in this situation. Narcotics are contraindicated in patients receiving monoamine oxidase inhibitors.

Inhalational Analgesics

A number of general anaesthetic agents produce analgesia when inhaled in subanaesthetic concentrations. For example, nitrous oxide in a concentration of 50% is equivalent to 15 mg morphine. *Nitrous oxide* in this concentration produces progressive loss of pain sensation and loss of consciousness in the *first stage of anaesthesia* (stage of analgesia). In the *second stage* (stage of excitement) the patient becomes unconscious, experiences dreams, and may exhibit violent activity in response to stimuli. Other signs of this stage include irregular respiration, uncontrolled eye movements, coughing and

sometimes vomiting. The *third stage* is that of surgical anaesthesia.

The effect of inhalational agents will be enhanced by prior narcotic administration. In addition, there is usually further reduction of pain because of the attention given by the patient to breathing on the mask (distraction effect). Inhalation analgesia, although self-administered, must be supervised by a nurse or medical attendant (figure 41.10).

(a) *Nitrous oxide/oxygen.* These gases are supplied in cylinders in liquid form under pressure. At the lower pressures supplied to the patient they become colourless gases, which are absorbed from the lungs into the blood stream and are carried to the brain, where the nitrous oxide affects the cells of the pain centres. Nitrous oxide is useful for *analgesia in late labour and delivery* in a 50-70% concentration with oxygen.

Its *advantages* are as follows: reasonable analgesia, nontoxic and nonirritating to the respiratory passages, quickly absorbed and eliminated, no unpleasant after-effects, uterine contractions unaffected (no prolongation of labour or postpartum atonicity), vomiting rare, no untoward effect on subsequent anaesthesia, and flexibility due to easy alteration of gas concentration.

The *disadvantages* are the requirement of a machine to deliver the gas and the disorientation and excitability of some patients if stage 2 levels of anaesthesia are reached. Occasionally, patients will not use the mask because of a feeling of suffocation or because of the disorientation produced. With the 50% gas:oxygen mixture, a third of patients will have unsatisfactory pain relief.

Figure 41.10 Self-administration of 50% nitrous oxide/oxygen mixture late in the first stage of labour. The patient sleeps between contractions but rouses and breathes on the mask when the contraction begins. Fear and pain are also dispelled by kindness and comfort provided by the attendant midwife.

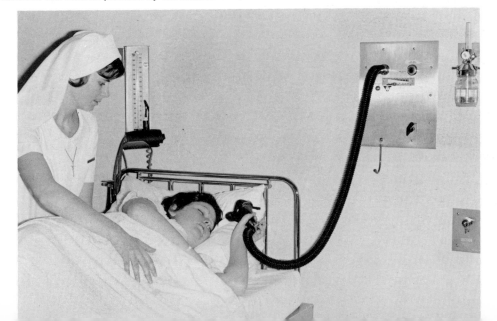

Typical nitrous oxide/oxygen machines. In most large hospitals, the gas and oxygen are supplied from remote storage tanks to an 'in the wall' machine (figure 41.10). Most machines, including 'off the wall' types (figure 41.11) work on an intermittent flow principle, delivering gas only 'on demand' — that is, when the patient inhales from the mask.

Routine checks of instrument. (i) *Cylinders.* See that they are in the proper place and fitting properly on the yolk and washer. The gauge indicates the amount of gas in the cylinders. The cylinder valve should be opened and closed before the cylinder is attached to the machine, and opened fully before use by the patient. Oxygen cylinders when full register 14,000 kPa (2,000 lb/sq inch), nitrous oxide cylinders 5,000 kPa (750 lb/sq inch). Oxygen cylinders must be changed before the pointer reaches 0, those for nitrous oxide when the pointer drops below 1/6 full. Cylinders must not be changed when the machine is in use and only one cylinder of each gas should be open at the one time. (ii) *Reducing valve.* The top gauge should read 60–70, and the machine must not be used if the gauge reads otherwise. (iii) *Check valve.* This should move freely with inspiration on the mask. If sticking, clean with ether. (iv) *Expiratory valve.* This must not be screwed down, otherwise the patient would rebreathe waste gases. (v) *Tubing and face mask.* These should be checked for kinking and patency, and fit, respectively.

Modern machines have 2 special safety features — firstly, automatic admission of room air if the oxygen supply is reduced or cut off, and secondly, an associated warning whistle. Most machines can be used for emergency oxygen administration by simultaneously pressing the emergency oxygen button on the front panel and the exhale valve button on the handpiece.

In larger centres, nitrous acid and oxygen are

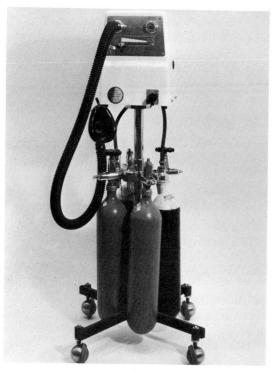

A

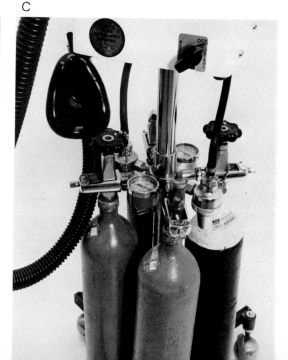

B

C

Figure 41.11 The CIG Mid-O-Gas trolley model is a mobile unit and is used in hospitals where the 'in the wall' or 'on the wall' models are not available. **A.** View of complete machine. **B.** Close-up view of front panel showing built-in humidifier and emergency oxygen button (on the left). The oxygen: nitrous oxide ratio is varied by means of the lever under the printed scale. The machine is set so that the minimum oxygen concentration that can be delivered is 30%. The master control switch (bottom right) turns on both gases simultaneously. **C.** Close-up view of cylinders and valves.

supplied from 'banks', comprising large cylinders or bulk containers. The reserves of gas are indicated in the gas storage room and on the walls in different parts of the hospital.

(b) *Methoxyflurane (Penthrane)*. This agent is a colourless, sweet-smelling, nonflammable, volatile liquid; it gives a somewhat better quality of analgesia than nitrous oxide and trichlorethylene (Trilene) with less nausea and vomiting, but is more expensive. Unlike nitrous oxide, it is soluble in body tissues and the effects are more prolonged. There is a rather wide degree of acceptance of the volatile inhalational agents in different parts of the world.

The advantages of this technique are similar to those of nitrous oxide/oxygen. It has little effect on uterine contractions or the fetus and does not complicate subsequent anaesthesia; it has few serious side-effects, the main problem being in patients with major renal impairment (for whom it is not advised). It has a bronchodilator action, which facilitates respiration. Because it is more pungent than nitrous oxide, the patient should be instructed to take several shallow breaths initially to accustom herself to the odour. The optimal concentration is 0.35%. *The apparatus.* This was developed in Cardiff and is somewhat similar to the Tecota Mark 6 Trilene inhaler. The equipment (figure 41.12) consists of an inhaler, inhaler outlet connector, antistatic corrugated tubing, face mask, and key filling device. Another special device, the 'pin safety system', ensures that filling can only be effected from a Penthrane bottle. The inhaler itself should be checked each 6–12 months. If the machine is left standing idle, a cork or other stopper should be placed in the outlet port to reduce evaporative loss.

(c) *Trichlorethylene (Trilene)*. This agent was formerly quite popular, but is now less commonly used. It tends to have a cumulative effect, depressing the mother, uterus, and baby. Occasionally, cardiac arrhythmias occur which may prove fatal. It must not be used in closed circuit with soda lime because of the formation of poisonous breakdown products. Administration is through either a Tecota Mark 6 or Emotril machine, the concentration of the gas being 0.35%–0.5% in atmospheric air.

General Remarks on Inhalational Analgesic Techniques

(i) *Familiarity of the patient with the apparatus.* Far better results will be obtained if the patient has been taught about the apparatus and its use in antenatal classes and early in labour. (ii) *Supervision by the midwife.* Correct functioning of the machine must be checked and the patient instructed and supervised until she is both confident and proficient. A correctly-fitting mask is essential, otherwise proper triggering of the check valve will not occur, and the gas mixture will be diluted with room air. The correct concentration is selected which produces adequate analgesia, whilst retaining the patient's cooperation. The proportion of nitrous oxide ranges from 50–70%. (iii) *Timing of administration.* This may be intermittent or continuous. With nitrous oxide, full analgesia only occurs 25–35 seconds after inhalation is started and is maximal in about 35–40 seconds. Hence, to be effective, inhalation *ideally should start 20–30 seconds before the contraction.* Since inhalational techniques are used mainly in the late first and second stages of labour, this may be practicable if contractions are occurring regularly. In the second stage, the patient begins bearing down soon after the contraction starts and this is a further reason to commence mask breathing *before* the contraction actually occurs. At the

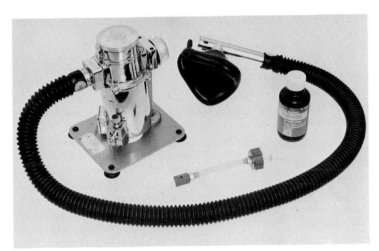

Figure 41.12 The Cardiff inhaler is automatically temperature compensated and pre-set to deliver 0.35% Penthrane vapour in air. Safe, adequate analgesia is induced and maintained by self-administration.

height of the contraction, the patient is encouraged to take a deep breath, hold it, and bear down. When the presenting part is crowned, the patient should breathe continuously on the mask and stop pushing.

Methoxyflurane and trichlorethylene should be inhaled initially for a period of 5–10 minutes, and thereafter with each contraction. Later, due to build up in the tissues, inhalation may only be needed every 3–4 contractions and cessation is usually advisable when the second stage is well established.

If the *continuous technique* is used with nitrous oxide, a concentration between 30–50%, given via a nasal catheter, will be adequate. If disorientation, restlessness, or unconsciousness should occur, the concentration should be reduced. The concentration of Penthrane is fixed at 0.35%, and that of Trilene ranges between 0.35–0.50%.

It should be remembered that prolonged deep breathing will wash out carbon dioxide from the patient's lungs and produce an alkalosis; this affects uteroplacental blood flow because of shunting, resulting in fetal acidosis, which in turn may unfavourably affect the affinity of oxygen to haemoglobin in fetal red cells.

Approximately two-thirds of patients obtain complete or substantial relief of pain with either nitrous oxide or Penthrane. The figure will be higher with closely supervised patients making maximum use of the technique. The alternative method of pain relief is some form of local or regional analgesia — paracervical, caudal, epidural or spinal block. *Causes of failure* include faulty working of the apparatus (2 or 3 inhalations by the attendant will clarify this), faulty technique by the patient, or an unsuspected obstetrical complication (obstructed labour). After use, the mask should be washed with soap and water after a disinfectant solution has been applied.

LOCAL ANALGESIA

A local analgesic drug is one which produces *temporary blockage of impulses along the nerve.* To anaesthetize an area the nerves in that area itself may be blocked (perineal infiltration for episiotomy, paracervical block) or alternatively, the nerves may be blocked at some more distant point (pudendal nerve block; caudal or lumbar epidural block). Nerve fibres conducting pain are more easily blocked than those carrying most other sensations — hence low concentrations of drug produce analgesia (only pain fibres blocked), and high concentrations also produce complete muscle relaxation (both sensory and

motor fibres blocked). Commonly-used drugs include lignocaine, lasting 60 minutes; mepivacaine, lasting 100 minutes; and bupivacaine, lasting 100–200 minutes. Because of its possible adverse effect on uteroplacental blood flow, the use of adrenaline (epinephrine) is not commonly used.

Nerve Pathways

An understanding of local analgesia requires an appreciation of the causes of pain in labour and the disposition of the nerve fibres carrying pain sensation. The areas of distribution and *intensity of pain* in the various stages of labour are shown in Figure 41.13. (i) *Uterine pain* (e.g. muscle contractions) is felt in the lower abdomen and back. Sympathetic afferent nerves pass upward mainly to the thoracic segments 11 and 12 and there is some contribution also to T10 and L1. This pain is abolished by lumbar or high caudal epidural block (figure 41.14). (ii) *Cervical* pain (dilatation) is felt in the lower back and hypogastrium. The impulses are carried by sympathetic afferent nerves to T11 and T12. Parasympathetic afferent nerves from the cervix and the pelvic floor pass backward to sacral segments 2, 3 and 4. Pain is abolished by caudal or lumbar epidural block, or paracervical block. (iii) *Vaginal and perineal* pain (stretching) is felt at the site. Somatic afferent nerves run mainly in the pudendal nerve to sacral segments. Pain is abolished by epidural block, pudendal nerve block, or local infiltration.

Spinal Nerve Block

The analgesic agent is injected *intrathecally* into the cerebrospinal fluid bathing the nerve fibres. Although this technique is relatively easy, serious sequelae occasionally occur (infection, neurological damage) and postspinal headache is not uncommon; there is less flexibility than with the epidural approach. Its main usefulness is in the provision of pelvic analgesia for an urgent midcavity delivery.

Epidural Nerve Block

In many centres more than 30% of patients receive epidural analgesia for pain relief in labour (see Chapter 16). The local analgesic is injected extrathecally into the epidural space (figure 41.14). The extent of the analgesia is determined largely by the volume and concentration of drug injected. To control the pain of late labour, a block of the segments T10–L1 is adequate, whereas for Caesarean section, a higher block — T8 or even T6 is needed; for delivery, a block downwards to involve the sacral nerves is necessary. (i) The requirements for the

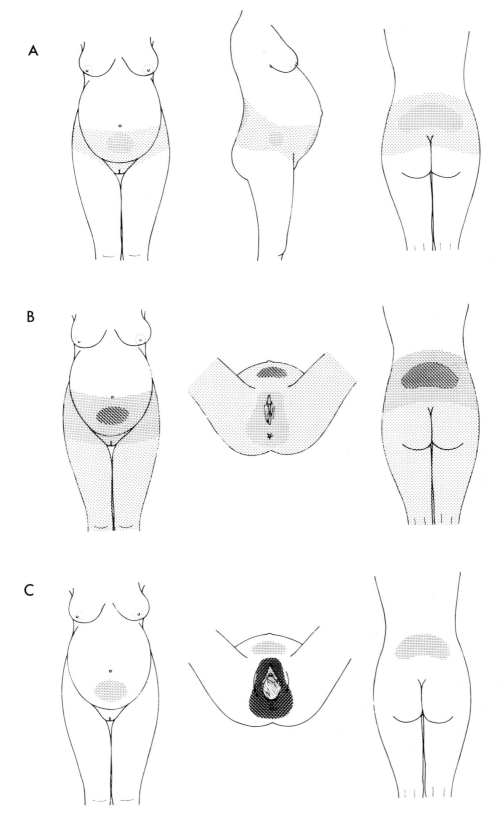

Figure 41.13 Distribution of pain in the various stages of labour. Density of stippling indicates intensity of pain. **A.** First stage. **B.** Late first stage and early second stage; uterine pain is the most intense. **C.** Late second stage and actual delivery; the perineum is the site of intense pain, the uterine pain being relatively reduced.

epidural tray are shown in figure 41.15. (ii) *Indications. Pain relief.* This is the prime indication and applies particularly to the nullipara and to patients with a low pain tolerance. Certain patients will specifically request this type of pain relief because of their own or other's experience with it. *Symptomatic heart disease.* The pain and distress of labour is relieved, and the bearing-down reflex abolished, thus avoiding the strain to the heart associated with expulsive efforts in the second stage (forceps or vacuum extraction being the preferred method of delivery) — however, extreme care is necessary if the patient has a fixed cardiac output (e.g. mitral stenosis, aortic stenosis, primary pulmonary hypertension). *Hypertensive disorders* (preeclampsia/eclampsia, chronic hypertension). The abolition of pain and blocking of vasomotor nerves both assist in control of the blood pressure. *Cerebrovascular disease.* Intracranial aneurysm and angioma are the usual indications. *Premature labour.* The need for narcotic analgesics which depress the fetus is avoided. *Incoordinate uterine action.* The elimination of pain, and thus fear and anxiety, often helps to normalize the activity. *Fetoplacental dysfunction.* Some have claimed this to be an indication, the babies being less acidotic at birth; others have shown that late deceleration patterns on the fetal heart tracing are more common with this form of analgesia. *Breech and twin delivery.* Opinions are also divided on the value of epidural analgesia in these conditions: the relaxation of the pelvic floor is advantageous, but the lack of stimulus for the patient to push can lead to a higher interference rate. (The patient can push (and empty her bladder), but because the sensation is lost she needs help to coordinate her efforts with the contractions). (iii) *Contraindications. Opposition by the patient. The presence of a uterine scar,* since warning signs of rupture may not be recognized. *Recent antepartum haemorrhage*: because compensatory vascular reflexes are partly abolished, sudden haemorrhage of even moderate degree may produce marked hypotension. *Cephalopelvic disproportion*: if moderate or marked disproportion is present, uterine rupture may occur — again because of the abolition of warning signs. *Sepsis* in the proposed area of operation. *Sensitivity* to local analgesic agents. *Anticoagulant drugs*, or *disseminated intravascular coagulopathy* (severe preeclampsia), these predisposing to haemorrhage in the epidural space. (iv) *Technique.* First, an *intravenous line* should be inserted to allow prompt treatment of hypotension should this occur. After the technique has been explained to the patient, she is placed in the left

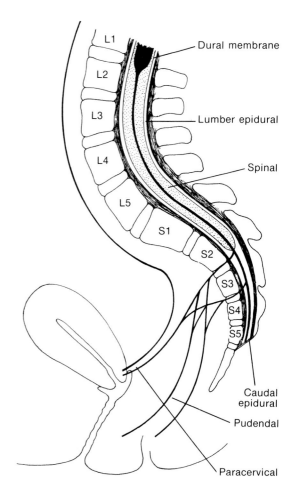

Figure 41.14 Sites used for nerve block. The word epidural defines the location of the injection relative to the spinal cord — it is outside the dura, the words lumbar and caudal describe the level of the spinal column at which the injection is inserted. A caudal epidural is inserted through the sacrococcygeal membrane outside the dura.

lateral position and an appropriate needle is inserted into the epidural space, taking aseptic and antiseptic precautions. If the continuous technique is to be employed, a fine sterile catheter is inserted through the needle and strapped in place. The required amount of analgesic (5–20 ml of 0.5% bupivacaine solution) is injected after it is certain that the needle has been correctly placed. The patient is nursed on her side to avoid aortocaval compression. (v) *Observations.* The blood pressure and pulse rate must be recorded at least every 5 minutes for 30 minutes after each injection, and the respiratory rate should also be observed. The higher the block the more likely is hypotension to occur. After this observation period, the patient may sit up or move around in bed, provided vital signs

Figure 41.15 Epidural tray. Needles from above downwards are Tuohy needle for lumbar epidural, trocar for Tuohy needle, glydin needle for caudal epidural, 16 gauge drawing up needle and lancet. The nylon epidural catheter is used only with the Tuohy needle.

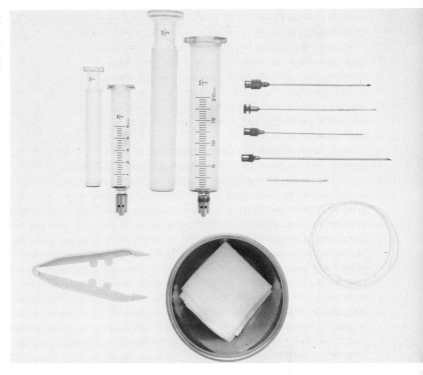

are satisfactory. (vi) *Complications.* These include accidental puncture of the dura, failure to locate the epidural space, puncture of an epidural vein causing haematoma, intravascular or intrathecal injection, kinking of the catheter, nerve damage, infection, and depression of uterine action. *Toxicity* results from overdosage and/ or intravascular injection. There is an initial stimulation (restlessness, tremor, convulsions), and this is followed by coma and respiratory arrest. Intravenous barbiturate may be necessary in the excitement phase, cardiovascular and respiratory support later. *Hypotension* may result from paralysis of sympathetic nerve fibres, aortocaval compression or a combination of both. This is remedied by placing the patient on her side, elevating the foot of the bed, oxygen, and by administration of intravenous fluid. *Total spinal block* results from the accidental injection of a large volume of solution into the intrathecal space. Complete motor, sensory and autonomic paralysis and marked hypotension occur. Artificial ventilation and vasopressor drugs must be administered immediately or death may occur. *Uterine hypotonia* occurs in 5–10% of patients, but usually activity returns in 15–30 minutes with continued relief of pain. *Collapse,* with marked hypotension and apnoea, may be due to a toxic effect of the drug or to an idiosyncrasy. Twitching of muscles or even convulsions may also occur. *Headache* may result from accidental or intentional puncture of the dura and leakage of cerebrospinal fluid, causing

loss of 'fluid buffering' of the brain. This complication is treated by insertion of an epidural block at a higher level; after delivery Hartmann solution is infused into the epidural catheter. The patient should be nursed flat, adequately hydrated (oral and intravenous fluids) and if the headache persists, nonnarcotic analgesics should be administered (aspirin, codeine). An epidural blood patch (injection of 10 ml of maternal blood) may be performed if the headache persists beyond 48 hours. *Fetal heart slowing or irregularity* has been observed in a small number of patients; it may be due to maternal hypotension, high maternal levels of analgesic, or even fetal puncture. *Loss of sensation* may occur in the bladder (causing overdistension); an indwelling urethral catheter is inserted if this occurs. *Loss of the bearing-down reflex* associated with reduced muscle tone results in a higher incidence of assisted delivery (greater than 50%). Drowsiness may result from absorption of the drug into the blood stream. *Neurological sequelae* may occur from direct injury or haematoma formation.

Although the majority of the above complications are rare, they point to the *need for experienced personnel in this type of analgesia.* (vii) The *advantages* of epidural analgesia lie in its efficiency (complete or substantial relief of pain) in 90% or more of patients. In addition, the patient is alert and cooperative, and there is a reduced risk of inhalation of vomitus. The fetus is rarely affected and the acid-base status is usually better than is the case with other analgesic methods. (viii) *The disadvantages* include the need for skilled personnel, the occasional serious complications indicated above, the tendency to slow the labour for a time, the increased incidence of operative vaginal delivery, intraoperative nausea, vomiting or restlessness in some patients, and the greater demand on staff time.

In *Caesarean section*, epidural analgesia has a number of *advantages* over general anaesthesia — participation of the parents in the birth, early handling of the baby and breast feeding, better postoperative pain relief, earlier mobility, less gastrointestinal stasis, no chest problems, less fever, the mothers are not as tired or depressed, thromboembolism is less common, and it is safer with such medical complications as asthma and diabetes; *blood loss* is less than with general anaesthesia. *Disadvantages* are that the method may fail, the patient feels pain and may require a general anaesthetic to be administered. It is technically more difficult to extract the infant's head from the uterus, especially if a Pfannenstiel incision is used, because the patient's abdominal muscles may not be completely relaxed.

Epidural narcotic administration has been found unsatisfactory.

Paracervical Block

The majority of pain-carrying fibres from the uterus and cervix pass through the paracervical tissues. Thus, satisfactory pain relief during the later stages of cervical dilatation can be obtained by the procedure of paracervical block. Approximately 6–10 ml of 0.25% bupivacaine is injected just beneath the mucosa of the vagina in each lateral fornix. A Kobak or other suitable needle is used. A continuous technique using catheters in each paracervical region has been described, but in practice this is rarely done. The paracervical block is relatively easy to perform, although when the needle is inserted, the vaginal vault tends to be pushed upward, and the analgesic solution delivered in the region of large venous plexuses, with the risk of intravascular injection or haematoma formation. Furthermore, the procedure is suitable only for first stage pain, and there is technical difficulty if the fetal head is well down in the pelvis, with the further risk of injection into the scalp. *Contraindications* include fetal distress, patient receiving anticoagulant therapy, and vaginal infection. The supine position should be avoided. Unfortunately, there are persistent problems with fetal bradycardia, acidosis and even death, due to a direct action of the drug on maternal uterine vessels, causing marked constriction, with reduction in uteroplacental blood flow.

Pudendal Block

This is a common technique, used for vaginal manipulative procedures. Either the Kobak needle is used per vaginam (figure 41.16) or less commonly, the approach to the ischial spine (and thus the pudendal nerve) is made through the perineum; the approach is usually dictated by the level of the presenting part. Lignocaine, 10–20 ml of a 0.5–1% solution, is usually employed, the nerve being blocked as it passes behind the ischial spine. The 3 other nerves supplying the perineum may require additional local infiltration — the ilioinguinal and genitofemoral nerves anterolaterally, and the perineal branch of the posterior cutaneous nerve of the thigh posteriorly. If the operative procedure is likely to be difficult — for example, a mid-forceps rotation — more extensive analgesia is required. It should be appreciated that the term 'block' is often a misnomer — the analgesia being inadequate on one or both sides. Verification of the analgesia should therefore precede manipulative intervention.

Perineal Infiltration

The most common form of local block is that for making and repairing an episiotomy or repair of a vaginal and/or vulval laceration. Usually, 10 ml of 1% lignocaine is infiltrated beneath and beside the area to be anaesthetized. As with any

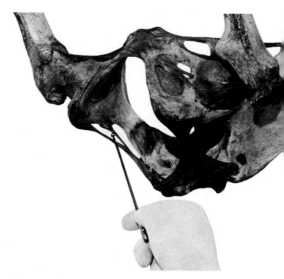

Figure 41.16 Pudendal nerve block by direct transvaginal approach to the ischial spine using the Kobak guarded needle — the needle protrudes 5 mm beyond the bead at the end of the sheathed introducer. The nerve alternatively may be reached by insertion of a lumbar puncture needle through the perineum, midway between ischial tuberosity and fourchette, directing it towards the ischial spine by a finger in the vagina.

local infiltration, care is always taken to ensure that the needle is not in a blood vessel, by applying the aspiration test before the solution is injected.

Abdominal Decompression

This procedure, pioneered by Heyns in South Africa, consisted of the application of a negative pressure (20–50 mm Hg) by means of a vacuum pump connected to a cage which was placed over the mother's abdomen. Apart from relief of pain, it was claimed that labour was significantly shortened, fetal oxygenation improved, and fetal intelligence enhanced. This historical note is included so that the reader will remember that the pain associated with uterine contractions in labour is significantly due to resistance of the abdominal musculature to the forward movement of the uterus — in grand multiparas with lax abdominal walls, one can sometimes see the uterus 'stand up' during contractions; these patients typically have efficient uterine action and precipitate labours.

Transcutaneous Electrical Nerve Stimulation (TENS)

This technique was originally used for the treatment of chronic pain. Recently it has been used both for the pain of labour and operative procedures (figure 41.17). It probably works on the principle of jamming other sensory inputs (including pain), although initiation of *endorphin* release or that of other naturally occurring opiate substances may also be involved.

Acupuncture

This method of pain relief has been extensively evaluated in the People's Republic of China, where together with narcotic drugs and local analgesia it is used for Caesarean section. Acupuncture seems to be a similar modality to transcutaneous nerve stimulation although it involves insertion of needles through the skin.

GENERAL ANAESTHESIA

'The application of anaesthesia to midwifery involves many more difficult and delicate problems than its mere application to surgery. New rules must be established for its use, its effects upon the action of the uterus, upon the state of the child, and on the puerperal state of the mother'.

Sir James Y. Simpson

Ever since 1847, when Simpson introduced chloroform into obstetrics, general anaesthesia

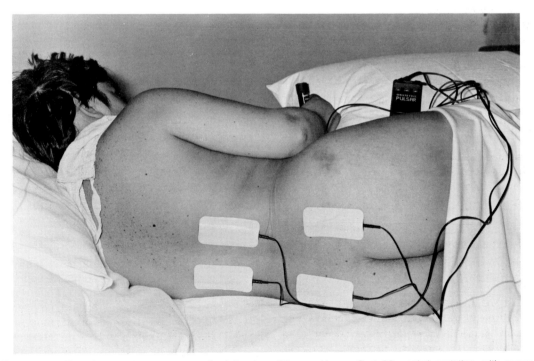

Figure 41.17 Use of transcutaneous nerve stimulation in a 27-year-old para 0 at 36 weeks' gestation, with severe backache in early labour. The upper pair of electrodes are applied at T10–L1 (uterine pain), and the lower pair at S2 –S4 (cervical pain). The 9 volt battery unit has a hand control which enables the patient to boost the intensity of the pulsed current output during a contraction. This method can be used with other forms of analgesia and is claimed to have an analgesic effect comparable to about 100 mg of pethidine.

has been recognized as a hazard for the pregnant patient, and, despite 'new rules', avoidable maternal deaths still occur from this cause. Unlike narcotic analgesics or local analgesics, general anaesthetics depress some of the vital protective reflexes of the body (those guarding the pharynx and larynx, and those maintaining the circulation).

Since a number of obstetrical anaesthetics are performed as an emergency in women who have recently had a full meal or who have suffered circulatory collapse, the potential for trouble can be appreciated.

Other factors of significance with general anaesthesia include the tendency to *greater blood loss* during operative procedures, the more difficult recovery period, and possible adverse effects on infant bonding.

Indications

(i) *Disorders of early pregnancy.* Abortion requiring curettage, ectopic pregnancy, insertion of cervical suture, hysterotomy. (ii) *Breech presentation* — in occasional cases where external cephalic version without anaesthesia has failed. (iii) *Major vaginal manipulative procedures.* Mid-pelvic arrest requiring rotation and forceps delivery. (iv) *Caesarean section.* (v) *Obstetric catastrophes* — ruptured uterus; uncontrolled postpartum bleeding. (vi) Manual removal of a retained placenta.

Premedication

Atropine, 0.6 mg intramuscularly, is given 30 minutes preoperatively, or in emergencies immediately preoperatively by the intravenous route. An alkali mixture is given orally — e.g. magnesium trisilicate, 15–30 ml.

Types

(i) *Spontaneous respiration* (mask anaesthesia). A potent inhalational agent such as halothane or ether is used to maintain deep anaesthesia. The patient breathes spontaneously, but recovery is slow and nausea and vomiting are common, the central nervous system being quite depressed. This type of anaesthetic is indicated when other facilities are unavailable or the procedure is relatively minor, since fetal respiratory depression and uterine relaxation (predisposing to postpartum haemorrhage) are more common. The reasons for avoiding mask anaesthesia in pregnancy or labour are: possible difficulty in airway control, regurgitation and inhalation of gastric content, and the effect of volatile agents on the uterus (relaxation, lack of response to oxytocic drugs). (ii) *Controlled respiration.* Muscle tone and movement are depressed by appropriate drugs (muscle relaxants) while sleep and analgesia are maintained by an agent such as nitrous oxide. Some patients complain of being aware of the operation, usually when the concentration of nitrous oxide is below 50%; the additional use of a volatile agent in low concentration (e.g. halothane 0.5%) up until the time of delivery will overcome this problem. Recovery is prompt since the central nervous system is not very depressed. Rapid induction and recovery reduce the risk of inhalation of vomitus.

Care of the Unconscious Patient

(i) *Constant supervision* until the patient can recognize surroundings and attend to her needs. (ii) Clear airway to be maintained: mucus and vomitus must be cleared immediately to prevent aspiration. Usually an airway will be in place; if not it should be inserted to prevent the tongue falling back. (iii) *Posture.* Lateral or semiprone with the head down. (iv) Oxygen is administered by mask (6–8 litres/minute) if the patient is anaemic or cyanosed. (v) *Vital signs* are recorded and charted.

Major Complications

(a) Inhalation of gastric content

This is more likely in the obstetric patient because of the emergency nature of many anaesthetics (full stomach), the inhibition of gastric emptying by the pain of the uterine contractions, the pressure of the gravid uterus on the stomach, and the relaxation of the less competent cardiac sphincter by the anaesthetic or the dorsal position. This may result in either blockage of the bronchi by large food particles or chemical pneumonitis (Mendelson gastric aspiration syndrome), the latter being characterized by intense bronchospasm and impaired pulmonary function.

Prevention. (i) *Diet during labour.* No solid food should be given once active labour has commenced. If labour persists for longer than 12 hours, intravenous fluids and calories must be administered. A regimen to combat the high acidity of the stomach contents should be instituted. Once labour is established all patients should be given an alkali preparation (e.g. *magnesium trisilicate*, 15 ml) orally every 2 hours; 30 minutes before a general anaesthetic the patient is given 15–30 ml of the same preparation, and turned from side to side, so that the alkali will mix with stomach contents. *Sodium citrate* (30 ml of a 0.3 mol/l solution) is a nonparticulate but strong tasting antacid used in some centres; other agents employed are cimetidine which inhibits gastric secretion of acid, and meto-clopramide (Maxolon) an antiemetic which also speeds gastric emptying if the patient has not received narcotic drugs which inhibit this action. (ii) *Anaesthetic technique.* Appropriate equipment should be available and in working order (suction, laryngoscopes, endotracheal tubes, tilting table); the lithotomy position should be avoided during induction; a wedge should be inserted under the patient's right side to avoid aortocaval compression; preoxygenation should be implemented (to improve maternal and fetal blood oxygen concentrations providing a safeguard in the event of any hypoxic episode, such as a failed or difficult intubation) and the nurse or anaesthetic assistant should apply pressure to the cricoid cartilage during the induction phase to close the oesophagus which lies posteriorly (*Sellick manoeuvre*), until the cuff on the endotracheal tube is inflated.

Management. (i) Intubation and endotracheal suction, bronchoscopy if solid material aspirated. (ii) Oxygen is given by mask to maintain good colour. (iii) Bronchodilator drugs to counteract bronchospasm. (iv) Hydrocortisone in large doses–local and intravenous (1–2 g). (v) Artificial ventilation if required. (vi) Intravenous therapy, correction of acidosis. (vii) Antibiotics.

(b) Circulatory collapse/cardiac failure

The usual *causes* are loss of blood (perhaps associated with a traumatic delivery) or less commonly asphyxia, dehydration from vomiting or prolonged labour, severe sepsis, vagal inhibition, supine hypotension, anaesthetic agents, thromboembolism, and preexisting cardiopulmonary disease.

Prevention. The above conditions are usually readily preventable — for example, the effects of haemorrhage are minimized by prevention of anaemia by good antenatal care, and rapid intravenous fluid replacement; asphyxia by avoidance of anaesthetic induction difficulties and hypoventilation.

(c) Respiratory failure

This may result from obstruction by the tongue, secretions, gastric content, or spasm of the larynx. If central, the cause may be drugs, blood loss, cardiac arrest, or pulmonary embolism.

(d) Cardiac arrest

See Chapter 54.

EFFECTS OF ANAESTHETIC AGENTS ON THE FETUS

The factors affecting placental transfer of a drug are: concentration gradient across the placenta (in turn influenced by degree of protein binding, blood pH and temperature, red cell binding capacity), lipid solubility, degree of ionization, placental circulation, dose and route of administration.

Most of the agents described in this section will directly affect the fetus to some extent. In addition, indirect effects may result from drug-induced alterations in maternal physiology (changes in uterine, cadiovascular, or respiratory function), or untoward complications (inhalation of gastric content).

The *premature baby* is less able to handle drugs because of immaturity of such organs of metabolism and excretion as the liver and kidney, and is less able to protect against their effects because of immaturity of physiological response.

In general, the major effect of hypnotic, analgesic, and anaesthetic drugs is respiratory depression, which is proportional to the duration of use and dose of the agent(s). Recent studies have shown a much wider spectrum of effect than was previously appreciated, such as poorer temperature control, appetite, sucking strength, reflex activity, and visual fixation. In some infants and with some drugs, the effects may persist for months.

RECORDS

The importance of accurate ordering, dispensing, and recording of drugs is emphasized, both by medical and nursing staffs. Because of the great variety of drugs, their often multiple use, and side-effects, there is a significant risk of mishap and perhaps medicolegal action.

chapter forty-two

Mechanism of Normal Labour. Conduct of Normal Delivery

OVERVIEW

In the majority of patients, the mechanism of labour follows a set pattern. The progressively increasing contractions first efface, and then dilate the cervix, and at the same time drive the presenting part through the birth canal. The process in the human is not as simple as in most animals, because of changes related to the erect posture (figure 2.11). The birth canal forms a 90° angle from the inlet to the outlet (the curve of Carus) and this, plus its length and relatively narrow dimensions, seldom permit the parturient an easy time — at least for the first experience.

To follow the mechanism of labour intelligently requires a knowledge of the anatomy of the maternal pelvis and fetus (Chapter 2) as well as an ability to palpate accurately, both abdominally and vaginally.

The mechanism of labour is described as a series of steps, but the process is a continuous one, at least until the actual delivery. The first essential is *descent*, and this is progressive with each contraction. As with cervical dilatation, there is a phase in the second half of labour when descent is more rapid. As the head meets increasing resistance it is forced to flex (*law of the lever*), presenting a progressively smaller diameter until maximum flexion has been attained.

The length of the birth canal is 9–10 cm (measured from the midpoints of the brim and outlet). Since this is the diameter of the fetal head, it can be appreciated that it will be *engaged* when it is half way down the birth canal — i.e. the presenting part has reached the ischial spines and the maximum diameter has passed the brim. The next movement of the head is *internal rotation* to bring the occiput anterior, allowing it to finally *extend* during the process of birth.

After delivery, the head may undergo 2 movements — *restitution* to return it to its natural relation to the shoulders, and often an additional *external rotation* as it follows the shoulders which rotate into the AP diameter of the pelvis prior to delivery of the trunk.

The appropriate conduct of delivery has undergone much reappraisal in the past decade or so. Major debate has centred on the *place of delivery* (hospital, birthing centre, home) (figure 42.1), *position for delivery* (traditional Western-style, birthing bed or chair, or squatting), and *amount of assistance* provided (minimal to fully controlled). The philosophy of 'gentle birth', in a family-centred atmosphere has done much to remove some of the depersonalizing aspects of the birth process. It should not be forgotten, however, that the unexpected complication is never far away during delivery, and mistakes may exact a heavy price.

DEFINITIONS

(i) *Lie*: the relation of the long axis of the baby to that of the uterus; usually longitudinal, but may be oblique or transverse. (ii) *Attitude*: the relation of the fetal head and limbs to the trunk, usually one of flexion, but may be extension (figure 42.2). (iii) *Presentation*: the part of the fetus which is lowermost in the uterus and presents on vaginal examination. (iv) *Position*: the relation of a part of the fetus, known as the denominator, to one of the 6 defined areas of the pelvic brim. (v) *Denominator*: an identifiable bony landmark chosen for each presentation of the fetus; the occiput is the denominator for ver- tex presentations. (vi) *Station*: the level of the presenting part in relation to a specified part of the maternal pelvis — usually the brim for abdominal palpation, and the *ischial spines* for vaginal examination.

A *review of the anatomy* of the *bony pelvis* and the *fetal skull* as well as the *muscular pelvic diaphragms* should be made at this point. *In summary*, the birth canal is made up of the bones of the true pelvis and the ligaments which bind them together, together with the associated muscular and fascial supports. The canal is curved gently from behind forward, about 90° (the curve of Carus) (figure 2.13). At the brim

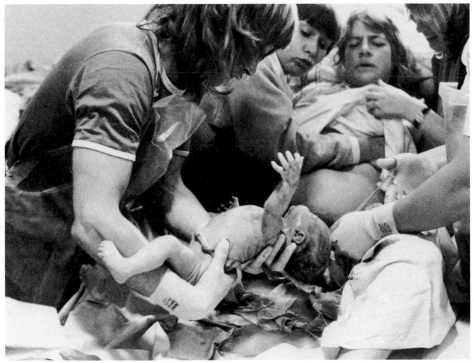

Figure 42.1 A father holds his newborn daughter who he has delivered (with the midwife standing watchfully nearby) in a family birth centre. The patient is witnessing her delivery, and is receiving the support and encouragement of her female friends. (Courtesy of Dr Michael Kloss).

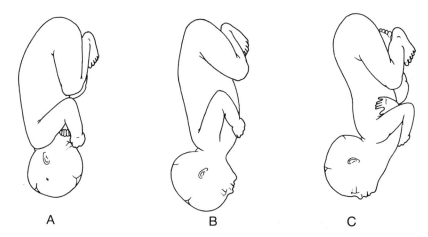

A   B   C

Figure 42.2 Attitude of the fetus. **A.** Vertex presentation: the head is fully flexed and the suboccipitobregmatic diameter (9.5 cm) presents. The occiput is the denominator. **B.** Brow presentation: the head is partly extended and the mentovertical diameter (14 cm) presents. **C.** Face presentation: the head is fully extended and the submentobregmatic diameter (9.5 cm) presents. The chin (mentum) is the denominator.

the widest diameter is the transverse; at midpelvis it is the oblique; and at the outlet it is the anteroposterior. The fetal skull, when fully flexed, is almost spherical in outline if viewed from below, since equal diameters are presenting in the 2 planes — the *biparietal and suboccipitobregmatic* (each measuring 9.5 cm). However, the head is not fully flexed until quite late in labour, so that an oval shape presents — the shorter biparietal diameter in one plane and the longer occipitofrontal (11–12 cm) or suboccipitofrontal (10 cm) in the other. This is why the head tends to lie in a transverse (occipitolateral) position at the brim (more often to the left), an oblique position in the midpelvis, and an anteroposterior position at the outlet.

CARDINAL MOVEMENTS (figure 42.3)

(i) *Descent.* Descent of the fetal head into the pelvis has already occurred in most nulliparas in the later weeks of pregnancy. In parous patients, significant descent only occurs after labour com-

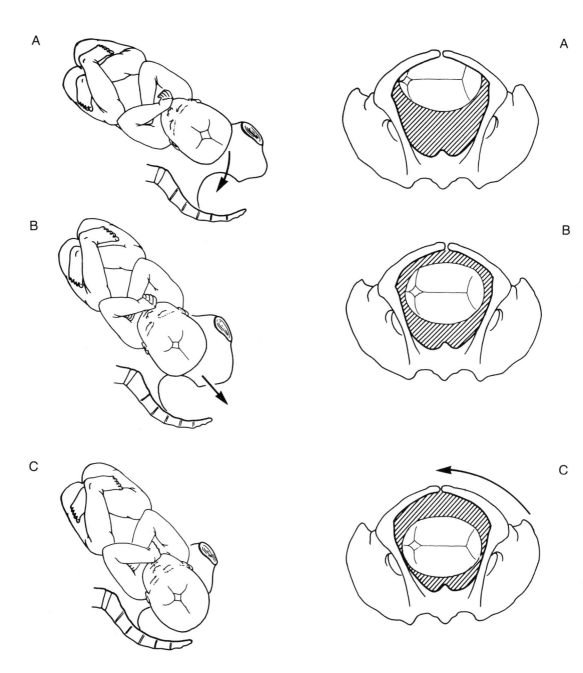

Figure 42.3 The mechanism of delivery from the left occipitolateral position (LOT). This is an explanation of the steps or movements the fetus undergoes to negotiate the birth canal. Each step is illustrated by paired diagrams of the pelvis viewed laterally and of the head as palpated from below during vaginal examination. **A.** The head enters the pelvic brim with the posterior parietal bone presenting. Both fontanelles are shown at the same station as would be the case if flexion was incomplete. **B.** Lateral flexion of the head on the neck enables the head to descend and engagement has occurred. The head is now synclitic (see figure 42.4). **C.** Further lateral flexion allows descent of the head past the pubic symphysis; 90° internal (anterior) rotation of the occiput is required. **D.** The occiput has rotated 45° towards the front. The shoulders have rotated with the head which is not always the case. The sagittal suture lies in the right oblique diameter of the pelvis. **E.** Internal (anterior) rotation of the occiput is complete. Further descent has occurred. The sagittal suture lies in the anteroposterior diameter of the outlet. The head now begins to extend. **F.** Birth of the head is due to extension with the pubic symphysis acting as fulcrum; 45° restitution will now occur. **G.** Restitution of the head is due to the twist on the neck (due to internal rotation) being undone. Had the shoulders not rotated 45° with the head (see D, above), restitution would have been through 90°; 45° external rotation will now occur. **H.** External rotation of the head is due to internal (anterior) rotation of the shoulders. This movement does not occur if internal rotation of the head is unaccompanied by movement of the trunk — as the shoulders are already in the anteroposterior diameter of the pelvis (see figure 42.5). Traction on the head directed posteriorly releases the anterior shoulder from beneath the pubic symphysis.

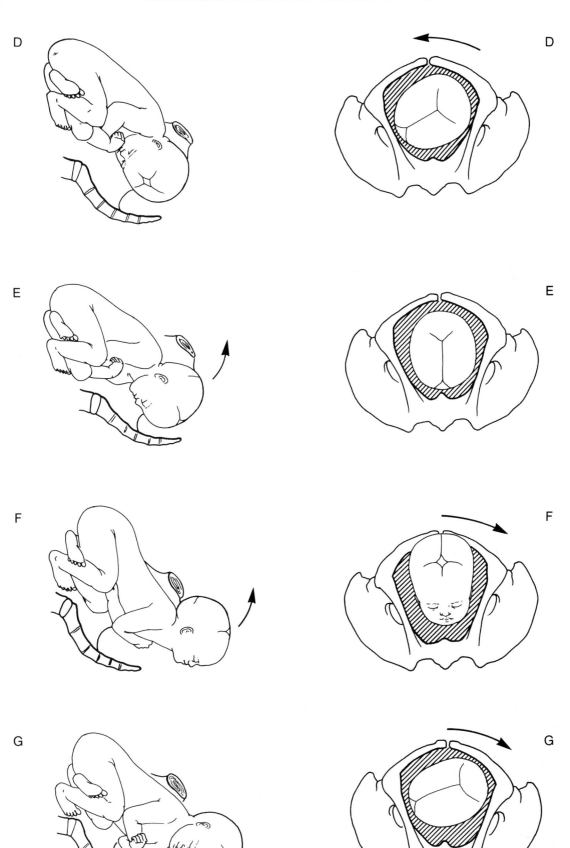

H

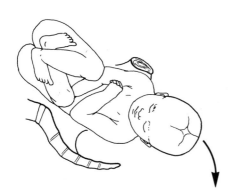

H

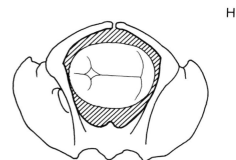

mences. *Descent occurs because of the contractions of the uterus* which push the fetus down and at the same time stretch and draw up the muscle fibres of the lower uterine segment. Descent is continuous throughout labour unless an insuperable obstruction is present. After the membranes rupture, the uterus acts more directly on the fetus (fetal axis pressure), driving the head down more efficiently through the lower birth canal.

(ii) *Engagement* is not strictly a mechanism — that is, it is not a movement that is made by the head (figures 6.8 and 42.4). Rather, it is a happening at a certain point in the descent of the head, when the *maximum diameters of the head have passed through the pelvic brim*. It may, like descent and flexion, occur even before labour has started, especially in the nullipara, *although this is not the rule (20–25%)*. It is, nevertheless, a crucial event in labour, since it is now highly likely that vaginal delivery will occur.

(iii) *Flexion.* This again is a continuous process throughout labour, and probably depends on the *principle of the lever*, a result of the fact that the articulation of the head with the spine is nearer to the occiput than the sinciput. If equal resistance is applied to the oncoming head, more force is exerted on the side of the longer arm (i.e. the sinciput) and so it gives way more easily (i.e. flexion occurs). With full flexion, the posterior fontanelle is almost in the centre of the area outlined by the cervix, and a much more favourable diameter presents (suboccipitobregmatic).

(iv) *Internal rotation.* This means *rotation of the head inside the pelvis*, as opposed to external rotation which occurs after the head is born (figure 42.5). The main cause probably lies in the peculiarities of the shape of the birth canal (90° forward curve) and the easier fit of the suboccipital area of the fetal head behind the symphysis pubis, together with the fact that the outlet of the pelvis is oval with the long axis in the AP diameter. A contributing factor is the forward and inward slope of the pelvic diaphragm (levatores ani), although in the majority of cases on X-ray study the head has already rotated or commenced to rotate before the pelvic floor is reached, and for practical purposes, the

A

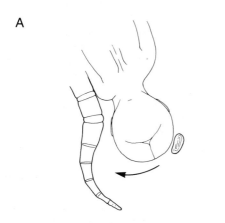

B

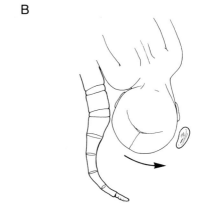

Figure 42.4 The head is synclitic when the sagittal suture lies midway between sacral promontory and pubic symphysis. **A.** The head descends and engages in the pelvis by lateral flexion when the posterior parietal presents. **B.** Asynclitic rocking back and forth of the moulded head enables negotiation of the pelvic brim when there is cephalopelvic disproportion (true conjugate inadequate for biparietal diameter).

A   B   C

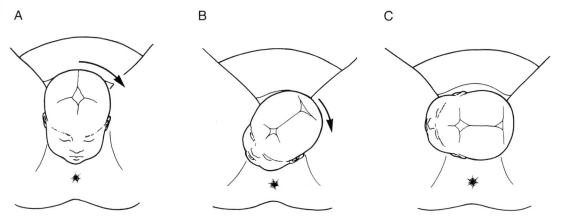

Figure 42.5 Restitution and external rotation from the LOA position. **A.** The head is born by extension and restitutes 45° to undo the twist on the neck. **B.** The head externally rotates a further 45° in the same direction as restitution, due to internal rotation of the shoulders through 45°. External rotation, although named for the head, is due to the shoulders and if prevented by the accoucheur can result in impacted shoulders. **C.** The face is directed laterally and the shoulders now lie in the anteroposterior diameter of the pelvic outlet.

head is tranversing a curved canal in which such structures as the pelvic diaphragm are smoothed out. Usually, the rotation is anterior, that is, the denominator (the occiput in this case) swings from LOT to LOA, and finally to the direct OA position. When the pelvis cannot accommodate the occiput anteriorly (narrow forepelvis), the sinciput rotates anteriorly resulting in an occipitoposterior position.

(v) *Extension*. The *head remains flexed until the leading part reaches the perineum. As the head is crowned it follows the natural forward inclination of the birth canal and extends*, the lower border of symphysis pubis acting as a fulcrum (figure 42.6). It follows that the occiput will appear initially, and as the process of extension continues, the vertex, forehead, and finally the face will appear from beneath the posterior part of the vulval ring.

(iv) *External rotation*. The *initial phase of external rotation of the head is called restitution and is simply the undoing or reversal of the head twisting which had taken place as described under internal rotation*. The movement usually happens quite quickly after the head is delivered, and may not be noticed if the accoucheur is not observant. The direction of movement of the occiput will be to the side of the back and the amount of rotation will indicate the direction in which the spinal column is facing and the diameter in which the shoulders are placed. In the present case, the restitution will be to the left since the fetal head started as an LOT, and will be 90° (or 45° as explained in the legend to figures 42.3 D, G and H when the shoulders rotated 45° as the head rotated 90°). *The second phase of external rotation is caused by rotation*

of the shoulders which naturally carry the head with them. In anterior positions of the occiput, the external rotation of the head is in the direction of restitution and is about 45°; in transverse positions, the shoulders stay in the AP diameter, and so no second phase rotation of the head occurs; finally in posterior positions, the external rotation of the head is opposite to the direction of restitution, usually 45° forwards (table 52.1). The basic fact is that *the shoulders are delivered in the AP of the outlet*, and the occiput is at right angles, hence it must be in the LOT or ROT position as the shoulders are delivered.

It is essential that these mechanisms be followed on the model, starting from anterior, transverse and posterior positions of the occiput, imparting internal rotation of the head, allowing restitution after delivery of the head, and watching the movement of the head as the shoulders are brought into the AP of the outlet from each of the above positions, both left and right.

(vii) *Trunk delivery*. Because of the curve of the birth canal, the *anterior shoulder appears first*, and with further downward fetal axis pressure exerted by the uterus, the posterior shoulder follows the forward sweep of the canal and appears at the fourchette. The *remainder of the trunk is born by the process of lateral flexion* or sideways bending of the spine. The initial movement, freeing the anterior shoulder is usually assisted by downward and backward pressure on the head by the accoucheur (figure 42.3 H). *This means that the full bisacromial diameter (12.5 cm) does not transverse the vulval ring*, the shorter acromiohumeral diameter (10 cm) presenting. This is important in reducing the incidence of posterior vulval tears.

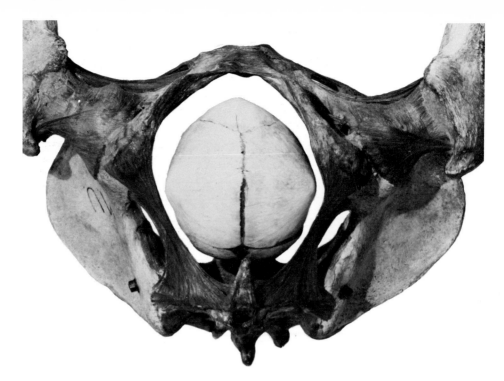

Figure 42.6 The position of the fontanelles and sagittal suture before birth of the head by extension of the neck. The posterior fontanelle is readily palpable anteriorly, but because the head is well flexed, the anterior fontanelle is situated out of easy reach in the hollow of the sacrum. The bones and ligaments of the pelvic outlet are shown.

CONDUCT OF NORMAL DELIVERY

Although vaginal delivery is usually a straightforward procedure, it is vital that a routine be developed and adhered to as closely as possible, otherwise vital steps may be omitted, particularly if a complication arises.

Preliminaries

A normal *delivery tray* should be set up in readiness when the patient enters the second stage. The instruments, drapes, apparel and dressings are shown in figure 42.7.

A hypodermic tray is also prepared for infiltration of the perineum (20 ml 1% lignocaine) if episiotomy is necessary.

A *bassinette* is made ready with warm blankets. The patient should empty her bladder shortly after the second stage has begun. If she is unsuccessful, and the bladder is distended, *catheterization* under strict asepsis should be carried out. The vulval and surrounding areas (pubis, thighs, perineum) should be washed and a clean gown and leggings put on.

Position of the Patient

(i) *Modified dorsal.* The patient lies on her back, preferably in a semisitting position, the knees are flexed, and the legs are widely separated. This position is suitable for routine delivery of the multipara, where no difficulty is anticipated. If the second stage is very rapid, there is often not time for more elaborate positioning.

(ii) *Squatting.* There has been recent enthusiasm for this oldest of positions. It is more physiological than the other positions, allows better pushing by the mother, and is associated with a widening of the pelvic outlet.

(iii) *Lithotomy* (figure 42.8). This position (perhaps modified in a birthing chair) is often used for nulliparas, in whom an episiotomy and repair is likely to be required. In this position it is easier to pick up and hold the chin, since there is better access to the anococcygeal area. Most prefer this position if the delivery is to be by *forceps* or vacuum extraction, since assessment of position is easier than if the patient is in the left lateral position. Its disadvantages are that the patient is at greater risk if inhalation of gastric contents occurs during anaesthesia or if she vomits during delivery.

(iv) *Left lateral* (figure 42.9). The patient lies on her left side, her head towards the centre of the bed and her buttocks at the edge; the legs are partially flexed. The upper leg is held by an assistant or is suspended from a suitable overhead attachment. The accoucheur either places her left arm around the upper leg (figure 42.9 A) or the delivery is conducted with the hands in front of the vulva.

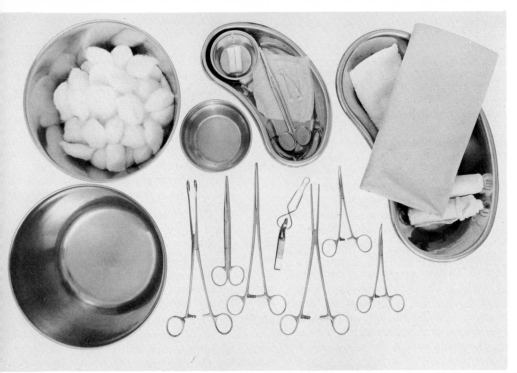

Figure 42.7 Normal delivery tray. Large bowls contain cotton wool swabs and 0.1% aqueous chlorhexidine solution. The small bowl will contain lubricant (chlorhexidine cream) for use prior to vaginal examination. The small kidney dish contains eye swabs in sterile water and clamp, gauze and scissors for cord. The large dish contains drapes, combined perineal pad and packs for use during repair of episiotomy. Instruments from the left are sponge forceps, episiotomy scissors, cord clamp, towel clips (seldom used), second cord clamp, and 2 curved artery forceps.

The *advantages* of this position are good control of the head, both in maintenance of flexion with the left hand (figure 42.9 B), and a controlled descent by the right hand, which picks up the chin easily. The perineum is thus guarded more securely, and a more favourable diameter passes the vulval ring because of *maximal flexion*, and fewer lacerations will occur. The position is safer from the viewpoint of inhalation of vomited or regurgitated material. The *disadvantages* of the position include the need for an assistant to hold the leg, greater difficulty in draping the patient and in maintaining the drapes, and the need to shift the patient to her side and then back again for the third stage and perineal repair should this be necessary.

The *disadvantages* of the other positions over the lithotomy and left lateral positions are that there is poorer control of the chin as the head is crowning, *delivery of the shoulders is more difficult*, it is more difficult for the operator than either the lithotomy or left lateral positions, and sterility is more difficult to maintain. When there is *shoulder dystocia* (impacted shoulders) the dorsal position is most unfavourable because downward traction which is required to free the anterior shoulder from beneath the symphysis pubis (figure 49.11) is prevented by the bed — the lithotomy position although less popular and

less comfortable, does not have this important disadvantage.

Recently, Dr Michel Odent has advocated an uninhibited and spontaneous approach to normal delivery where the mother chooses any position she wishes, changing it at will throughout labour and delivery (figures 42.10 and 59.1A).

Scrubbing Up

The factors determining the duration of the second stage have already been discussed. Although experience is usually the best guide as to the imminence of delivery, a check of the above factors will give a good indication. One is much more likely to be caught unawares by the multipara. Here, the duration of the second stage in previous labours is often helpful. Both premature and delayed scrubbing up may result in a breakdown of the antiseptic/aseptic routine.

Procedure. A clean apron, cap and mask are put on. Antiseptic lotions for swabbing and for the accoucheur's hands are prepared and the delivery packs are opened or the sterile cover removed from the delivery tray. The hands and forearms are scrubbed with a brush, under running water for 2–3 minutes using an antiseptic soap or emulsion. Several rinsings are advisable. Donning of a sterile gown and gloves completes the preparation.

Delivery

Antisepsis/Asepsis. (i) *Swabbing.* Cotton wool swabs soaked in antiseptic solution are grasped in sponge-holding forceps and the 'operative' area systematically swabbed. Usually, the insides of the thighs, the pubis and then the vulva are swabbed on one side and this is repeated on the other. Finally, an additional swabbing is made through the middle of the vulva. Different solutions are employed in different hospitals. Aqueous chlorhexidine 0.1% is commonly used for this purpose. (ii) *Draping.* This will depend on the position of the patient and hospital practice. Usually, separate drapes for the leg, abdomen, and buttock areas are employed, often supplemented with a larger window-type drape which excludes all of the field except the area from pubis to coccyx. Towel clips are placed to maintain the drapes in position which is the simplest from the viewpoint of the accoucher in training.

Delivery of the head. The position of the accoucheur will depend on the position of the patient. The following description will apply to delivery in the dorsal position.

The left hand is placed so that the fingers are spread over the vertex, usually with the base of the hand applied to the back of the occiput. This will maintain flexion of the head. The chin is secured by the right hand (covered with a sterile towel or gauze pad), feeling in the space between anus and coccyx. (When the head is crowning, the chin will be felt as it slips beneath the coccyx with contractions (figure 42.8 A)). The degree of extension of the head is controlled by the left hand, while the right hand prevents the chin slipping back, and allows controlled descent. As the occiput descends under the symphysis pubis, extension occurs and progressively the forehead, nose, mouth and finally chin emerge from beneath the posterior ring of the vulval opening (figure 42.8 B). Tension in the perineal area is reduced if the thumb and middle finger are placed on the outer lateral aspects of the vulval ring and brought towards the midline, pushing the ring backward and posteriorly; this also assists the ring to slip over the baby's head. If the perineum is tight, the chin may need freeing by slipping the index finger under the baby's mandible and elevating it. A pad should be placed over the anus, but the perineum must remain in clear view. Mucus is removed from the baby's mouth and nose.

Cord around the neck. A finger of the left hand is run up past the occiput to ascertain whether the cord is looped around the neck (it is in 25–30% of patients). If it is present, it is drawn down over the head; other loops are treated similarly. If there is undue tension, 2 clamps are placed on the cord about 2–3 cm apart and the cord is cut between them. The release of additional loops can be achieved quite easily by unwinding the clamped ends around the neck. Occasionally, the loop is quite loose and it can be slipped easily over the shoulder.

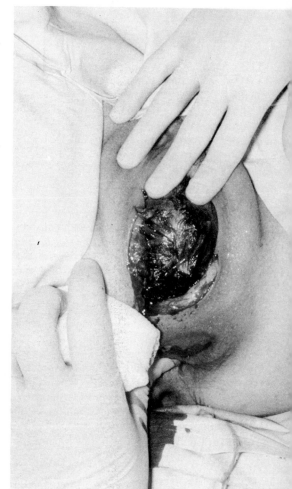

A

Figure 42.8 Normal delivery in the dorsal or lithotomy position has the advantage that the patient does not need to be moved for repair of an episiotomy. Also the position is more suitable for forceps delivery should this prove necessary. The main disadvantage is that it is more difficult to pick up the chin and control delivery of the head. **A.** This patient was a primigravida aged 21 years whose labour had lasted 7 hours. A right mediolateral episiotomy has been cut. Flexion of the head is being maintained. There is marked caput formation.

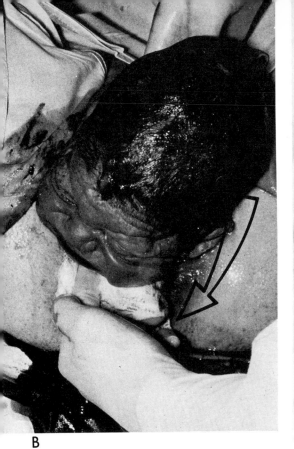

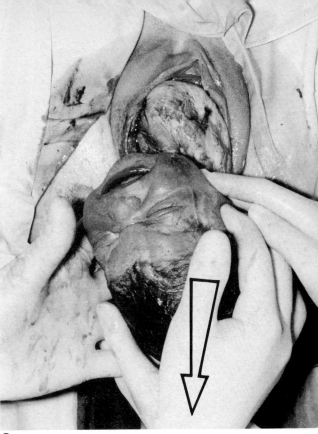

B

C

D

B. The head is born; the perineal pad protects the face from faecal contamination. Restitution through 45° has undone the twist on the neck. **C.** Overemphasis of external rotation (90° instead of the usual 45°) has been necessary to achieve complete rotation of the shoulders into the AP diameter of the pelvic outlet. The anterior shoulder is being released from beneath the symphysis pubis by traction directed posteriorly. The supervisor indicates the direction and degree of traction required — hence the extra pair of hands. **D.** The posterior shoulder is delivered by lateral flexion of the trunk in an anterior direction. Note that the overemphasis of external rotation is no longer applied and so the head faces laterally. **E.** The baby is born and held head downwards. He is covered with vernix and is very slippery; it is necessary to hold his head as shown since his weight could cause his feet to slip from the grasp of the other hand.

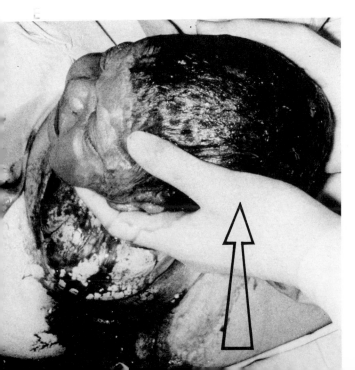

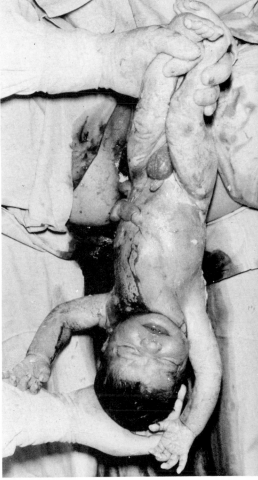

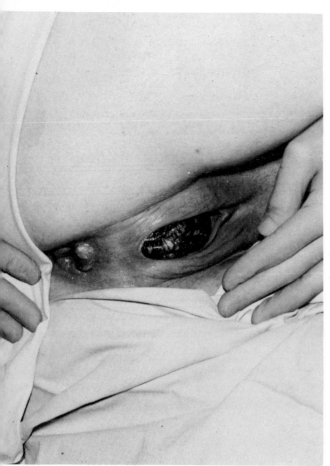
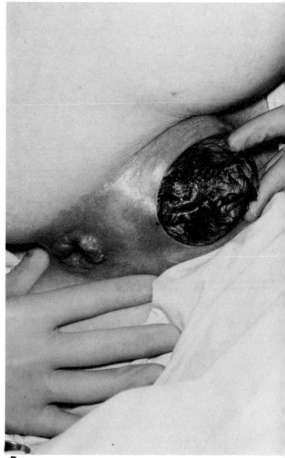

A   B

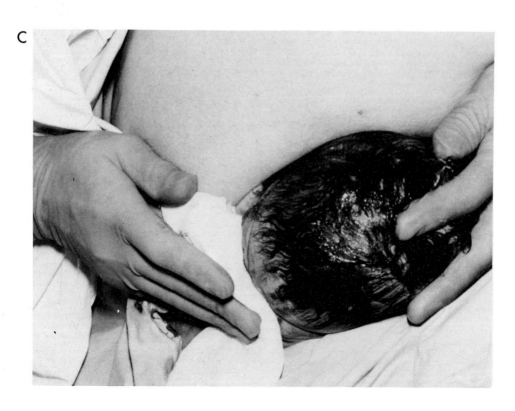

C

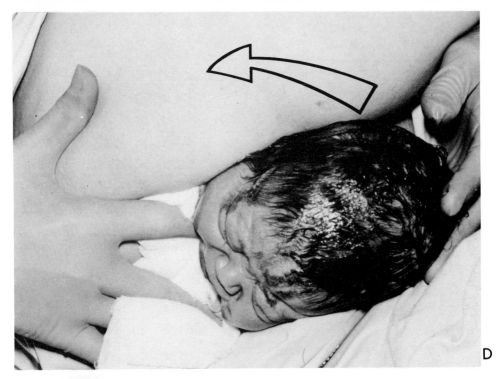

D

E

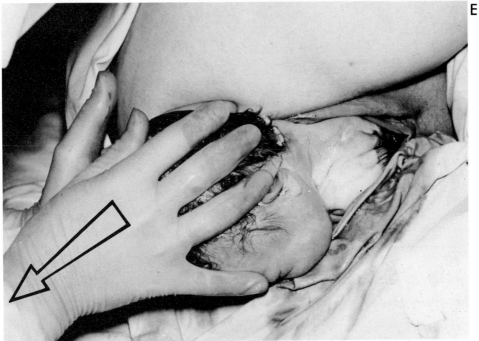

Figure 42.9 Normal delivery. The left lateral position is most suitable for teaching as the fetal chin is easier to grasp. Other advantages are lesser risks of postural hypotension and inhalation of vomitus. **A.** The patient, a primigravida aged 17 years, is swabbed and draped. The head is on view 45 minutes after the membranes ruptured and 15 hours after the onset of labour. **B.** The hands are in position to pick up the chin and maintain flexion (ensuring smallest AP diameter of head) by pressure on the occiput using either palm or fingers — avoid pinching maternal tissues anteriorly. Delivery is imminent as the perineum bulges during a contraction and the anus gapes; at this stage faeces soil the operative field unless the lower bowel has been emptied early in labour. The perineum is infiltrated with 1% lignocaine (10–15 ml) and an episiotomy incision is made. Flexion is maintained and sudden emergence of the head prevented. **C.** The head is being born slowly, by extension, between contractions. The accoucheur now controls the delivery and the patient is encouraged to breathe from the mask — uncontrolled expulsive efforts at this stage may result in perineal tearing and cerebral damage to the baby. **D.** As brow and orbital ridges appear, the perineal pad is used to push the perineum away from the face. The eyes are swabbed and the nose freed of mucus. The arrow indicates the direction in which the occiput will restitute. **E.** The head has undergone 90° combined restitution and external rotation and is being flexed to check that the anterior shoulder is beneath the symphysis pubis. Loops of cord if present would be drawn over the head or slipped over the shoulder if loose, or cut between clamps if tight. The anterior shoulder is delivered by lateral flexion of the trunk towards the sacrum. Here the shoulders lie in the AP diameter; rotation is not needed and traction alone will effect delivery.

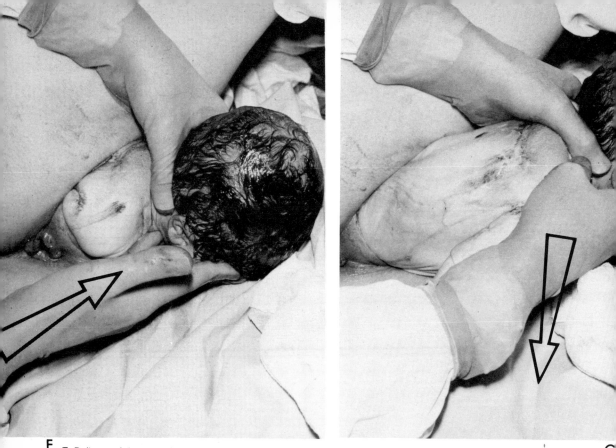

F | G

F. Delivery of the posterior shoulder by traction in the direction of the birth canal and lateral flexion of the trunk towards the maternal abdomen. The episiotomy is needlessly extended if the posterior shoulder is delivered too rapidly. With the posterior shoulder freed, the baby is grasped around the back of the neck. Pressure by a finger in the infant's axilla helps maintain lateral flexion of the trunk and provides traction to facilitate delivery of the shoulder. **G.** Delivery of the trunk. There is no need for continued lateral flexion as the diameters are smaller — there is no resistance to emergence of buttocks and feet. When the baby is born to the umbilicus, the head is lowered and the left hand readied to grasp the feet when they appear. **H.** The baby is held upside down to avoid inhalation of fluid since respiration usually commences at this time. The nasopharynx is aspirated to remove liquor, mucus, and blood. **I.** The mother is given either IV ergometrine (0.5 mg) or IM Syntometrine (1 ml) either at this stage or with delivery of the anterior shoulder. Note how the patient's wrist has been flexed to hold the vein stationary to facilitate insertion of the needle.

H | I

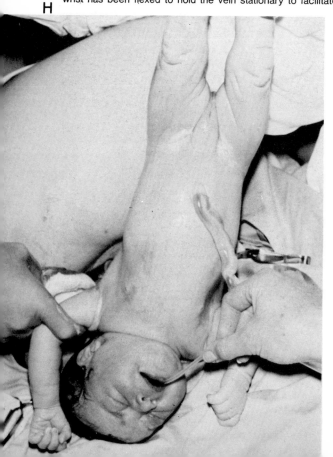

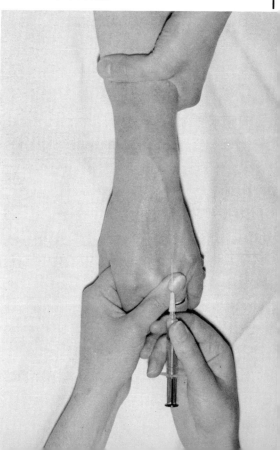

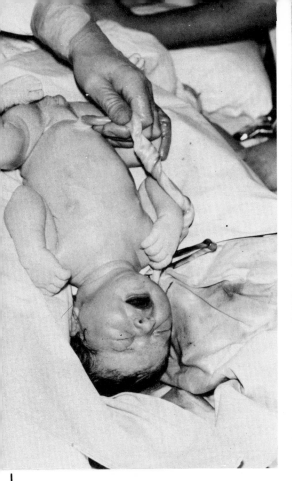
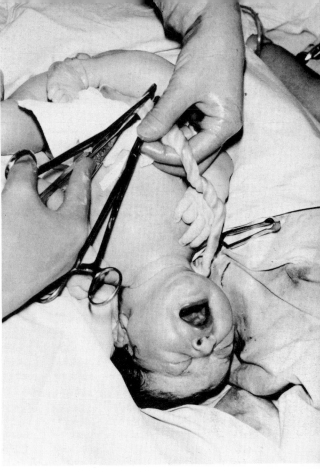

J

K

J. The mother has been turned into the dorsal position and the cord is checked for pulsations. **K.** The cord is divided between clamps, or, alternatively, when pulsations cease, the cord is clamped close to the baby's umbilicus using the plastic device shown in figure 42.7. **L.** The baby is handed to an attendant who wraps her in a warm sterile cloth, attaches identification bands to both wrists, and gives her to the mother. This baby weighed 3,470 g.

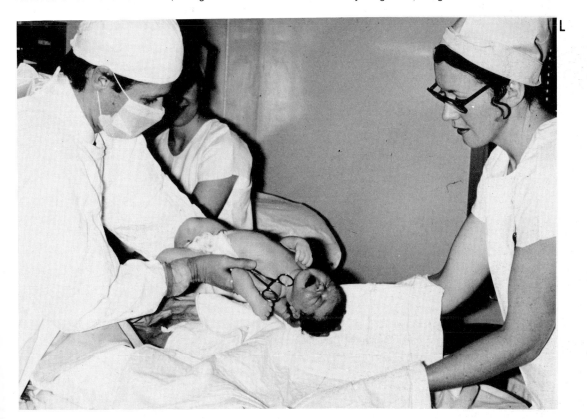

L

Delivery of the trunk. *Delivery of the shoulders* is a time of danger to the perineum and as much care should be taken as with delivery of the head. Usually the anterior shoulder slips from under the symphysis pubis with the next contraction, or it can be assisted by downward and backward traction of the head (figure 42.8 C). This should not be forcible, because of the risk to the brachial nerve plexus (*Erb paralysis*). If difficulty is experienced, the index finger may be slipped into the posterior axilla and traction exerted. If this is not successful, assistance should be obtained immediately. Usually an episiotomy will enlarge the vulval ring sufficiently to release the shoulder, but on rare occasions one may be faced with shoulders which are impacted at the pelvic brim (see Chapter 49).

After the anterior shoulder is freed, the direction of traction is more in the line of the lower birth canal — upward and forward. Further gentle steady traction allows the posterior shoulder to emerge over the perineum (figure 42.8 D). The latter structure should be watched carefully during this time.

The rest of the birth follows easily. It is usually best, when the shoulders are delivered, to change the hold on the baby's head, the right hand securing it behind the neck, while the left hand grasps the feet at the ankles (figure 42.8 E).

Some babies are thickly covered with vernix and quite slippery — they should *never be held with only one hand*, and always placed so that a fall would be harmless if the grip is lost.

Care of the Baby

The postdelivery management of the baby is discussed in Chapters 59 and 62.

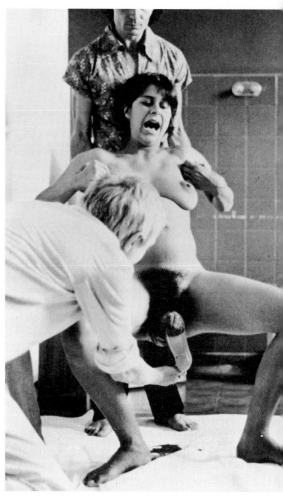

Figure 42.10 Spontaneous normal delivery (with intact amniotic sac) in a standing-squat with the mother supported under the arms and shoulders while she flexes her knees slightly and bears down. This variety of natural birth has the advantage that the position relaxes the adductor and perineal muscles. (Courtesy of Dr Michel Odent, Pithiviers Hospital, France).

chapter forty-three

The Third Stage of Labour

OVERVIEW

The third stage of labour is the period from the delivery of the baby to the delivery of the placenta. Separation of the placenta usually occurs quickly after birth of the baby because of the marked reduction in size of the uterus. Descent then occurs, first into the lower segment and then into the vagina. Bleeding from the ruptured uteroplacental blood vessels is mainly controlled by compression of the vessels by the retracted and contracting uterine muscle fibres ('*living ligatures*'); a *rapidly-acting coagulation process* is also important. Routine administration of *oxytocic drugs* further curtails bleeding by preventing the relaxation which usually occurs between contractions. The type and route (IV or IM) of the oxytocic is dictated by such factors as past history, amount of bleeding, level of blood pressure and whether nurses (midwives) are allowed to administer drugs by the IV route in the absence of a medical practitioner.

The essence of third stage management is alertness to the *signs of separation and descent of the placenta* and patience in *refraining from premature interference* unless this is dictated by the amount of bleeding which is occurring; *always pass a catheter if separation fails to occur after one attempt at Brandt-Andrews method of delivery of the placenta.*

The less experienced attendant is advised to look in advance for signs of potential difficulty, especially a history of third stage problems (*postpartum haemorrhage, manual removal of the placenta*) or a uterus which is scarred by previous surgery (especially Caesarean section); referral of such a patient is indicated.

Placental delivery is now managed by the Brandt-Andrews method of *controlled cord traction*; former procedures of pushing down on the uterus (Dublin method) or its vigorous squeezing (Crede method) have largely been abandoned. After delivery, a *careful inspection and recording is made of the placenta, membranes and cord.*

The fourth stage of labour is the somewhat ill-defined period of immediate postdelivery recovery. *It is important that careful observation and monitoring be continued for 2–4 hours in view of such potential hazards as bleeding from the genital tract*, rapid fluctuation in *blood pressure*, and early septicaemia. This is an ideal time for the wife and husband to enjoy their baby together and lay the foundation for a firm and lasting bond between them.

DEFINITION

The period from the delivery of the baby to the delivery of the placenta. This is normally completed within 5–10 minutes.

NORMAL PHYSIOLOGY

Studies have shown that *uterine contractions* in the third stage continue with the same strength and frequency as before — that is, *55–65 + mm Hg at intervals of 3–4 minutes.* The combination of such contractions and the reduction of surface area of the uterine cavity after birth of the baby causes the placenta to be sheared off the uterine wall — *that is, it separates.* Circulation continues for a short time in the umbilical cord and in the placenta. When the baby starts breathing, the *increase in oxygen in the blood causes the ductus arteriosus, ductus venosus, and umbilical arteries to contract and pulsations cease in the umbilical cord.* By this time the placenta is usually free in the uterine cavity. There is some *retroplacental bleeding* as the placenta tears off the uterine wall, severing the arteries and veins from the uterine bed, and this also aids in the separation process. With further contractions, the placenta is forced first into the lower segment, then the vagina and finally is expelled.

There are *2 main mechanisms* of placental delivery (figure 43.1). (i) *Schultze.* Here the *shiny fetal side* comes first. The placenta turns inside out like an umbrella in a gale, and appears at the vulva with the membranes following.

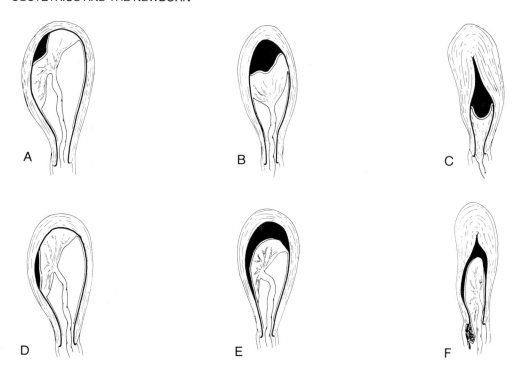

Figure 43.1 Mechanisms of placental delivery. **A B C** — Schultze mechanism: the retroplacental clot turns the placenta inside out and the shiny fetal surface presents as it enters the vagina. **D E F** — Matthews-Duncan mechanism: the placenta slides out edge first showing the fleshy cotyledons of the maternal surface as it appears at the vulva.

Usually, there is little or no bleeding until after the membranes have delivered, since the retroplacental blood clot is still retained. (ii) *Matthews-Duncan.* Here the *maternal side* is seen first; this is rough and composed of many discrete segments (cotyledons). Usually bleeding occurs before the placenta is delivered.

There is probably little significance in these 2 different mechanisms; it is likely that they depend largely on the original site of attachment of the placenta — the higher in the uterus it is, the more likely it is to *balloon down* (Schultze), the lower it is, the more likely it is to *slide down* (Matthews-Duncan).

The membranes are not separated either by reduction in uterine size or bleeding. Usually, it is the *weight of the placenta* and blood clot, or *traction* exerted by the accoucheur that is responsible (figure 43.2).

Control of haemorrhage is by the *normal coagulation processes* associated with any wound (release of thromboplastins, platelet aggregation, fibrin formation) together with the so-called '*living ligatures*' formed by the interlacing bundles of muscle in the uterine wall, which as a result of the marked reduction in the uterine size, twist and compress the vessels. The importance of the first mechanism is shown, however, by the failure of the contracted uterus to stop bleeding if there is a failure of coagulation.

Special conditions. (i) In *breech presentation* it is likely that placental separation is partial or complete by the time the trunk of the fetus is born. (ii) In *multiple pregnancy* there is a reduction in uterine size after the first baby is born, with the possibility of premature separation. This is less likely than with breech birth, since the amniotic sac(s) of the succeeding fetus(es) maintains some control over the degree of shrinkage at the placental site.

DISTURBANCES TO THE NORMAL PHYSIOLOGY

The process as described is less efficient if there has been a preceding *disorder of uterine function* (incoordination, constriction ring), or the uterus has been grossly *overdistended* (polyhydramnios, multiple pregnancy), or *paralysed* by certain anaesthetic agents (ether, halothane), or the *accoucheur fiddles* with the postpartum uterus causing irregular, uncoordinated contractions and *partial separation* with escape of blood from the retroplacental clot. Another type of disturbance is related to the administration of *ergometrine* (ergonovine) which causes a tonic contraction of the whole uterus: this hastens placental separation and controls bleeding. However, it is more physiological to give oxytocin and ergometrine together intramuscularly, since

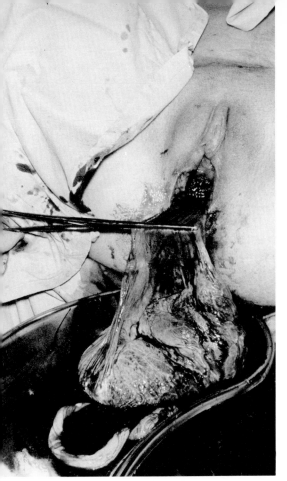

Figure 43.2 The trailing membranes are detached from the uterine wall and delivered complete by careful traction with a see-saw action. A cord clamp with transverse serrations (Rochester Peane) gives a good grip without tearing the membranes which should be grasped close to the vulva.

the oxytocin is faster-acting (than ergometrine) by this route and causes a physiological, peristaltic type of uterine activity which delivers the placenta to the lower segment or vagina before the tonic action of the ergometrine occurs. This reduces the incidence of a retained, separated placenta. *At Caesarean section*, the placenta is usually manually removed immediately, so that bleeding from the uterine incision can be controlled rapidly by suturing. *Abnormal adherence of the placenta (placenta accreta)* to the wall of the uterus (previous surgery, placenta praevia) will prevent the normal separation through the decidual layer of the endometrium.

MANAGEMENT

Proper management of the third stage is of vital importance in minimizing postpartum haemorrhage, retained placenta, maternal morbidity, and maternal death. At the outset, it must be stated that there is not complete agreement on such matters as to which oxytocic drug to give, the route of administration and when, and which

technique should be adopted for delivery of the placenta. Each hospital has its own procedures and these must be learnt and carried out.

General

It is most important to study carefully the patient's *reproductive history*. If there has been a previous problem in the third stage (haemorrhage, manual removal, curettage) or previous Caesarean section, the patient is in a high risk category. The same applies if she has a placenta praevia, coagulation problem, or anaemia in the current pregnancy.

Normal Conduct

General. After the baby has been delivered and attended to, the cord is doubly clamped 1–2 cm from the baby and divided: a longer length of cord (4–5 cm) is left if the baby has erythroblastosis and an exchange transfusion may be required. *The optimum time of clamping is 30–60 seconds after birth*: this will provide some 80 ml of extra blood to the baby. Excess blood volume in the baby can be a disadvantage, producing *polycythaemia* and *hyperviscosity*, with such attendant problems as respiratory distress, heart failure, jaundice, convulsions and apathy. The uterus is palpated through the sterile abdominal drape, and a note made of its size (possibility of an undiagnosed twin), consistency, and contractions. *If there is no undue bleeding it is not massaged or prodded.* A sterile basin or bedpan is placed against the perineum; this serves to contain the umbilical cord and to enable blood loss to be assessed. The cord is drawn down until resistance is felt. If there is an episiotomy it should be compressed with a gauze pad if free bleeding is occurring from the cut edges. Aseptic and antiseptic precautions must not be relaxed. If laboratory studies are needed for rhesus disease, cord blood should be collected into appropriate tubes (plain: group, Rh; sequestrene: haemoglobin, Coombs test; lithium heparin: bilirubin). Cord blood may also be required in certain maternal disorders (syphilis, sickle cell anaemia, thalassaemia and thrombocytopenic purpura).

Oxytocic. The most physiological and safest drug is Syntometrine (oxytocin 5 units, ergometrine 0.5 mg) given intramuscularly after the birth of the child and palpation of the uterus to exclude a second twin. The blood pressure must be checked before the oxytocic is given: *ergometrine is usually contraindicated* in patients with elevated *blood pressure* and in those with *heart disease* (especially mitral stenosis). An alternative to ergometrine is *oxytocin alone*, 5 units intramuscularly. Ergometrine by intravenous injection, whether given before or after the anterior shoulder has been born, may have significant side-effects (nausea, retching) or hazards (hypertension, cardiac irregularity) and is usually reserved for special indications (previous third stage labour problems, particularly haemorrhage).

Placental separation and descent. The signs are classically as follows: (i) show of blood, (ii) lengthening of the cord (at least 5 cm), (iii) rise in height of the fundus (from 2–3 cm below the umbilicus to 1–2 cm above), (iv) uterus assumes a more globular shape and greater mobility. These signs may occur with partial separation and may not all be present when complete separation has occurred.

Placental delivery. After separation, delivery of the placenta is most physiologically and painlessly effected by the *Brandt-Andrews technique of controlled cord traction*. The essentials of this method are as follows. The cord is reclamped near to the vulva and steadied with one hand while the other hand is used to push the uterine fundus upwards (figure 43.3). This will indicate if the placenta has separated, since the cord will not then follow the upward movement of the uterus. If separation has occurred, a combined movement is made of downward and backward traction on the cord and *upward displacement of the uterus, provided that the latter is firmly contracted.* The abdominal hand is the controlling factor since it holds the fundus and prevents the possibility of *inversion of the uterus* — this only occurs when cord traction is performed with the uterus relaxed and unprotected. The cord of the mature baby will tolerate a strain of 6 kg (range 2–11 kg) before rupture occurs (usually at the point of placental insertion). *If the placenta does not advance* there are usually only 2 possibilities — it is *still attached to the uterus* (perhaps only partially) *or it has become incarcerated* (trapped) in the tightly contracted uterus. In such cases,

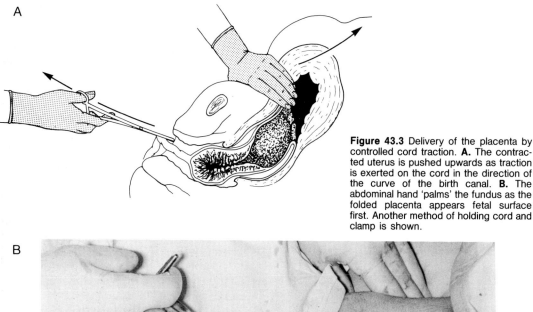

A

Figure 43.3 Delivery of the placenta by controlled cord traction. **A.** The contracted uterus is pushed upwards as traction is exerted on the cord in the direction of the curve of the birth canal. **B.** The abdominal hand 'palms' the fundus as the folded placenta appears fetal surface first. Another method of holding cord and clamp is shown.

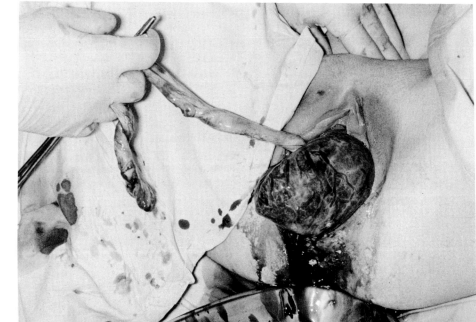

B

the attendant must be patient and repeat the procedure at intervals of some minutes, resisting the temptation to massage the uterus if bleeding is not excessive. If the umbilical cord vessels are congested, the clamp can be removed and the blood drained out. This reduces the size of the placenta and in addition, the risk of tranfusion of trapped fetal blood to the maternal circulation is much reduced. If there is delay in delivery of the placenta, *catheterization* is performed, *since uterine contractions are more effective when the bladder is empty*. This simple measure usually results in prompt separation and descent of the placenta. When the placenta is delivered, attention is given to the *membranes*. Usually they will strip readily from the uterine wall and will follow the placenta. If they begin to tear, the placenta should be rotated to cause a bunching up of the membranes near the vulva; a wide clamp is then applied and a steady traction exerted (figure 43.2). Experienced assistance must be sought if the placenta is not delivered within 10 minutes — earlier if bleeding is excessive. The further management of these complications is considered later.

An *alternative method* of placental delivery is the so-called *Dublin method* (figure 43.4). Here the *contracted uterus is used as a plunger* to push the placenta downwards from the lower segment or vagina. This method is satisfactory if carried out properly, but is often abused by the use of too much force, causing pain to the mother and stretching of the supports of the uterus.

If there has been an operative delivery, immediate removal of the placenta may be undertaken to reduce blood loss from the uterine wound in the case of Caesarean section or the episiotomy in the case of vaginal delivery.

In some situations, *routine exploration of the uterus* will be undertaken — previous uterine surgery, operative delivery, prolonged, difficult or precipitate labour, suspicion of a uterine malformation or rupture.

Inspection of the placenta. It is most important to examine the placenta in a careful and systematic fashion.

(i) *The maternal surface* is studied after fresh clots are removed from the surface. Any break in the regular arrangement of the cotyledons should be looked for, since this may indicate that part of the placenta is still attached to the uterine wall. Occasionally, one or more of the cotyledons may be torn during the process of separation, but when the placenta is cupped in the hands, the pieces will come together to form a smooth, continuous surface. Later confirmation is made when the placenta is washed under gently running water — if a piece is missing, free villi may be seen floating in the deficient area. Apart from missing areas, a check is made for *infarctions, old clot* (usually in a depressed area) indicating an episode of abruption, whitish-yellow areas of *calcification*, angiomas or other *tumours*, or partial *molar change* (the 2 latter conditions are rare). (See colour plates 16, 18, 19 and 33.)

(ii) *The fetal surface* is shiny, since it is viewed through the amnion. The course of the umbilical vessels is studied — they should all disappear into the substance of the placenta. If a vessel runs to the edge of the placenta and the membranes there are ragged or absent, the presence

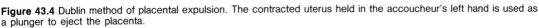

Figure 43.4 Dublin method of placental expulsion. The contracted uterus held in the accoucheur's left hand is used as a plunger to eject the placenta.

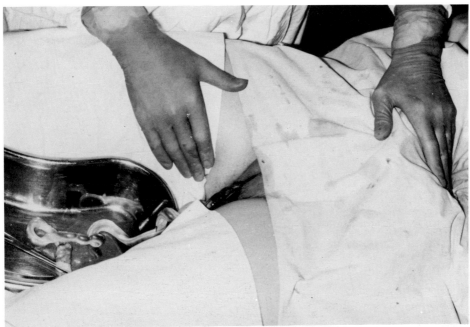

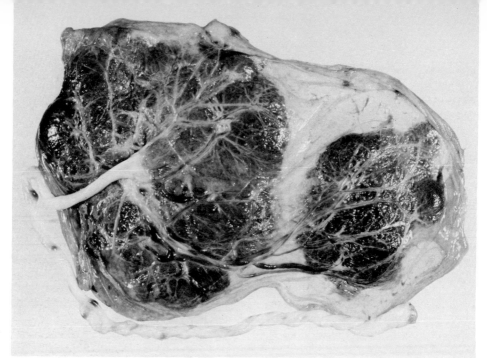

Figure 43.5 Fetal surface of a placenta succenturiata. Several large vessels pass across the membranes to the succenturiate lobe. The condition is termed vasa praevia when such vessels pass over the region of the internal os.

A

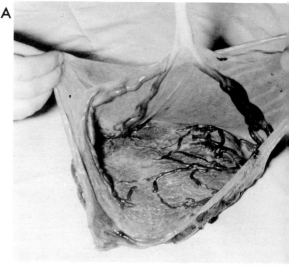

of a *succenturiate lobe* should be suspected (figure 43.5). *Velamentous insertion* is the name given to the cord which runs in the membranes before entering the placenta (figure 43.6). It occurs in about 1% of term pregnancies, more often in multiple pregnancies, and frequently in abortions. It is mainly of interest because of the risk of rupture of the intramembranous portion of the vessels, should they be in front of the presenting part (*vasa praevia* — colour plates 84 and 85). Placental location or formation is often abnormal, and infarction may be present. Hence, small for dates infants are commoner. It is thought to be due to errors at the implantation stage or unequal expansion of the fetal sac. Occasionally a nodular appearance may be seen (*amnion nodosum*), which is associated with oligohydramnios (figure 21.3). Whitish areas are common in the subchorial region and these usually represent fibrin deposition, not infarcts. The weight and dimensions of the placenta are recorded (figure 43.7), together with the time of its delivery and any significant anomaly which has been observed.

B

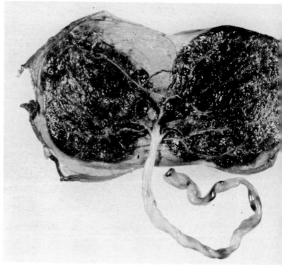

Figure 43.6 Velamentous insertion of the cord. **A.** This cord inserted 10 cm from the nearest placental edge. The membranes are held to demonstrate the vessels and fetal surface of the placenta. **B.** A bipartite (2-lobed) placenta with velamentous insertion of the cord.

(iii) The *membranes* are inspected for completeness. Ideally, there is a circular hole where the fetus emerged and the membranes are otherwise complete. The distance of the hole from the edge of the placenta indicates how close the placenta was to the internal os — if less than the length of the lower uterine segment then the placenta was partially praevia (*figure 1, Appendix IIIA*). *Often the membranes are 'ragged', that is, incomplete.* In such cases, an estimate should be made of how much of the membranes remains in the uterus. The membranes may insert on the surface of the placenta rather than at its edge (*circumvallate placenta*) and this should be recorded (figure 43.8); in this condition the placenta is unusually thick but has a reduced diameter, as though excessive regression of chorionic villi had occurred, with later extension of the remainder beyond the original edge of the placental disc. *Placenta membranacea* is the converse and much less common condition, where the chorionic villi persist over most or all of the circumference of the chorion, the placenta being wide but thin (figure 43.9 and colour plate 149). A very rare but interesting condition is absence of a complete membranous sac, the fetus being '*extrachorial*', perhaps as a result of long-standing premature rupture of the membranes (figure 43.10).

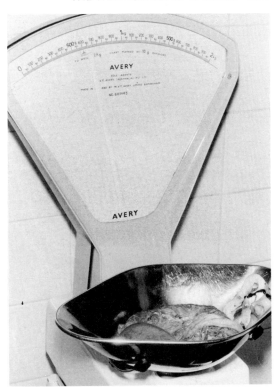

Figure 43.7 A self-indicating counter scale such as this should be used to document accurately the weight of the placenta — the largest of all endocrine glands, with an average weight of 600 g at term.

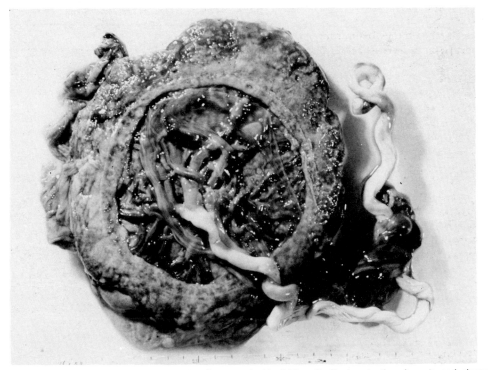

Figure 43.8 Circumvallate placenta; the amnion forms a double fold as it attaches to the placenta and obscures the vessels at the outer rim of the fetal surface. A mild accidental haemorrhage occurred at 38 weeks' gestation.

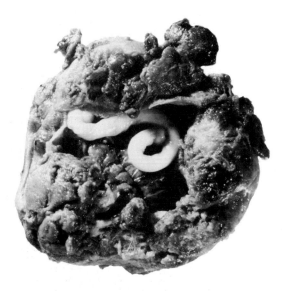

Figure 43.9 Placenta membranacea; the chorionic villi have persisted over the entire surface of the gestation sac. This is a rare variety of placenta praevia.

The length of the cord is then measured. When the cord contains only 2 vessels, the infant has about a 20% risk of congenital malformation, especially of the genitourinary and gastrointestinal systems, and should be carefully examined with this in mind (figure 65.14).

The incomplete placenta. If part of the placenta is missing or a succenturiate lobe is suspected, exploration of the uterus should be made (colour plate 33). If this is not done, there is a high risk of later bleeding, infection, and uterine subinvolution.

Examination of the birth canal. A gentle but thorough inspection is made for *injuries to the* (iv) *The umbilical cord* should be inspected for *vulva and vagina*, especially tears in the region true or false knots, amount of Wharton jelly, of the vulval ring. Occasionally, the epithelium staining by bilirubin (blood group incompati- may be intact but a haematoma may have devel- bility) or meconium (placental insufficiency), the oped in the deeper tissues. After operative presence of 3 vessels (in 1 in 350 patients there vaginal deliveries, or if bleeding is abnormal, the is only 1 artery rather than 2 — table 65.3), and whole length of the vagina and the cervix must any other anomalies such as varices, constric- be inspected. An empty bladder and the assist- tions or haematomas (figures 43.11 and 43.12). ance of a finger in the rectum will enable a better

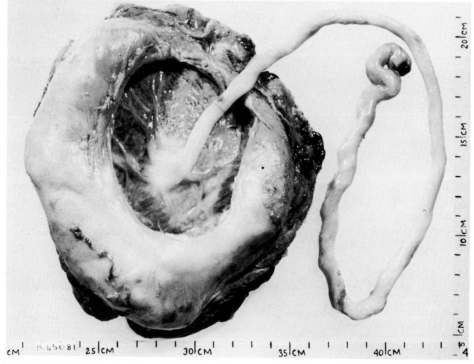

Figure 43.10 Placenta, membranes and cord (400 g) which were attached to an extrachorial fetus, born by assisted breech delivery at 30 weeks' gestation, 8 weeks after premature rupture of the 'membranes' had occurred. The infant survived! Histologically the free edge of fused chorion and amnion had a continuous epithelial lining, confirming that the membranes formed only a partial covering for the fetus.

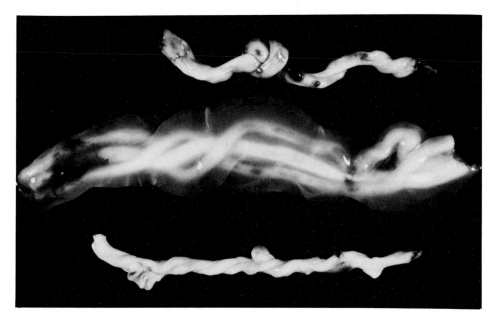

Figure 43.11 True and false knots of the umbilical cord. The middle cord had oedematous, transparent Wharton jelly although the baby was alive and well (no fetal hydrops or maternal diabetes). This rare specimen shows how umbilical vessels spiral around each other and how a twist of one causes a knuckle that simulates a knot.

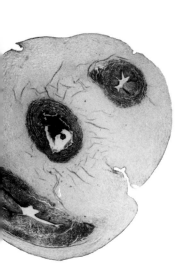

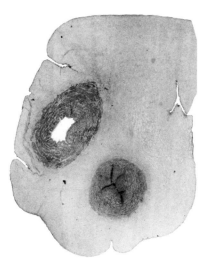

Figure 43.12 Cross-section of a normal cord and one containing a single umbilical artery (magnification X 8); in the latter case the mother had severe preeclampsia and the infant was growth retarded and had an imperforate anus (figure 65.14A).

delineation of bleeding into deeper pelvic tissues. The empty contracted uterus will feel quite firm, mobile, and the fundus will usually lie 3-4 cm below the umbilicus.

Repair of episiotomy or birth canal injury is carried out as soon as possible (see Chapter 45). Rapid cooling of the patient may occur, and she should be adequately covered before and during such procedures.

Further care. The *patient is cleaned* of all blood, and attention is given to the perianal area which may have become soiled by faeces. The *fundus is checked* to see that it is firmly contracted and any remaining clots are expelled from the vagina by gentle Dublin expression. Squeezing the fundus should *not* be done unless it is soft and high in the abdomen, since this disturbs the clot over the placental site and may cause fresh bleeding to occur. A *sterile pad* is placed over the perineum and the bed linen changed. If the patient has not had a general anaesthetic, a drink and light refreshment is given. If the baby does not require cot care, the mother is *allowed to nurse*. *She should rest on her side rather than on her back,* since the uterus then remains forwards; when the uterus falls into a retroverted position, the uterine veins may become distended and oozing may occur from the placental site (figure 43.13).

Routine observations of temperature, pulse rate, and blood pressure are made, the frequency depending on whether the preceding labour was normal or complicated. *Inspection of the perineal* pad and *palpation of the uterus* should be made every 15 minutes until a patient has left the labour ward, which is usually about 2 hours after the delivery. The *urine is checked for protein* as preeclampsia can occur for the first time late in labour or within a few hours of delivery. The *baby's condition* is similarly checked. The patient will usually appreciate some time alone with her husband and baby, allowing the *bonding* process to strengthen; *she is often tired and should then be allowed to sleep.* Many practitioners routinely prescribe sedation after delivery to minimize the risk of postpartum hypertension and eclampsia. *Many of the problems of the puerperium (psyche, breast feeding) can be prevented by restful sleep* after an often exhaustive time in labour and hours of lost sleep.

Special Problems Requiring Observation

Haemorrhage or shock. A close watch must be kept on the vital signs (pulse, respiration, blood pressure, peripheral circulation, urine output) if shock has occurred before or after delivery. Attention must also be given to the supervision of *intravenous fluid* administration and any *special drugs* that may have been ordered. The rare but serious complication of *amniotic fluid embolism* may manifest itself by delayed bleeding due to hypofibrinogenaemia. The patient must remain in the labour or recovery room until vital signs are stable.

Anaesthetic complications. After general anaesthesia (Caesarean section), the patient must be placed *on her side* and a *clear airway provided until she is fully awake.* Occasionally, inhalation of gastric content or some other anaesthetic complication may have occurred. Particular attention must be paid to observations of *respiratory rate* and the patient's *colour*.

Preeclampsia, eclampsia, or hypertension. The third stage represents a *dangerous period* for these patients — the stimulus of painful contractions, the effort required for expulsion of the baby, the augmentation of blood volume from the contracted uterus (especially after ergometrine) all tend to elevate the blood pressure; levels above 140/90, 10 minutes or more after delivery, must be reported. *Proper treatment will avert eclampsia or cerebral haemorrhage, either of which may prove fatal.*

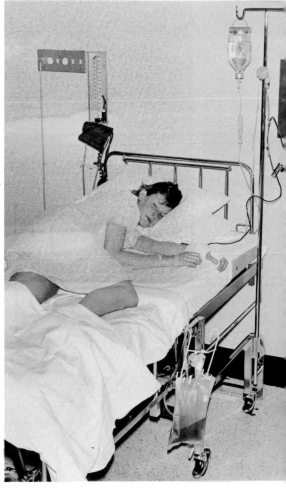

Figure 43.13 The lateral position is comfortable and tends to maintain the contracted uterus in the anteverted position. After forceps delivery of a 3,790 g infant this patient required vaginal packing to control severe haemorrhage from vaginal lacerations. The indwelling catheter was required until the pack was removed 16 hours later.

Medical disorders. These conditions are described in separate chapters. However, the rapid physiological changes occurring at the time of delivery should be remembered, and special care given to patients with such conditions as cardiac disease and diabetes mellitus.

Voiding. The recently delivered mother may find voiding difficult as a result of the trauma of delivery, and if the bladder appears full on palpation or there is excess blood loss from the birth canal, *catheterization* is advisable.

Rhesus testing. If the mother is rhesus negative, blood should be taken for laboratory tests (plain tube: blood group and antibodies; sequestrene: Kleihauer test).

OPERATIVE PROCEDURES

chapter forty-four

Induction of Labour

OVERVIEW

In some 5–25% of pregnancies, there comes a time when the fetus and/or mother would be better off if delivery was effected. The wide range is explained by different practices in different communities regarding elective induction of labour at 40 weeks' gestation, or 40 weeks plus 7–10 days, when there is no bona fide maternal or fetal indication. If the situation is one of considerable urgency, Caesarean section is normally undertaken; in less pressing circumstances, the onset of labour is brought about by one or more procedures to stimulate the uterus e.g. *rupture of the forewaters,* administration of *intravenous oxytocin by infusion,* or administration of *prostaglandin.* Before 28 weeks, the procedure is termed therapeutic abortion: if the abdominal approach is used, the procedure is termed a hysterotomy. A knowledge of the state of mother and fetus and the velocity of deterioration in this state gives a valid basis for the type and timing of the intervention. Neglect in the observance of these ground rules has led to women's action groups questioning the scale of labour induction, and in particular, its use for the convenience of the hospital and/or its staff.

Preeclampsia, prolonged pregnancy and *fetal growth retardation* are the 3 major indications and together they account for more than 50% of inductions (table 44.1). A variety of other disorders may compromise the mother and baby. In the past decade the incidence of induction has more than trebled, largely as a result of *elective inductions* performed at 40–41 weeks' gestation in patients with a well effaced cervix and cephalic presentation, the head having entered the pelvis. This practice is well established and favoured by many patients and obstetricians. However, it is never justifiable to perform an elective induction when maturity of the fetus is in doubt, its life being at the mercy of the mother's memory (menstrual data, date of quickening). The decision as to when to terminate requires experience and judgement, and should not be an arbitrary one. Inducing too early or too late carries penalties which are sometimes severe for the mother and baby.

The introduction of *prostaglandins* to clinical practice, particularly their local use to ripen the cervix, has removed one of the major difficulties of labour induction. Long induction-delivery intervals or even failure of the procedure are now uncommon, with a corresponding reduction of such associated problems as amnionitis and fetal infection.

Stimulation of uterine activity is never without risk — this is as true for prostaglandins as it was for all earlier oxytocic agents (pituitary extract of the past (Pituitrin), modern synthetic oxytocin (Syntocinon)) and is true for *all routes of administration.* Ideally, continuous fetal heart monitoring should be performed in any patient receiving an oxytocic agent to avoid fetal death due to uterine hypertonus, this having already occurred with vaginal prostaglandins as it did with previous oxytocic agents.

Amniotomy is the safest and most effective method of induction of labour. When labour is not established within 4 hours, an intravenous infusion of oxytocin should be commenced — 5 units/litre in nulliparas and 2 units/litre in multiparas; the rate of infusion commences at 10–20 drops/minute and is increased in 3 increments to 60 drops/minute; an increase in the concentration of the oxytocic agent is required in about 50% of nulliparas, but in fewer than 10% of multiparas. The advantage of withholding oxytocin at the time of amniotomy is that it is often unnecessary — also when contractions are strong it is much less frightening to the observer (risk of uterine hypertonus and/or rupture) when they are initiated by the powers of Nature!

A pregnancy is usually terminated when its continuation poses an undue threat to the well-being of the mother or fetus. Before the 26–28th weeks, the pregnancy is terminated usually for reasons of maternal risk; after the 26–28th weeks, the fetus is considered potentially viable and the procedure is more likely to be carried out for fetal or combined fetal and maternal indications. After 28 weeks, the procedure is termed induction of labour; before this, it is termed *therapeutic abortion*.

When induction of labour is undertaken, consideration must be given to 2 opposing sets of variables: the risk of maternal and/or fetal morbidity or death if the pregnancy continues, against the *risk of prematurity*, coupled with the possible *complications of the induction*, if the pregnancy is terminated.

INCIDENCE

Induction of labour is required in 5–25% of pregnancies, the latter figure being representative of a maternity hospital receiving nonbooked and emergency cases, the former being representative of a nonselected obstetric practice. As mentioned above the higher figure is heavily weighted by many patients and practitioners being reluctant to allow pregnancy to proceed past the estimated date of confinement (full term).

TIMING OF INDUCTION

One of the essentials of antenatal care is to establish the maturity of the fetus in the first half of pregnancy to enable proper timing of induction of labour or elective Caesarean section *if* these procedures become indicated later in pregnancy. Hence the need for all patients to note prospectively the date of quickening, and for ultrasonic verification of fetal maturity no later than 18–20 weeks' gestation when menstrual data and clinical estimation of uterine size do not correspond.

Correct timing is more likely if consideration is given to the following: (i) accurate diagnosis of the complication, (ii) a knowledge of the natural history of the complication, (iii) the status of the mother, (iv) the status of the fetus (oestriol or other function test), and finally (v) the effect of treatment.

INDICATIONS

At least 50% of inductions will be for one or more of the following conditions: *preeclampsia, prolonged pregnancy, fetal growth retardation/ distress, hypertension.* It should be emphasized that these conditions do not automatically warrant induction of labour — the severity of the condition, the condition of the fetus, and the favourability of the cervix etc must be carefully assessed. A list of the indications at a large maternity hospital is shown in table 44.1. In this series the decisions to perform amniotomy were made by a number of obstetricians with a wide range of opinion and clinical expertise.

Induction *at 40 weeks' gestation without other reason* is a 'social indication' and risks the unnecessary hazard of prematurity, for the reliability of the menstrual data, especially in this era of postpill conception, is in doubt in 20–30% of patients.

TABLE 44.1   INDICATIONS FOR SURGICAL INDUCTION OF LABOUR

	Number*	%
Preeclampsia	2,039	20.5
Prolonged pregnancy	2,023	20.3
Elective	1,374	13.8
Fetal growth retardation/placental insufficiency	921	9.2
Poor weight gain/weight loss	743	7.4
Hypertension	517	5.2
Spurious labour	207	2.0
Antepartum haemorrhage	120	1.2
Diabetes	91	0.9
Rhesus isoimmunization	86	0.8
Other or not stated	1,817	18.2

* Representing 9,938 consecutive inductions at a major teaching hospital — an incidence of 24.2%

(a) *Preeclampsia.* Moderate or severe degrees of this disease are uncommon if antenatal care has been adequate. If the condition is present, induction is usually indicated when there is (i) persistent proteinuria (1–7 days, according to severity), (ii) uncontrolled hypertension (diastolic pressure over 100), (iii) period of gestation beyond 37 weeks, (iv) evidence of fetal growth retardation or impaired fetoplacental function tests.

The advantages of induction before 40 weeks' gestation for the milder forms of preeclampsia (generalized oedema with mildly elevated blood pressure), particularly in the young nullipara, are often outweighed by such disadvantages as the difficulty of establishing labour and the risks of intrauterine infection. Attention to dietary measures — particularly a reduction of all forms of carbohydrates (including fruit) and an increase in vegetable roughage — and the selective use of bed rest will often enable induction to be postponed or avoided.

(b) *Hypertension with or without renal disease.* Similar remarks to the above may be made, particularly where the younger nullipara is concerned. Induction of labour before 40 weeks' gestation is seldom easy in such patients. Most patients can now be controlled with rest, sedation, and the selective use of hypotensive agents. Induction before full term should be reserved for those patients in whom induction appears easy and those presenting evidence of *placental insufficiency.*

In patients with *renal disease,* the prognosis is determined largely by the degree of elevation of the blood pressure and the blood urea at the start of the pregnancy. Proteinuria *per se,* even if in large amounts (nephrotic syndrome), has little effect on fetal prognosis. As with hypertension, each case must be considered individually, preferably with the help of consultation early in pregnancy. Occasionally, pregnancy represents a threat to the mother because of renal infection, usually the result of mechanical obstruction to the urinary tract or a renal calculus. Progressive renal damage may also occur in uncontrolled or poorly controlled preeclampsia or hypertension.

(c) *Prolonged pregnancy.* In the vast majority of patients with uncomplicated prolonged pregnancy (42 weeks or beyond) the fetus will come to no harm. Where placental insufficiency supervenes, there is almost always evidence of liquor absorption and its staining by meconium. This is reflected in loss of weight of the patient. The rate at which this change can take place has not been studied fully and because of this, induction of labour must often be performed empirically. However, in the younger nullipara with an unfavourable cervix, unless there is positive evidence of placental failure, induction should be deferred and the patient seen twice weekly and carefully assessed, preferably with the aid of cardiotocography, fetal kick charts and/or amnioscopy, and perhaps ultrasonography (to assess the amount of liquor etc).

Needless to say, corroborative evidence of fetal maturity should be obtained where possible (regularity and normality of the menstrual cycle, uterine size in the first trimester, and the time of quickening). Prolonged pregnancy increases the risk of the fetus in patients with such conditions as preeclampsia and hypertension.

(d) *Fetal growth retardation/placental insufficiency.* This is diagnosed when there is failure of the normal increase in maternal weight, girth, and fundal height; uterine hypertonus and diminution in liquor volume; reduced fetal movements, low urinary or plasma oestrogen levels; abnormalities on cardiotocography.

(e) *Elective induction.* As stated above this practice is not recommended, but must be listed because it has become established practice. When there is doubt about fetal maturity, and when there is no absolute fetal or maternal indication for induction, amniocentesis should be performed to confirm fetal pulmonary maturity. (lecithin: sphingomyelin ratio greater than 2:1).

(f) *Spurious labour.* This is not a bona fide indication for induction. It is often acted upon in the patient who comes into hospital at full term $\pm$ 7 days with contractions that fade away. It is recommended that such patients be sent home after checking fetal well-being by cardiotocography.

(g) *Antepartum haemorrhage.* (i) With *abruptio placentae* of moderate or severe degree, rupture of the membranes is indicated to reduce intrauterine tension and to start labour, after the mother has been resuscitated by blood transfusion, and blood coagulation failure, if present, has been corrected. In lesser degrees of abruption, induction will usually depend on the degree of involvement of the placenta, as evidenced by clinical findings. Some patients with little more than a mild haemorrhage (albeit repeated) may have placental abnormalities (circumvallate type), and recent work has indicated that placental failure is more common in this group. (ii) Where the bleeding is caused by a *placenta praevia* there is rarely any fetal disturbance as a result of diminished placental reserve, and induction of labour is seldom necessary for the latter reason. Rupture of the membranes may be indicated if labour has commenced, the placenta does not cover the os, and bleeding per vaginam is not copious.

(h) *Diabetes.* Induction of labour is performed electively at about 38 weeks' gestation to minimize the risk of intrauterine death near term. The presence of complications (preeclampsia, hypertension, renal disease, fetal distress, unstable disease etc) may indicate earlier induction or elective Caesarean section.

(i) *Rhesus isoimmunization.* This has become a less common indication due to prevention by administration of anti-D gamma globulin to nonisoimmunized rhesus negative mothers who give birth to rhesus positive infants.

(j) *Premature rupture of the membranes.* The period of gestation at which active interference is warranted depends to some extent on the presence of associated conditions such as preeclampsia, the estimated size of the fetus, and the presence or absence of amnionitis. Generally, if the pregnancy is 35–37 weeks or more, induction is indicated.

TABLE 44.2   INDICATIONS FOR SURGICAL INDUCTION OF LABOUR BEFORE 36 WEEKS' GESTATION

	Number*	%
Preeclampsia	120	55.0
Fetal death in utero	31	14.2
Fetal malformation	20	9.1
Rhesus isoimmunization	16	7.3
Fetal growth retardation	10	4.5
Accidental haemorrhage	8	3.6
Acute polyhydramnios	3	1.3
Other	10	4.5

* Represents 2.2% of surgical inductions (218 of 9,938) performed in one hospital

(k) *Miscellaneous.* This group comprises fetal death in utero, fetal malformations, acute poly-hydramnios etc. The large number of cases in this category shown in table 44.1 is explained by failure of the operator to record any indication for the procedure in the patients' case notes!

Only about 2% of surgical inductions are performed *before 36 weeks' gestation*. Table 44.2 illustrates that induction of labour before certain fetal viability is performed only for definite clinical indications. Table 44.3 is included for the reader's perspective to give an overview of the complications, mode of delivery and perinatal mortality rate in a series of almost 10,000 inductions of labour.

CONTRAINDICATIONS

(i) *Cephalopelvic disproportion*, unless slight, including the nullipara with a high head; (ii) *abnormal presentation* (with the possible exception of face or breech); (iii) *unstable lie* — risk of cord prolapse; (iv) *fetal distress* — Caesarean section would be indicated; (v) *placenta praevia*; (vi) *cord presentation*; (vii) *vasa praevia*; (viii) *invasive carcinoma of the cervix*.

PATIENT ASSESSMENT

Great care is necessary if there is antepartum haemorrhage, grand multiparity, previous uterine scar, history of rapid labour, breech or face presentation, and a patient less than 153 cm tall.

Before induction of labour by any method, certain preliminaries must be undertaken. (i) *Explanation of the procedure* to the patient to allay apprehension. (ii) Careful *examination of the abdomen* to assess the amount of liquor, nature of the presenting part and its station in the pelvis, and the fetal heart rate pattern. Particular thought should be given to the patient with a *high, mobile presenting part* before proceeding to induction. Since placenta praevia and

TABLE 44.3   DATA FROM A SERIES OF 9,938 CONSECUTIVE SURGICAL INDUCTIONS OF LABOUR

	Number	%
Prolapse of the umbilical cord	22	0.2
Multiple pregnancy	136	1.3
Epidural analgesia in labour	1,882	18.9
Prolonged labour (>24 hours)	204	2.0
Rupture of the uterus	7	0.07
Birth-weight < 2,500 g	447	4.5
Manipulative delivery	2,897	29.1
Forceps	2,027*	20.4
Caesarean section	753*	7.5
Breech	117	1.1
Postpartum haemorrhage	519	5.2
Genital tract infection	118	1.1
Stillbirths	111	1.1
Hypoxia/preeclampsia	58	
Congenital malformations	22	
Accidental haemorrhage	12	
Erythroblastosis	4	
Other	15	
Neonatal deaths	71	0.7
Hyaline membrane disease	37	
Congenital malformations	24	
Other	10	

* Incidences of forceps delivery and Caesarean section in the total hospital population were 26.1% and 11.3%, respectively (table 16.3)

prolapse of the cord are both likely in this situation, the patient should have been fasted for 4 hours and a theatre should be available if required. At the start of the procedure, vaginal examination should be carried out. The state of the cervix will be assessed and the presenting part confirmed. An idea of the *likelihood of induction success* can be gained from the *Bishop score* (cervical dilatation and effacement, each graded 0-3, station of presenting part 0-3, cervical consistency and position, each graded 0-2). A score of 9 or more favours induction success, remembering that cervical dilatation will exert the greatest influence; effacement and consistency of the cervix and station of the presenting part will exert about half this effect; cervical position, the remaining parameter, will exert the least effect. If the score is 4 or less, only pressing indications should be allowed and then some form of cervical ripening (a local prostaglandin gel, Foley catheter, or laminaria tent) should precede the amniotomy. Even with Bishop scores of 5-6, there is usually a longer interval before

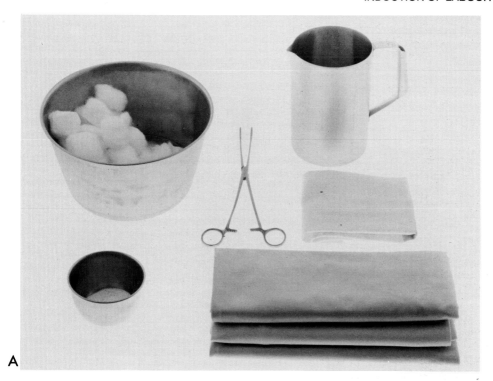

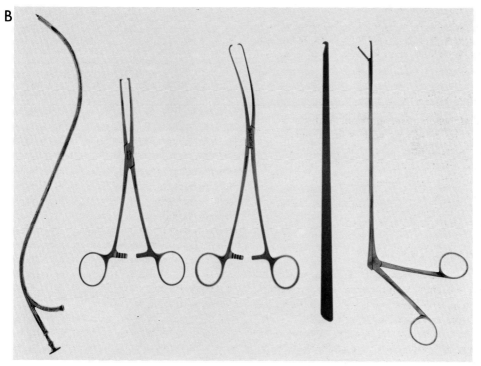

Figure 44.1 Instrument tray for artificial rupture of the membranes. **A.** The tray as set up by the central sterilization department in the hospital. The large bowl contains swabs and 1 in 1,000 aqueous chlorhexidine solution for washing down the vulva with sponge holding forceps; the small bowl contains 1% chlorhexidine cream; the small towel is for drying hands before donning gloves; the drapes are placed under the buttocks and to cover thighs and abdomen. The jug, although shown here, is available in a separate sterile pack when required for collection of liquor via a Drew Smythe catheter. **B.** Range of instruments used in order from left to right: Drew-Smythe catheter with obturator, Kocher forceps, vulsellum, AmniHook and alligator forceps. Each instrument is available in a separate sterile pack. Most obstetricians favour the alligator forceps once conversant with its use. The Drew-Smythe catheter is used when there is an undilated cervix or high presenting part.

the onset of labour, a higher failure rate, a longer labour, greater likelihood of operative delivery and a higher infection rate. The rare conditions of *vasa praevia* and *cord presentation* may be found.

Amnioscopy is used by some as an adjunct to amniotomy, the advantages claimed being detection of vasa praevia and cord presentation, greater accuracy, and greater patient comfort.

ARTIFICIAL RUPTURE OF MEMBRANES (SURGICAL INDUCTION)

This is the prime method of induction of labour, because of its reliability.

Instrument tray. The instruments and materials used are shown in figure 44.1.

Pain relief. This may vary from reassurance when the cervix is partly dilated and favourable, to effective analgesia where the cervix is undilated, hard and uneffaced. Frequently, nitrous oxide/oxygen or pethidine (100 mg IM) with or without a tranquillizer (Phenergan, 25 mg IM) is satisfactory.

Asepsis. Careful asepsis is more vital here than with almost any other surgical procedure, because of the possibility of a prolonged induction-delivery interval and the relative ineffectiveness of chemotherapy as far as the fetus is concerned. Pathogenic organisms, particularly anaerobes, are more often present than absent in the vagina, and particular care must be taken in swabbing out the vagina with a suitable antiseptic.

Membrane rupture (figure 44.2). Stretching the cervix and sweeping the membranes from the lower uterine segment probably enhance the likelihood of success (*prostaglandin release from decidua*) and make the procedure easier. The instrument used for the rupture depends on the preference of the operator; one of the specially designed instruments (AmniHook) is shown in figure 44.1 together with the other instruments in common use. Rupture of the *hindwaters by the Drew-Smythe catheter is less effective,* equally prone to cause infection, and carries the particular danger of placental separation and possibly damage to the lower uterine segment — it has the advantage of being an easier instrument to insert when the cervix is not effaced, the curve of the instrument allowing it to be passed up the cervical canal like a Hegar dilator, and then behind the head; with hindwater rupture the liquor can be collected into a container without contamination, for estimation of volume and colour (meconium). If there is a greater than normal amount of liquor, the hand should be kept in the vagina and the liquor released slowly with the presenting part being pushed into the pelvis from above. The use of the amnioscope has been referred to above. After the procedure, a check for *cord prolapse* is made, and the *fetal heart is listened to.* Further checks on the fetal heart are advisable each 10–15 minutes for the next hour. In some centres, an intrauterine catheter will be inserted to monitor contractions and a scalp electrode to monitor fetal condition.

Bed rest. Unless there is a specific indication for the patient to be in bed (preeclampsia) she should be ambulant, because labour will ensue earlier and prolapse of the cord is less likely. The bladder is preferably emptied every 2–4 hours until delivery.

A   B

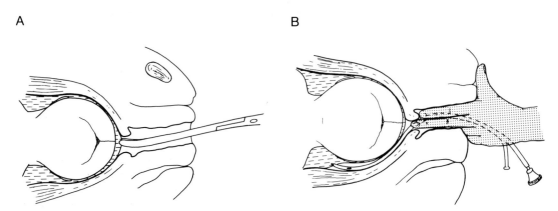

Figure 44.2 Techniques of amniotomy. **A.** Rupture of the forewaters with a vulsellum. The cervix is 2–3 cm dilated and the forewaters are within easy reach. The instrument is held against the head as it is closed in order to grasp and tear the chorion and amnion. The hole is then enlarged with the forefinger to allow further escape of liquor. **B.** Rupture of hindwaters with a Drew-Smythe catheter. The middle finger of the left hand is used to direct the catheter into the cervical canal — the handle is then depressed so that the catheter passes around the fetal head and enters the pool of liquor around the neck.

Chemotherapy. As far as the fetus is concerned, there is nothing to lose and much to gain by the employment of chemotherapy if delivery is not within sight after 12 hours. To achieve adequate levels in the fetal blood stream, twice normal doses should be given until delivery. Because of poor maternal absorption, oral therapy is most unreliable once labour has commenced. Cover will be necessary for both aerobic and anaerobic organisms. If the patient is undelivered 24 hours after amniotomy, a high vaginal swab should be taken for microscopy and culture, and chemotherapy commenced.

Failure of induction after membrane rupture. If labour has not commenced after 2–6 hours, depending on circumstances, an intravenous oxytocin infusion should be commenced unless contraindicated on other grounds. Many obstetricians routinely combine an oxytocin infusion with amniotomy to shorten the induction-delivery interval, minimize the risk of infection and maximize the probability of daytime delivery. As stated above, we prefer to wait about 4 hours after rupture of the membranes before commencing an oxytocin infusion — this avoids many infusions with their risks of uterine hypertonus and fetal hypoxia, and the pressure on nursing staff to monitor a forest of infusion sets in busy delivery suites. Serious consideration should be given to Caesarean section if the patient is not delivered within 24–36 hours of amniotomy. Indications for this operation may be aggravation of the preexisting complication, a fresh complication (such as fetal distress), or a problem related to the induction.

OXYTOCIN

Stimulation of the uterus with oxytocin is less effective when the membranes are intact and therefore it is usually only *primarily* indicated when the membranes have spontaneously ruptured after the 35th–37th week, there is a fetal death in utero, or there is some other contraindication to forewater rupture. Even with fetal death in utero we consider that rupture of the membranes should precede oxytocin infusion — to minimize the risk of coagulation failure caused by entry of thromboplastin into the maternal circulation. It has a role in cervical ripening, equivalent to local prostaglandin (though less easy to use).

All methods involving the administration of oxytocin suffer from the fact that there is an extremely wide variation in sensitivity from patient to patient (approximately 500-fold).

Assessment of uterine sensitivity. The following factors will usually be associated with a decreased sensitivity to oxytocin: (i) intact membranes, (ii) earlier gestation period, (iii) low parity, (iv) unfavourable cervix (firm, uneffaced, undilated, posteriorly placed — '*sacral cervix*'), (v) nonirritable uterus.

Technique of Administration

(i) *Intravenous infusion method.* The concentration is decided upon according to the above factors and will, in the first instance, usually be of the order of 2 to 5 units per 1,000 ml infusion fluid. An electrolyte-containing solution (e.g. Hartmann solution) is preferable to 5% dextrose because it reduces the risk of *water intoxication*. The addition of an ampoule of a suitably coloured solution for identification (vitamin B) is advisable. Alternatively, the oxytocin infusion pump line is inserted into the Hartmann solution drip line. A 20-gauge intracath needle inserted into a vein on the forearm provides the patient with maximum comfort and mobility. A *microdrip apparatus* delivers approximately 60 drops per ml, and provides a safer and more manageable infusion rate, because a smaller volume of fluid is infused. The rate in mU/minute can be calculated simply. For example, 5 units of oxytocin per 1,000 ml = 5 mU in 1 ml. If the microdrip apparatus delivers 60 drops/ml and the rate is 60 drops/minute, then 5 mU/minute will be delivered; at 15 drops/minute, only 1.25 mU/minute will be delivered, which is a good starting dose. Normal drip sets often have only 15–20 drops/ml, so that 3 to 4 times the above rates will be delivered at similar drip rates/minute.

The most important phase of the operation is the first ½ to 2 hours of the infusion. Critical observation of the fetal heart and uterine response at this time provides a valuable guide to the further management of the infusion.

In the *absence of contractions* it is standard practice to commence at 15–20 drops/minute and increase in 3 increments at intervals of 15–30 minutes to a maximum of 60 drops per minute. Thereafter, the oxytocin concentration is quadrupled and the rate is resumed at 10 drops/minute; alternatively, the concentration may be doubled and the rate halved. The rate is increased until *regular contractions of moderate intensity are occurring every 2–3 minutes* — timing of contractions being from the beginning of one contraction to the beginning of the next. In multiparas it is seldom necessary to increase the initial concentration (2 units/litre) of the infusion; in nulliparas about 50% require an increase in the initial concentration (5 units/

litre). Accurate infusion rates may be obtained with a drip monitor or one of the varieties of *infusion pump* which are available. Some of the latter are provided with fail-safe devices which turn off the machine and activate an alarm should the uterine pressure or fetal heart rate deviate from the normal range.

During the infusion, the drip rate and nature of contractions should be assessed every 15 minutes. The *fetal heart rate* should preferably be monitored continuously, or failing that, every 15 minutes. The *maternal pulse rate* is checked every 15 minutes, the *blood pressure* hourly and the *temperature* every 4 hours (evidence of infection). The vulval pad is observed every 15 minutes for evidence of haemorrhage or passage of meconium. If the contractions are occurring at intervals of less than 2½ minutes the rate of the infusion should be slowed; if there is *fetal or maternal distress*, or *vaginal bleeding*, the infusion should be discontinued and the situation reported immediately.

It is preferable to commence oxytocin infusions in the morning; during the night the patient should be sleeping, and a nurse is less often available for the careful observation of the patient that is necessary. In the nullipara, particularly, a critical assessment should be made (including cervical examination) in the midafternoon to ascertain what progress has been made. This in-progress assessment is even more important if the infusion is being repeated on a subsequent day.

Failure to establish labour usually indicates an insensitive uterus and the need for higher dosages of oxytocin, provided the fetal heart is satisfactory. Occasionally, reassessment will reveal that the forewaters are not fully ruptured.

The procedure may have to be abandoned because of *fetal or maternal distress*, or if satisfactory progress is not being made in cervical dilatation or descent of the presenting part. Anxiety on the part of the patient and/or obstetrician may sometimes be a contributing factor to termination of the procedure. The importance of adequate rest, sleep, hydration, and caloric intake during the induction period should be stressed.

(ii) *Buccal tablet method.* The buccal route has the advantage of ease of administration and patient acceptance. However, it is less efficient than intravenous oxytocin and less safe — a number of uterine ruptures have been reported with the method; because of this the buccal route is no longer used in many centres. Similarly, the *intranasal spray method* and *intramuscular* method of administration of oxytocin are no longer used — because the drug cannot be 'turned off' if uterine hyperactivity occurs, and uniform dosage (rate of absorption) cannot be ensured via these routes.

PROSTAGLANDINS

The prostaglandins are 20-carbon prostanoic acid derivatives, and 4 basic groups exist (A, B, E, and F). Each of these is further subdivided into 1 or 2, depending on the number of saturated bonds between the carbon atoms, and alpha or beta, depending on their spatial arrangement. Only the E_1, E_2 and F_2 compounds are of obstetrical interest. Each has a stimulating effect on uterine muscle. Apart from this intrinsic effect, prostaglandins have been shown to cause oxytocin release from the posterior lobe of the pituitary gland. The routes of administration can be oral, intravenous, extraamniotic, intraamniotic, or high vaginal. Since oxytocin is more dependent on gestational maturity, prostaglandin is preferred for inductions before 35–37 weeks in patients with low Bishop scores, and where the fetus is dead or anencephalic. Advantages of prostaglandins, apart from the above, include absence of water retention, specific cervical ripening effect and effectiveness via a number of different routes. The main disadvantage is the much narrower therapeutic range.

Cervical Preparation
When the Bishop score is 4 or less, vaginal application of prostaglandin (1–3 mg E_2 gel or pessary) the evening prior to induction will usually ripen the cervix sufficiently to facilitate both artificial rupture of the membranes and the onset of labour. In such cases, the fetus should be monitored for 2–3 hours after application. The application can be repeated the next morning if the criteria for amniotomy are not met. The technique is particularly valuable where a long and difficult labour is undesirable (cardiac disorder, breech presentation, previous Caesarean section, dysmaturity). With this technique, Caesarean section for failure of the induction should be no more than 1–2%.

In the extraamniotic infusion, a 30 ml size 12 or 14 Foley catheter is placed inside the cervix, inflated and a 250 µg/ml strength solution is infused at a rate of 3 ml/2 hours. This is preceded by a 1 ml test dose. This method should not be used in the presence of local infection, in patients with a uterine scar, or in those where the uterus appears irritable.

Induction of Labour
The concentrations of the 2 most commonly used compounds are 5 µg/ml (PGE$_2$) and 50 µg/ml

(PGF$_2$ alpha). This is equivalent to approximately 40 mU/ml of oxytocin. The intravenous infusion rate for PGF$_2$ alpha usually ranges from 2.5 to 25 μg/minute, that for PGE$_2$ being 1/10th of this, due to its greater potency. The same technique and precautions are used as for the oxytocin infusion. Experience indicates that the success rate is similar in the different groups, other factors being much more decisive (maturity of the fetus, parity, station of the presenting part, state of the membranes, and cervical 'score').

Prostaglandins may also be administered *orally*, the 0.5 mg tablet of PgE$_2$ is repeated at 30-60 minute intervals until labour is established. Although the oral route, as with oxytocin, is more dangerous than the intravenous route, a major advantage is the freedom from the infusion; this allows a greater degree of mobility with a resultant decrease in overall oxytocic and analgesic requirement and better fetal condition. Great care is required in assessment and supervision of the labour; there is a greater risk in the parous patient (rapid delivery, damage to the birth canal, fetal hypoxia). Newer, more potent preparations are now appearing commercially, but their effect on the fetus has not been fully evaluated.

The main *side-effects* of prostaglandins are nausea and vomiting (5-20% of IV infusions according to dose), diarrhoea, hot flushes, and phlebitis at the site of infusion. These effects are far more likely with the higher doses used for induction of abortion in the period from the 12th to the 20th weeks of pregnancy. Great care should be exercised if the patient gives a history of asthma or raised intraocular tension or if there is a scar in the uterus. Increases in uterine tone and prolongation of contractions should be looked for carefully. Since prostaglandins have no antidiuretic action, unlike oxytocin, they are preferred for patients with renal and heart disease, and where high doses of oxytocin would be needed (e.g. early fetal death).

OESTRADIOL

In trials on nulliparas, this compound in a dose of 150 mg has a comparable action to 4 mg of PgE$_2$. It is thought to act by an effect on the cervix (increase in collagenase and thus a softening) and perhaps also by facilitating natural oxytocin and/or prostaglandins. It has few unwanted side-effects.

FOLEY CATHETER

In patients in whom the *cervix is unfavourable*, good results may be obtained by the insertion of a 30 ml Foley catheter, through the cervix, and then inflating it. Labour usually ensues within 6-12 hours, when the bag is expelled. An extra-amniotic prostaglandin infusion (1-3 μg/ml) may be used concurrently. This technique, and the use of laminaria tents, although much less expensive than prostaglandin, increases infectious morbidity of both mother and baby.

COMPLICATIONS OF INDUCTION

Abnormalities of the fetal heart rate, especially if early in labour, usually point to the need for Caesarean section. Unaccounted distress of the patient, perhaps with nausea or vomiting, may indicate impending obstruction or a severe form of uterine incoordination, or even uterine rupture; vaginal bleeding during the course of infusion, as with the above, calls for its immediate cessation and careful review of the situation.

Precipitate delivery and/or uterine rupture. These are the major problems related to oxytocin administration. They will be seen most often where (i) there is inadequate supervision, (ii) the route of administration and dose of oxytocic is not optimal, and (iii) the patient has been poorly selected (disproportion, grand multiparity, scarred uterus).

Fetal asphyxia. In 3-5% of labour inductions there will be fetal heart irregularities associated with uterine hypertonus. This tendency is aggravated in patients having epidural analgesia. Although the uterine overactivity may not lead to rupture, there is often severe reduction of oxygenation to an already compromised fetus. If the intrauterine pressure between contractions exceeds 12 mm Hg, the infusion should be ceased to avoid impairment of placental blood flow and ensuing fetal distress.

Amniotic fluid embolism. This is a rare complication, and usually follows uterine hyperactivity and a tear in the lower uterine segment. Contractions should not occur at intervals of less than 3 minutes.

Infection. This may have serious consequences for both mother and fetus. In the mother, pelvic infection may result in future sterility or other morbidity. In the fetus, intrauterine infection may result in death or severe neonatal morbidity.

Postpartum haemorrhage. There is a tendency for uterine atony, leading to primary postpartum haemorrhage, after labours induced with oxytocin. Because of this it is advisable to maintain the oxytocic infusion for at least 1 hour after delivery — with this regimen the incidence of

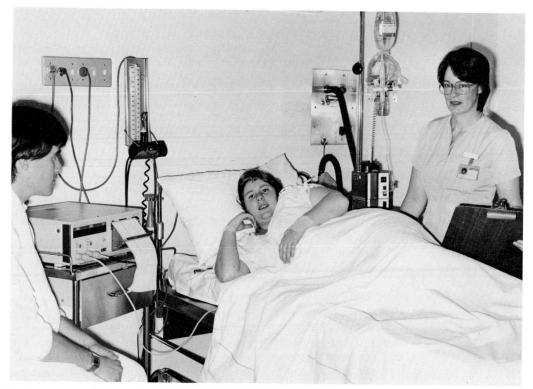

Figure 44.3 Induction of labour because of spontaneous rupture of the membranes at 37 weeks' gestation. Note peristaltic pump for control of the rate of infusion of the oxytocin solution. The fetal heart rate and uterine activity are being monitored by cardiotocography.

postpartum haemorrhage is the same (5.2%, table 44.3), as in the total hospital population (5.2%, table 16.1).

Miscellaneous complications. Damage to the lower uterine segment or placenta by the Drew-Smythe catheter has already been referred to. Direct trauma to the cervix is unusual and seldom troublesome. The problem of the vasa praevia has also been mentioned. *If bleeding follows amniotomy, the blood should be tested for fetal haemoglobin.*

Prolapse of the umbilical cord occurs with a frequency of approximately 0.1–1.0% (table 44.3); its occurrence can be minimized by attention to technique, particularly where there is a poorly-fitting presenting part at the time of induction.

Since oxytocin has an *antidiuretic action*, particularly in high doses (> 20 mU/minute), sodium and water retention may occur if the infusion is continued for more than 12 hours. In such cases, the fluid balance should be watched

carefully, or preferably the infusion should be recommended on the following day.

Unanticipated prematurity of the infant is now usually avoided by careful attention to history, obstetric examination, and special tests such as ultrasonic measurement, and liquor studies (surfactant level). *Jaundice* is increased if oxytocin has been used for induction.

MONITORING

Since, in many cases, induction of labour is undertaken because the fetus is at risk, it is logical that the fetal condition be monitored as intensively as is practical (preferably by continuous heart rate study, figure 44.3), and such stresses as uterine overactivity avoided (preferably by a continuous uterine pressure recording). The perineal pad should be checked for meconium staining at least every hour. Because of these requirements, the number of inductions by infusion in any one day in the labour ward should be rationalized.

chapter forty-five

Episiotomy

OVERVIEW

The incidence of episiotomy — the most *common of all operations* — will depend upon the obstetrician's philosophy of management of delivery — and the patient's approval of these attitudes. Those who favour almost routine episiotomy believe that when the head is safely accessible (on perineum) there is *no value in delay* — such practitioners stress that 10–15% of stillborn infants die just before birth without there having been previous evidence of distress. There is in addition an equal proportion of neonatal deaths due to unsuspected intrauterine hypoxia. The fetal heart rate is not usually monitored in the minutes before delivery — episiotomy ± low forceps delivery when the head is low could reduce the number of perinatal deaths and minimize the risks of hypoxia, so improving the *intellectual quality of survival*. This philosophy is opposed by those who favour *natural birth* with a minimum of interference. *An episiotomy wound is always painful*, but if properly repaired the long-term result (coital function) may be superior to that when episiotomy was deliberately avoided and the perineum remained intact. There can never be controlled clinical trials to settle this important issue, for episiotomy versus no episiotomy is not a simple option — a policy of no episiotomy can result in a sudden, uncontrolled perineal tear and few agree with the statement that a 'clean tear, is better than a careful incision?' It is preferable to have a temporarily painful perineum after delivery, due to an episiotomy wound, than a gaping introitus with absent perineal body due to excessive stretching and 'ironing out' of the perineum to facilitate delivery!

Episiotomy is usually regarded as a minor procedure and its performance and repair in clinical practice are often delegated to those who are relatively inexperienced and not always familiar with the anatomy of the region; this may lead to a less than satisfactory result.

As mentioned above there is current debate concerning the almost routine performance of episiotomy in the nullipara, the proper moment for its execution and its optimum siting. Some women's action groups place this operation in the category of 'ritual' surgery, and claim that the cost/benefit is insufficiently considered and that more can be done in the antenatal period to prepare the lower birth canal for the baby's exit without recourse to incisional or traumatic enlargement. This is obviously a matter that should be discussed with the patient in the antenatal period. The position adopted at birth, method of pushing, and control during delivery will also influence the frequency of episiotomy.

In practical terms, it should be remembered that *significant blood loss may occur from the episiotomy wound*, particularly if made too early. It can be a source of *much discomfort* in the early healing phase; *haematoma formation, wound breakdown*, and *infection* may further complicate the procedure.

Surveys of patients 3–6 months after delivery have revealed a significant number with persisting *dyspareunia* and symptomatic *vaginal relaxation* as unwanted reminders of the birth experience.

DEFINITION

An incision made in the perineum and vagina that enlarges the introitus and lessens the curve of the birth canal to facilitate the birth of the baby.

OBJECTIVES

(i) *To avoid undue pressure on the baby's head* and *facilitate delivery* when an inelastic perineum is delaying the second stage of labour. (ii) *To hasten delivery* when fetal distress or maternal exhaustion are present. (iii) *To enlarge the introitus* and reduce the curve of Carus. This avoids lacerations and bruising of the vagina, suburethral tissues and perineum; an episiotomy is easier to repair than a laceration and is less prone to infection.

INDICATIONS AND INCIDENCE

Episiotomy should be considered in the following circumstances: (i) When a tear of the perineum appears inevitable with 'crowning' of the head or during forceps delivery. (ii) All breech deliveries. (iii) When a premature baby is to be delivered. (iv) Delay in the second stage due to an inelastic perineum. (v) Fetal or maternal distress and prolonged labour if the head is on the perineum. (vi) Previous vaginal repair or third degree laceration. (vii) Prior to vaginal or intrauterine manipulations (mid-forceps, manual rotation of the head, internal version and breech extraction,

and delivery of impacted shoulders). (viii) Face to pubis delivery (either spontaneous or with forceps).

The *incidence* ranges from 0–90% in the nullipara, depending on geographic locality and the accoucheur's philosophy (see overview). The overall incidence is approximately 30– 40%. The operation usually needs to be repeated in subsequent deliveries because scars do not stretch.

TISSUES CUT BY THE EPISIOTOMY INCISION

(i) Vaginal epithelium and perineal skin. (ii) Colles fascia and bulbocavernosus muscle. (iii) Superficial and deep transverse perineal muscles. (iv) External anal sphincter (sometimes). (v) Levator ani muscle if the incision is extensive. Usually the muscle is displaced upwards away from the scissors as the head stretches the perineum. (vi) Ischiorectal fossa fat may be exposed in deep incisions.

TYPES (figure 45.1)

(i) *Median*. Not favoured unless the accoucheur is experienced, since extension through the anal sphincter may occur and result in a third degree tear. (ii) *Mediolateral* is the recommended variety. (iii) *J-shaped*. The incision starts in the midline and swings laterally to avoid the anal sphincter.

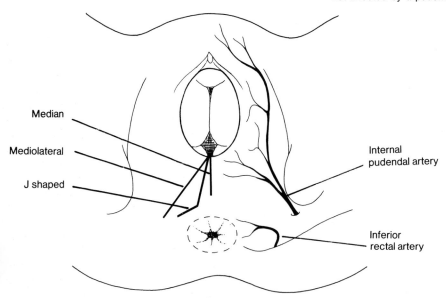

Figure 45.1 Types of episiotomy incision. If the incision extends past the anus it enters the area innervated by the perforating cutaneous nerves which are not affected by a pudendal nerve block.

Median

Mediolateral

J shaped

Internal pudendal artery

Inferior rectal artery

A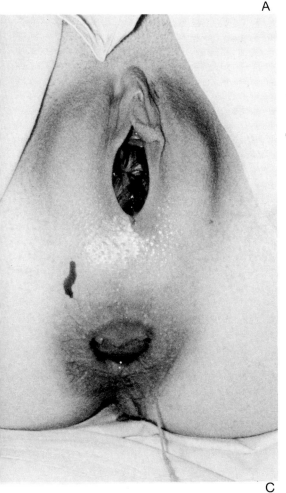

B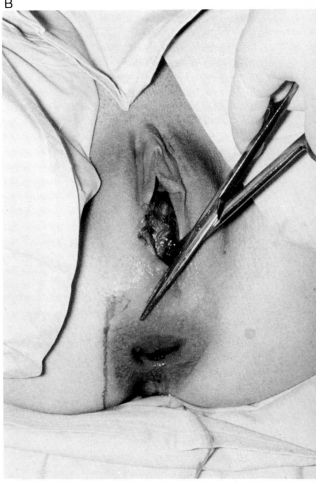

C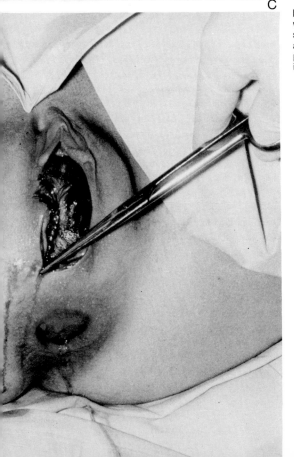

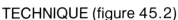

Figure 45.2 Technique of episiotomy. **A.** Local analgesia was provided by perineal infiltration (trickle of blood marks site of injection) when the head bulged the perineum. Note anal dilatation during a contraction. **B.** The scissors are in position at the fourchette. **C.** The incision being made during a contraction.

TECHNIQUE (figure 45.2)

Before episiotomy is carried out it is important to explain to the woman the reason for the procedure and what is involved. Regional analgesia is provided by local infiltration or pudendal nerve block (0.5–1% lignocaine), and this will also serve for the repair of the incision: 20 ml is the maximum safe volume which should be employed. A finger should be inserted into the vagina to *guard the fetal head* during local infiltration of the perineum; when the perineum bulges downwards during a contraction (figure 45.2) it is very thin and often the needle penetrates into the vagina. In the past when the patient was well sedated and breathing nitrous oxide, local analgesia was often dispensed with, when the perineum was stretched and thin. This practice caused unnecessary pain and understandable resentment by patients. *An episiotomy is always painful if local analgesia is not used.*

There are occasions however, when an episiotomy must be cut without the benefit of local analgesia e.g. perineal tear imminent with the patient pushing uncontrollably in strong labour.

The incision is made when the head bulges the perineum, since it is easier to judge the proper length, the anal sphincter is displaced, and blood loss is less.

One blade of the scissors is inserted inside the vagina with the cutting angle resting on the fourchette. This is important, since with the patient in the left lateral position it is easy for the scissors to slide up onto the right labium majus. Aim for a point midway between anus and ischial tuberosity and make a single cut during a contraction (figure 45.2).

If delivery is not immediate, control bleeding from the cut edges by firm pressure with a gauze swab while awaiting the next contraction. Occasionally, control of a bleeding point may require an artery clamp and ligature.

A median episiotomy should only be employed if the accoucheur is experienced. If extension to the rectum should occur (3–15% depending on the type of delivery) and repair is inadequate, the patient will suffer *rectal incontinence* and possibly *fistula formation*. This is more likely if the subpubic angle is narrow, the baby large, the delivery precipitate, and the vaginal part of the incision inadequate. The advantages of this technique are less bleeding, greater ease of repair, less pain during healing, and a lower incidence of subsequent dyspareunia.

REPAIR (figure 45.3)

The main *principles in repair* are to obtain haemostasis, align the edges anatomically, and not suture too tightly.

The patient is placed in the lithotomy position. The thighs should not be excessively abducted as this accentuates retraction of the lateral side of the wound and makes approximation difficult, and in addition may be uncomfortable for the patient. The operative field is swabbed, draped and well illuminated. Perineal infiltration with lignocaine 0.5–1% through the cut surface of the wound is performed if not already inserted. Absorbable sutures (chromic catgut 2/0 gauge) are used throughout.

The first step is the repair of the vaginal epithelium, and for this a continuous suture is used. A gauze pack is introduced into the vagina to aid exposure — it has an artery forceps attached so that it is not overlooked and left in the vagina. The structures to be sutured are identified and vaginal lacerations sought. Any arterial spurters

are clamped and ligated, but oozing from epithelial and skin edges is controlled by the pressure applied by the sutures. Haemostasis is imperative, otherwise extensive bruising and *haematoma formation* can occur, with the subsequent complications of *pain*, *infection*, and *disruption of the wound*. A forceps may be attached to the apex of the vaginal incision to ensure that it is visualized and sutured, otherwise bleeding may continue from it. Greater speed and better haemostasis are the advantages of a continuous suture, but interrupted sutures are favoured by many. Sutures are placed at about 1 cm intervals and a good bite of epithelium and submucosa is taken to obliterate dead space. Vaginal lacerations are also repaired. Sutures should not be tied too tightly because of the swelling which occurs in the following 24–48 hours. Three markers should be used for accurate opposition: the vaginal apex, the hymen and the mucocutaneous junction.

Occasionally the episiotomy incision extends high up the vagina, usually due to difficulty with the delivery of the *shoulders*. If the upper limit of the vaginal incision cannot be seen, a stitch is inserted as high as possible and tied; traction upon this stitch then exposes the upper limit of the incision which is sutured.

The second step is approximation of the perineal muscles. Interrupted sutures are used which control bleeding and reduce dead space, thus preventing haematoma formation. Usually 3 sutures are sufficient. The aim is to achieve good approximation with a minimum of buried catgut. The anatomical distortion inevitable with the mediolateral incision should be allowed for as the lower elements of the levator ani muscle and the bulbocavernosus muscle are sutured. The ultimate strength of the repaired pelvic floor depends mainly upon this layer.

The perineal skin is loosely approximated, the sutures being inserted 1 cm from the wound edges to give adequate apposition and to lessen the risk of their tearing out. It is preferable to commence anteriorly, since this facilitates accurate realignment of the wound edges. If the sutures start posteriorly, reconstitution of the perineal wedge tends to obscure unsutured tissue near the fourchette. The last few stitches are important for they prevent excessive scar tissue formation and future dyspareunia. Alternatively, a subcuticular suture may be used for the skin closure.

A vaginal examination ensures that no pack remains; *rectal examination* excludes stitches in the rectum and anal canal and *replaces prolapsed haemorrhoids* if present.

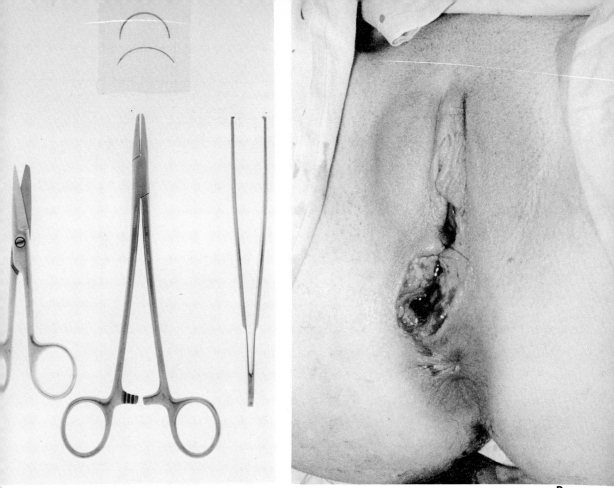

Figure 45.3 Repair of episiotomy. **A.** The instrument tray carries suture scissors, needle holder, toothed forceps, needles and swabs. The round-bodied needle is used for the vaginal epithelium and muscle layer. The skin is sutured using the cutting edged needle. **B.** The vaginal incision has been sutured from apex down to the introitus. **C.** Interrupted sutures have been inserted in the perineal muscles. **D.** After approximation of the skin edges, rectal examination is carried out to exclude the presence of sutures in the rectum or anal canal.

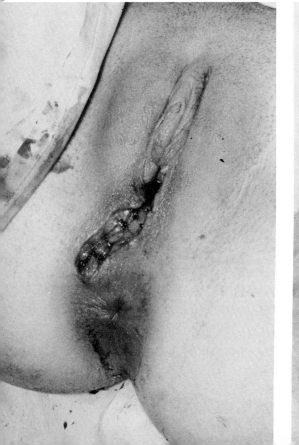

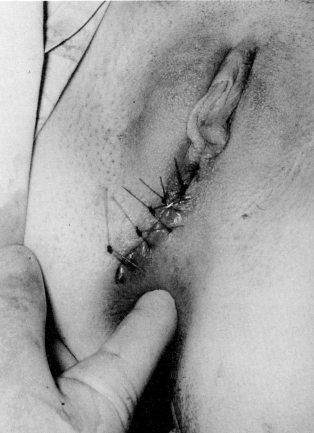

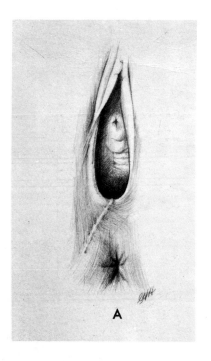

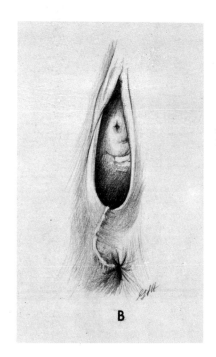

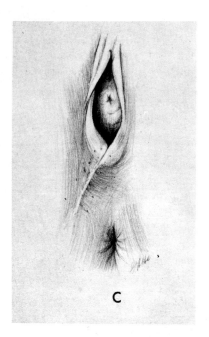

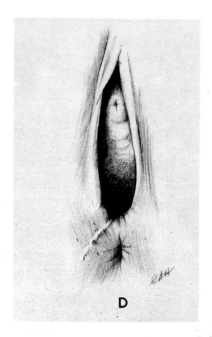

Figure 45.4 Results of episiotomy. **A.** The desired anatomical 'return to normal' result. **B.** Resultant scar when there has been a 'hockey stick' extension of the episiotomy into anal skin. **C.** Skin bridge: the perineum has been advanced by suturing the labia minora together. **D.** Rounded perineum with loss of perineal body due to failure to repair the deep layer. The result is that the bladder is exposed to coital thrust which often results in urinary symptoms. Failure to repair a torn anal sphincter may result in faecal incontinence. (From Beischer NA Med J Aust 1967; 2:189–195).

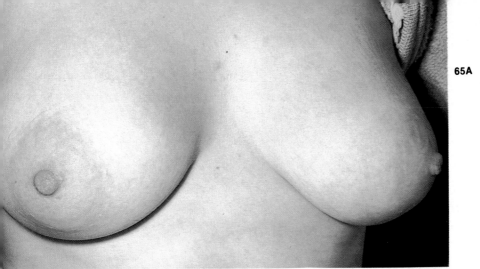

65A

Plate 65A A 24-year-old primigravida (weight 60.8 kg) at 8 weeks' gestation. She had noted swelling and tenderness of her breasts and nipples. Like most women she has not developed Montgomery follicles (colour plate 41).

Plate 65B The same patient showing engorgement of the breasts on day 5 of the puerperium. Note marked striae gravidarum and pigmentation. Her weight had increased to 78 kg at 38 weeks' gestation when Caesarean section was required for obstructed labour.

Plate 65C Her infant weighed 4,000 g at birth. Here, on day 5, he shows mild physiological jaundice. Like his mother he was blood group A rhesus positive.

Plate 65D Six weeks after birth the pigmentation of the linea nigra persists but the striae are somewhat less livid. The abdominal wall remains lax in spite of exercises. The Pfannenstiel incision has healed well. The mother's weight is 61.6 kg; the baby is fully breast-fed and weighs 5,600 g.

65B
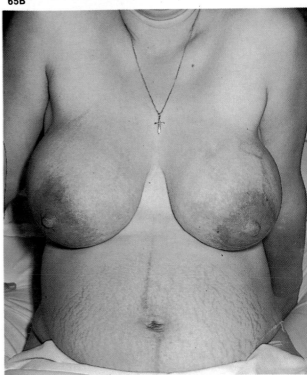

65C
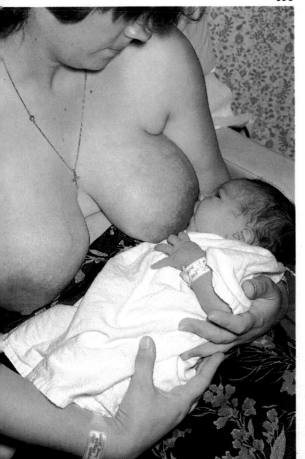

65D
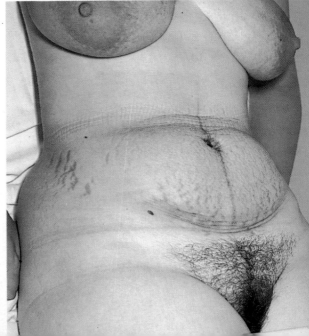

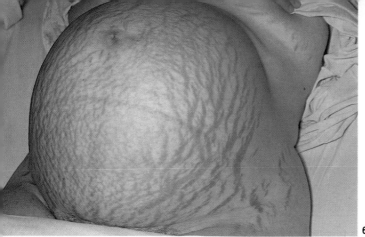

Plate 66A Primigravida (weight 102.6 kg) with twin pregnancy at 37 weeks' gestation, hospitalized because of preeclampsia. She has prodigious striae of abdomen, thighs and breasts.

66A

66B

Plate 66B She delivered spontaneously at 37.2 weeks, 5 hours after amniotomy. The fetal surface of the single placenta which weighed 1,145 g is shown. There are 2 succenturiate lobes and partial velamentous insertion of each umbilical cord.

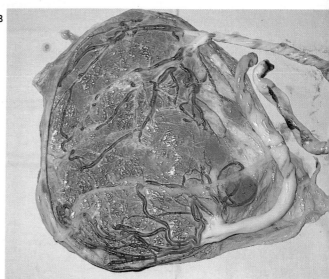

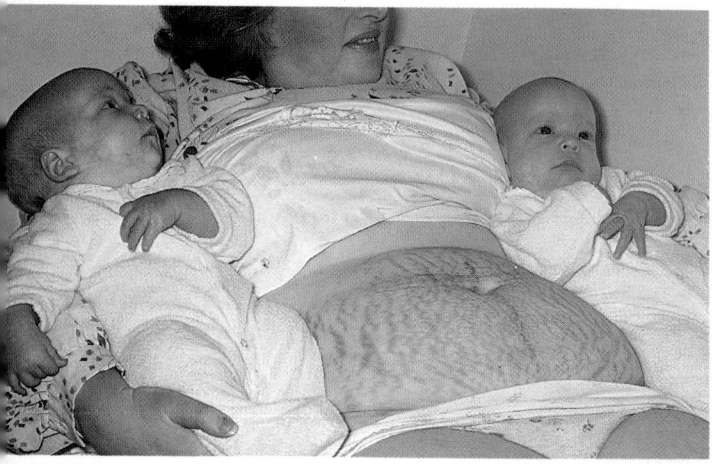

66C

Plate 66C The birth-weights of the identical twin boys, shown here aged 7 weeks, were 3,090 g and 2,610 g.

66D

Plate 66D Six months after delivery the patient has returned to her prepregnancy weight (84 kg). Her abdomen remains lax and the striae have not faded appreciably since the postnatal visit.

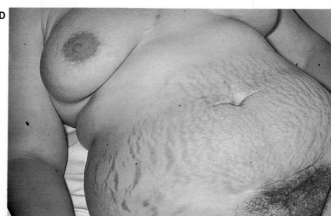

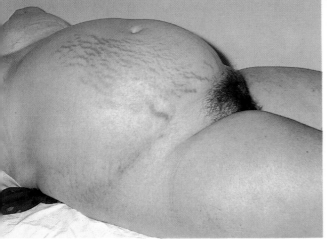

Plate 67A A 25-year-old primigravida (weight 94.8 kg; weight gain during pregnancy, 13 kg) at 34 weeks' gestation. Note scars of reduction mammoplasty. Striae are marked and are located, as is usual, mainly below the level of the umbilicus.

67A

67B

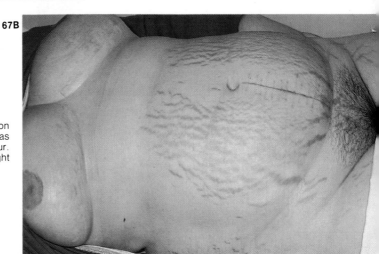

Plate 67B Appearance of striae gravidarum on day 9 of the puerperium. Caesarean section was performed because of fetal distress in labour. The infant was a healthy female, birth-weight 3.180 g.

68A

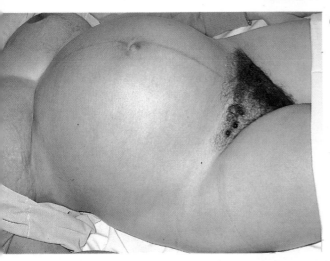

Plate 68A A 25-year-old primigravida (weight 65.8 kg; weight gain during pregnancy, 16 kg) with gestational diabetes at 39 weeks' gestation. Note scars of reduction mammoplasty and absence of striae, although her abdomen has undergone considerable stretching. Caesarean section was performed because of obstructed labour. The infant was a healthy male, birth-weight 3,760 g.

68B

Plate 68B At the postnatal visit 7 weeks after delivery, the Pfannenstiel incision is well healed. The baby is bottle-fed. Abdominal muscle tone has returned to normal. The variation in susceptibility to striae remains an enigma that interests all pregnant women and their obstetricians. Most women try to prevent striae by rubbing oil and/ or vitamin E preparations into the skin during pregnancy. These measures are not discouraged, but are probably ineffective although they do relieve the itching induced by stretching.

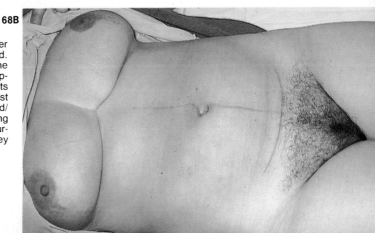

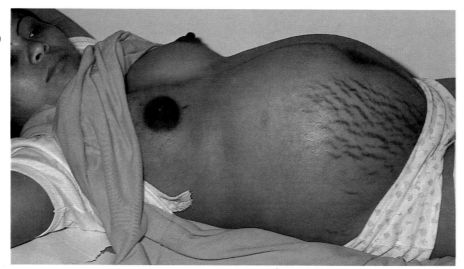

Plate 69 Unusually deeply pigmented striae gravidarum at term, in a 26-year-old primigravida, born in the Phillipines. The incidence, distribution, degree and colour of striae seem unrelated to racial origin or skin colour. They are associated with primigravidity, multiple pregnancy and excessive weight gain, which presumably share an endocrine influence. This patient had a mid-forceps delivery at 40.6 weeks of a male infant, birth-weight 3,690 g.

Plate 70 Triplets at 35 weeks' gestation in a 25-year-old para 2. The midline scar was that of an ovarian cystectomy. She delivered 4 days later after a 3-hour labour; assisted breech delivery (male, birth-weight 2,610 g), breech extraction (identical twin male, birth-weight 2,140 g) and internal version and breech extraction (female, birth-weight 2,195 g). The fused placentas weighed 1,340 g. The mother has regained her shape and the triplets, now aged 5 years, have thrived.

Plate 71 Acute polyhydramnios (incidence 1 in 4,000 pregnancies, 1 in 50 twin pregnancies) at 24.1 weeks' gestation in a 30-year-old para 2. This condition virtually only occurs with uniovular twins at 20–28 weeks' gestation, although there are exceptions (colour plate 12). This complication has a perinatal mortality rate of almost 100%, because the mother is too ill (abdominal pain, dyspnoea, oedema) for conservative management and the infants are too immature for survival. Usually only 1 amniotic sac (of the bigger twin) is polyhydramniotic; in this patient, both sacs contained in excess of 5,000 ml of liquor. The birth-weights were twin 1, 880 g, twin 2, 360 g; the placenta weighed 750 g. Acute polyhydramnios accounts for about 15% of the perinatal mortality in twins (Weir PE et al Br J Obstet Gynaecol 1979;86: 849-853).

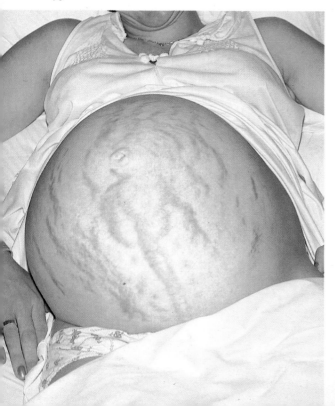

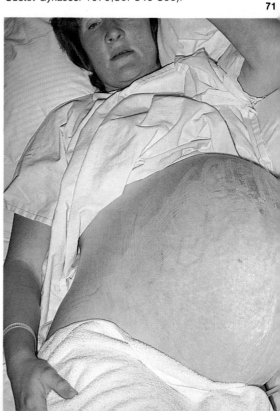

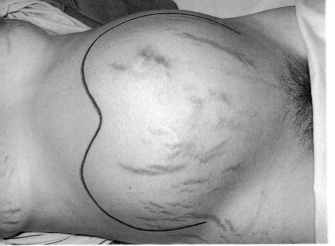

Plate 72 Bicornuate uterus (diagnosed by antenatal inspection and palpation, confirmed at manual removal of the placenta) and unusual size and distribution of striae, on breasts and abdomen, in a 17-year-old primigravida. She is shown at 38.2 weeks' gestation, weight 54.2 kg, weight gain only 5.2 kg since the first antenatal visit at 6.5 weeks' gestation. She was delivered at 39.3 weeks of a female infant, birth-weight 3,100 g.

72

73

Plate 73 Healed striae can be mistaken for surgical incisions and vice versa. Always ask the patient what operations she has had. The suprapubic skin fold in a plump patient often conceals the scar of a Pfannenstiel incision. This 41-year-old para 2 shows the scars of appendicectomy (28 years ago), hysterectomy (6 years ago), exploratory laparotomy for pancreatitis (2 years ago), and striae on abdomen and breasts dating from her first pregnancy 17 years ago.

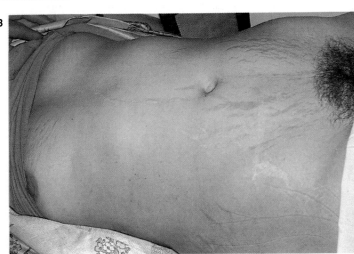

74A

Plate 74A New, mainly suprapubic striae in a 30-year-old para 1 at 40 weeks' gestation. Her weight is 74.6 kg; weight gain during pregnancy was 4.8 kg. The birth-weight of her first child, now aged 3 years, was 3,900 g. Normal delivery at 41 weeks resulted in a male infant, birth-weight 4,250 g.

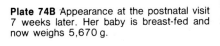

74B

Plate 74B Appearance at the postnatal visit 7 weeks later. Her baby is breast-fed and now weighs 5,670 g.

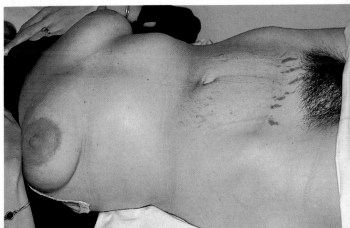

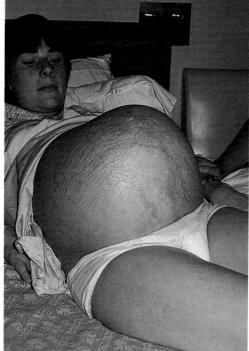

75A

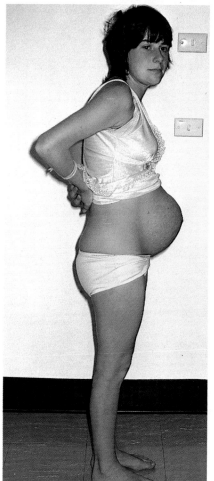

75B

Plate 75A A rhesus isoimmunized, 25-year-old para 1 with triplets at 32.4 weeks' gestation. She came into labour 3 days later and was delivered vaginally of 3 living boys, all direct Coombs positive; the first weighed 2,200 g, had a cord haemoglobin of 9.0 g/dl and required 1 exchange transfusion; the second weighed 2,415 g, had a cord haemoglobin of 11.7 g/dl and required 1 exchange transfusion; the third weighed 2,530 g, had a cord haemoglobin of 13.0 g/dl and required phototherapy alone. This picture shows the uterus protruding through a gross divarication of the rectus abdominis muscles.

Plate 75B Two days after delivery the patient's abdominal wall sags through the separated rectus muscles. Her weight had increased from a prepregnant 50.8 kg to 82.3 kg at 32 weeks.

75D

Plate 75C On day 2 of the puerperium, bowel peristaltic waves are visible through her thinned abdominal wall, the rectus muscles being displaced laterally.

Plate 75D Seven months after delivery the patient has regained her muscle tone, although her abdominal skin has not yet completely taken up the slack. Her weight is 50.8 kg. Her triplet sons are also in splendid health. This patient had no 'stretch marks' in her first pregnancy which resulted in a female infant, birth-weight 3,850 g. The folds of subumbilical loose skin may never take up in spite of regained muscle tone, especially in thin women, and many resort to plastic surgery to restore their confidence when wearing bikinis.

75C

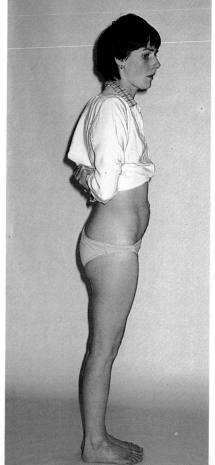

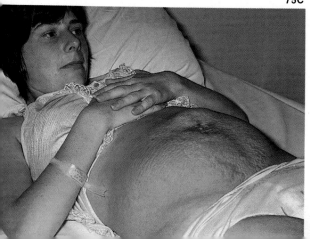

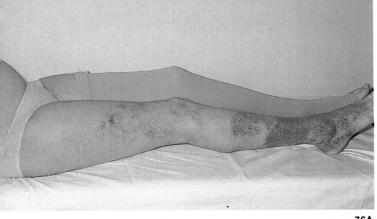

Plate 76A Varicose veins in a 32-year-old para 2 at 32 weeks' gestation. Her varicose veins first became apparent in her second pregnancy, almost disappeared after delivery, but returned early in the present pregnancy and became progressively worse. She is not obese (61.2 kg). The surgical stockings as shown on the left limb relieved the aching in her legs but not that in her vulval varicosities. She had a normal delivery at 41.5 weeks' gestation of a 3,530 g healthy infant. A small perineal tear required prompt suturing to control bleeding from varicose vulval veins.

76A

76B

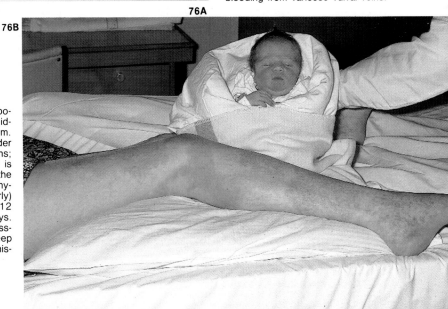

Plate 76B Superficial thrombophlebitis extending from groin to mid-calf on day 1 of the puerperium. There is a wide band of red, tender skin overlying the thrombosed veins; this is due to inflammation which is noninfective in origin, although the patient may have pyrexia and tachycardia. Aspirin orally (1g 6-hourly) relieved redness and pain within 12 hours and was continued for 8 days. Anticoagulant therapy is not necessary unless there is associated deep venous thrombosis or a previous history of thromboembolism.

76C

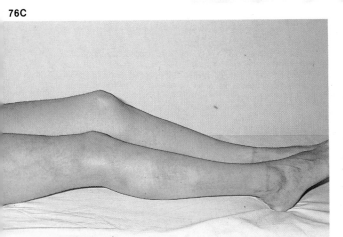

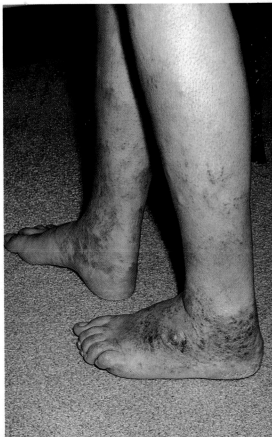

Plate 76C Appearance at the postnatal visit 6 weeks after delivery. As is usual, the varicosities have improved, but not quite returned to the prepregnant condition. She has no symptoms and surgical treatment was not advised. Her husband plans a vasectomy to avoid her risk of thromboembolism with oral contraceptive therapy.

Plate 77 More disfiguring varicosities in a 28-year-old para 2 at 28 weeks' gestation. She complained of nocturnal cramps (not necessarily due to the varicose veins) and aching legs. She is not obese (60 kg), but has a strong family history of varicose veins. She also has large, aching vulval varicosities. The veins subsided after a normal delivery at 41 weeks. At the postnatal visit the veins were still obvious, but the patient was not bothered by them.

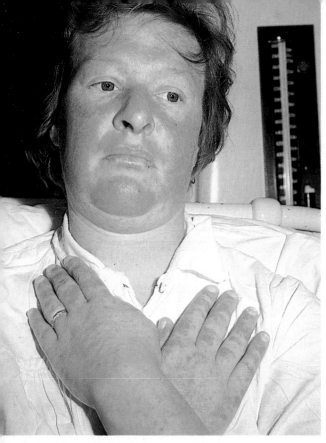

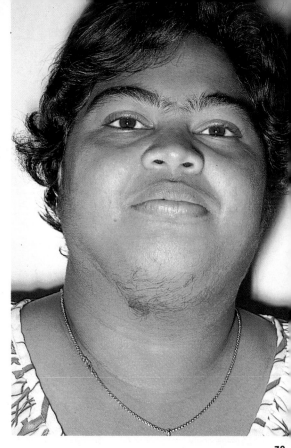

78

Plate 78 This 28-year-old primigravida presented at 30 weeks' gestation with systemic lupus erythematosus and severe preeclampsia (epigastric pain, blood pressure 170/125, proteinuria 20 g/l). She had a past history of acute nephritis when aged 14. Labour was induced; forceps delivery resulted in a 1,200 g infant who died aged 36 hours of hyaline membrane disease. Prednisolone, 5 mg tds, controlled the lupus, a disease which, even with corticosteroid therapy, has high maternal and perinatal mortality rates.

79

Plate 79 This 29-year-old para 2 developed hirsutes early in her second pregnancy. The condition improved after delivery but recurred in her third pregnancy. Glucose tolerance testing at 34 weeks revealed gestational diabetes. At Caesarean section, a healthy 2,800 g female with normal genitalia was delivered, and on routine inspection, an irregular enlargement of the left ovary was noted. The ovary was biopsied and histology revealed a luteoma, the likely cause of the androgen excess.

Plate 80 Herpes gestationis affecting a 22-year-old primigravida with a twin pregnancy and preeclampsia. The generalized rash appeared at 34 weeks and responded to corticosteroids. She was delivered of healthy male infants (2,680 g and 2,130 g) at 35 weeks' gestation after induction of labour because of increasing severity of preeclampsia. This skin disease is rare (1 in 5–10,000 pregnancies), unique to pregnancy and of unknown aetiology. It resolves soon after delivery and may recur in successive pregnancies. Because of the increased risk of intrauterine death, fetal condition must be carefully assessed (oestriol values, cardiotocography), and labour induced when the fetus is mature.

80

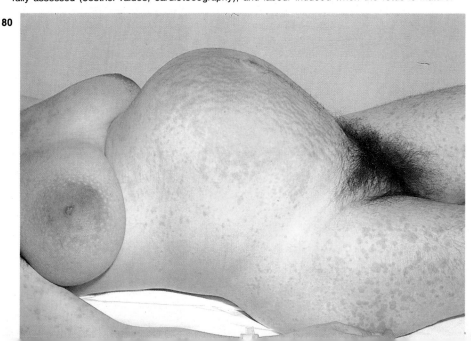

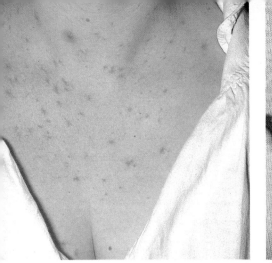
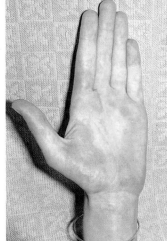

81A   81B

Plate 81A Numerous spider naevi in a 23-year-old para 1 at 34 weeks' gestation; she also had reddened ('liver') palms. The lesions began to appear at 23 weeks, but were not noted in her first pregnancy. Her glucose tolerance test was normal in spite of her obesity (106 kg). She developed generalized pruritus at 30 weeks which persisted in spite of antihistamine therapy. Liver function tests were normal except for an elevated serum alkaline phosphatase. Because of the increased risk of intrauterine death (2–4%), regular cardiotocography was performed and labour was induced at 38 weeks; normal delivery resulted in a 3,970 g, healthy male infant. (Courtesy of Dr David Abell).

Plate 81B Palmar erythema in a 25-year-old nullipara at 38 weeks' gestation. She was delivered 1 week later of a 2,600 g healthy male infant. Seen in 2–4% of patients, liver palms (and soles) are associated with spider naevi and generalized pruritus of pregnancy, and are probably related to oestrogen-induced alteration of hepatic function.

82

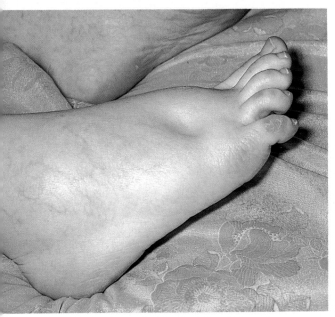

Plate 82 Gross pitting oedema in a 34-year-old para 7 with iron deficiency anaemia (haemoglobin 7.8 g/dl, serum iron 4.3 mmol/l (normal 10–30)) at 38 weeks' gestation. She had normal renal function tests, although she had developed hypertension and gross generalized oedema in all 8 pregnancies. Labour was induced at term because cardiotocography showed reduced fetal reserve; 3 hours later the patient had a precipitate delivery of a healthy female infant weighing 3,400 g.

Plate 83 An unusually long, thick, intact operculum passed by a 26-year-old primigravida immediately before the head came on view. Cervical elongation accounts for the impressive dimensions of this specimen. It is surprising how seldom an intact operculum is seen in obstetric practice.

83

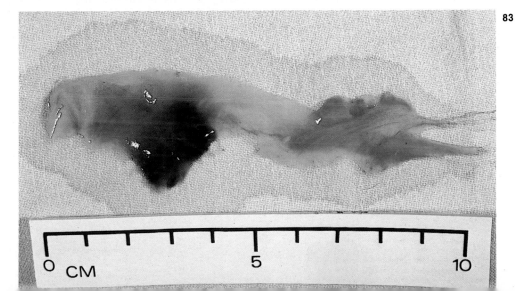

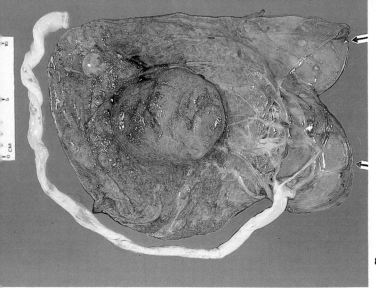

Plate 84 Vasa praevia. The patient was a 23-year-old para 1. At 37 weeks' gestation she reported that fetal movements had ceased after she lost 'a cupful' of bright blood vaginally. The Apt test was positive. Amniotic fluid did not drain vaginally until 2 hours later, when, presumably, the amnion ruptured. The infant was stillborn, birth-weight 3,100 g. Note velamentous insertion of the umbilical cord and succenturiate lobe. The arrows show the ends of the torn vessel from which the fetus bled to death. Usually, bleeding from a vasa praevia occurs late in the first stage of labour when the vessel is torn as the membranes (chorion and amnion) rupture.

84

85

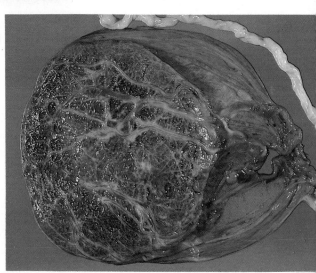

Plate 85 Vasa praevia from a 28-year-old para 1 admitted with irregular contractions and spontaneous rupture of the membranes at 39 weeks; 12 hours later she had a sudden painless haemorrhage (200 ml) and the fetal heart became unrecordable; the cervix was 3 cm dilated; 4 hours later she delivered a stillborn infant, birth-weight 3,390 g. Note velamentous cord insertion and torn vessel adjacent to the hole in the membranes. The perinatal mortality rate is high (50–80%) with vasa praevia, even if diagnosed quickly when haemorrhage occurs.

86

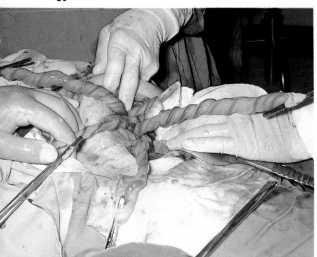

Plate 87 Uterine scar dehiscence with bleeding beginning at the ends of the wound. The intact amniotic sac bulges between the bladder and upper edge of the uterine tear. The patient, a 26-year-old para 1, was a retarded epileptic who had a Caesarean section for fetal distress in her first pregnancy. Laparotomy was performed when fetal distress (bradycardia and loss of beat to beat variation) occurred in early labour, at 41 weeks' gestation. The infant was born in good condition, birth-weight 4,155 g. Blood loss was minimal!

Plate 86 Umbilical cords of quintuplets (4 males, 1 female; birth-weights 1,000 g, 1,085 g, 1,115 g, 835 g and 975 g) seen at emergency Caesarean section at 28.5 weeks' gestation. The patient conceived following ovulation induction with gonadotrophins. The fused placentas weighed 1,640 g.

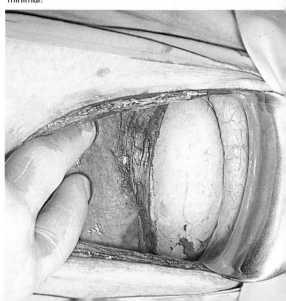

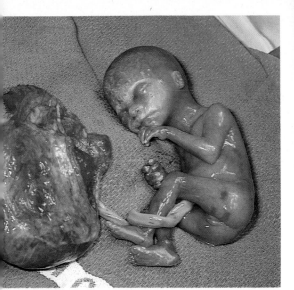

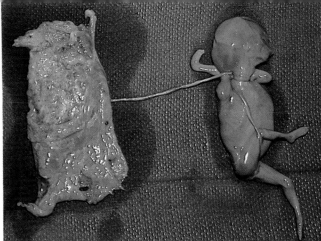

88　**Plate 88** Down syndrome at 18.4 weeks' gestation; the 280 g female fetus and placenta are seen after hysterotomy, performed when chromosome studies on amniotic fluid cells, obtained by amniocentesis at 17 weeks, revealed trisomy 21. The 40-year-old mother has 1 living child, born by Caesarean section, who has Down syndrome. The recurrence risk of trisomy 21 is only slightly greater than that for the general population (1 in 100 for patients aged 40–44 years).

Plate 89 Spontaneous abortion of this conceptus **89** occurred at 16 weeks' gestation after bizarre cord entanglement caused intrauterine death. Note that the cord tightly constricts the neck. Although present in 25–30% of births, cord loops around the neck seldom cause serious intrauterine hypoxia. Most second trimester abortions are due to cervical incompetence, premature rupture of the membranes, polyhydramnios, uterine and fetal malformations, and infections.

90

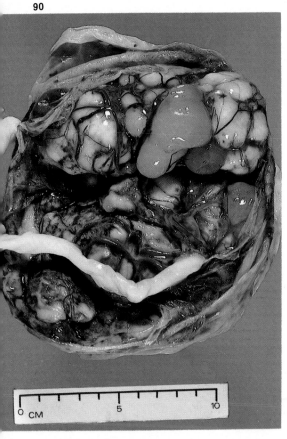

Plate 91 This 29-year-old para 1 developed lower abdominal pain at 39 weeks' gestation and collapsed. Her uterus was rigid (major degree of concealed placental abruption). Amniotomy was performed before resuscitation was commenced and blood coagulation failure excluded, a mistake that nearly cost the patient her life. Two hours later, the patient was delivered of a stillborn infant (birth-weight 4,100 g) and then had a torrential postpartum haemorrhage, as shown here — the measured blood loss was 3,870 ml!

91

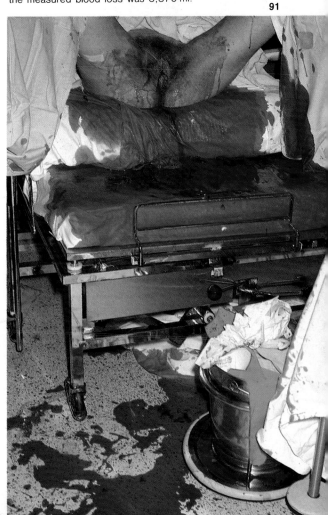

Plate 90 Idiopathic placental insufficiency. A 32-year-old primigravida came into spontaneous labour at 36 weeks' gestation and 9 hours later was delivered of a living, severely growth retarded male infant, birth-weight 1,970 g. The placenta weighed 400 g and the fetal surface shown here had multiple white masses and 3 gelatinous areas thought to be tumours. The maternal surface showed white infarcts. Histology showed extensive degeneration within areas of infarction, but no abnormal trophoblastic proliferation.

Plate 92A Cephalopelvic disproportion in a multigravida with a large fetus presenting occipitoposterior. She had a mid-forceps delivery of a 3,445 g infant in her first pregnancy after induction of labour at 37.5 weeks' gestation for gestational diabetes; the baby developed severe respiratory distress and survived after a stormy illness, punctuated by a pneumothorax. Here, at term in her second pregnancy, she weighs 93.8 kg, has gross generalized oedema and hypertension (150/110). Gestational diabetes has again developed. Note oedematous striae and indentation from pressure of the fetal stethoscope. Amniotomy was performed after implementation of a pre-eclampsia sedation regimen. After 6 hours' labour, there was no progress and Caesarean section was performed. (The duration of her first labour was 9 hours).

92A

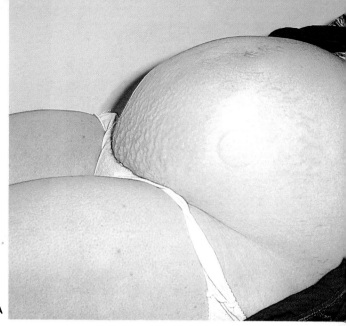

92B

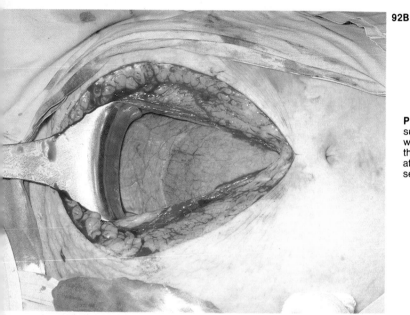

Plate 92B The retractor in the midline subumbilical incision exposes Bandl's ring where loosely attached peritoneum over the thinned lower segment joins that firmly attached to the muscle of the upper uterine segment.

92C

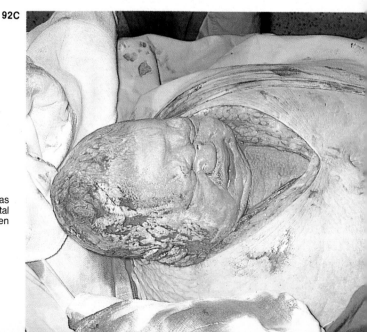

Plate 92C The lower uterine segment has been incised transversely and the large fetal head, directly occipitoposterior, has been delivered by manual extraction.

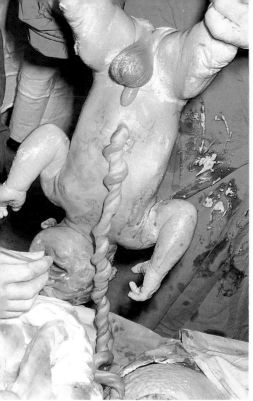

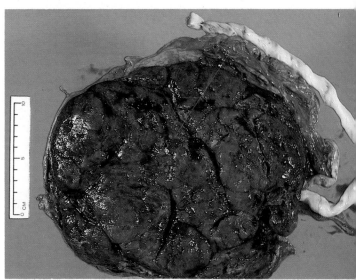

Plate 92D The baby is very large (birth-weight 5,100 g). His nasopharynx is aspirated of secretions and blood from the uterine incision. He is blue because respiration has not commenced. Note the thick cord and copious protective coating of vernix caseosa.

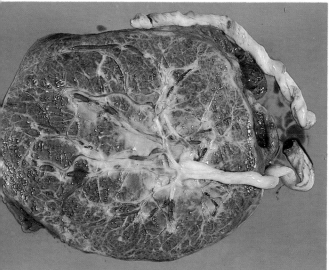

92D **92E**

Plate 92E Maternal surface of the huge placenta (26 × 20 cm) which weighed 1,060 g. The most common cause of a large placenta is a large baby, not diabetes mellitus, erythroblastosis or multiple pregnancy!

92F

92G

Plate 92F Fetal surface of the placenta showing normal insertion of the umbilical cord.

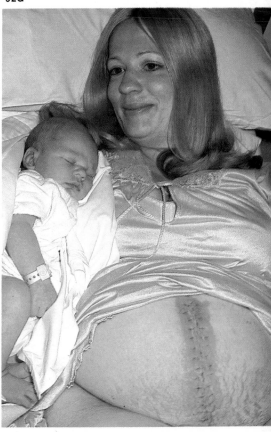

Plate 92G Eight days after delivery the radiant mother is seen with her healthy son. Her weight is already 14 kg less than at her last prenatal visit. The wound is well healed but coloured with the antiseptic 2% solution of mercurochrome. The striae are still oedematous. Her glucose tolerance had returned to normal when retested 6 weeks' postpartum. The moral of this tale is to consider the possibility of disproportion when a multigravida, especially if obese, does not labour well — she usually requires Caesarean section, not epidural analgesia and infusion of oxytocin to enhance labour.

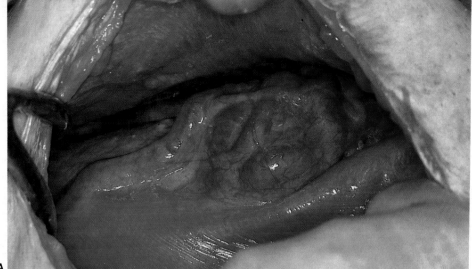

93A

Plate 93A Group of distended ovarian and uterine veins, lateral to the left round ligament (showing the marked hypertrophy that occurs in pregnancy), in a 39-year-old, para 4, gestational diabetic, before removal of the baby at repeat elective Caesarean section at 38 weeks' gestation. There is marked dextrorotation of the uterus.

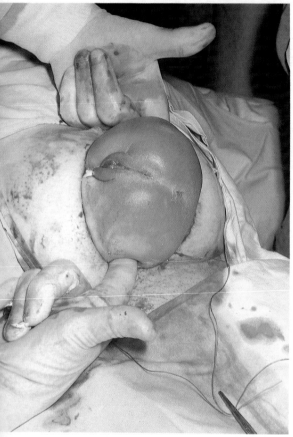

93B

Plate 93B Bilateral groin traction delivers the buttocks and extended legs of the female infant presenting as a frank breech. A suture has been placed in the midline of the lower uterine segment to allow ready identification of the edge of the incision after delivery.

Plate 93C Traction on the legs delivers the trunk and brings the shoulders into the wound.

93C

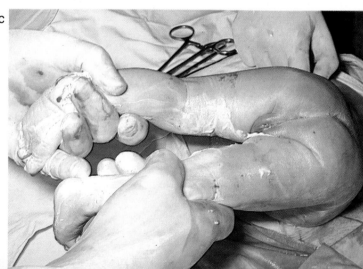

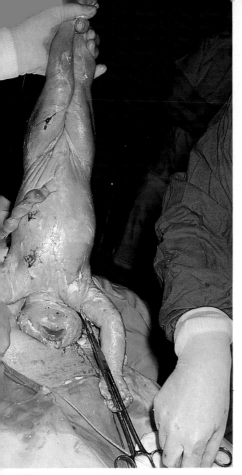

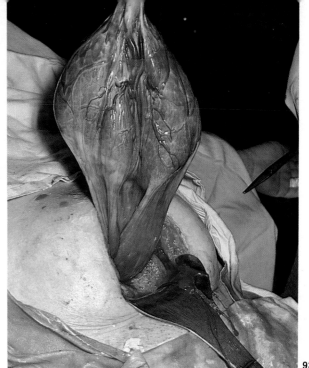

93E

93F

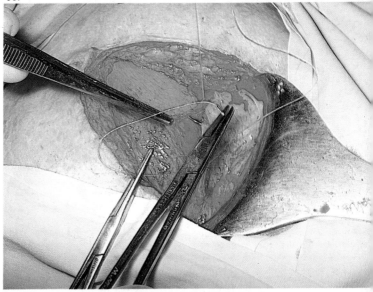

93D

Plate 93D The child is born, her nasopharynx and mouth are aspirated and, after division of the doubly-clamped umbilical cord, she is handed to the paediatrician. Her birth-weight was 3,380 g.

Plate 93E Cord traction separates the placenta and trailing membranes; the firm attachment of the latter to the decidua is well seen at this stage of the delivery.

Plate 93F Two rows of continuous chromic catgut sutures have closed the transverse incision in the lower uterine segment. The incision in the uterovesical fold of the peritoneum is being sutured.

Plate 93G Before closing the abdomen, the ovaries are routinely inspected to exclude tumours. Note that the veins between Fallopian tube and round ligament (arrows) are no longer distended as they were before delivery (colour plate 93A).

93G

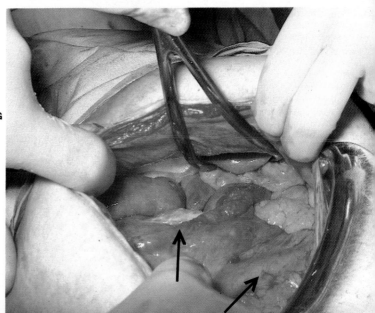

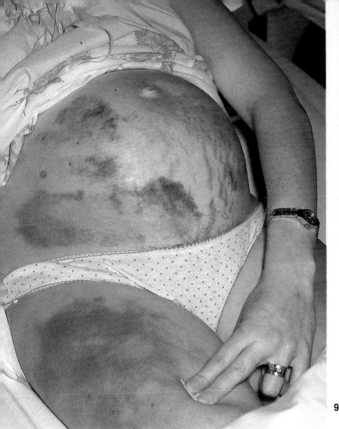

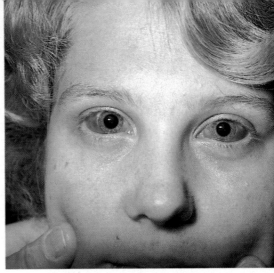

Plate 95 Bilateral subconjunctival haemorrhages in a 25-year-old primigravida who responded with unusual vigour when urged to 'push' in the second stage because of fetal distress (bradycardia and passage of meconium). She had a precipitate delivery of a vigorous, growth retarded (birth-weight 2,350 g at 40 weeks) male infant. This photograph was taken 6 days after delivery when the haemorrhages, which were painless, had already subsided; thereafter they resolved rapidly.

94

96

Plate 94 Bruising at the sites of subcutaneous heparin injections in a 26-year-old para 1 who was found to have primary pulmonary hypertension at 30 weeks' gestation. Subsequently, it was learned that her mother had died of the same condition. She was delivered uneventfully of a living infant, birth-weight 2,290 g, at 35 weeks' gestation, but went into heart failure on day 8 of the puerperium and died 24 hours later in spite of intensive care. The moral is that serious cardiovascular disease may remain unrecognized until late in a second pregnancy yet cause heart failure and death.

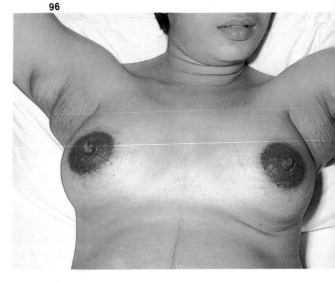

Plate 96 Bilateral axillary breasts in a lactating 27-year-old, para 1 Malaysian 5 days after normal delivery at term. She was unaware of the accessory breast tissue before delivery, although one of her sisters had required excision of axillary breasts noted during her first lactation. At the postnatal visit 5 weeks later, the accessory breasts were smaller, but still troublesome enough for the patient to request their removal.

97

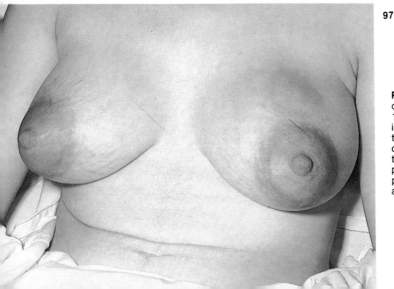

Plate 97 Abscess in the upper lateral quadrant of the left breast in a lactating 26-year-old para 1, 7 weeks after normal delivery at term. A radial incision was made over the fluctuant centre of the reddened area and 35 ml of pus escaped. A drain tube was inserted. Breast feeding continued. Antibiotics usually cause resolution and prevent abscess formation if commenced promptly at the first signs of infection (redness and localized tenderness).

If there is *persistent oozing* from an episiotomy wound and/or vaginal lacerations after repair, haemorrhage can usually be controlled by insertion of a *gauze pack* (10 cm × 2 metres) into the vagina. This is removed 12–24 hours later. If a pack is used, an *indwelling catheter* is inserted because the pack will occlude the urethra and prevent voiding. If packing is required, an antibiotic should be prescribed.

CARE IN THE PUERPERIUM

(i) *Analgesia* is needed for the first 48–72 hours. Pain is greater with larger episiotomies and much external suturing, long second stage, operative delivery, and perineal bruising. An air cushion makes sitting more comfortable. If the episiotomy is large, an icepack applied several times during the first hour will reduce oedema and bruising. (ii) Four-hourly *perineal toilets*; the application of spirit should be avoided for it causes pain. (iii) *Dusting powder* applied after bathing keeps the wound dry. *Advice* is needed regarding care of the wound after toilet activity. Patients should be cautioned against disregarding the call to empty the bowels (because of the fear of pain), since this will lead to greater eventual difficulty. (iv) *Radiant heat* lamp for 5 minutes 2–3 times per day is used if the wound is moist, infected, or painful. (v) *Smears and cultures* are taken and chemotherapy commenced if infection develops. (vi) If the *wound breaks down*, it should be resutured with nonabsorbable material after thorough cleansing.

COMPLICATIONS

Blood loss in excess of 300 ml occurs in 5–10%; this is usually related to larger episiotomies in the nullipara or if varices are present; making the incision too soon will also increase the loss. If a significant haematoma forms, it should be evacuated, haemostasis secured, and resuture carried out.

Infection is relatively uncommon considering the nature of the area: it usually takes the form of a stitch abscess or infected haematoma; occasionally, infection of the ischiorectal fossa may occur and there may be a major problem, with fasciitis and myonecrosis.

The anatomical result of episiotomy repair is not always satisfactory. Emotional as well as anatomical factors influence the functional result, and provision of adequate advice regarding contraception is important in this context. About 40% of patients subsequently experience *dyspareunia*; usually this is temporary and of minor importance, but in 5% the symptom is severe and persistent. Mostly this problem is due to introital narrowing, asymmetric repair, or granuloma formation. Two of the common mistakes made in repair of episiotomy wounds or vaginal lacerations are shown in figure 45.4.

Temporary *loss of libido* is a common symptom after childbirth, regardless of whether or not an episiotomy has been performed. Although there is great variation of practice and opinion, much marital disharmony is caused by the male wishing to resume coital activity too soon after parturition.

chapter forty-six

Forceps and Vacuum Extraction

OVERVIEW

Unfortunately, the mother is not able to deliver the baby unaided in all labours; in some, eventual delivery would be possible, but at an unacceptable risk. The assistance of forceps or vacuum extraction is usually needed if the mother or baby is showing distress or the second stage of labour is prolonged. These indications are often interpreted according to somewhat subjective criteria, and this, together with rather wide variations in the level of obstetric sophistication, explains the range in incidence rates — e.g. from 5 to 30% or more. The incidence of forceps has risen with the increase in popularity of epidural analgesia because of incomplete rotation of the head.

Neither of the above instruments is intended to overcome significant obstruction — Caesarean section is the correct option here. Each is particularly useful, however, in minor obstruction, especially that due to the maternal soft tissues, and also in correcting the position of the baby's head (e.g. from occipitoposterior or occipitolateral). The selection of instrument is often due more to tradition and individual training than to unique advantages.

For other than outlet forceps (head on the perineum), a degree of skill is required to diagnose cephalopelvic relationships, and to execute the application, the rotation (if needed), and the extraction without harm to mother or baby. Another skill lies in knowing when not to undertake this type of delivery. The cardinal sin is failing to give up before harm has been done: one advantage of the vacuum extractor (at least in the case of the mother) is that it usually tells you when this point in time has arrived.

A close review of the patient should be undertaken at the 36-week visit and at the start of labour, looking for features that would unfavourably influence labour, and trying to assess its likely outcome.

FORCEPS

The forceps, first brought into use in the 17th century by the Chamberlens, a Hugenot family, represent one of the milestones in obstetrical practice. There have since been a large number of modifications to the original instrument, the major departure in concept being the vacuum extractor. Each instrument is designed to expedite the safe delivery of the baby from the mother's birth canal.

INCIDENCE

There is a very wide range according to variation in facilities available and different philosophies of practice. At one extreme is the United States of America where, in some centres, the majority of deliveries of nulliparas are by forceps; at the other are some undeveloped countries where the use of forceps would be exceptional. Where there is a real indication, the incidence ranges from 5–15%. The relative increase in nulliparas and the popularity of epidural analgesia in some centres have increased the rate; in the latter case largely because of a greater incidence of failed internal rotation of the head in late labour.

INDICATIONS

The classical indications for forceps delivery are given below. The less experienced operator should think carefully about embarking on the procedure if the following 'danger signals' are present: head still palpable abdominally, gestation 43 weeks or more, baby large, much moulding, prolonged first and/or second stage, significant back pain.

(i) *Delay in the second stage of labour.* This is the most common indication. Usually there has been a difficult or prolonged labour in a nullipara; preceding this there has often been late engagement of the head and slow dilatation of the cervix. Second stage delay results from maternal fatigue or inability to relax the pelvic floor muscles, an unyielding perineum, or a poorly positioned head (posterior or deep transverse arrest), or one which is larger than normal. The contractions weaken, the progress of the baby slows or stops, and the maternal bearing down efforts become less effective. In some patients the reduced bearing-down efforts are caused by epidural analgesia. The *usual time limits for the second stage are 1 hour for nulliparas and 30 minutes for multiparas*, although it should be remembered that these are merely guidelines and will depend on the condition of the mother and fetus as well as the nature and progress of the labour.

(ii) *Prophylaxis.* It is often advantageous to *shorten the second stage of labour* even though no distress is yet apparent. There is advantage to the mother in such conditions as hypertension, preeclampsia/eclampsia, cardiac or other serious medical disorders — deterioration in the condition thus being prevented. Similarly, if the fetus is considered to have a reduced reserve, reduction of the stress of the second stage often results in the birth of the baby in a good, rather than in a distressed condition. Some believe that routine early forceps delivery results in less damage to the maternal pelvic tissues and less trauma for the baby.

(iii) *Fetal distress.* In approximately 10% of stillbirths, fetal death occurs minutes before birth, usually unexpectedly, due to acute placental insufficiency, probably caused by placental separation late in the second stage of labour. Because of this, delivery should never be delayed when the head is safely accessible. When the head is on the perineum, local analgesic should be injected and delivery effected by episiotomy and forceps if necessary. This is the modern philosophy of obstetrics, and minimizes the harmful effects of fetal hypoxia late in labour. The baby is more likely to become distressed during the second stage of labour, probably as a result of the cumulative effect of the hypoxia imposed by the frequent, strong contractions occurring at this time, and the added pressure resulting from bearing-down efforts. Apart from the slowing of placental circulation during contractions, there is considerable pressure on the baby's head as it passes deeper into the birth canal. The distress may also be due to other causes such as placental failure, occult cord prolapse, or intraamniotic infection. The classical features are a fetal heart rate above 160 or below 120/minute, a drop in rate in association with a contraction (especially at the end of the contraction — *type 2 deceleration*), and the presence of meconium in the liquor. A fall in scalp blood pH below 7.20 indicates a condition of acidosis secondary to hypoxia.

(iv) *Maternal distress.* Distress of the mother is not easy to define; usually there are both physical and psychological components. Typically, the *pulse rate* is persistently above 100/minute, the *urine volume* is reduced (less than 30 ml/hour) and *acetonuria* is present; there may be elevation of the *temperature* above 38.5°C, and the patient looks pale and tired. These signs of maternal distress are due to dehydration, ketosis, and possibly infection. The patient's behaviour will often indicate that she has reached the end of her psychological resources (increasing restlessness and disquiet, low pain threshold, and requests for something to be done). This state of affairs is now seen much less commonly, because of antenatal preparation, better physical and psychological support during labour, and earlier termination of labour than occurred 10 or 20 years ago.

(v) *Miscellaneous.* Forceps are often applied to *the aftercoming head of the breech*, to facilitate delivery and protect the head if the baby is small (colour plate 32). Special forceps (Piper) are sometimes used, especially in the USA. At *Caesarean section*, forceps may be used to deliver the baby's head through the uterine incision.

TYPES OF FORCEPS DELIVERY (figure 46.1)

(i) *Outlet.* The head has reached the pelvic floor, the position is anterior and the scalp can be seen without parting the labia. (ii) *Mid-forceps.* The head is engaged (maximum diameter has passed the pelvic brim), and the lowest part of the head has reached or passed the ischial spines, but rotation to the anterior position may not have occurred and descent as described for 'outlet forceps' has not occurred. (iii) *High forceps.* The head is not engaged.

The incidence of *outlet forceps* differs considerably from place to place and from one operator to another, according to the concept of prophylactic value of this procedure; it may range from 5-75% of deliveries. Mid-forceps delivery, on the other hand, is not performed without specific indication, as given above, and the incidence is usually 5-10% of deliveries (table 16.3). *High forceps application is never used except in the unusual case of the second twin*, and perhaps by a specialist in a situation where the head has been engaged, but pushed up by an inexperienced person, usually in an attempt at manual rotation.

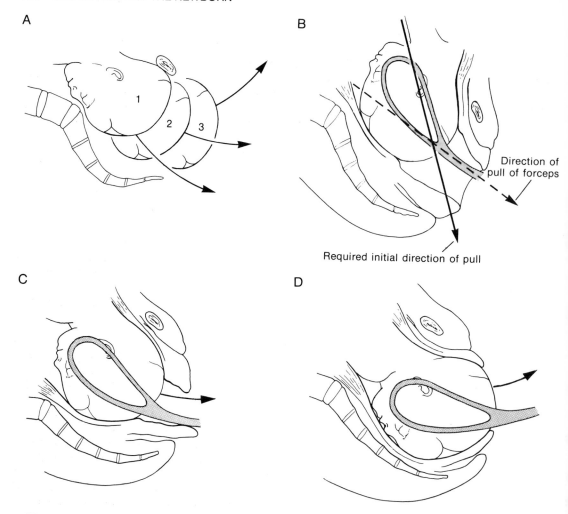

Figure 46.1 Types of forceps delivery and direction of traction. **A.** Station of the head for mid-forceps (1), low forceps (2), and outlet forceps (3), deliveries. The arrows show how the direction of traction must change as the head descends, in order to follow the curve of the birth canal. **B.** Axis traction is an attachment to the handle or blades of the forceps used to achieve traction in the direction of the curve of Carus when the head is just engaged (the difficult mid-forceps shown here is the highest station from which forceps delivery would be performed). **C.** The usual type of mid-forceps delivery: the lowest part of the head is past the level of the ischial spines. The forceps grasp the occipital region and extend onto the cheeks. **D.** Outlet forceps: the greatest diameter of the head is past the narrow pelvic plane. Delivery is completed by extension of the head around the symphysis pubis.

GENERAL DESCRIPTION OF THE INSTRUMENT

The obstetric forceps consists of 2 pieces, joined together by a locking mechanism. Each piece has a *handle* and this is connected to the *blade* by the *shank* (figure 46.2). The *lock* is usually situated at the junction of the handle and shank; it is usually of fixed type, but may be sliding, as in Kielland forceps. There is often a projection at the lower end of the handle called the *shoulder*, which is used for assisting traction and/or rotation of the baby's head. The blades of the forceps, which are applied to each side of the head, are usually open (fenestrated). In all forceps there is a *cephalic curve* which fits the con-

tour of the baby's head, and a *pelvic curve*, which allows for the concave shape of the sacrum. In forceps primarily designed for rotation of the head (e.g. Kielland forceps), the pelvic curve is minimal. By means of the cephalic and pelvic curves, each forceps blade can be designated as left or right, according to which side of the maternal pelvis it is applied.

In some forceps, there is an additional *axis traction device* which is attached to the end of the handle (Neville Barnes) or to the blades (Milne Murray). In some forceps the blades do not cross when locking, but remain parallel (Shute forceps). The Laufe forceps are similar to the Kielland instrument in some respects (length, sliding lock, handles, and shank (except the locking hinge)), and similar to the Barton instrument in other respects (no pelvic curve, thinner blade, hinge incorporated in one blade). The blades have a more rounded cephalic curve, adapting to the nowadays less moulded head. In the Luikart modification, the blade is solid, but has a pseudofenestration on the inner (cephalic) surface. The types of forceps in common use are illustrated in figure 46.2.

TECHNIQUE OF FORCEPS DELIVERY

Prerequisites. (i) Cervix fully dilated, (ii) head engaged, favourable position and presentation (vertex: occipitoanterior unless using Kielland or similar forceps; face: mentoanterior), (iii) membranes ruptured, (iv) adequate analgesia, (v) empty bladder. Factors to consider in the likely difficulty of the procedure include size of baby/ maternal pelvis, duration of labour, moulding, station, position and flexion of the head. The patient should be fully informed of the reason for the procedure and what is involved.

Nursing details. The consent form for operation must be signed. Dentures and hairpins are removed. Leggings are applied, and premedication (atropine, 0.6–1.0 mg s/c) given if ordered.

Instruments and Drapes (colour plate 25)

Technique. The patient is usually in the *lithotomy position* and full antiseptic preparations and draping are carried out; precaution against the supine hypotensive syndrome (pelvic tilt) may be indicated as for Caesarean delivery. *Anaesthesia* may be local (perineal infiltration, pudendal nerve block, or epidural), or general (Chapter 41) depending on the station and position of the head, and the anticipated difficulty of the procedure. *The bladder is catheterized* and the urine volume measured. With the help of antiseptic obstetric cream, a careful examination is made to determine the state of the membranes, dilatation of the cervix, presentation, station and position of the head, the presence of caput and

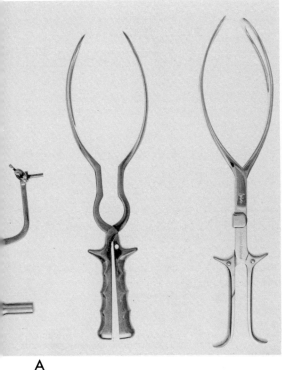

A

Figure 46.2 Forceps in common use. **A.** Neville Barnes forceps and axis traction attachment are shown on the left and Kielland forceps on the right. The cephalic curve of the blades is similar in each. The different locking mechanisms are shown. **B.** Lateral view showing that Barnes forceps have a much larger pelvic curve than Kielland forceps.

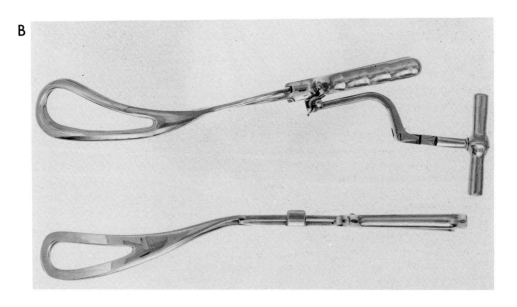

B

moulding, the tightness of fit of the head in the pelvis, and finally, the general size and architecture of the pelvis.

Outlet forceps. Here the blades are simply applied to the sides of the baby's head — the left blade being inserted first. A check is made that the forceps are applied correctly and symmetrically. If this is the case, the 2 blades come together and lock easily (figure 46.3); the sagittal suture lies midway between the blades and parallel to them. Minor rotation may be necessary to bring the sagittal suture to the anteroposterior position. In most patients an *episiotomy* is made before the forceps delivery is commenced. Steady traction is exerted, usually for 15–30 seconds, to simulate the strength and frequency of the uterine contractions. The direction of traction is in a forward and downward direction, following the direction of the birth canal. The fetal heart should be listened to between contractions. Although some slowing occurs as a result of head compression, the rate should return to normal after cessation of traction and release of compression. Persistence of bradycardia indicates fetal distress, or perhaps the entanglement of a loop of cord in the forceps, although this is rare and usually only occurs with more complicated

applications. As the head bulges the perineum, the direction of traction is changed. An episiotomy is usually carried out at this stage if not already performed. The blades are carefully removed as the head is about to pass through the expanded vulva, and the rest of the procedure is carried out as for a normal delivery (colour plates 25–28) — some practitioners prefer to deliver the head with the forceps still applied, since extension and further descent can be readily controlled; then the blades are removed so that the shoulders (which often cause some difficulty) can be delivered.

Mid-forceps. This operation may be relatively simple if the head has rotated beyond the transverse, if it is well engaged, and there is no significant disproportion between head and pelvis. On the other hand, if these conditions do not apply, considerable skill and experience may be required if the baby is to be born in good condition and the mother's soft tissues are not to suffer damage. The inexperienced operator should beware if the pregnancy is prolonged, the baby appears large, the head not deeply in the pelvis, the labour prolonged, and back pain troublesome during the labour.

The general procedure is similar to that

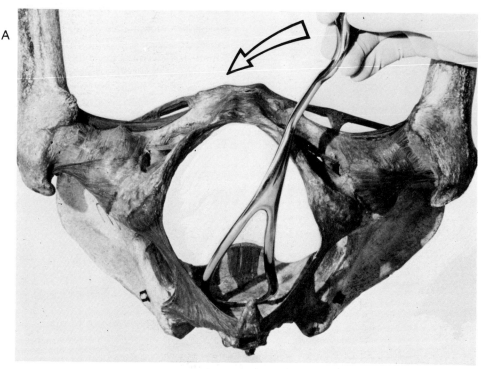

Figure 46.3 Technique of forceps application. **A.** Introduction of the left blade. The handle is rotated through a wide circle to avoid trauma by the blade as it rotates into position around the head.

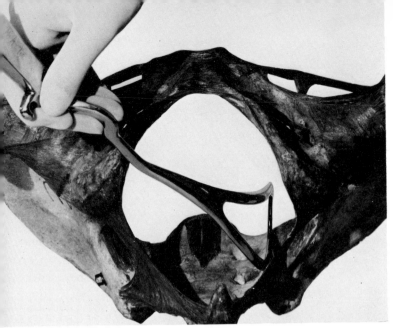

B. The handle is lowered and the blade passes the fetal cheek and temple.

B

C

C. The blade in position when applied to the head with its pelvic curve coinciding with that of the birth canal.

D

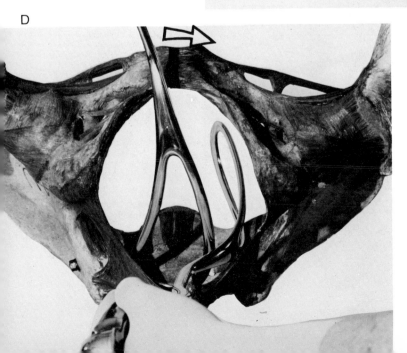

D. Introduction of the right blade which is inserted in the midline.

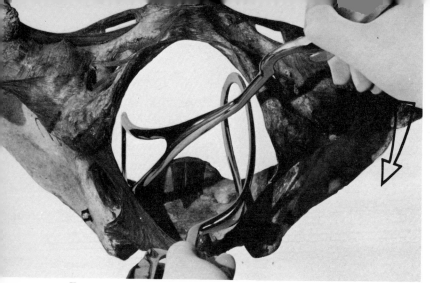

E. The blade passing fetal cheek and temple.

E

F

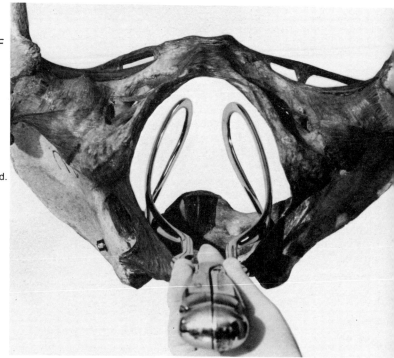

F. The forceps in position and locked.

G

G. The widest diameter between the blades grasps the biparietal diameter and the tips overlie the fetal cheeks. The head is well flexed (posterior fontanelle readily palpable).

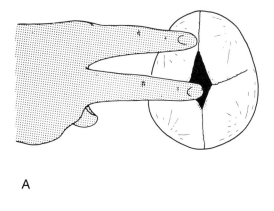 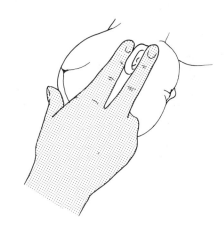

Figure 46.4 Diagnosis of position of the head. **A.** The anterior fontanelle is readily palpated when the head is deflexed unless there is much caput or moulding. **B.** When the position is occipitolateral, the ear is palpable beneath the pubic symphysis. The root of the ear indicates whether the occiput lies to the left or to the right.

outlined in the outlet forceps, the main difference being in the rotation of the fetal head. *The first essential is an accurate appraisal of station, flexion, and position.* This is aided by the usual measures of palpation of sutures and fontanelles. If there is any uncertainty, additional *palpation of the ear and occipital ridge* is essential (figure 46.4). Rotation of the head is achieved either manually after achieving maximum flexion (perhaps aided by abdominal rotation of the anterior shoulder) or by means of forceps. If *manual rotation* is performed, the head is held in the anterior position and the forceps blades are applied (figure 46.5). Great care is necessary to ensure that they are symmetrically placed on the baby's head, since this is the key to successful delivery and a baby in good condition. *Traction is often much greater than that required for outlet forceps.* Because of the higher station in the pelvis, the correct direction of pull is aided by exerting downward pressure on the shanks of the forceps with traction (Pajot manoeuvre) or applying the *axis traction apparatus.* If forceps rotation is to be attempted, a large episiotomy is usually made and the Kielland or a similar instrument employed (figure 46.6). The blades are applied to the fetal head in the posterior or occipitolateral ('transverse') position, usually by 'wandering' the anterior blade over the baby's face (the sinciput being smaller than the occiput offers less resistance to the forceps blade as it is rotated into position), and directly applying the posterior blade, care being taken not to cause a vaginal laceration by pressure of the forceps blade against the sacral promontory. The handles of the instrument are pushed downward against the perineum and the occiput is rotated to the front by means of a rotational force

TABLE 46.1   CLINICAL DETAILS IN A RECENT SERIES OF 10,714 FORCEPS DELIVERIES IN A TEACHING HOSPITAL

	Number	%
Incidence	10,714 in 40,982 deliveries	26.1
Nulliparas	7,446	70.0
Fetal distress	4,458	41.2
Epidural analgesia	3,867	36.0
Low-forceps	6,322	59.1
Mid-forceps	4,392	40.9
Delivery from:		
occipitoanterior position	7,626	71.1
occipitolateral position	1,029	9.7
occipitoposterior position	2,059	19.2
Birth-weight		
2,500 g and below	754	7.0
4,000 g and above	1,083	10.0
Manual removal of placenta	823	7.6*
Postpartum haemorrhage	853	7.9**
Perinatal mortality	188	1.7

* Overall hospital incidence 4.3%; ** overall hospital incidence 5.2%

applied to the shoulders on the blades (figure 46.7).

If traction fails to achieve the desired result, a check is made to see whether the position of the head has been determined accurately, the cervix is fully dilated, or there is unsuspected contraction of the lower pelvis.

Table 46.1 summarizes the clinical details in a large series of forceps deliveries in an Australian teaching hospital. The following points are noteworthy:

1. The high *incidence of forceps delivery* in this series (26%) is in keeping with modern obstetric

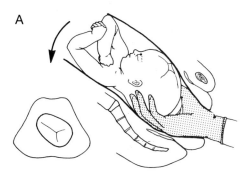

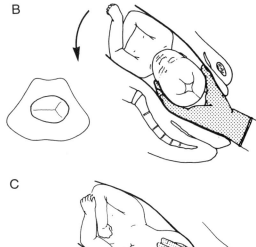

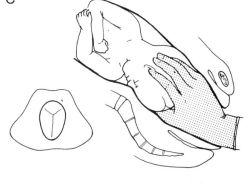

Figure 46.5 Manual rotation of the occiput from the left occipitoposterior position. **A.** The cervix is fully dilated and the head is engaged. General anaesthesia is preferred. The right hand grasps the occiput. **B.** The head has been rotated to the left occipitolateral position. **C.** The head has been rotated to the occipitoanterior position with the inevitable loss of station as it was disimpacted. Forceps delivery can now be performed — this is a high forceps delivery and is dangerous even when carried out by an experienced obstetrician.

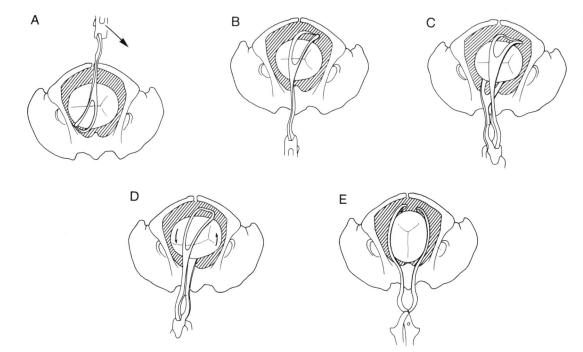

Figure 46.6 Forceps rotation from the left occipitolateral position. **A.** The anterior (right) blade is applied by rotating ('wandering') it around the sinciput. It is usually easier to apply the anterior blade first. The handle is lowered as the blade is introduced. **B.** The anterior blade of the forceps is in position, applied cephalically. The pelvic curve of the forceps is at right angles to that of the birth canal. **C.** The posterior (left) blade is inserted directly, care being taken to avoid pressing against the sacral promontory, as this can cause extensive vaginal laceration. **D.** Anterior rotation of the occiput with forceps has commenced. **E.** The occiput is anterior and now the pelvic curve of the forceps coincides with that of the birth canal.

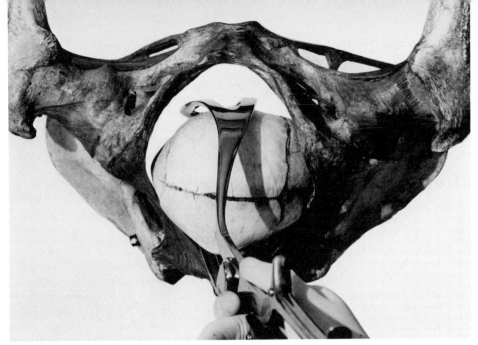

Figure 46.7 Kielland forceps applied to a head (somewhat deflexed) in the right occipitolateral position. This instrument has only a small pelvic curve and so forceps rotation is less likely to cause vaginal laceration.

philosophy, that delivery should be performed when the head is *safely accessible*, even in the absence of fetal or maternal distress or delay in the second stage of labour.

2. *Nulliparas* had a much higher incidence of forceps delivery than multiparas — they comprised 40% of the obstetric population and 70% of those having forceps deliveries.

3. The high incidence of *fetal distress* (41%) is expected since it is one of the 3 classical indications for forceps delivery (with delay in the second stage and maternal distress). More intensive monitoring of the fetal heart rate in labour was probably a contributing factor.

4. The relatively *high incidence of mid-forceps delivery* (10.7% of all deliveries and 40.9% of all forceps deliveries) is explained by strict use of the following definitions:
   (a) a low-forceps is when the head is on view and the occiput anterior,
   (b) a forceps delivery is never low if *rotation of the head*, either manually or with forceps, is required.

Forceps to the *aftercoming head* in a breech delivery is usually a mid-forceps, and accounted for 10% of the mid-forceps deliveries in this series.

As stated earlier in the chapter, increased use of *epidural analgesia* in labour results in more mid-forceps deliveries because of failure of rotation of the occiput and reduced maternal expulsive effort in the second stage of labour.

5. In this series when the head arrested in the

occipitolateral position (deep 'transverse' arrest), *forceps rotation* was performed in 90% of patients, usually with Kielland forceps; *manual* rotation was used in 10% of patients.

When the head arrested in the *occipitoposterior position* forceps rotation to occipitoanterior was performed in 80%, manual rotation to occipitoanterior in 6%, and in 14% the patient was delivered face to pubis i.e. *persistent occipitoposterior*.

6. The incidences of *manual removal of the placenta* and *primary postpartum haemorrhage* were approximately double that in the total hospital population.

Face presentation. The same principles apply as with vertex presentations; however greater care is necessary to avoid damage to the facial structures during placement of the blades.

Brow presentation. Manoeuvres have been described for conversion of brow to either vertex or face with forceps. This requires considerable experience, and most operators would adopt manual methods or resort to Caesarean section, according to circumstances pertaining in the particular case.

TRIAL OF FORCEPS

Here, the operation is done in the *operating theatre*, set up for Caesarean section should the forceps delivery fail. Those in favour of this procedure claim that there is less tendency to exert undue force, the operator desisting sooner than would be the case if the delivery was conducted in the labour room. The opponents claim that the need for trial forceps indicates a lack of predictive ability on the part of the operator. It is our opinion that there are sufficient imponderables in some mid-pelvic arrests to justify the procedure.

FAILED FORCEPS

This is to be distinguished from the above. Usually, there is a combination of inexperience of the operator, failure to observe the necessary conditions, failure to appreciate the station and position of the head and/or the presence of unusual complications (large baby, or an abnormality such as hydrocephaly, pelvic tumour, constriction ring of the uterus, or outlet contraction). The management consists firstly of accurate assessment; thereafter, a decision is usually made between Caesarean section, appropriate forceps management, allowance of a further period of labour, or a destructive operation and vaginal delivery.

TABLE 46.2 RESULTS IN 75 CASES OF FAILED FORCEPS IN A LARGE TEACHING HOSPITAL

Incidence	0.7% of all forceps deliveries
Method of delivery	
Caesarean section	56
Forceps	16
Internal version and breech extraction	2
Normal	1
Ruptured uterus treated by hysterectomy	1
Perinatal mortality	4

Table 46.2 shows the clinical data associated with 75 cases of failed forceps in one institution. 'Failed forceps' was diagnosed if an attempt at an instrumental birth had, at any time in that labour, been unsuccessful in achieving vaginal delivery. Therefore, all cases of *trial of forceps* not resulting in vaginal delivery were included. Failed forceps was usually followed by Caesarean section (56 cases); 16 had a successful forceps delivery, usually by a more experienced practitioner; 2 internal versions and breech extractions were performed, and 1 patient delivered spontaneously when labour was allowed to continue! Analysis of these cases revealed that failure was due to inability to recognize or correct an *occipitoposterior* or *occipitolateral* position, *excessive fetal size* (in 15 birth-weight exceeded 4,000 g), or to an *incompletely dilated cervix*. There were 7 cases of failed *vacuum extraction*, 3 of which involved attempted delivery of the *second twin*.

It was concluded that *general anaesthesia* rather than epidural analgesia is often required for difficult mid-forceps deliveries. The dangers of internal version in singleton pregnancy were illustrated by the case of uterine rupture requiring hysterectomy. Two of the 4 *perinatal deaths* were avoidable — the others were the result of hydrocephaly and conjoined twins.

FORCEPS INJURIES

Mother. The usual injuries are to the soft tissues. *Tears of the cervix and vagina* occur in 15–20% of forceps rotations and are related to the manipulations and the shearing stress associated with rotation of the fetal head; the *postpartum haemorrhage* and *manual removal* rates are about doubled (table 46.1). Also forceps delivery is associated with a high incidence of *episiotomy*, and often the incision extends high into the vagina during the delivery, resulting in a difficult repair and considerable blood loss. Occasionally, *uterine rupture* may occur; lower segment injuries are more likely if applications are made before full dilatation of the cervix. There may be *damage to the fascial supporting tissues of the uterus, bladder and rectum*, or even direct injury to these structures. *Nerve* and *joint* injuries usually result from attempts to overcome cephalopelvic disproportion. *Infection* is more likely because of tissue damage, blood loss, and lapse of aseptic technique. *Retention of urine* may result from bruising of the bladder base and urethra.

Baby. The most serious injuries result from incorrect application of the forceps. This causes abnormal stresses within the skull, and rupture of large veins, often producing fatal *intracranial haemorrhage*; 5–10% of babies suffer some birth asphyxia if delivered by midcavity forceps (mostly due to preexisting conditions). In 5–10% of such operations there will be some difficulty with delivery of the shoulders (*shoulder dystocia*, colour plate 140). Also, direct damage to structures such as the eye, nose and ear is more likely (colour plate 143). *Fractures of the skull* or facial bones also are likely (colour plate 144). Occasionally, pressure of the forceps blade on the *facial nerve* as it passes forwards in front of the ear causes temporary paralysis of that side of the face. Abrasions are not uncommon, but these heal quickly. Entanglement of the cord between the forceps blade and the fetal head has been mentioned. Damage to the vertebral arteries may occur with rotation of the fetal head, leading to central nervous system damage.

VACUUM EXTRACTION

The purpose of the vacuum extractor is similar to that of the obstetric forceps — namely, to assist nature in delivery of the baby. Simpson in 1794 is credited with designing the first instrument of this type, but it was not until relatively recently (1954) that Malmstrom in Sweden perfected and introduced it into clinical practice.

In some countries, the vacuum extractor has almost entirely replaced the forceps; in others, it is hardly used at all.

INDICATIONS

In general, these are the same as for forceps. The instrument cannot be used in face presentations or for the after-coming head in breech deliveries, or for the immature baby. Most would consider that, if fetal distress is acute, forceps rather than vacuum extraction is to be preferred because of the lessened delay. For prophylactic use, delay in the second stage, maternal distress, and fetal distress that is not acute, the extractor is equivalent to the forceps. The instrument has a useful place in delivery of the second twin if fetal distress has occurred, since the head is often high and the cervix no longer fully dilated. In areas where symphysiotomy is practised, the vacuum extractor can be used to guide the head away from the bladder base. The restrictions applying to full dilatation of the cervix are not so important as with the obstetrical forceps, since the suction cup will fit through an undilated cervix. Those favouring the instrument claim this to be one of its advantages, particularly in the multipara, where cervical dilatation is more easily achieved. Thus, Caesarean section might be averted. *This does not mean that it is ever safe to use the vacuum extractor when the head is not engaged.* The technique does not require general anaesthesia, and if excessive force is used, the cup will pull off, minimizing the danger to both mother and baby.

GENERAL DESCRIPTION OF THE INSTRUMENT (figure 46.8)

The principle of use is that a suitably-sized metal (or silicone rubber) cup is applied as near the occiput as possible (to maintain flexion during traction) and a vacuum is created inside the cup by means of a hand or electric pump. Ideally the cup should be placed over the posterior fontanelle symmetrically i.e. the sagittal suture is evenly overlapped on either side by the cup. The suction draws the loose scalp of the fetus into the cup in the form of a chignon or bun. Traction is then applied by means of a chain attached to the cup. The cups are of stainless steel and there are 3 sizes — 4 cm, 5 cm, and 6 cm (the smallest cup is usually restricted to use in the second twin; the 5 cm cup is more manoeuvrable and is best for posterior and lateral positions). The traction chain is passed through the hole in the base of the cup and through the rubber pressure tubing which is attached to the cup (figure 46.8). The chain is prevented from slipping through the cup by an attached metal disc. The other end of the traction chain is attached to a metal handle by a pin which passes through one of the links in the chain. A longer length of pressure tubing passes from the traction handle to the source of suction. A pressure gauge indicates the pressure developed in the system. A number of new versions of the instrument have recently been introduced.

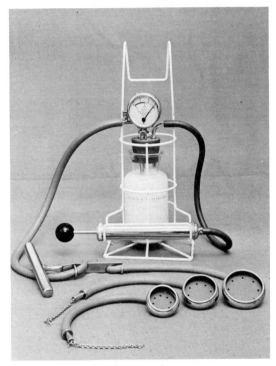

Figure 46.8 Components of the vacuum extractor: hand pump, vacuum bottle, gauge, handle, and rubber tubing (with traction chain inside) attached to the suction cup.

TECHNIQUE

The preparations are the same as for forceps delivery. The correct size of cup is chosen according to the size of the baby, and the apparatus is assembled and connected to the suction. The efficiency of the pump and connections are tested by occluding the cup with the palm of the hand. The introitus is gently dilated manually and the cup, lubricated with obstetric cream, is inserted into the vagina — preferably at the time

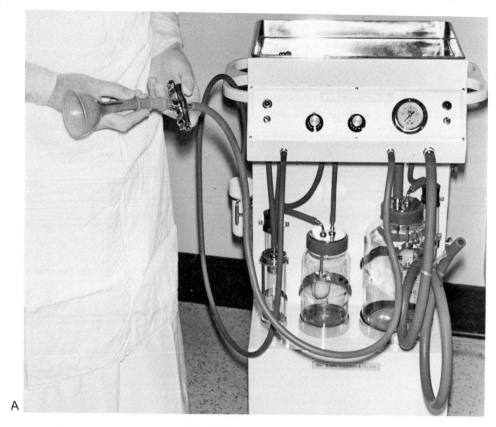

A

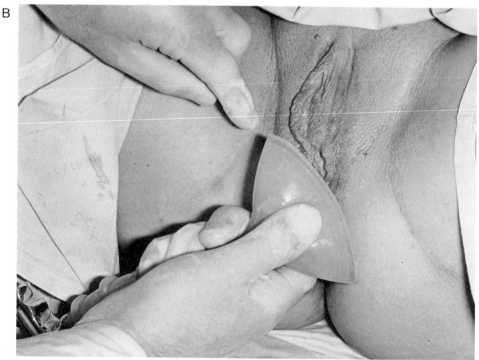

B

Figure 46.9 Assembled vacuum extractor using the silicone rubber cup introduced by Kobayashi (Red Cross Maternity Hospital, Tokyo). **A.** The cup is ideal for outlet forceps delivery of infants of 36 weeks' maturity or more, using continuous suction at 73 kPa (550 mm Hg) pressure. **B.** The cup is compressed to minimize trauma before it is introduced into the vagina. **C.** After cutting an episiotomy, traction is applied in the direction of the curve of the birth canal. **D.** The head is delivered by extension around the subpubic arch, being controlled by the extractor — the third hand belongs to the medical student who will complete the delivery. (Courtesy of Dr Kevin Barham).

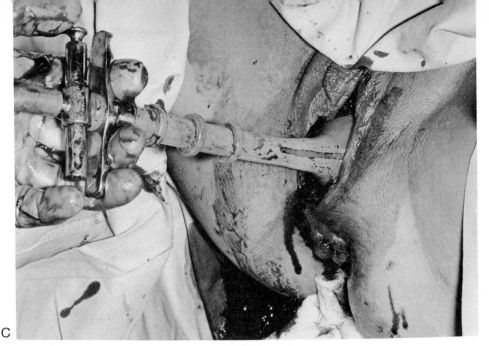

C

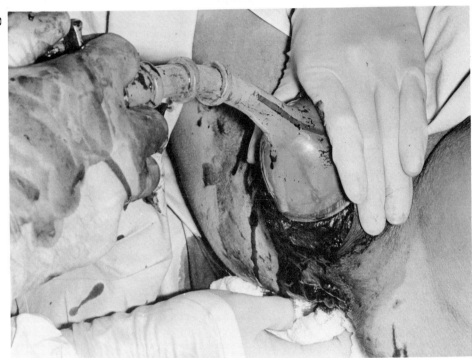

D

of a contraction. The cup is applied as near to the posterior fontanelle as possible and held there while suction is applied. Perhaps the single most important factor in safety and success is placement of the cup in the proper area of the fetal skull. The pressure is decreased until a negative pressure of 0.7–0.8 kg/cm² is achieved (0.5 kg/cm² if the baby is premature). Use of the soft cup introduced by Takashi Kobayashi of Japan to minimize trauma of the fetal scalp is shown in figure 46.9. Modifications have been made to the design of the metal cup to prevent it lifting at one edge when pulling at an angle, which is difficult to avoid when the head has arrested in an occipitoposterior position in the midpelvis (figure 46.10).

After checking that no part of the vagina or cervix has been drawn into the cup, a series of tractions are made, coinciding with the contractions of the uterus if these are occurring normally. The thumb and index finger of the non-pulling hand monitor the application of the cup on the head and the latter's descent. Traction is stopped if the cup lifts or a hiss of air occurs

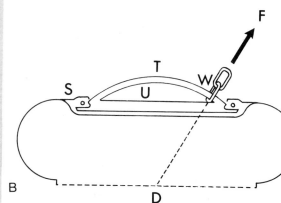

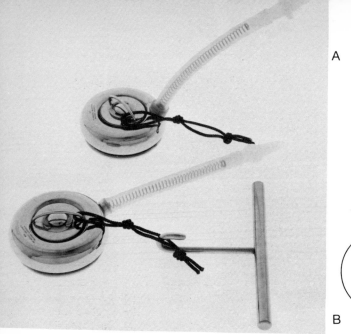

Figure 46.10 New method of traction for the vacuum cup which allows the direction of pull to be in the curve of the birth canal in deliveries from the midpelvis. **A.** Photograph of cups for anterior and posterior positions of the occiput, traction cord and traction handle. **B.** Cross-section of cup. T: 2 mm metal rod curved to form the perimeter of a circle about D; this rod is mounted on a plate U. U: a circular plate which rotates against its bearing S. W: a ring which slides on T along the perimeter of the circle with its centre D. This mechanism allows 2 planes of movement and ensures that the line of traction is always through D (range 60°). (From O'Neil AGB et al. Aust NZ J Obstet Gynaecol 1981; 21:24–26).

(indicating a break in the vacuum). When the head has passed through the introitus, the suction is released, the cup removed and the remainder of the delivery completed normally. The scalp is examined for any abrasions and the baby is given 1 mg of vitamin K_1.

As long as the application is made in the occipital region, no particular regard is paid to the position of the fetal head in the pelvis, in contradistinction to forceps delivery — the *occiput, if not already anterior, rotates to the front spontaneously during descent.*

Failed Vacuum Extraction

Initial difficulties may be experienced in attaining adequate suction. Generally, there is either a faulty pump, blockage of the tubing which has not been cleaned properly, leakage of air at one of the connections, or collapse of the tube due to perishing. If adequate suction is obtained, but the *cup slips off*, the reasons may be inadequate time given to establishing formation of a chignon in the cup, inclusion of soft parts under the rim of the cup, traction at too great an angle to the insertion of the cup, and excessive traction. If delivery is not accomplished with 3–4 pulls, consideration must be given to an alternative method. There should be a definite advance with each pull and in midcavity applications the head should be on the pelvic floor after the second pull. Reasons for failure of descent include disproportion, poor site

of cup application, and wrong direction of pull.

The cup should not be applied more than twice. If these rules are adhered to, delivery of the head should rarely take more than 12–15 minutes.

As with forceps, there may be unexpected complications making traction difficult. The general failure rate lies between 2–10%, according to experience, and the number of applications made before full dilatation of the cervix.

INJURIES

Mother. Injuries are rare with the extractor, this being one of its major advantages over the forceps. Frequently, no analgesia is required, which may further reduce the probability of complications.

Fetus. It has been estimated that the fetal intracranial pressure is only 1/10–1/20 of that developed with forceps extraction. Thus, asphyxia is reduced. However, a greater distortion may be produced and this may offset reduction in pressure that is obtained. The most troublesome injury is *abrasion to the scalp*; the frequency of *cephalhaematoma is also increased* (tables 66.1 and 66.2). Unlike the obstetric forceps, the vacuum extractor does not guard the fetal head from direct injury by pressure against the bony pelvis during delivery. Retinal haemorrhage and electroencephalographic abnormalities are other reported complications.

chapter forty-seven

Caesarean Section

OVERVIEW

Few subjects have generated as much controversy as the place of Caesarean section in modern obstetrics. One or 2 decades ago, most obstetric hospitals would have a section rate of 5% or less; in many hospitals the rate now approaches 20% or even higher. This is partly the result of an increase in the safety of the operation, and partly a response to the desirability of producing a child as near to normal as nature intended.

The doubling/trebling of the Caesarean section rate in the past decade which has occurred in most centres is due to more operations being performed for *previous Caesarean* (30%), *dystocia* (30%), *breech presentation* (15%) and *fetal distress* (15%). Labours associated with these problems are now more likely to be terminated by Caesarean section on *humanitarian grounds* (quality of survival of mother and child). Because 'previous section' heads the list of indications for Caesarean section (37%, table 47.1), the *trial of labour finesse* in patients with a uterine scar has an increased importance, since a higher proportion of vaginal deliveries in these patients is perceived as the only way to halt the ever increasing incidence of Caesarean section.

Labour after Caesarean section is allowable in about 30-40% of patients with a uterine scar, and vaginal delivery results in 50-70% at the price of uterine rupture in about 1% (table 47.2).

Changes in practice should always be evaluated. Rising rates of Caesarean section should be questioned in terms of fetal results and risks to the mother. The *maternal mortality rate* is estimated to be about 80 in 100,000 patients having Caesarean section (table 14.1). Perinatal mortality rates are easily calculated but the justification of an increased Caesarean section rate is likely to be on the improved *quality of survival of the infant* — this information is not readily available but must not be overlooked in the Caesarean section argument. Finally, the *perinatal mortality rate associated with Caesarean section* (currently about 24 per 1,000; table 16.3), cannot be expected to fall when the increased rate takes in more of the fetuses at greatest risk (prematurity ± breech presentation, severe preeclampsia, premature rupture of the membranes, antepartum haemorrhage).

The *lower segment-type operation* is now almost universal, with the *classical procedure* reserved for a few well-defined indications. Maternal mortality reports continue to describe deaths associated with Caesarean section — some largely related to antecedent problems, a few to the anaesthetic and some to the operation itself. *Epidural analgesia* is increasingly popular (table 47.3) particularly with the parents: the opportunity to be more involved with the birth and to nurse the baby in the first moments of life are important positive factors. Another trend supported by parents is the *presence of the father in the operating theatre* so that the couple can share the birth together.

The vogue for *sterilization* at the time of Caesarean section has lessened with advent of the laparoscopic technique. The patient is often not in an adequate frame of mind to make such a decision at this time and the first 4-6 months of life can be dangerous for the infant (e.g. cot death).

Careful medical and nursing care after the operation will lessen the potential complications that can arise and will hasten the mother's return to normality.

Counselling as to her obstetrical future should not be omitted.

Currently there is debate concerning the place of *repeat Caesarean section*. Most authorities now accept that it is not necessary if the previous section was lower segment in type, the postoperative uterine healing uneventful, the indication nonrecurring, the patient has been assessed by a specialist, and is under careful supervision in labour. Conduction analgesia during labour is usually avoided since it may remove a *warning of scar rupture*. Manual assessment of the scar after delivery is helpful in immediate and future management.

Other areas of dispute include the place of section in *breech delivery*, *fetal distress* and *placental abruption*: these are considered further in the relevant chapters.

DEFINITION

Caesarean section is the surgical technique whereby the fetus is delivered through an incision in the uterus.

INCIDENCE

There is a rather wide variation depending mainly on the nature of the practice at a particular hospital. For example, the rate will be higher if the hospital admits many emergency patients from smaller units, or if there is a larger number of private as opposed to clinic patients, or if the socioeconomic class of the patient is low; the general *range is from 5–25%*.

TYPES OF OPERATION
Lower Segment

This is by far the commonest technique (98%). The approach is nearly always a transverse one through the lower uterine segment after opening the peritoneal cavity (figure 47.1). Rarely, the extraperitoneal approach is used.

Upper Segment

This was the only type of operation used for several centuries, hence the term 'classical section'. The operation is abdominal transperitoneal, and the incision is made in the upper part i.e. body of the uterus (figure 47.2).

INDICATIONS

These may be recurring or nonrecurring. A *recurring* indication is a severely contracted pelvis, since a live baby could not be born any other way, and things will be the same in the next pregnancy. A *nonrecurring* indication is a major degree of *placenta praevia* in a patient with a normal pelvis. One may also make a distinction between *absolute indications*, as given above, and *relative indications*, where vaginal delivery is feasible, the choice often depending on philosophical approach rather than absolute requirement. Examples of the latter include previous section without a recurring indication apart from the uterine scar but with a breech presentation at full term.

The operation may be performed *electively*, as for example in a patient with a known pelvic contraction; or as an *emergency*, as for prolapse of the umbilical cord. The decision to undertake Caesarean section is based on a careful assessment of factors in the *history* (age, parity, years married, living children, infertility), *examination* (general diseases, disorders of pregnancy, relative size of fetus and birth canal, progress of fetus and labour), and *special tests* (pelvimetry, fetal well-being). The final factor is experience, which indicates the most likely outcome on the basis of previous similar cases.

A

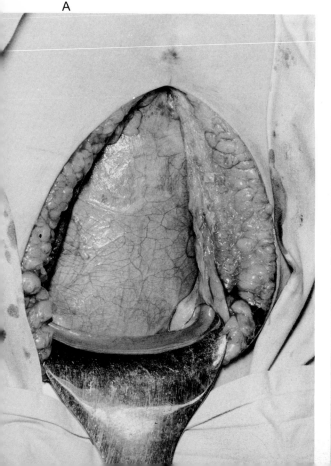

B

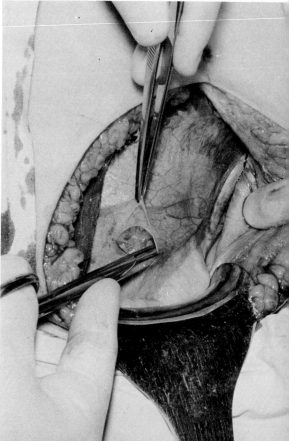

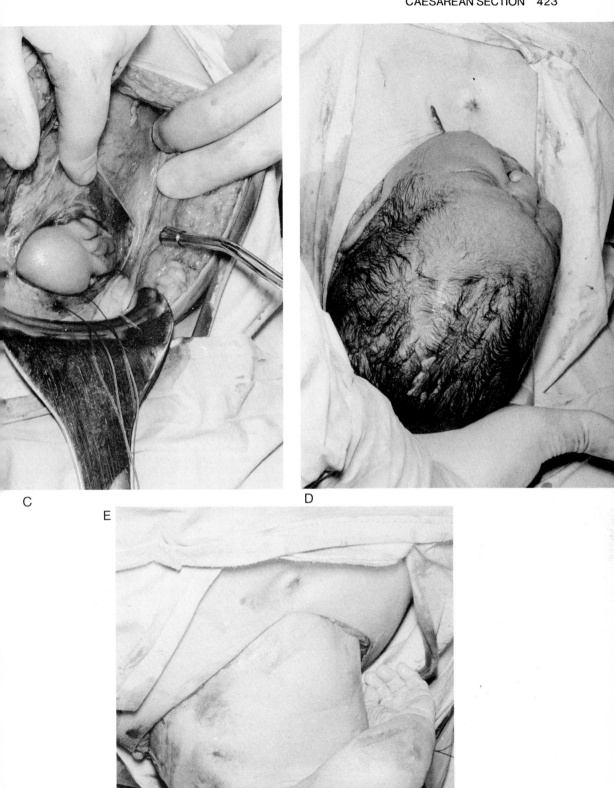

C

D

E

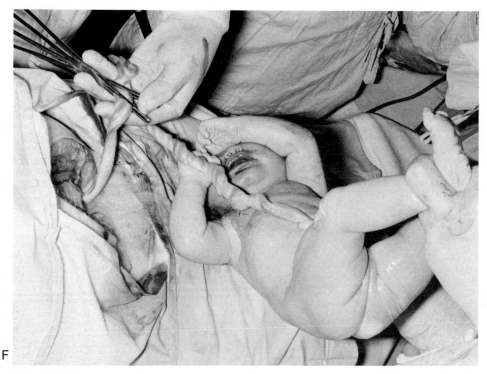

F

Figure 47.1 Lower segment Caesarean section, performed in a primigravida with maternal distress and obstructed labour, due to posterior position of the occiput. The infant weighed 3,870 g. **A.** Midline subumbilical incision exposes upper and lower uterine segments. **B.** The loose peritoneum (uterovesical fold) covering the lower segment is displayed before being cut transversely. The bladder bulges upward from beneath the retractor. **C.** The lower segment has been incised and the lower edge is held in the midline by a suture. The head is not engaged. Fat fetal cheek and lips bulge into the wound. **D.** Manual delivery of the head; a right occipitoposterior position is confirmed. **E.** Large vernix-coated trunk is delivered by fundal pressure and traction on the head. **F.** The infant is held, head dependent, to prevent inhalation of liquor amnii. The nasopharynx is aspirated, the cord clamped and cut, and the paediatrician takes the baby. **G.** The placenta is delivered by cord traction, the anaesthetist having given ergometrine 0.5 mg intravenously as the baby was born. **H.** The lower segment has been sutured in 2 layers and the continuous suturing of the peritoneum has begun. The left ovary, Fallopian tube and round ligament are shown. **I.** The uterovesical peritoneal fold has been sutured. The ovaries and tubes are inspected for pathology, haemostasis is checked and abdomen closed.

G

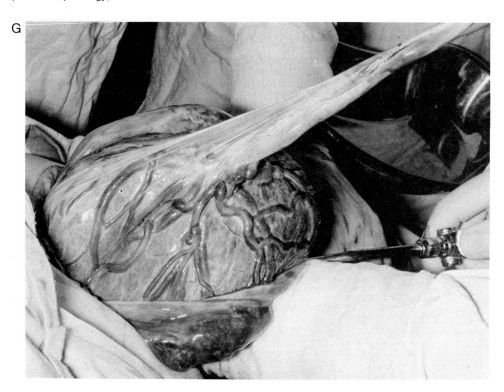

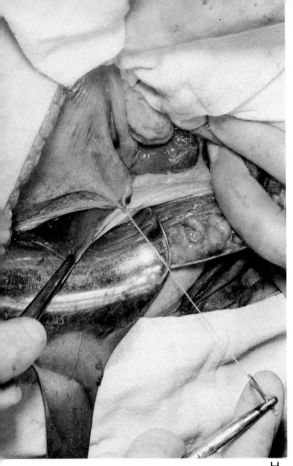

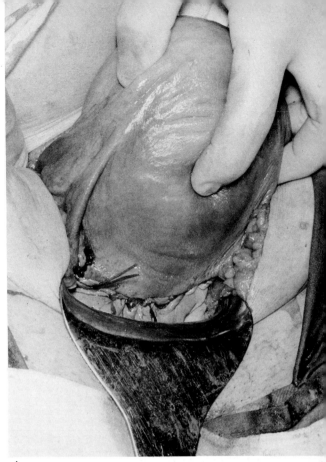

H   I

Figure 47.2 In a classical Caesarean section the thick muscle of the upper uterine segment is incised vertically in the midline.

When the labour is advanced, the main decision may rest between Caesarean section and operative vaginal delivery, for example, by forceps or vacuum extraction.

The incidence of the different indications for Caesarean section is given in table 47.1. The section rate for the series of 4,633 cases shown in the table was 11.3%, and the *perinatal mortality* associated with it was 24 per 1,000 (table 16.3). There were 46 *classical Caesarean sections*, the main indications for which were transverse lie, placenta praevia and poorly-formed lower segment associated with prematurity (table 47.3). There were only 36 *Caesarean hysterectomies* performed, the main indications being haemorrhage (17) (placenta accreta ± placenta praevia 5), rupture of the uterus (7), and technical difficulties with repair (6).

The main indication for Caesarean section was the presence of a uterine scar (36.7%). The other common indications were *dystocia* (21.9%), *fetal distress* (19.5%), *malpresentation* (11.3%) and *antepartum haemorrhage* (4.4%). It should be noted that distinction between *obstructed labour* and *incoordinate uterine action* as main indications for Caesarean section is somewhat artificial as these complications tend to occur together. It should also be noted that obstructed labour was often associated with *fetal distress*, which in turn was often associated with *fetal growth retardation* and *preeclampsia*, although the latter is seldom by itself an indication for Caesarean section. It is interesting to note that *malpresentations* account for only about 1 in 10 decisions to perform a Caesarean section. In about *30% of patients there was more than one* indication — for example, it is common for a patient to have a *posterior position*, large baby, abnormal shape or size of the pelvis, incoordinate uterine action with finally fetal distress occurring when there is also evidence of *obstructed labour* (retraction ring, head jammed in the pelvis with gross caput and moulding, and with an oedematous anterior lip of cervix).

Table 47.1 shows that *placental abruption* is seldom the primary indication for Caesarean section. Likewise in *multiple pregnancy* the primary indication for the Caesarean section is usually a *malpresentation* (footling breech, transverse lie), or a previous Caesarean with known pelvic contraction, rather than the twin pregnancy itself (table 53.2).

REPEAT ELECTIVE OPERATION/ TRIAL OF LABOUR

In a number of centres, there is a philosophy of 'once a Caesarean, always a Caesarean', i.e. all future deliveries should be by the abdominal route. This dictum is attributed to *Dr E. Gragin* (1916), at a time when the section rate was only about 1% and most were by the classical technique! Many now believe that the risk of subsequent serious scar rupture is so low that provided the pelvis is adequate, the condition is nonrecurring, and the hospital facilities are good, a trial of labour is proper. If there has been a previous vaginal delivery, the case is further strengthened. Such patients must be handled at specialist level, since many fine points in obstetrical judgement are likely to arise. Common nonrecurring indications where trial of labour is feasible are fetal distress, preeclampsia, uterine inertia/incoordination, breech and other malpresentations, and antepartum haemorrhage. Even when cephalopelvic disproportion is the initial indication, some 40% are able to deliver vaginally in a subsequent pregnancy. The overall success rate for attempted vaginal delivery is about 65% (nonrecurring 75%, recurring 30–40%).

In most hospitals a conservative policy is adopted and vaginal delivery is favoured when there has been a previous section for a nonrecurring indication (e.g. *fetal distress*, *placenta praevia*). A *trial of labour* (*trial of scar*) is also permissible in a patient who had a previous Caesarean performed because of obstructed labour, if *X-ray pelvimetry* shows the pelvis to be of normal dimensions; however, such patients are less likely to achieve vaginal delivery. Trial of labour following Caesarean section is a safe procedure, only when conducted in an appropriate hospital setting with close surveillance of the labour. In general, *epidural analgesia* and augmentation of labour with *intravenous oxytocin* are contraindicated in such patients — signs of *obstructed labour* may be overlooked, resulting in a greater risk of *uterine rupture*. Patients who have had a previous vaginal delivery, either before or subsequent to a Caesarean section, are more likely to have a successful trial of scar resulting in a normal vaginal delivery.

Favourable conditions are required for a trial

TABLE 47.1   INDICATIONS FOR OPERATION IN A RECENT SERIES OF 4,633 CAESAREAN SECTIONS IN A TEACHING HOSPITAL

Main indication		Number	%
Repeat Caesarean section		1,702	36.7
Primary Caesarean section			
Dystocia		1,018	21.9
Obstructed labour/ contracted pelvis	727		
Incoordinate uterine action/failed induction	231		
Failed forceps	60		
Fetal distress		907	19.5
Distress alone	327		
Distress plus intrauterine growth retardation	278		
Distress plus obstructed labour	226		
Distress plus preeclampsia	76		
Malpresentations		525	11.3
Breech	351		
Transverse/unstable lie	88		
Brow/face	44		
Cord prolapse/ presentation	42		
Antepartum haemorrhage		207	4.4
Placenta praevia	190		
Abruptio placentae	17		
Diabetes		48	1.3
Multiple pregnancy		38	0.8
Rhesus isoimmunization		10	0.2
Miscellaneous		178	3.8

of labour to succeed in a patient with a Caesarean section scar; preferably, labour should begin *spontaneously* and progress normally with delivery achieved within 8–12 hours. Rupture of the membranes before the onset of contractions, failure of the head to engage, or of the cervix to dilate progressively are unfavourable signs and indicate that repeat Caesarean section will be required. Table 47.2 shows the results obtained in a series of 2,298 patients who had had a previous Caesarean section. A *repeat operation was performed electively in 66%* and 34% had a trial of labour; the trial was successful, resulting in *vaginal delivery in 76% of patients.* However, it should be noted that in this series, the incidence of *uterine rupture was 1%* and 1 infant was stillborn because of this complication. It was concluded that *continuous monitoring of the fetal heart rate* was necessary in such labours (colour plate 87), which should not be allowed to continue for more than 12 hours, or be enhanced with intravenous administration of oxytocin.

Caesarean section is rarely indicated if the *baby is dead,* but if there is also a major degree of placenta praevia, a difficult malpresentation, or double monster, this approach is safer for the mother. If the mother is very recently dead (0–10 minutes), *postmortem Caesarean section* may be done (always classical).

The *classical operation* has been superseded because bleeding is greater, the peritoneal cavity is more readily contaminated, there is a greater likelihood of later bowel adhesions and ileus; subsequent rupture is more likely and usually more serious. The lower segment operation does not have these disadvantages to the same degree, but it is slightly more difficult, *bladder injury is more likely,* and *haemorrhage may be severe* if the uterine vessels are damaged by lateral extension of the incision during extraction of the fetus.

PARENTS ATTITUDES TO CAESAREAN SECTION

A number of questions have arisen in recent years in relation to Caesarean birth. The father of the child often requests that he be allowed in the theatre for the birth. This enables the couple to share the experience if conduction analgesia is used or to relate the experience if general anaesthesia is used. In many centres this request is not being met — in others the father is allowed to be present only when the operation is performed under regional analgesia.

One of the major concerns is the marked difference in section rates between centres — from 5–10% in some to 25% in others. The rate

TABLE 47.2   LABOUR AFTER CAESAREAN SECTION

Number of patients with previous Caesarean		2,298
Repeat elective Caesarean section	1,520	(66.1%)
Trial of scar	778	(33.8%)
Vaginal delivery	595 (76.4%)	
Emergency Caesarean	183 (23.5%) (7*)	

* Cases of uterine rupture

in private practice is usually significantly higher than in clinic practice. A similar situation exists in relation to repeat section. The strong feeling of some parents is evidenced by the formation of such groups as *Caesarean Prevention Movement* and *Vaginal Births after Caesareans.* Questions that are being raised are informed consent information, alternative options, obstetrician's attitude to Caesarean delivery and intervention in general, and the raised cost factor.

Caesarean birth is looked on by many mothers as a relief and means of providing a healthy infant; others, however, feel great disappointment and perhaps a sense of failure in not achieving a normal vaginal birth. In many cases, guilt, anger and depression may offset perceived advantages of the Caesarean route because of interference to the mother's care of the newborn.

Epidural analgesia has become much more popular; not only does it allow the mother psychological participation in the birth, but the complications inevitable to general anaesthesia are avoided. Table 47.3 shows the recent rapid increase in the use of epidural analgesia for Caesarean section. This table also shows the recent trend to deliver more *very small* (less than 2,500 g or before 36 weeks' gestation) and *very large* (over 4,000 g) infants by Caesarean section. This table also shows the increasing popularity of the *Pfannenstiel incision* (colour plates 67 and 68).

Table 47.4 illustrates the change in perinatal mortality rates associated with Caesarean section with the operation being performed more often for low birth-weight infants. It is seen that as the Caesarean section rate increased there was a disproportionate rise in the number of *neonatal deaths* from complications of prematurity (hyaline membrane disease). With this trend to deliver more high risk premature infants by Caesarean section, the perinatal mortality rate associated with the operation has increased, although the overall perinatal rate, over the same interval, improved in this particular hospital from 29.7 to 22.6 per 1,000 births.

TABLE 47.3 SOME STATISTICS ASSOCIATED WITH CAESAREAN SECTION IN A LARGE TEACHING HOSPITAL

	1971–1974	1975–1977	1978–1980
No. of Caesarean sections	1,214	1,513	1,906
Before 36 weeks' gestation	71 (5.8)	79 (5.2)	194 (10.2)
Birth-weight < 2,500 g	128 (10.5)	143 (9.5)	246 (12.9)
Birth-weight > 4,000 g	100 (8.9)	167 (11.0)	214 (11.2)
Epidural analgesia	—	50 (3.3)	366 (19.2)
Pfannenstiel incision	—	562 (37.1)	1,024 (53.7)
Blood transfusion	167 (13.7)	164 (10.8)	156 (8.2)
Classical incision	—	22 (1.5)	24 (1.3)
Ruptured uterus	7	9	6
Caesarean hysterectomy	10	13	13
Maternal death	1	2	1

Figures in parentheses are percentages

TABLE 47.4   CHANGING INCIDENCE OF CAESAREAN SECTION AND ASSOCIATED MORTALITY RATES IN ONE LARGE TEACHING HOSPITAL

Year	Caesarean section		No. of maternal deaths	No. of stillbirths	No. of neonatal deaths	Perinatal mortality rate (per 1,000)
	Number	Incidence				
1971–1974	1,214	9.3%	1	11	27	31
1975–1977	1,513	11.4%	2	8	22	20
1978–1980	1,906	12.9%	1	7	37	23
1981–1983	2,299	14.4%	—	11	32	19

PREPARATION FOR CAESAREAN SECTION

For elective operations, the patient is usually admitted the day before, and routine admission procedures are carried out — history, examination, and special investigations, such as urine and blood tests. Skin and bowel preparation is similar to that for any abdominal operation. Wound infection rates are significantly lower if a depilatory cream is used for hair removal or alternatively, *shaving is deferred* until just before surgery.

A sedative is usually ordered to ensure a restful sleep. Formerly a disposable enema was given the night before operation, but this practice has been discontinued and is in fact contraindicated if the patient has had an antepartum haemorrhage or if placenta praevia is suspected (high presenting part). It is beneficial for a *physiotherapist* to see the patient before operation. No food or fluids are given for the 6 hours before operation.

The patient is dressed in a clean gown, leggings, and cap. Dentures should be removed, placed in a clean container marked with the patient's name, and an entry made to this effect. An identification tag is placed on the patient's wrist. Usually a catheter is placed in the bladder before the patient is sent to theatre and taped in place. Some obstetricians prefer to pass a catheter in theatre after the patient has been anaesthetized — this causes her a minimum of discomfort and ensures that the bladder is empty (unless it is of the Foley type, an indwelling catheter can slip out of the bladder into the urethra!).

Premedication, usually atropine, 0.6–1.0 mg, is given subcutaneously 30 minutes before operation; in some cases, especially if there is an emergency, the anaesthetist will give the atropine intravenously.

Two units of *blood are cross-matched* if an above normal loss is expected (e.g. placenta praevia); otherwise, in many centres the blood is typed and screened for unexpected antibodies and cross-matched only if required. About 10% of patients will require a *blood transfusion* because of excessive haemorrhage at Caesarean section (table 47.3).

The chart, with *signed consent form* and any X-ray films must accompany the patient. NB: It is not mandatory for the husband to sign his wife's sterilization form in the United Kingdom.

Alimentation and gastric contents. In labour, if there is a likelihood that Caesarean section may become necessary, food and oral fluids should not be administered. If a recent meal has been taken, the stomach may be emptied by the passage of a large bore tube; however, this is distressing to the patient and perhaps to the baby also and trained anaesthetists can overcome the problem by employing the Sellick manoeuvre at the time of induction. An alkaline mixture such as *magnesium trisilicate* 15–20 ml taken orally will neutralize the acid in the stomach which is particularly harmful to the respiratory tree if aspirated; the addition of an anticholinergic drug is desirable.

Oxygen. Should be administered by mask in the ward and during transport if indicated by the condition of the mother and baby.

Explanation. The procedure should be explained adequately to the patient and reassurance given concerning her own and the baby's well-being. *The husband is also informed* of the need and reasons for Caesarean section.

Transport. Care must be taken that no injury occurs to the patient when moving on and off the trolleys or during transport. A nurse will accompany the patient and wait with her until she is wheeled into the theatre. Whilst being transported and waiting, the patient should *lie on her side.*

Induction of anaesthesia. The person assisting the anaesthetist will assist with cricoid pressure during intubation (*Sellick manoeuvre*) if requested by the anaesthetist and should ensure that the *suction apparatus* is in proper working order. The patient's gown should be lifted away from the abdomen and her arms placed by her side or folded across her chest and secured by her folded gown. The operation is performed with the patient lying partly to one side to avoid the harmful effects (to both mother and fetus) of *postural hypotension.* Epidural analgesia is popular with many couples since the mother is conscious of the birth experience and can nurse the baby as soon as resuscitation has been effected. There is less physiological upset to the mother and bonding and breast feeding are facilitated. The mother suffers less from nausea and drowsiness and the baby is not as slow to initiate respiration.

Once the patient is anaesthetized, *calf stimulators* are applied to minimize the risk of venous thrombosis and thromboembolism — they are not used when the Caesarean is performed under *epidural analgesia.*

Intravenous infusion. It is advisable that an intravenous infusion be commenced if not already running. Blood loss at Caesarean section is often unpredictable, and may be heavy. In addition, the resulting haemoconcentration and trauma predispose to thromboembolism. Solutions of 5% dextrose, unless given slowly, cause maternal and fetal hyperglycaemia and acidosis and balanced salt solution is preferable at this stage.

Instruments. The instruments and drapes required are those for any abdominal operation, together with special requirements for Caesarean section: abdominal retractor (1), curved retractor (1), midwifery forceps (1), curved scissors (2) (fine and medium), straight scissors (2), Green-Armytage forceps (6), tissue forceps (Allis) (4), needle holders (2), sucker and tubing, diathermy, needles, sutures, sponge forceps (8), towel clips (6), scalpel handles (3), scalpel blades, curved artery forceps (12), straight artery forceps (6), toothed dissecting forceps (2) (fine and medium), plain dissecting forceps (1), swabs (12) and packs (6) (should have a radio-opaque strip).

Suction for anaesthetist, operator, and baby.

Resuscitation of the baby. Usually a special table is set aside for the paediatrician and nurse assistant to manage the infant after birth (figure 47.3). The requirements are as follows: suction, laryngoscope (infant), endotracheal tubes and introducer, oxygen with mask and catheter fittings, cord ligatures or clamp, syringes (2 ml and 10 ml), needles, ampoules of sodium bicarbonate, naloxone, vitamin K_1, and means of providing warmth for the baby.

TECHNIQUE OF OPERATION
(colour plates 92 and 93, figure 47.1)

After the patient is anaesthetized, she is placed in partial Trendelenburg position and the right hip is elevated to relieve pressure of the uterus on the great vessels. The abdomen is prepared with a suitable antiseptic solution (e.g. alcoholic hexachlorophane solution), and drapes are applied. A vertical or transverse approach is made through the lower abdomen and bleeding vessels are clamped and diathermied or ligated with fine plain catgut (000). A moist pack, tagged with an artery forceps, is sometimes placed in each paracolic gutter beside the uterus to minimize the escape of blood and liquor into the peritoneal cavity. The lower segment is exposed with the aid of a curved retractor and the loose peritoneum over it cut with curved scissors (figure 47.1). The peritoneum is usually reflected downwards, carrying the bladder with it. The muscle of the lower segment is incised with a scalpel in a tranverse direction, the level being at the greatest diameter of the presenting part. Curved scissors are used to extend the incision laterally; use of the fingers to enlarge the

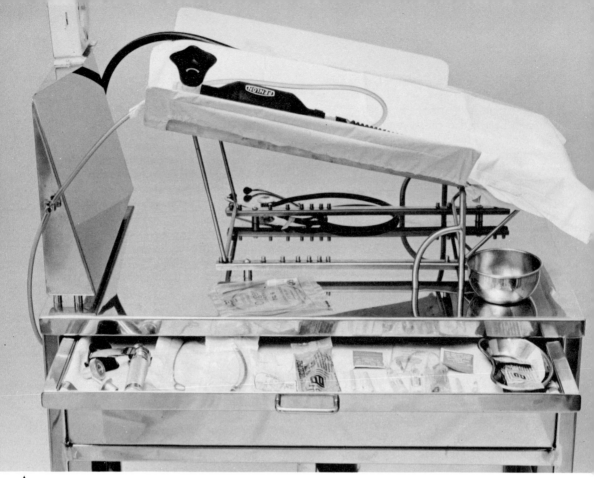

A

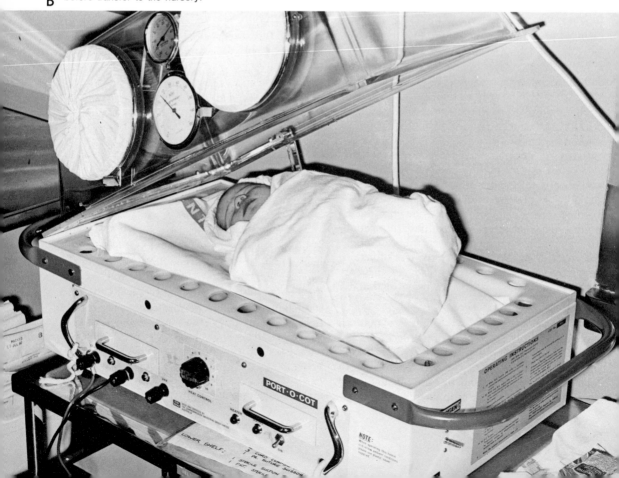

Figure 47.3 A. Resuscitation equipment for the newborn infant includes facilities for nasopharyngeal aspiration, oxygen administration, warming (by overhead radiant heater not shown in this photograph), and administration of drugs. **B.** Following resuscitation the infant has been placed in a transport incubator (oxygen, heat, suction and visibility provided) before transfer to the nursery.

B

incision is not recommended since healing of the muscle is less satisfactory. At this point, some operators prefer to place a marking suture, absorbable or nonabsorbable, in the lower flap for later identification (figure 47.1C).

As much liquor and blood as possible is removed with the sucker, in order to prevent aspiration by the baby. The retractor is removed and the baby is delivered either manually or with forceps. The baby's oropharynx and nose are aspirated, and the cord is clamped and cut. The nurse or doctor will take the baby in a sterile wrap to the resuscitation table, where the usual procedures will be carried out (figure 47.3).

Prophylactic antibiotics may be given at this stage by intravenous injection, especially if the patient has been labouring with ruptured membranes for more than 6 hours, or if other risk factors for infection are present (obesity, anaemia, low socioeconomic status, multiple vaginal examinations/fetal monitoring by scalp electrode).

Forceps, usually the Green-Armytage type, may be applied to the edges of the uterine incision for traction and to control bleeding. After an oxytocic has been given (ergometrine, Syntometrine, or Syntocinon), the placenta is removed, and the placental site is explored. A finger or cervical dilator is passed down through the cervical canal to ensure adequate patency. One or 2 rows of chromic catgut or polyglycolic sutures (0 or 1) on a round body needle are used to close the uterine incision; the first is usually continuous, the second continuous or interrupted. Additional sutures may be required to control bleeding. Some operators prefer to place stay sutures initially at each end of the incision; the ends of catgut used for each layer are held with artery forceps until the next layer is inserted. The peritoneum is closed with catgut (0). Packs are removed and a count is made of instruments and packs. If this is correct the abdomen is closed in layers, usually chromic catgut (0 or 1) for the peritoneum, chromic catgut (1) or polyglycolic for the rectus sheath, plain catgut (0) for the subcutaneous fat layer, and silk (3/0), prolene or clips for the skin.

The skin is dressed with an aerosol antiseptic spray and left open, or closed with sterile paraffin gauze and a dry dressing, or closed with a gauze soaked in alcoholic chlorhexidine and a pad and strapping applied. The *catheter*, if still indwelling, is usually removed and any *clot in the vagina* removed with a sponge on a holder or digitally.

Difficulties

Adhesions from a previous section or pelvic surgery may render access difficult. The poorly-formed lower segment is more common early in the third trimester, and may necessitate a vertical incision. Jamming of the fetal head deep in the pelvis should be recognized before operation and dislodged gently upward at the time of catheterization. Difficulty in delivery of the head may also result from an incision placed too high or too low in the lower segment; fundal pressure will assist in the latter case. Occasionally, the incision has been too small and will need to be enlarged (preferably by stretching with the fingers).

The Classical Operation

This is required in *1-2%* of Caesarean sections (table 47.3) usually for *transverse lie* of the fetus, *failure of development of the lower segment* (prematurity ± breech presentation), dense adhesions, presence of *large veins* over the lower segment (*placenta praevia*), *constriction ring*, invasive carcinoma of the cervix, and as an emergency after death of the mother. The classical operation is likely to be performed more often than formerly because more very premature infants (26–32 weeks' gestation) are being delivered by Caesarean section — in these pregnancies the lower segment is often poorly formed, especially when there is the combination of *fetal growth retardation, oligohydramnios and breech presentation*.

Additional Procedures

Hysterectomy. This is required in about 1 in 130 patients who have a Caesarean section (table 47.3) — the operation (*Caesarean hysterectomy*) is undertaken more often in some centres where it is performed electively as a means of *sterilization*. The usual indications are *uterine rupture*, inability to *control haemorrhage* from the lower segment incision, *placenta accreta* (often praevia accreta) and tumours (hydatidiform mole in the elderly multipara, carcinoma of the cervix). Occasionally hysterectomy is required for secondary postpartum haemorrhage either in patients who have delivered vaginally or following Caesarean section. The operative procedure differs in no way from that used in the nonpregnant woman. The only additional instruments required are clamps for the paracervical ligaments (colour plate 23).

Sterilization. To save an additional operation, sterilization is often performed, if indicated, after completion of the section, the patient and her husband having previously provided well considered written consent. *About 8-10% of patients have sterilization performed* at the time of repeat Caesarean section. The technique of tubal occlusion is discussed in Chapter 56.

POSTOPERATIVE CARE

In the recovery room the patient is nursed on her side until fully conscious, and is then transferred to the postnatal ward.

Observations of the patient's colour, conscious state, pulse rate, blood pressure, respiratory rate, and vaginal loss should be recorded as for any major surgical procedure: every 15 minutes for the 1–2 hours spent in the recovery room, then half-hourly for 4 hours, and thereafter every 4–8 hours. If the loss from the vagina is greater than normal, more frequent observations are necessary. If *epidural analgesia* has been used the sensation in the feet should be checked.

An *intravenous infusion* is always running, and so orders are required concerning rate and type of infusion required. Special fluids (plasma, blood, fibrinogen) may be required if haemorrhage has been serious. The drip rate, absence of tissue infiltration, and level in the flask should be checked every 1–4 hours. Usually nothing is given by mouth for 24 hours, apart from ice to suck or sips of fluid. The infusion is discontinued after 24–48 hours when the patient is tolerating fluids orally.

If the *catheter* has been left in the bladder after operation it will either be allowed to drain continuously or released 4 or 6-hourly. The freedom of drainage, adequacy of output and security of fixation of the catheter to the thigh should be checked 4-hourly. If the catheter has been removed and the patient is unable to void, she must be recatheterized with careful asepsis if simpler measures fail.

Pethidine 100 mg or Omnopon 10–15 mg will be given IM every 3–4 hours as required for pain; many patients do not ask for pain relief but it should be offered (up to 36 hours postoperatively). If epidural analgesia has been used there will be a pain free period after recovering consciousness. At night a sedative is often helpful in addition.

Oxygen is given routinely in some hospitals in the recovery room; in others it is only administered if the patient's condition is abnormal.

Physiotherapy. Active and passive leg movements, deep breathing and coughing, and later abdominal exercises are encouraged at least every 2 hours. This is important in the prophylaxis of postoperative complications such as *thromboembolism* and *atelectasis/pneumonia*. Pelvic floor exercises ensure a quicker return to normal of the lax and stretched pelvic musculature. The mother will normally be allowed up the day after operation and will be able to shower on the second or third day.

The mother should be allowed to nurse the baby as soon as she is fully conscious and may feed the baby for short periods on the 1st day. She should be warned that the milk may come in a day or so later than is the case after normal vaginal delivery.

If the bowels have not opened by the 3rd day, an aperient is usually given night and morning until this is remedied.

Antibiotics are not usually given as a routine, but are advisable if a factor predisposing to infection is present — e.g. rupture of membranes for more than 6 hours. In such cases, a drug or drugs covering both anaerobic and aerobic organisms should be used.

A routine *haemoglobin estimation* is made on the 3rd day.

Other nursing measures are the same as for general puerperal and routine postoperative care. The abdominal sutures or clips are removed on the 5th–7th day, according to circumstances.

COMPLICATIONS

Immediate complications for the *mother* include those related to the anaesthetic (drug overdose, hypoxia, aspiration of gastric content), or the operation (haemorrhage, damage to bladder or bowel), or the condition necessitating operation (hypertensive disease, diabetes, uterine infection). *Subsequent complications* include infection (abdominal wall, uterus, urinary tract, chest) thromboembolism, ileus, haemorrhage and wound infection, wound dehiscence. Local infection is related to the duration of membrane rupture and labour, number of pelvic examinations and the skill of the operator (haemostasis etc).

Distant complications are mainly *uterine rupture* in a subsequent pregnancy (colour plate 87), *adhesion formation* and *intestinal obstruction*.

The baby may be adversely affected by the operation itself, for example, hypoxia from the supine hypotensive syndrome if the mother is not positioned properly, hypoxia from overdose of drugs or anaesthetic agent given to the mother, or because she is under-or overventilated. There may be excessive bleeding before the baby is delivered or difficulty may be experienced in extracting the baby from the uterus if the abdominal or uterine incision is too small. *Respiratory distress* is more common in the premature baby; this may be related to the fact that amniotic fluid is not squeezed out of the lung as in vaginal delivery (*wet lung syndrome*). Chiefly, however, the baby will suffer from the condition responsible for the section, such as *growth retardation, antepartum haemorrhage,* or *obstructed labour*. In many cases, the baby will be premature and suffer from the complications related to that condition. It is not surprising that the Apgar score of the baby is often less than that in vaginal deliveries. The major avoidable error is to undertake elective section before the fetus is mature.

Mortality rates are given for both the mother and baby, but so often it is difficult to separate the contribution of the operation itself and the underlying cause — e.g. in the series of 4,633 Caesarean sections shown in tables 47.1 and 47.2 there were 4 maternal deaths; 2 were from obstetric causes (eclampsia complicated by massive cerebral haemorrhage (1), preeclampsia complicated by coagulopathy and renal failure (1)) and 2 from associated conditions (disseminated malignant melanoma (1),lupus nephritis/renal failure (1)); none of these 4 deaths occurred as a result of the anaesthetic itself. The general maternal mortality rate ranges from 40–100 per 100,000 Caesarean sections, being mainly the result of haemorrhage, sepsis, thromboembolism or anaesthetic accident (see Chapter 14). This rate is significantly higher than the overall maternal mortality rate (10–40 per 100,000 births) and 4–5 times higher than that of vaginal delivery (10–20 per 100,000 births), which is why high Caesarean section rates are not encouraged.

For elective operations, the mortality to the fetus should be no greater than after vaginal delivery. More accurate prediction of fetal lung maturity has markedly lessened the incidence of death from *hyaline membrane disease*. If babies already dead are excluded, the perinatal mortality rates in the series of 6,932 Caesarean operations shown in table 47.4 were *2.4% for primary operations* and *0.8% for repeat (elective) operations*. As stated earlier in this chapter, the neonatal death rate associated with Caesarean section will depend upon the number of operations performed before 36 weeks' gestation (breech presentation, premature rupture of the membranes, antepartum haemorrhage, preeclampsia) (table 47.3). If complete uterine rupture occurs, 30–40% of babies will die; if the rupture is incomplete, the figure is usually below 10% (see Chapter 54).

DISORDERS OF LABOUR

chapter forty-eight

Fetal Distress

OVERVIEW

The subject of fetal distress has assumed great importance in obstetrics because of the concept of *quality of life — i.e. life without handicap.* Although this is not always attainable in our current state of knowledge, avoidable factors are receiving much attention. The first questions that must be answered are: what is fetal 'distress' and what does it mean? Basically, it is a signal from the fetus that it is under stress. The significance depends on many factors — duration of the stress (minutes–weeks); its nature (hypoxia, sepsis, trauma, drugs), and its severity. *It may indicate the normal reaction of a healthy fetus or a near terminal response* (figure 23.1); it may also be a sign that the fetus has a serious congenital malformation (e.g. neural tube defect) or intrauterine infection.

Although there has been a great accrual of knowledge of fetal physiology and responses to stress, the *instruments of measurement are still imperfect* in terms of providing a description of how much difficulty the fetus is experiencing and what reserves are available should a conservative course be adopted. While this state persists, the spectre of fetal brain damage will haunt the obstetrician and encourage more radical treatment options. It is probable that the pendulum has overswung in this direction in recent years. *Nonetheless, the introduction of cardiotocography antenatally and continuous fetal heart monitoring in labour has made an enormous contribution to the assessment of fetal well-being and decising-making regarding timing and method of delivery.*

Another dilemma concerns the *place of confinement.* Although the popularity of *home birth* is not great in most developed countries (1–5%), for it to receive general endorsement, there must be an affirmative reply to the question — can fetal distress in labour be predicted? It would seem that the answer to this is no.

Cost benefit considerations usually emerge when screening procedures are discussed. Each labour ward must decide who should be *monitored*, how this should be done, and what interpretive policies will be followed. Protocols along these lines lessen the confusion that surrounds some of current-day monitoring.

The increasing *desire of the patients to enter into decision-making* can place additional stress on the health care attendant — particularly with the currently popular philosophy that there is too much interference in the labour process (monitoring may be perceived to be part of this).

In the majority of patients, fetal distress arises because of *hypoxia* — there being many obstacles in the path of the haemoglobin and its captive oxygen before the latter can be delivered to the fetus. *Before labour*, degenerative changes in the placenta and associated blood vessels play a major role (Chapter 23); *during labour*, the interruption to blood flow in several related areas is paramount (uterus, placenta, umbilical cord).

The *effects on the fetus* of such insults are becoming codified, and this information will be of increasing value as a basis of decision-making as further knowledge accumulates, particularly with computer assistance. Currently, most attention is given to fetal heart rate behaviour and blood sampling for *detection of acidosis* (an inevitable result of significant hypoxia).

Accidents to the umbilical cord are of sufficient frequency and gravity to merit special attention. *Prolapse* of the cord requires immediate remedy if the baby's life is to be saved. Other cord accidents (*entanglement and knotting*) will present as do other causes of hypoxia.

The *Apgar score* at 1 and 5 minutes after birth is usually taken as a measure of fetal distress during labour; however, hypoxia is only one cause of a low Apgar score, and thus long-term correlations are not very precise.

FETAL DISTRESS

DEFINITION

An impairment in the oxygenation and/or nutritional state of the fetus, revealed on clinical and/or investigational study. It may be acute (prolapsed cord, placental abruption), subacute (hypertonic uterine action), or chronic (placental insufficiency).

INCIDENCE

This differs rather widely according to accepted definition and the intensity of monitoring in labour. Between 15 and 20% of fetuses will show clinical evidence of distress before delivery (meconium in the liquor, heart rate below 120 or above 160 beats per minute or both), and 25–35% of those in whom continuous heart rate monitoring is used (table 48.1).

TABLE 48.1   RESULTS OF CONTINUOUS INTRAPARTUM FETAL HEART RATE MONITORING IN 7,858 OF 28,058 CONSECUTIVE LABOURS

	%	
Incidence	28.0	
Stillbirths	0.19	
Neonatal deaths	0.45	
Abnormal heart rate pattern	34.6	
Early deceleration (type 1 dip)		50.0
Late deceleration (type 2 dip)		10.0
Tachycardia		25.0
Bradycardia		15.0
Caesarean sections	11.8	
Obstructed labour		44.5
Fetal distress		36.4
Incoordinate uterine action		9.0
Malpresentation		4.1
Antepartum haemorrhage		3.4
Severe preeclampsia		1.8
Prolapsed cord		0.7

TABLE 48.2   CAUSES OF FETAL DISTRESS

1. *Mother*	Hypotension or shock from any cause
	Cardiovascular disease
	Anaemia
	Respiratory depression or disease
	Malnutrition
	Acidosis and dehydration
	Supine hypotension syndrome
2. *Uterus*	Excessive or prolonged uterine activity
	Vascular degeneration
3. *Placenta*	Vascular degeneration and infarction
	Premature separation
	Primary hypoplasia.
4. *Cord*	Compression (knot, entwinement)
5. *Fetus*	Infection
	Malformation
	Haemorrhage
	Anaemia

Figure 48.1 Postural (supine) hypotension syndrome. Transverse section of abdomen in late pregnancy illustrating that the pressure of the uterus and contents is most likely to compress the inferior vena cava (and aorta) when the patient lies on her back; cardiac output increases 10% when the patient turns to the right lateral position and 20% when turning to the left lateral position — the preferred position for rest in pregnancy.

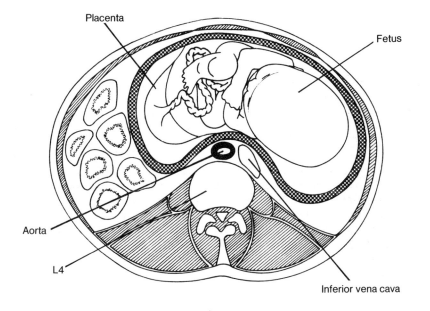

AETIOLOGY

The causes of fetal distress are summarized in table 48.2. They may be present before the onset of labour (especially maternal disorders and placental pathology) or occur during labour (especially uterine, umbilical cord and fetal factors). In a large minority of patients, there is no obvious cause for the distress. Distress after birth is considered in the neonatology section.

The Mother

Maternal oxygenation. An inadequate oxygen content of the maternal blood may result from poor gas exchange in the lungs (poorly administered anaesthesia, lung pathology), cardiac failure, or anaemia. A reduction in the pressure at

which the blood is delivered is seen in such conditions as fainting and the *supine hypotensive syndrome* (where it is usually transient — figure 48.1), shock (where it may be prolonged), and epidural analgesia.

Maternal nutrition. A suboptimal level of nutrients in the mother's blood may result from poor intake, poor absorption, or diseases of such vital organs as the liver and pancreas.

Uterus

The most important factor is *abnormal uterine action of the hypertonic type.* Since the pressure in the uterine wall during a contraction is greater than that in the uterine and umbilical vessels, it follows that, if the contractions are too close

Figure 48.2 Cord complications A. Knotting of the umbilical cord around the ankle caused death of this 3,040 g infant; the mother, a 33-year-old para 3, reported cessation of movements at 36 weeks' gestation. The fetal heart was inaudible and vaginal examination showed marked overlap of the parietal bones. Labour was induced by amniotomy and spontaneous delivery occurred 4 hours later, 2 days after the movements had ceased; note the degree of maceration. Cord entanglement is an uncommon cause of intrauterine death (see colour plate 89). **B.** True knot in the umbilical cord photographed fortuitously at repeat Caesarean section (the photographer was present to record dehiscence of the uterine scar). The patient was a 32-year-old para 3 diabetic, and cardiotocography had shown loss of beat to beat variation. The infant was born in good condition.   A   B

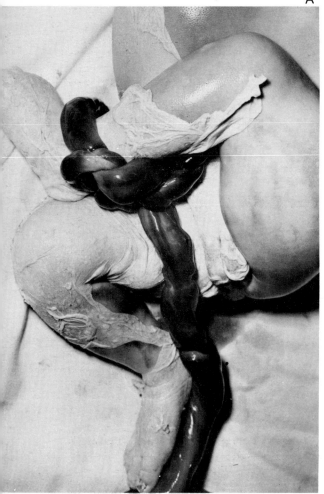

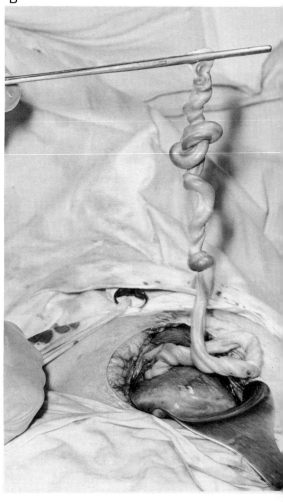

together or stronger than normal (above 60–80 mm Hg), too little blood will pass to and from the area of exchange, which is the intervillous space of the placenta. The general effect of uterine contractions is to produce an acceleration of the fetal heart in the earlier part of the contraction and a deceleration toward the end.

Placenta

This is the organ of exchange between the mother and fetus. The placenta has a definite life span, and if pregnancy is too prolonged, senescence will occur. As elsewhere in the body, the arteries become diseased (atherosis and sclerosis) in the presence of such conditions as *hypertension, preeclampsia, diabetes and chronic renal disease*. This restricts the amount of blood reaching the placenta. If the uterine vessels are affected, there is a greater likeihood of thromboses in the intervillous space. These changes can be seen as *infarcts* in the placenta after delivery — reddish-brown homogeneous areas when fresh, later becoming pale and fibrotic (colour plates 18 and 19). Premature separation of the placenta from the decidual lining of the uterus occurs mainly in the last trimester; this diminishes the placental reserve in proportion to the *degree of the abruption* (figures 19.2 and 19.3; colour plates 15 and 16).

Occasionally, when the *area of the placenta is suddenly reduced* (rupture of membranes in a patient with polyhydramnios or delivery of the first twin), there may be some compromise in blood flow.

In some patients, the *placenta is poorly formed*, even early in pregnancy, and the area of exchange (intervillous space and villous area) is never normal.

Umbilical Cord

This is the final supply link to the fetus, and blood flow may be diminished or cut off by entanglements about the body of the fetus, knotting, presentation, or prolapse (figure 48.2 A and B). The cord is looped around the fetal neck at least once in 20–25% of deliveries and 1% have a true knot (figure 48.2B) — these seldom cause fetal death in utero before the onset of labour (unlike cord entanglements (figure 48.2A)) since the knot tightens only when the contractions cause descent of the head (figure 51.8 C and D).

Fetus

There are a number of conditions in the fetus, as in the mother, that may cause signs of distress. Apart from placental inadequacy, there may be distress due to *infection*, cardiac disorders (*con-*

genital malformation), *anaemia* (erythroblastosis, bleeding into the mother's or a twin's circulation (colour plates 47 and 46)), or shock (haemorrhage from a vasa praevia (colour plates 84 and 85)).

ASSESSMENT

The *well-being* of the fetus during labour *is assessed* basically by *clinical*, *electronic* (fetal heart behaviour) and *biochemical* (oxygen, acid-base of capillary blood) means; *ultrasound* (movement, breathing activity) is used in some units.

Cardiotocography

Pathophysiology. Changes in fetal heart rate depend mainly on the interaction of the following variables — *direct and reflex activity of the autonomic nervous system and the degree of oxygenation of the fetal vasomotor centre and heart.* Thus, pressure on the fetal head as it enters the pelvis or during external cephalic version will stimulate the vagus nerve and cause slowing of the heart rate; so will pressure on the umbilical cord. Mild hypoxia causes an *acceleration* of the rate initially, but as the oxygen lack (and the *degree of acidosis*) increases, both the centre in the brain which governs heart action and the heart muscle itself are affected and the heart slows.

Clinical significance. The normal and abnormal features on cardiotocography have been discussed in Chapters 13 and 23.

There is as yet insufficient data to allow a precise significance to be attached to the different cardiotocographic parameters in terms of actual fetal condition. The variables are many — e.g. *tachycardia, bradycardia, acceleration, deceleration, beat to beat and baseline variation*, and *sinusoidal activity*. An abnormality may occur alone or in a number of combinations; in addition, there is a wide variation in degree of the abnormality and its duration. One of the major problems is that it is often difficult to be sure whether the change observed is representative of a healthy fetus reacting satisfactorily to stress or a severely compromized fetus with little reserve. Overall, there is an uncomfortably high number of false positive and false negative tests, with a rather variable and not very satisfactory predictive value.

Computerization of the data, with immediate reference to stored information for comparison, will maximize the value of cardiotocography and other indices used in the prediction of fetal distress.

Electrocardiography

In addition to the fetal heart rate pattern analysis, the *ECG* itself may be used. Features characteristic of hypoxia are looked for in the configuration of the complex. During marked variable deceleration (intermittent cord compression) the P wave is biphasic or absent and the PQ interval may be longer or shorter depending on the amount of drop in rate; less consistent (50%) are changes in the ST segment and T waves (depression).

The above changes can be best followed if there is a continuous fetal heart monitor in the labour ward. If this is not available, *the importance of following the heart rate in the period after the contraction is emphasized.* The fall in rate and its duration reflects fairly well the decrease in placental reserve. Counting with a simple instrument employing the Doppler principle is usually quite efficient.

Echocardiography

This is a new technique, based on the sonar principle, that allows investigation of the fetal heart structure and function. This is especially useful if the cardiotocographic findings suggest the presence of congenital heart disease. Indices such as chamber dimensions, stroke volume, ejection fraction, and anatomical changes during systole can be assessed.

Acid-Base Status

In Chapter 36, a description was given of the means whereby energy was obtained for the different functions of the body. In essence, oxygen is used in the energy-producing cycle, and carbon dioxide is the end product which is eliminated by the lungs. If the supply of oxygen is inadequate, a less efficient energy-producing mechanism is switched in (the *anaerobic glycolytic pathway*), and the end products are *lactic acid* and *pyruvic acid*, which cannot be eliminated as simply as carbon dioxide. These acids can be neutralized by several 'buffer' systems in the body, but when these become saturated, a state of progressive *metabolic acidosis* occurs, i.e. there is a fall in the pH in the tissues. If unrelieved, vital enzyme and membrane transport functions fail and the cells die. The degree of acidosis can be measured reasonably accurately with the technique of *fetal blood sampling* (usually scalp, occasionally buttock).

This procedure is usually *indicated when fetal distress is suspected* on the basis of either clinical findings (oligohydramnios, meconium staining of liquor, poor fetal movements) or investigations (cardiotocography, fetal breathing pattern).

The tray required for the procedure is shown in figure 21.7. The position and preparation of the patient is the same as that described under 'Surgical Induction of Labour'. After cleansing of the vagina, an appropriately-sized amnioscope is inserted gently through the cervix until the presenting part comes into view. The area in view is wiped clean and is sprayed with ethyl chloride. A sample of capillary blood is obtained by piercing the scalp with a small disposable blade and drawing the blood into a fine plastic tube treated to prevent clotting. If a coincident acidosis is suspected in the mother, a sample of her blood should also be taken for analysis.

The *normal pH value is 7.35* (range 7.45-7.25); the more depressed the reading below this, the more likely is the baby to be suffering from hypoxia. A value *below 7.20 is definitely pathological* and calls for close review; if the level has fallen to 7.10, the fetus is in considerable danger, and death is common at about pH 6.8.

Amniotic Fluid Quantity and Meconium Staining

Passage of meconium occurs because asphyxia stimulates the vagus nerve, which supplies the gut. This is observed in some 10-15% of patients. If the colouration of the liquor is green the hypoxic insult is recent — very recent if the meconium is formed. With time, the colour changes to a yellowish-brown. The amount of amniotic fluid with which the meconium is mixed broadly parallels the adequacy of placental function. Very little liquor heavily admixed with meconium suggests that the fetus has little in reserve.

Fetal Breathing

Normally, the fetus will spend 30% of the time in breathing activity (range 10-60%). If hypoxic, the breathing episodes will be briefer and gasping may occur.

Postnatal Features

Pallor (asphyxia pallida) results from the shunting of blood from peripheral, less essential parts of the body (vasoconstriction), in order to preserve the vital centres.

Respiratory distress. The formation of surfactant in the lungs is curtailed by hypoxia, and both atelectasis and hyaline membrane formation are more common (respiratory distress syndrome). *Meconium aspiration.* Asphyxia stimulates gasping by the fetus in utero particularly after 34-36 weeks; if meconium is present in the liquor, it tends to produce a severe pneumonitis because of its irritating chemical action.

Summary

With hypoxia, there is generally a change in the fetal heart rate pattern before there is a fall in blood pH. Thus, the *fetal heart rate* is used for primary monitoring, particularly in patients with risk factors, and if the pattern is abnormal, *scalp blood pH* is estimated at intervals until the baby is born or the deterioration is such that labour is terminated. Scalp sampling can only be done at intervals, although it predicts more accurately the condition of the fetus at birth (Apgar score).

There should be a full and accurate estimate made of the fetal condition and an assessment of the urgency of the situation — i.e. fetal reserve, rate of deterioration, and the amount of uterine work required until delivery can be accomplished.

MANAGEMENT

(i) Look for possible causes (prolapsed cord). (ii) *Remove the cause* if possible: correct maternal factors (e.g. anaemia, dehydration, caloric lack, hypotension, hypertonic uterine activity — e.g. reduce oxytocin if indicated or give tocolytic agent). (iii) Give *oxygen* by mask to the mother (6 litres/minute). (iv) Turn the mother on her side to improve uterine blood flow. (v) Anticipate operative intervention (cross-match blood, anaesthetist, paediatrician) and/or a depressed baby (paediatrician). (vi) If the scalp pH is less than 7.15, immediate delivery is indicated; between 7.15 and 7.20, the maternal pH should be measured, and the fetal pH is repeated; if above 7.20, continue routine observations and repeat if progress is unsatisfactory or fetal heart rate abnormalities are present. If Caesarean section is indicated and an operating theatre is not available, ritodrine, 6 mg given IV over 2–3 minutes, will reduce the hypoxia of the uterine contractions.

The measures taken after delivery are discussed in the chapter on asphyxia and resuscitation of the newborn infant (Chapter 62).

PROGNOSIS

The outcome of the baby with fetal distress is quite variable, because of the *multiplicity of causes* (e.g. hypoxia, trauma, sepsis, drugs, congenital anomaly). One of the surprising things is the *resilience of the majority of such infants*; for example, in a recent study, cerebral palsy occurred in only 1% of infants severely asphyxiated at birth (Apgar score 0–3 at 5 minutes). The

following are useful *prognostic features* of postanoxic encephalopathy: level of consciousness, neuromuscular control (tone, posture, stretch reflexes, myoclonus), complex reflexes (sucking, Moro, oculovestibular, tonic neck), autonomic function (pupils, heart rate, gastrointestinal motility), electroencephalography, and finally, duration of the clinical disturbance.

TABLE 48.3 INDICATIONS FOR CONTINUOUS INTRAPARTUM FETAL HEART RATE MONITORING IN A SERIES OF 7,858 CASES

	%
Preeclampsia/hypertension	20.3
Meconium in liquor	16.8
41 weeks' gestation or more	13.6
Low oestriol excretion	9.1
Abnormal fetal heart rate	6.5
Weight loss at term	3.6
Antepartum haemorrhage	3.1
Epidural analgesia	1.4
Routine	11.5
Miscellaneous	13.6

For the reader's perspective tables 48.1 and 48.3 have been included to show the indications and results of *intrapartum fetal heart rate monitoring* in a large teaching hospital. Note that: (i) The incidence of monitoring was 28% — the frequency varies from one institution to another and depends upon the proportion of high risk pregnancies, and the extent to which monitoring of low risk pregnancies is practised. (ii) The main indications were clinical evidence of fetal distress and hypertension/preeclampsia which together accounted for 43% of cases. (iii) The Caesarean section rate of patients monitored was 11.8% which was similar to that in the overall hospital population (12.3%) and indicates that continuous fetal heart rate monitoring need not result in a higher Caesarean section rate. Indeed, when fetal distress is further investigated by fetal scalp pH studies, the Caesarean rate may be reduced by indicating patients in whom it is safe, from the fetal point of view, to allow labour to continue. (iv) The incidence of abnormal fetal heart rate patterns was 35% — only 10% of these showed critical reserve (late decelerations) which requires prompt delivery; the common abnormality was early decelerations, many of which occurred in the later stages of labour due to head compression. (v) The perinatal mortality rate was 0.6%. There are occasions when the clinical detection of an abnormal fetal heart rate, or the presence of meconium in the liquor, occurs too late to allow delivery of a living infant. It may be that *routine*

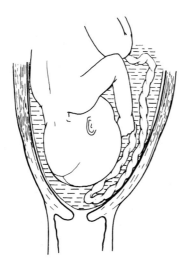

Figure 48.3 Cord presentation; the membranes are intact.

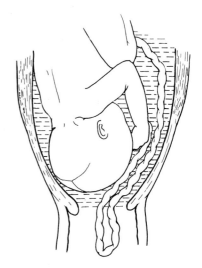

Figure 48.4 Prolapse of the cord in labour, with the cervix almost fully dilated.

external fetal cardiotocography when patients are admitted in labour would allow selection of those who require *continuous monitoring*, with further improvement in overall perinatal results. Such a programme is expensive and further controlled trials are required to determine if such a regimen is worthwhile.

UMBILICAL CORD ACCIDENTS

PROLAPSE

Definition
The cord lies beside the presenting part (occult prolapse) or below it (frank prolapse), the membranes having ruptured. The condition may or may not be preceded by *cord presentation*, where the cord is similarly placed but the membranes are still intact (figures 48.3 and 48.4).

Incidence
This ranges from 1 in 200–1 in 500 deliveries (cephalic presentations, 0.2–0.4%; breech presentations, 2–4%). Occult prolapse occurs in about 0.5% of labours.

Aetiology
Any condition preventing normal apposition of the presenting part to the lower uterine segment at the time of rupture of the membranes. A long cord is usually only a contributory factor to those listed below. The condition is more common in labour, since it is then that rupture of the membranes usually occurs. Prolapse may occur

because the baby is already distressed, the cord becoming slack and sinking down. *Fetus*: malpresentations (40%) (breech, especially footling; transverse and oblique lie; less commonly face and brow); multiple pregnancy (15%); malformations, prematurity (20%). *Amniotic fluid*: polyhydramnios (5%). *Placenta*: praevial position (5%). *Uterus*: fibroids, congenital malformation, laxity. *Pelvis*: contraction (10%). *Attendant*: artificial rupture of membranes, intrauterine manipulation.

Table 48.4 shows the associated clinical conditions in a series of 118 cases of cord presentation or prolapse — the incidence was 0.3% (1 in 372 pregnancies); 1.9% for *breech presentations* (33 of 1,673) and *3.3%* in cases of *multiple pregnancy* (19 of 571).

TABLE 48.4   CONDITIONS ASSOCIATED WITH PRESENTATION AND PROLAPSE OF THE UMBILICAL CORD IN A SERIES OF 118 CASES

	Number
Breech presentation	33
Surgical induction of labour	21
Multiple pregnancy	19
Antepartum haemorrhage	9
Unstable lie	6
Polyhydramnios	5
Face presentation	4
External cephalic version	1

Diagnosis
Presentation of the cord may be diagnosed if the examiner is alert; the characteristic soft, pulsatile

nature of the cord is felt through the membranes (figure 48.3). *Prolapse* (figure 48.4) should be excluded by *immediate vaginal examination when the membranes rupture in the presence of any of the aetiological factors listed above* i.e. *breech presentation, multiple pregnancy, unstable lie, high presenting part, polyhydramnios,* or the onset of *fetal distress* (passage of meconium, fetal heart rate abnormalities). Occasionally, the cord may pass through the introitus and its presence is reported by the patient. Usually, there is a pronounced slowing of the fetal heart, and auscultation is therefore necessary in all patients when the membranes rupture or if meconium-stained liquor is observed. Unsuspected presentation or prolapse may be detected by the application of pressure to the uterine fundus and presenting part: the cord compression results in a drop in fetal heart rate. Cord compression typically results in an early or variable deceleration of the fetal heart rate during a uterine contraction.

Management

Prevention

The main factor in prevention is avoidance of *artificial rupture of the membranes* when the presenting part is not fitting well into the lower uterine segment (table 48.4).

Early Detection

This depends on a constant awareness of the possibility; occasionally, a cord presentation will be detected, and this will allow appropriate measures to be taken. Cord prolapse occurs outside the labour ward in 15–25% of patients; the patient should be encouraged to attend early in labour (especially if the presentation is breech or not fitting well into the brim). With an increasing number of labours being monitored electronically, there is often an early warning of cord presentation and occult prolapse.

Active Treatment

Treatment is immediate delivery when the fetus is alive and mature — if not deliverable vaginally the emergency measures outlined below are implemented.

Emergency measures. (i) Summon medical aid; it is likely that an anaesthetist and paediatrician will be needed also. (ii) The patient is placed in the knee-chest or exaggerated Sims position. (iii) The presenting part is pushed upward to relieve pressure on the cord (sterile gloved hand in the vagina); this is continued

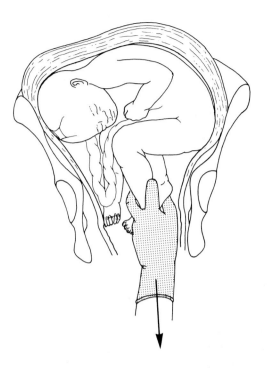

Figure 48.5 Compound presentation of cord, arm and feet with the cervix fully dilated. This is an indication for internal version and breech extraction, as shown here, but only when cephalopelvic disproportion can be excluded.

until delivery of the baby is commenced. (An alternative method consists of running 500–1,000 ml of sterile normal saline into the bladder through a No 16 Foley catheter while the presenting part is being held up; this keeps the presenting part away from the lower uterine segment and cord, and also helps by inhibiting contractions). (iv) The cord is replaced in the vagina if prolapse to the exterior has occurred. (v) Oxygen is administered to the mother by mask. (vi) Explanation and reassurance are given. (vii) Blood will be required for urgent cross-matching if Caesarean section is to be performed (about 50% of patients with mature pregnancies — table 48.5). An injection of *ritodrine* (6 mg in 10 ml normal saline over 2–3 minutes intravenously) will usually abolish uterine activity. *If the cervix is not fully dilated, Caesarean section is performed unless the fetus is dead or very immature* (table 48.5). If the cervix is fully dilated, delivery is expedited in the most appropriate manner — *episiotomy, forceps application, or breech extraction* (figure 48.5) if the patient does not immediately deliver spontaneously.

Failure to detect pulsation usually indicates fetal death, but confirmatory absence of heart sounds or electrical activity must be obtained.

Table 48.5 illustrates the method of delivery and fetal results in the series of 118 cases referred to previously. The perinatal mortality rate was 22.8%, and was 13.5% in those pregnancies which had reached 28 weeks' gestation. Note that the Caesarean section rate was highest (55%) in the pregnancies which had reached 37 weeks' gestation — yet on the other hand, when the diagnosis was made, *45% of patients in this series were suitable for immediate vaginal delivery.*

TABLE 48.5   CORD PRESENTATION AND PROLAPSE. FETAL OUTCOME ACCORDING TO MATURITY AND METHOD OF DELIVERY

Method of delivery	20–27.6 weeks	28–36.6 weeks	37 weeks and more
Normal	4 (4)	3 (2)	3 (1)
Forceps	1 (1)	4 (1)	18 (3)
Breech	10 (8)	14 (4)	11 (1)
Caesarean	—	11 (1)	39 (1)
Total	15 (13)	32 (8)	71 (6)

Figures in parentheses denote perintal deaths

Prognosis

This depends on a number of factors: period of gestation, duration of prolapse, strength of uterine contractions, stage of labour, presentation, rapidity and efficiency of first-aid and definitive treatment. The perinatal mortality rate is approximately 15–20% in teaching centres, but up to 50% in isolated centres; these figures can be halved if corrected for such conditions as fetal malformation and immaturity. If the hypoxia has been significant, the surviving infant may have symptoms relating to cerebral damage. Some 2–4% of stillbirths and 1–2% of neonatal deaths are due to cord prolapse.

The danger to the mother of hasty operative intervention should be mentioned — anaesthetic complications, postpartum haemorrhage, and sepsis are all more common.

ENTANGLEMENT

Incidence

Cord around the baby's neck is relatively common — 20–30%. One loop of cord around the neck occurs in about 20%, 2 loops in 2.5%, 3 loops in 0.5%, more than 3 loops in 0.1%. Cord around the body is present in 1–2% (figure 48.2A).

Aetiology

There is generally an excess of fluid and/or a long cord, and the occurrence is probably related to freedom of fetal movement. Tangling is common (20–25%) in *monoamniotic uniovular* twins (figure 53.2 A and B).

Complications

There is often some compromise to umbilical blood flow if the cord is tight, and a variable deceleration pattern is seen if cardiotocography is being carried out in labour. Apgar scores are usually lower, but cord entanglement is only rarely a cause of stillbirth (figure 48.2A). Occasionally, the disposition of the fetus in utero is disturbed by the effect of the cord traction (e.g. deflexion or malpresentation) or the head fails to progress in labour.

SHORT CORD

This has many of the features of cord entanglement. The shortening may be absolute (e.g. less than 30 cm) or relative, due to looping around the fetus.

Features include fetal distress, fetal death, placental abruption, breech presentation, delayed onset of labour and occasionally cord rupture.

KNOTTING

Incidence

0.5–1.5%; the incidence is similar (about 1%) in aborted fetuses, indicating its occurrence as early as the first trimester.

Aetiology

Similar to entanglement, usually occurring accidentally due to fetal activity. The condition occurs more often in male fetuses. The nearer the knot is to the fetus, the earlier the occurrence in the pregnancy. Usually the knot does not tighten until descent of the presenting part occurs in labour (figure 48.2B).

Complications

Fetal distress occurs in 15% of patients and 1-minute Apgar scores are lower. The perinatal death rate is increased 5 times.

chapter forty-nine

Dystocia

OVERVIEW

Unfortunately, the passage of the baby through the birth canal at the end of pregnancy is not always plain sailing; dystocia will occur in 2-4% of all labours and in 4-8% of nulliparous labours. Hindrances include *abnormal functioning of the uterus*; abnormal *resistance to dilatation of the cervix*; abnormalities in *size, position* or *presentation of the baby*; and finally, narrowing of the *birth canal*. Careful examination in late pregnancy will reveal indications of all but the first of these problems.

In labour, close observation of the major determinants of success is necessary — namely, the *uterine contractions, dilatation of the cervix*, and *descent of the presenting part*; the condition of the fetus and mother are also monitored, particularly where the labour is becoming prolonged. These findings are documented in the *partograph*. Deviations from the normal course of labour are reflected in this graphical analysis of labour, and indicate firstly that labour has deviated significantly from normal (crossing the alert line) and later, that intervention is necessary before damage occurs to the fetus and mother (crossing the action line). There is a good relationship between cervical dilatation rate (both initial and average) and delivery outcome. For example, if the initial rate is 1 cm per hour or more, there will be a spontaneous vaginal delivery in over 95%; if less than 1 cm per hour, 60% will require operative vaginal delivery or Caesarean section. *Cephalopelvic disproportion* must be excluded in any labour which is not progressing satisfactorily despite adequate contractions. Often there is a combination of *dysfunctional labour* and some *deflexion* of the fetal head, causing a larger diameter to present. Considerable clinical acumen (experience, careful and skilled assessment, intuition) is often required in the management of labour dystocia.

Acceleration of the labour can usually be effected by the use of a carefully supervised *oxytocin infusion*: the stronger, more effective contractions often tip the scales in favour of descent, flexion, and then forward rotation of the fetal occiput.

Fetal condition should be monitored continuously by cardiotocography when labour is enhanced with an oxytocic infusion. *Augmentation of labour* has special hazards (uterine hypertonus causing fetal hypoxia ± uterine rupture) when used in *multiparas* and/or when combined with *epidural analgesia*.

Because of the current active approach to dystocia, very long labours are now uncommon — Caesarean section is performed if oxytocin and other measures do not correct the failure of cervical dilatation and descent of the presenting part within a defined time limit (4-6 hours). This operation has largely replaced difficult and traumatic midcavity extraction procedures.

The *monitoring of fetal well-being* by electronic and biochemical means has helped to define the timing and optimum route of delivery.

A particular type of obstructive dystocia is *impaction of the shoulders*. This complication can often be anticipated, but if not, it requires a precise plan of action if the baby's life is to be saved.

DEFINITION

Dystocia is abnormal or difficult labour; prolongation is usual.

Although there are many reasons for this, it is convenient to consider 2 main groups: dysfunctional labour (the powers) and disproportion (passenger and passages).

UTERINE MUSCLE DYSFUNCTION (table 49.1)

The major *criteria for normal uterine action* during labour are fundal dominance, synchronization in the spread of the excitation wave, progressive increase in amplitude, duration and frequency of contractions, and finally, relaxation between contractions. In *dysfunctional labour*, the above criteria are not met. Inevitably, there will be an *impairment in descent of the presenting part and/or dilatation of the cervix.*

TABLE 49.1   TYPES OF ABNORMAL UTERINE ACTION

1. Hypotonic activity
   - (a) Primary hypotonia (primary uterine inertia)
   - (b) Secondary hypotonia (uterine exhaustion)
2. Hypertonic activity
   - (a) Coordinate uterine action
     - (i)   Precipitate labour
     - (ii) Retraction ring (obstructed labour)
   - (b) Incoordinate uterine action
     - (i)   Hypertonic lower uterine segment
     - (ii)   Constriction ring (local tonic contraction)
     - (iii) Uterine tetany (generalized tonic contraction)
     - (iv)   Cervical dystocia   Primary
                                     Secondary
     - (v)   Spurious (false) labour

HYPOTONIC ACTIVITY

Here the uterine contractions are weak and/or occur infrequently; if tocographic measurements are being made, the pressures will be below 30 mm of mercury. The net result is that the work performed by the uterus is less than normal.

Primary Hypotonia (Primary Inertia)

The contractions are abnormal throughout labour; the *condition is more common in nulliparas,* but strangely, may also occur in patients who have had a number of labours. This dysfunction is usually manifest as prolongation of the latent phase (cervical effacement).

It may result from sedatives or analgesics given too early in labour, a carry-over of inhibitory processes existing during pregnancy (progesterone dominance, lack of adequate levels of oxytocin and prostaglandin), poor spread of the contractile wave in the uterus or a poor response of the muscle to that excitation, or inhibition of normal processes as a result of fear and anxiety of the patient (stimulation of the sympathetic nervous system and release of adrenalin). In some patients, the uterus may be handicapped by *overdistension* or *lack of a well-fitting presenting part* to stimulate the lower uterine segment and cervix.

Secondary Hypotonia (Uterine Exhaustion)

This is a protective action taken by the uterus against rupture (usually in the nullipara) and occurs when there is a serious block to progress (disproportion); it may also occur in prolonged labours and at the end of labour, when the patient is tired and in need of fluid and calories, as well as sleep.

HYPERTONIC ACTIVITY

Uterine Action Otherwise Normal

This is the reverse of primary hypotonic inertia; there is a rapid spread of the excitation wave over the uterus and strong coordinated contractions occur. The work done by the uterus is greater than normal and the labour is often classified as *precipitate* (lasting less than 4 hours). It should be observed, however, that not in all rapid labours is there hypertonic activity; in some patients, usually those of higher parity, the speed is due to a lower resistance of the birth canal (bony pelvis, pelvic and perineal musculature).

Uterine Action Disordered (incoordinate uterine action)

The wave of contraction does not start normally in the fundal region and spread downward, and successive waves are often variable in amplitude, duration, and frequency. As a result, the normal peristaltic action, which is essential for evacuating the contents of a hollow muscular organ such as the uterus, does not occur. There is often an increase in resting (basal) tone between contractions. A special type is the *hypertonic lower uterine segment* (reversed polarity). An extreme form occurs when there is a localized spasm of one part of the uterus — the *constriction ring.* Not infrequently, the cervix is noted to be unyielding and firm and the term *cervical* dystocia is applied; in most cases, this probably represents a failure in normal softening of the connective tissue matrix, although in some cases, a mechanism similar to that occurring in constriction ring (localized spasm) may involve the muscular tissue of the cervix. Excessive rigidity may also be due to ageing or previous surgical procedures to the cervix. Usually the presenting part is low in the pelvis and the uterine muscle polarity is normal.

A further form of hypertonic activity is that known as *uterine tetany* (generalized spasm). Classically, this is seen after *ergometrine administration*. Unlike oxytocin, this drug acts unselectively on the uterus causing all muscle fibres to contract simultaneously (loss of normal fundal dominance). In addition, because of the continued stimulus of the drug, there is no proper relaxation — that is, the tone of the muscle remains very high. Another cause is *abruptio placentae*, where the extravasated blood acts as a persistent stimulus to muscle contraction. Occasionally, in patients with *disproportion* (e.g. shoulder presentation) the contractions increase progressively in strength and frequency as the uterus endeavours to overcome the obstruction, until one contraction runs into another and tetany results.

Spurious (false) *labour* occurs when the patient is distressed by contractions but cervical effacement and dilatation do not occur — backache is often present. After sedation the contractions usually fade away; when labour recommences (days or weeks later) the contractions are usually coordinate and progress normally.

DIAGNOSIS

Much of the basic work establishing the normal patterns of uterine activity was made with small, sensitive pressure catheters attached to recording machines. A fair idea of the strength of uterine contractions can be obtained clinically by palpation of the abdomen. This can be supplemented by sensitive pressure transducers recording from the abdomen or from the interior of the uterus (via a fine polyethylene catheter after the membranes have ruptured).

Differentiation of hypotonia and hypertonia presents little difficulty. *Incoordination* is usually inferred because of the failure to progress in spite of adequate activity and absence of cephalopelvic disproportion. It is a disorder seen particularly in the nullipara; associated features are a high anxiety state, *posterior position of the occiput*, a significant amount of *pain early in labour, often felt in the back and present between contractions.*

CLINICAL SIGNIFICANCE

Hypotonic Uterine Activity

There is prolongation of labour and the chief problems here are the *risk of infection* (particularly if the membranes are ruptured), and *deterioration in the patient's morale*. The latter is more related to anxiety and impatience than physical stress (which occurs with hypertonic incoordinate activity).

Hypertonic Uterine Activity

In coordinate hypertonic action the strong contractions may cause *fetal hypoxia*, firstly because the uteroplacental blood flow is shut off for a longer period, secondly because there is insufficient relaxation between one contraction and the next for proper exchange of blood gases and nutrients between the fetal and maternal circulations, and finally, the abnormal pressure exerted on the fetal head as it is forced through the birth canal reduces blood flow to the vital centres of the brain. The latter may also cause tearing of intracranial structures, resulting in haemorrhage. *Damage to maternal structures* (cervix, vagina, and perineum) is likely because of the rapidity of the birth; postpartum haemorrhage is often associated.

Incoordinate Activity

The main problem is fetal hypoxia. Labour is prolonged as a result of the inefficient action and this progressively reduces the fetal reserves. In the type designated as *hypertonic lower uterine segment* (reversed polarity), there is a higher than normal pressure exerted on the fetal head by the lower uterus, with disturbance to the cerebral circulation. The risk of *intraamniotic infection* rises as the duration of labour increases. Incoordinate activity is exhausting for the mother because of the longer duration of labour and the often associated troublesome *back pain*.

Constriction ring usually occurs after the uterus has been contracting for a long period and is more common if *manipulative procedures* (e.g. attempt at external cephalic version in labour) have been carried out. The ring is usually between the fetal head and trunk, but may occur anywhere in the uterus. Progress of labour and descent of the fetus come to a standstill. If the umbilical cord is caught in the ring, severe asphyxia or death may occur; the pressure effects are greater if the membranes are ruptured. A diagnostic feature of constriction ring dystocia is that the *presenting part usually recedes (loses station) during a contraction.*

In *cervical dystocia*, there is a similar pattern — labour contractions are strong, but there is very slow cervical dilatation (figure 49.1). This condition is less serious for the baby, unless labour is significantly prolonged. Often the cervix is directed posteriorly (sacral) and there may be associated cephalopelvic disproportion, usually due to an occipitoposterior position. Rarely, if the condition is neglected, the posterior cervical lip becomes gangrenous due to pressure between the fetal head and the sacral promontory, and detaches (figure 49.2).

Figure 49.1 Cervical dystocia may be primary or secondary to cervical surgery (cautery, conization or amputation). The thinned-out cervix may be visible at the introitus. If treatment is delayed, annular detachment of the cervix may occur.

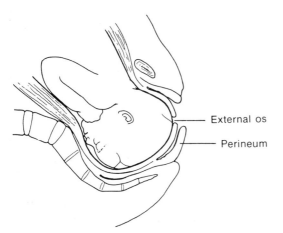

External os

Perineum

MANAGEMENT

Hypotonic Activity

If this is the result of excessive or early medication, the patient is rested and then is observed in the early first stage room where she can sit or walk about. If persistent, an *intravenous infusion of oxytocin* is commenced. A careful assessment should be made of the cervix, and the station, attitude, and position of the presenting part; amniotomy is not indicated if the labour is still in the latent phase.

Secondary hypotonic activity requires a *careful assessment* of all facets of the labour — powers, passenger, passages — to determine whether any other abnormality, *particularly disproportion*, exists. Also, the general condition of the patient must be assessed — has she had adequate rest, sleep, analgesia and nutrients? Improper conduction analgesia may be responsible. These aspects should be corrected if necessary. *Many of these patients will have minor disproportion*, with or without malpositions (usually posterior position of the occiput) or minor deflexion attitudes (vertex or bregma presentations). Improved uterine activity is often sufficient to produce normal anterior rotation and/or flexion of the head, and thus *oxytocin infusion is the treatment of choice (acceleration of labour) if significant disproportion has been excluded*. Amniotomy alone is usually not effective. If satisfactory progress has not occurred in 2–6 hours, depending on circumstances, Caesarean section is indicated.

Figure 49.2 Almost complete annular detachment of the cervix — an obstetric mishap of the past (Melbourne, 1955). A 44-year-old para 2 was given intramuscular injections of oxytocin to induce labour at 42 weeks' gestation. She came into 'strong labour' and 4 hours later delivery occurred with both anterior and posterior cervical lips outside the vulva; i.e. delivery occurred through the haemorrhagic posterior lip of the cervix when the external os was only 5 cm dilated. The infant was alive and well, birth-weight 4,380 g. This posterior lip of cervix shown here (9 × 5 × 3 cm) became detached — haemorrhage necessitated blood transfusion and suture of the cervical tear in theatre under general anaesthesia. At the postnatal check the cervix was well healed, but had a large tongue-like anterior lip! (Courtesy of Dr John Fliegner).

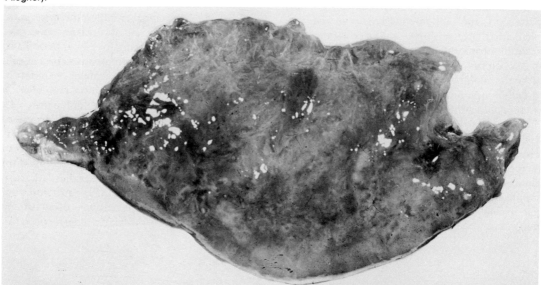

Hypertonic Activity

Hypertonic coordinated labour. The process is often over before the diagnosis is made, since there is usually a 'precipitate delivery' as well. If delivery appears imminent before the patient has reached the delivery room, no attempt should be made to prevent the baby's egress from the birth canal since this is more dangerous to the baby (because of head compression) than birth in unprepared circumstances.

Hypertonic incoordinate activity. This is the most difficult problem to manage. It is important to maintain the patient's morale by frequent attendance, sympathy, encouragement, and explanation. *Intravenous fluids containing glucose and electrolytes* are usually needed, and careful attention must be paid to observations of the mother and fetus (including close fetal heart monitoring). It is wise to take vaginal smears for microbiological examination, and prophylactic antibiotics should be given after about 10 hours of labour if delivery does not appear to be in sight. *Pain relief* is important, particularly from the *backache* that often persists between contractions; *epidural analgesia* is most helpful, giving the patient relief from pain and the ability to rest and sleep. Again, there may be an element of *disproportion* or malapplication of the presenting part to the cervix, as in posterior positions. *Oxytocin infusion*, while less successful than in hypotonic inertia, is worth a trial, with the provisos already given. The infusion rate should be 1–2 mU/minute for the first 30 minutes and this is increased by 1 mU/minute half-hourly, with careful observation of uterine activity before each increase (both basal tone and contraction peak). Caesarean section will be indicated if delivery is not within sight in 4–6 hours or there is significant fetal distress.

Constriction ring is seldom diagnosed except when difficulty is experienced at the time of operative delivery. At times, a clear depression in the abdomen can be made out at the site of the ring if the patient is not obese. The cervix and lower segment remain relaxed below the ring, even during a contraction. The condition is treated usually by *deep anaesthesia* with one of the volatile agents such as ether or halothane, assisted with inhalation of a capsule of *amyl nitrite*. Caesarean section (with the incision placed longitudinally in the uterus) may be required.

In *cervical dystocia* the cervix usually dilates slowly, and this may be assisted by manual dilatation at the time of pelvic examination, under gas and oxygen analgesia. Incision is rarely if ever indicated.

A *retraction ring* is seen when the uterus labours against obstruction (figure 52.4); the management is that of the cephalopelvic disproportion — by forceps delivery after rotation of an occipitoposterior position, or by Caesarean section. *Uterine tetany* requires prompt treatment to avoid fetal death from hypoxia, and possibly uterine rupture — general anaesthesia and delivery by forceps if conditions are suitable, otherwise by Caesarean section. *Spurious labour* is treated by sedation, reassurance, exclusion of cephalopelvic disproportion and fetal distress — labour usually progresses normally when it becomes established.

VOLUNTARY MUSCLE DYSFUNCTION

Two sets of voluntary muscles are involved in the birth of the baby: (i) those involved in *pushing* the presenting part through the lower birth canal during the second stage — the '*secondary powers*' (diaphragm, abdominal wall) and (ii) those of the pelvic and perineal diaphragms which must *relax* to allow the passage of the baby. The importance of the proper coordination of these muscles (*contraction of the former and relaxation of the latter*) in the successful delivery of the baby is not always appreciated.

The secondary powers may be weakened through nonuse, high parity, diastasis recti or because of poor cardiac or respiratory function. Also, some patients have a poor idea of directing expulsive effort towards the perineum, where it is most effective. Spinal and epidural anaesthesia depress the expulsion reflex.

Of more importance is the inability of many patients, particularly nulliparas, to relax the pelvic outlet musculature during the second stage. This is partly because the necessary coordination has not been achieved, but mostly because the pain produced by each descent of the presenting part causes reflex contraction of these muscles. These patients don't have the ability to 'let go', and a vicious circle of pain, spasm, further pain, is initiated. The condition can often be foretold when pelvic examination is carried out earlier in the pregnancy: this either produces reflex spasm or the patient is unable to actively relax the pelvic floor and perineum. Preventive treatment consists of antenatal exercises under the supervision of a physiotherapist. Considerable help in the birth process is given by graduated dilatation of the vaginal opening during the antenatal period. With the use of a suitable lubricant (e.g. wheat germ oil), the vulval ring is stretched by fingers placed inside the vagina (perineal massage). Apart from making the birth easier, the likelihood of a long and difficult second stage is reduced, as is the need for episiotomy or other operative procedures. If these measures are not successful, pudendal block and forceps delivery are usually required.

CEPHALOPELVIC DISPROPORTION

The second major cause of difficult labour is disparity in size between the birth canal and the fetus which must pass through it. It is convenient to consider these in turn.

AETIOLOGY

The Birth Canal

Bony pelvis. The different physiological shapes and pelvic measurements are described in Chapter 2. A contraction of one of the major diameters may be defined as *mild* if it is 1 cm less than normal, *moderate* if 1–2 cm less, and *marked* if more than 2 cm less than normal. If more than one diameter is contracted, the above figures are adjusted downwards. Approximately 5–10% of patients have a mild contraction and 2–5% a moderate or marked contraction. Although a general impression can be obtained from clinical examination of the pelvis, accurate assessment requires radiographic pelvimetry.

Types of contraction. The pelvis may be narrowed in one or more of the 3 main planes — the brim, the midpelvis, and the outlet.

The contraction usually represents a general diminution of one of the 4 basic pelvic types: *gynaecoid* (round), *platypelloid* (flat), *anthropoid* (long oval), or *android* (heart-shaped). If the gynaecoid pelvis is contracted, usually most diameters are equally affected; in the other types of the pelvis, the greatest difficulty will arise in the diameter already relatively shortened: platypelloid — the AP diameter of the brim; anthropoid — the transverse diameters; and android — all diameters, but more evident at the midpelvis and outlet.

In rare circumstances, the pelvis may be *distorted in shape.* (i) *Rachitic.* Rickets in childhood causes an exaggerated flattening of the pelvis due to a downward and forward projection of the sacral promontory; the transverse diameters and outlet are often normal. (ii) *Scoliotic.* Poliomyelitis and other causes of scoliosis such as tuberculosis of the spine, are now very rare. The pelvis in such cases is usually asymmetrical, and the degree of contraction not marked. (iii) *Coxalgic.* Here, diseases of the hip joint in infancy (epiphyseal disorders or tuberculosis) cause an asymmetry of the pelvis. Again, gross forms of these diseases are now very rare. (iv) *Traumatic.* The usual injury arises from *motor vehicle accidents in which the pelvis is fractured.* The most troublesome deformity arises from lateral injury, when the head of the femur is driven into the cavity of the pelvis (figure 49.3). (v) *Congenital.* In the *Naegele*-type pelvis there is asymmetric contraction on one side due to maldevelopment in the region of the sacroiliac joint; in the *Robert*-type pelvis the condition is bilateral, the pelvis appearing as a narrow wedge in outline. *Congenital hip dislocation* is now usually recognized and treated before the flattening characteristic of this condition occurs. In *spondylolisthesis* the fifth lumbar vertebra slides over the first piece of the sacrum, so impinging on the anteroposterior diameter of the pelvic inlet. *Assimilation pelvis* is a congenital anomaly; in high assimilation the fifth lumbar vertebra is incorporated into the sacrum giving it 6 pieces instead of 5, producing a deep pelvis which is more difficult for the fetus to negotiate. (In low assimilation the reverse occurs, the first piece of the sacrum becoming a sixth lumbar vertebra, and the pelvis is shallower than normal).

Figure 49.3 Two years previously this patient was in a motor car accident and suffered severe injury, including fractures of the pelvis (pubis, ischium, and iliac crest) and intraperitoneal and extraperitoneal rupture of the bladder. This film at 38 weeks shows distortion of the left side of the pelvis. A living infant (2,950 g) was delivered by elective lower segment Caesarean section. The operation was difficult because of adhesions between bladder, uterus and anterior abdominal wall.

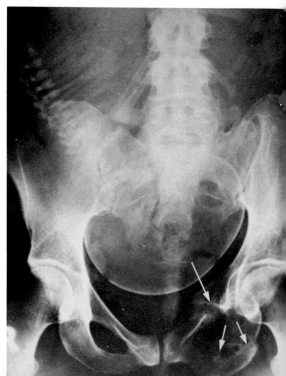

A

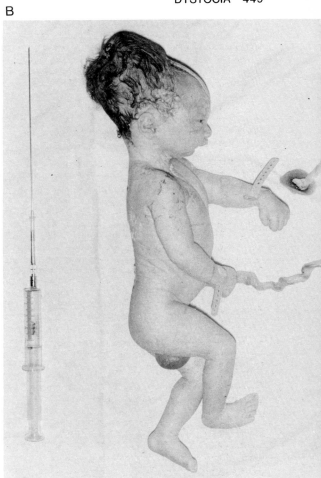

B

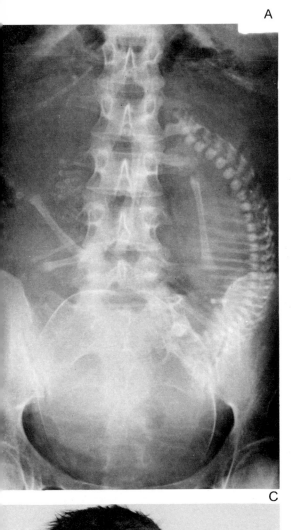

C

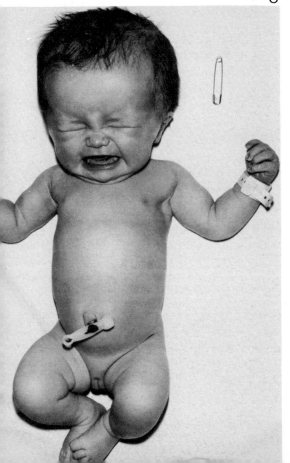

D

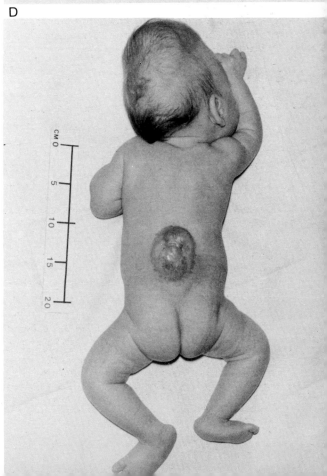

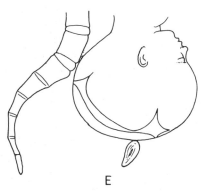
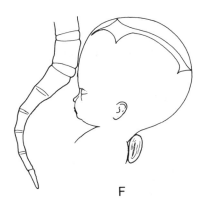

E

F

Figure 49.4 Hydrocephaly usually develops in late pregnancy, but the first signs may not occur until the first months of infancy. **A.** Major degree of hydrocephaly in a primigravida at full term. Labour was induced by amniotomy and an oxytocin infusion; 1,000 ml of cerebrospinal fluid was aspirated through the huge anterior fontanelle seen here as an extensive bony defect. Forceps delivery was performed 3 hours after amniotomy. **B.** The infant was stillborn. He weighed 3,750 g not counting the 1,000 ml of cerebrospinal fluid. There was no polyhydramnios. The wide bore lumbar puncture needle and syringe used for aspiration is shown. **C.** This baby was huge (birth-weight 4,850 g) and hydrocephalic (head circumference 47 cm — normal 35 cm). In labour the breech presented and obstruction occurred at the level of the pelvic brim. At Caesarean section the trunk and limbs were delivered, and cerebrospinal fluid was aspirated through the posterior fontanelle before the head could be extracted. Neurosurgery was performed on the 4th day of life after this photograph was taken. **D.** This hydrocephalic baby with associated spina bifida and meningomyelocele, weighed 2,790 g at birth, and was born by mid-forceps delivery, the head not being unduly large. In labour, a hydrocephalic head can be confused with a moulded, large, normal head and if in doubt one should never perforate the skull. The sad sequelae of survival in this case were intellectual impairment, talipes, recurrent urinary infections and paralysis of the lower limbs. This photograph was taken when the child was 10 weeks old. **E.** Vertex presentation. The head can be needled via the maternal abdomen or through the cervix. Sometimes the head collapses spontaneously in labour; if it does not, obstruction must result. **F.** Breech presentation is favourable when there is hydrocephaly as the trunk can be held to steady the head during perforation through the palate. Note large fontanelles and wide sagittal suture.

Figure 49.5 Conjoined twins (thoracopagus or chest to chest). Their combined birth-weight was 3,550 g. They were born by Caesarean section at 36 weeks' gestation, after attempted forceps delivery of twin 1 (left side of photograph) had failed. Vaginal delivery is possible when the attachment is by a wide pliable skin fold. Note single umbilical cord and attachments of chest and abdominal wall; there was a common heart, pericardium and diaphragm. Even if born alive, successful surgical separation would have been impossible.

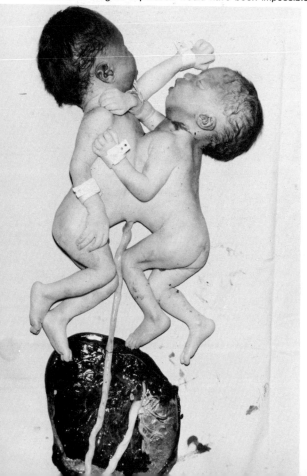

Soft Tissues. The *uterus* may be responsible (e.g. nonpregnant horn of a double uterus, fibromyoma, cervical scarring), or the *ovary* (benign or malignant neoplasm), or the obstruction may arise in one of the nonreproductive pelvic structures.

Fetus

The fetus may contribute to disproportion because of abnormal growth, or alternatively, because of the presentation of an abnormal diameter to the birth canal (colour plates 45 and 54). (i) *Abnormalities of growth* include general enlargement of the fetus (genetic causes; prediabetic or diabetic mother; colour plate 53); or local anomalies (hydrocephaly, tumour, ascites, figure 49.4 and colour plate 56). Conjoined twins form a special group, as does locking of normal twins (figure 49.5 and colour plate 50). (ii) *Presentation of an abnormal diameter.* Here the size of the fetus is within normal limits, but the lie (transverse, oblique) or presentation (brow) is abnormal (figure 49.7). *Compound presentation* describes the situation where there

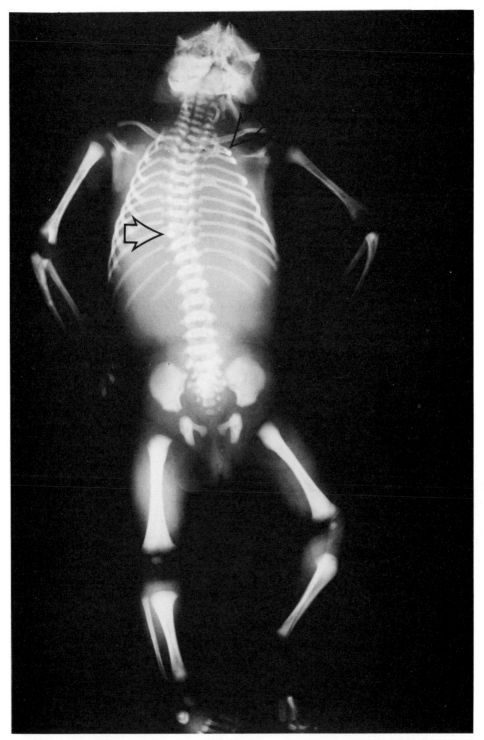

Figure 49.6 Anencephaly can cause dystocia if the small cranium slips through an incompietely dilated cervix. Never pull on the head, but await full cervical dilatation when spontaneous delivery will occur. This fetus was born at 34 weeks and had unusually well developed distal femoral epiphyses for this maturity. Oestriol excretion of 7 μmol (2 mg)/24 hours led to the diagnosis. There was no polyhydramnios. As well as the deficient cranium, this post mortem X-ray shows a right hemivertebra at T9 and left upper rib anomalies.

is an associated prolapse of hand and/or foot in a cephalic presentation or hand(s) in a breech presentation. It occurs in about 1 in 1,000 deliveries and is more common in multiple pregnancy, premature birth, and other instances of poor application of the presenting part to the pelvis (colour plate 141). The diagnosis may be suspected if the presenting part remains high and deviated from the midline and there is protraction of the active phase of labour.

DIAGNOSIS

History

If the patient has had previous children, there will usually be a history of *prolonged labour*, *operative interference*, and perhaps *birth trauma*

(intracranial injury, retarded development, spasticity or even perinatal death). In such cases, it is possible that *pelvimetry* has already been carried out. The *birth-weights* of previous children should be ascertained. The medical or obstetrical history may suggest diabetes. Other factors in the maternal history that should be elicited include serious childhood illnesses (bone disorders), injuries to the pelvis, and poor socioeconomic state during childhood (rickets).

General Examination

Examination should be directed to stature, posture, spinal and pelvic symmetry, and gait. Evidence of childhood diseases such as tuberculosis, poliomyelitis and rickets should be sought. Dur-

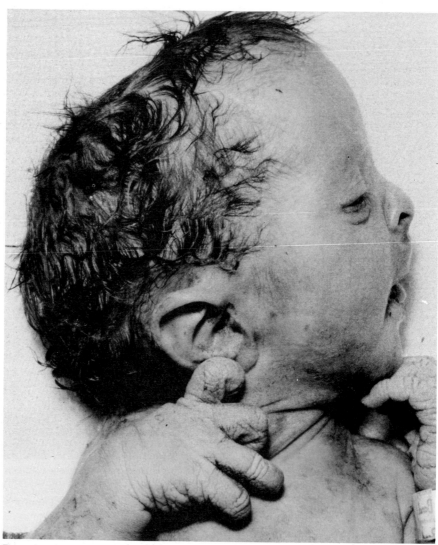

Figure 49.7 This meconium-stained infant was born by Caesarean section and shows the typical moulding of a brow presentation in obstructed labour. The head (neck) remains partly extended. The infant was small for dates (2,560 g at 41 weeks) and shows the other signs of placental insufficiency. In her following 2 pregnancies the mother had vaginal deliveries of infants weighing 4,100 g and 3,820 g.

ing pregnancy, polyhydramnios might suggest the possibility of a malformation such as hydrocephaly. The fetus may be palpably large and this finding should always be taken seriously (approximately 1% of Caucasian women will have babies weighing 4,500 g or more at birth and Caesarean section will be required in at least 25% of these; shoulder dystocia will occur in a further 10–15%; colour plate 140). If the presentation is abnormal, this may be detected during pregnancy or perhaps only when pelvic examination is performed in labour.

Pelvic examination should be performed routinely at the first antenatal visit and a careful assessment of the pelvis made. If it is considered that a contraction exists, radiographic pelvimetry can be arranged between the 36th–37th weeks; in late pregnancy a better idea of cephalopelvic relationships can be obtained with a film taken while the patient is standing. *Pelvic contraction should be suspected in all patients less than 152 cm tall.* Occasionally, pelvic examination is difficult at the first antenatal visit, particularly in nulliparas, and if this is so, it is usually repeated at the 34th–36th week of gestation. Suspicious features on vaginal examination include a palpable sacral promontory, poor sacral curvature, prominent ischial spines, narrow sacrosciatic notches and subpubic angle, and reduced intertuberous diameter. The presence of soft tissue tumours of the uterus (fibromyomas), ovary (benign or malignant neoplasms), or surrounding structures should also be detected on pelvic examination. Occasionally, malformations of the genital tract will be found that could cause dystocia (bicornuate uterus, vaginal septum). Ultrasonic investigation may be helpful in doubtful cases.

During labour, the features of obstruction to progress will occur (see later).

MANAGEMENT

Specific Aetiologies

Pelvic contraction. Unless a Caesarean section has been carried out in a previous pregnancy, a decision concerning the management of the delivery is delayed until the results of the pelvimetry are known later in pregnancy. The patient is usually managed normally if the features on history and examination are not confirmed on pelvimetry. For minor and moderate degrees of pelvic contraction and if no other abnormality such as cardiac disease is present, a *trial of labour* is undertaken. For marked pelvic contraction, or moderate contraction plus another abnormality, elective Caesarean section is usually carried out.

Soft tissue tumours. The management of potentially obstructive soft tissue lesions requires individual consideration. All *ovarian tumours*, if more than 4–5 cm in diameter, should be removed between the 14th–18th weeks. *Uterine fibroids* are usually in the upper segment of the uterus and move out of the pelvis as pregnancy advances. They are not removed during pregnancy; either a trial of labour or Caesarean section is indicated, depending on circumstances. The *nonpregnant horn* of a bicornuate or double uterus is managed similarly. A *vaginal septum* which is likely to obstruct labour is often excised during pregnancy rather than during the second stage of labour because obstruction usually occurs and occasionally the septum is avulsed, causing extensive vaginal laceration.

Enlarged fetal diameter(s). If the infant is normal, but oversized, a trial of labour is usually allowed. Caesarean section is more likely if the mother is diabetic. The treatment of the anomalous fetus must be individualized; the management of malpresentations is considered in Chapters 50 and 51. A conservative approach is best employed in compound presentation, since the prolapsed extremity tends to slip back as the presenting part descends; in the less common vertex:foot presentation, obstruction is likely and Caesarean section is usually necessary.

Technical Procedures

Caesarean section has been described in Chapter 47. Elective section is carried out between 38 and 39 weeks. If there is any doubt about the maturity of the baby, liquor amnii is taken for estimation of the L/S ratio.

Trial of labour is carried out where disproportion is suspected but is not of a major degree; usually the patient is a nullipara. The requirements are as follows. The presentation must be *cephalic*, the labour must begin *spontaneously*, and be conducted in a hospital where adequate facilities exist for the observation of the patient and performance of operative vaginal delivery or Caesarean section should either of these become necessary. Pelvic assessment when the membranes rupture, and at intervals thereafter, coupled with critical assessment of progress, are important. The conduct of the labour otherwise differs little from normal (figure 49.8); it is prudent, however, to cross-match blood and commence intravenous fluids early.

Not infrequently, difficulties arise only when labour has been in progress for some time; either the patient has had no antenatal care, or suspicious features were not noted on routine examination. *The following features during labour are*

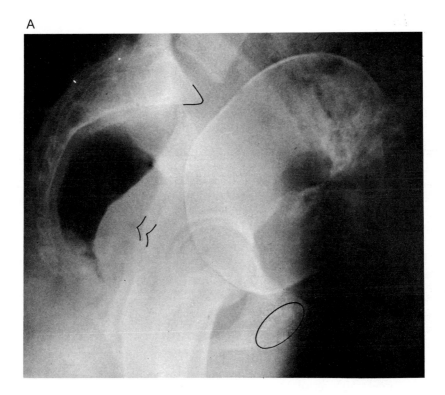

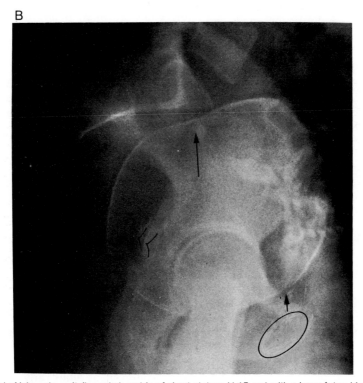

Figure 49.8 Trial of labour in an Italian primigravida of short stature (145 cm) with a large fetus (4,000 g). **A.** At 41 weeks X-ray pelvimetry, performed because of a high head, showed nonengagement and mild pelvic contraction (true conjugate 10.5 cm, transverse diameter of brim 12.3 cm, bispinous 9.9 cm, available AP of outlet 10.4 cm). **B.** Labour began spontaneously the following day when the membranes ruptured; 24 hours later this lateral X-ray showed that the head was engaged and reached 1.5 cm below the level of ischial spines. There was considerable moulding; 1 cm of sinciput was palpable abdominally. Epidural analgesia was commenced.

C

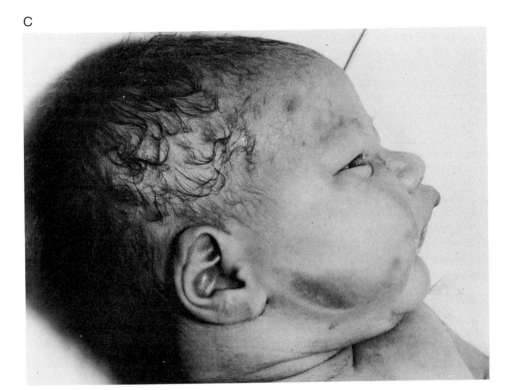

D

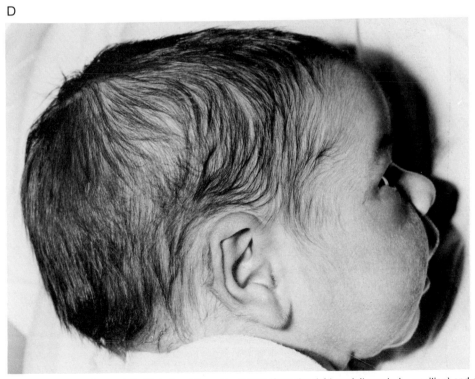

C. Two hours later the cervix was fully dilated and forceps rotation (from the right occipitoposterior position) and delivery were performed. This photograph, taken shortly after birth, shows caput and moulding and the mark on the cheek of the accurately applied forceps blade. **D.** Appearance of the baby 2 days later. In her next pregnancy the mother had a spontaneous normal delivery at 40 weeks of an infant weighing 3,250 g.

regarded as unfavourable. (i) *Early rupture of the membranes.* Prolapse of the cord or a fetal limb may occur, amnionitis and fetal pneumonia are more common, and fetal hypoxia may occur because of reduction in placental area and early head compression. Pelvic examination is always carried out at this time and progress critically assessed (effacement and dilatation of the cervix, nature of the liquor, application of the cervix to the presenting part, station, flexion and position of the presenting part, caput and moulding, 'tightness of fit', movement of the presenting part with a contraction). (ii) *Inefficient uterine action.* This may occur primarily, probably because of the poor application of the presenting part to the pelvis and lower uterine segment, or after labour has been in progress for some time, probably because uterine action fails in the face of the obstruction. (iii) *Slow dilatation of the cervix.* This is often a feature in such patients,

again due to poor application of the presenting part to the cervix. The cervix hangs down loosely like a sleeve and may be oedematous. (iv) *Poor descent of the presenting part.* Careful assessment (particularly abdominal) of the station of the fetal head will reveal that both occiput and sinciput remain palpable, and descent is slow. (v) *Fetal distress.* The effort of the uterus to overcome the obstruction, together with the pressure of the contracted pelvis on the fetal skull, often cause fetal distress. This may be aggravated by intrauterine infection which results from premature rupture of the membranes. (vi) *Maternal distress.* If the labour is prolonged, maternal distress may occur. (vii) *Changes in the presenting part.* Moulding will increase progressively; caput also increases, but is a less reliable sign, since it also occurs excessively with incoordinate uterine action. (viii) *Changes in the upper-lower segment ratio.* As labour becomes obstructed, the

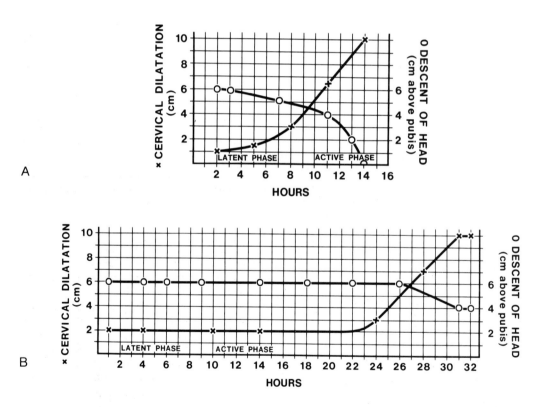

Figure 49.9 Graphic recording of cervical dilatation and descent of the head in labour. **A.** Normal labour at 40 weeks' gestation in a nullipara. The active phase of cervical dilatation commenced after 8 hours and full dilatation was achieved 6 hours later. The head descended steadily during the active phase of labour, culminating in a spontaneous vertex delivery. Note that in most normal labours vaginal examination is not performed, assessment of progress relying upon abdominal palpation of descent of the head. **B.** Partograph of a 28-year-old primigravida who had amniotomy at 40 weeks' gestation for hypertension. An intravenous oxytocin infusion was commenced 4 hours later and resulted in incoordinate labour, without cervical dilatation (prolonged latent phase); the infusion was discontinued and after 4 hours sleep, coordinate contractions occurred with progress to full cervical dilatation after an active phase of about 10 hours' duration. The head descended 2 cm in the active phase but remained 4 cm palpable abdominally in spite of 1 hour of bearing down in the second stage of labour; at this time there was a retraction ring, and vaginal examination showed extreme caput and moulding, with a persistent occipitoposterior position. Caesarean section was performed; the infant was in good condition, birth-weight 3,815 g. Vaginal examination to assess progress is indicated when the patient requires her second dose of analgesic and is mandatory before epidural analgesia is commenced, and 2–4 hourly thereafter.

upper segment becomes excessively retracted and thus smaller, while the lower segment becomes excessively expanded and thinned. The junction is demarcated by *Bandl's retraction ring*, and can be detected on inspection as it rises up into the abdomen (figure 52.4).

OBSTRUCTED LABOUR

A point needing emphasis is the danger of *lack of progress*. This may occur in a labour that is not technically prolonged, but may be more damaging (especially to the fetus) if it is neglected. When there has been no true descent of the presenting part despite adequate contractions, the labour is said to be *obstructed*; this is usually diagnosed when lack of progress is found at 2 successive examinations at least 1 hour apart. *However, the diagnosis may be obvious, without further observation, if the clinical picture is complete.*

The partograph (figure 49.9) is very helpful in providing a visual record of cervical dilatation and descent of the presenting part. As the latter becomes jammed in the pelvis, the slopes of the 2 curves will flatten, passing first the 'alert line' and some time later, the 'action line' (figure 40.4).

Obstruction can be relative or absolute. Usually labour has been prolonged and the features described above develop, culminating in *arrest of descent* and/or rotation of the head, extensive formation of *caput* and *moulding*, the presence of a *retraction ring* and usually there is an *occipitoposterior position* (figure 52.4); there is often *fetal* and *maternal distress*. Delivery should be effected either by forceps rotation if conditions are favourable, or by Caesarean section if they are not.

It should be noted that *obstructed labour can develop rapidly in multiparas* — beware of the multipara who has poor contractions, and whose pulse rate is rising — she often has a larger infant than you anticipated; she requires careful assessment and perhaps Caesarean section — *not oxytocic infusion* for incoordinate uterine action! (colour plate 92).

PROLONGED LABOUR

There has been a significant change in attitude to prolonged labour. In former times, one would see labours lasting 48 hours or even longer in statistical reports. Opinion has now hardened that there should be a very good reason for allowing a woman to labour longer than 24 hours, and proponents of the 12-hour oxytocin-aided labour have recently put forward a strong case.

FIRST STAGE

Definition

Properly, this would be a duration beyond 2 standard deviations from the norm, the latter being taken as 8–10 hours in the nullipara and 6–8 hours in the multipara; for convenience, however, *24 hours is chosen*. Usually, all parturients are considered together, although a limit of 18 hours is more logical for the multipara.

Incidence

Approximately 5% of nulliparas and 1% of multiparas have a prolonged labour (table 49.2).

TABLE 49.2   RESULTS OF 1,136 PROLONGED LABOURS (MORE THAN 24 HOURS' DURATION) IN 41,982 CONSECUTIVE CONFINEMENTS

		%	
Incidence		2.8	
Primiparas	5.2		
Multiparas	1.0		
Prolonged pregnancy		10.4	(6.0)
Occipitoposterior position		33.5	(10.6)
Fetal distress		52.8	
Primary postpartum haemorrhage		4.9	(4.4)
Birth-weight above 4,000 g		10.4	
Delivery			
Spontaneous		29.2	(62.6)
Forceps		48.2	(26.1)
Caesarean section		22.5	(11.3)
Stillbirth		1.6	(1.2)
Neonatal death		1.6	(1.4)

Figures in parentheses denote incidences in total population (table 16.1)

Aetiology

Very often there is more than one factor involved. Abnormal uterine action is the predominant factor in 50% of patients, relative fetal causes in 25% (i.e. normal baby but abnormal position or presentation), absolute fetal causes in 20%, and birth canal causes in 5%. It should be noted that prolonged labour is by no means always associated with *cephalopelvic disproportion*; in many cases, the patient is labouring between 32 and 38 weeks' gestation, *incoordinate uterine activity* being the cause of the delay.

Maternal Complications

(i) *Metabolic derangement* occurs because very little is absorbed from the gut by the patient in labour, and unless adequate intravenous replacement of fluids, calories, and vitamins is made, maternal distress will follow, as evidenced by elevation of the pulse rate and temperature, oliguria, ketonuria, and proteinuria. This is an ideal setting for shock, particularly if another insult is added, such as trauma, infection, or haemorrhage. (ii) *Mechanical.* The possibility of uterine rupture has been discussed already. Other disasters, such as vesicovaginal fistula which is a possible sequel to neglected obstructed labour, should not occur. (iii) *Psychological.* The patient usually becomes progressively disturbed the longer labour progresses: this is the result of a combination of factors — anxiety, pain, metabolic upset, loss of sleep, and perhaps intrauterine infection. (iv) *Infection.* The barrier effect of the cervical mucus plug and the fetal membranes is lost once active labour commences. Microorganisms, which are prevalent in the vagina, pass upward into the amniotic cavity and cause an amnionitis, with later spread to the uterus and parauterine tissues.

Fetal Complications

(i) *Metabolic.* The fetus will be affected by any metabolic upset in the mother, particularly if fluids and calories are restricted. (ii) *Mechanical.* The main problem is compression of the fetal head by the lower uterine segment and bony pelvis; this reduces blood flow to the brain as moulding becomes more marked and damages the lower part of the brain stem as it is forced downward. (iii) *Oxygenation* is impaired because of the effect of uterine contractions, which intermittently shut off uteroplacental blood flow. This is accentuated if contractions are prolonged. If the cord is low-lying or entangled around the baby's body, this may be another cause of hypoxia. (iv) *Infection.* The baby inhales the infected liquor and this causes a pneumonitis; spread to other sites may follow (meningitis, pyelonephritis). (v) *Delivery.* There is a relationship between difficult labour and difficult delivery; protracted deceleration phase and delayed second stage are especially significant. (vi) *After the birth,* there may be asphyxia and a low Apgar score, feeding difficulty, hypoglycaemia, and traumatic injury to contend with (colour plates 143 and 144).

Management

The prime need is to know *why* the labour is prolonged. It may be reasonable to persist if the uterus is hypotonic, but disastrous if obstruction is present. (i) *Specific management* depends on the cause. (ii) *General management* is similar to that outlined under the normal care of the patient in labour. (iii) *Special measures.* Attention is given to vital signs, both maternal and fetal, fluid balance, intravenous fluid and calories, rest and sleep, analgesia, and psychological support. The time of rupture of the membranes must be noted and reported; a vaginal examin-

ation will be carried out to eliminate cord prolapse and to assess carefully the pelvic findings. Showering, sponging, and cooling with a fan or air-conditioning prevents the patient from getting hot and bothered. Sitting the patient out of bed as well as ambulation usually improve the quality of uterine activity and descent of the presenting part. Catheterization may be necessary if the patient is unable to void satisfactorily. *Antibiotics,* preceded by a vaginal smear, should be commenced at 12 hours if the labour looks like being prolonged. To achieve satisfactory levels in the fetus, the dose should be 2–3 times normal, given parenterally. A broad spectrum antibiotic covering anaerobes as well as Gram-positive and Gram-negative aerobes is required. *Pain relief.* Conduction analgesia (epidural) is suitable for patients with disordered uterine action of the hypertonic or normotonic type. It is suitable if there are mechanical difficulties associated with a *posterior position* of the occiput, but great care is necessary if true cephalopelvic disproportion exists. The complete analgesia provides a welcome relief to the mother and allows a refreshing sleep at night. An *oxytocin infusion* is indicated in hypotonic inertia. In some centres, it is given even if contractions seem adequate, but are thought to be disordered, in order to force a conclusion within 4–6 hours. If facilities are available, *fetal cardiac monitoring* should be carried out. *Assessment of progress.* The main parameters are *descent of the presenting part,* assessed abdominally and vaginally (and if necessary, radiographically) (figure 49.8), and *dilatation of the cervix.* The features described earlier in this section (membranes, liquor, cervix, presenting part, pelvis) are assessed in order to formulate further management. A *partograph* showing rate of dilatation of the cervix, is very useful in charting the progress of the labour (figure 49.9). In the active phase of labour, the rate of dilatation should be 1.0–1.2 cm per hour in the nullipara and 1.2–1.5 cm per hour in the multipara. The curve for descent of the presenting part is hyperbolic rather than the sigmoid shape which describes cervical dilatation (figure 40.4); descent in the active phase should be 1 cm or more per hour. Preparations should be made for a possible instrumental delivery, neonatal resuscitation, and an abnormal third stage.

Table 49.2 illustrates that prolonged labour is often associated with *fetal distress* (50%), *occipitoposterior position* (35%) and a *large fetus* (10%) — the incidences of *forceps delivery* (50%) and *Caesarean section* (22%) are double that of the total population, and the *perinatal mortality rate* is increased to about 3%.

SECOND STAGE

Definition
A duration longer than 1 hour in a nullipara or ½ hour in a multipara.

Incidence
About 10% of all labours.

Aetiology
The same factors may operate as discussed for the first stage, namely abnormal uterine action, large fetal diameter, or obstruction in the passages. However, since the cervix is fully dilated and descent to the pelvic floor has usually been achieved, the precise causes are often different. Rather than primary disordered uterine action, we see more of the *secondary type of inertia* (uterine exhaustion). If a major increase in the fetal presenting diameters was present, obstruction would have occurred in the first stage. As far as the passages are concerned, we may be dealing with *outlet contraction*, but much more likely is spasm of the levator or pelvic diaphragms (because of pain and anxiety), plus a *rigid or tight perineum*. An additional consideration is the patient's voluntary effort. If the nerve endings in the pelvic floor are blocked by *conduction type analgesia*, the bearing-down reflex will be lost to a significant extent; an inefficient expulsive effort may also result from incoordination, exhaustion, weakness of the abdominal muscles, or a disabling condition of the heart or lungs.

Management
Prolongation of the second stage of labour signals the need for delivery. It is treated by timely forceps or vacuum extraction. Occasionally, if the fetus is in good condition, further delay is permissible if a degree of descent is obtained which allows a nontraumatic delivery rather than a more difficult procedure in the midpelvis (breech or forceps delivery).

Symphysiotomy is practised in some centres. It can be useful in delay in the second stage where there is some disproportion, including the aftercoming head of the breech. It is contraindicated if the baby is large or the mother obese (undue symphyseal separation), the baby small or dead, or there has been a previous Caesarean section.

SHOULDER DYSTOCIA (IMPACTED SHOULDERS)

Impaction of the shoulders is present when there is obstruction to the passage of the shoulders through the bony pelvis, the head having already been delivered. This complication is particularly important, since it can occur unexpectedly in cephalic presentations and *there may be no time to summon help*. The obstetric attendant should always be on guard for this emergency in any *obese or diabetic patient*, or one whose *labour is prolonged* despite good contractions. Impacted shoulders should not be confused with difficulty with the shoulders due to a *small head passing through an incompletely dilated cervix* — this can occur with anencephaly, microcephaly or fetal death with skull collapse. In this circumstance the head is *not delivered* but is in the vagina — treatment is to await full cervical dilatation when spontaneous delivery will occur — attempts to extract the fetus when the cervix is not fully dilated may result in rupture of the uterus. Difficulty with the shoulders during a *breech delivery* is due to a large baby or *extended arms* and is usually dealt with by the Lovset manoeuvre (see Chapter 50).

INCIDENCE
About 1 in 100 deliveries, but the figure is higher if lesser degrees are included.

AETIOLOGY
Obstruction may be due to: (i) Disproportion due to *large fetal shoulders* or a small *maternal pelvis* (especially a reduced true conjugate diameter), impaction occurring at the pelvic brim with the shoulders in the AP diameter of the pelvis. (ii) *Failure of rotation of the shoulders* into the AP diameter of the pelvis. Often this occurs as a complication of an *occipitoposterior position* — there being delay in the second stage of labour. The head is on view and forceps delivery is followed by impacted shoulders — the accoucheur can anticipate the problem since undue traction is required to deliver the head when it is well clear of the bony pelvis, the difficulty being due to impaction of the shoulders in the oblique diameter of the midpelvis.

CLINICAL FEATURES
The emergency occurs after the fetal head has negotiated the bony pelvis and has been delivered.

DIAGNOSIS
The head is born, often with difficulty, but the neck and shoulders fail to appear. The chin burrows into the maternal perineum when the occiput is anterior. Conditions causing confusion include compound presentation (hand lying

below the chin), incomplete cervical dilatation (anencephaly, macerated fetus), fetal trunk enlargement (ascites, tumour), and constriction ring.

TREATMENT

Prophylaxis

Macrosomia of the fetus should be suspected in the following circumstances: (i) maternal diabetes mellitus; (ii) maternal obesity and excessive weight gain in the pregnancy; (iii) history of large infants (above 4,000 g); (iv) history of shoulder dystocia in previous pregnancies; (v) suspicion of a macrosomic infant on clinical palpation; (vi) a large abdominothoracic: head ratio on ultrasonography; (vii) prolonged labour (especially a protracted second stage) despite good contractions.

If impacted shoulders is anticipated and vaginal delivery is contemplated, an experienced obstetrician, assistant, anaesthetist and paediatrician should be available.

Emergency

Initial measures. (i) Do a vaginal examination to exclude a limb beside the head and clear the infant's air passages thoroughly. (ii) Bring the patient to the edge of the bed/chair/delivery table. (iii) Cut a large episiotomy; this is not easy since the head is in the way. (iv) Let the head go, in case it has been externally rotated in the wrong direction, and the shoulders have not rotated; this occurs more commonly when the head has engaged in the posterior position, or during forceps delivery when the shoulder mechanism may fail to occur under general or local anaesthesia. *By rotation of the head in the correct direction and pulling posteriorly at the same time, the anterior shoulder should appear under the pubic arch* (figure 49.11). (v) Fundal pressure by an assistant, together with suprapubic pressure, may be helpful.

Later measures. If the above procedures fail, it must be realized that the fetus is in considerable danger. The choice of further management will differ with individual obstetricians and will depend on whether the patient is anaesthetized or not. If no anaesthetist is available, pethidine 50 mg may be given slowly intravenously to facilitate manipulations. (i) If it is considered that more forceful traction will injure the cervical spine (colour plate 145), the Willughby manoeuvre is carried out: the hand (right or left, whichever faces the occiput/fetal back) is inserted into the vagina posterior to the fetal head and 2 fingers are placed in and behind the axilla and

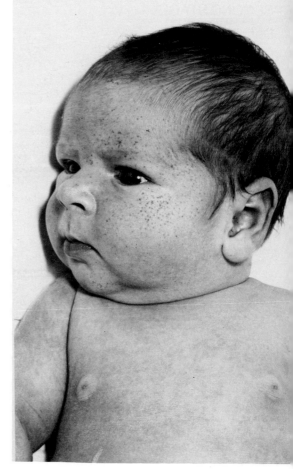

Figure 49.10 Infant (birth-weight 4,110 g) aged 24 hours with purpuric rash from asphyxia caused by impacted shoulders. Low forceps delivery was performed for delay in the second stage after an 8-hour labour in a 21-year-old para 2.

are used to rotate the shoulder (a similar principle to the Lovset manoeuvre). The anterior shoulder is freed from the symphysis pubis and can be delivered by traction on the head plus fundal and suprapubic pressure. (ii) If the above measure fails, *an arm must be brought down.* Generally, the posterior arm is easier to bring down because there is more room in the hollow of the sacrum to carry out manipulation. This is achieved by pressing in the antecubital fossa to release the arm, after which combined traction on the head and arm is sufficient to effect delivery of the shoulder. Once the shoulders are low enough, hook the index fingers of both hands into the anterior axilla and pull posteriorly to release and deliver the anterior shoulder. To give access to the anterior shoulder an assistant must exert traction on the head in a posterior direction. This type of delivery often causes an

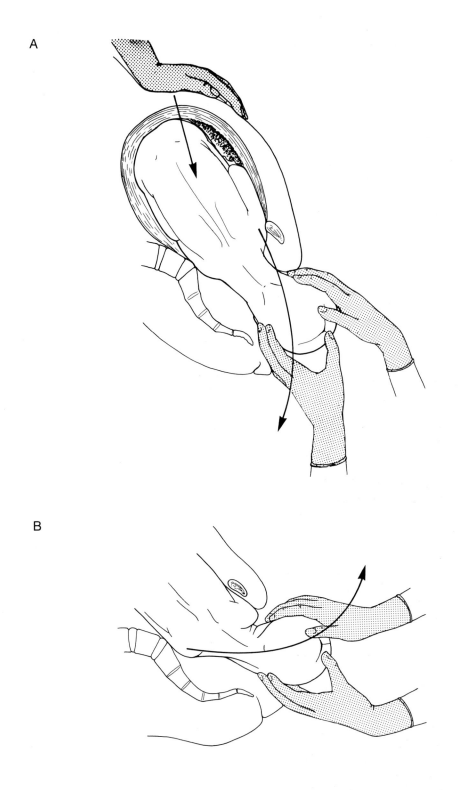

Figure 49.11 Treatment of impacted shoulders. **A.** Traction on the head in a posterior direction brings the anterior shoulder past the pubic symphysis into the pelvis. Note fundal pressure by an assistant. **B.** Traction is then applied in an anterior direction to bring the posterior shoulder into the pelvis.

Erb palsy or fracture of the clavicle or humerus (colour plate 140). (iii) If the above fails and the patient is not already anaesthetized, a general anaesthetic must be given and the baby extracted, with or without *cleidotomy*. The latter is not an easy procedure and there is a serious risk of fetal and maternal damage: the head is drawn down firmly towards the floor, the anterior clavicle identified, the skin over it incised with scissors, and a cutting instrument severs the clavicle and displaces the ends; the same procedure may be necessary on the posterior clavicle, the head being displaced upward.

After delivery, the episiotomy must be repaired, together with any cervical or vaginal lacerations that may have occurred (these are common unless the episiotomy is extensive). Manual exploration of the uterus may be indicated to exclude uterine rupture; in any case, a careful check on the condition of the mother must be kept for postpartum bleeding and infection.

The infant will usually require resuscitation, special observation, and possibly treatment for brachial plexus and skeletal injury — particularly fractures of the clavicle and humerus (colour plate 140 and figure 66.4).

PROGNOSIS

Fetal. Unless delivery is achieved within 5-7 minutes, the baby will die as a result of (i) asphyxiation, since the cord may be occluded and chest expansion is not possible even though inspiratory movements are attempted; (ii) pressure of tissues around the neck obstruct venous return to the heart (the baby's face and scalp become deeply engorged and cyanotic) (figure 49.10); (iii) premature placental separation. Injuries to the spinal cord and brachial plexus may occur (Erb C5, 6; Klumpke C7, 8) due to forceful attempts at delivery (colour plates 140 and 145).

Maternal. Severe maternal trauma, including uterine rupture, can occur if excessive force is employed.

chapter fifty

Errors of Fetal Polarity

OVERVIEW

There is much debate in current obstetrics on how the breech baby should be delivered — vaginally or by Caesarean section (colour plates 29–32 and 93). The present chapter assumes a decision in favour of an attempt at vaginal delivery has been made. The trial of labour finesse is inappropriate for breech delivery because it is too late to perform Caesarean section when cephalopelvic disproportion exists and difficulty occurs with delivery of the aftercoming head. *The possible need for Caesarean section is always reviewed after the onset of spontaneous labour to assess that conditions are favourable for vaginal delivery* (breech engaged, no cord or footling presentation, membranes intact, coordinate contractions). The main point of emphasis is that *breech delivery should only be undertaken by an experienced obstetrician* because of the disastrous consequences to the baby should the delivery go awry. An assistant is helpful if forceps are to be used for the aftercoming head; an *anaesthetist* may be required at short notice if difficulties arise in delivery of the head, and finally, a *paediatrician*, if available, should also be on hand in case the baby is asphyxiated and requires resuscitation. In the great majority of patients the birth is by an *assisted breech delivery*, with or without forceps to the aftercoming head. The remainder will be delivered by Caesarean section (if a significant problem arises during labour), *breech extraction* (if the birth needs to be expedited and conditions for delivery are favourable), or *spontaneously* (usually birth before the mother's arrival in the delivery room or rapid birth in a multipara).

Significant trends in labour management include assessment of the size of the fetus by ultrasonography, continuous electronic monitoring of the fetal heart rate and earlier resort to Caesarean section if fetal condition or progress of labour is giving concern.

The mechanism of labour in breech presentation differs in many respects from the situation when the head presents. For example, the presenting part may be a foot, knee, buttocks (*frank breech*) or buttocks plus feet (*complete breech*). The breech is not articulated like the head and is capable only of limited movement during its passage through the birth canal. When the baby is *premature* the head is much larger than the breech, and since it passes through the cervix last in breech delivery, this can create major problems with *entrapment in an incompletely dilated cervix*. A further difficulty is that the favourable fetal attitude of *universal flexion* tends to be broken up as the breech descends rather than reinforced as is the case with cephalic presentations.

The *umbilical cord* is at greater risk, not only of prolapse, but pressure against the presenting part in the final stage of labour and during delivery.

Finally, *moulding*, the mechanism whereby the head is able to squeeze, slowly and safely, through some tight spots, is denied the breech baby — the head having no more than 3–5 minutes to pass through the entire birth canal.

In view of the foregoing, it is not unexpected that the clinician seeks favourable conditions before selecting the vaginal route for delivery of the breech presentation. Overall *Caesarean section rates vary from 25–75% or more.*

During the labour itself, the principles of care are little different from those pertaining to cephalic presentations. A close watch is kept on the fetal condition and rate of dilatation of the cervix: deviations are usually dealt with more expeditiously (by Caesarean section).

Success of the delivery depends largely on a correct forecast of the *fetal and pelvic dimensions*, the normality of *uterine action*, and the availability of adequate skills (obstetric, anaesthetic, paediatric) and facilities. One of the major points in technique is to *maintain fetal flexion* by allowing the mother to push the baby out, or if traction is exerted, to maintain flexion by coordinated fundal pressure.

Vaginal breech birth will only be safe for the baby if carried out or supervised by an attendant who has mastered the art.

The *perinatal mortality rate* associated with breech delivery ranges from *5-20%* according to the facilities available (experienced obstetrician, anaesthetist, paediatrician, special care nursery) and the presence of *associated complications* (prematurity, premature rupture of the membranes, fetal malformations, placenta praevia, multiple pregnancy).

In transverse and oblique lies correction is usually easier than with breech presentation, but the conversion tends to be unstable due to the presence of such underlying factors as *polyhydramnios, lax abdominal muscles* and placenta praevia. If the correction remains stable, vaginal delivery can be anticipated, but, if not, Caesarean section is advisable; the latter procedure is also indicated if premature rupture of the membranes has occurred. A longitudinal incision in the uterus avoids the difficulty often complicating the lower segment transverse incision — an arm popping out which makes delivery of the rest of the baby very difficult. The *Caesarean section rate* in patients with transverse or unstable lie is about 60%. The *perinatal mortality rate is 5-15%* due mainly to prematurity, internal version, and prolapse of the umbilical cord.

BREECH PRESENTATION

General information concerning breech presentation and its management during pregnancy has been given in Chapter 26.

In order to follow labour and manage the breech delivery successfully, it is necessary first to study the underlying mechanism, since this differs appreciably from that where the head is presenting.

MECHANISM OF BREECH DELIVERY

Breech Movements

(i) *Initial station.* In nulliparas, especially if the legs are extended (*frank breech*), the breech is likely to be well in the pelvis at the start of labour. In other cases, the station is often higher than with a vertex presentation.

(ii) *Descent.* This occurs throughout labour, but again, the breech may remain relatively high until late in the first stage.

(iii) *Engagement.* The breech is engaged when the bitrochanteric diameter (distance between the greater trochanters of the femora, 9–10 cm) has passed the pelvic brim. *Engagement is much more difficult to assess than in cephalic presentation,* since there are no definable landmarks either on abdominal or vaginal examination. One can, however, gain a reasonable idea of the extent to which the breech has entered the pelvis.

(iv) *Internal (anterior) rotation.* In a right sacroanterior position (RSA), for example, the anterior hip (which is at a lower level than the posterior hip) rotates to the front, bringing the sacrum to face directly to the right. *It should be emphasized that it is not the denominator which*

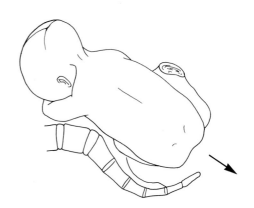

Figure 50.1 Mechanism of breech delivery. Engagement has occurred and with further descent to the pelvic floor the bitrochanteric diameter has rotated into the anteroposterior diameter of the pelvic outlet.

rotates to the anterior position, as in vertex and face presentations, but the anterior hip (figure 50.1).

(v) *Lateral flexion.* With further descent, the breech must now negotiate the curve of the birth canal, which corresponds to the curve of the maternal sacrum, coccyx and anococcygeal raphe. This requires a lateral bending of the lower part of the trunk as the anterior buttock stems under the symphysis and the posterior buttock swings forward past the posterior structures mentioned above (figure 50.2).

(vi) *Delivery.* The breech is delivered with the sacrum in the lateral position, since this is most appropriate to the outlet diameters (the bitrochanteric diameter lying in the AP diameter of the outlet), and to the *mechanism of birth by lateral flexion.* There is no 'caput' as such, although there may be congestion of the buttocks

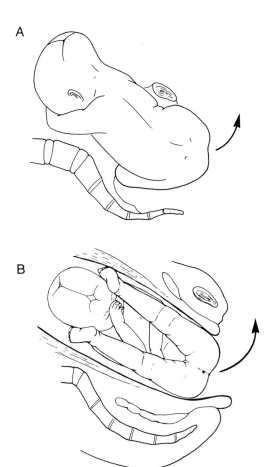

Figure 50.2 Birth of buttocks by lateral flexion of the trunk. **A.** The anterior buttock rotates around the symphysis and appears to 'climb up' from the mother's perineum. The shoulders have not yet engaged. **B.** Extended legs impede lateral flexion by splinting the fetal trunk. A wide episiotomy is required for the buttocks to negotiate the curve of the birth canal.

and perineal area (especially the scrotum in male babies, colour plates 29 and 30). If there is a footling or knee presentation, there may also be considerable swelling, cyanosis and perhaps ecchymoses.

(vii) *Restitution.* After the pelvic girdle is delivered there is usually a movement of the breech again toward the position it occupied in the pelvis — namely RSA, a turn of 45°. This is less constant than with vertex presentations, because the breech does not rotate as freely.

(viii) *External rotation.* In vertex presentations, this depends on movement imparted to the head after delivery by rotation of the shoulders into the AP diameter of pelvis. In breech deliveries, this movement, if it occurs, is quite late since the shoulders, which are its prime determinant, enter the pelvis only after the trunk is delivered. Usually the breech delivery is 'assisted', rather than being completely spontaneous, and this also affects restitution and external rotation.

Shoulder Movements

These are the same as for the breech. The bisacromial diameter (distance between the acromion processes of the scapulae, 10–11 cm) is in the same plane as the bitrochanteric diameter of the breech, and describes the same movements within the constraint imposed by the operator — i.e. descent, engagement in the pelvis, anterior internal rotation, lateral flexion, and delivery.

Head Movements

(i) *Descent.* This occurs much more rapidly than in cephalic presentations, usually taking no more than 2–4 minutes.

(ii) *Engagement.* Although the head enters the pelvis in the reverse manner, the same diameters of engagement pass the pelvic brim — the biparietal in one plane and the suboccipito-bregmatic in the other. However, with cephalic presentations, resistance and friction of the birth canal increase flexion, but in breech presentations, the opposite occurs and there is a *tendency to deflexion.* Thus, not infrequently it is the suboccipitofrontal or occipitofrontal diameter that has to pass through the pelvis. This deflexion is aggravated if the breech is extracted and minimized if explusion is by the efforts of the uterus and secondary powers of the mother, aided if necessary by properly exerted fundal pressure. Engagement usually occurs as the shoulders are passing through the vulval ring. Since the shoulders are delivered in the AP position, the head will engage as a ROT in the particular patient we are considering.

(iii) *Internal anterior rotation* will either occur spontaneously, or more probably the back will be turned to the anterior position by the accoucheur after delivery of the shoulders.

(iv) *Delivery.* The back of the baby's neck rests under the symphysis pubis and, while flexion is being maintained, the head is delivered over the perineum — the chin, face, and forehead appearing in succession, and finally the occiput passes from under the symphysis pubis.

Variations

Posterior and lateral positions. If the position is RSP or LSP, there is not a 135° rotation (3/8 circle) as in cephalic presentations, but only 45° (1/8 circle) to bring the bitrochanteric diameter into the AP of the pelvis. For lateral positions (RSL, LSL) internal rotation is not necessary.

If there is a rotation of the sacrum backwards after delivery of the breech (restitution to a posterior position), this must be corrected manually, otherwise the head will enter the pelvis in a posterior position, which is very unfavourable.

Knee and footling presentations. These usually do not alter the mechanism as described. The major exception is when the posterior leg presents. This causes the anterior buttock to be pushed over the symphysis pubis and arrested there. This is corrected either spontenously or manually by rotation of the sacrum more anteriorly, allowing the anterior buttock to descend.

Extended legs. The mechanism is essentially unchanged, but because the trunk is splinted, lateral flexion, which is necessary to follow the curve of the birth canal, is limited and thus labour tends to be slower (figure 50.2b).

Extended arms. The arms are normally folded across the chest, and are freed and delivered after each shoulder is delivered. In premature breech deliveries, which are not uncommon, the cervix may not be fully dilated by the relatively small breech and thus the arms may be pulled up beside the head in a manner similar to that which follows the drawing of a tight pullover over a child's head. Another cause is breech extraction, which *breaks up the attitude of flexion.*

MANAGEMENT DURING LABOUR

General Principles
The general care, observations, and management are similar to the description given for cephalic presentations. Maternal exhaustion is prevented by adequate explanation, pain relief, sleep, and fluids.

Fetal Assessment
In most cases, the diagnosis of breech presentation will have been made in the antenatal period. The special features on abdominal examination have already been described. *A careful assessment of fetal size* should be made and multiple pregnancy excluded. On vaginal examination, the consistency of the breech is quite different from the vertex, and should immediately bring the diagnosis to mind. Apart from confirmation of the presentation, a determination should be made as to whether the legs are flexed or extended, and whether the cord is presenting or palpable. Breech presentation must be distinguished from face and shoulder presentations, and anencephaly. The feet are distinguished from the hands by the presence of the

more prominent heel, the shorter digits, the straight line from digit 1 to 5, and the inability to separate widely the first and second digits. Finally, the foot cannot be straightened out fully. It should be remembered that occasionally a foot may lie alongside the head in cephalic presentations (compound presentation — colour plate 141).

The second stage of labour is diagnosed by the same criteria as used for vertex presentations. At this time, the anterior buttock usually becomes visible if the legs are extended.

Special Problems
Because the complete breech fits less well into the lower uterine segment than the head, the *membranes tend to rupture earlier* in labour. For the same reason, *cord prolapse* is more common (3% of all breech presentations, 10–15% if footling) and *should be excluded by sterile pelvic examination when the membranes rupture.*

Meconium staining of the liquor is not uncommon late in the first stage or in the second stage, when the breech is being compressed in the birth canal. If the meconium is formed and fresh, and the fetal heart is satisfactory, this is a normal happening. *If it occurs earlier in labour it has the same significance as in vertex presentations. Monitoring of the baby,* both by fetal heart rate pattern and buttock blood sampling is often advisable. Values for pH are higher than where the vertex presents, because there is less obstruction to the circulation because of the irregularity of the presenting part.

Monitoring of the progress of labour is especially important in breech presentation. A partograph should be kept and close attention paid to rates of cervical dilatation (1 cm/hour in the nullipara, 1.3 cm in the multipara). Augmentation of inefficient labour with oxytocin is a controversial issue, but seems reasonable if there is no disporportion and the labour is being carefully watched.

If the posterior leg is presenting and progress is not normal, it is usual to carry out a sterile vaginal examination and attempt to rotate the sacrum to the front, and so disengage the anterior buttock from the symphysis pubis.

It has been mentioned that the breech (especially if the legs are extended and the patient is a nullipara) negotiates the birth canal with difficulty during the second stage and at delivery because of the *need for lateral flexion of the trunk.* The second stage is thus often longer and there tends to be a faster deterioration in the condition of the fetus.

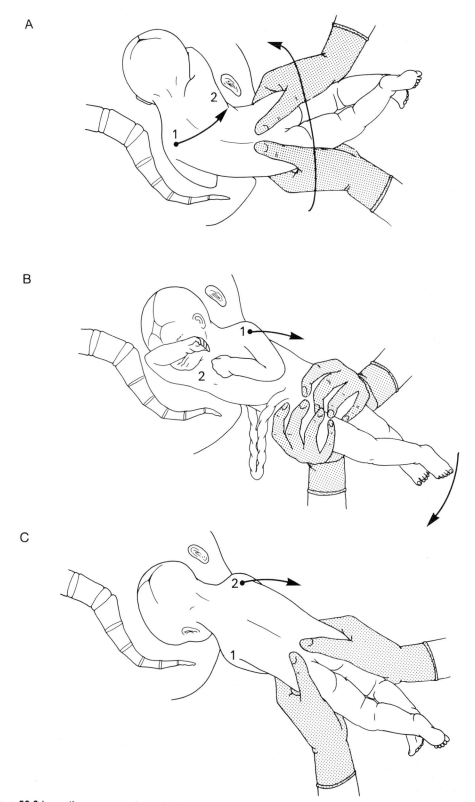

Figure 50.3 Lovset's manoeuvre is particularly useful for delivery of the shoulders when the arms are extended. **A.** The baby is rotated through 180° so that the posterior shoulder (1) becomes anterior and lies at a lower level in the pelvis (below the symphysis pubis). **B.** The anterior shoulder (1) is delivered and, whilst the back is kept uppermost, the body is rotated back 180° to bring the second shoulder (2) anteriorly below the symphysis. **C.** Delivery of the second shoulder (2) is accomplished.

BREECH DELIVERY

The usual method of breech birth is by *assisted breech delivery* and this will be described initially. In all cases, skilled supervision and assistance, an anaesthetist, and a paediatrician should be available.

(i) The patient should be briefed as to the situation, procedures to be undertaken, and her own role; a cooperative patient, with good morale, is very helpful in achieving a favourable outcome. (ii) The patient is placed in the lithotomy position. (iii) Antiseptic preparation as for normal delivery. (iv) Instruments and drapes as for normal delivery, with the addition of a sterile breech cloth. (v) Pelvic examination is made to assess the station, position, disposition of limbs, and pelvic size and shape. The bladder is emptied by catheter if necessary. (vi) Analgesia: usually perineal infiltration with 0.5% lignocaine, or pudendal nerve block; continuous epidural analgesia is preferred in many centres and may have been commenced during the first stage. (vii) *Episiotomy* is performed routinely in nulliparas when the breech is distending the perineum, in multiparas if the perineum is tight. The incision is best made after the anterior buttock is born, when the posterior buttock is distending the perineum and the breech is not retracting between contractions. It may be made earlier if there is a tight vulval ring. (viii) The breech is born by maternal expulsive effort. If the legs are flexed, they are freed as the breech passes through the introitus. With continued effort, the lower trunk is delivered to the level of the umbilicus. A loop of cord is grasped and gently pulled down. An assessment is made of the strength and frequency of pulsations. There should be no panic if the rate is slow, however, since this is often a reflex response to compression. (ix) A warm, moist cloth is placed over the buttocks and legs, and the baby grasped as shown in figures 50.3 and 50.7; grasping the baby's abdomen rather than the pelvic girdle is liable to cause serious injury to such structures as the liver and spleen. With the next contraction, the breech is pulled downward towards the floor and the *anterior shoulder* is delivered (colour plate 31). Then the arm is delivered by passing the hand over the shoulder and down the front of the humerus toward the elbow and exerting gentle, steady pressure. The *posterior shoulder* is delivered by swinging the baby upwards when it will sweep over the perineum posteriorly; the posterior arm is similarly freed. An alternative method of delivering the posterior shoulder is to rotate it to the anterior position by the *Lovset manoeuvre* (figure 50.3).

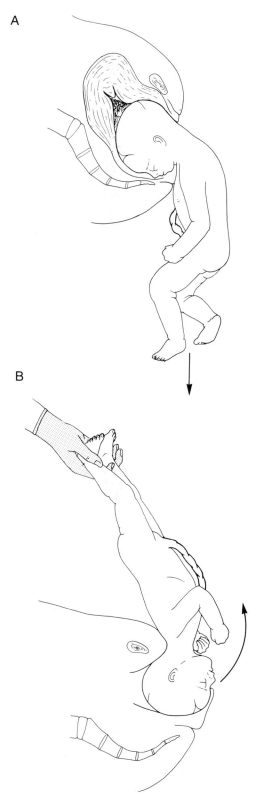

Figure 50.4 Burns-Marshall method of delivering the head. **A.** Baby hangs with back uppermost to flex and promote engagement of the head. **B.** The head is delivered by traction on the feet as they are swung upwards — the head is born by extension as it rotates around the symphysis.

A

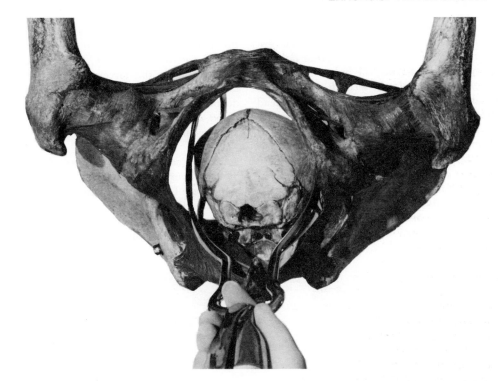

B

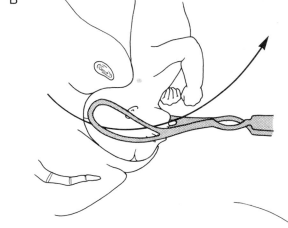

Figure 50.5 Forceps delivery of the aftercoming head. **A.** The occiput must be anterior (posterior fontanelle beneath the symphysis pubis). **B.** When the mouth appears the infant can breathe although the greatest diameters of the head are still negotiating the narrow pelvic plane and outlet.

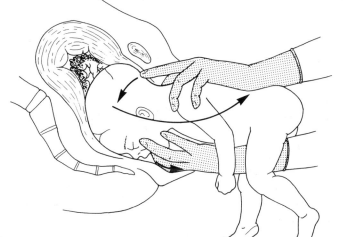

Figure 50.6 Mauriceau-Smellie-Veit technique for delivery of the head is particularly useful when deflexion has caused failure of engagement.

This technique is of more value if the posterior arm is above the head or behind it (nuchal position) or if the direct method fails. *After delivery of the shoulders and arms, the baby is allowed to hang downwards for 15–30 seconds* if there is no worry about his condition. This flexes the head and facilitates engagement in the pelvis. Usually, the hair-line will become visible (figure 50.4). (x) The preferred method of *delivery of the head* is to apply forceps. The blades are applied directly to the sides of the head, the baby having been lifted up over the mother's abdomen by the assistant, who also holds the arms out of the way. *This protects the baby's head, allows aspiration of the nasopharynx, and permits controlled delivery of the head without sudden decompression.* The delivery is no different from that with the vertex presenting. Gentleness is essential in placing the forceps blades. The baby's mouth appears early and with a sterile speculum depressing the perineum the assistant aspirates blood, liquor, and mucus from the baby's oro- and nasopharynx (figure 50.5 and colour plate 32).

Oxygen can then be administered if necessary. Slow delivery through the outlet is essential, since there has not been time for proper moulding of the head; with a rapid exit the compressed intracranial structures may suddenly expand, resulting in tears and haemorrhage.

A

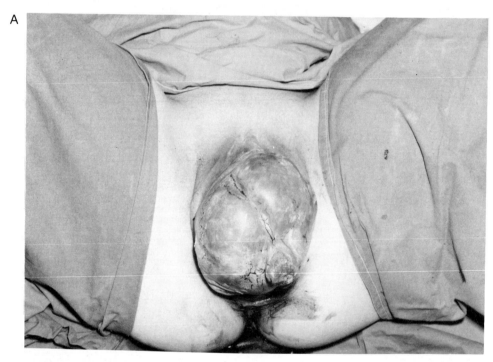

B

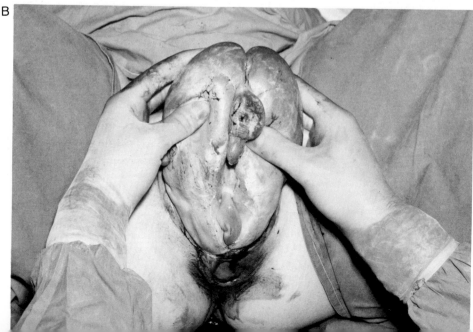

C

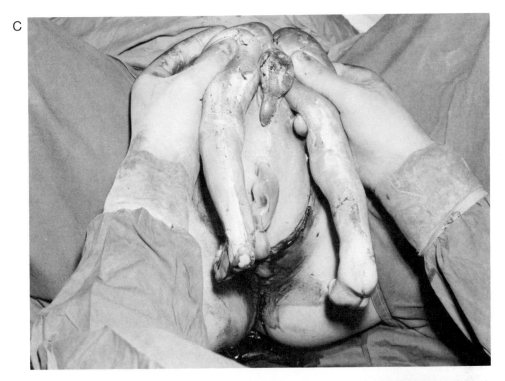

D

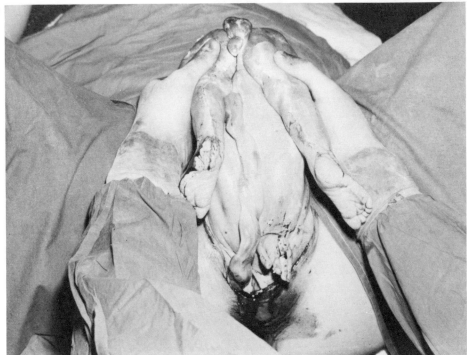

Figure 50.7 Bracht method of breech delivery. **A.** With each contraction the posterior hip rolls over the perineum and the sacrum rotates laterally to bring the bitrochanteric diameter into the anteroposterior diameter of the pelvic outlet. When the buttocks are born they rotate upwards, bringing the sacrum anterior. **B.** The body and extended legs are held together with both hands maintaining the upward and anterior rotation of the body. **C.** With the baby's back directed against the mother's symphysis, the feet pass over the perineum. **D.** The hands and arms appear over the perineum having been tucked in under the chin.

E

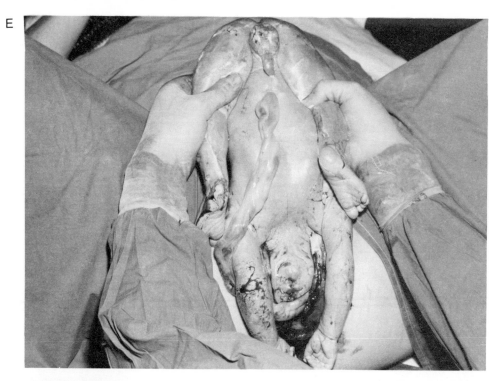

F

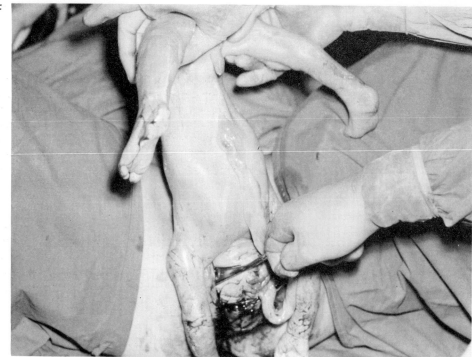

E. Spontaneous simultaneous delivery of the elbows succeeded by arms with the bisacromial diameter in the transverse of the pelvic outlet. **F.** An attitude of extreme extension now produced by curvature of the baby's back allows the head to pass through the outlet in its most favourable diameter, guarded by forceps. (Courtesy of Dr Max Jotkowitz).

The head may also be delivered by the manual (classical) technique (Mauriceau-Smellie-Veit). The baby is placed on the accoucheur's arm, straddling it with arms and legs; flexion of the head is maintained by the middle finger placed in the baby's mouth and the ring and index fingers beside the nose on the alveolar ridge. The index finger of the other hand pushes on the region of the occiput to further increase flexion. The head is delivered by drawing the body downward and then forward over the mother's abdomen (figure 50.6).

In variations of this technique, there may be assisted downward suprapubic pressure by an assistant, and this may be coupled with lateral rotation of the head in the pelvis if the head has not engaged (Wigand-Martin). Finally, Bracht described a manoeuvre whereby the feet are grasped and the body drawn high up onto the maternal abdomen: the symphysis acts as a fulcrum about which the fetal occipital region rotates (figure 50.7). This is only suitable if the head is engaged.

Preparations should always be made for an infant who may have suffered from hypoxia; otherwise the routine care of the baby is as previously described.

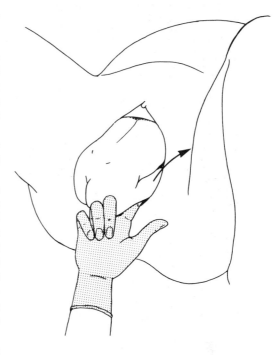

Figure 50.8 Pressure behind the knee flexes the anterior extended leg which then delivers.

Difficulties during Delivery

If the breech has distended the perineum, it is rare that delivery to the umbilicus does not follow, especially if episiotomy has been performed. *Extended legs* are delivered by pressure in the popliteal fossa to produce flexion and the foot is grasped (figure 50.8). *Groin traction* may be necessary if the breech does not descend easily to the perineum.

If further progress is difficult, fetal ascites or abdominal tumour may be suspected (and confirmed by intrauterine palpation), or a constriction ring might have developed. *Difficulty with the shoulders* may occur if the baby is large or the arms have become extended. Lovset's manoeuvre is usually employed (figure 50.3). Extended arms may also be dealt with by the 'classical' method whereby a hand is introduced into the vagina and each forearm is swept in an arc over the baby's face (it is usually easier if the posterior arm is delivered first). *Most problems are experienced in delivery of the head, mainly through failing to maintain flexion.* Disproportion may be present due to unsuspected pelvic narrowing, a large fetus, or hydrocephaly. An experienced operator is required to overcome these difficulties.

If the baby is small or the presentation footling, the trunk may slip through a *cervix which is not fully dilated.* An experienced doctor may be able to push up the cervix, especially in a multipara; or forceps may be applied if a hand can be introduced inside the cervix (this manoeuvre is dangerous to mother and child). Pulling on the legs is useless and only tightens the cervix around the baby's neck. If the cervix is thin it can be cut; alternatively, induction of general anaesthesia will allow cervical dilatation.

Deviation from an uncomplicated assisted breech delivery depends on such factors as the efficiency of the labour, the parity of the patient, and the size of baby and pelvis. In some patients, virtually no assistance will be required apart from support of the baby and keeping it warm; in others, guidance and traction will be required at most stages, e.g. the breech, shoulders, arms, and head.

Breech Extraction

The indications and conditions for this procedure are similar in principle to those described for forceps delivery. In general, progress has slowed or ceased in the second stage of labour, or there is an indication to hasten the second stage because of distress of the fetus or mother. Since the procedure involves major manipulation, anaesthesia (epidural or general) is necessary. Further, the cervix must be fully dilated,

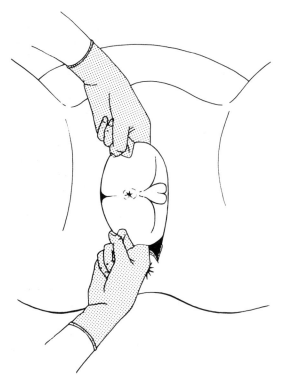

Figure 50.9 Delivery of extended legs by groin traction.

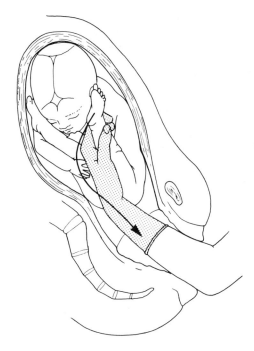

Figure 50.10 Pinard's manoeuvre is used when arrest of a breech with extended legs has occurred in the midpelvis. The breech must be disimpacted before the leg can be brought down. The manoeuvre is dangerous to mother and child and Caesarean section is preferred.

the breech engaged in the pelvis, and no significant disproportion present. Except for delivery of the second twin, Caesarean section is usually preferred to breech extraction for difficulties arising during the second stage, unless it is felt that the delivery will be an easy one.

Assessment. A careful examination is made to ascertain that the above conditions are present, to assess station, position, and disposition of the legs.

Breech delivery. The breech may be delivered in one of several ways. (i) *Groin traction* (figure 50.9), where the index fingers are placed in one or both groins. (ii) *Leg traction*, either directly, if a foot or leg is presenting or after the hand has been inserted into the uterus to *bring down a leg* by Pinard's manoeuvre (figure 50.10). The anterior leg is brought down for reasons previously described. With further traction the other leg is delivered. The further procedure is similar to that described under assisted delivery, except that the baby is delivered by the operator rather than by maternal expulsive efforts. One of the most important aspects of breech extraction is to prevent deflexion of the head, which tends to occur naturally with this presentation. The

most effective means for this is to maintain pressure on the sinciput from above during traction. Some patients with epidural analgesia may be able to cooperate in assisting with delivery of the trunk and head once the breech has been delivered.

Caesarean Section

Abdominal delivery may be necessary during labour as a result of fetal distress or failure of progress (descent or dilatation). Usually, less stringent criteria are adopted in the selection of patients for section than is the case where the vertex is presenting.

PROGNOSIS

Maternal

The morbidity and mortality is slightly higher in breech deliveries, mainly because of the associated manipulations required and the possibility of tears, haemorrhage and infection; there are also the risks of anaesthesia should this be required.

Fetal

There are 4 problems: the *breech delivery* itself, *associated obstetrical complications, prema-*

turity, and *fetal malformation* (which may have been the cause of the breech presentation). The mortality ranges from 5–10% in series excluding emergency cases.

In a series of 1,645 breech deliveries in a teaching hospital during the 10 years 1971–1980, almost 1 in 5 (308 or *18.7%*) were due to *multiple pregnancies. The perinatal mortality rate was 17.2%* in this series, which included emergency admissions. *Prematurity* and *major fetal malformations* incompatible with life accounted for *more than 80%* of the perinatal deaths — in 160 of the 308 deaths (52%), delivery occurred before 28 weeks' gestation. During the 10 years the *Caesarean section rate* in this hospital for singleton breech presentations increased from 30% to 45%. If one considers only uncomplicated cases at term, the loss is little different than that for normal uncomplicated cephalic presentations (0.5–1% versus 0.25–0.5%).

The main dangers are *external cephalic version* antenatally (see Chapter 26); *asphyxia* from cord prolapse or pressure during delivery, or delay in delivery of the trunk or head); *intracranial haemorrhage* (lack of time for moulding, deflexion resulting from extraction, hasty delivery of the head, rapid exit from the birth canal); *prematurity* (associated pathology, such as placental abruption, premature rupture of membranes); *other trauma* (cervical spine and vertebral artery injuries, cerebellar damage as a result of excess pressure on the occipital bone, nerve palsies from excessive traction, damage to abdominal viscera and skeletal muscles from careless handling).

TRANSVERSE/OBLIQUE LIE: SHOULDER PRESENTATION

MANAGEMENT OF THE DELIVERY

The general features of transverse and oblique lie and their management during pregnancy have been discussed in Chapter 26.

There is no normal mechanism of labour, although small babies may occasionally be delivered by spontaneous evolution. Definitive steps must therefore be taken at 38–39 weeks to deliver the baby. The following treatments are available.

Caesarean Section

This is preferred in most nulliparas, in those with a suspected uterine malformation or pelvic tumour, pelvic contraction, premature rupture of the membranes, prolapsed cord, placenta praevia, infertility, and large infant.

Trial of Labour

If correction can be made fairly easily to a longitudinal lie, a conservative approach can be adopted — perhaps with Buist pads on either side of the abdomen if the lie is unstable. If this fails, Caesarean section is performed.

The situation where the diagnosis has not been made and the patient presents in well established labour needs separate consideration. The diagnosis can usually be made on abdominal examination, although if contractions are frequent and painful this may not be easy. On pelvic examination, the shoulder, torso, elbow, or hand will be felt and the condition must be distinguished from breech and face presentations, and also anencephaly.

If the shoulder presents, one can usually distinguish such landmarks as the scapula and its acromial process, the clavicle, and the axillary fossa. The acromion is used as the denominator to indicate the baby's position although it is of less relevance than in other presentations, where there is a definable mechanism of labour.

If the fetus is alive and not grossly premature,

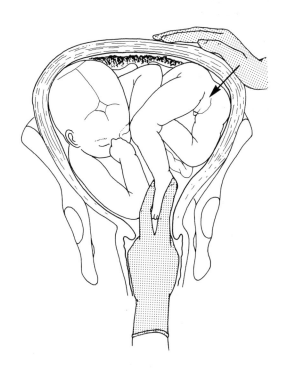

Figure 50.11 Bipolar (Braxton Hicks) version. This manoeuvre is used only when the fetus is dead or unlikely to survive because of prematurity.

Caesarean section (usually classical) is performed because of the high risk of rupture of the over-stretched lower uterine segment (colour plate 141). Occasionally, external version may be successful (especially in the multiparous patient) if the membranes are intact and the contractions are not too strong or frequent. Spontaneous delivery, if the lie is uncorrected, should never be relied upon ('spontaneous evolution'). *Internal version followed by breech extraction* is associated with a relatively high fetal mortality rate and the risk of uterine rupture (colour plate 23); it has virtually been abandoned for this condition.

If the baby is dead or abnormal, *bipolar or internal podalic version* may be attempted with the uterus fully relaxed under general anaesthesia (figure 50.11). This is best attempted only if the membranes have not been long ruptured and the baby is not large. Otherwise Caesarean section is the safest procedure. *Destructive operations* (e.g. amputation of arm or head and arm) are very rarely practised nowadays. The situation with the second twin is a special one and is considered in Chapter 53.

PROGNOSIS

In the series of 343 cases of transverse, oblique and unstable lie shown in table 16.3, the Caesarean section rate was 62% and the perinatal mortality rate 7.8%.

Maternal

It is now very rare for a mother to die from this complication — the main dangers are from associated conditions, especially placenta praevia, and the problems associated with Caesarean section (especially thromboembolism) and anaesthesia. Neglected labours may still occasionally cause uterine rupture in multiparas.

Fetal

The perinatal mortality ranges from 5-15%, largely due to associated conditions causing *premature labour; cord prolapse* and obstructed labour will claim further lives. In recent years, the rate has fallen considerably with more consistent antenatal care, hospital admission, timely Caesarean section, and fewer internal versions.

chapter fifty-one

Deflexion Attitudes of the Fetus

OVERVIEW

When the fetus presents cephalically there are *2 main factors that maintain the flexed attitude* of the head. The first, which acts throughout pregnancy and labour, is the normal *predominance of flexor tone* in the baby, which is seen not only in the relation of head to chest, but in relation to the limbs and trunk (colour plate 4). Occasionally, either in vertex or breech presentations, this is reversed and a predominant extensor tone exists ('flying fetus', colour plate 51). The second factor usually comes into operation in late pregnancy and more especially in labour; it depends on the fact that the atlantooccipital joint, on which the head flexes and extends on the trunk, is not centrally placed at the base of the skull — it is more towards the back. If a simple principle learnt in geometry is recalled — *the law of the lever* — it will be appreciated that when the head meets with resistance, flexion is automatic and progressive, according to the strength of that resistance; the reverse is seen when the resistance is in the opposite direction as in breech delivery.

Minor deflexion attitudes are not uncommon and occur characteristically where the fetal occiput is posterior (the head extends as it drops back to fill the hollow of the sacrum). With further deflexion, the bregma, brow, and finally the face will present.

Brow presentation is uncommon (about 1 in 700 deliveries), but should be recognized because *obstructed labour is usual* and Caesarean section is necessary in the majority of patients (table 51.1). *Diagnosis* before or early in labour requires a *high index of suspicion*, because of its rarity and absence of remarkable features on routine examination. There is often unsatisfactory progress in labour and careful vaginal examination will reveal the larger anterior fontanelle, root of the nose and orbital ridges in place of the occiput and posterior fontanelle. On abdominal examination, the rounded C-shaped contour is replaced by one which is more cylindrical and S-shaped.

If labour is progressing, a conservative approach is adopted, since spontaneous conversion to an occiput or face presentation may occur, or allow this to be effected by vaginal manipulation.

Face presentation occurs in approximately 1 in 750 deliveries, and again is usually caused by an increase in fetal extensor tone. *Diagnosis* is more easily made on vaginal examination because of the softness of the facial tissues; the abdominal findings are similar to those where the brow is presenting.

Because the presenting diameter (submentobregmatic) is similar to that in the fully flexed fetus (suboccipitobregmatic) there is a much *greater likelihood of vaginal delivery* than in brow presentation (table 51.1). The *denominator is the chin* rather than the occiput; the mechanism of labour is similar except that the *head is born by a process of flexion rather than by extension*.

If either of the above conditions is diagnosed, it is advisable to obtain *consultant opinion* because of the probability (brow) or possibility (face) of operative delivery (table 51.1).

AETIOLOGY

In major extension attitudes (brow, face), it is now thought that *abnormal extensor tone* is usually present (colour plate 101 and figure 51.1). Other aetiological factors include *tumours of the anterior fetal neck* (thyroid, branchial), *malformations* (anencephaly and iniencephaly) (colour plate 52 and table 51.1). In *cephalopelvic disproportion* the head is held up by the biparietal eminences and deflexion may occur, thus allowing the smaller bitemporal diameter (8 cm compared with 9.5 cm) to descend to a lower station in the birth canal. This, of course is ineffective, and does not resolve the mechanical problem. The mechanism is different with *posterior positions* and depends on the fact that the birth canal is not a simple vertical tube — rather it is curved and the entrance is inclined about 45° to the horizontal. The baby's head in

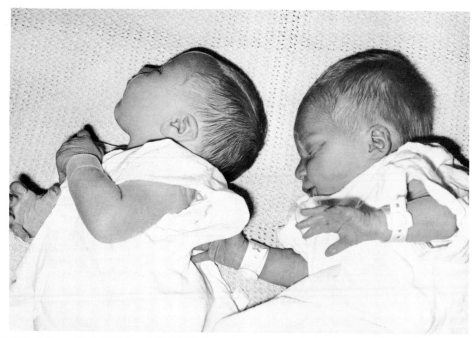

Figure 51.1 The baby on the left (birth-weight 3,370 g) was born as a brow by low forceps delivery after a 3-hour labour, when the head was 'on perineum'. This photograph taken 2 days later shows the prominent brow and persistence of extensor tone. The infant shown on the right (birth-weight 3,000 g) was born from the occipitoanterior position by mid-forceps delivery, and has a normally-shaped head. The moral is that forceps delivery of a brow is possible, without correction by flexion or extension, if the head is deep in the pelvis.

a posterior position naturally extends somewhat as it enters the pelvic cavity.

High parity (> 4) and *prematurity* are more common and sometimes the extended attitude is *accidental or incidental* — the fetus may have been stretching or 'looking about' when the membranes ruptured! Alternatively, if poly-hydramnios is present, a slight degree of exten-sor tone is allowed freer play.

TABLE 51.1   OVERVIEW OF FACE AND BROW PRESENTATIONS OCCURRING IN 40,982* CONSECUTIVE PREGNANCIES (TABLE 16.3)

	Face presentation	Brow presentation
Incidence	55 or 1 in 745**	60 or 1 in 683
Primipara	34%	45%
Multipara	65%	55%
Perinatal deaths	14 (25.4%)	—
Fetal malformations		
Anencephaly	9 (16.3%)	—
Hydrocephaly	—	2 (3.3%)
Delivery		
Spontaneous	49%	5%
Forceps	34%	30%
Caesarean section	16%	65%

* In this series 40% of patients were primiparas and 60% were multiparas

** Incidence of face presentation 1 in 890 pregnancies if cases of anencephaly are excluded

POSTERIOR POSITION OF THE OCCIPUT

Posterior position is mentioned in this chapter because of the *almost inevitability of some deflexion*; this will persist unless anterior rotation of the occiput occurs. A posterior pos-ition is observed in labour in some 15–20% of patients. Early in labour, this will be associated with some deflexion in attitude as the occiput moves downward and backward into the hollow of the sacrum. Successively larger diameters present as the head extends, culminating in the occipitofrontal (11–12 cm); because of this, the head tends to remain higher in the pelvis and less well applied to the cervix (so providing less stimulus to it). With coordinated contractions of good strength, the favourable influence of the lever principle will come into operation as the head descends; flexion will increase and forward rotation will occur, usually with normal delivery the outcome.

If additional unfavourable factors are present, such as poor or disordered uterine action, or dis-proportion unrelated to the deflexed attitude, arrest of the labour or at least very slow progress is probable.

A further factor affecting the outcome is the basic morphology or shape of the pelvis — if gynaecoid, normal anterior rotation is usual; if

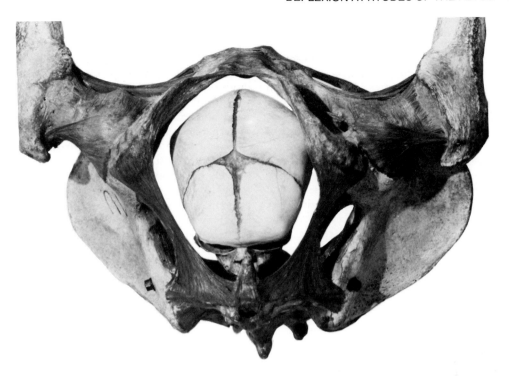

Figure 51.2 Anterior fontanelle (bregma) presentation may represent a stage in extension to a face, but when the head is deep in the pelvic cavity as shown here, complete extension is unlikely to occur, and brow presentation with obstructed labour usually results.

anthropoid or android, rotation may be slow or absent; in platypelloid pelves, posterior positions are not found.

This condition is discussed further in Chapter 52.

BREGMA (ANTERIOR FONTANELLE) PRESENTATION

A posterior position or any of the other factors favouring extension may be present.

Diagnosis

On abdominal examination, there is some *loss of the normal C-shape of the fetal contour*, making the uterus less rounded. On Pawlik's or deep pelvic grip, the head will be higher than normal and the occiput and sinciput will be felt with equal ease. On vaginal examination the larger anterior fontanelle (bregma) will be felt first, whilst the smaller posterior fontanelle will be difficult to reach or out of touch, depending on the dilatation of the cervix (figure 51.2).

Clinical Course

This usually follows that described for posterior positions. In some patients, the deflexion attitude represents a transient finding in the conversion of a vertex to brow or vice versa. The prognosis for vaginal delivery in the former case is poor, since the fetal head is usually deflexing in an attempt to present the more favourable bitemporal diameter to the pelvis.

Manual flexion is worth attempting if obvious disproportion is not present on vaginal examination. The thumb is placed on the sinciput and the fingers seek the ridge at the base of the occiput. If flexion occurs, an attempt is also made to help anterior rotation (if the occiput is not already anterior) with the fingers on the occiput or the edge of the lambdoid suture. This manoeuvre requires analgesia and a cervical dilatation of at least 5–6 cm.

BROW PRESENTATION

In this complication, the brow (area between the anterior fontanelle and root of the nose) forms the presenting part. It is *the most unfavourable of all of the deflexion attitudes* since the *large mentovertical diameter* (14 cm, figure 2.15) is presenting: in the mature fetus this is usually an insuperable bar to delivery.

Incidence

Excluding transient situations, this presentation occurs about once in 700 pregnancies (table 51.1).

Aetiology

A general discussion of factors affecting flexion and extension of the fetal head has been given. The importance of *primary extensor tone* in the fetus was emphasized (figures 49.7 and 51.1). In the series quoted, brow presentation was slightly more common in primiparas (table 51.1).

It is often overlooked that *shape as well as size of the fetal head* is as relevant to the mechanism of birth as is shape and size of the maternal pelvis. Brow presentation can be due to primary shape of the fetal head and in such a case normal delivery may occur; the mentovertical diameter is 10 cm rather than 14 cm because of the flattened occiput (scaphocephaly) (colour plate 104 and figure 51.1).

Diagnosis

The condition is diagnosed during pregnancy only in a small minority of patients, since some astuteness on the part of the attendant is required in view of the rarity of the condition. *Suspicion is often first aroused, especially* in the multipara, when the first stage of labour is prolonged and the baby does not seem overlarge. *On abdominal examination,* the rounded uterine contour becomes more cylindrical, and the paradoxical finding is recorded on Pawlik grip of the higher pole of the head on the side opposite to the limbs; the head itself often appears to be large because of the deflexion. Palpation of the fetal trunk is confusing: the chest is pushed forward and may be on the opposite side of the maternal abdomen to the breech (figure 51.3A). The fetal heart is often heard easily over the prominent chest. On *vaginal examination* (usually in labour, when the condition becomes recognized) the diagnosis may be difficult if the cervix is not well dilated. Only the central forehead may be felt, with the frontal suture running across it. However, on further palpation, this suture will run into the larger anterior fontanelle at one end, and will finish at the root of the nose at the other. If the fingers proceed laterally from the nose, the orbital ridges will be felt (figure 51.3B).

Clinical Course and Management

During pregnancy. Brow presentation usually indicates the need for radiographic pelvimetry, unless a large baby has been delivered previously. A diagnostic review of other detectable

A

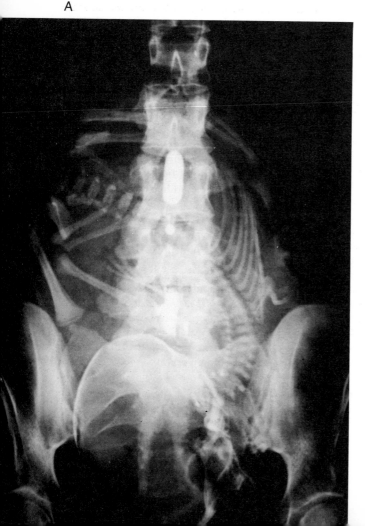

B

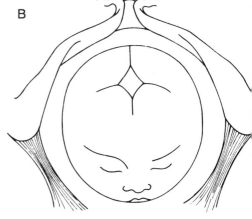

Figure 51.3 Brow presentation. **A.** X-ray at 41 weeks in a primigravida with disseminated sclerosis; a previous myelogram accounted for the contrast media in the spinal canal. The fetus was growth retarded (2,850 g) and died early in labour. The cord was tightly looped 4 times around the neck and probably was responsible for extension of the head. **B.** Bony features — bregma, root of nose, and orbital ridges — palpable on vaginal examination in labour.

aetiological factors is made. Since correction may occur, a trial of labour is allowed provided the pelvis is no more than mildly contracted. Otherwise, elective Caesarean section is performed at about 38 weeks.

During labour. A successful outcome may occur in the presence of favourable factors (good contractions, preservation of membranes, satisfactory descent of the head, and dilatation of the cervix). Often the brow may correct or be corrected to a vertex or face during the course of labour. If reasonable progress can be made with such a large diameter presenting (mentovertical, normally 13–14 cm) anything less should be much simpler. If the above favourable factors are not realized, *Caesarean section* is performed.

As mentioned earlier, the diagnosis is often made because of *delay in the first or second stages of labour*, perhaps when secondary arrest has occurred or failure of descent of the head is observed on abdominal examination. In such patients, a careful vaginal examination is carried out and a note is made of the state of the membranes and liquor, dilatation of the cervix and its application to the presenting part, the station of the head, the position of the anterior fontanelle and root of the nose, degree of caput and moulding, pelvic capacity, and finally the degree to which the head seems free or jammed in the pelvis. Resort is usually also made to X-ray pelvimetry if there appears some prospects of vaginal delivery (colour plate 102). If the latter course is elected, careful assessment of progress by abdominal and vaginal examination is made.

Correction may be attempted later in the first stage or in the second stage either manually or occasionally with Kielland forceps. Whether to convert to a face or vertex is determined by which manoeuvre will result in the denominator becoming anterior — the occiput or chin. For example, it is preferable to extend the head further to produce a mentoanterior position than to flex it and produce an occipitoposterior position. Vaginal delivery after *conversion of a brow to a face or vertex presentation* is a difficult and hazardous intrauterine manipulation — 2 of the 7 cases attempted in the series shown in table 51.1 resulted in 'failed forceps' with delivery ultimately being effected by Caesarean section. *Forceps delivery* may be performed when the brow is deep in the pelvis (below the level of the ischial spines), all other necessary conditions being fulfilled; this applies in about 30% of cases (figure 51.1 and table 51.1).

The procedure of *internal version is seldom if ever performed*, because of the risks to the mother and baby.

Prognosis

The overall *perinatal mortality* for this condition is about 5% (2–3 times normal); with early diagnosis and appropriate treatment, it should be little greater than normal, although the possibility of hydrocephaly exists (table 51.1). The labour is usually longer, and because of this and the increased head compression there is a greater risk of cerebral anoxia and attendant complications. Prolapse of the cord, obstetric manipulations, and intrauterine infection are also more common.

The mother is at risk from operative interference (vaginal manipulation or Caesarean section), attendant anaesthesia, and the risk of uterine rupture if the condition is neglected. The *Caesarean section rate* is 50–70% (table 51.1).

FACE PRESENTATION

This is the most extreme form of deflexion, and, because of this, a favourable diameter again presents to the pelvis — the submentobregmatic (9.5 cm), which is the same as the most favourable diameter when the head is fully flexed — the suboccipitobregmatic.

Incidence

Even when cases of *anencephaly* are included the condition is slightly less common than brow presentation, occurring about once in 750 deliveries (table 51.1).

Aetiology

The main factors have already been discussed. Unless a distinctive cause such as anencephaly or tumour of the fetal neck is present, the usual cause will again be heightened extensor tone (colour plates 51 and 52, figures 51.1 and 51.4). In a minority of patients, an underlying cephalopelvic disproportion will be present. Three or more loops of cord around the neck can also cause extension of the head (figures 51.3 and 51.8D).

Diagnosis

As with brow presentation, the diagnosis will be made only in a minority of patients before the onset of labour. The *abdominal findings* described under brow presentation are present in an exaggerated fashion. The fetal outline can now best be described by an S rather than a C. It is easy to mistake the prominent fetal chest for the back and the occiput for the sinciput. The deep groove between fetal back and occiput is, however, characteristic. Before labour is well established and the head is fully extended, it tends to be high in the pelvis and prominent on

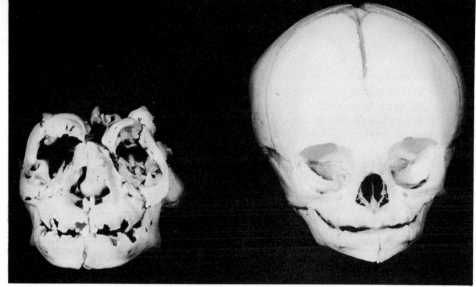

Figure 51.4 Frontal view of the skulls of an anencephalic and normal full term infant. Because the anencephalic has no cranium, cephalic presentation must always be as a face.

Figure 51.5 Face presentation. **A.** Abdominal examination reveals a high head; the diagnosis is confirmed when X-ray pelvimetry is performed because of this. **B.** X-ray showing an S-shaped fetal spine (and incidentally a well-marked lower femoral epiphysis). **C.** Nose, mouth and orbital ridges are the features on vaginal examination. These may be mistaken for anus and sacrum of a breech, or for the open cranium of an anencephalic fetus, especially when there is caput formation. It should be noted that in each of the 3 figures the position is different.

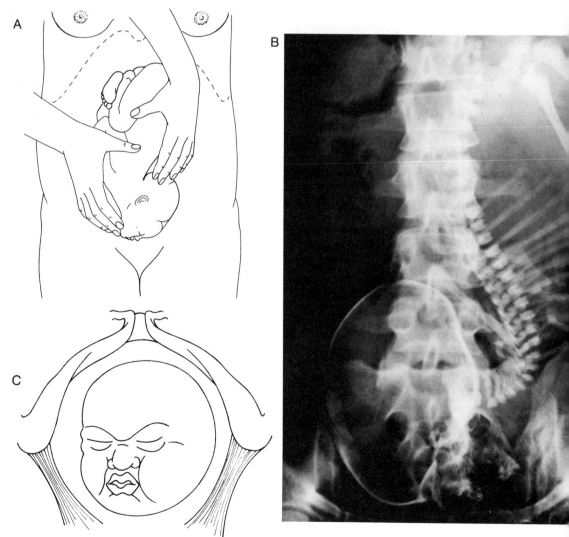

abdominal examination (figure 51.5). The fetal heart is again heard easily over the prominent chest, often near the midline. As with brow presentation, the finding of limbs on the side opposite to the supposed sinciput is a suspicious feature. *On vaginal examination*, the findings may again be quite confusing if the cervix is not well dilated. A partly soft, partly firm, irregular contour will be noted which is easy to confuse with breech presentation, anencephaly, and transverse lie. The most useful landmarks are the orbital ridges, the nose, and the mouth and alveolar ridges. Unless a caput has formed, the general consistency is much firmer than in breech presentation.

If in doubt, prodding should not be vigorous because of possible damage to the baby's eyes; radiographic or ultrasonographic examination will often be necessary (figure 51.5).

Clinical Course and Management

(a) *During pregnancy.* If a face presentation is suspected in pregnancy an ultrasound study is carried out, since in more than 10% of cases *anencephaly* will be present; other aetiological features such as a tumour of the neck may be seen. A reappraisal is made of the pelvis and a pelvimetry ordered if contraction is suspected.

As with brow presentation, a decision is made regarding the need or otherwise of Caesarean section, the usual indications being pelvic contraction and fetal distress in labour. Normal labour will be allowed in 90–95% of patients.

(b) *Labour.* The general *mechanism of labour* is similar to that in vertex presentations, except that the chin rather than the occiput is the denominator, progressive extension rather than flexion occurs, and at delivery there is again the opposite mechanism — *birth is by flexion of the head, not extension.*

In figure 51.5A a right mentotransverse position is revealed by abdominal palpation. The following is the mechanism of labour in this position.

(i) *Descent* of the head. (ii) *Extension* of the head as it meets progressively greater resistance in the birth canal. (iii) *Anterior rotation* of the chin. (iv) *Engagement* as the biparietal eminences pass through the pelvic brim; the chin is at the level of the coccyx and the head is much deeper in the pelvis than in vertex presentations at the time of engagement (two-thirds compared with one-third). (v) *Delivery.* With further descent the face distends the perineum and the head is born by flexion, the front of the neck rotating around the bottom of the symphysis pubis (figure 51.6). (vi) *Restitution* occurs as with vertex presentations; in this case the chin rotates back to the mother's right side to assume a normal relation with the shoulders and trunk. (vii) *External rotation.* The shoulders are already in the anteroposterior diameter and usually remain in this position — the anterior shoulder is delivered first, followed by the posterior; the remainder of the delivery is the same as that described in vertex presentation.

Figure 51.6 Face presentation: mechanism of delivery. **A.** The chin is anterior and has descended until the fetal hyoid bone is at the level of the symphysis pubis. **B.** The head pivots on the symphysis pubis and is born by flexion. The chin appears first, followed by the nose, brow, vertex, and occiput.

A

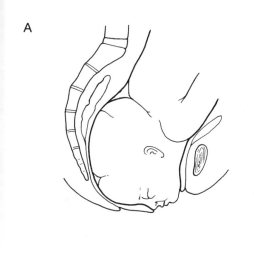

B

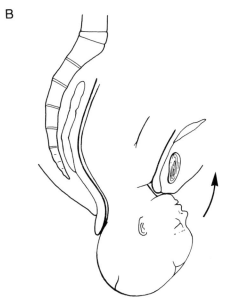

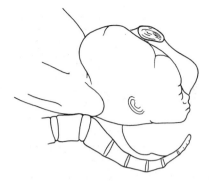

Figure 51.7 Persistent mentoposterior position: delivery can occur only if the chin rotates anteriorly.

(c) *General care of the patient.* The labour is usually longer than normal, probably as a result of the poorer fit of the face in the lower uterine segment, poorer moulding, and the fact that full extension is less easily achieved than full flexion. The progress of labour is followed by abdominal and if necessary, vaginal examination.

Care should be undertaken at the time of vaginal examination not to injure the baby's eyes with antiseptics or careless palpation. A pelvic examination is indicated when the membranes rupture. Otherwise the management and labour is similar to that described for the patient with a normal vertex presentation.

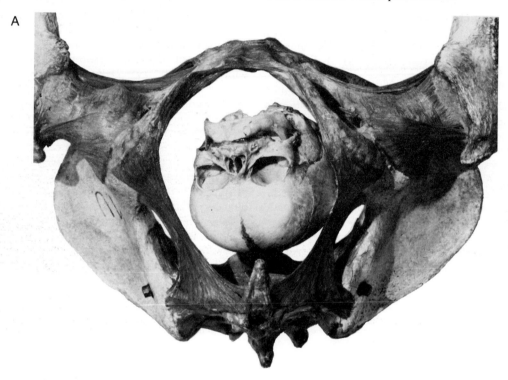

A

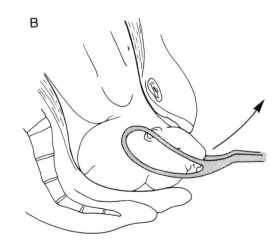

B

Figure 51.8 Face presentation and forceps delivery. **A.** Right mentoanterior position, head engaged, conditions suitable for forceps application and delivery. **B.** Forceps applied; the tips of the blades lie over the ears. The arrow indicates the direction of traction for delivery by flexion of the head.

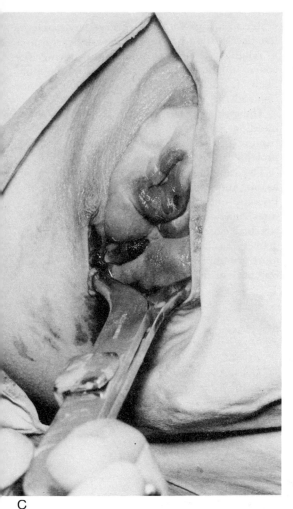

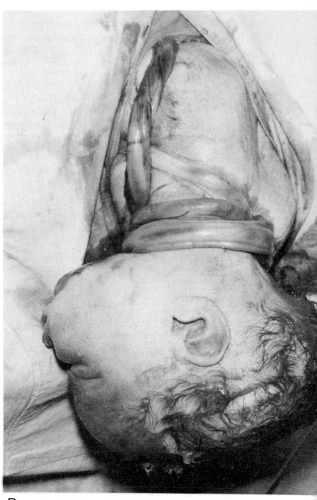

C

D

C. Delivery with Kielland forceps and large episiotomy after rotation from the mentoposterior to mentoanterior position shown here. The mother was aged 17 years and at 42 weeks' gestation; the fetus weighed 3,220 g and died 4 hours after the start of labour, which lasted 17 hours. **D.** The cause of the intrauterine death and the face presentation was 3 tight loops of cord around the neck. Anoxia occurred with descent of the head in labour and tightening of the umbilical noose. Note extreme caput and moulding.

(d) *Delivery*. The usual preparations are made and an episiotomy is performed under local analgesia if the perineum is tight. As the chin rotates around the symphysis pubis, the brow, vertex, and occiput will in turn sweep over the perineum. Unlike in the vertex presentation, there will be no chin to pick up below the coccyx, only the top of the baby's head. After delivery of the head, the rest of the baby is managed as in a normal birth. There is usually a caput of some size involving the soft facial tissues and this is very disfiguring if marked (as in long labours): the face is swollen and blue, and the eyes are closed; there are often subconjunctival haemorrhages. The mother should be informed that these changes will resolve quickly and completely.

Vaginal manipulative assistance (manual rotation and/or forceps assistance) will be required in many of those with mentotransverse and mentoposterior positions because of failed rotation. *Spontaneous delivery* occurs in about 50% of cases, forceps delivery is required in about 35% and Caesarean section in about 15% (table 51.1).

Complications and Prognosis

It has been mentioned that face presentation *may reflect an underlying disorder*. The most serious is *anencephaly*, and the couple should be told of this beforehand, to lessen the shock which would otherwise occur after delivery. *Tumours of the neck* are rare, and can be managed satisfactorily by medical or surgical means depending on their nature.

In some patients, the face presentation is the

end result of a deflexed attitude resulting from *cephalopelvic disproportion*. Pelvimetry or unsatisfactory progress in labour may indicate the need for Caesarean section.

If there is a *mentoposterior position*, mento-anterior rotation will occur only in a minority of patients. In the remainder, delivery is impossible, since the head cannot extend any further to traverse the curve of Carus (figure 51.7). Rarely, if the baby is small, it may be delivered in this position, but normally Caesarean section is necessary if manual or forceps rotation is not applicable or too difficult. Correction of a mentoposterior position by forceps or manual rotation, followed by forceps delivery, is always a dangerous intrauterine manoeuvre because the head cannot be engaged in this position (figure 6.8) — in most cases Caesarean section is pref-

erable to a high forceps delivery. A variable or late deceleration pattern of the fetal heart rate is a relatively frequent observation during the course of labour. The larger the baby, the more likely is the need for operative interference (figure 51.8).

The risk of *maternal injury* and postpartum bleeding is higher for the above reason. Early rupture of the membranes predisposes to cord prolapse and intraamniotic infection.

The caput over the face causes *the baby* no harm, and rapidly subsides within 48 hours. Pressure or damage to the anterior neck structures may occur, and the baby should be watched closely for any breathing problems if delivery has been difficult. Low Apgar scores are more common when a mentoposterior position was present during labour.

chapter fifty-two

Errors of Fetal Position

OVERVIEW

It is necessary, in the understanding of the progress of labour, to be able to describe the orientation and level of the presenting part in the pelvis. In the case of cephalic presentations in which there is a normal degree of flexion present, the occiput is used as the denominator to relate to the maternal pelvis. *The way in which the head enters the pelvis is determined largely by the shape of the brim.* The *shape of the head* is also relevant, although this factor is often ignored in descriptions of the different mechanisms of labour. In general, the transverse diameter of the brim exceeds the anteroposterior diameter by 2 cm or so, and this favours *lateral positions* of the occiput because the outline of the incompletely flexed head is oval rather than round. In 15–20%, *posterior positions* will be favoured. By contrast, the pelvic outlet is widest in its anteroposterior diameter, and thus *rotation of the occiput to the anterior* will occur, since the rounded contour of the maximally flexed head will again become oval as it deflexes in the process of birth.

The presence of an occipitoposterior or occipitolateral position early in labour is a fact for noting rather than for immediate concern. However, the *potential for difficulty* exists: the posterior position is usually associated with some *deflexion* as the occiput accommodates to the roomier posterior pelvis (hollow of the sacrum). This alone may be enough to hold up the head because of the greater diameter of engagement (suboccipitofrontal or occipitofrontal). The situation may be aggravated by *pelvic contraction* of some degree and/or *inefficient uterine activity*. Usually this nexus is broken by the normal augmentation of uterine activity as labour progresses: flexion increases, descent to the pelvic floor occurs, and internal rotation of the occiput follows. Unfortunately, the outcome may not be so favourable. The *occiput may stick where it is, rotate only to the lateral position,* or *rotate to the direct posterior position*; the 2 former situations always require rescue — either by vaginal manipulation (rotation and forceps delivery) or Caesarean section if conditions are unfavourable for vaginal delivery.

Methods now exist to calculate the work performed by the uterus in labour and studies uniformly demonstrate that *more work is required if the position is initially posterior.* Thus the patient needs greater *moral and physical support*, and particular attention to pain relief.

The *lateral (transverse) position* may exist de novo or represent a failed rotation of an initially posterior position. The presenting part is usually lower in the pelvis ('*deep transverse arrest*'), but similar manipulative assistance to that described above may be necessary.

Statistics show that *Caesarean section* is more often carried out in the patient with a malposition; often the latter is the final straw in a situation which may include lowered placental reserve, an obstetric complication such as preeclampsia, or a specific labour problem such as *pelvic contraction* or *incoordinate uterine action*.

OCCIPUT POSTERIOR

The occiput of the fetus lies posterior to the transverse diameter of the pelvic brim in about 15-20% of patients at the onset of labour. In about 60% of these the posterior position represents little more than a normal variation in the cephalic mechanism. In such cases, there is normal rotation of the occiput to the anterior position during the first stage of labour and an uncomplicated delivery. *In the remaining 40% (i.e. about 6–8% of all labours) the malposition has an importance out of proportion to its incidence, for it is associated with, if not the direct cause of, the majority of difficult and prolonged labours.* Because of the deflexion of the head which normally follows, the mechanical problem is intensified because of the larger diameter (occipitofrontal 11–12 cm) which presents. If an occipitoposterior position and contracted pelvis coexist, the following classical sequence of events often results: high head at term, poor fit in lower uterine segment, prolonged pregnancy (especially nulliparas), premature rupture of the membranes, less efficient uterine action, prolonged and perhaps obstructed labour, intrauterine infection, maternal and fetal distress, high incidence of forceps delivery and Caesarean section, and finally, increased fetal and maternal morbidity and mortality.

Another component of the occipitoposterior syndrome is the short-coupled individual ('dystocia dystrophia' syndrome), who has a contracted, abnormally-shaped pelvis (android, anthropoid).

Aetiology

The most likely and logical explanation for the posterior position is that of mutual configuration — that is, the larger posterior segment of the head fits better into the larger posterior segment of the maternal pelvis. This is particularly so where the heart shape of the pelvis is exaggerated (android type). In addition, the normal anterior rotation may be impeded if the transverse diameter of the pelvis is reduced (anthropoid type — figure 2.12). The occipital protuberance of the baby is often accentuated and this may determine the normal mechanism of flexion which usually precedes internal rotation.

If the placenta is situated anteriorly in the uterus, a posterior position of the baby is favoured, since the baby tends to face towards the placenta.

Diagnosis

Inspection. Often there is a hollowing of the lower abdomen and a protrusion of the upper abdomen (due to loss of fetal curvature). *Subumbilical flattening* is more noticeable in labour during contractions.

Palpation. Fetal limbs are palpable anteriorly, and the fetal back and shoulder are out toward the flank (figure 52.1). On suprapubic palpation, the occiput is felt to be deeper than the sinciput and often deflexed. When the occiput is directly posterior the smaller irregular sinciput is palpable and may be mistaken for the firm irregular outline of a breech with extended legs.

Auscultation. The fetal heart is often best heard in the flank (this is not a very reliable indicator, however).

Vaginal examination. The posterior fontanelle (and behind it the occiput) lies posteriorly. Because of *deflexion of the head*, the anterior

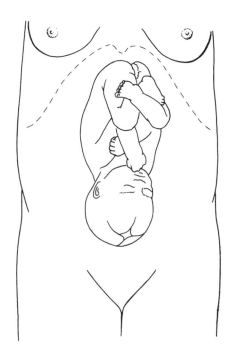

Figure 52.1 In occipitoposterior positions the anterior shoulder is well out from the midline and fetal limbs are readily palpable — this may cause a mistaken diagnosis of multiple pregnancy.

fontanelle may also be palpable and at the same level in the pelvis as the posterior fontanelle rather than higher up. The direction of the sagittal suture indicates whether it is an ROP or a LOP. If caput has obscured usual identifying landmarks (sutures/fontanelles), the ear or occipital ridge is sought.

Special investigation. Radiography or ultrasonography give an accurate picture of the position, but are rarely used for this purpose alone.

Mechanism of Labour

There are several possible outcomes, depending on such factors as the size and shape of the pelvis and fetal head, and the strength and coordination of uterine contractions.

(i) *Spontaneous anterior rotation* occurs in the late first stage of labour in 60–65% of patients, particularly where there are no unfavourable factors present (figure 52.2). In these patients delivery will usually be spontaneous or assisted by forceps (plus episiotomy) if delay occurs in the second stage or there is fetal or maternal distress. The mechanism is similar to that outlined in the mechanism of normal labour (Chapter 42). It should be noted that *restitution of the head after delivery may occupy 3/8ths of a circle if the*

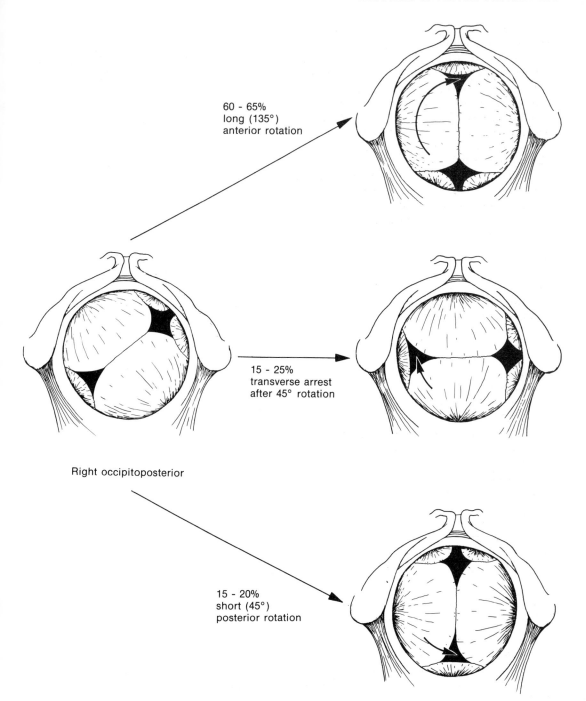

60 - 65%
long (135°)
anterior rotation

15 - 25%
transverse arrest
after 45° rotation

Right occipitoposterior

15 - 20%
short (45°)
posterior rotation

Figure 52.2 The results of complete and incomplete rotation of the occiput from the ROP position are shown. Transverse arrest may be due to incomplete anterior rotation from a posterior position, or the occiput may have been in the transverse position from the outset of labour.

trunk is still in the posterior position. Often, however, the shoulders rotate 45° (into the AP diameter) or 90° (into the opposite oblique diameter) and restitution then occurs through 90° or 45°, respectively (table 52.1).

(ii) *Posterior rotation* results in delivery face to-pubes (*persistent occipitoposterior*) and occurs in 15–20% of posterior positions, ie. 1.5-2% of all births, this figure including both spontaneous deliveries and those effected with forceps (table 16.3). Here the mechanism is different in a number of respects. In early labour, descent, flexion, and engagement occur as for the occipitolateral

or anterior positions. When the head reaches the pelvic floor, however, the internal rotation of the occiput is posterior rather than anterior (1/8th of a circle), so that it comes to lie in the hollow of the sacrum (direct occipitoposterior; occipitosacral). As the head reaches the perineum, maximum flexion is obtained and the brow and then the face is applied to the symphysis pubis in front (figure 52.3); this is in contrast to the back of the neck in occipitoanterior deliveries. The perineum is distended by the occiput which is directed forward by the lower curve of the birth canal. *Birth is by extension* as in anterior pos-

TABLE 52.1   CHECK CHART SHOWING THE DIRECTION AND DEGREE OF INTERNAL ROTATION, RESTITUTION AND EXTERNAL ROTATION OF THE OCCIPUT, IN RELATION TO ITS INITIAL POSITION

Position of occiput	Internal rotation (before delivery)		Restitution (after delivery)		External rotation
Left occipitolateral (transverse)	→	90°	←	90°	NIL
Left occipitoanterior	→	45°	←	45° ←	45°
Left occipitoposterior*					
— long anterior rotation, shoulders stationary	→	135°	←	135°	→ 45°
— long anterior rotation, shoulders rotation 90°	→	135°	←	45° ←	45°
— short posterior rotation (delivery as POP)	→	45°	←	45° ←	45°

* The 3 possible mechanisms of delivery from the LOP position are shown

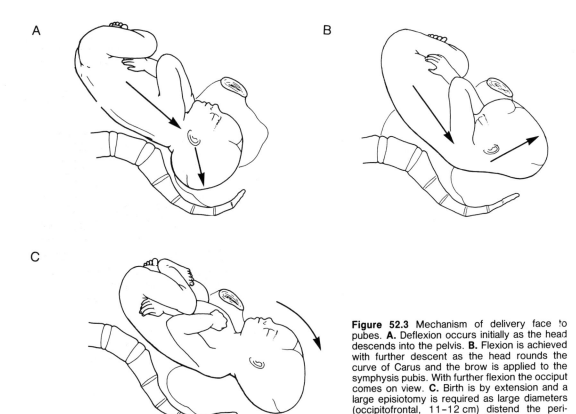

Figure 52.3 Mechanism of delivery face to pubes. **A.** Deflexion occurs initially as the head descends into the pelvis. **B.** Flexion is achieved with further descent as the head rounds the curve of Carus and the brow is applied to the symphysis pubis. With further flexion the occiput comes on view. **C.** Birth is by extension and a large episiotomy is required as large diameters (occipitofrontal, 11–12 cm) distend the perineum.

ition of the occiput, except that larger diameters extend the perineum, and so a large episiotomy is required to avoid perineal tears. Restitution usually occurs through 1/8th of a circle as the occiput turns to its former posterior position. External rotation of the head (a further 1/8th of a circle forward) is caused by the shoulders moving from the oblique to the AP diameter of the pelvis (table 52.1).

(iii) *Transverse (lateral) arrest* occurs in 15–25% of posterior positions. Here the long anterior rotation is held up, often because of an unfavourable pelvic shape (android pelvis, flat sacrum, prominent ischial spines), and other unfavourable factors such as a deflexed head of above average dimensions and/or hardness (prolonged pregnancy).

(iv) *Failure of rotation.* The head remains in the oblique posterior position, rotating neither to the front nor back. As with transverse arrest, there is often a combination of unfavourable factors present.

(v) *Extension.* Some degree of extension accompanies most posterior positions, partly because the convex maternal spine breaks up the normally flexed fetus, and partly because the *occiput extends backwards over the sacral promontory as it enters the pelvis.* If there is a greater than normal extensor tone in the baby or some

disproportion is present, further deflexion may occur to produce a brow or even a face presentation.

Management

In most patients no special measures are required, since a favourable outcome can be anticipated. Recent work suggests that, in the nullipara, oxytoxin may be helpful during labour if uterine activity is subnormal. Prolonged and difficult labour may occur however, and special attention should be given to provision of adequate *sedation and hydration; intravenous fluids* prevent dehydration of the mother and reduce the risk of fetal acidosis and distress. Obviously, care must be taken that cephalopelvic relationships are properly assessed, and the progress of the mother and baby are carefully monitored. A pelvimetry may have been ordered if there has been failure of the head to enter the pelvis late in pregnancy.

If the head is not fitting well, a *pelvic examination* is indicated when the membranes rupture.

First stage delay. This is managed as outlined in Chapter 49. *Caesarean section* may be necessary if there is significant fetal distress and/or lack of progress (figure 53.4).

Figure 52.4 A 25-year-old primigravida seen before Caesarean section which was indicated by fetal distress (meconium in liquor, type 1 dips, tachycardia), incoordinate uterine action and obstructed labour due to an occipitoposterior position. Labour began spontaneously at 42.2 weeks' gestation. The patient required epidural analgesia for pain relief — 2 'top-ups' were given during the 18 hours of labour. Note the subumbilical flattening below the retraction ring. The catheter was required because the patient had been unable to void. Note also the wedge under the mattress to tilt the patient, thus minimizing the risk of vena caval occlusion. The infant was born in good condition, birth-weight 3,510 g. This is the most common clinical situation seen in patients having primary (first) Caesarean sections — the combination of posterior position, incoordinate and obstructed labour ± fetal and maternal distress.

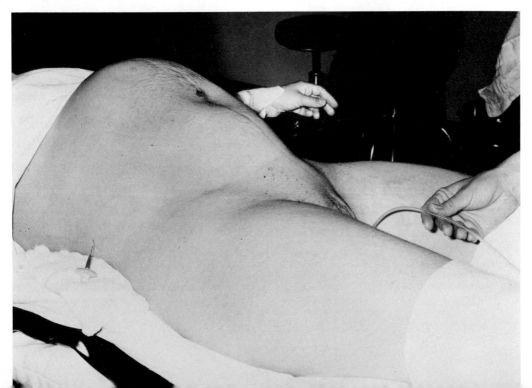

Second stage delay. This is likely if full anterior rotation has not occurred. There are a number of options available, depending on the abnormality present. (i) *Posterior rotation* (occipitosacral, face to pubes). This is best managed by a wide episiotomy, perhaps aided by forceps or vacuum extraction. (ii) *Transverse arrest.* Usually operative interference is necessary. The head is flexed manually and then rotated anteriorly (rarely posteriorly) either manually or with Kielland or similar forceps. (iii) *Failure of rotation.* This is managed as for deep transverse arrest. If the pelvis is adequate, the vacuum extractor may be used; if the cup is applied to the occiput, the instrument may be used for both rotation and extraction. (iv) *Extension.* The management of the extended head (bregma, brow, face) is discussed in Chapter 51.

Results

Table 16.3 shows the outcome in a series of 4,363 cases of occipitoposterior position diagnosed by vaginal examination in labour. *The incidence of posterior position in this series was 10.6%*; since anterior rotation often occurs uneventfully without need to assess the progress in labour by vaginal examination, the incidence of posterior position of the occiput at the onset of labour is likely to be 15–20%, as quoted earlier in the chapter.

In this series the methods of delivery were: spontaneous delivery *occiput anterior* (25%), spontaneous delivery *occiput posterior* (6%), *forceps delivery* (52%), *Caesarean section* (16%). The 705 Caesarean sections in this group of patients accounted for *25% of all primary (first) Caesarean sections performed in the hospital during the period concerned.*

In this series the *perinatal mortality* rate was 24 per 1,000 births.

OCCIPUT LATERAL (TRANSVERSE)

The occiput may be directed either to the left (LOL) or right (ROL) side of the mother's pelvis.

Aetiology

Transitory. In many cases, the occipitolateral position which is diagnosed on pelvic or other examination represents a phase in rotation from the posterior position; a further examination in 1-2 hours or less will confirm further rotation to the anterior position.

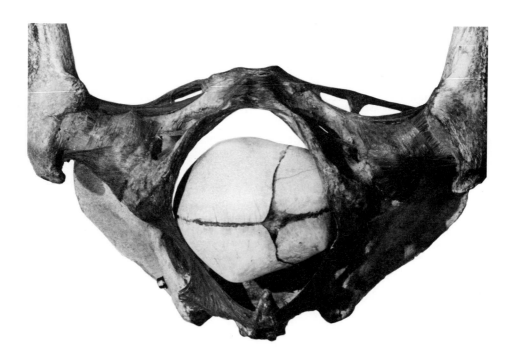

Figure 52.5 Deep transverse arrest: the head is below the level of the ischial spines, at which anterior rotation normally occurs. Failure of rotation may be due to deflexion rather than pelvic contraction. Occasionally the head rotates anteriorly during a contraction when on view, but usually, especially in nulliparas, forceps rotation and delivery are required.

Fixed. (i) *Arrest of anterior rotation of an originally occipitoposterior position.* The most likely cause is a combination of partial deflexion of the head and unfavourable size and/or shape of the pelvis. An android pelvis, narrowed anteriorly and with flattened sacrum, is often the cause. (ii) *Failure of anterior rotation of an originally occipitolateral position.* Usually in such cases there is some flattening of the pelvis, again with some deflexion of the head and/or unfavourable cephalopelvic relationships in the mid or lower pelvis.

Diagnosis
The features and diagnostic points are similar to those outlined under 'posterior position'. Of particular importance are the findings on *pelvic examination*, since it is mainly in late labour that difficulties arise. Examination on 2 occasions, 1–2 hours apart, is required to differentiate whether the occipitolateral position is transitory or fixed. Signs of *deflexion of the head* and *cephalopelvic disproportion* should be sought.

Mechanism
Spontaneous anterior rotation is the usual outcome. The occiput rotates to the OA position and is born normally by extension; restitution occupies one-quarter of a circle as the head reestablishes its normal relation with the trunk. The shoulders usually remain in the AP diameter, so there is no external rotation imparted to the head (table 52.1).

Arrest. The situation is similar, regardless of whether the occiput began in the posterior or lateral position (figure 52.5). Without assistance, obstruction to labour will occur, with probable serious sequelae to mother and fetus.

Management
Diagnosis of a transverse position before or early in labour requires no special treatment. If arrest is diagnosed, a decision must be made as to the best means of delivery. Usually, the os is fully dilated and the procedures described under 'posterior position' are carried out (i.e. manual or forceps rotation and assisted delivery, or vacuum extraction if the head is lower in the pelvis). In the later first stage, vacuum extraction may be attempted if delivery is urgent, and there is no disproportion; alternatively, *Caesarean section* is undertaken.

chapter fifty-three

Multiple Pregnancy

OVERVIEW

Although labour and delivery in multiple pregnancy is often no more taxing than that of the singleton pregnancy, the potential for unexpected problems is sufficiently great to require specialist attendance. With each increase in fetal number, the difficulties compound and the likelihood of operative delivery increases.

Labour is often premature (table 53.1), and although the active phase and second stage are longer than normal, this is more than compensated by a shortened latent phase.

Monitoring of each fetus in late pregnancy by cardiotocography ± ultrasonography is desirable. Anticipation of possible difficulties is the keynote in management: availability of an *anaesthetist* and operating theatre should the need for Caesarean section suddenly occur; an *intravenous line* is inserted once labour begins and *blood should be cross-matched* in case of postpartum haemorrhage; and 2 or more neonatologists should be available (according to the number of fetuses) because of the likelihood of *neonatal difficulties.*

In 75–85% of patients, twin 1 will be cephalic and spontaneous vaginal delivery can be anticipated (table 53.2); if epidural analgesia is used the need for instrumental assistance is increased.

The second twin should normally be delivered within 20 minutes and interference will be required if there is fetal distress or failure to progress — management options then include *internal version and breech extraction* or *vacuum extraction* if the head is presenting but high, *forceps* delivery if the head is engaged, *breech extraction,* or Caesarean section (rarely — table 53.2).

After delivery, the placentas and membranes should be examined carefully and documented to establish zygosity.

Internal podalic version is considered at the end of the chapter since in modern obstetrics this procedure is virtually restricted to the management of multiple pregnancy after the first child is born, with the exception of extraction of the baby at *Caesarean section* when the lie is transverse or the head high and mobile.

The general characteristics of multiple pregnancy, together with associated antenatal problems and their management have been discussed in Chapter 25.

As a general rule, patients with a twin pregnancy should be managed by an experienced obstetrician because of the potential problems involved. With triplets and higher orders, special unit care is mandatory.

Because almost 50% of stillbirths in twins occur after 34 weeks' gestation (table 53.1), fetal well-being should be monitored in late pregnancy to select patients requiring induction of labour or Caesarean section (see Chapter 25).

Labour

In many patients, labour progresses normally, the main differences being a shortened latent phase and a lengthened active phase and second stage: the overall length of labour is usually a little shorter than that in the mother with a singleton pregnancy. In the remainder a number of problems may arise. (i) *Prematurity* is the greatest worry, and care must be exercised in the administration of analgesic drugs that might depress fetal respiration. Epidural analgesia is thus often preferable, especially in the nullipara: this has the added advantage of facilitating manipulative procedures. Although the second stage of labour is longer and Apgar scores somewhat lower, the delivery is easier and there is less trauma to the babies. Caesarean section is more likely because of the increase in premature labour and for the other complications mentioned below. (ii) *Premature rupture of the membranes,* apart from precipitating labour, predisposes to the further complication of (iii) *prolapse of the umbilical cord* and (iv) *intrauter-*

TABLE 53.1 GESTATION AT DELIVERY IN TWINS COMPARED WITH LIVEBORN SINGLETONS, AND COMPARISON OF STILLBIRTH AND NEONATAL DEATH RATES IN TWINS 1 AND 2

Gestation at delivery	Twins (%)	Singletons (%)	Twin 1		Twin 2	
			Stillbirth (number)	Neonatal death (number)	Stillbirth (number)	Neonatal death (number)
Less than 28 weeks	7.1 (55.0)	0.5 (68.7)	8	23	8	21
28–32 weeks	11.2 (23.8)	1.4 (15.2)	5	16	4	14
33–36 weeks	26.4 (2.3)	4.6 (2.2)	6	3	3	4
37 weeks and more	55.1 (0.0)	93.3 (0.2)	2	—	8	—
Total	560	14,413	21	42	23	39

Figures in parentheses denote neonatal death rates (%)

TABLE 53.2 METHOD OF DELIVERY IN A SERIES OF 560 TWIN PREGNANCIES

Method of delivery	Twin 1		Twin 2	
	Number	%	Number	%
Spontaneous vertex	236	42.1	156	27.8
Forceps *	160	28.5	102	18.2
Breech **	85	15.1	221	39.6
Caesarean section ***	79	14.1	81	14.4

* 25% of forceps deliveries for twin 1, and 50% for twin 2 were mid-forceps
** Internal version and breech extraction was the method of delivery for 0.0% of first twins and 6.4% of second twins
*** There were 2 cases where Caesarean section was performed after vaginal delivery of the first twin (obstructed labour (1), failed breech extraction (1))

ine infection. (v) *Malpresentation* is more common with the second twin (table 53.2), and thus is more a problem with delivery than during labour. (vi) *Obstructed labour* may result from malpresentation or the very rare complication of conjoined twins (colour plates 45 and 50, figure 25.7). (vii) The *postpartum haemorrhage* rate is increased.

The weight of the uterus and its contents can be very considerable, and the patient should be nursed on her side, not only for comfort, but also to prevent pressure on the major blood vessels which lie behind the uterus (colour plates 70 and 75).

Other complications which typically arise during the antenatal course, such as preeclampsia, antepartum haemorrhage or anaemia, may also need appropriate management. *Induction of labour* may be necessary as with singleton pregnancies. If conditions are unfavourable, Caesarean section should be considered. Use of an oxytocic infusion to settle the head into the pelvis before rupturing the membranes is not recommended because of the risk of cord prolapse if the membranes rupture with the presenting part still above the pelvic brim. *Paediatric personnel* and *facilities* should be ready in advance and an *anaesthetist* warned that his services may be required at delivery. The usual course, if there are any problems anticipated with the babies, is for there to be a paediatrician for each baby delivered. An *intravenous infusion* should be set up and *blood should be crossmatched* (2 units). It is important that the presentation of the fetuses be determined early in labour, if necessary by ultrasonography or radiography if the latter is unavailable.

Heart rate monitors with dual channels for both fetuses are now available and this adds a desirable safeguard to care in labour. Usually the scalp electrode is used for twin 1 and the ultrasound transducer for twin 2.

Management of Delivery

If the first baby is presenting as a vertex, which is usual, no special precaution or interference is warranted. The delivery is allowed to proceed as for a singleton, unless there are indications for interference (delay; maternal or fetal distress). If the first twin is presenting by the breech again the delivery proceeds as for a singleton, unless unusual features are present.

After delivery of the first baby, the routine *oxytocic is withheld*, and the cord is clamped to prevent the twin transfusion syndrome wherein one twin becomes exsanguinated by bleeding into the circulation of the other (colour plate 46). Identifying tags should be placed on both ends of the divided umbilical cord.

Abdominal examination is now carried out to ascertain the lie, presentation, station, and position of the next baby. If not longitudinal, the lie is converted by external version. Provided the presenting part, vertex or breech, is in the brim of the pelvis, a vaginal examination is carried out and the *membranes of the second twin are ruptured*, first ensuring that there is no cord presenting. The liquor should be allowed to drain slowly, the hand remaining in the vagina. The presenting part is steadied over the brim while this is being done. *Normal contractions of the uterus will now expel the second twin*. It can be helpful for fetal cardiac monitoring to be continued until delivery is effected. If uterine action is unsatisfactory or there is delay (more than 10–15 minutes) either *oxytocin is given* (by intravenous infusion (10 u/l at 20 drops/minute) or intramuscular injection (4u)), or a breech extraction, forceps or vacuum extraction is carried out. There is no advantage in waiting, since perinatal mortality increases as a result of asphyxia (contraction of the placental site, possibly cord prolapse, and rarely placental separation). The necessity for gentleness must be borne in mind if the baby is premature, and adequate relaxation of the uterus is necessary if intrauterine manipulations are carried out.

Note that *the membranes should not be ruptured if the head presents and is above the pelvic brim*, because if cord prolapse occurs conditions are not favourable for either forceps delivery or internal version and breech extraction — it is preferable under this circumstance if there is an indication for delivery (delay or distress) to administer a *general anaesthetic* and perform *internal version and breech extraction*. This manoeuvre is required in about 6% of second twin deliveries (table 53.2).

After delivery of the last baby, ergometrine or Syntometrine is given, and the normal procedure for conduct of the third stage adopted. Although the combined placentas are larger than in a singleton pregnancy, separation is usually completed early. The usual problem is retention of the separated placenta. Brandt-Andrews technique is employed, assisted by maternal effort. Retention of the placenta and *postpartum haemorrhage* are managed along routine lines. In order to maintain the uterus in a firmly contracted state, 20–30 units of oxytocin are added to the intravenous infusion flask after delivery.

The placentas and membranes are examined carefully to determine the zygosity of the babies; this is usually evident from the number of membranes (amnion and chorion) separating the babies. Further identifying procedures may also be carried out (blood groups, hand and foot prints etc).

Unusual Complications of Delivery

Rupture of the second sac membranes before the first is diagnosed when routine pelvic examination reveals intact membranes of the presenting twin. If cord prolapse of this or the first twin occurs, Caesarean section may be necessary if the fetus is still alive. Delivery of the first placenta before the second fetus is born is serious if the 2 placentas are joined; immediate delivery of the second fetus is necessary because of abruption of the placenta. *Locking* and various forms of collision and impaction are very rare and require examination by an experienced clinician, usually under anaesthesia, and either manipulative untangling or Caesarean section. *Conjoined twins* may not be suspected before delivery; obstructed labour usually occurs, either before or after part of one twin has been born, and Caesarean section is usually the safest course for the mother (figure 25.7, colour plate 45). *Other indications for Caesarean section* include cord prolapse before the cervix is fully dilated, malpresentation of the first twin, significant disproportion, and previous Caesarean section. The incidence of Caesarean section is about 15% — approximately 50% higher in twin than singleton pregnancy (tables 16.3 and 53.2).

Failure to diagnose the second twin usually represents a lack of diagnostic skill before or during labour; the situation only becomes particularly serious if uterine palpation is omitted before routine administration of the oxytocic. Deep relaxant anaesthesia may then become necessary to allow extraction of the imprisoned fetus.

Prognosis

Morbidity and mortality is increased in both mother and baby. The causes of *perinatal mortality* are largely *prematurity* and its associated problems (asphyxia and respiratory distress), *intrauterine growth retardation, trauma,* and *malformations.* The perinatal mortality rate is approximately 10% — 3–8 times that for singletons; approximate figures according to birthweight are: < 1,000 g, 75%; 1,000–1,499 g, 20%; 1,500–2,499 g, 5%; 2,500 and above, 1–2%. The greatest loss occurs during the neonatal period, mainly from prematurity (hyaline membrane disease). In most series, the second twin has a worse outlook than the first, usually because of malpresentation, and the need for operative intervention. The more skilled this is, the more closely the figures approach one another (table 53.2). Although there is no significant difference between the mean birthweights of twin 1 and twin 2, the incidence of *respiratory distress* is increased 3–4 times in the latter. Both twin 1 and twin 2 have a high incidence of *intrauterine growth retardation* after 32–34 weeks' gestation, and this is especially so with twin 2 after 38 weeks' gestation (figure

25.8). The incidence of *congenital malformation* is increased 2–4 times in twin pregnancy (figure 53.1). *There is a significantly higher loss in monozygous twins* (2–4 times): this is related to (i) an increased incidence of fetal growth retardation, (ii) acute polyhydramnios (figure 25.12), (iii) congenital anomalies, (iv) cord accidents (figure 53.2), and vascular anastomoses between the placentas with circulatory imbalance (colour plate 46).

When more than 2 fetuses are present, the mortality rises very steeply (triplets, 30%, quadruplets, 50%).

Tables 53.1 and 53.2 give an overview of the method of delivery and perinatal mortality rates in a series of 560 patients with twin pregnancies managed in a teaching hospital. This series may exaggerate the importance of prematurity because of selective referral of patients in premature labour. However, the following points should be noted.

1. The proportion of twin pregnancies terminating *before 33 weeks* (18%) was much higher than in singleton pregnancies (1.9%) (table 53.1).

2. The *neonatal death rate* for twins was similar to singletons for any given maturity i.e. *a higher proportion of twins die because more are premature* (table 53.1).

3. The perinatal mortality rate for twin 1 (63 of 560) was virtually the same as for twin 2 (62 of 560) (table 53.1).

4. Two-thirds of twin deaths (81 of 125) were *neonatal deaths*, and 80% of all twin deaths occurred *before 33 weeks' gestation* (table 53.1) — hence the rationale of *rest in hospital between 28–34 weeks* for patients with multiple pregnancy.

5. Twins accounted for *24% of all neonatal deaths before 28 weeks' gestation* i.e. the contribution of multiple pregnancy to deaths from prematurity is monumental.

6. In this series of 560 cases the stillbirth rate was 3.9% and the neonatal death rate was 7.2%, giving a *perinatal mortality rate of 11.1%*.

7. During 1971–1980, twins accounted for *11.3% (125 of 1,100) of all perinatal deaths in the hospital*.

8. The incidence of manipulative delivery (forceps + breech) for twin 2 (58%) was higher than

Figure 53.1 A clinical diagnosis of twins warrants ultrasonography or radiography to confirm the diagnosis and to exclude malformations. Here both fetuses lie transversely and the uppermost is anencephalic — the bones of the vault are absent.

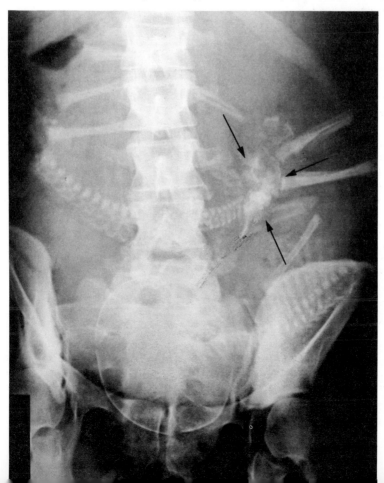

A

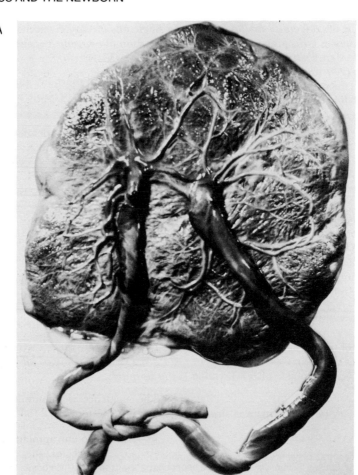

Figure 53.2 Cord entanglement or knotting is a special hazard (in addition to those of prematurity, placental shunts and malformations) for the monoamniotic variety of uniovular twins, causing death from hypoxia in 50–80% of cases. **A.** The knotted cords of unlucky stillborn twins. **B.** Braided umbilical cords of lucky twins — they survived the cord entanglement and fetal-fetal transfusion. (From Golan A et al Aust NZJ Obstet Gynaecol 1982; 22:165–167). The moral is that the second twin should be delivered immediately when there is a single amniotic sac.

B

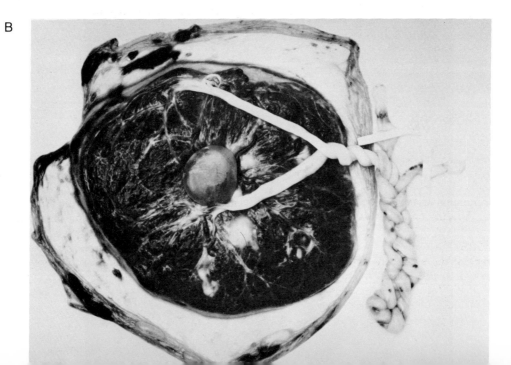

for twin 1 (44%); *breech delivery was more than twice as common for twin 2 than for twin 1* (table 53.2).

9. It is most uncommon for *Caesarean section* to be necessary for delivery of twin 2 after twin 1 has been delivered vaginally (table 53.2).

Table 53.3 illustrates the importance of breech presentation as a factor in the delivery of twins — especially second twins, 41% of which are delivered by the breech, either vaginally or by Caesarean section.

TABLE 53.3 INCIDENCES OF BREECH PRESENTATION AND DELIVERY IN 795 CONSECUTIVE TWIN PREGNANCIES

Method of delivery	Twin 1		Twin 2	
	Number	%	Number	%
Assisted breech delivery	94	11.8	123	15.4
Caesarean section	44	5.5	54	6.7
Breech extraction	10	1.2	98	12.3
Internal version and breech extraction	0	0.0	51	6.4
Total	148	18.6	326	41.0

Continuing Care

The care of twin babies (and higher orders of multiple birth) imposes a significant strain on the parents, especially the mother. Follow-up is therefore most important to ensure that there is adequate counselling and help with the many problems that may occur after leaving hospital — e.g. nutrition, adequate rest and sleep, breast feeding, and progress of the babies.

INTERNAL PODALIC VERSION AND BREECH EXTRACTION

The deliberate turning of the baby to the relatively unfavourable breech presentation is usually done to expedite delivery when the fetus is compromised. *After the version has been performed the baby is delivered by breech extraction.*

In modern obstetrics, internal version and breech extraction is seldom used for vaginal delivery of a singleton infant, unless the child is dead, or nonviable because of major malformation or extreme prematurity.

Indications

(i) Delivery of the *second twin if some complication has occurred* which threatens its well-

being (cord prolapse, placental separation, fetal distress, oblique or transverse lie which cannot be corrected) and when *the head is too high for safe forceps delivery.* The procedure is required for delivery of about 6% of second twins (table 53.2); it is seldom if ever required for the first twin since labour would not be allowed to continue if the lie was transverse (risk of cord prolapse), and it would be unlikely that the necessary conditions (full cervical dilatation) would be present without forceps delivery being feasible. (ii) The procedure is sometimes performed at *elective Caesarean section* (5–10% of cases); when the head is high and there is copious liquor it is easier to displace the head laterally and grasp a leg and then perform a breech extraction, than to deliver the child cephalically via the lower uterine segment incision. The procedure is not recommended if the head is in the pelvis, especially when the patient has laboured with ruptured membranes. It should be noted that *breech presentation is favourable at Caesarean section* — it is easier to grasp the breech than a head (except when there are extended legs deeply engaged in the pelvis); there is no curve of Carus for the head to negotiate at Caesarean section although the delivery of the aftercoming head can be difficult if the uterus contracts around the neck — similar to entrapment of the head by the cervix in delivery of the premature breech infant. A special indication for delivery of the infant by internal version and breech extraction at Caesarean section is when there is an *anterior placenta praevia*; here the bleeding (low pressure, venous) is controlled by tamponade by the thigh and body of the child during delivery — as in bipolar version (figure 50.11) which was introduced by Braxton Hicks to control bleeding from placenta praevia. (iii) *Transverse or oblique lie* in the multipara whose membranes are intact or recently ruptured, and the fetus is of normal or small size. (iv) *Prolapse of the umbilical cord* in the multipara with the fetus of normal or small size. (v) In the past, internal version was used as an alternative to Caesarean section, when attempts to correct a brow presentation, or to rotate the head in a mentoposterior position, had failed.

Necessary Conditions

These are the same, in several respects, as those for forceps delivery — the *cervix must be fully dilated*, the *pelvis adequate*, and the *anaesthesia sufficient to relax the uterus* for the required intrauterine manipulations (*ether* or *halothane* relax the uterus; the usual voluntary muscle relaxants used by anaesthetists do not). *The membranes must be intact or recently ruptured*

— i.e. the uterus must not be tightly wrapped around the fetus because efforts to perform the version is then likely to cause uterine rupture (colour plate 23).

Technique

The same position, preparation, aseptic technique and instruments tray is needed as for forceps delivery. General anaesthesia is necessary. A paediatrician should be in attendance.

The hand which corresponds to the side on which the fetal limbs are placed is inserted fully into the uterus and a foot secured, preferably the anteriorly placed one. One foot is enough to pull upon, but the *manoeuvre is easier if both can be grasped.* The head is deflected to one side to facilitate this. The leg is then drawn down through the cervix and vagina and the head and trunk manoeuvred into a longitudinal position with the abdominal hand. With intermittent traction, assisted by pressure on the fundus to maintain an attitude of flexion, the baby is delivered as described under 'Breech Extraction' in Chapter 50. The crucially important point is to *prevent deflexion of the head*, which tends to occur because of the direction of pull and because the uterus is not aiding in the expulsion (and thus keeping the fetus flexed).

After delivery, a careful *inspection is made for tears* to the upper vagina and to the cervix. The nurse should be prepared for this possibility, by having adequate swabs, sponge-holding forceps for the cervix, vaginal retractors and suture materials available.

Preparations should be made for *resuscitation of the infant*, should this be required.

Complications

(i) *Maternal.* Uterine rupture, lacerations of the cervix or lower birth canal, haemorrhage, and shock.

(ii) *Fetal.* Intracranial haemorrhage and asphyxia.

Prognosis

The perinatal mortality and morbidity is acceptable if the procedure is used only for multiple pregnancy and at Caesarean section. We do not consider that the possible need of internal version (transverse lie of second twin) is a reason for elective Caesarean section in multiple pregnancy; likewise the dangers of breech delivery or breech extraction are not so great that elective Caesarean section is required when the second twin presents by the breech.

Table 53.4 illustrates that internal version and breech extraction has an acceptable perinatal mortality rate when performed by trained personnel for delivery of the second twin — the 3 deaths (5.9%) were from malformations or complications of prematurity.

TABLE 53.4   INDICATIONS FOR INTERNAL VERSION AND BREECH EXTRACTION IN 795 TWIN PREGNANCIES

Internal version and breech extraction		Number	%
First twin		0	0
Second twin		51	6.4
Indications			
Transverse lie	20		
Prolapsed arm/shoulder	9		
Cord presentation/prolapse	5		
Compound presentation	5		
High vertex	4		
Placental separation	2		
Elective	6		
Perinatal mortality		3	5.9
1 anencephalic			
1, 26 weeks' gestation (birth-weight 870 g) died on day 2 from hyaline membrane disease			
1, 28 weeks' gestation (birth-weight 1,030 g), acute polyhydramnios, died on day 27 from hyaline membrane disease			

chapter fifty-four

Postpartum Haemorrhage and Shock

OVERVIEW

Postpartum haemorrhage and shock will always be a part of obstetrics. Such haemorrhage occurs in *3–5% of pregnancies* and accounts for *about 10% of maternal deaths* (table 14.1). The *essential principles of management are to be prepared, to diagnose the problem with accuracy, and to act without procrastination* in implementing the sequence of steps necessary to control the bleeding. The 2 main causes of bleeding are *retained placental tissue* and *birth canal trauma*; with routine use of oxytocic drugs in management of the third stage of labour *uterine atony* is seldom the cause, and *coagulation disorders* are quite uncommon (1 in 1,500 deliveries). In general, *trauma* is to be expected predominantly in the primipara, in whom *lacerations* and operative interference are much more likely; *placental retention*, on the other hand, may complicate any delivery.

It is not always easy to tell whether one is going to have a small or a big problem: sometimes very brisk bleeding (e.g. from vessels in the placental bed or those involved in a cervical tear) ceases within a few minutes; at other times it continues, and demands cool, logical, and decisive action. Decisions that must often be made include the need for blood replacement, consultation with an expert, and exploration of the genital tract (usually under anaesthesia), after exclusion of blood coagulation failure. Firm *bimanual compression* of the uterus often gives the accoucheur a well-needed breathing space, and may convert an unmanageable situation to a manageable one.

Although there are high risk pregnancies where postpartum haemorrhage should be anticipated (previous postpartum haemorrhage, chorioamnionitis, prolonged labour, placenta praevia, Caesarean section, multiple pregnancy), *most cases occur unexpectedly*. This unpredictability of primary postpartum haemorrhage is the *main maternal hazard of home confinement*.

Obstetric shock may in nature be other than haemorrhagic — e.g. *cardiogenic*, where there is primary failure of a diseased heart; *neurogenic* and *anaphylactic*, where there is paralysis and increased permeability of small blood vessels; and finally, *septic*, where there is toxic spoiling of wide areas of the body, including the cardiovascular system.

Increasingly, the shock may be due to causes outside the pregnancy — e.g. *motor vehicle accident*.

PRIMARY POSTPARTUM HAEMORRHAGE

Primary postpartum haemorrhage is defined as bleeding of 500 ml or more from the birth canal in the first 24 hours after delivery of the baby. It should be emphasized that *blood loss is almost always underestimated clinically* (by ⅓–½). This is because the blood which soaks garments, drapes, and bed linen may not be included, and allowance is not made for the fact that a clot does not represent the amount of blood lost, because the serum is not included. Primiparas lose significantly more than multiparas, largely because of the greater number of episiotomies performed — this increases blood loss by an average of 100–150 ml. Major postpartum haemorrhage is a potential cause of maternal death unless diagnosis and treatment are prompt.

Incidence

This ranges from 3–5% of *vaginal deliveries* (table 54.1); the rate is higher in the nullipara and when labour is induced. However, the average blood loss at *Caesarean section* is 800–1,200 ml which necessitates *blood transfusion* in 10% of patients (table 47.3). The amount of bleeding is considerably less (400–600 ml) when the operation is performed under *epidural analgesia*. In the People's Republic of China all Caesarean sections are performed under *acupuncture* plus local analgesia and the average blood loss is reported to be less than 250 ml!

There are *4 major causes* of primary haemorrhage.

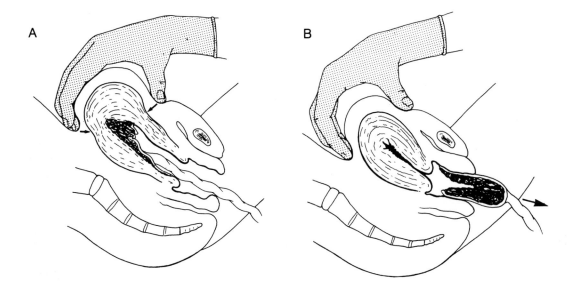

Figure 54.1 Crede expression of the attached placenta. **A.** The contracted fundus is squeezed between thumb and fingers to separate the placenta. **B.** The placenta is squeezed from the uterus and pushed out of the vagina. This manoeuvre often causes considerable pain and is not recommended.

1. RETAINED PRODUCTS OF CONCEPTION

Nonseparation and retention of part or whole of the placenta is the most common cause of postpartum haemorrhage (figure 54.1). Arteries and venous sinuses in the placental bed are not constricted as would normally occur (Chapter 42) and, in addition, the presence of the retained material inhibits general contractility of the uterus.

Diagnosis

Where the whole placenta, or a large portion is retained, the diagnosis is obvious. Difficulty might arise, however, if there is a small cotyledon retained (especially if the placenta is ragged) or if there is an additional (succenturiate) lobe (colour plate 33). On occasions, large segments of retained membrane may act in the same way as a cotyledon.

Management

The chief problem is when to explore the uterus. Often, placental retention is caused by the ergometrine given at the time of delivery (figure 54.2), and if active bleeding is not occurring, a period of 10–20 minutes may be allowed to elapse, when a further attempt may be made to remove the placenta by external means. It should be appreciated, however, that blood loss is usually proportional to the time the placenta remains in the uterus. If this fails, or continued

Figure 54.2 Placenta separated, but retained by oxytocic-induced constriction of muscle in upper uterine segment. Haemorrhage continues; controlled cord traction or manual removal required.

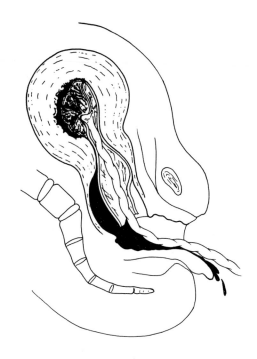

bleeding indicates earlier interference, an intra-venous infusion should be started, blood cross-matched (at least 2 units), and preparations made for operative intervention.

Manual removal of the placenta is usually carried out under regional or general anaesthesia. The *incidence* of the procedure is 2–5% (table 16.3), excluding cases where the detached placenta, caught in the cervix by an ergometrine-induced contraction, is removed digitally. Fresh sterile gloves, gown, and drapes should be used. The fingers are brought into the shape of a cone and the hand follows the umbilical cord into the uterine cavity. An assessment is made of the degree of adherence of the placenta and the site of attachment. The fingers are then inserted at one edge of the placenta, with the external hand on the abdomen exerting firm counter-pressure. With sweeping movements, the placenta is stripped from the wall of the uterus (figure 54.3). It is important that the procedure should be carried out gently and methodically, the operator having a clear mental picture of the disposition and extent of the placenta on the uterine wall. Occasionally, the placenta may be morbidly adherent to the uterus (placenta accreta), either wholly or in part. In such cases, a plane of cleavage will not be found, and the risk of uterine rupture is high. This condition may occur spontaneously, but is more common where there has been trauma to the uterus (previous curettage —

especially postpartum, previous manual removal, previous Caesarean section or uterine operation, or implantation of the placenta in the lower segment). Another rare condition, constriction ring, may incarcerate the placenta and require relaxation by anaesthetic agents or amyl nitrite. The cavity of the uterus should be explored, finally, either before or after the placenta is withdrawn from the uterus. The procedure is similar if smaller portions of the placenta are retained — a large blunt curette may be used to remove small fragments and membranes.

Careful inspection of the removed placenta is mandatory, and a check of the birth canal is made to exclude tears, which may coexist. Usually, an additional injection of an oxytocic is given.

If *placenta accreta* is present (1 in 2–3,000 deliveries), surgical intervention is usually required. Bleeding may be controlled by *uterine or internal iliac artery ligation*, but *hysterectomy* may be necessary in some patients, particularly if rupture of the uterine wall has occurred during attempted removal.

2. TRAUMA

Any disruption of the birth canal may cause excessive bleeding, because of the great vascularity of this region during pregnancy. In general, tears of the uterus and upper vagina are

A

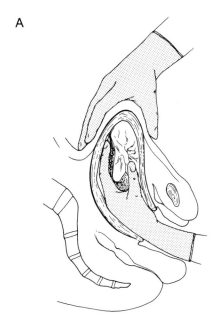

B

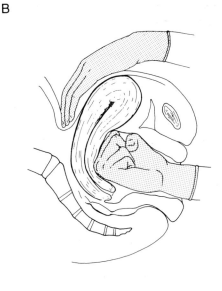

Figure 54.3 Manual removal of the placenta. **A.** The placenta is palmed as the fingers separate it from the uterine wall. The abdominal hand steadies the uterus and allows the correct plane of cleavage of be found. **B.** Bimanual compression is an effective method of controlling haemorrhage from an atonic uterus. After manual removal, if the empty uterus is flaccid and haemorrhage persistent, the compression is maintained until the effects of the general anaesthetic wear off — the uterus then responds to oxytocic drugs and contracts normally.

more serious, because of the larger vessels that may be torn and the difficulty in gaining access to them. The common sites of bleeding are the introitus, especially the posterior fourchette region, and the upper vagina and cervix.

Tears of the birth canal are more likely in the following circumstances: failure to cut an episiotomy, rapid labour, premature bearing down efforts, large baby, and obstetrical interference — forceps (especially other than outlet), internal version, impacted shoulders, and destructive operation. On occasions, the haemorrhage may be concealed as a result of bleeding into the pelvic or perineal tissues (haematoma formation). A special situation exists with trauma from *motor vehicle and allied accidents*. In addition to possible major damage to the head and chest, the pregnant uterus may pose particular hazards — placental abruption and/or rupture from direct trauma, and avulsion of the internal iliac vessels (figure 23.1). Additional injuries to be considered include splenic and hepatic rupture and damage to the bony pelvis.

The *diagnosis* of traumatic bleeding is easy if the lesion is low in the birth canal, but can be quite difficult if it is in the upper vagina, cervix or uterus, because of the problem of adequate exposure.

Uterine Rupture

Although this complication can occur before labour (usually from a previous classical Caesarean section or other uterine scar), it is most convenient to consider it in relation to postpartum haemorrhage.

Incidence ranges from 1 in 1,000–4,000 deliveries (table 16.1), depending on the geographical area (the latter figure reflects the incidence in a modern maternity hospital). Regardless of cause, there is a predominance of multiparas affected.

(a) *Uterine scar.* Vertical scars (classical Caesarean section, hysterotomy) are much more likely to rupture (figure 54.4). The transverse scar tends rather to dehisce, leaving a central window; this may extend laterally, however, with the potential for serious bleeding from ruptured uterine vessels at the side of the uterus (colour plate 87). Rupture is far less common after operation on the nonpregnant uterus (myomectomy, sterility procedures). It should be remembered that perforation of the uterus (often unrecognized) at the time of curettage or manual removal of the placenta might also leave a weak scar. *Factors predisposing* to rupture include poor technique of repair of uterine incisions,

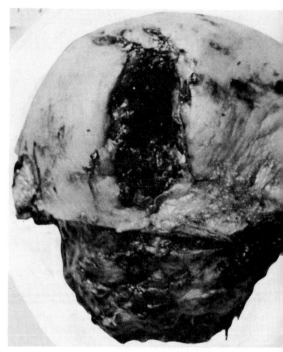

Figure 54.4 Complete rupture of the uterus occurred in labour at the site of a previous classical Caesarean section scar: subtotal hysterectomy specimen.

faulty haemostasis leading to haematoma formation, and infection. *Factors precipitating* rupture include uterine overdistension (multiple pregnancy, polyhydramnios) and dystocia.

The clinical picture is often different in rupture of upper and lower segment scars, and depends on the size of injured blood vessels. *Upper segment rupture* is nearly always a dramatic event — sharp, tearing type of pain, faintness or collapse, bleeding from the birth canal, and signs of intraperitoneal bleeding, perhaps including shoulder-tip pain. Fetal death is usual. The fetus may be felt separately from the uterus in the abdomen. By contrast, *lower segment rupture* is usually less dramatic, because of the thinner muscle, less vascularity and retention of the fetus in the uterus (figure 54.5). The patient complains of an ache or pain in the lower abdomen, and labour contractions often slow or cease. There is often evidence of fetal distress (colour plate 87). The diagnosis may be made only at the time of repeat Caesarean section or at manual removal of the placenta and/or during exploration for postpartum haemorrhage (figure 54.6).

Management. Preventive measures include admission to hospital at 37–38 weeks, particularly if the scar is vertical and the uterus is overdistended. *Oxytocin* should be administered only under the most careful supervision. Version

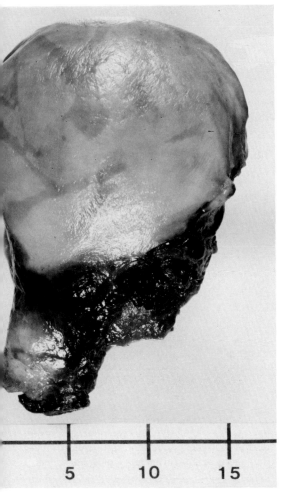

Figure 54.5 Total hysterectomy specimen from the patient shown in figure 54.13. Complete rupture of left lower uterine segment had occurred as a result of internal version and breech extraction. The left broad ligament contained a massive haematoma which had burst into the peritoneal cavity.

is usually contraindicated. *Early warning signs* are scar tenderness, lower abdominal pain between contractions, trickle of blood per vaginam, unexplained decrease in contractions, unexplained lack of progress, and rise in pulse rate or fall in blood pressure.

Treatment. Apart from the usual measures for haemorrhagic shock, the control of this complication often requires hysterectomy. Repair may be undertaken if the patient is anxious to have further children.

(b) *Obstructed labour.* Ruptures due to this cause are now few in number, as a result of better management of labour and fewer prolonged labours. In the great majority of cases, the patient is a multipara, and the fetus is either significantly larger than previously or presents with an unfavourable diameter (brow presentation).

The clinical picture is nearly always dramatic — abdominal pain, collapse, vaginal bleeding, cessation of labour. These features may only be evident after delivery, if the rupture has occurred in the second stage. The tear usually starts in the overdistended lower segment, but often extends laterally to the region of the uterine vessels (figure 54.5).

Management. *Preventive measures* include recognition of cephalopelvic disproportion either before labour commences or during labour before obstruction occurs. *Early warning signs* are the presence of very strong contractions, rising pulse rate, a distressed patient, pain between contractions, lack of descent, and a distended and tender lower uterine segment.

Treatment is similar to that for major scar rupture.

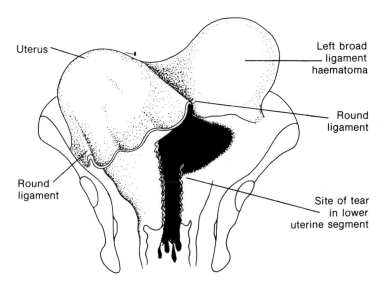

Uterus

Left broad ligament haematoma

Round ligament

Round ligament

Site of tear in lower uterine segment

Figure 54.6 This rupture of the left lower uterine segment is 'incomplete' as the broad ligament peritoneum is intact. The tear has extended through cervix into the vagina and there is copious vaginal haemorrhage. The uterus is displaced to the right by the broad ligament haematoma.

(c) *Oxytocic drugs.* There has been a marked reduction in the number of ruptures from this cause since the replacement of the intramuscular route by carefully controlled oxytocin infusion for the induction of labour. The modern trend to 'accelerate' labour with oxytocin to prevent a duration longer than 12 hours, or to overcome inertia, may see a resurgence in the number of ruptures (particularly in multiparas), since cephalopelvic disproportion is not always easy to pick by less experienced personnel. Other causes of rupture include lack of proper supervision during the administration of the oxytocin, use of oxytocin (or prostaglandin) concentrations which are too high, and failure to cut back the drip rate when the acceleration phase of labour has been reached.

The clinical features, warning signs and treatment are similar to those described for obstructed labour.

(d) *Operative trauma.* Rupture from this cause before the onset of labour occurs only exceptionally, e.g. *external cephalic version* usually in the presence of a uterine scar. *Internal version* is now almost restricted to delivery of the second twin and this former major cause has almost entirely been eliminated (figures 54.5 and 54.13). *Breech extraction* of the single fetus is hazardous because intrauterine manipulation may be required to deliver the legs or arms (colour plate 23). *Mid-forceps* delivery with rotation of the head is now probably the commonest cause. Often there is an unsuspected disproportion — usually of fetal origin (large baby, malformation). Another serious condition is *placenta accreta*; this is usually partial and is related to implantation of the placenta over a previous Caesarean section scar or in the lower segment (placenta praevia-accreta). When the placenta is morbidly adhered to the uterine wall, attempts at manual removal often result in tearing of the uterus, which adds to the amount of bleeding.

The classical clinical feature is heavy, continuous bleeding which follows closely on the procedure.

The treatment is again hysterectomy after resuscitation; repair of the rupture may be possible in selected cases.

Prognosis of uterine rupture. That for lower segment scar rupture is usually good, both for the mother and fetus, since the baby is not usually ejected from the uterus as in an upper segment rupture. In the latter, the fetal loss is very high, although occasional saves will be made if laparotomy is performed quickly. The prognosis for the mother depends on the adequacy of resuscitation and skill of the operator in the performance of the often difficult surgery. Hysterectomy, if necessary, will remove future prospects of childbearing.

Hypofibrinogenaemia is a condition that may complicate uterine rupture. In some patients, the trauma itself is enough to release sufficient thromboplastic material into the circulation, or the formation of local massive clot may consume fibrinogen; in other patients, the rupture allows the amniotic fluid to gain access to the circulation, and this acts as a source of thromboplastin.

Damage to bladder or ureter may occasionally occur, either as a result of extension of the uterine rupture (usually because the bladder is adherent to the lower segment after a previous Caesarean section), or as a complication of the surgical procedure. In such cases, an indwelling catheter will be inserted which will stay in for at least 7–10 days. The continued patency of the catheter must be checked by charting the urine volume every 4 hours; if there is a decrease, blockage of the catheter is likely, and an immediate report must be made to the doctor in charge.

Cervical and Vaginal Lacerations

The characteristic feature is a steady loss of bright red blood, which commences soon after delivery of the baby. Unless the uterus is also damaged, it is firmly contracted. These features help to distinguish traumatic and placental site bleeding.

In such a situation, repair of the laceration must be carried out before too much blood has been lost; a doctor must be called if not in attendance. If the loss is heavy, *bimanual compression* should be employed (vaginal hand pressing firmly against the front of the cervix and lower segment, abdominal hand pressing the back of the uterus downwards and forwards against the vaginal hand) (figure 54.3b). *Packing* may be used as an emergency, but must be properly performed (figure 54.7). In this situation it often wastes time and blood, and bimanual compression is preferable.

Preparations will include blood for crossmatching, materials for intravenous infusion, suture tray, a set of sponge forceps, vaginal retractors, extra swabs, sucker (additional to that required by anaesthetist and paediatrician) and spotlight. An anaesthetic may be required if the repair is not straight forward.

Technique of repair. The vaginal walls are well retracted by an assistant and a systematic inspection is made of the vagina and cervix. If the bleeding is from a vaginal laceration, it is closed

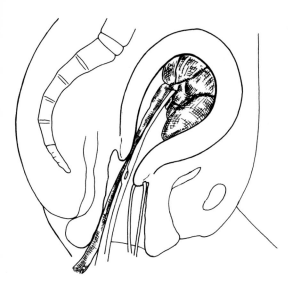

Figure 54.7 Packing the uterus is more effective for secondary postpartum haemorrhage or postabortal haemorrhage than for primary postpartum haemorrhage, irrespective of the cause. Wide ribbon gauze (10 cm) is used and is removed after 12–24 hours.

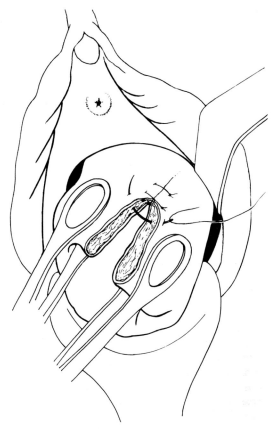

Figure 54.8 Repair of a cervical tear is necessary only when bleeding continues, and this is very uncommon. Sponge forceps grasp the cervix; a retractor is usually necessary for adequate exposure.

with a continuous chromic catgut suture (No. 0 or 1). If the bleeding is from a cervical laceration, the cervix is grasped with 2 or more sponge forceps and drawn down until the apex of the tear is visible. A suture is placed just beyond this for secure haemostasis and the repair is completed with either a continuous or interrupted suture (figure 54.8).

If the bleeding is coming from inside the cervical canal, it is likely that its origin is from the placental site or a tear in the uterus; exploration will determine this.

Vulval Lacerations

These will be evident on inspection. Repair is effected in 1 or 2 layers as for episiotomy (figure 54.9).

Third Degree Tear

Here, the tear extends posteriorly to involve the anal canal and possibly the rectum also.

Causes. (i) Labour — precipitate, birth before admission, (ii) baby — large or unfavourable diameter presenting (face to pubis), (iii) delivery technique — failure to maintain flexion and thus presentation of the most favourable diameter of the fetal head; failure to control the rate of expulsion of head or shoulders; and failure to perform episiotomy where indicated, (iv) perineum — scarred, thin (v) pelvis — android, subpubic angle narrow, (vi) patient — uncooperative.

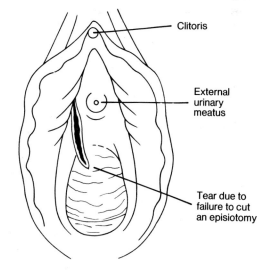

Clitoris

External urinary meatus

Tear due to failure to cut an episiotomy

Figure 54.9 Tear of the vestibule due to sparing the perineum — the occiput strikes against the ischiopubic bones as the head recoils from the perineal musculature. The area near the clitoris and urethral meatus is very vascular, and careful suturing is required.

Management. Prevention is usually possible — an informed, cooperative patient, proper delivery technique, and timely episiotomy. *Treatment.* The repair should be carried out by an experienced person. Each layer should be carefully identified, and sutured, and haemostasis secured. The retracted ends of the external sphincter of the anus must be identified and approximated after the anal mucosa has been sutured. Then the vaginal epithelium and perineum are sutured as in repair of an episiotomy (figure 45.3).

Haematoma Formation

The bleeding in this case is *into the tissues*, rather than external. It is often associated with lacerations of the uterus or vagina, due to retraction of vessels and continued bleeding, but may result from tearing of vessels beneath the intact surface. Other causes include failure to secure haemostasis when lacerations are being repaired, and direct trauma with the needle at the time of pudendal nerve block (colour plate 34).

The degree of discomfort to the patient is proportional to the size of the haematoma; if large, severe pain is experienced (classically perirectal) and shock may result.

Treatment. If the haematoma is accessible, the patient's convalescence will be shorter and more comfortable if an incision is made, the clot evacuated, bleeding point(s) ligated, and the cavity closed in layers. When the haematoma is high in the vagina (above the levator ani muscles) treatment should be conservative.

Blood transfusion and antibiotic therapy may be required.

3. UTERINE ATONY

Before oxytocic drugs were given as a routine during the third stage, uterine atony was easily the most common cause of postpartum haemorrhage, particularly since many patients also had chloroform or ether for the actual delivery. This cause is now much less common. It may still arise if a *volatile anaesthetic*, such as ether or halothane, has been given to provide relaxation for intrauterine manipulations, or other uterine relaxing drugs have been used (beta blockers, magnesium sulphate). Also, there are occasions when the *baby is born outside the delivery room* — such as at home, in the taxi, or the hospital lift. The inhibitory effect of a *retained placenta or cotyledon* has already been mentioned. A number of other factors may interfere with normal uterine retraction: full bladder, incoordinate uterine action, uterine sepsis, fibromyomas, exhaustion (as from a prolonged labour), and high parity. Sometimes, the oxytocic drug is given subcutaneously, rather than intramuscularly or intravenously as intended, and its onset of action will be delayed; this prolongation will be accentuated if the patient is in shock and the peripheral circulation is poor. Overdistension of the uterus by twins or polyhydramnios has been mentioned as a cause, but in such cases it is probable that other factors are more important.

If the response to conventional agents (ergometrine, oxytocin) is inadequate, intramuscular (or intramyometrial) injection of one of the newer prostaglandins may give dramatic results.

4. COAGULATION DEFECT

In obstetric practice, disseminated intravascular coagulation is easily the most common cause of failure of blood clotting. The clinical conditions predisposing to this complication are severe abruption of the placenta (60-70%), a dead fetus retained in utero for longer than 4 weeks, severe preeclampsia, amniotic fluid embolism, extensive tissue damage, and shock. In some cases of otherwise unexplained bleeding, there may be an exaggeration of the normal process of placental or systemic intravascular coagulation. If any one of these conditions is present, blood clotting must be assessed. This can be done clinically by placing 5 ml of blood in a plain tube and gently inverting it every minute; if a firm clot does not form within 6-8 minutes, hypofibrinogenaemia is likely and blood should be sent to the laboratory for more accurate testing of the fibrinogen level. Occasionally, other conditions such as thrombocytopenic purpura, leukaemia, and von Willebrand disease may present with postpartum haemorrhage (see Chapter 34).

PLAN OF ACTION IN PRIMARY POSTPARTUM HAEMORRHAGE

(i) *Anticipation of the high risk patient.* The *history* is important, particularly previous postpartum haemorrhage or manual removal of the placenta, multiple curettage, operations on the uterus, high parity, antepartum haemorrhage, haemorrhagic tendency, or chronic anaemia. *Examination* may reveal conditions likely to lead to operative delivery: malpresentations or malpositions, multiple pregnancy, prolonged and difficult labour, or structural uterine abnormalities. The *haemoglobin value* should have been checked within 4-6 weeks of delivery to discover the anaemic patient. (ii) An *intravenous infusion* in progress and cross-matched blood available is a wise precaution in the high risk patient. (iii) The rules of conduct of the third stage should be observed — do not thoughtlessly or impatiently fiddle with the uterus. (iv) If brisk bleeding is occurring, the dose and route of the oxytocic that was administered should be checked. On no account must the patient be left; a senior member of the nursing staff and the doctor should be called. (v) *Check the uterus to ensure that it is contracted*; massage should be done evenly and firmly. Massage (rubbing up the fundus) will quickly cause the uterus to contract and control the bleeding — hence the popular dictum that '*an empty contracted uterus will not bleed*', the only exception to the rule being the presence of blood coagulation failure. (vi) Check the lower birth canal for obvious bleeding — especially from the episiotomy site or vaginal tears; apply pressure or a clamp to the bleeding point. (vii) *The bladder should be emptied by catheter* — this usually promotes separation and delivery of the placenta if it is retained. (viii) A further attempt is made to deliver the placenta if it is still in the uterus — by controlled cord traction or the Dublin method of fundal pressure if the cord has been avulsed. If it has been delivered, it is rechecked carefully for completeness and the presence of a hole in the membranes which might indicate a missing succenturiate lobe. (ix) A further dose of oxytocin may be given (5–10 u of Syntocinon and/or 0.25–0.5 mg ergometrine intravenously or intramuscularly). (x) If the bleeding is continuing, preparations must be made for *general anaesthesia* and *manual removal of the placenta* or *exploration for damage* higher in the birth canal: for the latter, a suture tray with adequate retractors, sponge holders and swabs, and gauze roll (10 cm) is necessary. A good spotlight is essential. An anaesthetist and additional assistants should be called. Bimanual compression, properly applied, will conserve blood while the above preparations are being made (figure 54.3b). If a serious problem seems likely, thought must be given to consultation/transport/operating theatre as indicated. (xi) Blood loss should be measured and clotting noted. (xii) Blood should be taken for cross-matching and laboratory coagulation study. (xiii) An intravenous infusion must be commenced. If the blood loss exceeds 1,000 ml, a litre of glucose-saline or Hartmann solution is given, followed by dextran or plasma; blood is given when it becomes available. (xiv) If the patient is showing symptoms and signs of shock, elevate the foot of the bed. (xv) The patient must be given a simple explanation of what is happening and the management proposed. The doctor will notify the husband or nearest relative as a rule. (xvi) Monitoring of vital signs must be commenced and appropriately charted. (xvii) Further management will depend on the findings.

INVERSION OF THE UTERUS

In this rare complication (about 1 in 20,000 deliveries), the fundus of the uterus descends through the cervix and lies either in the vagina or outside the introitus. The placenta is usually still adherent, either totally or partially. This condition is now extremely rare with the routine use of oxytocics and the Brandt-Andrews method of placental delivery.

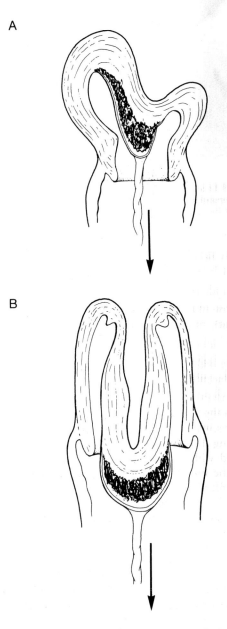

Figure 54.10 Inversion of the uterus is usually due to pulling on the cord when the uterus is atonic (no oxytocic given). **A.** The inversion is beginning — note fundal dimple. **B.** Partial inversion: the fundus has passed through the cervix and is in the vagina.

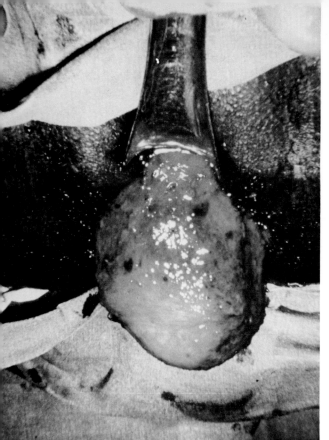 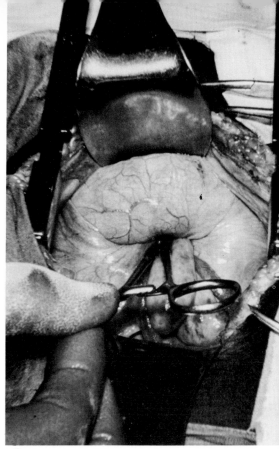

A   B

Figure 54.11 Inversion of the puerperal uterus. **A.** The uterus inside-out between the Negro patient's thighs. **B.** Appearance at laparotomy — forceps indicate the inverted fundus. **C.** The uterus and adnexa after correction of the inversion. Note that the ovaries lie on the posterior aspect of the broad ligaments. (Courtesy of Dr Christopher Orr).

C

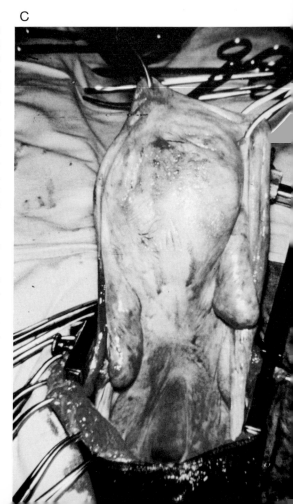

It may occur spontaneously (usually when the placenta is implanted at the fundus) as a result of a sudden rise of intraabdominal pressure (expulsion of placenta by the patient coughing or vomiting), or may be the result of gross fundal pressure and/or pulling on the cord when the uterus is relaxed and/or during manual removal of the placenta (figure 54.10). A large mass is felt or seen (figure 54.11) and there is no uterus palpable in the abdomen. The only condition which simulates inversion is a submucous fibromyoma projecting through the external os — this can be confused with partial inversion (figure 54.10B) where the fundus may still be palpable abdominally. Bleeding may or may not be excessive, but shock is common if the uterus is not quickly replaced.

After shock has been corrected by intravenous therapy, an attempt is made to replace the uterus manually: with the fundus in the palm of the hand, strong upward pressure is exerted to place the uterine ligaments on the stretch; if this is maintained for 3–5 minutes the fundus will usually recede upwards as the ring widens. It is then pushed upwards with the clenched fist. The placenta if still attached to the fundus is manually removed *after* the inversion has been replaced — it provides a firmer fundus to press upon and lessens the risk of uterine rupture. Alternatively, *O'Sullivan's hydrostatic method* may be used: here sterile saline at body temperature is run into the upper vagina while the forearm occludes its egress below; the vagina balloons, the ring stretches and the fundus returns to its normal position. If the constricting ring feels tight, it may be relaxed with a slow intravenous bolus of 2 g of *magnesium sulphate*. Rarely, abdominal surgery may be necessary; the inverted fundus is drawn up by toothed forceps applied stepwise (figures 54.11B and C).

SECONDARY POSTPARTUM HAEMORRHAGE

Definition
Bleeding in excess of normal lochial loss after the first 24 hours postpartum and until the end of the puerperium.

Incidence
Ranges from 0.5 to 1.5% (table 54.1).

TABLE 54.1   POSTPARTUM HAEMORRHAGE STATISTICS IN 36,349 CONSECUTIVE VAGINAL DELIVERIES*

	Primary	Secondary
Incidence	4.4%	1.3%
Blood transfusion	38.1%	30.2%

* Hysterectomy was required in 5 of 1,632 patients with primary postpartum haemorrhage and 7 of 505 patients with secondary postpartum haemorrhage

Aetiology
Usually dissolution of thrombi at the placental site or areas of trauma, and/or subinvolution and/or retained pieces of placenta or membrane. The usual site is the cornual area where attachment to myometrium is more likely. Rarely, a placental polyp may form and result in heavy bleeding up to several years later. *Infection* is likely if pieces of tissue remain in the uterus, since these form a favourable nidus for bacteria. Rarely, the bleeding may result from *fibromyomas* (especially the submucous variety); lacerations (particularly if infected); carcinoma of the cervix; choriocarcinoma (usually after the second month); and too early coitus. As with primary postpartum haemorrhage, general bleeding disorders may present in this manner. In approximately half the patients, the cause is obscure.

Diagnosis
If the cause is in the lower birth canal it will be detected easily, but otherwise the diagnosis will not be made unless curettage is carried out and the tissue submitted for histological study.

Clinical Features
Secondary bleeding may be preceded by a history of ragged placenta or membranes, offensive and/or persistently red lochia, subinvolution of the uterus, and unexplained temperature elevation. The amount of blood loss ranges from that of a menstrual period to an amount sufficient to precipitate shock. It occurs most commonly between the 5th–15th days of the puerperium.

Management
Careful inspection of the placenta and membranes after delivery, adequate repair of lacerations, and prevention of infection will all minimize later trouble. Subinvolution of the uterus should alert the attendant to the possibility of retained material. If the patient has demonstrated the warning signs outlined above, she should be instructed to report any loss after discharge from hospital.

Treatment of the bleeding episode may be conservative if it is small in amount and settles with *rest* and chemotherapy. *Curettage* (figure 54.12) should not be performed routinely, since the uterus is often friable and may be perforated, for which hysterectomy may be required. Ergot preparations are probably of little value given orally; they should be administered parenterally if indicated. Speculum examination will determine whether the bleeding is coming from the uterus, or from an infected laceration in the lower birth canal. The latter may need suturing. If the bleeding occurs before the episiotomy is properly healed, the latter can be reinforced by including it in a generous encircling suture, otherwise it may break down during examination and curettage. A vaginal swab is taken for microbiological study, and *chemotherapy* commenced even if the patient is afebrile, since *endometritis is usually present*. Except when bleeding is heavy or persistent, chemotherapy is more important than curettage.

In the series of 505 patients shown in table 54.1, 30% received a *blood transfusion*, and *curettage* was performed in 60% because of heavy or persistent haemorrhage. Secondary postpartum haemorrhage often occurs after the patient has been discharged home. Only the more severe cases result in the patient's readmission to hospital and inclusion in the above statistics — this accounts for the high incidences of curettage and blood transfusion in this group of patients.

Emergency treatment may be necessary —

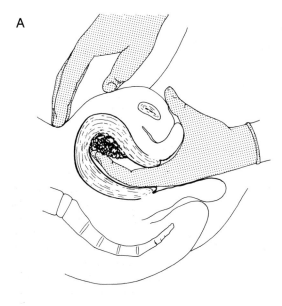

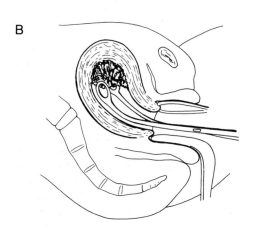

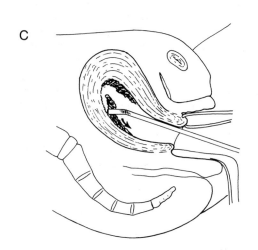

uterine massage, bimanual compression, and intravenous ergometrine (0.5 mg) or intramuscular Syntometrine (1 ml); this is followed by blood transfusion if required. It is important that blood loss is measured accurately. Only exceptionally will such measures as hypogastric/uterine artery ligation or hysterectomy be necessary (see footnote to table 54.1).

OBSTETRIC SHOCK AND RESUSCITATION

Shock may be defined as a state of decompensation between the heart and vascular system, manifested by inadequacy of normal perfusion of the organs of the body.

AETIOLOGY

The organs of the body receive blood at a certain pressure which brings vital substances such as oxygen and nutrients, and carries away waste products such as carbon dioxide and lactic acid. For this to be effective, it is necessary to have a balance between the following: (i) a heart pumping blood at the required pressure, (ii) an adequate volume of blood in the circulation (usually 4.5–5.5 litres), (iii) a normal degree of tone in the blood vessels. Shock occurs when one or more of these systems is significantly deranged.

Cardiogenic
The heart may fail because of rheumatic valvular disease (usually chronic), or because of a coronary occlusion or myocarditis (usually acute). There will then not be enough pressure in the system to provide life support for the cells in the different parts of the body.

Hypovolaemic
The blood volume is decreased most rapidly and obviously by haemorrhage (abortion, ectopic pregnancy, mole, antepartum and postpartum haemorrhage). It should be remembered, however, that equally serious falls in volume may occur if the patient is not taking fluids by mouth,

Figure 54.12 Methods used to remove retained placental products from the uterus in the treatment of secondary postpartum haemorrhage or bleeding due to incomplete abortion. **A.** Curage — use of fingers as in manual removal of the placenta: fingers are blunt and least likely to rupture the uterus. **B.** Sponge forceps are used to grasp placental tissue and dislodge it in one piece with minimal blood loss. **C.** Curettage is required to remove smaller pieces of placenta and to ensure that the uterus is empty.

or they are not being absorbed (hyperemesis gravidarum, prolonged labour, ileus after Caesarean section). The same effect may occur if the blood volume is normal, but there is an inadequate return to the heart, a characteristic of the supine hypotensive syndrome where the heavy gravid uterus falls back and obstructs the inferior vena cava, or where the pulmonary circulation is blocked by an embolus (blood clot, amniotic fluid debris, air).

Neurogenic

The blood vessels are normally in a 'tonic state', resulting from the balanced activity of the 2 divisions of the autonomic nervous system (sympathetic and parasympathetic). In normal conditions, the capacity of the system balances the blood volume within it. When there is an *over-activity of the nerves which relax the blood vessels* (parasympathetic), as described above, the reservoir becomes much enlarged and the pressure drops. Other things may directly dilate blood vessels — the hormone *progesterone*, produced in large amounts by the placenta (primarily to inhibit the muscle of the uterus), also relaxes the muscle in the wall of blood vessels, and explains why fainting is commoner in pregnancy. In *anaphylactic shock*, the mechanism is similar to neurogenic shock, the peripheral vasodilation and increased capillary permeability resulting from liberated vasoactive substances (bradykinin, histamine).

In the conditions of *neurogenic shock*, there is stimulation of the nerves which depress the heart and blood vessels (vagus and other parasympathetic nerves) usually by an intense visual or painful stimulus. The most familiar example is the person who faints at the scene of an accident, although not injured. The condition of uterine inversion after delivery produces shock even though little blood has been lost, because of pain and overstimulation of the visceral nerves supplying the uterus and adnexa. The same applies to major trauma to the genital tract.

Septic

In severe infections, (septic abortion, chorioamnionitis, pyelonephritis, puerperal infection, ruptured viscus) the bacterial toxins may affect the blood vessels (endotoxin shock) either directly, or indirectly by disturbing the centre for autonomic nervous system control in the brain.

In many cases, more than one factor is involved. For example, a patient with severe pre-eclampsia may have had an artificial rupture of the membranes, laboured unsuccessfully for a long period without intravenous fluids, and then required a Caesarean section which resulted in excessive blood loss; also, intrauterine infection may have followed the amniotomy and long labour. Here, there is a metabolic disorder and an infection which are damaging to blood vessels and cells, loss of body fluid as a result of the long labour, and bleeding at the time of Caesarean section.

PATHOPHYSIOLOGY

The basic problem is that there is not enough blood flow (carrying oxygen and nutrients) in the capillary vessels supplying vital organs. This has 2 major consequences. (i) *Hypoxia* of the tissues initially depresses their function and if unrelieved eventually causes their death. They are forced to work anaerobically, which produces an excess of lactic and pyruvic acid ('metabolic acidosis'), and this further depresses the heart and other vital centres. (ii) *Coagulation of the blood* in the smaller blood vessels results from the hypoxia and slowing of the flow, and is hastened if thromboplastins are released at the same time (trauma, abruptio placentae, amniotic fluid embolism, infection). This disseminated intravascular coagulation (DIC) adds to the hypoxia of the tissues.

Unless the shock is treated in time, it becomes 'irreversible', and the patient will die.

Compensatory Mechanisms

(i) *Sympathetic nervous system*. As the pressure falls in the large arteries and veins there is an activation of the sympathetic nervous system (which includes the adrenal medulla). Blood is shunted away from nonvital areas such as the skin (coldness and pallor), kidney (oliguria), and muscles; and the heart is stimulated (tachycardia). If the position is not corrected, the intense vasoconstriction adds to the problems by contributing to tissue hypoxia and intravascular coagulation. (ii) *Fluid retaining mechanisms*. The same stimuli as described above activate 2 further mechanisms — antidiuretic hormone release from the posterior lobe of the pituitary gland, and aldosterone release from the adrenal cortex, both of which help the kidney to conserve water. (iii) *Fibrinolytic system*. This is activated in conditions of shock (plasminogen-plasmin), and this is responsible for clearing the intravascular thrombi which have formed.

CLINICAL FEATURES

These largely reflect the activity of the compensatory mechanisms as described above.

Tachycardia is usual in volume depletion

shock and the pulse is weak and difficult to feel. The rate usually reflects the severity of shock: for example mild, 80–99/minute, moderate, 100–119/minute, marked, 120–139/minute, critical, 140/minute or over. The reverse occurs (bradycardia) in neurogenic shock. Skin pallor is usual, but there is much variation in people normally, and pallor may be intense where the condition is not serious (fainting). A better sign is pallor of the lips — if noticeable, there is significant anaemia or blood loss. Skin temperature is usually low, but may depend on room temperature. A fall in blood pressure is usual, and is a reflection of the degree of shock, remembering that it may be very low in temporary upsets such as fainting and the supine hypotensive syndrome. If the shock is mild the systolic pressure is usually 100 or more; moderate, 85–99; marked, 70–84; critical, below 70. Cyanosis is rare unless the lungs are affected (pulmonary embolism) or the heart is failing. Respiration may be initially faster and shallower, later deeper and irregular. Nausea and vomiting are relatively common as are periods of restlessness. Urine output is usually low (< 30 ml/hour).

TREATMENT

Only the principles of management will be discussed, since the treatment of the individual conditions is discussed elsewhere in the book.

General

(i) All *vital signs* of the mother must be measured and recorded accurately. In addition, such observations as fetal heart rate, uterine contractions, fluid balance, blood loss, blood clotting, and conscious state must be included. (ii) Reassurance and explanation, gentle handling of the patient, and avoidance of panic. (iii) *Laboratory tests.* Full blood study, coagulation profile if indicated, serum electrolytes and creatinine, bacteriological and acid-base studies.

Replacement of Circulating Blood Volume

Prevention of dehydration where possible; otherwise replacement with a solution determined by caloric and electrolyte requirements. Further blood loss must be stopped. Initial replacement, 1–2 litres of glucose 5% in water, normal saline, or Hartmann solution. This will rapidly replace much of the lost blood volume without danger of transfusion reactions and will lower the blood viscosity which is often high in shock. If blood is then available, it should be given, otherwise 1 or 2 bottles of a colloid solution (soluble plasma protein substitute (SPPS), Haemaccel, or dextran) until cross-matching has been effected. Unmatched blood may occasionally be necessary in desperate situations; it is preferable to use blood of the patient's own group and Rh type, rather than group O Rh-negative blood. In general, the infusion needle should be wide bore (16 gauge or wider), placed in a large vein, and the solution given under pressure. If the anticipated transfusion is very considerable (2–3 litres per hour), microfiltration and warming of the blood is recommended, and calcium gluconate, bicarbonate, fresh frozen plasma and platelets may need to be added; fresh frozen plasma may also be needed in DIC, liver disease, and clotting factor deficiencies. If anaesthesia and surgery are likely, an extra 20% (1,000 ml) of the blood volume (5,000 ml) should be allowed for, and the same applies if the loss is continuing. Two intravenous infusion lines may be necessary. Raising the foot of the bed and bandaging the legs will temporarily help by increasing the supply of blood to vital centres. The amount of transfusion fluid required in a straightforward situation can usually be gauged by response of vital signs and urine flow. Hyperosmotic saline (200–400 ml of 7.5% solution) is often very effective in increasing blood pressure and urine flow and improving the conscious state.

In complicated cases, *central venous pressure* (CVP) measurement is very helpful to allow assessment of the correct volume of fluid replacement. A wide bore (15 gauge) catheter is inserted into one of the large intrathoracic veins leading to the heart (via the median basilic, subclavian, or external jugular). This is connected to a manometer (figure 54.13) and an infusion apparatus with a 3-way tap. To measure CVP the manometer is filled from the infusion flask and the latter is then switched out so that the manometer is in line with the central vein. The saline in the manometer will fall and then oscillate (respiratory effect). The height of fluid in the manometer above the midaxillary line equals the CVP and this indicates if fluid is required. In general, a value of 0–5 cm water (or saline) indicates hypovolaemia; 6–10 cm indicates possible hypovolaemia and a trial administration of fluid; 11 cm or more indicates normovolaemia, hypervolaemia, or heart failure, and further fluid is not required. This set-up requires close supervision, since negative pressures can be created (the catheter is intrathoracic); air embolism can occur if the infusion bottles are not watched closely or the apparatus comes apart. Other complications include vein trauma, catheter embolism, lung trauma, and hydrothorax.

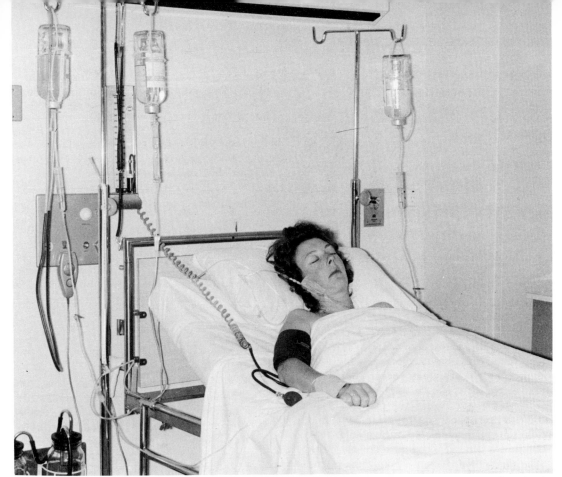

Figure 54.13 A patient receiving intensive care after hysterectomy for uterine rupture caused by internal version for delivery of a second twin. A central venous infusion and pressure monitor is in position, in addition to intravenous infusions in each arm. She required an 8,000 ml blood transfusion.

Vascular Tone

Vasoconstrictor drugs, such as dopamine (5–10 µg/kg/min), noradrenaline and angiotensin, have been used to exaggerate nature's vasoconstrictive response; however, it is less dangerous and more physiological to replace circulating blood volume. *Vasodilator drugs*, such as isoprenaline and chlorpromazine, are used to offset the vasoconstrictive response and lessen tissue hypoxia; if they are employed, early and adequate replacement of circulating volume is required.

Hypoxia

Oxygen should be administered by mask, not intranasally, since the latter method is relatively ineffective.

Coagulation Failure

If the blood does not clot normally, hypofibrinogenaemia is usually present. Fresh frozen plasma (or cryoprecipitate, 0.2 u/kg) is given, and perhaps heparin, which will prevent further coagulation in the microcirculation.

Chemotherapy

This will be necessary in massive doses if the shock is due to sepsis; cover must be provided against both aerobic and anaerobic organisms. The exact choice of antibiotic will be determined by the severity of the infection, patient allergy, organism if known, and urinary output. For methicillin-resistant staphylococcal infections, vancomycin, 1g 12-hourly IV is recommended. To combat endotoxic shock, particularly that due to E. coli infection, freeze dried human plasma rich in antilipopolysaccharide IgG is given; this binds to the endotoxin.

Analgesia

Pethidine (IM or IV injection) or a similar narcotic is needed if there is haemorrhage or trauma.

Mannitol

This is an osmotic diuretic and is useful in the early phase of oliguria or where red cell haemolysis has occurred (abortion complicated by Clostridium welchii infection or incompatible blood transfusion).

Hydrocortisone

Adrenal cortical hormones are used to assist the circulation and combat the effect of stress.

Other Measures

Assisted ventilation, or therapy for cardiac arrest may occasionally be necessary; digitalization may be required for cardiac failure.

AMNIOTIC FLUID EMBOLISM

Incidence

1 in 50,000 deliveries.

Clinical Features

Amniotic fluid enters the maternal circulation, usually through a small tear in the lower uterine segment. The initial symptoms are dyspnoea and cynosis, together with pallor, chills, restlessness, and perhaps convulsions. Shock usually follows rapidly, and death may occur before any effective treatment can be applied (colour plate 62). In less severe forms, the patient survives, but the thromboplastin contained in the amniotic fluid results in disseminated intravascular coagulation and a general bleeding tendency ensues.

The *differential diagnosis* comprises pulmonary thromboembolism, acute anaphylaxis, acute myocardial failure, Mendelson syndrome, eclampsia. If the presentation is one of coagulation disorder, other causes of disseminated intravascular coagulation should be looked for as well as Von Willebrand disease and thrombocytopenic purpura.

Treatment

This comprises oxygen by mask, assisted respiration if necessary, intravenous morphine, hydrocortisone, atropine, papaverine, and heparin by infusion (20,000–40,000 units); digitalis, aminophylline, lasix, and isoprenaline may also be needed. Coagulation factors may need replacement (fresh frozen plasma). *Bleeding due to uterine rupture may necessitate hysterectomy.* If CVP remains high, rotating tourniquets and perhaps venesection may be helpful.

TRANSFUSION COMPLICATIONS

LEAKAGE INTO TISSUES

If the needle or cannula is dislodged from the vein, the infusion fluid will run into the tissues. This should be detected by regular inspection of the infusion site and if present the infusion will need to be reinserted elsewhere or discontinued.

If the infusion is used as a vehicle for drug therapy, its proper functioning merits special care.

PHLEBITIS

There is a reddened, painful induration over the vein. The infusion should be changed to another site and local therapy and analgesics given.

EMBOLISM

Air embolism usually occurs when an infusion is being given under pressure and a watch is not kept on the fluid in the giving set: this may be fatal. Parts of the apparatus, especially plastic catheters, may enter the circulation if they are damaged and break off, or if they have not been fastened securely.

REACTIONS

Haemolytic

The blood is incompatible with that of the patient. Pain in the arm, neck or back occurs early, together with restlessness, nausea, rigors and pyrexia; headache and tingling in the limbs may also be present. The red cells are haemolysed, producing free haemoglobin in the blood and urine, and later jaundice. The renal tubules are blocked by red cell debris, and oliguria is common. The complication is particularly dangerous if the patient is anaesthetized, since a larger amount of the blood may be given (she cannot complain of pain etc). Potential seriousness of such reactions emphasize the need for the greatest care in checking that the right blood goes to the right patient. A common cause for error is when 2 patients with the same name are in the hospital at the same time.

The transfusion must be ceased immediately and the matter reported. All bottles must be kept for checking and urine samples measured hourly. The kidneys may be stimulated with mannitol, 100 ml of a 20% solution intravenously; ethacrynic acid, 50 mg; and a 5% dextrose load (2,000 ml). Sodium bicarbonate 300 meq is given intravenously.

Pyrogenic

These are rare now that improvements have been made to fluids and tubing. They are manifest by pyrexia, shivers, anxiety and restlessness. The infusion should be discontinued temporarily and the complication reported. If it is not due to haemolytic reaction, the infusion may be continued slowly after administration of ephedrine, antihistamines, and an analgesic. If symptoms have not settled in 30 minutes, the infusion is discontinued.

Allergic

This reaction occurs later, and apart from the usual features of pyrexia and rigors, there is urticaria, oedema of the face and neck, and perhaps dyspnoea and cyanosis. The infusion is stopped and again an antihistamine drug and ephedrine is given, together with hydrocortisone.

Overload and Citrate Intoxication

These are both rare in obstetric practice.

Viral Agents

Viral hepatitis is causing increasing concern. Apart from its greater incidence, it is now appreciated that anicteric hepatitis occurs 3–4 times as frequently as the icteric form. Other agents such as *cytomegalovirus* may also be present and ideally should be screened for when a blood transfusion is given to a pregnant woman or her baby.

UNUSUAL SEQUELAE OF OBSTETRICAL HAEMORRHAGE AND SHOCK

Sheehan Syndrome

Sheehan, a pathologist in England, reported in 1937 that there was often necrosis of the anterior lobe (and rarely the posterior lobe) of the pituitary gland in women who had died after labours complicated by severe haemorrhage and shock. The majority of patients had had postpartum haemorrhage, but in others there was antepartum haemorrhage, shock associated with dystocia, long labours, Caesarean section, or eclampsia. It was postulated that as a result of the shock there was a spasm of the vessels supplying the pituitary gland. More recently, it is believed that the cause in many patients is disseminated intravascular coagulation, causing infarction of the gland.

The earliest clinical manifestation is failure of lactation, then amenorrhoea; gradual diminution in function of the thyroid and adrenal glands follows (lethargy, loss of libido, feeling of cold, decrease in hair growth, coarsening of skin and hair). If the condition is not recognized and treated, serious ill-health or death may occur.

Asherman Syndrome

This condition may be confused with the above in the early stages because in both there is amenorrhoea and infertility following major haemorrhage in pregnancy. In this condition, however, the defect is localized to the uterus and results from over-vigorous curettage of the uterine cavity in an attempt to control bleeding. This removes the lining, the walls adhere and the cavity is obliterated to a greater or lesser degree. Some 50% of such patients are infertile, and of those who become pregnant, only a minority achieve an uncomplicated term delivery.

CARDIAC ARREST

Definition

Cessation of effective myocardial contractions and cardiac output (no pulse or heart sounds): this is associated with loss of consciousness, respiratory arrest, dilating pupils, cyanosis, pallor, and finally death if the condition is not quickly relieved.

Incidence

Approximately 1 in 5,000–10,000 pregnancies.

Aetiology

(i) *Hypoxia during anaesthesia.* The induction phase of the anaesthetic is most dangerous because the patient is often paralysed and has lost protection of her airway (cough reflex), and such problems as *difficulties in intubation* and aspiration of gastric contents (Mendelson syndrome) may cause severe hypoxia. (ii) *Electrolyte imbalance/acidosis.* This may result from a progressive deterioration in condition or a more acute episode (e.g. hypercapnia). (iii) *Rapid blood loss or shock.* (iv) *Drug or anaesthetic overdose or anaphylaxis.* (v) *Vagal inhibition,* especially in association with inversion of the uterus or manipulation of the uterus at Caesarean section. (vi) *Amniotic fluid embolism* which can occur during labour or at elective Caesarean section due to raised intrauterine pressure during extraction of the baby — acting in combination with *preexisting cardiac disease* or with one or more of the above factors. (vii) *Air embolism.* (viii) *Cerebrovascular accident.*

Diagnosis

Rapid diagnosis is crucial to survival without neurological damage. Sudden loss of consciousness (or deepening of the unconscious state plus profound *hypotension* if under anaesthesia), absence of heart beat and pulsation in a major vessel (e.g. carotid), together with *cyanosis* and/or *pallor*, and loss of *pupillary reflex* immediately suggest the diagnosis. *Cardiac irregularities* may precede the arrest. If the patient is undergoing an operative procedure, it may be observed that the blood is ominously '*dark*'; the *jugular venous pressure* rises and, if being monitored, *ECG changes* appear.

Management

Prevention. The high risk patient should be recognized — cardiac disease, patient taking cardioreactive drugs, prolonged labour, general anaesthesia especially if the patient is vomiting or likely to be difficult to intubate (short, thick-necked individual). The general condition of the patient should be maintained — particularly where biochemical imbalance is likely (vomiting, diabetes mellitus, prolonged labour). It is important that *anaemia* should be recognized and corrected, particularly before *anaesthesia*. The latter is rarely a simple procedure in the pregnant woman — *the problem of regurgitation of stomach contents and consequent pulmonary and aspiration is everpresent.*

Treatment. *Do not panic* but always call for *assistance.* The following immediate measures should be applied, singly or together. (i) *Cease any drug or anaesthetic* that is being administered. (ii) *Establish an airway* — give positive pressure 100% oxygen by mask or tube (if available); mouth to mouth resuscitation may be necessary; the artificial ventilation is maintained at a rate of 12–20/minute. (iii) *Establish circulation.* Thump the sternum vigorously twice (this may convert asystole to sinus rhythm). *External cardiac massage*: the patient is placed on a firm flat surface and heart emptying is effected by intermittent depression of the lower sternum — using both hands the sternum is depressed 2–4 cm at a rate of 60 times per minute. (iv) *Elevation of the legs* will aid venous return and assist cardiac filling and circulatory efficiency. (v) An *electrocardiogram* is taken as soon as available: external *defibrillation* may be required. (vi) Supportive therapy may include *intravenous crystalloids*, colloids or blood; bicarbonate (100 ml 4.2% initially, then 100 ml every 10 minutes) to combat acidosis; drugs to combat cardiac arrhythmia or to stimulate cardiac action (*adrenaline 1 ml of 1 in 10,000* repeated if blood pressure is not maintained and followed by an intravenous infusion (1 ml of 1 in 1,000 added to 1 litre of Hartmann solution)). Other drugs that may be used include *cardiac stimulants* (isoprenaline, calcium, dopamine), *antiarrhythmics* (lignocaine, procainamide) and *potassium*.

Appropriate *intravenous fluids* are administered: blood and/or volume expanding solution, colloid for anaphylaxis; care is necessary not to overload the circulation, especially if the patient has preexisting cardiac disease.

After normal cardiac action has returned, the patient is shifted to an *intensive care unit* or special area for further cardiac monitoring ± respiratory support. If the patient is undergoing surgery, a decision must be made as to the most appropriate course of action to terminate the procedure.

In the newborn, the usual cause of arrest is hypoxia. After nasopharyngeal aspiration, the lungs are ventilated with oxygen by mask. Sufficient pressure is then applied by 2 fingers over the midsternum to depress it 2 cm, the rate being 120–130/minute.

NORMAL PUERPERIUM

chapter fifty-five

Anatomy and Physiology: Normal Care

OVERVIEW

The puerperium is the *6-week period* which follows childbirth. The latter is the climax of the months of pregnancy, whereas the puerperium is the beginning of many challenges (emotional and physical) and adjustments to be faced by the new parents.

The puerperium is a time of *return to normal of the mother's altered anatomy, physiology, and biochemistry*; a time of *nurturing the baby* through the difficult early weeks of life (including, hopefully, the establishment of breast feeding); and finally, a time of *family bonding* — thus begins the ultimate phase of human emotional maturity.

One of the major phenomena of the puerperium is *involution*. No longer necessary, the enlarged uterus, the expanded blood volume, and the many other body systems supporting the baby and placenta return to their prepregnancy state. These adjustments are made relatively quickly — thus there is a major *diuresis* in the early postpartum days as the unwanted body fluid is excreted by the kidneys, and a *negative nitrogen balance* as the catabolism of unwanted tissue occurs. Because of its occurrence in the great majority of subjects, *emotional instability* in the first postpartum week can be looked on as a natural process related to the stresses of parturition and the subsequent physiological and biochemical upheavals. Some changes take longer to return to normal, e.g. the relaxation of smooth muscle; abnormalities of function in relation to this progressively improve — constipation; varices of the legs, vulva, and anal canal; hydronephrosis and hydroureter. The *last major function to return* is *ovulation* and *menstruation*.

Because of the rapid changes which are taking place in the early puerperium, it is necessary that a close watch be kept on the vital signs of both mother and baby. Thereafter, the processes of normal involution should be followed.

The *advantages of breast feeding* will have been explained to the parents and one of the major endeavours of the medical attendant should be to make this work, despite the difficulties which may arise. The mothering role takes time and it is vital that emotional support, information, counselling, and physical care be given unstintingly.

Patients requiring greater attention include those with poor social support (e.g. single mothers), physical and emotional health problems, and low nurturance levels.

Physical discomforts may upset the patient — afterpains, haemorrhoids, breast engorgement, episiotomy and Caesarean section wounds, and explanations regarding the cause and temporary nature of these should be given and analgesia provided. *Adequate sleep and rest are important.*

Before the mother is discharged from hospital with her baby, the medical team should be confident that she has the information and support necessary for the difficult weeks ahead.

DEFINITION

The puerperium (Latin *puer* = infant) is the period from completion of the third stage of labour to the return to the normal nonpregnant physiological state, 6 weeks later.

PHYSIOLOGICAL CHANGES

Reproductive Tract

Essentially there is a return to the nonpregnant condition, this process being known as *invol-* ution. The main cause of the change is withdrawal of the hormones elaborated by the placenta (especially oestrogen and progesterone). Apart from lactation, there is a reversal from tissue build-up (anabolism) to tissue breakdown (catabolism). Thus, the unwanted bulk of muscle fibres in the uterus is diminished; the weight drops from 1,000 to 60 g and the size from $15 \times 12 \times 8$ cm to $8 \times 6 \times 4$ cm in the space of 6–8 weeks.

The uterine fundus is about at umbilical level on the day after birth, 4–5 finger-breadths above the symphysis pubis on day 5, and by 10–14 days the fundus is no longer palpable abdominally (figure 55.1). The placental site soon becomes only a small depression and the uterine lining is restored. The passage of dissolved blood clot and then exudate (serum and lymph) from the uterus is responsible for the lochial discharge. This is initially red (*lochia rubra*) and lasts for 2–14 days, then serous (*lochia serosa*, 5–20 days), and finally white (*lochia alba*, 4–8 weeks). Although persistence of lochia rubra beyond the 14th day may be seen with no evidence of other abnormality, it should raise suspicion of retained products or other pathology.

The cervix may be seen at the introitus if the uterine supports are weak, or if undue traction has been exerted on the cord or placenta, or the fundus has been pushed down forcibly from above during the third stage. It is floppy, bluish-red, and there is often a lateral laceration. It involutes along with the uterus, so that by 2–3 weeks the internal os is closed. Similar changes occur in the vagina.

Because of the liberal blood supply of the area, *episiotomy and laceration repairs* have usually healed in 5–7 days.

The abdominal wall and perineal muscles regain their tone after several weeks; the rectus muscles may, however, remain separated in the midline (diastasis recti) (colour plate 75).

Breasts. Enlargement of the breasts occurs gradually throughout pregnancy under the influence of oestrogen (duct system) and progesterone (alveoli), with the assistance of

Figure 55.1 Rate of diminution of fundal height during the puerperium. By day 10–14 the uterus is impalpable abdominally in the absence of retained placental tissue or membranes, endometritis, and fibromyomas, all of which delay involution.

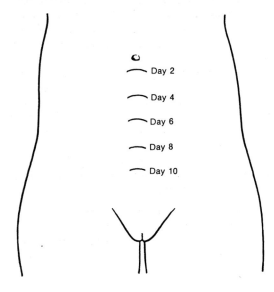

somato-mammotrophin (also called human placental lactogen — HPL), these hormones all being secreted by the placenta. With the sharp drop in hormone levels after birth, it is probable that the inhibition of the lactogenic hormone, *prolactin* (from the hypothalamus-pituitary gland) is released and milk secretion occurs. Initially, the secretion is thick and yellow and is called *colostrum*. It contains little or no casein, about 15% lactalbumin and lactoglobulin, a high percentage of fat, and is also rich in antibodies. This process is accompanied by *vascular engorgement* for the first 2–4 days, and this is usually more marked in primiparas. The main stimulus to further secretion is *suckling*, which acts by emptying the lactiferous ducts.

The stimulation of the nipple and areola also causes a 'let-down' of milk as a result of nervous impulses passing to the posterior lobe of the pituitary gland, causing the release of oxytocin which contracts the *myoepithelial* cells lining the lactiferous ducts and sinuses (figure 60.1). (A further role of oxytocin is that of facilitating uterine involution — the patient often notices uterine cramps ('afterpains') at this time). The breasts often feel hard and lumpy in the first few days as a result of both rapid filling of glandular elements and vascular engorgement. The process of lactation is considered more fully in Chapter 60.

Ovulation occurs in a minority of patients who are breast feeding, although this is very unusual before the 10th week. If lactation is suppressed, the first ovulation usually occurs within 7–10 weeks.

The Blood

The blood volume returns to nonpregnant levels and there is reduction in flow to the heart, kidneys, etc, but an increase to the breasts because of the demands of lactation. The excess water is eliminated through the kidneys in the first few days of the puerperium. The general appearance of the patient often changes markedly as a result of this fluid loss, particularly in those with pre-eclampsia or eclampsia (colour plates 9 and 10). There is a return to normal of the red and white blood cell numbers. *The blood becomes more coagulable* due to liberation of clotting factors and a decrease in fluidity of the plasma (*increased viscosity*).

Renal Tract

The *diuresis* resulting from the body's loss of fluid early in the puerperium has been mentioned. This sometimes coincides in the first 12–24 hours with an inability of the patient to void (usually as a result of perineal injuries, oedema, bruising of the urethra and bladder neck, and bedpan difficulty), and *bladder distension* may result, requiring catheterization. *Lactosuria* is present during the early phase of lactation, and the glycosuria of pregnancy disappears. Small amounts of protein may be present in the urine for the first 72 hours. The dilatation of the renal pelvis and ureters (physiological hydronephrosis and hydroureter — figure 37.1) slowly decreases over the ensuing 4–6 weeks.

Gastrointestinal Tract

The patient is quite thirsty in the early puerperium. Apart from the diuresis, there has usually been a greater or lesser degree of dehydration in labour, and perspiration is greater, both sensible and insensible. The gastrointestinal tract gradually regains its normal absorptive and contractile function. Constipation is common for 3–4 days as a result of dehydration, low oral intake, lack of tone, and sometimes reflex inhibition of defaecation by a painful perineum. After Caesarean section, intravenous fluids should be continued until bowel sounds are normal; too early feeding of the mother may result in a troublesome ileus.

Psychological State

There is frequently an *emotional lability* (swing of mood) in the puerperium, especially in the first week (about 80%). The joy and sense of achievement after delivery is often followed in a few days by depression or melancholia, usually with fits of crying (*postpregnancy blues*). This is seen as a reaction to the physical and mental stress of childbirth, together with the marked readjustments in fluid and electrolyte balance, the breakdown of tissue components, and the alteration in hormone levels (withdrawal of oestrogen and progesterone). A deeper depression is seen in 5%, and a frank psychosis in about 0.3% (see Chapter 28).

MANAGEMENT

Immediate

The patient is kept in the labour ward until *vital signs are stable*, the blood pressure is satisfactory (below 150/90 if prior hypertension or pre-eclampsia; above 100/60 if prior haemorrhage or shock), bleeding has ceased, and there are no other abnormalities needing close observation. During this time, the mother should be allowed to cuddle the baby, and if she intends to breast-feed, a short period of suckling is of mutual benefit. Fluids according to choice are provided. Visitors are limited to the husband and immediate relatives (parents, other children, siblings).

After Transfer to the Postnatal Ward

Observations

Vital signs. Temperature and pulse rate are often raised for some hours after delivery, with a gradual return to normal; the respiratory rate is little altered. Abnormal changes may reflect disorders associated with labour complications (e.g. haemorrhage) or new pathology (e.g. puerperal sepsis). Observations are made 4-hourly for 24–28 hours then twice daily, unless abnormal (temperature 38°C (100°F or over) or pulse rate 90/min). If the blood pressure is elevated, it should be checked at least 4-hourly initially, then twice daily.

The *uterine fundus* is palpated and perhaps measured, and a check is made that the patient is emptying her bladder adequately. The colour and amount of the *lochia* should be recorded; frank blood loss should be reported. Inspection of the *breasts* will reveal early signs of nipple cracking or inflammation and abnormal engorgement. A check of the *legs* should be made for deep vein thrombosis — tenderness in the thigh or calf, swelling, or temperature difference.

The *mental state* of the mother should be noted and signs of depression or instability reported. The cleanliness and healing of the *episiotomy* or any lacerations should be checked.

General Measures

Diet. Unless the patient is recovering from an operation (Caesarean section) she will be able to tolerate the usual ward diet which should be high in protein and vitamins. Adequate fluids are also important.

Hygiene. Swabdowns of the perineum are necessary every 4–6 hours when the patient has an episiotomy or an indwelling catheter, until she is ambulant and showering. An *infrared lamp* to the perineum is soothing and hastens healing, particularly if there is an episiotomy wound which is soggy or infected. It is used routinely twice daily for the first 48 hours when the patient has an episiotomy, unless she has a haematoma or swollen wound, when *ice packs* are used. The lamp is also used after *salt baths* which are given when the perineal wound is moist, infected or tender. Vulval pads, if used, should be changed when soiled and also after vulval toilet or bathing.

Pain relief. Measures may range from an aspirin mixture to morphine or omnopon, depending on the antecedent history (e.g. episiotomy, Caesarean section). Strong analgesics are rarely required after 48 hours. *Afterpains* are caused by strong *uterine contractions*, which are in turn caused by *oxytocin* liberated from the pituitary gland in response to suckling; they are more common and stronger in *multiparas*. The reason for these should be explained to the mother; occasionally analgesia (e.g. aspirin) is required. Uterine cramps may also be caused by retained pieces of placenta or membranes. Sitz baths and a heat lamp help to relieve the pain of episiotomy and speed healing.

Sleep. As a result of strangeness of surroundings, thoughts or worries about the baby or home, discomfort of the perineal repair, ward noise, etc, the mother may find sleep difficult. The attendant should ensure that discomforts and anxieties are handled appropriately, and if necessary a hypnotic should be prescribed as a temporary measure since the mother is unlikely to cope adequately if she has a significant sleep deficit; furthermore, this may be the forerunner of serious psychological decompensation.

Visitors. Only the husband or close relative should be allowed for the first 48–72 hours. Thereafter, screening is necessary to exclude those with infections.

Physiotherapy. Deep breathing, together with abdominal, pelvic floor and leg exercises, should be encouraged to prevent thromboembolism and also chest complications, particularly if general anaesthesia has been used. Such exercises should be continued daily, until examination is carried out at the postnatal visit. The patient is encouraged to get out of bed on the second day (*early ambulation*) and to go to the toilet and bathroom.

Bladder. The bladder may become overdistended early in the puerperium as a result of urethral bruising, reflex inhibition from perineal or abdominal wounds, or temporary paralysis following epidural analgesia. If simple measures fail, *careful catheterization under aseptic conditions* should be carried out; if residual urine is high (more than 90 ml), the catheter should be left in place for 24 hours. The mother should be warned that there will be a *diuresis* postpartum so that she will not be concerned by the frequent trips to the toilet. All women catheterized during or after labour should have a mid-stream urine specimen sent for laboratory study 2 days later.

Bowels. Usually the bowels will have opened by the third day. If not, aperients (milk of magnesia or senna tablets) and stool softeners (Coloxyl, Agarol) are advisable. This may be followed by a suppository or small enema if constipation persists. If there has been a tear involving the rectum, a low residue diet is usually ordered for 6–7 days until healing has occurred. *Haemorrhoids* may be troublesome (figure 57.1) and can be relieved by astringent preparations (cold compresses of witch hazel or magnesium sulphate) together with suppositories given at night.

Emotional support. The attendant should remember the patient's tendency to emotional lability in the first week of the puerperium and should be careful when making remarks about her progress or that of the baby, since these remarks are often magnified out of all proportion by the mother. The nurse must adopt a supporting and sympathetic role, and refrain from criticism. She must do her best to allay the patient's worries and fears and give encouragement in the early, sometimes difficult days of establishment of breast feeding.

Breasts. Routine care of the breasts includes cleansing before and after each feeding and perhaps the use of an emollient cream, such as lanolin or a proprietary preparation. If *expression* is necessary, it may be effected either manually or by means of a breast pump (premature or frail babies, or abnormalities of the nipple, such as inversion or fissuring). A check should be made to see that the mother has a good supporting bra. *Cracked nipples* are additionally treated by heat lamp, an antibiotic ointment, and tincture of benzoin.

If lactation is to be suppressed, a 14-day course of *bromocriptine* tablets (2.5 mg bd) may be given; some give no medication and rely on the cessation of lactation in the absence of breast stimulation. Active treatment lessens engorgement and discomfort, but is expensive.

Education. The mother should receive full instructions concerning the care of the baby — the articles of clothing and bedding required, bathing, hygiene, technique of breast or bottle feeding, causes of crying after feeding, care of the umbilicus and buttocks, napkin management, normal and abnormal stools, amount of sleep desirable, weighing and weight gain, and the significance of such things as withdrawal vaginal bleeding, breast enlargement, birth marks, and physiological jaundice.

She usually wishes to be reassured about the baby's normality and progress with feedings and weighings.

There are a number of other subjects that may arise: infant feeding problems (excess crying, vomiting, wind and colic, failure to suck well or gain weight, abnormal bowel motions and sore buttocks) (Chapters 60 and 61), resumption of sex relations (see below), family planning (Chapter 56), visits to maternal and child welfare centres, and *maternal health worries* (sore nipples, sore or inflamed breasts, abnormal vaginal bleeding or discharge, pelvic pain, urinary difficulties).

Postpartum sexuality. Since there may be significant changes to sexual functioning in relation to childbirth and subsequent child care, this subject should be discussed with the mother before discharge from hospital. The following topics form a useful framework.

(a) *Sexual feelings and response.* In the first 2 months, the sexual response is often slower and less intense. This may be related to a transfer of emotional interest to the baby, *hormonal changes* (low sex steroids, high prolactin), *poorer vaginal lubrication*, and general *fatigue*. Some couples will notice significant vaginal laxity; for others, the episiotomy repair will provide a more acceptable fit.

(b) *Resumption of intercourse.* If the perineum is intact, coitus is often resumed within 2–3 weeks. With an episiotomy or repair of a perineal tear, there may be discomfort for 4–8 weeks or even longer. Mothers who are breast feeding tend to initiate intercourse earlier, although breast tenderness and milk loss at orgasm are minor problems.

The mother is given an appointment for *postnatal review* 4–6 weeks after she leaves hospital; the *baby* should also attend if conditions such as nystagmus, birth marks, umbilical or inguinal hernias have been noticed. The mother is advised to continue taking *iron tablets* for 2–3 months, especially if there has been a postpartum haemorrhage or she is breast feeding. Although lochia rubra usually ceases during the second postpartum week, some patients bleed intermittently for 6–8 weeks, and because of this have difficulty recognizing when menstruation has returned. *These patients require a haemoglobin estimation*; if the bleeding is heavy, *curettage* is performed to diagnose causes such as retained placental tissue or (rarely) choriocarcinoma (colour plate 40) (Chapter 54). If there has been a suturing of the perineum (episiotomy, tear), instructions are given concerning its further care (including mirror inspection). The value of continuing perineal and pelvic floor exercises is stressed.

If the patient has been troubled by *haemorrhoids* after delivery, these should be checked at the time of hospital discharge; if not resolved, dietary advice (adequate fluid and fibre intake), Sitz baths, local preparations, and rest periods are advised — if *rectal bleeding* persists, investigation to exclude a large bowel tumour is indicated (sigmoidoscopy, barium enema). A laxative may be required if *constipation* persists in spite of dietary measures.

The patient is encouraged to report any difficulties arising between hospital discharge and the 6-week postnatal check. Telephone checks, home visits, group sessions, lay group help (e.g. Nursing Mothers' (or similar) Association) can all help the new family during this difficult period.

Postnatal Visit

A *history* is taken of the progress of the mother and baby since leaving hospital and reports of visits to health care personnel noted. The attendant should be aware of the many stresses experienced by the mother at this time — lack of sleep and round the clock feeding, cleaning, and dressing the baby; to this may be added general household chores and, if there are other children, messes, noise and inadvertent destruction, and finally, social isolation. Such mothers may need temporary support, periods of total free time for relaxation, exercise etc. *Major psychiatric problems may surface after the mother has left hospital*, and she should be questioned as to how well she is coping, what family support is available, whether she is feeling depressed, how much her partner is involved in the parenting and how well he is coping in this role.

General and pelvic examinations are performed to exclude the presence of hypertension, vaginitis, cervical erosion, uterovaginal prolapse or subinvolution of the uterus. During speculum examination a *cervical smear* is taken to exclude subclinical carcinoma if this investigation has not been performed within 12 months or minor changes had been reported at the previous examination. Advice is given regarding the possibility of temporary *dyspareunia* if the patient has had an episiotomy or vaginal laceration, or *decreased sexual responsiveness*. Vaginal dryness is common because of the inhibitory effect of prolactin on the ovaries if the woman is breast feeding; a suitable lubricative jelly should be prescribed. *Backache* is a significant problem in at least 10% of patients and is usually due to *sacroiliac strain* from poor posture and loss of tone in abdominal musculature. Usually exercises are helpful; occasionally referral to a physiotherapist is necessary and if pain persists other *orthopaedic causes* must be excluded.

A decision is reached regarding the method of *birth control* to be practised (Chapter 56). Other health measures (e.g. vaccinations for the baby) should be discussed.

chapter fifty-six

Family Planning

OVERVIEW

The ability of a couple to restrict the number of their offspring to their particular ideal number has been termed '*the fifth freedom*' by Sir Theodore Fox, a former editor of the Lancet. This ideal number is quite an individual matter, ranging from none to perhaps 10 or more. It depends on such factors as strength of parental instinct, career, and socioeconomic circumstances.

The *benefits of family planning* are many. The health and well-being of the family unit are maintained at an optimal level, since the parents are able to cope — physically, psychologically, and economically. The children have a better opportunity of developing in a loving and contented atmosphere.

Contraception after childbirth requires special consideration, since traditional methods are often unsuitable. If the woman is *fully breast feeding*, she is unlikely to ovulate because of the inhibition of ovulation by the elevated levels of prolactin (nature's contraceptive).

Protection can usually be assumed in any woman up to 6 weeks after third trimester delivery, since ovulation does not resume before this time.

The method chosen will depend on a number of factors — whether or not the patient is breast feeding, whether the couple wish to space or terminate childbearing, individual preference etc. The subject of contraception should be discussed before the patient leaves hospital and implemented at the 6-week postnatal visit where relevant.

For the woman who is breast feeding, the usual recommendation is a low dose, *progestin-only pill* ('minipill'). For the remainder, the first choice is usually a combined oral contraceptive. The *intrauterine device* is satisfactory but preferably should be left until uterine involution is complete (6 weeks). The *cervical mucus method* is often difficult in view of the prolactin-induced atrophic changes in the vagina and the uncertainty of the return of ovulation. If a *diaphragm* has been used in the past, it is likely that a larger size will be necessary, and hence the patient should be remeasured to determine this.

In the past, *sterilization* of the female was often carried out in the early puerperium. This is now done only if the indication is pressing; experience has shown that change of mind is not unusual, even in the weeks or months after delivery, and, furthermore, the child may be lost as a result of cot death or other cause. The introduction of laparascopic sterilization, with reduction of time spent in hospital, has lessened the advantage of postpartum sterilization. The latter also has the disadvantages of a higher failure rate and increased incidences of complications due to haemorrhage and infection.

BASIC CONCEPTS

Fertility is defined as the ability to conceive and bear children — the opposite of infertility. The fertile period of life lies between puberty and menopause, although fertility at each extreme is much reduced because of the lessened frequency of ovulation. After the age of 15, the woman's fertility rapidly reaches a peak and only after the age of 30 is there a decline, which is more rapid after the age of 40. The male is capable of fertilization at or soon after puberty; the decline occurs later than in the female and is much more gradual.

Fertility in the menstrual cycle. With isolated intercourse, the chance of becoming pregnant depends mostly on the stage of the menstrual cycle. *The most fertile period is when ovulation occurs (at about the 12th–14th day in a 28-day cycle).* When 3 or 4 days on each side of this are exceeded, the risk of pregnancy is markedly diminished.

Theoretical points of attack. (i) *Preventing ovulation* by inhibiting the hypothalamus or pituitary gland, or the ovary itself; (ii) *preventing the sperm from gaining access to the cervix*, and thus to the uterus and Fallopian tube; (iii) *occluding the genital ducts* in the female or male; (iv) *preventing implantation* of the fertilized ovum in the uterus.

Features of the ideal contraceptive method.

The most desirable feature is of course efficacy, i.e. *prevention of pregnancy*. This is usually measured by the *Pearl index* (number of unwanted pregnancies during 100 years of exposure). This is obviously a concept for assessing efficacy in large numbers of women over shorter periods of time; a more recent concept is the *life-table method*. The Pearl index for women in the natural state is about 40–50; that is, if they were blessed to live for 100 fertile years they would have a child about every second year if no precautions were taken. A very reliable method will have an index less than 1; a satisfactory index is 2–3; tolerable, 4–5; figures above this are usually unacceptable. *Safety* is also important; freedom from unwanted children is little cheer if it is accompanied by ill-health or even the risk of death. *Side-effects* are related to the factor of safety, but the majority are annoying rather than dangerous. Tolerance to the side-effects of family planning methods varies just as does tolerance to other annoyances. Acceptance of the trouble involved in applying the method is again an individual matter; what is a hardly-noticed routine for some is intolerable to others.

Other factors influencing choice.

Probably the most important factor is *which partner is the most responsible*, or worried about the consequences. Often the process is agreeably worked out after full discussion. The responsible partner may change with time, influencing factors being age, added maturity, number of children, and chance events such as discussions with friends. *Cultural and religious* factors are often strong determinants of choice; methods which flourish in some societies, languish in others. *Governments* may influence methods by the nature of decrees. The *frequency of intercourse* is related to the libido (sex drive) of the couple (itself partly related to age), the duration of marriage, and other factors such as occupational mobility of one of the partners; the range is from several times per day to once a month or less. It would be tedious to apply a mechanical method in the former case, and hardly necessary to use a method giving all-the-time protection in the latter. *Cost* does have some relation to method choice, since some methods are significantly more expensive than others.

The Next Child

After delivery, there are a number of considerations which may influence the couple in relation to having another child and which should be mentioned in counselling.

Coping. Coping strengths differ as do other demands which the mother may have (e.g. education, work). Some couples will have low personal resources, poor stress resistance, and little or no family/social support.

Enjoying parenthood. Some parents wish to have 2–3 years when they can devote most of their time to the baby and enjoy the early growing up period. In addition, studies suggest that a minimum period between the birth of siblings is necessary for their emotional and intellectual development.

Adverse childbirth experience. The pregnancy, labour, or postnatal experience may have been unusually taxing or unpleasant, and the couple may be put off having another child until the mental and physical scars have healed.

Economic factors. Here, long-term factors are particularly important, and involve such considerations as housing, schooling, employment, and way of life. Close spacing of children enhances companionship and sharing, but conflicts are more common and personal development of each sibling perhaps less.

METHODS IN COMMON USE
(table 56.1)

Generally, methods may be classified as either temporary or permanent. In the former, protection lasts only as long as the method is applied and fertility is restored when it is discontinued.

Hormonal Preparations

The oral hormone contraceptive preparations are the most reliable of the available methods. There are several types in use.

(i) *Combined.* These contain 30–50 μg of oestrogen — either ethinyl oestradiol or mestranol (a closely related substance) and a progestin (there are a variety of these according to the manufacturing company). There are usually 21 active tablets, the remainder being an inert substance such as lactose. Withdrawal bleeding takes place within 2–3 days of finishing the active tablets; because ovulation is inhibited, menstruation is usually painless.

The *efficacy is very high* (Pearl index 0.2–1.5 according to the reliability of the patient and other less well understood factors such as absorption of the contents of the pill from the bowel). The major side-effect is *thromboembolism*, which can be fatal. With present dosages, this is excessively rare, but such preparations are

TABLE 56.1   PRESENT-DAY CONTRACEPTION METHODS

	Hormone Methods				
Class	Combined oral contraceptive	Minipill	Depot Progestin injection	Progestin-containing vaginal ring or subcutaneous implant	Postcoital contraceptive
Composition	Oestrogen + progestogen	Progestogen	Esterified progestogens, e.g. medroxy progesterone acetate	Silastic device containing polymerized steroids	Oestrogen, progestin or oestrogen/ progestin
Stage of development	Routine use	Routine use	Routine use in many countries	Routine use in many countries	Routine use
Advantages	Very high reliability	Very high safety	Long-term activity 3–6 months	Long-term activity	High reliability if given in sufficient dose for 3–5 days after coitus
Major disadvantages	A very small proportion of users prone to serious sequelae (e.g. thrombo-embolic disease)	Less reliable than the combined OC (failure rate 2–5/100 woman years). Irregular bleeding in some women	Irregular bleeding in some users; irregular release of hormone	Irregular bleeding in some users; irregular release of hormone	High doses needed — oestrogens produce nausea and vomiting; irregular bleeding
How it works	Inhibition of ovulation due to hormone effect on hypothalmo-pituitary axis	Direct action on cervical mucus, rendering it impenetrable to sperms; partial inhibition of ovulation	Inhibition of ovulation by feedback mechanism plus direct action on cervical mucus	Inhibition of ovulation by feedback mechanism plus direct action on cervical mucus	Direct action on uterus preventing nidation

contraindicated in subjects at risk. There are many minor side-effects, again less common with the more recent low dose preparations. *Oestrogen effects* include nausea, cervical mucus discharge, chloasma, fluid retention, blood pressure rise, change in blood hormone levels (thyroid, adrenal), and in the function of some organs such as the liver. Progesterone effects are few and less significant.

In the *triphasic formula*, lower hormone doses are involved.

Many side-effects of preparations such as these are difficult to evaluate (fatigue, nervousness, headache, insomnia, nausea, cramps), since they may also appear when the patient is taking control (placebo) tablets with no active ingredient.

(ii) *Progestin only*. The progesterone is usually given in tablet form which is taken continuously (minipill). Several synthetic progestins are used

(norethisterone 350 μg; norgestrel, lynestrenol etc). This method is somewhat less efficacious — Pearl index 1.5–5.0 — but is acceptable and safe. The major drawback is cycle irregularity in some patients. Other formulations include injections of a depot preparation every 3–6 months, or incorporation of the progestin in a vaginal ring, intrauterine device, or subcutaneous silastic capsule.

Compounds containing oestrogen act mainly by *inhibiting the release of follicle stimulating hormone (FSH)* from the pituitary gland by negative feedback inhibition (prevention of the secretion of FSH releasing factor from the hypothalamus). Progesterone compounds *inhibit luteinizing hormone (LH)* in the same way, but this is not consistent with the low dosages now used, and they probably act mainly by *changing the character of the mucus* in the cervical canal to make it thicker and impermeable to sperms.

Intrauterine devices			Spermicides & barrier	Rhythm
Medicated IUD	Copper IUDS	Inert plastic IUDS	Spermicides	
Plastic IUD with a progestogen incorporated into the polymer	Plastic 'T' or '7' shape with copper wire wound around the stem; oval 'multiload'	Plastic coil or loop	Foams, jellies, cream, vaginal suppositories, and aerosols containing spermicidal detergents or metals	
Clinical trials	Routine use	Routine use	Routine use	Routine use
Enables a small device to be used which should lower discontinuance rate due to pain	Higher success rate than inert devices; also can use a smaller device	Safe if correctly inserted; semipermanent once in place	Safe	No medication required
Ectopic pregnancy, limited life of the device; higher cost	Ectopic pregnancy; needs replacement after approximately 2–4 yr as copper is released at 50 μg/day	Ectopic pregnancy	Should be used in conjunction with barrier methods (cap or condom) during unsafe period	Less reliable; psychological difficulties
Local action on uterus and cervical mucus rendering sperm penetration difficult; foreign body effect	May be associated with cationic antagonism of zinc in certain local enzyme systems; foreign body effect	Foreign body effect (infiltration of polymorphonuclear leucocytes into endometrial cavity preventing blastocyst development)	Antispermatozoal effect; immobilizes sperm in the ejaculate	Avoidance of coitus at time of probable ovulation

Preparations of this type are useful if the patient is breast feeding (since milk yield is unaffected), and also if oestrogen side-effects are troublesome or expected.

Occasionally (about 1% of users) the inhibition of the hypothalamus/pituitary system may be prolonged after the pill has been stopped, sometimes for several years. Ovulation stimulating drugs may then be required if further children are desired.

(iii) *Morning after.* If unprotected intercourse has taken place, pregnancy may be prevented if a 5-day course of ethinyl oestradiol, 0.05 mg bd is taken. More recently, postcoital progestins (e.g. norgestrel) have proved effective.

Intrauterine Devices

It has been known for a very long time that foreign objects placed in the uterus prevent pregnancy. However, it has only been in the past few decades that design and material improvements have allowed widespread application.

There are probably several modes of action of the device — it may affect transport of the (fertilized) ovum in the tube, act directly on the uterine wall by abrasion or prevention of decidual formation, create an unfavourable environment because of its composition (especially metallic content of copper and zinc), or create a hostile response in the uterus (phagocytic cells or lysozymes).

The intrauterine device is associated with a lower mortality rate (1–10 deaths per million women-years of use) than the oral contraceptive, but its morbidity is higher. It is also less effective as a contraceptive, does not prevent pregnancies outside the uterus, and may further compromise fertility by causing low grade *pelvic inflammation*.

Types of compound. There are many, but at present 4 are mainly used (figures 56.1 and 56.2). (i) *Copper Multiload.* This is a plastic device with a central, copper-bearing plastic stem to which are attached 2 flexible plastic arms. Of currently used devices, it most nearly conforms to the 'ideal' configuration. It has relatively low symptom, removal, expulsion, and pregnancy rates. (ii) *Copper 7 or T.* The shape of the device is as suggested by the name. There is again a winding of fine copper wound on the central stem. These devices are somewhat less effective (Pearl index 1.5–2.5), but are easy to insert in the uterus because of their narrower shape. (iii) *Plastic loop.* This is still in common use. It is relatively easy to manufacture in large quantities and is thus the cheapest of the 3 devices. All of the above devices have a nylon 'tail' projecting through the cervix which enables the patient to check that the device has not been expelled; the tail also facilitates removal, when or if this becomes necessary. It has the disadvantage that it can act as a *path for ascending infection.* (iv) *Grafenberg ring.* This was introduced in 1928. The German silver composition contributed to its efficacy, because other metallic substances, including copper, were mixed with the silver. This is still used in some centres. It

lies entirely within the uterus and requires special instruments for insertion and removal.

There is a variety of other devices in use throughout the world, but most are variations on the above types. The recent trend is to incorporate different types of medication in the device to enhance the contraceptive effect (progesterone) or reduce side-effects.

Insertion of the IUD (figure 56.2). No anaesthesia is usually required, although in nulliparous or apprehensive patients, local analgesia to the cervix is given either by paracervical block (5 ml of 0.5% lignocaine to each lateral fornix) or topical analgesia to the endocervix. *Even though the risk of uterine infection is small, many regard nulliparity as a contraindication to IUD insertion.*

If the insertion is not being performed after abortion or delivery, the time chosen is usually the last day of the menstrual cycle — the os is relatively open and the patient is certainly not pregnant. A *careful vaginal examination* is made to assess the size and position of the uterus, and to detect any pathology present. *Sterile precautions* are used. The patient is in the dorsal position and a self-retaining bivalve speculum is used to expose the cervix. The vagina and cervix

Figure 56.1 A. The popular mechanical contraceptive devices: measuring rings, rubber diaphragm, and condom; the 3 sizes of Grafenberg ring together with special forked inserter and hooked remover; Lippes loop with special introducer. **B.** Close-up view of copper-T, copper-7, multiload-Cu 250 and Lippes loop. Both the copper-T and copper-7 carry 200 sq mm of exposed electrolytic copper wire coiled around the vertical limb. The multiload-Cu 250 provides a minimal copper surface area of 263 sq mm and is the preferred IUD: no push-rod is required to insert this device, since the fins on the transverse arms catch against the endometrium as the introducer is withdrawn; average results after 1 year: pregnancy rate 1%, expulsion rate 10%, removal rate 9% and continuation rate 80%.

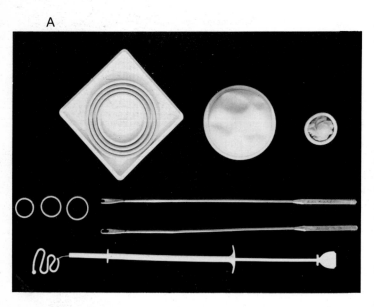

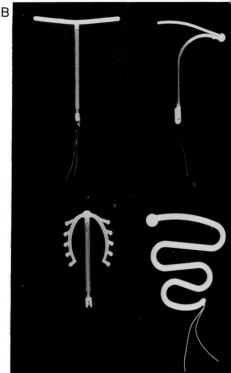

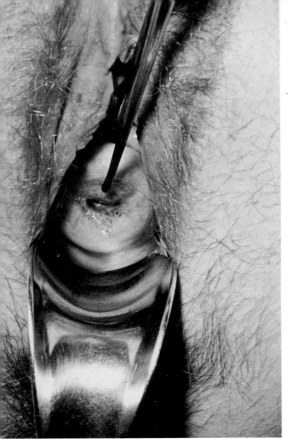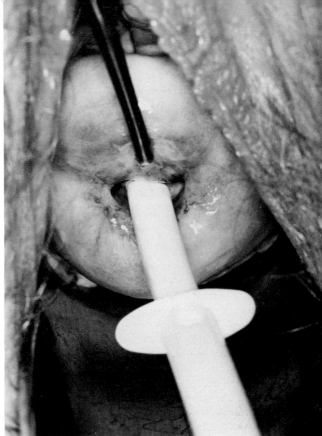

A   B

Figure 56.2 Insertion of a Lippes loop. **A.** The cervix is exposed with a Sims speculum and steadied by a tenaculum with the patient in the dorsal or left lateral position. Some operators prefer a bivalve speculum. Note that this patient has a 'sharkmouth' cervix due to bilateral tears during delivery. **B.** With the loop pulled into the inserter, the latter is introduced into the uterus which had already been sounded for depth and direction, after bimanual palpation had checked that the uterus was in the anteverted position. **C.** Position of inserter, with only bulbous tip of the loop showing, illustrated in a fresh hysterectomy specimen, before the loop is pushed from the inserter with the push-rod. **D.** Intrauterine position of the loop after being pushed free from the inserter. The inserter is withdrawn to expose the tail which is cut as long as possible to facilitate palpation by the patient and perhaps to minimize the risk of being drawn into the uterus during coitus (orgasm) or in early pregnancy.

C   D

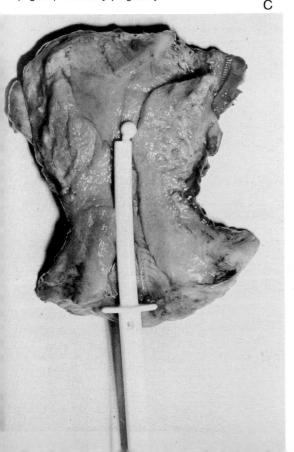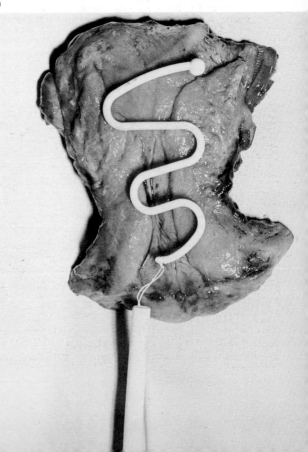

are cleansed with an antiseptic solution, the anterior lip of the cervix is grasped with a vulsellum forceps or tenaculum and a sound is gently passed into the cavity to determine its size and direction. The sterile device is then removed from its pack and inserted into the uterus. The device should lie easily in the cavity, without discomfort to the patient and the tail should project through the external os (figure 56.2).

Advantages. The major advantage is the prolonged protection without the need for daily motivation by the patient; the efficacy is less than that of the combined oral contraceptive, but superior to other methods.

Complications. These are greater than with the oral contraceptives, but are steadily being reduced with improvements in technology. (i) *Expulsion.* If unnoticed this is serious because of the high pregnancy risk. Over a period of 1 year it would occur in 5–10% of patients, and relates to such factors as relative size of uterus and device, uterine irritability, technique and time of insertion, parity, initial insertion or reinsertion, and time in the uterus. (ii) *Pregnancy.* With the newer devices this is 1.5–3%; with older devices, up to 5%. It is more common when the device has been expelled unknown to the patient. Ectopic pregnancy is not prevented and this is a major disadvantage in the younger patient desirous of more children. (iii) *Bleeding.* Usually there is an increased flow on days 3 and 4, rather than on days 1 and 2. Anaemia is thus more common. This is more likely in the early months of use and often settles down. (iv) *Pain, cramping.* Some 5–15% of patients are worried by this symptom; again, it usually settles in most patients. (v) *Infection.* Significant infection should be rare (1–2%) if insertion is not made in the presence of infection or under unsterile circumstances. It is probable that most infections are gonococcal and can be present subclinically at the time of insertion or be acquired afterwards. Many would consider that any risk of infection which results in blocked Fallopian tubes is unacceptable in single or nulliparous patients. (vi) *Uterine perforation.* This may occur, albeit rarely. When recognized, the device should be removed either with the laparoscope or by laparotomy. Obviously, the patient will not be protected if the device is not in the uterus. (vii) *Removal* is necessary in 5–10% of patients in the first year because of one or other of the above complications. If pregnancy occurs, the risk of abortion is increased (30%) and is said not to be further increased if the device is removed in early pregnancy. Deliberate removal may also follow a decision by the couple to plan another

pregnancy, or to change to another method. There is no effect on future fertility unless infection occurs. *Lactation is unaffected*, unlike the case with some of the hormonal preparations.

Recent trends include the incorporation of medications to prolong the effective life of the device (up to 10 years) and to reduce bleeding; improved size and shape to conform to the uterine configuration; improved instrumentation and insertion techniques.

Barrier Methods

Here, there is a chemical or mechanical barrier against the spermatozoa.

(i) *Progestational compounds.* These probably act by the formation of a barrier in the cervical mucus, as already discussed.

(ii) *Chemicals.* Spermicidal creams, foams, tablets or jellies may be inserted into the upper vagina before intercourse. Their efficacy varies rather widely (Pearl index 3–15), according to the sophistication of the compound and patient, and consistency of use. Like all of the barrier methods requiring active and repetitive use, the system may break down because of the 'getting carried away' effect. A vaginal applicator is used for creams and foam preparations.

(iii) *Diaphragm.* This is a moulded rubber device (figure 56.1A) which fits behind the cervix, covers it, and is tucked up behind the symphysis pubis (figure 56.3). The correct size is determined beforehand by means of a set of measuring rings which range from 50 to 90 mm (figure 56.1A). After delivery, particularly the first, it is necessary to remeasure the patient because of the stretching of the birth canal: this should be deferred until the 6-week postnatal visit when involution is complete. The patient must be taught how to insert the diaphagm by means of a model and a check made that she is able to position it correctly. The most common mistake is to place the upper end in the anterior rather than the posterior fornix, leaving the cervix uncovered. Usually, it is recommended that a spermicidal cream be used in conjunction with the diaphragm, being placed both on the dome, which will come in contact with the cervix, and around the rim. If used properly the efficacy is satisfactory (Pearl index 4–8), but the method is not suitable if further children are really not desired, or contraindicated because of medical conditions.

(iv) *Condom.* This is used by the male, repetitively each time intercourse occurs. It consists of a thin rubber sheath at the end of which is a reservoir to collect the ejaculate (figure

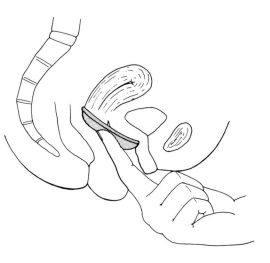

Figure 56.3 Insertion of diaphragm. The forefinger is used to check that the cervix is covered by the rubber dome.

56.1A). It may be used in conjunction with vaginal chemical methods, particularly at mid-cycle, when the risk of pregnancy is high. Whereas the diaphragm can be fitted well in advance, the condom is fitted immediately before intercourse (i.e. after erection) and disturbs the rhythm of the act to an unacceptable extent for many people. Again, if used properly, the efficacy is in the satisfactory range (Pearl index 3-6), although the method is open to a number of pitfalls if too much is asked of it.

Rhythm Methods

These are practised particularly, but not exclusively, by Roman Catholics. Essentially, the method is based on the fact that ovulation occurs on the 12th–14th day of a 28-day cycle. If a certain number of days are set aside on either side of this to allow for normal variations in the exact day of ovulation and for survival of the sperm and ovum in the birth canal, a reasonable efficacy can be achieved. The longer the period of abstinence in the middle of the cycle, the safer will be the method. Refinements consist of the patient plotting a basal body temperature graph to pin-point the ovulation day more accurately (mainly of value in retrospect since the temperature rises only after ovulation has occurred), or examining her vagina to detect 'mucus days', which indicate that oestrogen levels are high and will soon trigger ovulation (by LH release). The mucus is secreted by the cervical glands and is clear and slippery, like raw egg white. After ovulation, it again becomes thick, opaque and tacky — 'dry days'. Unfortunately, in up to 30% of women, there is no clear-cut mucus pattern or it is variable from cycle to cycle. The details of mucus observation method of Billings are shown in figure 56.4. A recent method utilizes the

detection of uteroglobin by means of a vaginal probe; this is an indirect measure of ovulation.

The only side-effects are pregnancy, and psychosexual problems related to the abstinence (which must be practised at the very time (ovulation) when nature's call to coitus is strong).

The Pearl index varies widely (4–15) according to the number of safe days set aside and the lengths to which the person is prepared to go to establish ovulation more accurately. The greatest difficulty lies in the tendency for occasional menstrual cycles to be significantly shorter or longer than average, and since these cannot be predicted in advance in patients with fairly normal cycles, failure is apt to result. Particular difficulties surround its use in the postpartum months because of the irregular return of ovulation and the atrophic condition of the vagina (prolactin effect) in breast feeding women. Vaginal infection and discharge makes identification of mucus days more difficult, as does recent intercourse. Lack of cycle regularity is more marked in the declining reproductive years when a further pregnancy is less welcome. In younger couples, particularly those with a high libido, the period of abstinence proves troublesome.

A partial rhythm method is used by some couples, whereby precautions other than abstinence (usually a barrier method), are taken at mid-cycle ± 4–5 days.

The value of a temperature chart is that the mid-cycle rise in temperature (*due to progesterone from the corpus luteum*) indicates that ovulation has occurred; hence postovulation safe days are identified. The temperature chart does not identify preovulation safe days, although it is claimed that the mucus observation method does.

Coitus Interruptus ('Withdrawal')

This is one of the most ancient methods known to man. It is best for emergency situations where precautions have either not been thought of or are not available. It is, however, usually most unsatisfactory for the female partner, whose orgasmic ability (climax) often lags behind that of the male in any case, and furthermore, it is not a particularly safe method — yet it is used as the only means of contraception in some cultures, even in developed countries where socio-economic factors are irrelevant.

Therapeutic Abortion

In this procedure, the pregnancy is terminated by medical or surgical means (figure 56.5), usually only up to the 28th week (see Chapter 18).

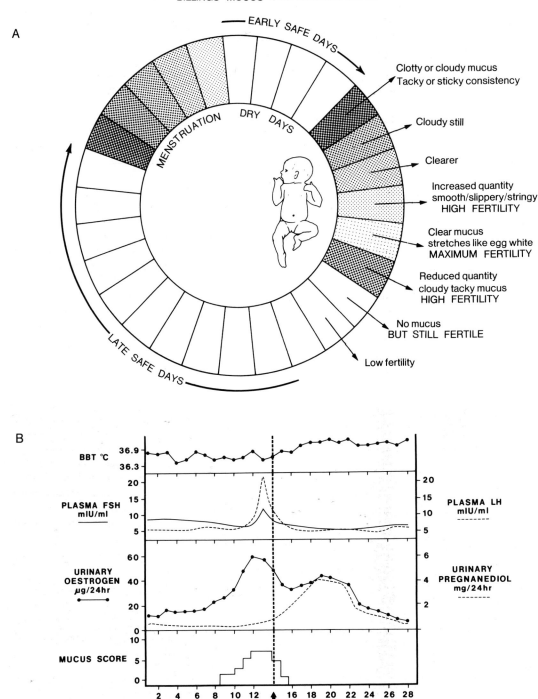

Figure 56.4 A. Billings mucus identification chart used to help patients identify the type of cervical mucus which is felt in the vagina each day. This illustration is merely a guide since the mucus consistency will not necessarily follow the exact pattern or length of days indicated here. Observation of change in mucus enables approximately 50% of women to have 6 days' warning of impending ovulation. **B.** Basal temperature, plasma follicle stimulating hormone and luteinizing hormone, urinary oestrogen and pregnanediol excretion, and cervical mucus score during the normal menstrual cycle. Time of ovulation is shown by the vertical dotted line. Cervical mucus is rated on volume and characteristics (dry sensation (1), yellow or white minimal (2), yellow or white sticky (3), cloudy becoming clear (4), thinner more stretchy (7), stretchy, lubricative clear (7), wet slippery (9)). The urinary oestrogen peak occurs 36 hours before ovulation which is triggered by the LH surge. Progesterone from the corpus luteum causes the temperature rise and also inhibits cervical mucus production and changes its characteristics. (Courtesy of Professor James Brown).

Sterilization

The procedure of sterilization is not usually regarded as reversible, although some of the methods are more 'permanent' than others.

Definition. The rendering of the male or female sterile by operative or other techniques (e.g. radiotherapy) applied to the essential organs of reproduction.

Indications. The procedure is indicated when a future pregnancy is liable to be harmful, physically or mentally. In each case a decision is reached on the basis of the age of the patient, her social and economic circumstances, the number of children she has to look after, the severity of the medical disorder, its behaviour in previous pregnancies, and its known natural course. There are many conditions that might be aggravated by pregnancy or render a woman less capable of withstanding the stress of pregnancy and child bearing.

The more important of these are as follows. (i) *Medical disorders*: hypertension, chronic renal disorders (glomerulonephritis, pyelonephritis), cardiac disease, diabetes mellitus, malignant disease, chronic pulmonary or liver disease. (ii) *Psychiatric disorders*: gross subnormality, schizophrenia, and other psychoses. (iii) *Obstetrical disorders*: previous uterine rupture or multiple Caesarean sections, thromboembolism, recurrent fetal malformation, severe rhesus iso-immunization, or hereditary disorders (haemophilia, Tay-Sachs disease, congenital blindness).

Techniques. The methods used all have one aim — prevention of successful implantation of the fertilized ovum.

(i) In the *female* hysterectomy and/or bilateral oophorectomy is 100% effective and permanent. The same result may be obtained by irradiating the ovaries. If ovarian function is destroyed, however, it may have adverse medical and psychosexual effects. Alternatively, the Fallopian tubes may be removed, or divided and ligated. A number of techniques have been described and the approach can be made either abdominally or vaginally. The modern technique is to occlude permanently the inner half of the Fallopian tube via the laparoscope (figure 56.6). The occluding device is usually a clip or small plastic ring; diathermy coagulation carries greater dangers (e.g. bowel burns) and is now less favoured. An emerging technique is the use of a fast-setting plastic introduced into the tubes via a hysteroscope.

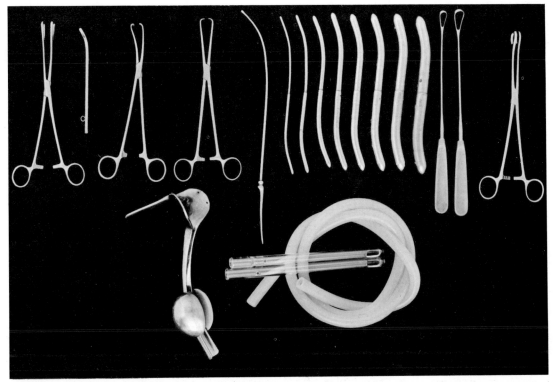

Figure 56.5 Instruments used at curettage, in order from left to right: sponge holding forceps, metal catheter, vulsellum, tenaculum, uterine sound, Hegar dilators, 2 sharp curettes and ovum forceps. Below are shown the Auvard self-retaining speculum and plastic tubing and glass cannulas used for suction curettage.

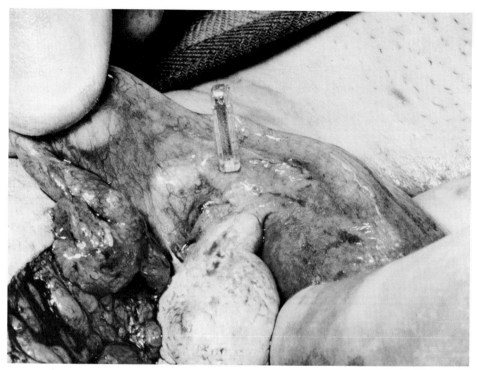

Figure 56.6 Plastic Hulka clip applied to the isthmus of the Fallopian tube. It has a metallic spring and destroys only a 3 mm length of tube. Before application of the clip, both medial and fimbrial ends of the tube are inspected to ensure that the round ligament is not mistaken for the Fallopian tube. (Courtesy of Professor John Leeton).

(ii) In the *male*, the operation of vasectomy is performed. In this technique a small incision is made under local analgesia at the base of the scrotum and the vas is identified, separated, divided and ligated. Additional procedures are often carried out to make the operation more reliable — excision of a segment of the vas, fulguration, interposition of a fascial barrier etc.

PRECAUTIONS AND COUNSELLING

Since ensuing sterility may be irreversible, careful evaluation of the couple is important. The possibility of after-effects, both psychological and sexual, should also be considered. The following are essential prerequisites. (i) Both husband and wife understand completely the nature of the operation and the likelihood of its effects being permanent. (ii) A consent form containing this information must be signed by the patient and preferably also by her husband. (iii) The possibility of pregnancy in some cases, albeit slight, should be explained. (iv) Preferably, the marriage should be stable and both parents satisfied with their present number of children. Medical, psychological, sexual, and social problems should be discussed, and any misconceptions in either partner rectified. The patient also should be reassured that sexual activity will not be affected.

DISORDERS OF THE PUERPERIUM

chapter fifty-seven

Puerperal Disorders

OVERVIEW

The puerperium places many demands on the new mother. There may be a *carry-over of problems from the pregnancy and labour*, and after delivery, *further major adaptations* are necessary.

Both genital and urinary tracts are prone to *infection* because of the nature of the labour process; defences are breached because of loss of tissue integrity, trauma, blood loss, examination and instrumentation, and the possibility of nonviable tissue remaining to provide a nidus for bacterial growth. With major operative procedures (e.g. Caesarean section), other avenues of infection are opened. The other common site of infection is the breast (mastitis, colour plate 97). An accurate diagnosis can usually be made after careful history and examination. This is of some importance, since the major infecting organisms are usually different in each site and if antibiotic therapy is required, it should be appropriate. The effect of the antibiotic on the newborn should be remembered if the patient is breast feeding.

The complex support system built up over the 9 months of pregnancy to support the fetus undergoes rapid involution in the puerperium. There is a dramatic loss of body water and this is followed by catabolic products of uterine muscle breakdown; the levels of hormones produced by the placenta fall precipitously. There is, in addition, the changes necessary for lactation, particularly the liberation of oxytocin and prolactin and beginning of milk synthesis. Against this background, it is not surprising that some destabilization occurs to the mother's psyche. A disorder affecting the majority of women is *dysphoria or mood lability* — 'the blues'. It usually resolves by the end of the first week, but if not handled properly can lead to much distress. A more serious psychological upset is termed *temporary postnatal depression*. *Frank psychosis* — e.g. schizophrenia, is very uncommon (incidence 1 in 300).

Thromboembolic disorders are more likely to occur in the puerperium because of the amount of tissue breakdown (thromboplastin generation), increased platelet activity, and haemoconcentration. These conditions are considered in Chapter 34.

In the *miscellaneous conditions*, there are 2 problems related to the delivery — *haemorrhoids*, which result from general venous engorgement (progesterone effect) exacerbated by pushing during the second stage, and *anal fissure* which follows overdistension of the anal margin as the head is crowning. Both conditions cause major discomfort and inhibit proper bowel function.

Because there is some diminution of immune activity during pregnancy, *autoimmune disorders* tend to ameliorate; during the puerperium, *exacerbations* are common, and these should be anticipated. An allied problem concerns the *drug treatment* of certain diseases (e.g. diabetes mellitus with insulin, epilepsy with anticonvulsants); significant modifications are often required (usually *dose reduction*) in the puerperium because of different metabolic conditions.

The very important problems that may arise in relation to *infant feeding* are considered in Chapters 60 and 61.

PUERPERAL INFECTION

The *definition* of a puerperal infection is when the *temperature reaches 38°C* (100.4°F) *on any 2 of the first 14 days after abortion or delivery.*

The general aspects of infection have been discussed in Chapter 27. It was emphasized that the puerperal patient is more liable to a number of infections — genital tract, Caesarean wound, breast, renal tract, chest.

GENITAL TRACT

Incidence
After vaginal delivery, 1–3%; after Caesarean section, 10–50% depending on a number of factors, such as social class, time of membrane rupture and length of labour.

Aetiology
(i) There is a loss of protective epithelial cover at the placental site. (ii) Pieces of *placental tissue*, membrane or clot may be retained and serve as a nidus of infection. (iii) There is usually some bruising or trauma to the tissues. (iv) Blood loss and/or preexisting anaemia lowers resistance. (v) *Premature rupture of the membranes* may allow ascent of the normally-present vaginal pathogens and/or such organisms may be introduced in the course of examinations or operations.

Source of Infection
(i) *Lower genital tract.* A variety of organisms particularly *anaerobes* (streptococci and bacteroides), can be cultured from the genital tract of all pregnant women and some of these are potentially pathogenic. Normally, the patient is living in a balanced state with these, but when there is trauma, blood loss and the presence of dead tissue the balance is upset and the bacteria gain control. (ii) *Bowel.* Typically E. coli, other Gram-negative bacilli and faecal streptococci. These may already be inhabitants of the vagina as a result of poor perineal or sexual hygiene, or may have been transmitted at the time of labour or delivery by inadequate attention to antisepsis and asepsis. (iii) *Attendants.* The most serious pathogens are the staphylococci and haemolytic streptococci. These are usually carried on the hands or in the nasopharynx. (iv) *Environment.* Hospitals always have a reservoir of pathogenic organisms from other infected patients and these are carried in the air as dust and droplet particles or on utensils and linen. A wide variety of organisms is carried in this way. (v) The husband or consort may be the reservoir for specific infections such as gonorrhoea or syphilis.

Diagnosis, Clinical Features and Treatment

(a) *Lower genital tract.* Here the infection is usually visible, the most obvious example being an *infected episiotomy wound*; the classical features of reddening, swelling and tenderness are present. If the infection is marked or has occurred in a haematoma, breakdown of the wound may occur. Gonorrhoea is often unsuspected, its detection usually resulting from a positive culture being obtained from the baby's eyes (gonococcal conjunctivitis).

Management. (i) A swab is taken for microbiological study (smears and culture). (ii) Frequent bathing with antiseptic solution or hypertonic saline packs. (iii) Heat lamp every 2–4 hours (see Chapter 55). (iv) Antibiotics if infection produces constitutional effects (fever, malaise). (v) An infected haematoma may require evacuation. (vi) Analgesics if required. (vii) Breakdown of an episiotomy or laceration may require suture when the infection is controlled.

(b) *Upper genital tract.* Often a distinction is made between infections in the uterus, adnexa (Fallopian tubes and ovaries), and parametrium. In reality, the clinical signs depend largely on the virulence of the organism and the mother's defence reaction to it. In more severe infections, there may be spread *upward* to the Fallopian tubes and ovaries (salpingo-oophoritis), *outward* to the parametrial cellular tissue (*parametritis* or *cellulitis*), and, if more extensive, the peritoneal cavity will be involved (pelvic or general *peritonitis*). *Septic pelvic thrombophlebitis* is an occasional sequel; if acute, pain may be marked and an acute abdominal process simulated.

In virtually all cases, the infection begins in the uterus (*endometritis*) in relation to the raw placental wound site, or in pieces of remaining dead tissue (placenta, membranes, clot).

Clinical presentation. Typically, there will be a history of premature rupture of membranes, a long labour, temperature elevation in labour, operative interference, incomplete secundines, and perhaps anaemia. Before the rise of temperature is detected, there may be constitutional effects (malaise, anorexia, headache, aches and pains, sweating or chills), an offensive, heavy vaginal loss, or lower abdominal discomfort or pain. In other patients the only complaint may be that she is feeling hot and flushed. If the infection is virulent or more widespread, particularly involving the pelvic peritoneum, or abscesses have formed, the patient will obviously be quite ill. The temperature is usually 39–40°C, the pulse rate 110–140/minute, and the above-mentioned constitutional and local symptoms will be more marked. Rarely, the infection may be life-threatening. If *general peritonitis* is present, there will be ileus, abdominal pain, tenderness and rigidity, with vomiting, dehydration and prostration, together with sweating and chills. *Septicaemia* and *pyaemia* represent an invasion of the blood stream by organisms or purulent material. Constitutional symptoms predominate and if the organism is virulent, collapse (septic shock) and death may follow.

Management. Prophylaxis. (i) Adequate diet and *prevention of anaemia.* (ii) Prevention of exhaustion, dehydration, and starvation during labour. (iii) Strict observance of the rules of antisepsis and asepsis, especially if multiple vaginal examinations are performed in labour. (iv) Gentleness in all operative obstetric procedures. (v) Minimizing blood loss, and prompt *blood transfusion* when indicated. (vi) Intervention during labour only when indicated. (vii) Removal of retained products and clot which are a nidus for infection.

Active treatment. (i) Elicit a careful history of predisposing factors. (ii) An examination is made by speculum; high *vaginal* and/or *uterine swabs* are taken for microscopy and culture, the *genital tract is inspected*, and the nature of the discharge is noted. A *bimanual examination* is carried out to check the uterus, adnexa, cellular tissues and pelvic peritoneum for swelling and/or tenderness. A *blood culture* is taken if the infection is severe or septicaemia is suspected. *Septic ovarian vein thrombosis* is a difficult entity to diagnose: a tender, linear, adnexal-lumbar mass is suggestive and confirmation is usually possible with computed tomography. (iii) *Chemotherapy* is commenced — the drug selected usually depends on individual or collective (hospital) choice. The main factor affecting this, as well as the dose and route of administration, will be the severity of the infection. The agent(s) must have the minimum capability of controlling anaerobes (both bacilli and cocci) and faecal flora; an additional agent may be required for resistant staphylococci etc. Recent studies suggest that mycoplasma infections are not uncommon in the puerperium; tetracycline is necessary for such infections. (iv) Observations of pulse, blood pressure and temperature, fluid balance, vaginal discharge, and constitutional effects will be necessary. (v) Intravenous fluids are given if the infection is serious, or if the patient is nauseated or vomiting. (vi) Pain is relieved by *analgesic* drugs; *psychological support* is also important,

since the pain and fever tend to make the patient upset and/or depressed.

If *septic shock* is present, special measures such as *central venous pressure monitoring*, drugs to support the heart and circulation, and adrenal cortical hormone may be necessary. Where abscess formation has occurred, surgical drainage will usually be needed.

BREAST INFECTION (see Chapter 60)

URINARY TRACT INFECTION

Renal tract infection is one of the commoner causes of puerperal pyrexia.

Aetiology

The changes in the renal tract in pregnancy have been described in Chapter 37. There is a stasis of urine and during labour and delivery there is often bruising of the base of the bladder and urethra. The lower urethra is always colonized by bacteria and the *catheterization* which may be required during labour or the third stage unavoidably introduces such microorganisms into the bladder. Stasis of bladder urine is increased by difficulties in voiding after delivery as a result of hypotonicity of the bladder, oedema of the bladder neck or reflex inhibition from the pain of perineal or abdominal wounds. Often in such patients there is an abnormally high residual urine after voiding. Patients with preexisting *bacteriuria* are more likely to have an overt infection. An association with conduction analgesia (e.g. epidural) has been reported.

Clinical Features and Management

The features are little different from those already described when such infections occur during pregnancy (Chapter 37). A history will often be as described above and this, together with loin pain, frequency and dysuria, and the presence of turbid urine, will suggest the diagnosis.

A *mid-stream urine specimen*, obtained preferably after cleansing of the vulva by the nurse and placement of a sterile tampon in the lower vagina, is sent for microscopy and culture. Occasionally, a catheter may need to be passed if the patient is unable to void, or a high residual urine is suspected.

Specific and supportive treatment is similar to that outlined in Chapter 37. If there has been a previous episode of infection, an appointment for an *intravenous pyelogram* should be made at the postnatal visit, when the physiological hydronephrosis has disappeared.

PUERPERAL PSYCHIATRIC DISTURBANCES

Traditionally, psychiatric disturbances in the puerperium have been subdivided into 3 categories: (i) *mild*: dysphoria (the 'blues'); (ii) *moderate*: temporary postnatal depression; and (iii) *severe*: psychosis — usually depression or schizoaffective disorder.

General aspects of psychiatric disturbance in pregnancy have been considered in Chapter 28. It is important to be aware of the nature of puerperal mental illness, since failure to foresee and treat promptly causes unnecessary suffering to the mother and perhaps major damage to the family unit. The conditions listed represent clinical entities, but deterioration to the more serious condition may occur.

DYSPHORIA

Incidence
Postpartum blues occurs in 20–80% of patients, depending on sociocultural conditions and the criteria used for diagnosis.

Aetiology
The exact basis is unknown, but probably is largely *metabolic* because of its fairly regular occurrence. Major postpartum changes include an abrupt fall in the levels of adrenocortical hormone and placental hormones (oestrogen, progesterone, HCG, HPL), a significant loss of body water, and breakdown of unwanted tissue (e.g. uterine muscle).

Clinical Features
The upset usually occurs between the 4th and 10th postpartum days. Characteristic features are lability of mood (*euphoria*, *tearfulness*), anxiety, some confusion and forgetfulness, irritability, tiredness, inability to relax, and insomnia).

Management
Counselling. Early in the puerperium, the subject of postpartum mood change should be brought to the patient's attention, and its frequent occurrence, likely metabolic-endocrine basis, and temporary nature emphasized. If the patient is tense and anxious, a mild tranquilliser may be ordered and a sedative at night if insomnia is troublesome.

TEMPORARY DEPRESSION

Incidence is 5–10%.

Aetiology
This may represent a mixed group — some patients having a *depression* related to disappointments arising out of the pregnancy (failure of labour, baby of the wrong sex or with poor/malformed features) or other life aspects, others having an *endogenous depression* of a mild-moderate nature. In either case, a *careful history* should alert the attendant to the possibility.

Clinical Features
Significant features in the *history* include *past psychiatric difficulties*, major menstrual problems, poor relationship to parents or husband/partner, lack of social contacts/help, major problems in the pregnancy, labour, or puerperium (including a sick or premature child, feeding difficulty).

The problem may surface at any time from delivery up to 3–4 months. Prominent symptoms include fatigue, insomnia, withdrawal from relationships with the baby and husband, loss of confidence, psychomotor slowing with inability to organize herself or surroundings.

Management
As with temporary dysphoria, much can be done by *anticipation* of the problem. *This is important since the conditions may not become apparent until after the mother has left hospital.*

It should be part of postpartum care to ascertain risk factors which might indicate later psychiatric decompensation — e.g. previous history, pregnancy and puerperal problems, ongoing difficulties, and adequacy of home environment and support. This should again be looked at critically at the 6-week postnatal visit. The mother often does not have sufficient insight into her changed behaviour, and if a problem is suspected, discussions should be held with close relatives.

The basic treatment involves *counselling* — insight into the problem, her personality and relationships, coping strategies with reorientation towards the maternal role (schedule rearrangement, extra help), adequate rest, sleep, and exercise; *bonding facilitation* if this is fragile or poorly developed (if necessary in a special family and behavioural therapy unit); and *referral for specialist care* if the need arises.

PSYCHOSIS

Major psychotic disorder is rare in pregnancy (2–3 in 1,000); about a third of these occur in the puerperium. The vast majority are depressive in nature. Psychiatric referral is necessary in this group (Chapter 28). Decisions must be made regarding antipsychotic drug therapy, hospital admission, care of the baby and whether breast feeding is safe or otherwise.

OTHER DISORDERS

A number of other conditions may affect the puerperal patient. *Preexisting problems*, either *obstetrical* (e.g. preeclampsia/eclampsia, ante-partum haemorrhage, sepsis, operative delivery) or *medical* (e.g. hypertension, diabetes mellitus, epilepsy, asthma) will require special care. These, and conditions such as postpartum haem-orrhage and shock, urinary tract and postanaes-thetic complications are discussed in separate chapters.

THROMBOEMBOLISM

Thrombophlebitis is the term given to the inflammatory reaction, usually in superficial leg veins, which is associated with thrombosis of those veins (colour plate 76). *Phlebothrombosis* is a similar process, but inflammation is mini-mal, the deeper veins tend to be involved and the clot tends to break off and form emboli which travel to the lung (pulmonary embolism), often with serious or even fatal results. A thromboem-bolic process should be suspected in any puer-peral patient with an otherwise undiagnosed low-grade fever. The condition is discussed in Chap-ter 34.

MISCELLANEOUS DISORDERS

Haemorrhoids

It has been mentioned that there is a general dilatation of veins during pregnancy resulting from the placental hormone, progesterone. Engorgement of the haemorrhoidal plexus of veins at the lower end of the bowel is further aggravated by the tendency of the pregnant patient to be *constipated* and thus to strain when emptying her bowels, and more particularly by the pushing required during the second stage of labour and delivery (figure 57.1). Bleeding, pro-lapse, and thrombosis are common compli-cations. *Bleeding*, although common during pregnancy, is rarely serious and settles in the puerperium. *Prolapse* should be corrected immediately, preferably after bed rest in the head down position and application of cold and astringent packs. If reduction is not successful, the anal ring should be dilated to 4 fingers under local analgesia (lignocaine 1%, 10–15 ml; hyalu-ronidase 150 u). *Thrombosis* is always painful and requires analgesics and surgical attention.

Prophylaxis is important — prevention of con-stipation by adequate fluids and a diet rich in

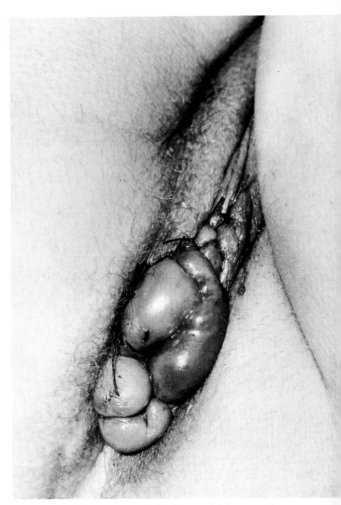

Figure 57.1 Oedematous painful haemorrhoids are not uncommon in the puerperium and occur within 24 hours of delivery. A too-tightly sutured episiotomy incision contrib-uted to the swelling in this patient. The prolapsed haemor-rhoids should be replaced after episiotomy repair and after bowel actions.

fibre foods such as bran and cereals; replacement of prolapsed haemorrhoids promptly; and avoid-ance of fruitless, pushing-down efforts in the second stage of labour if progress is very slow.

Anal Fissure

This is a small fissured ulcer at the mucocutaneous junction of the anus. It usually arises at delivery when the skin splits posteriorly and is reopened each time the bowels are used. A vicious circle is often produced — bowel actions are withheld because of the pain and the stool hardens causing greater damage when the bowel eventually opens. The fissure is seen if the patient is asked to bear down and the buttocks are separated gently.

Treatment consists in the application of a

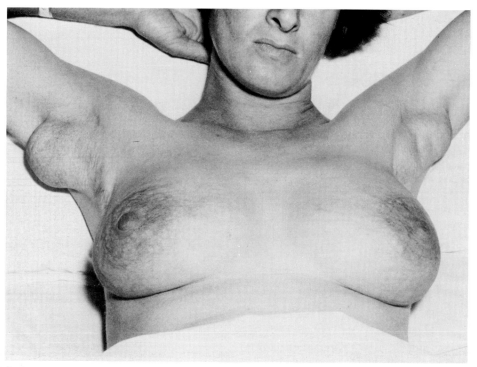

Figure 57.2 Bilateral axillary accessory breasts in a lactating multipara 3 days after delivery. The lumps were a nuisance and an embarrassment and were therefore ultimately excised.

compound *suppository* or ointment containing an analgesic, astringent, and antiseptic. If this, together with a laxative, does not result in cure, anal *dilatation* may be required as already described.

NONINFLAMMATORY BREAST DISORDERS

Accessory Breast Tissue

Accessory breast tissue is usually in the axilla and has no connection with the breast and usually has no separate nipple (figure 57.2 and colour plate 96). The lump is often quite uncomfortable for a number of days, while lactation becomes established, but then resolves and causes minimal discomfort in about 50% of cases, even although lactation continues. The condition occurs in all degrees (incidence about 1–2%) and surprisingly may not be recognized during the first or second lactation. In many patients the lumps are an embarrassment and excision is required (figure 57.2 and colour plate 96).

Breast Engorgement, Inverted and Cracked Nippled — see Chapter 60

THE NEWBORN

chapter fifty-eight

Fetal Respiration and Circulation

OVERVIEW

Improved knowledge of the fetal respiratory and circulatory systems and of the changes that occur at birth have given a better understanding of the transition from an aquatic to an air breathing existence. This in turn has provided an appreciation of the *persistent fetal circulation syndrome*, the *intrapulmonary and extrapulmonary shunting of blood associated with pulmonary pathology* and the problems associated with *failure of the ductus arteriosus to close*. Techniques have been developed to lower the pulmonary blood pressure and to close the ductus arteriosus, thus *reducing the need for assisted ventilation* and lessening the risks due to the complications of this aggressive method of management.

INTRODUCTION

The fetus is totally dependent on the placenta for nutrition and respiration. This organ is more than an annoying afterbirth to be recovered, inspected, weighed, measured and disposed of by the midwife. With the fetus and mother it is part of a biological trinity, each component requiring an independent developmental normality, but sharing an interactive dependence. The lungs of the fetus do not function as organs of gas exchange and, until the placenta becomes separated at birth, they are airless structures with a minimal blood flow (estimated at 4% of the cardiac output). How different is the situation following the first breath when the total cardiac flow must circulate through the now airfilled and vascular organs. The fetus is dramatically transformed from an aquatic existence to dependence on the oxygenated atmosphere. Failure to adjust to these changes leads quickly to disability or death. *The first minutes of life are truly more hazardous and associated with a greater mortality than any other period in an individual's existence.* An appreciation of the cardiorespiratory physiology of the fetus and newborn infant is important in understanding a number of related disorders of the newborn.

THE FETAL CIRCULATION

Oxygenated blood from the placenta traverses the umbilical vein and then passes to the inferior vena cava through the *ductus venosus* (figure 58.1). Dye studies reveal that the flow of this highly oxygenated blood (65% saturation) from the inferior vena cava enters the heart and splits on the free edge of the interatrial septum. The major part passes directly through the *foramen ovale* into the left atrium, thence via the left ventricle into the aorta and the arteries of the head and arms. It must be remembered that the oxygen saturation of the blood is less in the fetus than in the adult and fetal function is adapted to this situation. The smaller stream flows with the oxygen reduced blood from the superior vena cava into the right ventricle. From here it passes into the pulmonary artery and is then directed

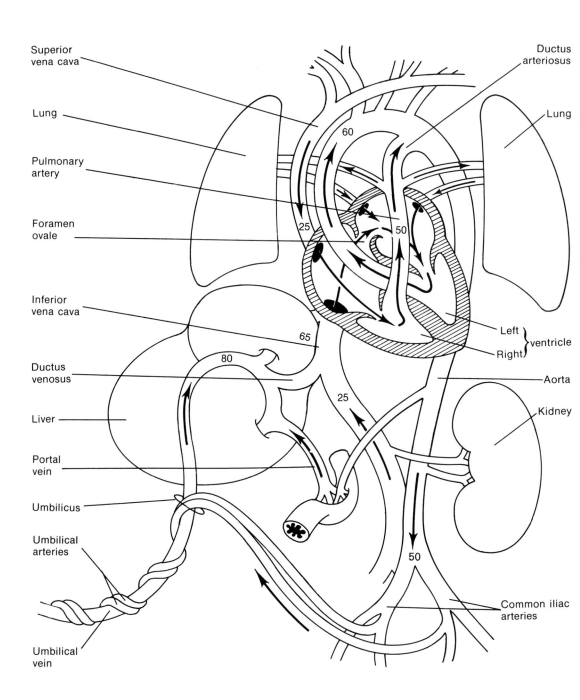

Figure 58.1 The fetal circulation. The figures give the oxygen saturation of the blood at the points indicated.

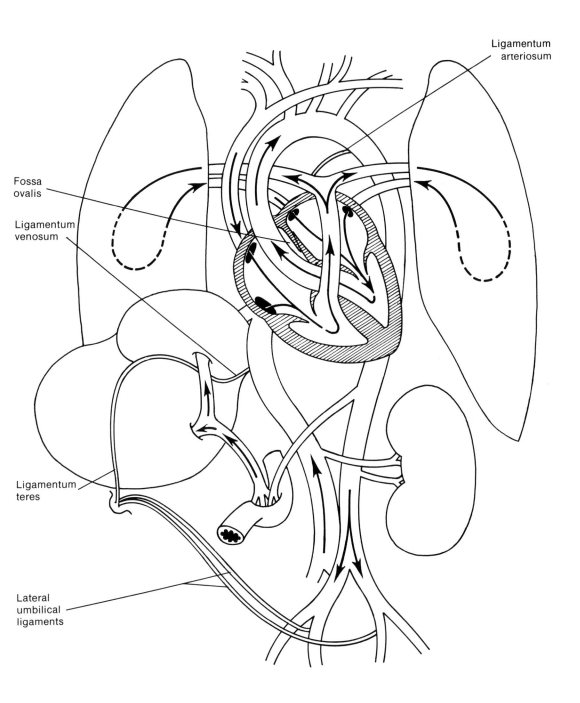

Ligamentum
arteriosum

Fossa
ovalis

Ligamentum
venosum

Ligamentum
teres

Lateral
umbilical
ligaments

Figure 58.2 Normal circulation in the newborn infant. The closed channels of fetal life are named.

through the *ductus arteriosus* to the aorta rather than into the lungs. This less oxygenated blood (50% saturation) is carried in the descending aorta to the lower body. The umbilical arteries are given off from the iliac arteries (which arise at the bifurcation of the abdominal aorta) and pass in the abdominal wall to emerge at the umbilicus and then run in a spiralling fashion about the umbilical vein in the loose mucoid supporting tissue in the umbilical cord (Wharton jelly); they complete the fetal vascular circuit by ramifying into smaller tributaries in the placental substance.

The passage to the placenta of oxygen-reduced blood in the umbilical arteries and the emergence of oxygen-enriched blood in the umbilical vein is equivalent to the pulmonary circulation in the adult.

CIRCULATORY CHANGES AFTER BIRTH

After birth, profound circulatory changes occur, although the final adjustments may continue for days to weeks. The first change is expansion of the lungs with air, and with the first breaths the pulmonary vessels are uncoiled, resulting in a great reduction in resistance to the flow of blood to the lungs; this in turn causes a fall in pressure on the right side of the heart and closure of the foramen ovale. At the same time there is *a rise of oxygen tension* in the blood. This results in *release of prostaglandins* which cause contraction of smooth muscle in the wall of the ductus arteriosus and effect its physiological closure. The 'adult' circulatory pattern (figure 58.2) is thereby attained.

CIRCULATORY PROBLEMS AFTER BIRTH

Persistent Fetal Circulation Syndrome

Here the lungs are normal, but the pressure in the pulmonary vascular tree fails to drop as expected. The result is an infant who continues to shunt blood away from the lungs and hence is cyanotic and dyspnoeic, although the chest radiograph appears normal. Associated with this syndrome are *hyperviscosity, hypocalcaemia, hypomagnesaemia, acidosis, hypoxia, infection, shock* and a *genetic tendency*. The principles of management are to determine the causal or associated factor and treat it. If the pulmonary blood pressure still fails to drop, drugs which exert a pulmonary hypotensive effect such as tolazoline hydrochloride (Priscol) and sodium nitroprusside dihydrate (Nipride) can be used.

Shunting Associated with Primary Pulmonary Pathology

Primary pulmonary pathology (e.g. hyaline membrane disease, pneumonia and meconium aspiration) results in either failure of the pulmonary vessels to uncoil and/or constriction of the uncoiled vessels, with resultant failure of the pulmonary vascular pressure to fall or return of the pressure to the high levels typical of fetal life. The result is shunting of blood through the foramen ovale away from the lungs. Hypoxaemia occurs, with reopening of the ductus arteriosus and worsening of the shunt. The result is a severely cyanotic and hypoxic infant. Treatment is aimed primarily at correction of the respiratory problem and secondarily at correction of the pulmonary hypertension.

chapter fifty-nine

Routine Care and Common Disorders

OVERVIEW

The 2 major aims of routine care are firstly to minimize adverse influences on the infant and secondly to detect problems sufficiently early to prevent them becoming serious. *Routine care must be continually evaluated* to eliminate deleterious techniques and improve existing ones. An example of this is the change in attitude towards *selection of infants for transfer to special care nurseries.* Separation of the mother from the infant may lead to *difficulties in bonding,* and appreciation of this problem has resulted in more strict criteria being established for admission of infants to a special care nursery. The modern aim is to keep newborn infants with their mothers whenever possible (colour plates 98–100).

The *neonatal period* is defined as the *first 28 days* of life. Death is not uncommon during this period, but it should be noted that the first 24 hours claims 75% of those who die. In this chapter the requirements for and care of an apparently normal infant are considered in detail. It is important to anticipate the birth of an infant who may require more specialized care at/or after birth. Resuscitation is discussed in Chapter 62 (Asphyxia and Resuscitation) and care of the high risk infant after birth is discussed in Chapter 64 (Immaturity and Disorders of Growth).

CARE BEFORE BIRTH

The condition of the fetus is assessed regularly during labour by noting the regularity or otherwise of the *fetal heart rate* and the presence or absence of *meconium-stained liquor.* In certain cases, *cardiotocographic* recording of the fetal heart and *fetal scalp blood pH* measurement are carried out by the obstetrician.

Preparations are made to receive the baby. (i) A warmed cot with *warm* blanket wraps in the delivery room. (ii) The suction apparatus is tested and availability of suitable sterile suction catheters is confirmed. (iii) The oxygen source and flowmeter are tested and availability of suitable sterile catheters capable of administering intranasal oxygen is confirmed (a 6 French gauge catheter with 1 end hole is recommended). (iv) *A resuscitation trolley* or area should be near at hand with equipment and drugs necessary for intensive resuscitative procedures if needed (figure 47.3). Items required include an infant laryngoscope and blade, endotracheal tubes ranging in size from 2.5–4.0, endotracheal introducers and connections, positive pressure oxygen apparatus (e.g. Penlon bag, or usual anaesthetic bag and mask), syringes, needles, ampoules of sterile 50% glucose, 8.7% sodium bicarbonate, naloxone hydrochloride (Narcan), vitamin K_1 (Konakion), and umbilical catheters.

A warmed blanket is at the foot of the bed with 2 labels attached. These labels bear the mother's details and are attached to the infant's wrists. These labels are shown to the mother and verified verbally with her before and after the infant's birth.

CARE AT BIRTH

In normal births, immediate nursing by the mother is beneficial for bonding (figure 59.1A), and suckling assists placental separation and delivery.

Aspiration of the mouth is performed as soon as the head is born and then the nose and eyes are wiped clean with a moist swab. After the birth is completed, the baby is held head down to allow secretions to gravitate into the pharynx which is again aspirated; *all suction should be of brief duration.*

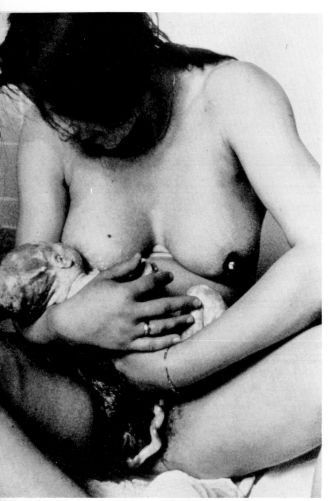

A vitamin K_1 preparation (1 mg Konakion) is injected intramuscularly and the baby is wrapped in the warmed sterile wrapper.

Identity labels are attached to the infant's wrists and these are verified with the mother before the baby is taken from the delivery room. *Footprinting* is another way of identifying a particular infant.

CARE AFTER BIRTH — LABOUR WARD

The baby is placed in a *warmed cot* on his side and a cord dressing is applied. He is covered with 2 blankets and an additional external source of heat, such as an overhead radiant heater, an electric blanket or hot water bottle (scalding of the infant's skin may occur if it is in direct contact with the hot water bottle) may be necessary.

The baby should be *observed* in the cot for *at least 1 hour* for signs of cyanosis, excessive mucus secretion, or abnormal behaviour. The *airways* are kept clear and the *umbilical stump* frequently inspected for oozing.

About 1 hour after delivery, if the infant's condition is satisfactory and his temperature is above 36°C, he is inspected, cleansed and the parameters of growth are recorded.

Figure 59.1 Examination of the fontanelle for size and tension.

A **Figure 59.1A** Mother suckling her newborn baby, having sat down after delivery in the supported squatting position (figure 42.10). Bonuses are bonding and placental separation by a naturally-induced surge of oxytocin. (Courtesy of Dr Michel Odent).

The optimal time for clamping (or tying) the cord is not known for certain. Late clamping of the cord results in an additional volume of blood reaching the infant. This may result in hyperviscosity, jaundice and cardiorespiratory, neurological and renal problems. The extra blood specifically aggravates jaundice in premature infants and in those with erythroblastosis, so early clamping of the cord is advised in such infants. In the asphyxiated infant, early clamping allows rapid transfer of the child for resuscitation purposes. After clamping the cord, it is cut and inspected to ascertain that 3 vessels are present (when 2 vessels only are present, the risk of an associated major fetal malformation is 20–25%).

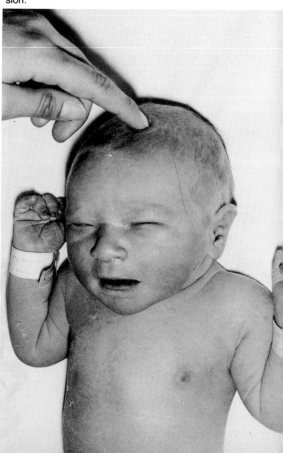

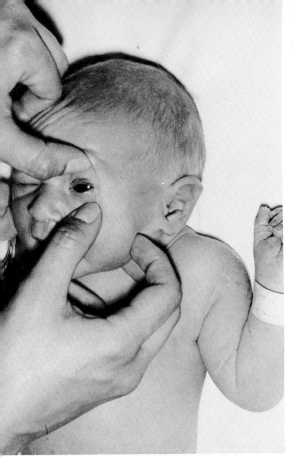

Figure 59.2 Checking that the eyes are present and normal.

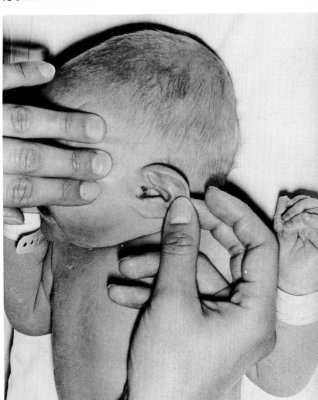

Figure 59.3 Inspection of the ears for symmetry, correct placement, absence of malformations, and patency of the canal.

Figure 59.4 Examination of the mouth to exclude cleft palate.

Figure 59.5 The apex beat must be counted for a full 60 seconds to obtain the correct rate.

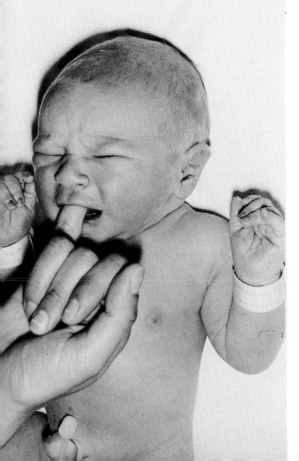

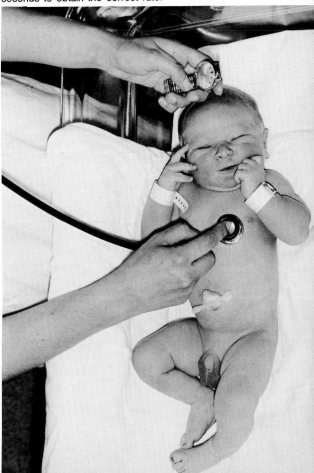

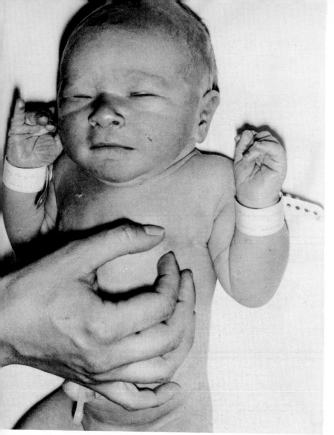

Figure 59.6 The size of the 'breast button' is helpful in estimation of the infant's maturity.

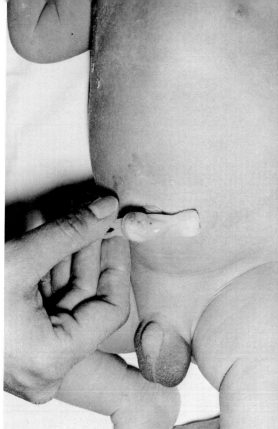

Figure 59.7 The cord is inspected for the number of vessels present. Make sure the cord is securely clamped and that no bleeding can occur.

Figure 59.8 Inspection of the genitalia; no hypospadias is present and both testes have descended.

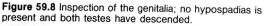

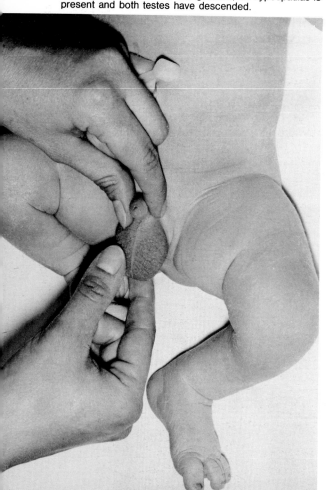

General inspection. To prevent the child from becoming cold, the general inspection should be performed rapidly but methodically, preferably under an infant warmer. One aims to discover the presence of malformations, evidence of injury, or difficulties the child may be experiencing in the adaptation to extrauterine life. The examination begins at the top of the child, and progresses downwards (figures 59.1–59.10).

Cleansing. Using individual disposable equipment, and sterile swabs, the infant is cleansed in warm water. Particular attention is paid to the flexures and creases. The infant is then gently dried with a towel. Currently no antiseptic lotions other than alcohol impregnated swabs (Mediswabs) are in use in the United Kingdom.

Measurements. The naked infant is *weighed* and *measured* (it takes 2 staff members to do this (figures 59.12–59.14). The average full term infant weighs about 3,500 g, the average crown-heel length is 50 cm and the average head circumference is 35 cm. For length measurement, the child is placed either in a suitable measuring device or on a flat surface. A tape is held alongside the baby, the crown of the infant's head is

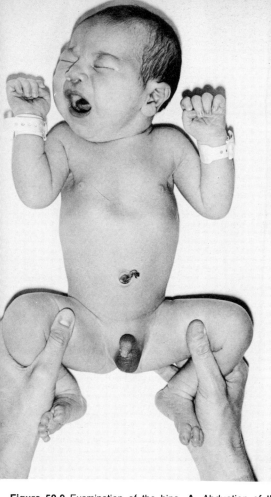

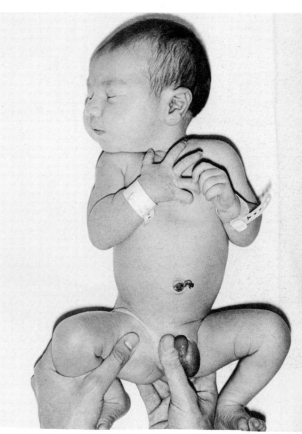

B

Figure 59.9 Examination of the hips. **A.** Abduction of the hips may be limited in children suffering from congenital dislocation of the hips. **B.** One hand steadies the pelvis, and the other grasps the flexed leg and is used to abduct and adduct the thigh; note any jerk.

Figure 59.10 The anus is inspected for patency.

Figure 59.11 Cleansing the newborn infant with a limited amount of an antiseptic solution.

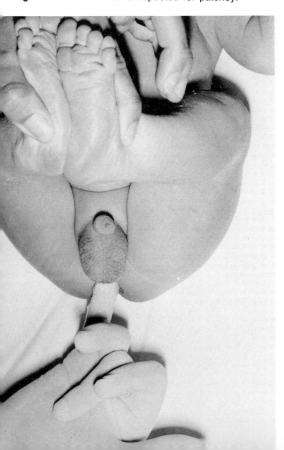

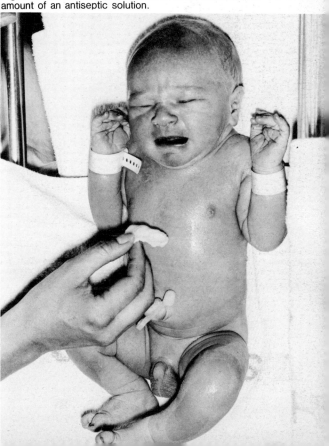

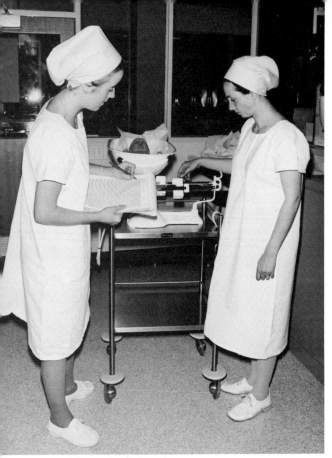

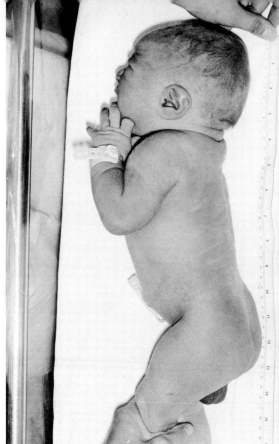

Figure 59.12 The weight of a newborn infant should be checked by two trained members of the staff.

Figure 59.13 One method of measuring the crown-heel length.

Figure 59.14 Measurement of the head circumference.

Figure 59.15 With the arrival of a new infant to the nursery, particulars of name and sex are checked by the attending postnatal nurse.

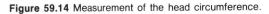

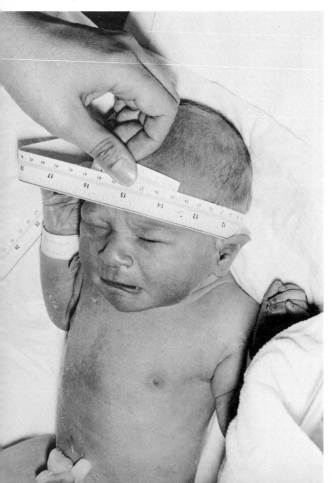

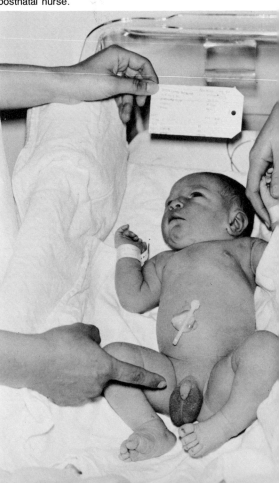

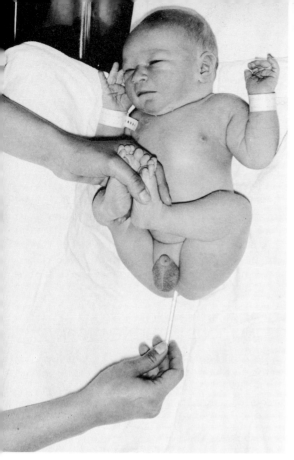

Figure 59.16 Checking the temperature of a child recently arrived in the nursery.

aligned to the top of the tape, held there, then both legs are straightened at the knees to get the total crown-heel measurement (figure 59.13). The head circumference encompasses the parietal eminences, the forehead and the occiput (figure 59.14).

Transfer to the postnatal nursery is generally carried out at the same time as the mother's transfer. Before this is done, all particulars of name and sex are checked with the labour ward records and the infant's temperature is taken and recorded.

CARE AFTER BIRTH — NURSERY

On arrival in the postnatal nursery, all particulars of name and sex are again checked by the postnatal nurse (figure 59.15). The baby is received into a warmed cot and the body temperature is recorded (figure 59.16): if below 36°C, it is checked hourly until over 36°C.

It must be emphasized that *newborn babies need careful handling*; they are still in the process of making the necessary adjustments to extrauterine life.

It has been customary to send any baby born by an abnormal delivery (forceps, Caesarean section, or breech delivery), to a special care nursery. Experience has shown that not all such infants require special care and hence a selection of those deemed likely to require such care is required — e.g. all premature infants and those requiring special management. Some may only require observation for 24 hours. When considered to be well enough, they are transferred to the postnatal ward. Each baby should be examined by a doctor within 24 hours of birth.

Temperature and respirations. The temperature and respiration are recorded once and subsequent observations are performed only if the initial measurements were abnormal. Initial temperature is taken per rectum (figure 59.16) and thereafter per axilla. When recording the latter, the thermometer must be kept in position for at least 3 minutes. If the temperature is below 35°C, the true temperature is recorded on a low reading thermometer; if the temperature is not above 36°C after 3 hours, the infant is placed in an insul-cot for warming.

Cord care. The umbilicus is an *open wound* and serves as an important portal of entry of infection. Cleansing of the cord is not routinely performed, but care must be maintained to keep the cord dry. No antiseptic or dressings are applied to the cord.

Feeding. See Chapters 60 and 61 on breast and artificial feeding.

Routine cleaning. The baby is cleansed daily with soap and water. This is done in the infant's cot to prevent cross-infection.

Urine. Most infants urinate within 24 hours of birth. Often they do so at birth and this should be recorded on the neonatal chart. Thereafter, urine is passed about 4 times a day in the first 4 days, and this gradually increases to about 10 times per day at 10 days of age.

The pink deposit sometimes seen on the napkin is caused by urates and should not be mistaken for blood. Placentally insufficient babies pass less urine initially and may not urinate for up to 36–48 hours. However, the doctor should be notified if the infant has not voided within 30 hours of birth; one must then exclude dehydration and urinary tract obstruction (e.g. posterior urethral valves).

Stools. Meconium is passed for the first 2–3 days. Then the infant passes a *transitional stool* that is a mixture of green-black meconium, milk-curd and sometimes a little mucus. By the end of the first week, if the infant is breast-fed, the stools are soft, yellow, acid, and nonoffensive.

Initially these stools are passed with each feeding, but later they become less frequent, firmer, and darker in colour. The artificially-fed infant has less frequent, darker and firmer stools.

Weighing. The infant is weighed at birth, and on day 4 and then on alternate days until discharged. Thereafter weighing is performed weekly by the health visitor. Normal infants lose up to 10% of their birth-weight due to poor food intake, and urine and meconium loss. Thereafter, the infant gains weight and has usually regained his birth-weight by the 10th day. The average infant *gains approximately 300 g per week. Excessive* initial weight loss must be reported to the doctor who will examine the baby to eludicate the reason.

Clothing. This is *changed daily* or more frequently if required. In hospital, a gown and singlet with cuddle blanket is usually sufficient to keep the baby warm. When wrapping the infant, remember the infant *needs room to breathe and move*, and a tight restrictive wrapping can cause harm by inhibiting chest expansion.

Buttocks. Initially, sticky meconium is cleansed with a *sterile oily lotion.* Thereafter the baby's buttocks are washed with *warm water and dried. Zinc cream* is applied after all changes. Sore buttocks should be treated at once.

Vomiting. This is common in the newborn period and can be due to a variety of causes.

Observation and charts. It is important to chart observations accurately. All treatments are charted, as well as the volume of feedings and how these are taken. Any departure from normal behaviour must be reported at once.

Domicile. There are 2 possibilities.

(a) *Rooming-in.* Here the baby stays with the mother and is cared for by her. It has the following advantages: (i) the mother gets to know her baby, interprets his cries, and at the end of her hospital stay, handles him with confidence, (ii) the mother may demand feed the baby when he is hungry, and (iii) the risk of cross-infection is greatly reduced. For general welfare of mother and baby, rooming-in is the best method, but a tired mother should have the opportunity to refuse and be allowed as much rest as possible.

(b) *Communal nursery.* Here the baby is cared for by the nursing staff and is only brought to the mother for feeding. However, each infant must have his own personal requisites, and *communal baths and change tables should never be used.* There should be adequate facilities for hand washing and disposable hand towels must always be used.

Discharge advice. Before discharge, the mother is shown how to bathe her baby and how to make up artifical feedings. She is also given details of any medications (e.g. vitamins) and general care (e.g. care of the umbilical stump if this is still adherent, and circumcision dressings).

On discharge the mother will receive daily visits from the community midwife for a minimum of 10 days to a maximum of 28 days. Thereafter the infant's progress will be assessed by health visitors at the local child health clinic. At these clinics, medical, nursing and support services are available.

COMMON 'PHYSIOLOGICAL' CONDITIONS IN THE NEWBORN

Engorged breasts. The infant's breasts become tense and hard (figure 59.17) and exude watery milk fluid (figure 59.18). No treatment is required, since the condition subsides spontaneously.

Hydrocele. Common in male infants and generally disappears by about 6 weeks of age.

Pseudomenstruation. Female infants may have a blood-stained vaginal discharge. It is a withdrawal phenomenon from maternal hormonal influence (oestrogen action on the uterus) and needs no treatment.

Vasomotor instability. Mottled skin, blue hands and feet, with good colour elsewhere and lasting only a few minutes is due to vasomotor instability. It is more common in premature infants.

Naevus flammeus. This is a V-shaped redness of the upper forehead extending onto the eyelids and frequently present on the occiput and nape of the neck (colour plate 59). These areas are not raised and fade spontaneously without treatment. They are due to fine telangiectatic blood vessels and are most obvious when the infant cries due to flushing of the vessels with blood.

Milia. These are white spots located on the nose and occasionally on the forehead and are due to retention of secretions in sebaceous glands (figure 59.19). They disappear about 2 weeks after birth. Presumably these spots have the same composition as vernix.

'Mongolian blue-spot'. These are blue patches which are found over the lower spine, buttocks and legs. They are common in babies whose parents are of non-Caucasian origin, and eventually disappear. The mother may have to be reassured that they are not due to bruising.

Figure 59.17 Engorged breasts.

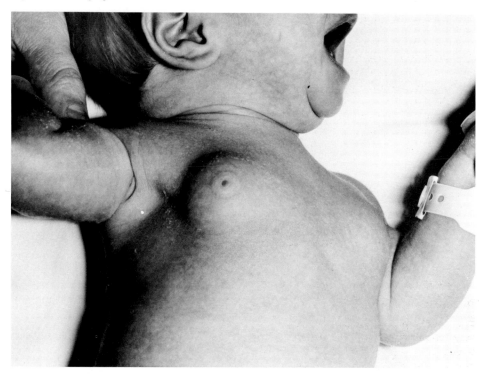

Figure 59.18 'Witch's milk': watery fluid exuding from a physiologically engorged breast when it was subjected to gentle pressure.

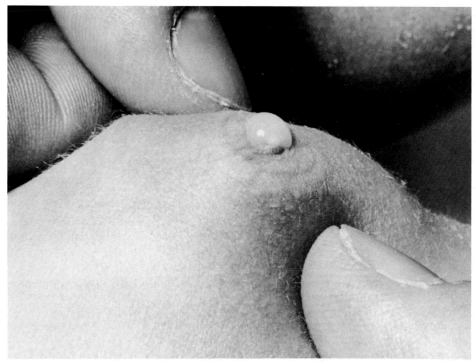

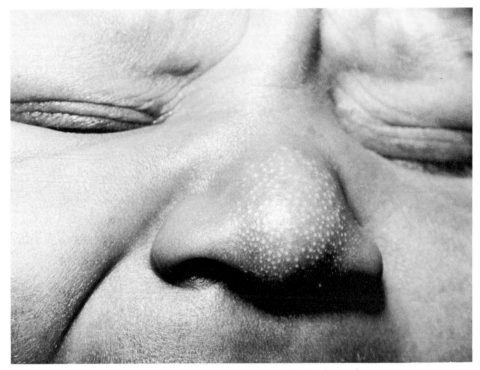

Figure 59.19 Milia: these spots are often mistaken for pustules by the mother.

Figure 59.20 Sucking-blister.

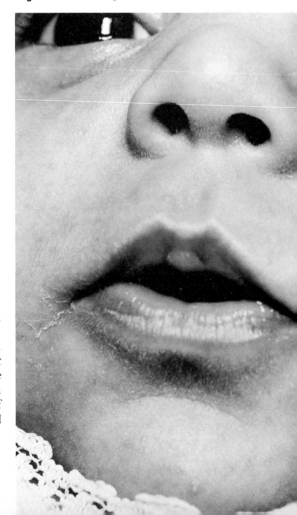

Sucking-blister. This may be seen on the upper lip (figure 59.20). It is harmless and disappears in time without scarring.

Vaginal skin tags. Redundant tags of mucous membrane often protrude from the vulva. These shrink over the ensuing weeks.

Cranial cyanosis (infants with blue heads and pink bodies). The cyanosis stops abruptly at the junction of the head with the trunk. It is due to delay in delivering the shoulders after the head is born during which time the chest is compressed. A cord looped tightly around the neck can cause the same picture. The condition disappears after several days without treatment.

COMMON DISORDERS IN THE NEONATAL PERIOD

Vomiting

This is a common symptom in the newborn and usually the cause is a simple one. If however, there is a *serious underlying condition*, there will be additional features *such as excessive weight loss, copious vomitus or a green colour to the vomitus*. Remember that gastric acidity is high in the newborn baby and may cause scalding of the face, particularly if the fluid is not removed immediately and the linen changed.

Nonserious Causes

(i) *Gastric.* There may be an irritation of the lining of the stomach due to swallowed blood or meconium, excessive amounts of normal gastric mucus, or trauma to the gastric mucosa by excessive aspiration at birth and thereafter. The treatment is gentle gastric lavage with warm sterile water. Occasionally an oral sedative such as sodium phenobarbitone is required.

(ii) *Feeding technique.* The rate of feeding may be too rapid or too slow, there may be a failure to 'bring up wind' or the volume of feeding may be too large.

Serious Causes

(i) *Cerebral irritation.* This is often due to hypoxia or birth injury. Treatment of the underlying cerebral condition is necessary (see Chapter 66).

(ii) *Infection.* Vomiting is frequently an early presenting symptom of infection in the newborn, especially of the *urinary tract*.

(iii) *Intestinal obstruction.* The vomitus usually contains bile and the infant characteristically has *abdominal distension, constipation and weight loss*. The condition is usually confirmed by radiography and requires surgical correction.

(iv) *Oesophageal atresia (tracheo-oesophageal fistula).* This congenital abnormality should be diagnosed early. It is invariably associated with polyhydramnios. Therefore, all infants born of mothers who have had polyhydramnios during their pregnancy should have a 10 French gauge catheter passed into the stomach. Patency of the anus and rectum should also be elicited by passage of an oiled catheter.

(v) *Oesophageal reflux.* A relaxed cardiac sphincter leads to regurgitant vomiting often streaked with blood and mucus. Oesophageal reflux is more common in premature infants. This condition is treated by sedation, propping the infant upright, and thickening the feedings (e.g. alginic acid compound-Gaviscon granules) (colour plate 137). The condition is self-corrective and only very rarely requires surgical intervention. Indications for surgical consultation are persistent poor weight gain and severe haematemesis.

(vi) *Pyloric stenosis.* This condition usually does not manifest itself until the infant is 3 weeks old. The vomiting is projectile and gastric peristalsis is marked. After the diagnosis is confirmed, the infant is treated surgically (Ramstedt operation). In maternity hospitals, this condition is seen in the special care nurseries among premature babies.

(vii) *Hypoglycaemia* may present with vomiting and must be excluded as a cause in the vomiting newborn infant.

Abnormalities of the Stools

Diarrhoea. This is defined as the passage of more than 3 extra stools per day above the infant's usual number, the condition persisting for 48 hours or more (see Chapter 67). Since the concentrating ability of the kidney of the newborn infant is poor, diarrhoea may rapidly produce dehydration and electrolyte disturbances.

Clay-coloured stools. These occur if there is obstruction of the bile ducts.

Melaena stools. The passage of blood in the motions may be due to ingested maternal blood or may be a manifestation of bleeding disorders in the neonate such as *haemorrhagic disease*. The *Apt* test will differentiate between maternal and fetal blood.

Grey or dark stools. These occur in babies who have commenced oral iron; the stools are often a little offensive.

Constipation. Defined as no stools passed for 48 hours and the stools are hard and dry. Causes: (i) *prematurity* — the meconium is thick and sticky and the infant may need the assistance of saline enemas or the passage of an oiled catheter to clear the bowel (colour plate 60); with this assistance, the bowel is usually cleared in 3 days; (ii) *imperforate anus* — should be obvious on examination (figure 65.14); (iii) *intestinal obstruction*; (iv) *underfeeding* — this can produce either small, dry, hard stools or frequent small green 'starvation stools'; the infant will be fretful.

Sore Buttocks

This is a common complaint and varies from redness to extensive excoriation. The skin of the newborn is delicate and particular care must be taken when cleansing and drying the buttock area. This applies especially to premature babies since their skin is much finer than that of babies born at term.

Causes: (i) infrequent changing of napkins; (ii) loose, frequent, acid stools due to either *gastroenteritis* or unsuitable feedings containing too much sugar; (iii) cleansing the skin with the napkin and not with the cotton wool provided; (iv) napkins washed in unsuitable detergents and insufficiently rinsed; (v) infection caused by the fungus, Monilia albicans (colour plate 131).

Treatment. (i) Try to ascertain the cause and correct if possible; (ii) change napkins frequently; (iii) wash the buttocks well with soap, rinse, and thoroughly pat dry; (iv) expose buttocks to sunshine or dry heat; make sure that the baby is warmly wrapped and only the buttocks are exposed; (v) if the buttocks show evidence of monilial infection treat with an antifungal cream (Nystatin, Kenacomb or Pimafucort) or with aqueous gentian violet 1% twice daily. (vi) mercurochrome (2% aqueous paint) is also helpful in drying an excoriated area on the baby's buttocks when applied after exposure to sunshine or heat; (vii) other healing agents include zinc and castor oil cream, vaseline, barrier cream and a powder containing zinc, starch and camphor; the creams are valuable mainly because they provide a waterproofing barrier for the skin.

Urticaria Neonatorum

Although this sounds alarming it is not. It presents as an urticarial vesicular rash that has a reddened periphery. The lesions may be sparse or dense. The central vesicle may contain yellowish serum if the baby is jaundiced and often the vesicles contain pus. However, the pus is sterile on culture. The rash subsides spontaneously without treatment in about 3–4 days.

Conjunctival Infection

This can be either bacterial, viral, or chemical and manifests itself as a 'sticky eye' or a purulent discharge such as seen in gonococcal infections (colour plate 130) (see Chapter 67).

Oral Thrush See Chapter 67.

Scratching

Term and postterm infants often have long fingernails and scratch their eyelids, foreheads and cheeks with the fingers when thumb sucking (colour plate 105, figures 59.21 and 59.22). Scratch marks are an unsightly blemish and upset the mother. They are avoided by mittens or careful trimming of the nails.

Hirsutes

This condition is rare in mature infants (figure 59.23). The parents, who themselves are usually hirsute, can be reassured that the excessive hair will fall out within a few months of birth.

Circumcision

Although this is a procedure that is not generally recommended by paediatricians, there may be strong pressures for its performance. There are social factors 'all his brothers have been done, doctor', and religious rites (e.g. Jewish faith). The reason that the procedure is not recommended is because of the complications, which are haemorrhage, infection, ulceration and rare surgical catastrophes. The procedure is performed between days 6 and 9.

There are 3 basic techniques: (i) bone crushing forceps — no sutures used; (ii) 'Little Trim-

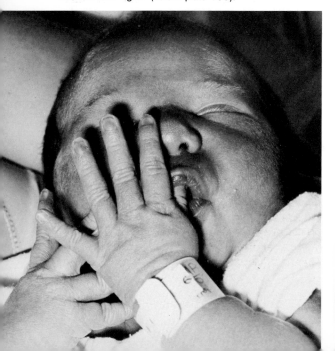

Figure 59.21 During thumb-sucking the baby often scratches the face with the fingers, especially when the nails are long (term or postterm pregnancy). The fingers knead the face (eyelids, brow, cheeks) while the thumb is sucked with vigour (colour plate 105).

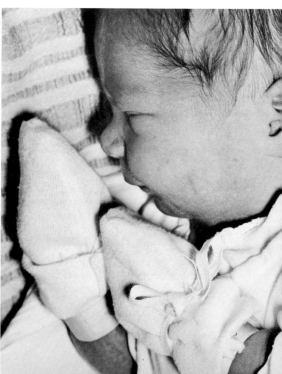

Figure 59.22 To minimize scratching, mittens are used to cover the hands or the fingernails can be trimmed.

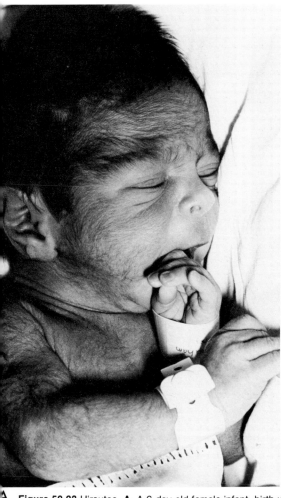
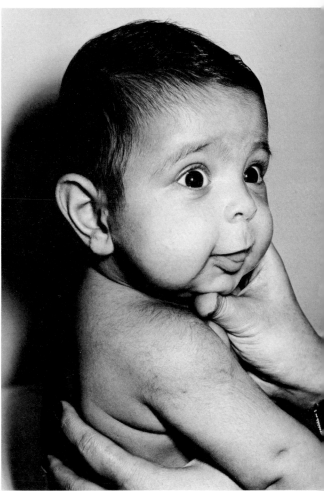

A   **B**

Figure 59.23 Hirsutes. **A.** A 6-day-old female infant, birth-weight 2,600 g, delivered at 38 weeks' gestation. The mother was a gestational diabetic of Syrian ancestry. **B.** At 4 months of age the excessive hair has largely disappeared and the infant no longer 'looks like a hairy monkey' (the mother's words!)

mer' with dome, which comes in various sizes — this is also a crushing technique with no sutures used; (iii) Spencer Wells artery forceps are used to separate the foreskin from the glans of the penis; the foreskin is incised and trimmed and the wound is sutured with fine catgut (figure 59.24).

After the operation, the area is dressed with dry ribbon gauze and on this is dropped compound tincture of benzoin. This is then left to dry and this original dressing is left in place for 4 days. On the outside, another dressing is wrapped (usually an unravelled cotton wool ball is adequate). This outside dressing is changed when necessary.

On return to the nursery the baby has a notice on his cot to remind everyone that he was circumcised that day. The wound is inspected frequently for oozing and if necessary more compound tincture of benzoin is dropped onto the *original dressing*. The baby is sponged, not bathed. On discharge, the mother is advised that the original dressing should not be removed until the fourth day after the operation. On the fourth day, the baby is placed in the bath and the dressing is soaked off. A few drops of castor or olive oil may be dropped onto the original dressing the night before it is due to be removed. For the next 6 days the mother dresses the wound with vaseline gauze and cotton wool, changing this as necessary. The sterile vaseline gauze dressings should be supplied to the mother on discharge from hospital.

Contraindications: (i) hypospadias — the skin is retained for use later in the definitive repair; (ii) an infant too ill to stand the procedure; (iii) prematurity; (iv) bleeding disorders; (v) mother on oral anticoagulants and breast-feeding the infant; (vi) local infection; (vii) jaundice.

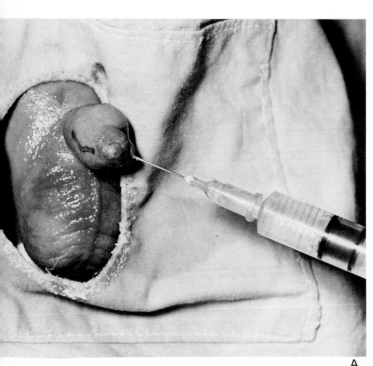
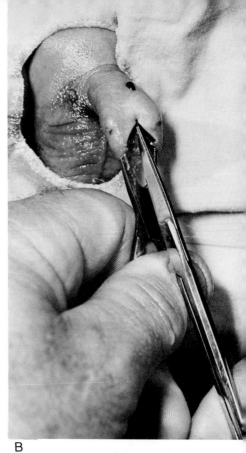

A   B

Figure 59.24 Circumcision. **A.** To minimize pain, 1% lignocaine hydrochloride (Xylocaine) is injected into the prepuce although this distorts the tissues and makes it more difficult the judge the correct amount of skin to be excised. **B.** A longitudinal dorsal slit is cut along the prepuce to allow retraction of the prepuce. **C.** The prepuce has been retracted and separated from the glans to which it was adherent. A circumferential excision of the prepuce is then performed; 3–4 fine catgut sutures are inserted to secure haemostasis and appose the thicker outer layer to the inner layer of the prepuce. **D.** The area is dressed with dry ribbon gauze onto which compound tincture of benzoin is dripped. The dressing is left undisturbed for 4 days.

C   D

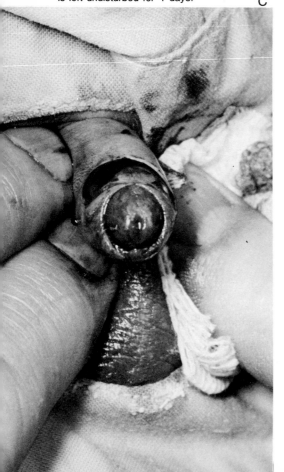
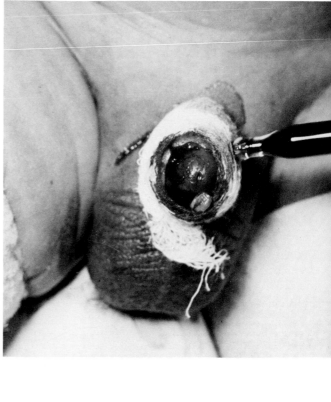

chapter sixty

Breast Feeding

OVERVIEW

Until relatively recently, survival of mankind was totally dependent upon successful breast feeding. After the second world war breast feeding became less popular, and there was a decline in both the proportion of women wishing to breast-feed and the length of time breast feeding was continued. Breast feeding, however, confers both short-term and long-term advantages. Short-term advantages are *reduced risks of infection and possibly also necrotizing enterocolitis*; long-term advantages are *improved mother-infant bonding, reduced incidences of infection and the sudden infant death syndrome*. Recent trends have been to encourage mothers to breast-feed and to ascertain why so many women fail to do so. Reasons for the latter relate particularly to the separation of the mother from her baby and the lack of encouragement. Separation is largely an *economically-determined factor*, particularly if the baby is left at home in family care rather than at the work place (which would favour continued breast feeding); variation in maternity leave provisions is a further important consideration. Recent surveys have stressed the importance women place on the *attitudes of health care professionals*: a positive and repeated message to the mother regarding breast feeding is often lacking in antenatal care. Such a *positive attitude towards breast feeding* should begin during the antenatal period. This should be reinforced in the first few days after birth when minor difficulties are common and when maternal emotional factors are most likely to erupt and result in a hasty decision to bottle-feed. *Perseverance in the first days of establishment of breast feeding*, by patient, midwife and medical practitioner, harvests a rich reward — a more contented mother, baby and hospital staff! Of major importance to success are *early and frequent suckling by the baby after birth* and *abolition of supplementary feedings unless medically prescribed*.

Those involved in the care of the mother and her baby should be aware of the anatomical and physiological principles underlying breast feeding, the composition of breast milk, and how it differs from cow's milk and other artificial preparations.

Lactation is preceded by development of the mammary glands during pregnancy, chiefly under the influence of oestrogen and progesterone. The abrupt fall in these hormones after birth allows the high circulating level of prolactin to initiate lactation. Continuance requires adequate stimulation of the nipple by the baby during the process of suckling: this reinforces *prolactin* release and also causes *oxytocin* release, important in milk let-down at the start of each feeding.

Major factors interfering with lactation include *psychological stress* in the mother, *breast engorgement, nipple problems*, and *mastitis*.

The *duration of feeding* is influenced by personal and cultural factors; the emotional and nutritional aspects should be understood as well as *techniques of weaning*.

There are many active groups of nursing mothers in the community who have launched a successful crusade for a return to breast feeding. In most countries, the great majority of women attempt to breast-feed and approximately 50% succeed in doing so for at least 3 months. However, although there is no doubt that breast feeding is the best way to feed the human infant, it must be remembered that *not all women wish or are able to breast-feed*. Hence, appropriate regimens of artificial feeding suitable for newborn infants are required.

INTRODUCTION

Breast milk is a complete food, adequate with respect to fluid requirements, protein, fat, carbohydrate, minerals and vitamins for all the needs of the rapidly-growing *term* infant for several months.

Success in breast feeding depends not nearly so much on the physical as on the *emotional state* of the mother. The nurse and the doctor can be of tremendous help in reassuring, instilling confidence, and helping to infuse a feeling of calmness, contentment and optimism when breast feeding is being established.

ADVANTAGES OF BREAST FEEDING

The infant. (i) Since the milk comes directly to the baby's mouth, the chance of transfer of infection to the child is greatly lowered. The milk also contains *maternal immunoglobulins* and immunocompetent cells that help the newborn infant resist infection. (ii) Mother's milk is naturally adapted to the infant's *digestion and nutritional requirements.* (iii) The close physical contact and the opportunity of mothering that breast feeding affords help to satisfy the infant's need for *love and security.*

The mother. (i) Breast feeding gives the mother a great deal of *emotional satisfaction and pleasure.* The suckling of the baby also enhances and stimulates the maternal instinct. (ii) Breast feeding aids in the *involution of the uterus*, the suckling of the baby at the breast stimulating uterine contractions (by *release of oxytocin* from the pituitary gland). (iii) It is convenient, and in comparison with artificial feeding, saves the mother much work, time, and money.

COMPOSITION OF BREAST MILK

The proportions are protein 1.5%, fat 3.5%, carbohydrate 7.0%, minerals 0.2% (total solids 12%), water 88.0%. The caloric value of breast milk is 20 calories (84 kJ) per 30 ml (1 ounce).

Protein. There are 2 proteins present in slightly different amounts, lactalbumin and casein. Lactalbumin contains all the amino acids essential for the baby. The casein of human milk has the important quality of forming a fine, flocculent, easily digested curd when coagulated, in contrast with cow's milk casein which forms a large, tough curd.

Fat. The chemical composition of the fat in breast milk results in fine droplets that are easily digested.

Carbohydrate is present in the form of lactose.

Minerals. All the minerals necessary for the baby are provided, but only a small amount of iron is present. If the baby is premature iron should be introduced at the 5th week after delivery.

ANATOMY OF THE BREAST

The breast is situated on the anterior chest wall between the second and sixth ribs, and extends from the sternum to the axilla.

External structure. The breast has an elongated tail going towards the axilla, known as the axillary tail of Spence. In the centre of the breast is an erectile structure about 0.5 cm in length — the *nipple*, the tip of which is indented by the openings of 15–20 lactiferous ducts. Surrounding the nipple is an area of loose skin about 2 cm in diameter (the areola) which is pinkish in colour. Within the areola are situated 18–20 *sebaceous glands* — *Montgomery follicles* (colour plate 41).

Internal structure (figure 60.1). The glandular tissue is divided into 15–20 lobes. Each lobe radiates outwards from the areola like the spokes of a wheel. Each lobe is subdivided into *lobules* which are made up of masses of milk-secreting units known as *alveoli*. The alveolar cells take up the substances they require to form breast milk from the maternal blood. The alveoli drain into intralobular ducts which unite to form *lactiferous ducts* which dilate as they pass towards the nipple to form the *lactiferous sinuses* (small reservoirs) (15–20) which are situated at the base of the nipple. From these sinuses the lactiferous ducts open onto the summit of the nipple. Extensive fibrous tissue and fat separate the lobes and support not only the glandular tissue but also the vessels, nerves, and lymphatics.

CHANGES DURING PREGNANCY

During pregnancy changes take place in the breast, preparing it for the function of lactation (colour plates 41–44 and 65). These changes are brought about by hormonal activity. Progesterone stimulates alveolar growth and oestrogen stimulates proliferation of the duct system.

(i) *Increased blood supply.* The veins over the breast become noticeable.

(ii) *Enlargement* occurs both of the breast (proliferation of lactiferous ducts and alveolar growth) and of the nipple.

(iii) The *areola enlarges* and becomes pigmented (more noticeable in brunettes).

(iv) *Montgomery follicles* are modified seb-

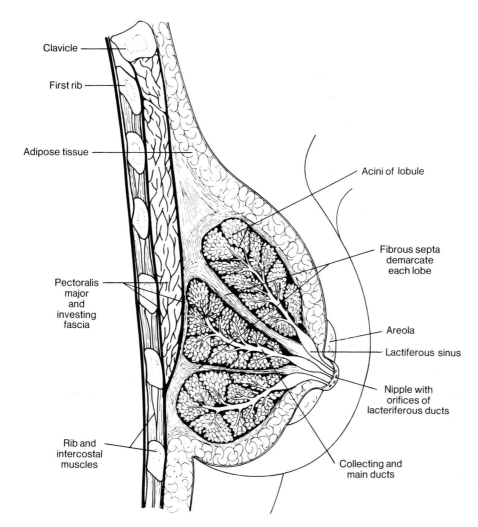

Clavicle

First rib

Adipose tissue

Pectoralis major and investing fascia

Rib and intercostal muscles

Acini of lobule

Fibrous septa demarcate each lobe

Areola

Lactiferous sinus

Nipple with orifices of lacteriferous ducts

Collecting and main ducts

Figure 60.1 Sagittal section through breast and anterior chest wall showing lobular architecture with breast segments being separated by fibrous septa. Main collecting ducts drain to lacteriferous sinuses lying beneath the areola.

aceous glands in the primary areola and they become more prominent. Their secretion keeps the nipple soft and pliable during pregnancy.

(v) *Colostrum* can be expressed.

(vi) *Striae* may appear during pregnancy and usually do so at the time of rapid enlargement of the breasts, often late in the first trimester. Surprisingly, striae are not caused by the rapid, often extreme enlargement which occurs with the onset of lactation.

THE PHYSIOLOGY OF LACTATION

The process of lactation can be considered to take place in 3 stages: the production of milk in the alveoli, the flow of milk along the ducts to the nipple, and the withdrawal of milk from the nipple by the baby.

During pregnancy the anterior lobe of the pituitary gland releases *prolactin* (lactogenic hormone), but production of breast milk is held in abeyance by inhibition of the action of prolactin by the high blood oestrogen level which is thought to act locally on breast tissue. After delivery, the level of oestrogen falls, allowing prolactin to initiate lactation (production of lactalbumin, casein, lactose). Stimulation of local nerve endings by the baby sucking in turn induces secretion of more prolactin and thus more breast milk.

The ejection of milk is helped by the hormone *oxytocin* released from the posterior lobe of the mother's pituitary gland in response to suckling; this is the basis of the let-down reflex. Oxytocin causes contraction of the *myoepithelial cells* which invest the mammary alveoli, forcing milk into the lactiferous ducts. (Oxytocin also causes uterine muscle contraction and so uterine pain is often experienced during breast feeding).

Colostrum. Breast milk is not formed immediately after delivery; for the first 2–3 days the secretion of the breasts is colostrum which is different from milk both in appearance and composition. It is yellow in colour, thicker in consistency, and is formed only in small amounts. Colostrum has a high protein content and a low content of fat and carbohydrate. The role of colostrum is in educating the digestive tract to its function of absorption, and providing immunoglobulins and immunocompetent cells to the infant.

'Coming in' of the milk. On the 3rd or 4th day, the secretion of the breast changes to breast milk. The breasts become full, sometimes tense and uncomfortable, and this is termed the 'coming in' of the milk. In some mothers, this does not occur; rather there is a slow increase over the first 3 weeks.

To maintain successful lactation, the necessary requirements are: (i) a mentally and physically healthy mother, (ii) an adequate and frequently repeated sucking stimulus to provide the neurohormonal reflex, (iii) a large blood supply to the breast.

ANTENATAL PREPARATION

When the mother first visits the antenatal clinic a history is taken of success or otherwise of previous breast feeding. An examination of the breasts is made, noting the following: the nipple — mobility, inversion, or retraction; the areola — for pigmentation; the breasts — increase in size which usually denotes growth of glandular tissue which is favourable; the skin — elasticity and thinness, which are favourable.

The general health of the mother should be maintained at as high a level as possible, with correction of any errors of hygiene. A *correct diet* is very important.

The advantages of breast feeding are brought to the notice of the mother and father, and she is encouraged to believe in her capacity to feed her baby. She should be given simple instruction in the physiological processes of lactation, so that she will have some idea what to expect after the birth of her baby.

Daily antenatal nipple care is not now thought to be essential. It should be left up to the mother whether to handle the breast or not antenatally. Applying lanoline cream to the nipples is of no proven value.

Flat or partially inverted nipples require no extra care, although with inverted nipples the wearing of a plastic nipple shield antenatally may be of some value (Meredith Breast Shields, formerly known as Woolwick Shields).

A well-fitting maternity brassiere should be worn. It should be made of firm material, be of the uplift design, have wide adjustable shoulder straps, back-lacing to allow for enlargement of the breasts, and front fastening to allow for breast feeding after delivery.

MANAGEMENT OF BREAST FEEDING

Breast feeding is a partnership between mother and baby, the most important period being the first few days of the baby's life. It is necessary that mother and baby should have learnt how to manage the suckling before the milk 'comes in'.

Wherever possible, *the baby is put to the breast soon after delivery* (figure 59.1A): this stimulates the release of oxytocin and prolactin from the pituitary gland, and facilitates early milk production by the mother.

TECHNIQUE OF BREAST FEEDING

The mother's hands are washed and the nipples are cleansed if ointment has previously been applied. She adopts a position of comfort — either sitting up in bed with the back supported (figure 60.2A), lying on her side, or sitting in a low chair. The baby (in this case a boy) should be awake, dry and comfortable, and loosely wrapped with the hands free. He is held securely and comfortably by the mother; he may be supported on a pillow if this is more comfortable.

The milk should be issuing from the nipple. The infant's mouth should be open, and the tongue protruded and curved. (At rest, the tongue is held habitually against the hard palate). The infant cannot see the breast: it is found by the 'seeking reflex' — that is, the head turns to the side of the cheek that is touched by the breast. The base of the breast is supported by the mother, and the nipple is 'fed' into the baby's mouth (figure 60.2B). It is important that not only the nipple, but some of the areola is taken into his mouth in order that he may have a firm grasp of the nipple. The gums will then lie over the lactiferous sinuses. The junction of the mouth and the nipple should be as airtight as possible as he closes his mouth about the nipple. If the angles of the mouth are open, the necessary vacuum for sucking is not created. The nose is kept clear of the breast by passing the finger from the base of the breast towards the nipple in the region of the baby's nose (figure 60.2C). Milk is then obtained by compression of the lactiferous sinuses and by suction.

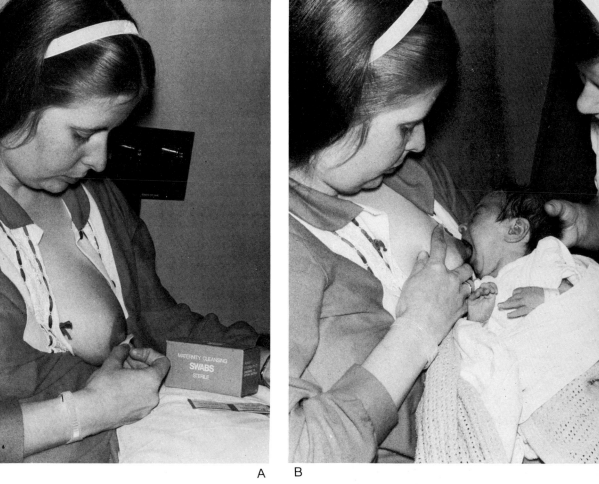

A   B

Figure 60.2 Technique of breast feeding. **A.** The nipples are cleansed (often this step is omitted). **B.** The nipple is fed into the baby's mouth. **C.** The nose is kept clear by pressure on the breast.

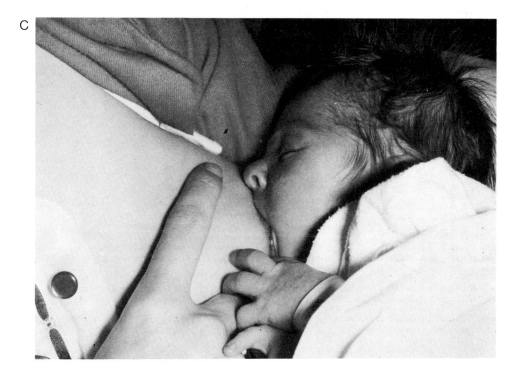

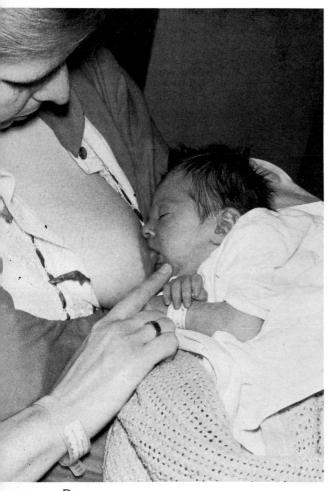

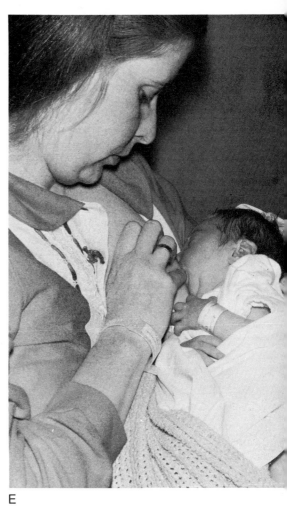

D

E

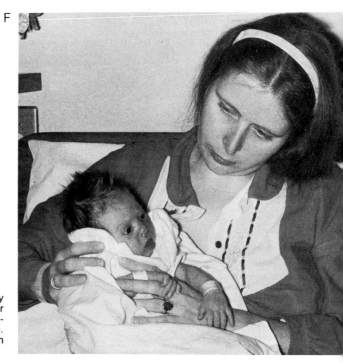

F

D. Detachment of the infant from the nipple by pressure on his jaw. **E.** Insertion of a finger breaks the sucking vacuum and prevents damage of the nipple when the infant is withdrawn. **F.** Bringing up the wind by gentle pressure on the infant's abdomen.

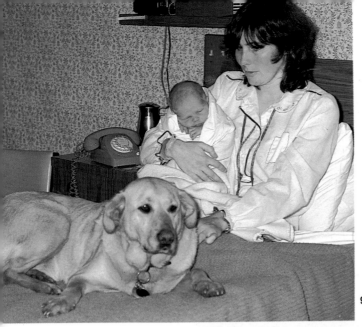

Plate 98 Blind (familial cataracts) 26-year-old para 1 with her healthy son (birth-weight 3,990 g) and devoted guide dog on day 7 of the puerperium. She had a forceps delivery at term following induction of labour because of preeclampsia. She breast-fed and bathed her infant and successfully retained her social independence. The dog lived in the hospital until discharged with the rest of the family 8 days after the confinement — there are occasions when hospital regulations should be waived! It took a few weeks for the dog to fully accept the baby.

98

99

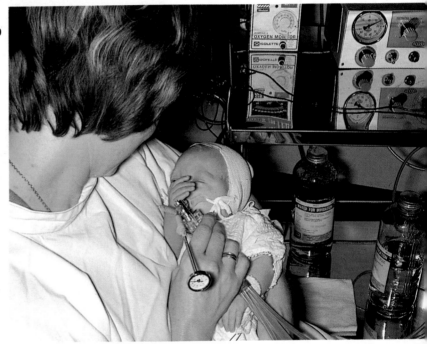

Plate 99 A 33-year-old para 3 cuddles her 14-week-old son (born at 27 weeks' gestation, birth-weight 880 g), 5 days before he died; apnoeic attacks had necessitated ventilatory support which resulted in bronchopulmonary dysplasia and finally cardiorespiratory failure. Bonding is not only necessary but possible even in critically ill premature infants requiring intensive management.

100

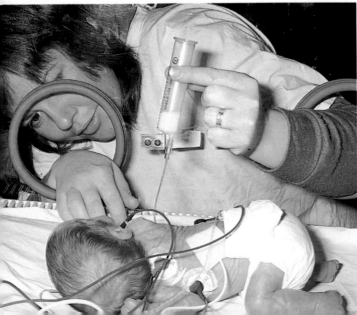

Plate 100 A 26-year-old para 1 tube feeds her 1,300 g 7-week-old baby, a second twin, birth-weight 890 g, born at 26 weeks' gestation (the first twin, birth-weight 550 g, died shortly after birth). This baby had required prolonged ventilatory support and ligation of a patent ductus arteriosus, but was discharged home at 'term', aged 13 weeks, weighing 2,590 g. The mechanical attachments shown here are the electrodes of the heart and respiratory rate recorders, the electrode of the transcutaneous oxygen monitor and the servocontrol sensor for regulation of the temperature of the incubator. Bonding was crucial to this mother who feared that her premature delivery was caused by a previous induced abortion.

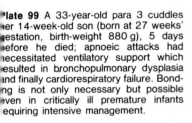

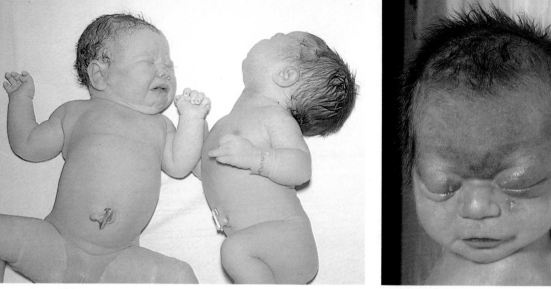

101

Plate 101 Two plump term female infants born on the same day. Note the difference in attitude. The infant on the left presented by the vertex and was born normally. The other, who was born by Caesarean section because of obstructed labour due to brow presentation, shows persistence of extension due to primary muscular tone (rather than a tumour of the neck or loops of umbilical cord).

102

Plate 102 Brow presentation can cause obstructed labour even when the fetus is small and the pelvis is of normal size. This infant (birth-weight 2,770 g) shows bruising due to extensive caput forming when she presented by the brow. The mother was a 24-year-old para 2. During early labour, vaginal examination revealed a left mentoposterior position; 5 hours later the cervix was fully dilated and the brow presented, orbital ridges and nose being palpable. Further flexion then occurred spontaneously with a normal occipitoanterior delivery resulting after a labour of 7 hours' duration.

103

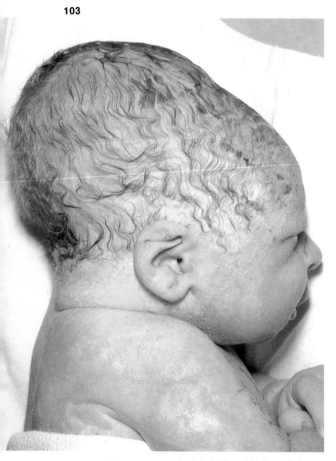

Plate 103 This baby weighed 3,250 g at birth and shows elongation of a normally-shaped head due to moulding. The occiput was anterior at amniotomy and at delivery.

104

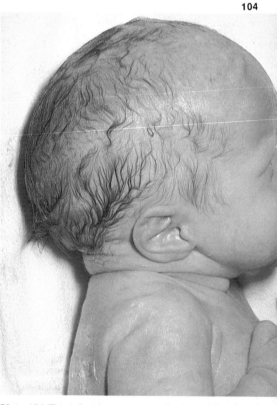

Plate 104 This infant has an unusually-shaped head such that brow presentation did not present unfavourable diameters; birth-weight was 2,960 g. His mother was a 28-year-old para 2. After a 7-hour labour, an anterior brow presentation was noted by palpation when the head came on view; spontaneous delivery occurred without flexion to the occipitoposterior position. A head of this shape explains how an infant of normal size can engage in the pelvis as a brow presentation.

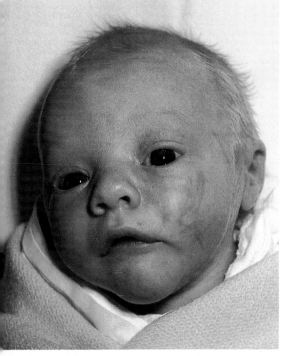

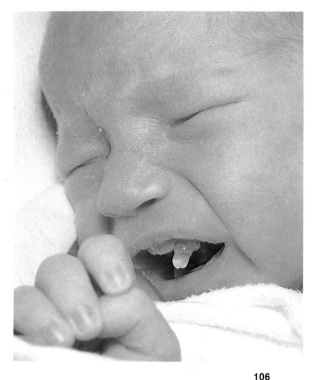

105

106

Plate 105 This male infant (birth-weight 3,260 g) is 5 days old and was born at 40.6 weeks' gestation. These marks were made by his long fingernails as he avidly sucked his thumb, and with equal vigour scratched his face and eyelids. Loosely-tied cotton mittens were used to prevent further scratching. Cutting the nails with scissors or filing them with the soft side of an emery board are safe and effective alternative methods. Scratches and long fingernails are hallmarks of postterm pregnancies.

Plate 106 Epulis of the left gum margin simulating a tooth in a 12-day-old male infant (birth-weight 2,900 g) born at 36 weeks' gestation. He is jaundiced (serum bilirubin 181 μmol/l) and refuses to suck. Histology of the lesion, which was excised without anaesthesia, showed a pyogenic granuloma. A true natal tooth is rare (1 in 3–5,000 births); it causes maternal discomfort during suckling, but is usually wobbly and readily extracted.

107

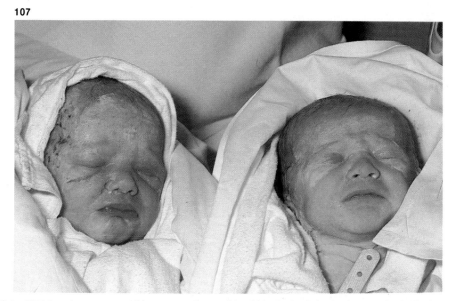

Plate 107 Mirror image naevus flammeus on the eyelids of identical twin boys photographed 15 minutes after birth. The mother was a 29-year-old para 2 referred at 36 weeks' gestation with preeclampsia. Labour was induced and spontaneous normal deliveries occurred 15 hours later. The birth-weights of the twins were 2,210 g and 2,710 g respectively; the placenta weighed 860 g.

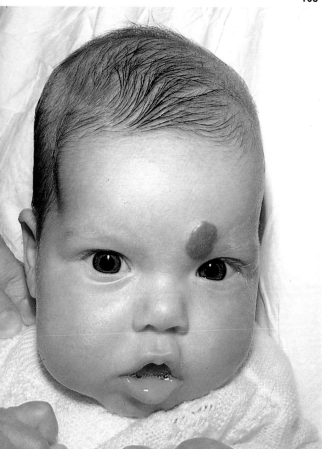

108

Plate 108 Strawberry naevus (capillary haemangioma) in a female infant aged 12 weeks, seen after the phase of rapid expansion which alarmed the mother. Although spontaneous regression occurs in more than 90% of cases by the age of 9 years, the mother could not be reassured and plastic surgery was requested.

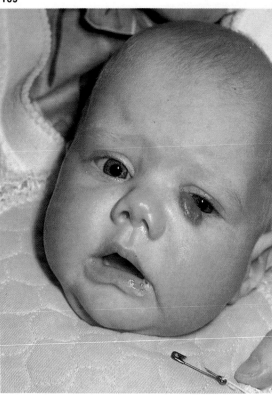

109

Plate 109 Strawberry naevus in a 16-week-old infant who at birth had shown the effects of severe placental insufficiency (birth-weight 1,990 g at 37 weeks' gestation, placenta 370 g). Although nature resolves the lesion with the best cosmetic result, the ophthalmologist advised conservative surgery to reduce the bulk of the lesion because it interfered with vision and could have resulted in blindness.

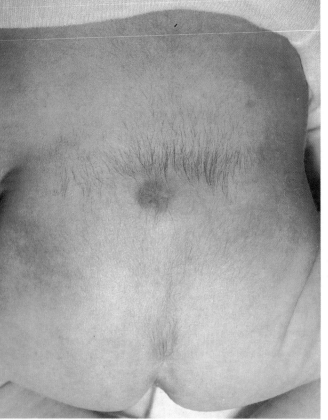

110

Plate 110 Small meningomyelocele with lower sacral nerve involvement in a 7-day-old infant, birth-weight 3,835 g. The area of telangiectatic skin was noted at birth. Such a lesion could be mistaken for a naevus, but its position suggested the possibility of a spina bifida. Careful examination revealed reduced perineal sensation; because of the possibility of urinary and orthopaedic complications, the infant was referred for specialist paediatric care.

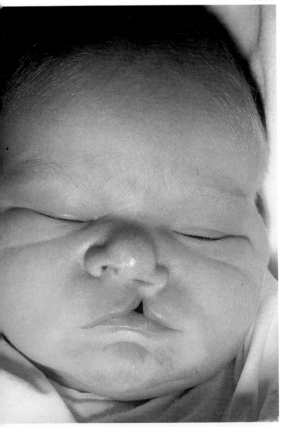

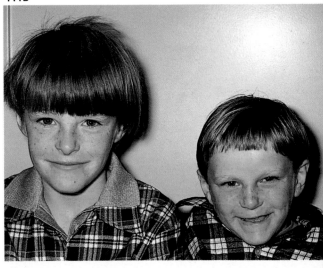

Plate 111A Unilateral cleft lip in a 5-day-old infant, birth-weight 3,620 g. Such lesions are repaired when the child is aged about 3 months or has reached a weight of about 5 kg. The risk of recurrence in a subsequent pregnancy is 2–10%.

Plate 111B The excellent result of surgery is seen 6 years later as the child poses with one of his elder, unaffected brothers.

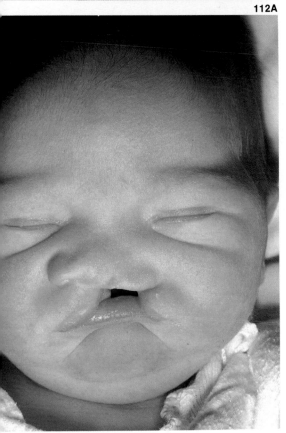

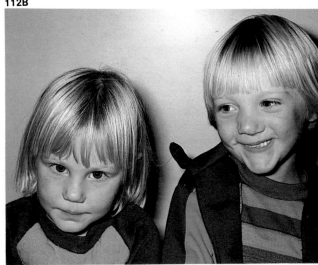

Plate 112A Unilateral cleft lip and associated cleft palate in a 2-day-old male infant, birth-weight 3,320 g. Surgical correction of these defects is staged; the lip is repaired when the child is 3 months of age and the palate is reconstructed when the child is aged 1–2 years. The risk of recurrence of cleft palate in a subsequent pregnancy is 2–17%.

Plate 112B The excellent result of surgery is seen 4 years and 9 months later as the child poses with his younger, unaffected brother.

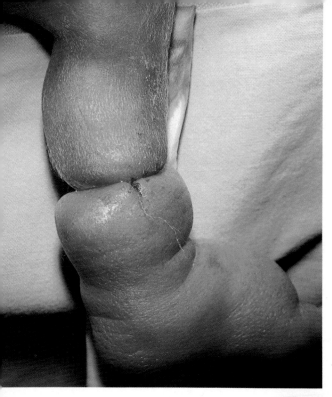

Plate 113 Medial view of the left leg of a 2-day-old female infant, a second twin, birth-weight 1,320 g, born by breech extraction at 32 weeks' gestation. Note gross oedema below the deep constriction caused by an amniotic band, at the level of which were transverse fractures of tibia and fibula. It is easy to believe such a lesion can cause prenatal amputation. The fractures healed and the oedema resolved uneventfully after a small longitudinal incision was made over the constriction. The amniotic band syndrome is rare (1 in 10–20,000 births). The band probably forms when the amnion ruptures and rolls into a cord, the fetus lying within the intact chorion, perhaps with associated oligohydramnios.

113

114

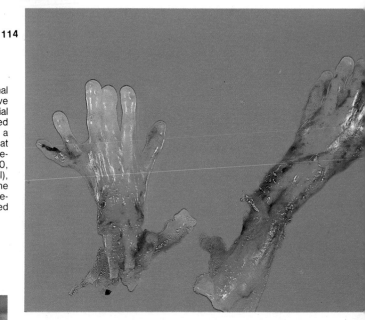

Plate 114 Hydatidiform mole and abnormal fetus. These horrible hands with impressive polydactyly were found when the material obtained by suction curettage was strained to collect tissue for histology. The mother, a 22-year-old primigravida, had presented at 16 weeks' gestation with severe pre-eclampsia (blood pressure 185/140, generalized oedema, proteinuria 20 g/l), hyperemesis and disproportionate uterine enlargement. Bilateral ovarian tumours, presumably theca-lutein cysts, were palpated after the uterus was evacuated.

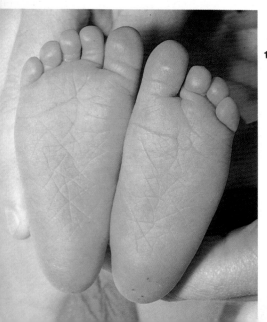

115

Plate 115 Unilateral limb malformations in a 1-day-old male infant, birth-weight 3,210 g. The left foot has only 4 toes and is smaller than the right. Search for associated anomalies showed the left leg to be shorter than the right; radiography revealed a short tibia and absence of the fibula.

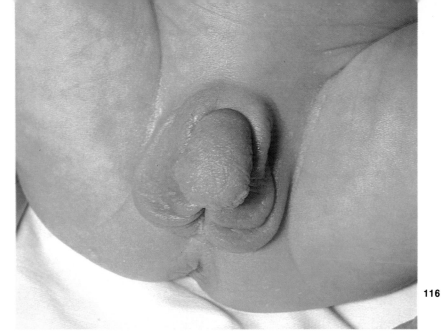

116

Plate 116 Ambiguous genitalia in a 8-day-old infant born at 38 weeks' gestation, birth-weight 2,690 g. The urethra opened at the base of the phallus, posterior to which were loose folds of skin without palpable testes. There was no vaginal orifice. Chromosome constitution was XY. Cystourethrography displayed a normal bladder and long urethra. On micturition, reflux occurred into a closed vagina. Laparotomy revealed a normal uterus, Fallopian tubes, a right gonad containing testicular tissue and a left gonad composed of connective tissue. It was decided to raise the child as a female and the genitalia were adjusted accordingly (clitorectomy, vaginoplasty, removal of gonads).

Plate 117 Anterior perineal (ectopic) anus in a 6-day-old female infant born at term of an 18-year-old primigravida; birth-weight was 3,130 g. Regular anal dilatation was the only treatment required. If stenosis occurs then anoplasty, with temporary colostomy, is necessary. The great variation in the normal anatomy of the female perineum is best seen during the second stage of labour, before cutting an episiotomy. When this infant in her turn becomes a mother, she will require careful mediolateral episiotomy, since there will be only a short distance between posterior fourchette and anterior margin of the anus.

Plate 118 Total epispadias, extrophy of the bladder and bilateral inguinal hernias in a 1-day-old male infant, born at 40 weeks' gestation of a 23-year-old primigravida. Restoration to 'normal' required a 5-stage series of operations. Following bilateral osteotomies to mobilize the pubic bones, the bladder was closed and ureteric implantations carried out. Next, the pubic bones were approximated in the midline over the repaired bladder and the abdominal wall skin was closed. The hernias were repaired when the infant was aged 2 months. Finally, when the infant was 30 months of age, and after urinary continence was established, the epispadias was repaired to near normal urethral and penile anatomy.

117

118

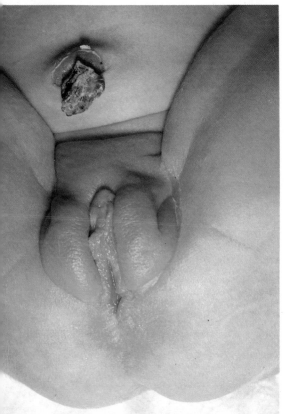

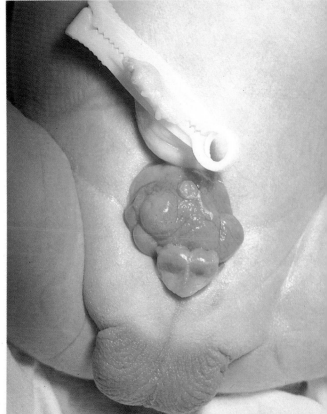

Plate 119 Like a newborn kitten, this tiny, female 2-day-old infant (birth-weight 570 g, born at 24.6 weeks' gestation) cannot open her eyes. She died aged 3 days. The mother, a 27-year-old primigravida, had several episodes of threatened abortion, developed premature rupture of the membranes at 23 weeks' gestation, then came into labour 13 days later. The terrible trilogy of second trimester troubles that account for more than 30% of perinatal deaths (due to prematurity with delivery before 28 weeks), and considerable maternal hazard (mainly from infection) are threatened abortion ± cervical incompetence, ante-partum haemorrhage and premature rupture of the membranes, individually or combined. In her next pregnancy the patient delivered a normal infant at term, after prophylactic cervical ligation at 16 weeks and several episodes of premature labour.

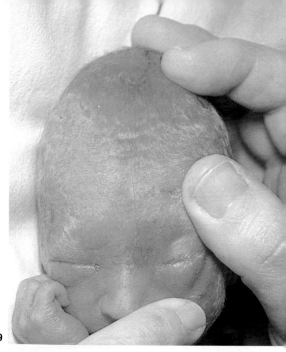

119

120

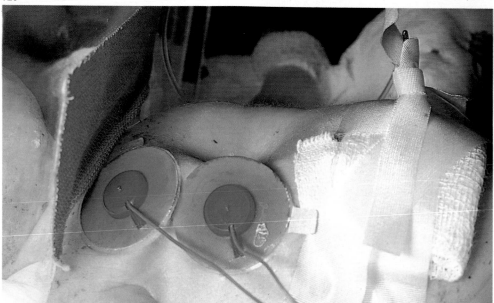

121

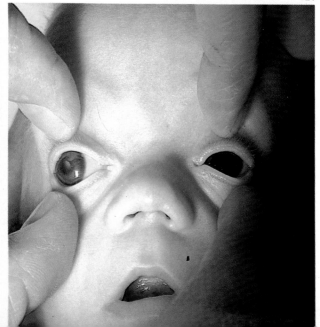

Plate 120 Extreme chest retraction in a 3-day-old female infant born at 29.4 weeks' gestation when spontaneous labour occurred following placental abruption. Birth-weight was 1,300 g. The child is receiving oxygen by means of a headbox, but nowadays, in a modern intensive care nursery, would be intubated and receiving ventilatory support. Also shown are electrodes and leads of cardiac and respiratory monitors and an umbilical artery catheter (for blood gas sampling). The child died shortly after this photograph was taken; autopsy confirmed that respiratory distress was due to hyaline membrane disease and pulmonary atelectasis, and also revealed an intraventricular haemorrhage.

Plate 121 Retrolental fibroplasia in a male infant aged 16 weeks who was born at 25.4 weeks' gestation, birth-weight 740 g. At 6 months of age he shows some of the sad sequelae of extreme prematurity. Note the grey mass showing through the pupil of the right eye which is blind because of associated total retinal detachment. In the left eye there is severe retrolental fibroplasia with possible progression to retinal detachment and complete blindness. There is also hydrocephaly and severe right cerebral atrophy. The mother had an incompetent cervix. A cervical stitch was inserted at 15 weeks, but premature rupture of the membranes occurred at 25 weeks and labour began 4 days later. The baby required ventilatory support for 45 days. Prematurity (and cervical incompetence) is a curse!

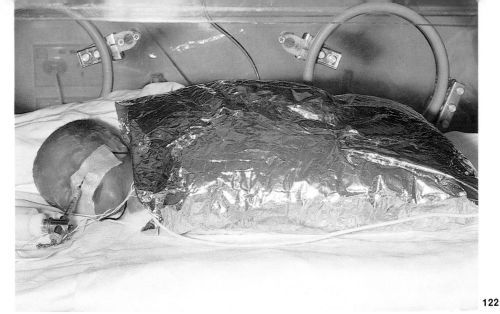

122

Plate 122 'Space rescue blanket' as used by astronauts is one method of heat conservation. This baby is one of uniovular twins born at 28 weeks' gestation when labour was induced because of maternal distress due to acute polyhydramnios. Birth-weight was 910 g. The child is shown aged 1 day, intubated and receiving ventilatory support. The baby died aged 7 days from complications of respiratory distress — pneumothorax, pneumomediastinum, bronchopulmonary dysplasia and pulmonary haemorrhage.

123

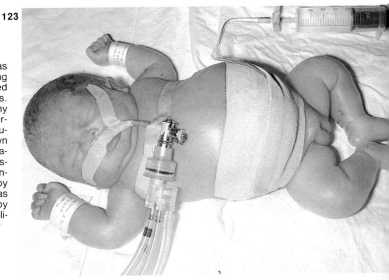

Plate 123 This hydropic 1-day-old infant was born at 32 weeks' gestation; 2 of her 3 living siblings (2 others were stillborn) had required exchange transfusions for erythroblastosis. Before labour was induced, cardiotocography had shown a sinusoidal pattern and late decelerations. The cord pH was 6.8. The baby was intubated immediately after birth and is shown receiving ventilatory support; abdominal paracentesis is in use to relieve distension and pressure on the diaphragm to improve lung expansion. In spite of exchange transfusion the baby died from pulmonary haemorrhage which was due to hypoxic heart failure and aggravated by the blood coagulopathy that so often complicates severe erythroblastosis.

124

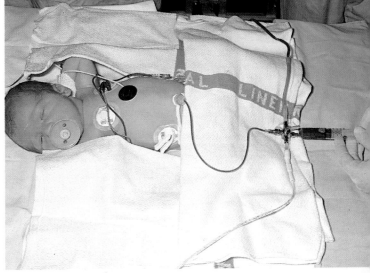

Plate 124 Exchange transfusion of a newborn infant (birth-weight 3,180 g at 37.5 weeks' gestation) found to have polycythaemia (packed cell volume 67%, haemoglobin 22.1 g/dl) when investigated because of tachycardia noted shortly after birth. Polycythaemia (PCV 65%) is associated in the short-term with respiratory distress and irritability and in the long-term, without treatment, there is approximately a 35% incidence of intellectual impairment. After a 20% blood volume exchange transfusion with SPPS (stable pooled protein solution), the haemoglobin value had fallen to 17.7 g/dl and PCV to 53%. Thereafter the infant's progress was uneventful. Note 4-way tap from SPPS to syringe, syringe to baby via umbilical vein catheter and from baby to waste. The black disc is the servocontrol sensor of the radiant heater above the cot, the other 3 being the cardiorespiratory monitoring electrodes.

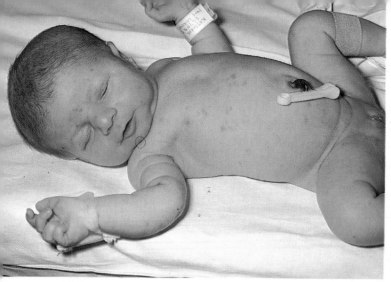

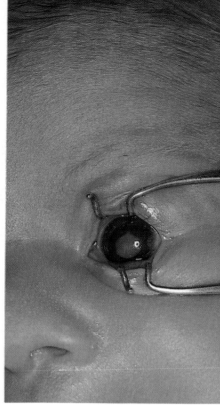

125A

Plate 125A Congenital rubella syndrome (purpuric rash, hepatosplenomegaly, bilateral cataracts, pulmonary stenosis, placental insufficiency) in a 1-day-old infant, birth-weight 2,110 g at 38.2 weeks' gestation. Rubella virus was isolated from throat swab, urine and leuco-cytes; rubella IgM antibodies (which do not cross the placenta) were detected in the infant's serum. The mother, a 28-year-old para 3, had subclinical infection early in the first trimester, probably at the time her other children had clinical rubella. During pregnancy there was clinical and ultrasound evidence of fetal growth retardation; Caesarean section was performed for fetal distress in labour. The moral is that all women should be immunized against rubella and ideally should have a blood test to confirm immunity before being at risk of conception.

125B

Plate 125B Cataract in the left eye displayed when the infant shown in plate 125A was aged 7 days. Rubella virus was isolated from both cataracts which were removed by needle aspiration. Contact lenses were fitted when the child was 8 weeks of age. The baby continued to excrete virus (positive throat swabs) for at least 4 months. Review at 8 months of age showed satisfactory progress. The risks of rubella embryopathy during pregnancy are as follows:— 1–8 weeks, 40–80% risk (malformations + microcephaly and mental retardation); 9–12 weeks, 20% risk (mainly deafness and brain damage); 13–16 weeks, 5% risk; 17–20 weeks, 1% risk (mainly retinopathy, rarely deafness and minor brain damage). Handicap due to rubella is rare when maternal infection occurs after 16 weeks' gestation.

126

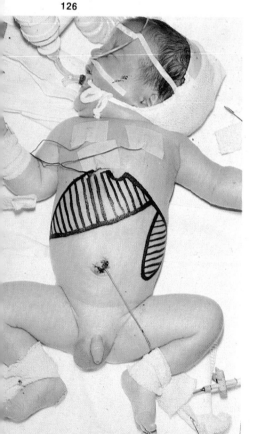

Plate 126 Cytomegalic inclusion disease in a 2-day-old infant causing jaun-dice, hepatosplenomegaly and pneumonitis necessitating intubation and ventilatory support. The mother, a 16-year-old primigravida, developed poly-hydramnios at 30 weeks' gestation; amniocentesis was performed at 32 weeks to determine the L:S ratio and perform amniography and fetography (fat soluble and water soluble radio-opaque dyes) to seek fetal malforma-tions. The liquor was yellow and cytomegalovirus was isolated from it. Obstructed labour required Caesarean delivery at 39.4 weeks; birth-weight was 3,500 g. Cytomegalovirus (CMV) was isolated from urine and saliva, and when the baby died aged 25 days, autopsy revealed the characteristic intranuclear inclusion bodies, especially in renal tubular cells. CMV is the most common intrauterine (transplacental) viral infection (1 in 200 births); only 5–10% of infected fetuses (diagnosed by viral excretion in neonates) have significant disease (hepatosplenomegaly, thrombocytopenia, purpura, jaundice, cerebral calcification with microcephaly, hydrocephaly or brain damage) in the first weeks of life. This infection is the most important cause of potentially preventable neurological impairment; human vaccination is still in the experimental stage.

Plate 127 This microcephalic infant was born at 39.4 weeks' gestation after labour was induced for mild preeclampsia. Her birth-weight was 2,590 g. The purpuric rash seen on the face simulates that due to hypoxia (impacted shoulders, umbilical cord looped tightly around neck), but is due to cyto-megalovirus infection which was proven by viral culture, then autopsy when the infant died aged 20 days.

Plate 128 Intrauterine death due to listeriosis. The mother, a 33-year-old para 2, developed abdominal pain and tachycardia at 21.1 weeks' gestation, followed by spontaneous rupture of the membranes and normal delivery of this slightly macerated fetus (birth-weight 480 g) showing a purpuric rash. Infection with Listeria monocytogenes is a rare cause of intrauterine death and neonatal meningoencephalitis (incidence 1 in 20,000 births). Ascend-ing infection from the genital tract involves the decidua initially, then results in fetal septicaemia probably as an intrauterine (rather than transplacental) infection. A heavy growth of Listeria was obtained from the placenta and fetal skin; autopsy showed miliary lesions with colonies of the organism in lungs and liver.

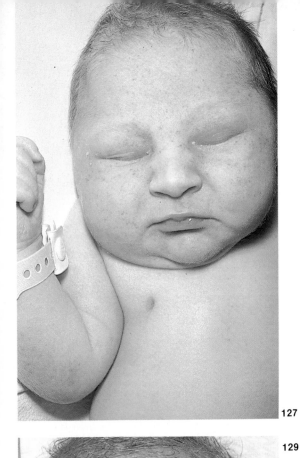

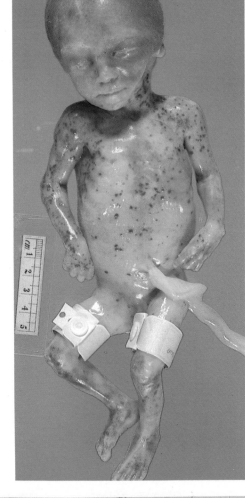

127

129

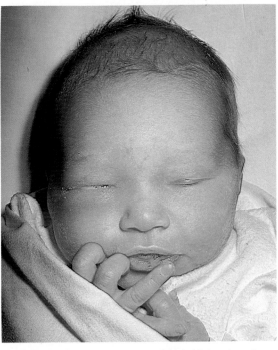

128

130

Plate 129 Erythema toxicum in a small for dates 13-day-old infant (birth-weight 2,150 g at 37 week's gestation). These lesions look like pustules, but in most cases no bacteria can be cultured from them. Histologically, aggregates of eosinophils are seen which is suggestive of an allergic aetiology. The baby was tremulous, plethoric and had a cyanotic attack; he was found to have hypoglycaemia and polycythaemia (haemoglobin 23.5 g/dl). Intravenous dextrose infusion and antibiotics resulted in rapid improvement.

Plate 130 Purulent conjunctivitis and periorbital oedema in a 6-day-old infant, born at term, birth-weight 3,190 g. An eye swab for microscopy and culture was negative but essential to exclude gonococcal and other bacterial infections. Response was rapid to chloramphenicol eye drops! Such lesions are often caused by Chlamydia which require special culture technique for identification.

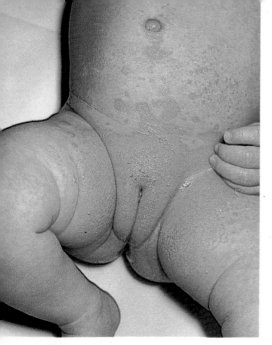

131

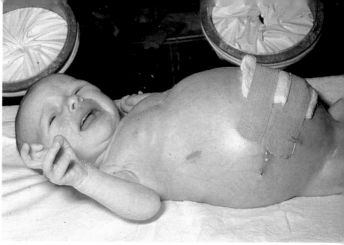

132

Plate 131 Monilial dermatitis in the napkin area of a 6-week-old infant. It is an intensely erythematous confluent plaque with a scalloped border and a sharply demarcated edge. It is formed by confluence of numerous papules which also stud the nearby skin as satellite papules which are the hallmark of monilial dermatitis. The clinical diagnosis can be confirmed by swab and culture — and looking for thrush in the infant's mouth. Perineal infection often occurs from faecal contamination. Nystatin cream effected a rapid cure.

Plate 132 Congenital neuroblastoma presenting at birth as an abdominal mass due to massive hepatic metastases. Most of these tumours arise from the adrenal glands or sympathetic nerve chains and 25% occur in the first year of life. Treatment is surgical — removal of the primary lesion plus chemotherapy ± irradiation. The prognosis is surprisingly good, with a 75% survival.

Plate 133 Prune belly syndrome (incidence 1 in 60,000 births) comprises dystrophy of abdominal wall musculature, urinary tract abnormalities and undescended testes. There is gross distension of the bladder, megaloureters and varying degrees of renal dysplasia — the latter determining the ultimate prognosis. An enlarged bladder can be identified by antenatal ultrasound, but decompression in utero is not recommended unless there is urethral obstruction.

Plate 134 Following Caesarean birth for fetal distress, this infant died aged 1 hour from respiratory failure due to a huge left posterior diaphragmatic hernia; colon, small bowel and spleen in the left pleural cavity have displaced the heart and mediastinum to the right and caused bilateral pulmonary hypoplasia. Because the pulmonary hypoplasia is irreversible, even prompt diagnosis and repair of the diaphragmatic defect cannot save such children. Small hernias often present when the baby is 3–4 days old and are amenable to surgery. As in 20–30% of cases of major malformations, this infant was small for dates (1,570 g at 38 weeks' gestation).

133

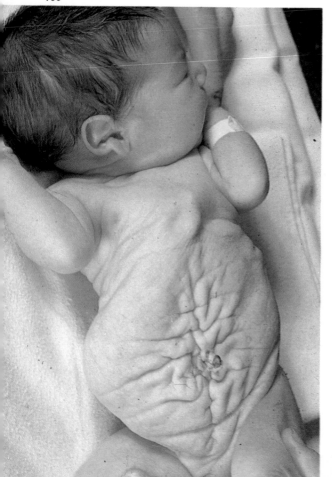

134

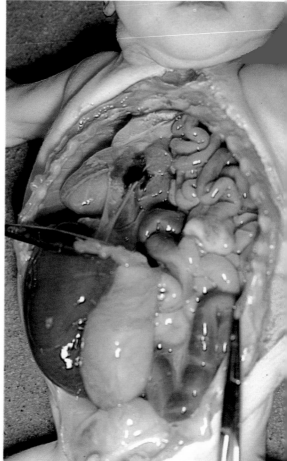

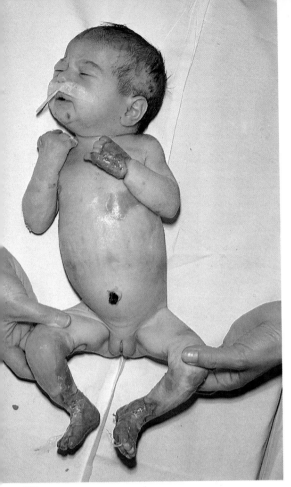

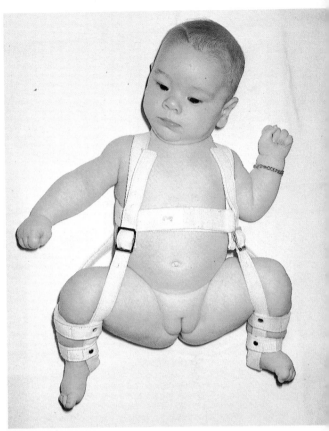

135

136

137

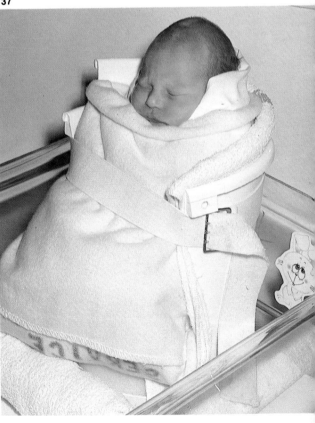

Plate 135 Epidermolysis bullosa in a 12-day-old small for dates infant, birth-weight 2,940 g at 41 weeks' gestation. This is a genetically transmitted group of skin diseases characterized by the formation of blisters due to minimal trauma. This infant has large lesions of the hands and legs that were present at birth. Note erosion of skin on the left chest wall due to pressure of the arm. Prognosis and genetic counselling is dependent upon accurate diagnosis which requires electron microscopy of skin to identify the lethal dominant form. Corticosteroid therapy may reduce scarring and stricture formation (e.g. of oesophagus). This child survived.

Plate 136 This infant had congenital dislocation of the left hip, the commonest of all major malformations, detected at the routine examination after birth. Treatment consisted of maintenance in the abducted position in this harness until the hip was normal clinically and radiographically. She is shown at the age of 12 weeks prior to removal of the harness; a cure has been effected which is the usual result if treatment is commenced soon after birth.

Plate 137 This 7-day-old baby (birth-weight 2,290 g at 32.4 weeks' gestation) has gastro-oesophageal reflux which is a common cause of vomiting, especially in premature infants. His jaundice responded to phototherapy. He is shown propped upright in a special 'propping bucket' which is used for 2–4 weeks until the regurgitation ceases. He was discharged home on day 32, weighing 2,790 g. Babies who tend to vomit after feedings are often nursed propped up even when there is no proven gastro-oesophageal reflux.

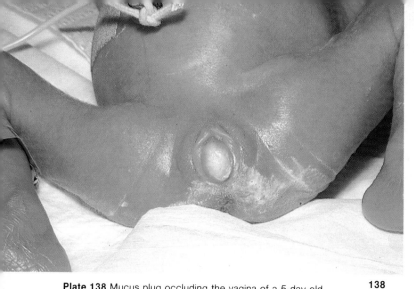

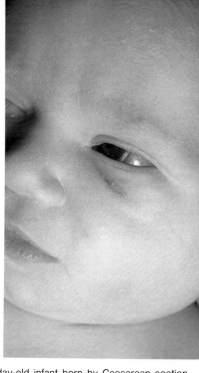

138

Plate 138 Mucus plug occluding the vagina of a 5-day-old jaundiced infant (birth-weight 1,220 g) born by breech delivery at 30 weeks' gestation; spontaneous labour had occurred following a mild placental abruption. These plugs occur in about 1 in 200 babies in special care nurseries. The plug disintegrates without treatment.

139

Plate 140 Total brachial plexus palsy due to impacted shoulders in a 4-day-old baby following difficult mid-forceps delivery. His birth-weight was 4,950 g. Complete resolution did not occur. The more common nerve palsies (total incidence 2 per 1,000 births) involve upper brachial plexus (Erb C5,6, 50%), facial nerve (45%), total brachial plexus (3%) and lower brachial plexus (Klumpke C7, C8, T1, 2%). They are associated with impacted shoulders, breech extraction and difficult forceps delivery. More than 90% recover completely, usually within a few days.

Plate 139 A 2-day-old infant born by Caesarean section performed because of obstructed labour due to a transverse lie. The delivery was difficult and the child sustained a right-sided Erb palsy and facial bruising of the type often seen after a difficult mid-forceps delivery. Subconjunctival haemorrhages also occur in infants having normal vaginal births. Spontaneous resolution occurs without treatment.

140

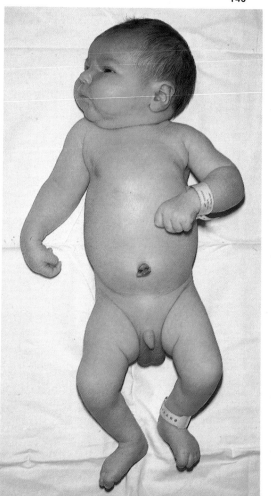

Plate 141 Compound presentation (breech and hands) accounts for the extensive bruising and oedema shown by this 2,320 g infant whose 24-year-old primigravid mother was admitted in premature labour at 32 weeks' gestation. This photograph was taken shortly after birth by Caesarean section. The next day a left Erb palsy was noted which resolved as the bruising subsided.

141

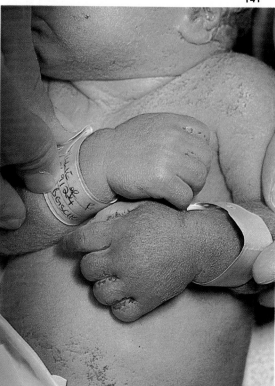

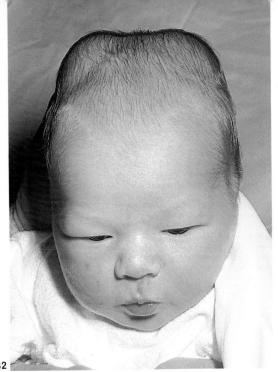

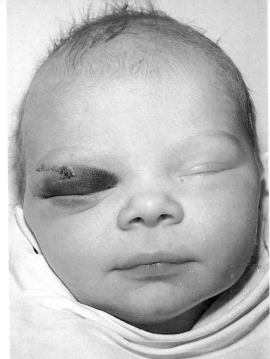

42

143A   143B

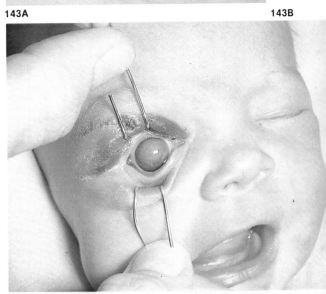

Plate 142 Bilateral cephalhaematomas in a 4-day-old male infant (birth-weight 4,170 g), born at 40.2 weeks' gestation by difficult mid-forceps delivery. Note the mild jaundice. The incidence of cephalhaematoma is related to the method of delivery (elective Caesarean 0.1%, normal 1–2%, forceps 5%, vacuum extraction 10%). In a series of 1,030 infants with cephalhaematomas, 10% had bilirubin values above 150 μmol/l (9 mg/dl), 5% required phototherapy for treatment of jaundice, 0.5% required exchange transfusion, and 0.5% required a simple blood transfusion.

Plate 143A Periorbital haematoma and jaundice in a male infant aged 4 days, birth-weight 4,090 g. He was born by Kielland forceps rotation and delivery from the occipitoposterior position. His mother was a 20-year-old primigravida.

Plate 143B Corneal opacity due to shearing of the cornea demonstrated by retraction of the eyelids. Antibiotic ointment was applied and in 2 weeks the cloudiness of the cornea had resolved. At the age of 3 years there was marked impairment of vision in the right eye.

Plate 144 Depressed fracture of the left frontal bone in a 1-day-old male infant, birth-weight 3,100 g. The mother was a 25-year-old primigravida with a contracted pelvis (transverse diameter of the pelvic brim 11.5 cm) who had a trial of labour and trial of forceps (Kielland) from the left occipitoposterior position. The baby also has a right facial nerve palsy. The fracture was elevated 4 days after birth. The child showed no signs of cerebral damage!

144

Plate 145 The feared complication of impacted shoulders. This spinal cord belonged to a male infant, birth-weight 3,850 g. The mother was a 23-year-old primigravida who had a mid-forceps delivery under general anaesthesia, after a 38-hour labour. There was great difficulty with delivery of the shoulders. The baby made no respiratory effort, was flaccid, and died after 14 hours of resuscitative care. There was no fracture of the skull or spine. The spinal cord shows a narrowed congested area 3 cm from its origin; section showed the area to be softened and haemorrhagic.

145

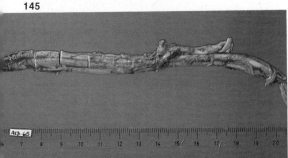

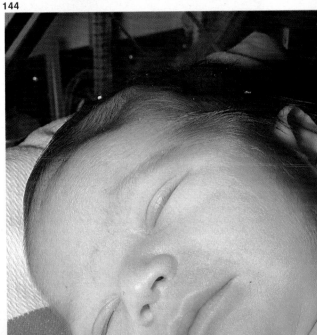

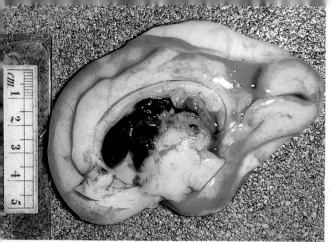

146

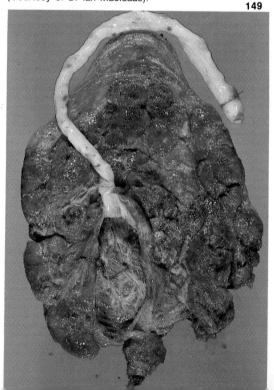

147

148

Plate 146 Extensive intraventricular and subarachnoid haemorrhage seen at autopsy in the brain of an 'undiagnosed' second twin, birth-weight 1,220 g, born by breech delivery after the onset of spontaneous labour at 28 weeks' gestation. The baby died aged 14 hours. Realtime ultrasound scanning has shown that intraventricular haemorrhage occurs within the first 24 hours of age in 30–50% of low birth-weight infants (below 1,500 g). The incidence is lower in infants born by Caesarean section although the cause of bleeding is hypoxic damage to the immature, thin-walled, fragile capillaries in the subependymal layer, the blood bursting into the ventricle. Intraventricular haemorrhage virtually occurs only in premature infants — there is no physical damage to falx or tentorium.

Plate 147 Necrotizing enterocolitis (incidence 2 per 1,000, 10 times more common when birth-weight is below 1,500 g, mortality rate 25%) in a 4-day-old female infant, birth-weight 1,595 g whose survival is doubly miraculous. Her mother presented at 32 weeks' gestation with severe preeclampsia and blood coagulation failure complicating hydatidiform molar degeneration of one-half of a single placenta. After uneventful initial progress, the baby developed abdominal distension and vomiting on day 4 and passed blood per rectum. Laparotomy revealed that the distal half of small bowel and proximal half of large bowel were gangrenous; jejunostomy and transverse colostomy were carried out after the affected segments had been resected. Both stomas were closed when the child was aged 12 months. At the age of 14 months the child is small (8 kg), but shows satisfactory physical and intellectual development. (Courtesy of Dr John Thorburn).

Plate 149 Placenta membranacea. The patient was a 22-year-old primigravida. Ultrasonography, performed at 30 weeks' gestation because of polyhydramnios and breech presentation, showed an extensive thin placenta attached to anterior, posterior and lateral uterine walls, completely covering the internal os (grade 4 or central placenta praevia); the patient was admitted to hospital! During the following weeks she had several minor episodes of painless vaginal bleeding. Lower segment Caesarean section was performed through the placenta at 37 weeks' gestation. The infant was born in good condition, birth-weight 2,630 g. The placenta weighed 590 g and extended over almost the entire surface of the chorion — it did not quite reach to the fundus. By what secret mechanism does Nature usually ensure normal development of the placenta without excessive atrophy or persistence of chorionic villi (figures 4.3, 4.5, 4.7 and 43.8, colour plates 1 and 84)? (Courtesy of Dr Ian MacIsaac).

149

Plate 148 Pulmonary interstitial emphysema due to attempted resuscitation of a 3,320 g hydrocephalic infant who died aged 3 hours from subdural and intraventricular haemorrhage (300 ml of cerebrospinal fluid was aspirated before mid-forceps delivery). Pulmonary air-leak (interstitial emphysema ± pneumothorax and pneumomediastinum) develops in 20% of infants with respiratory distress and is associated with a 3-fold increase in mortality. It occurs mainly in premature infants with hyaline membrane disease who require ventilatory support.

During the first 3 minutes, the 'let-down' reflex comes into operation, and it is for this reason that the baby obtains the greater part (90%) of his feeding in the first 3–5 minutes. The infant commences consecutive feedings at alternate breasts.

When the infant has finished feeding, he is carefully withdrawn from the nipple to prevent any trauma to it. This can be performed by gently pushing down on his jaw (figure 60.2D), or by inserting a finger into the angle of his mouth (figure 60.2E); both of these methods break the vacuum created by the sucking.

When changing from one breast to the other and at the conclusion of the feeding, the infant needs to be 'dewinded'. There are 2 methods. (i) The baby may be held upright over the mother's shoulder with his stomach, i.e. the upper left quadrant of the abdomen, resting against her shoulder while she exerts gentle intermittent pressure on the back by rubbing or patting. (ii) He is sat up on the mother's knee inclined a little forward. She places one hand over his stomach and with the other hand exerts gentle pressure on his back (figure 60.2F). Care should be taken that the pressure is exerted over the stomach and not just along the spine.

The infant is then placed lying on either side in the cot, with the head of the cot elevated if there is any tendency to vomiting.

In the early days of lactation, the breasts should be inspected after each feeding, and particularly after the last feeding at night.

The *signs of successful breast feeding* are: the infant is contented, sleeps well and is a good colour; tissue turgor is firm, weight gain is normal and there is an adequate number of wet nappies.

Breast Feeding Regimens

Self-demand. By this method, the baby is put to the breast, not at regular intervals, but when showing signs of hunger. With this method the baby is awake, eager and seeking for food, and so sucks more strongly, empties the breast easily and obtains more satisfactory feeding; furthermore, because of the strong stimulation of the breasts, lactation is more easily established. Demand feeding has been found to be the most satisfactory regimen for almost all infants. The baby usually adjusts to a regular schedule during the first few weeks. This is the method most commonly advocated at present in the United Kingdom.

Regular hours. In this method of feeding, the baby is first put to the breast as soon after birth as the condition of the mother and baby will allow. One then follows a regular regimen of 3–4 hourly feeding intervals. This method has many disadvantages to the infant — feeding times often bear no relationship to hunger, so babies fed at regular feeding hours tend to suck less satisfactorily than those fed according to the self-demand regimen. This feeding by the clock regimen is not recommended for most infants.

Test Feeding

Test feeding is a procedure whereby the amount of breast milk obtained by the infant is assessed. Test feeding gives helpful information if carried out over a 24-hour period, but isolated test feedings are of little value.

The infant is changed and weighed in his clothes. He is fed as the mother usually feeds him and is then reweighed in exactly the same clothing. The difference in weight equals the amount obtained at the breast (table 60.1).

TABLE 60.1 AVERAGE DAILY AMOUNT OF BREAST MILK (ML) OBTAINED BY TERM INFANTS

1st day	60–90
2nd day	120–180
3rd day	270
4th day	330
5th day	390
6th day	420
7th day	420
2nd week	510–540
3rd week	570
4th week	600

Hygiene of the Nursing Mother

The general health must be maintained, and the mother should, as far as possible, be kept free from anxiety and adequately rested.

Diet. The diet must be sufficient for the mother's own health, and at the same time supply all the elements necessary for the secretion of breast milk. The elements in which her diet is most likely to be low are *calcium and vitamins*. In recent years a high energy diet with frequent snacks between meals has been recommended to keep up the milk supply.

Rest and exercise. At least 8 hours sleep at night and 1 hour of rest during the day should be the aim. Exercise in the outdoors is beneficial.

Advice on Discharge From Hospital

When leaving hospital, the mother is instructed in points of general hygiene of the nursing mother, and the need for frequent visits to the health centre is emphasized, in order that the baby may be observed and weighed regularly, and that any difficulties with regard to the condition of her breasts or lactation may be resolved.

DIFFICULTIES IN BREAST FEEDING

The difficulties which may arise in relation to breast feeding during the first week of the puerperium are numerous and to the young mother they are often a major problem. These difficulties may be general or local, and may occur in the mother, the infant, or both. In general, apart from psychological factors, the principal impediments to successful breast feeding are to be found in anatomical or physiological abnormalities in the mother's breasts.

(A) MATERNAL DIFFICULTIES

THE BREASTS

Engorgement (figures 60.3 and 60.4)

This is a common condition which tends to occur on about the 3rd or 4th day; surveys have indicated that it is present in about 5% of women 48 hours after delivery, in 35–40% by 72 hours, and in 40–45% by 96 hours. Hormonal activity causes an increase in blood flow to the breasts and a sudden secretion of milk. Tension in the breast increases with resulting obstruction to the *venous and lymphatic vessels* and interference with the *flow of milk* along ducts. The problem may be accentuated by thick colostrum which tends to block milk ducts. Engorgement may also occur at any time during lactation if there is inadequate removal of milk from the breasts in cases where supply temporarily exceeds demand.

The condition may largely be prevented by the following measures. (i) The baby commences feeding from alternate breasts. (ii) The feeding is supervised by trained nurses and midwives in the early days. (iii) The baby is allowed unrestricted access to the breast.

For *mild engorgement* the following treatment is given. (i) Heat, in the form of a hot shower or bath. (ii) Expression of a little fluid before putting the baby to the breast to relieve the tension, and a further expression after the feeding. (iii) Analgesia — soluble aspirin 30 minutes before feeding. (iv) Support — a good brassiere to lift and support the breasts may be helpful.

In *severe engorgement* (figure 60.4) the following treatment is given in addition to the above. (i) An analgesic is usually necessary and

therapeutic ultrasound is often helpful. (ii) Alternating hot and cold compresses and warm oil packs between feedings is also helpful. (iii) *Persistent pyrexia signifies infection*, and the milk should be cultured, and antibiotics given.

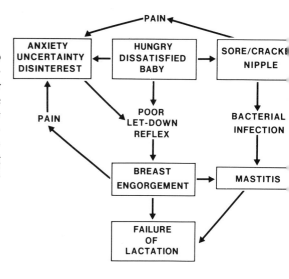

Figure 60.3 Interrelated factors which can result in breast engorgement, breast infection and failure of lactation.

Breast Infection

Mastitis

Aetiology. Inflammation of the breasts is usually secondary to cracking of the nipples and breast engorgement (figure 60.3). The organism (almost invariably the staphylococcus) gains entrance through the cracked nipple and multiplies in the stagnant milk. In some patients, infection occurs because of stasis of milk behind a blocked duct. Contributing factors include poor technique (breast engorgement, damage to nipple by the baby) and staphylococcal carriage by the baby.

Clinical features. The breasts are inflamed, hard, reddened and painful, there are enlarged glands in the axilla, and there is pyrexia, tachycardia and often malaise.

Management. Prophylaxis. Many infections can be prevented or minimized by proper hygiene, and stressing to the mother the need to avoid engorgement and nipple cracking. It may be necessary to take a nose and throat swab from the baby if it is suspected that colonization/infection has occurred.

When mastitis has occurred, an appropriate antibiotic is administered to the mother. There is no need to stop feeding from the infected side,

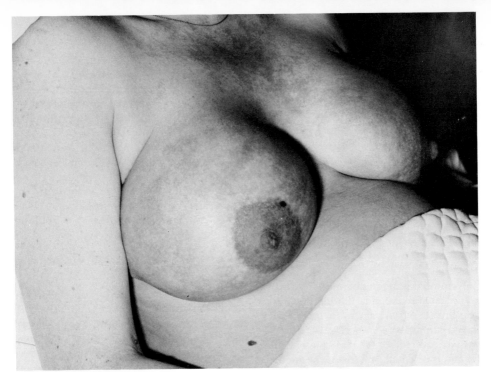

Figure 60.4 Severe breast engorgement on day 3 of the puerperium in a 27-year-old primipara. Her breasts were lumpy, hot and reddened as shown by the blotches in this picture. She was afebrile. There was more embarrassment than pain. Expression caused resolution but the patient decided to bottle-feed her infant. Fewer than 5% of patients have engorgement of such severity.

although the mother may find this too painful and the milk should then be manually expressed. A sample of milk should be sent for culture (this usually reveals penicillin-resistant staphylococci). Hot compresses may be helpful in stimulating milk flow.

Abscess

If mastitis is not treated correctly and promptly, an abscess may form (colour plate 97). The incidence has been reduced approximately 10-fold (from 3% to 0.3%) since the use of hexachlorophane cleansing of the baby (Chapter 59), this having reduced the incidence of staphylococcal colonization from about 70% to 30%. It should be remembered that in some 80% or more of patients with this complication the condition develops only after leaving the hospital, so that a prophylactic educational message regarding the early reporting of mastitis is wise. It is often said that the mother gets the infection from the baby, but in some cases the woman has not breast-fed the baby and the strain of staphylococcus is different in the mother and newborn.

The *diagnosis* of abscess in the breast may be difficult, since *fluctuation* is less easy to elicit than in other sites. If resolution of the induration does not occur with *chemotherapy, incision and drainage* is carried out. Ultrasonography is helpful in the difficult case to identify a collection of pus.

LACTATION

Overabundance

In this situation the breasts refill very quickly and the milk flows from the nipples between feedings. The baby receives his feeding too rapidly and is overfed. Overfeeding and feedings received too quickly will soon be evident by vomiting and the presence of abnormal stools; usually sore buttocks will result.

Treatment. The following techniques should be tried. (i) If the breast is so full that the infant has difficulty fixing on the nipple, express a quantity of milk before the infant commences feeding. (ii) Employ the principles of demand feeding.

Insufficient Supply

The most important cause is insufficient nipple stimulation. Milk is produced on a supply and demand basis. The problem is often seen where the mother is over-anxious and very tense or apprehensive, as is often the case in the elderly primipara. It often coincides with withdrawal from the new mother of help and she suddenly has to cope with her new baby, home and perhaps other children. She becomes over-tired and anxious and the milk supply dwindles. It is much more common than overfeeding. Other causes include poor mammary development, poor general health or anaemia, and poor stimulatory efforts by the baby.

The condition is recognized by: (i) a crying restless baby or in some cases a sleepy baby, (ii) failure to gain weight or weight loss, (iii) signs of dehydration (loss of skin turgor, scanty urine, constipation).

Treatment. (i) Stimulation is necessary; change baby to more frequent feedings and supervise each feeding until both mother and baby become more confident, (ii) allow adequate time for feeding; never rush or hurry the mother, (iii) the mother should be encouraged to relax completely several times daily: as she breathes out she should imagine the tension flowing out of her body and at the same time visualize the milk flowing down the ducts of the breast, (iv) privacy must be ensured and a relaxed atmosphere is necessary; fear or tension must be overcome, (v) rest at night and during the day is essential, otherwise the mother will not lactate satisfactorily, (vi) diet must contain all the essential foods and fluids, (vii) haemoglobin estimation may be of value to detect unexpected maternal anaemia, (viii) the contraceptive pill may have been commenced too early and this may reduce the supply in some women or affect the palatability of the milk, resulting in partial refusal by the baby, (ix) ensure that physical discomfort (e.g. painful perineum) is not inhibiting the let-down reflex.

Complementary feeding should only be advised in extreme cases because the baby may not have to work so hard to obtain milk through an artificial teat and thus may give up the breast in favour of the bottle.

NIPPLES

Inverted Nipples
The expectant mother should receive treatment during pregnancy. The mother wears Meredith (Woolwich) Breast Shields (colour plate 44). Some 10–15% of women have flat or inverted nipples.

Sore Nipples
The importance of nipple soreness is usually underemphasized. During pregnancy, tactile sensitivity of the nipple decreases significantly, but increases soon after birth of the baby. Over the second–fourth days after delivery, more than 80% of women experience some nipple discomfort; in about 50% of these it is moderate or extreme, usually when the baby attaches at the start of the feeding. In a significant number, however, the pain continues during the feeding. The major factor associated with nipple dis-

comfort is breast engorgement, and it has little relation to the duration of feeding. Nipple tenderness may be confined to one breast.

Treatment consists of: (i) More frequent *brief* feedings, (ii) feeding from the less painful side first, (iii) use of anhydrous lanolin on the nipples, (iv) exposure to the air — this can be achieved by wearing a suitable device under the bra to keep the clothing away from the sore nipple and allow the air to circulate around it, (v) exposure to sunlight for 1–5 minutes, (vi) vary the feeding position, (vii) keep the nipple area dry.

Cracked Nipples
If the excoriation is only superficial, use the lanolin-air-sunlight treatment already described. However, if the nipples are deeply cracked the baby is temporarily removed from the breast and the latter is gently expressed by hand. Heat can be applied to the cracked area and the nipple can be protected by use of a nipple shield.

Nipple Discharge
A reddish or brownish discharge from the nipple occurs in 1–3% of women: primiparas are more often affected and the discharge tends to occur at the colostrum stage. It may occur spontaneously or be due to breast massage/expression traumatizing delicate blood vessels, an intraduct papilloma, or very rarely, a duct carcinoma. Management consists in cessation of breast/nipple manipulation, continuation of feeding and referral if the condition persists.

Too Large or Too Small
A mismatch between the size of the infant's mouth and the nipples can make for difficulties with breast feeding (figure 60.5).

PSYCHOLOGICAL DIFFICULTIES

The mental attitude of the mother plays a major role in the success or failure of breast feeding. The mother must never be forced to breast-feed her baby if she does not wish to do so. Some women are over-anxious to succeed and this in itself worsens the situation, others again are uninterested, whilst others are too excitable. Such mothers require a great deal of understanding, patience, and help from the midwife and doctor if their problems are to be overcome.

(B) NEONATAL DIFFICULTIES

Absence of Sucking Powers
This may result from immaturity, cerebral injury, infection, congenital heart disease, or other

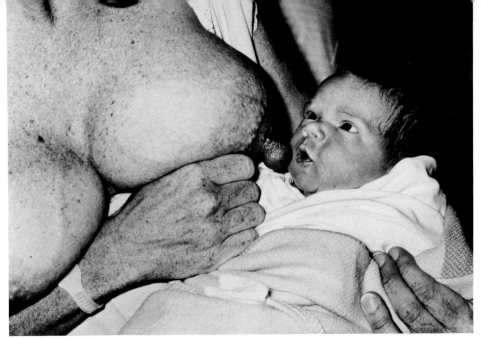

Figure 60.5 Huge enlargement of the nipples and moderate breast engorgement on day 7 of the puerperium in a 38-year-old para 3. The baby could not open her mouth wide enough to cope! The nipples were not sore. The milk supply was plentiful. The patient expressed and breast feeding was resumed successfully when the nipples became less swollen. The mother did not suffer this rare complication in her only other lactation 14 years previously.

debilitating illness. These babies require cot nursing and nasogastric feeding with expressed breast milk, until the sucking powers have developed or returned.

Anatomical Problems

(i) *Cleft palate and lip* (colour plates 111 and 112). Babies with such defects require to be fed with a spoon or special bottle with a cleft palate mouthpiece. Gavage feeding should be avoided since scarring may result, making repair of the abnormality more difficult.

(ii) *Micrognathia*, due to a poorly developed mandible. A nipple shield with a special type of long mouth piece may be used.

(iii) *Nasal obstruction*. The newborn baby breathes through his nose and any obstruction of the upper respiratory tract, whether it be due to infection or some organic obstruction, will create a problem and warrant treatment (see Chapter 65).

Infection

Local infection such as stomatitis may prevent an infant sucking.

Sleepy or Lethargic Infant

Some babies may be unduly sleepy following delivery. This may be caused by drugs given to the mother in labour or by neonatal jaundice. Commonly the baby is slow to learn to suck. This condition needs patience on the part of the mother who will need to put the baby on the breast frequently and may need to keep up the milk supply by manual expression. The baby may need to be awakened for feeding to avoid dehydration.

The Excitable Baby

The nervous, excitable baby requires a great deal of patience and gentle handling. Supervision throughout the feedings is necessary until the baby and mother become more confident.

Gastro-oesophageal Reflux

In some babies there is reflux of acid stomach content into the oesophagus leading to painful heartburn. This will be relieved by posture (raising the head of the bassinet) and antacid therapy (e.g. Mylanta) (colour plate 137).

Breast Refusal

Refusal of the breast by the baby is one of the most demoralizing experiences of the mother; this is all the more so if there is no apparent reason. It may occur at the initiation of breast feeding or after its establishment. Early refusal is most likely to be caused by errors of technique of mother and/or baby; later refusal indicates the need for a medical check, particular attention being paid to the ears, nose and throat. Some common causes and their management are summarized in table 60.2.

BREAST EXPRESSION

The methods of breast expression may be manual or mechanical, the latter being by means of

TABLE 60.2 BREAST REFUSAL

Causative factor	Examples	Management
Faulty technique of mother	Baby unable to breathe	Keep nose clear of breast; check whether upper lip occluding nostrils; ensure nostrils are clear
Faulty technique of baby	Inability to coordinate sucking, swallowing and breathing	
	Tongue over nipple	
	Restless	Prefeed handling kept to a minimum, feed in quiet surroundings
Engorged breasts and/or nipple problems		Prevention by early suckling/emptying
Too rapid flow of milk		Hand express till initial rush of milk ceases and/or posture feeding
Medical conditions in mother	Dietary problems	Identify and eliminate
	Menstruation	Reassurance of temporary nature
Medical conditions in baby	Oral moniliasis (thrush)	Nystatin, gentian violet 1% paint
	ENT infection	Appropriate treatment

a hand or electric pump. Manual expression is the method of choice, but some mothers find it difficult and tedious, and hence mechanical methods are used.

Manual Expression

After careful cleansing of the hands, the fingers are placed under the breast for support and the thumb on top (figure 60.6A); compression is applied between the thumb and fingers rhythmically about 30 times per minute working downwards towards the nipple. Occasional pressure with the palm of the hand to force milk towards the nipple is advantageous (figure 60.6B).

Hand Pump

The bulb is compressed and then placed firmly over the nipple and gradually released (figure 60.7A). This is repeated as often as necessary to empty the breast. Because of the possibility of trauma to the nipple with the bulb type of breast pump the Kaneson pump is now recommended (figure 60.7B).

Electric Pump

As before, the pump is placed over the nipple (figure 60.8); the power is switched on and intermittent suction begins.

SUPPRESSION OF LACTATION

Lactation may have to be suppressed either in the interest of the mother or because of the presence of some defect in the sucking mechanism of the infant.

INDICATIONS

(i) Perinatal death. (ii) The mother does not wish to breast-feed or the infant is being adopted. (iii) Severe breast problems such as inverted, cracked or hypersensitive nipples unresponsive to treatment. (iv) Puerperal psychosis. (v) Recently acquired maternal syphilis with an unaffected baby. (vi) Active maternal tuberculosis. (vii) To wean after breast feeding.

There are 2 important situations in which weaning should not be automatically and thoughtlessly advised.

(i) Low Birth-weight, Immature and Sick Infants

Although the infant may be unable to suck at the breast, many mothers are willing and able to express breast milk for their infants. Such a mother should be encouraged to express, for it is one way in which she can contribute to the baby's progress.

(ii) Maternal Drugs and Breast Feeding

Most drugs taken by the lactating woman appear in the breast milk but usually the infant receives less than 1% of the maternal dose. If the mother is receiving large doses of a potentially toxic drug, the advisability of breast feeding should be carefully considered. Heroin, anticonvulsants, anticoagulants and antithyroid drugs are potentially harmful to the infant (see Chapter 11).

MANAGEMENT

Where it is known that breast feeding is not advisable or desired from the commencement of the puerperium, a good supporting brassiere should be worn, and stimulation of the breast should be avoided; analgesic drugs may be necessary for painful engorgement. This conservative management is all that is required in the

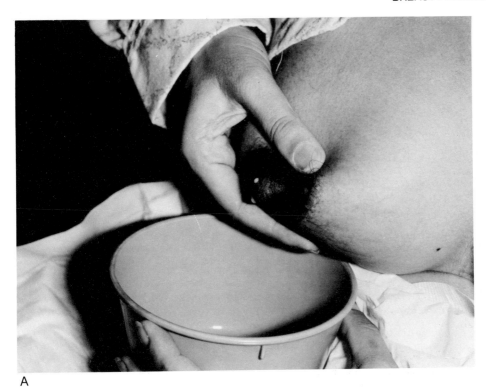

A

Figure 60.6 Manual expression. **A.** The lactiferous sinuses at the base of the nipples are squeezed between thumb and fingers. **B.** The breast is massaged towards the nipple.

B

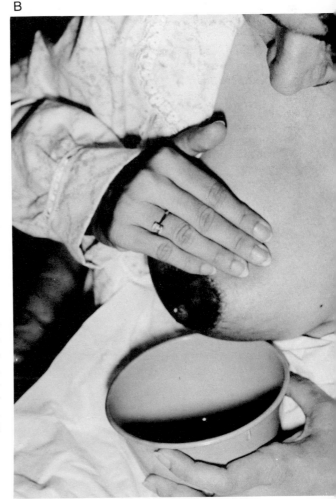

majority of patients. Oestrogen preparations carry some risk of venous thrombosis and pulmonary thromboembolism and are rarely used today. *Bromocriptine* (Parlodel) is the drug of choice if drugs are required to suppress lactation. Bromocriptine inhibits prolactin synthesis and its release from the anterior lobe of the pituitary gland. This drug is given for 10–14 days in a dose of 5 mg/day. Side-effects include hypotension, dizziness, nausea/vomiting, epigastric discomfort, nasal congestion, fatigue, and skin rash. In animals and probably in the human, prolactin enhances maternal feelings; bromocriptine may counteract this. An additional problem is that prolactin acts as a natural contraceptive; its suppression will result in an *earlier return of fertility*.

RELACTATION

For a number of reasons (low supply, sore nipples, fretful baby), a mother may cease breast feeding but then regret the decision and desire to resume lactation. The change of mind may be related to such factors as missing the closeness of the baby, formula disagreeing with the baby, new information regarding the advantages of breast feeding or changed circumstances (e.g. in the work place). Frequent suckling will help to reestablish a good milk supply.

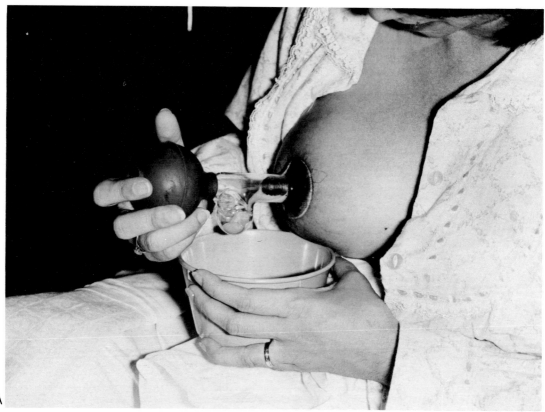

A

Figure 60.7 Hand pump. **A.** Bulb type of pump which although still in common use has the disadvantage that the degree of suction is not easy to control and so the nipple can be damaged. **B.** The Kaneson hand pump has the advantages of easy regulation of suction and interconversion to a feeding bottle by attachment of a teat.

B

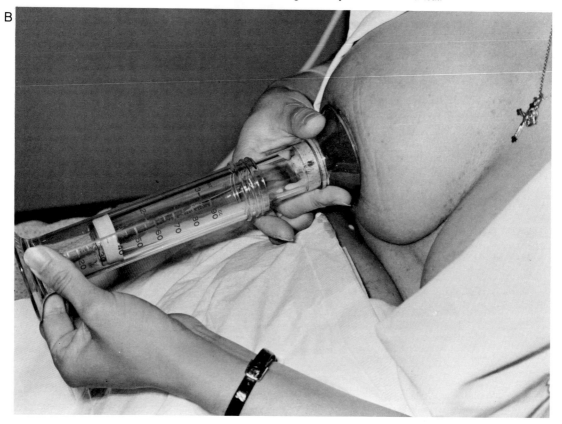

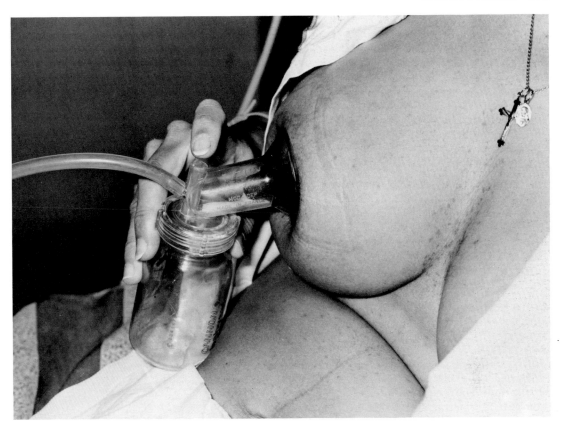

Figure 60.8 Electric pump being used on day 4 of the puerperium by a 30-year-old para 1 Chinese patient. Note that the finger is intermittently applied to the release port to regulate the duration and strength of suction.

chapter sixty-one

Artificial Feeding

OVERVIEW

When breast feeding is impossible or deleterious to mother or baby, some form of artificial feeding must be given. This usually means an artificial feed modified to mimic breast milk in terms of the protein, fat, carbohydrate and vitamin content. Manufacturers now claim that modern artificial feedings are 'humanized' (i.e. made to mimic human breast milk). However, this is a play on words because, in spite of the improvements due to modern technology, it remains different from the real thing.

INTRODUCTION

Although breast feeding is superior to artificial feeding for most mothers and babies, there are times when it is impossible or inadvisable. In such situations infants may be fed successfully with an artificial feeding. Whilst the sense of intimacy and togetherness fostered by breast feeding is most advantageous to both mother and baby, it must be remembered that a loving mother, even when she is using artificial feeding, can impart an adequate amount of security in her manner of handling her infant (figure 61.1). To this end the mother should simulate breast feeding as closely as possible.

Any artificial feeding to be successful must meet the following requirements: (i) it must be within the infant's digestive capabilities, (ii) it must yield sufficient calories for the infant's requirements, (iii) it must contain sufficient water to meet the baby's fluid requirements, and (iv) it must contain sufficient protein, fat, carbohydrate, mineral, salts and vitamins to meet the infant's nutritional needs. It is possible to fulfil these requirements in a variety of ways. Daily nutritional requirements for term and preterm infants are shown in table 61.1.

TABLE 61.1 DAILY NUTRITIONAL REQUIREMENTS PER KILOGRAM BODY WEIGHT

Nutrients	Infant	
	Term	Preterm
Calories	100	120
Fluid	150 ml	200 ml
Protein	2–2.5 g	2.5–3 g
Fat	4 g	6 g
Sodium	2 mmol	3–4 mmol
Potassium	2 mmol	3 mmol
Calcium	2 mmol	2 mmol
Phosphorus	1.3 mmol	1.3 mmol
Magnesium	0.4 mmol	0.4 mmol

Composition of Milk

For the first few days after birth of the baby, the secretion of the breast is colostrum. On the third or fourth day the secretion changes to milk which is intended by nature to provide the infant with both food and fluid. Cow's milk, like human milk, is composed of approximately 88% water and 12% solids, but the solids are differently disposed (table 61.2).

The calorific value of both human and cow's milk is 20 calories per 30 ml (1 ounce).

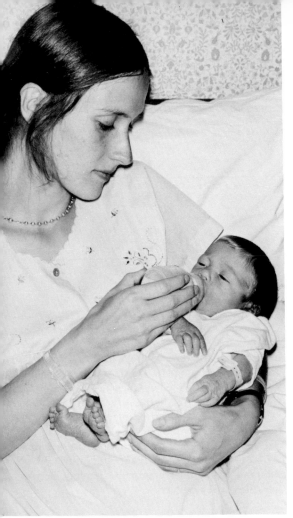

Figure 61.1 During bottle feeding the baby is held comfortably with the head well supported. The bottle is tilted so that its neck is full of milk to avoid undue sucking in of air. It is possible to obtain eye-to-eye contact during bottle feeding as it is with breast feeding, so furthering maternal-infant bonding.

tough curd which is difficult for the infant to manage, whereas breast milk casein produces a fine flocculent curd which is easily digested.

Fat. Although the amount of fat in the 2 milks is approximately the same, the chemical composition differs and the fat droplets are larger and more difficult to digest in cow's milk than the smaller droplets in human milk.

Carbohydrates. The sugar in both cow's milk and human milk is *lactose*, but it is present in a smaller amount in cow's milk.

Minerals. The mineral content in cow's milk is higher than that in human milk with the exception of iron. The artifically-fed baby may therefore require an *iron supplement*.

Vitamins. The vitamins are *reduced or destroyed* in preparing cow's milk feedings and mild deficiency may result, with failure of the infant to thrive. Severe deficiency is rarely seen in developed countries. (i) *Vitamin A.* Severe deficiency may cause damage to the eyes, mucous membrane, and skin. (ii) *Vitamin B.* Severe deficiency causes disorders of the skin, digestive and nervous systems. (iii) *Vitamin C.* Severe deficiency causes *scurvy*. (iv) *Vitamin D.* Severe deficiency results in *rickets*. Vitamin requirements for infants are shown in table 61.3.

Bacteria. Human milk obtained by sucking directly from the breast is practically sterile. Artificial milk is liable to contamination with bacteria from different sources and therefore care must be taken to ensure sterility during its preparation.

MILK FORMULAS

The normal term infant will thrive on a wide variety of feeding mixtures which include (i) Goldcap SMA powder and liquid, (ii) Whitecap SMA (Wyeth), Cow & Gate Premium, Babymilk Plus, (iii) Farley Ostermilk Complete Formula, Osterfeed Ostermilk 2 Improved Formula, and (iv) Milupa Milumil.

Protein. There are 3 differences between the proteins of the 2 milks. (i) The total amount of protein is much higher in cow's milk. (ii) The proportion of lactalbumin to casein is different, there being a larger proportion of casein in cow's milk. (iii) The physical state of the casein is different. When cow's milk is coagulated by the action of acids and rennin, it produces a large,

TABLE 61.2   COMPOSITION OF MILK FEEDS

	Breast milk	Cow's milk	Ostermilk Complete Formula	Cow & Gate Premium	SMA S26
Calcium (mmol per litre)	8.2	31.3	15.0	13.8	11.0
Phosphorus (mmol per litre)	4.8	31.0	16.2	12.9	10.7
Sodium (mmol per litre)	6.5	25.2	14.4	10.0	6.5
Protein (g per litre)	12	33	18	18	15
Fats (g per litre)	38	37	30	33	36
Carbohydrates (g per litre)	70	48	93	69	72
Energy (kilojoules per litre)	280	276	297	263	272
(kilocalories per 100 mls)	(67)	(66)	(71)	(63)	(65)

TABLE 61.3   VITAMIN REQUIREMENTS FOR INFANTS

	Vitamin A (units)	Thiamine hydrochloride (B_1) (mg)	Riboflavine (B_2) (mg)	Pyridoxine hydrochloride (B_6) (mg)	Nicotinamide (mg)	Vitamin C (mg)	Vitamin D (units)
		Vitamin B complex					
Recommended daily amounts for the first year of life	1,500	0.5	0.9	0.4	5.0	30	400
Amount contained in DHSS vitamin drops (10 drops; 250 µl)	1,400	—	—	—	—	43	571

These are essentially milk preparations containing approximately the same amount of protein as breast milk, with the fat content modified by the substitution of vegetable oils for butter fat, and with added vitamins. They attempt to imitate breast milk in constituents.

Prepacked Feedings

Prepacked infant feedings of different caloric value are available for hospital usage. These feedings have a shelf-life of a number of weeks and need not be refrigerated. In some hospitals the availability of these products has altered artificial feeding practices. Eventually it is expected that a wider range of disposable prepacked infant feeding systems will become available. It seems likely that these will become increasingly popular within hospital neonatal nurseries.

Selection of Formula

The newborn infant has a greater capacity for digestion and absorption of food than was previously accepted. In consideration of what type of food one should select for an infant, one must consider 2 aspects: the needs of the individual infant, and the wishes of the mother.

The premature but vigorous baby. Such infants are fed a 20 calorie per 60 ml formula from the first day of life at 60 ml per kg per day; the volume is then increased as shown in table 61.4.

Small for dates infants require calories to prevent the occurrence of hypoglycaemia. These infants are given 20 calorie per 30 ml formulas. It may be necessary to utilize a 24 calorie per 30 ml mixture from very early in life, but with care as necrotizing enterocolitis may be more common in infants fed with higher caloric milk preparations.

The *sick baby* or *weak premature infant* often requires parenteral infusion of 10% dextrose during the early days of life. When oral feedings are commenced, expressed breast milk or a simulated breast milk feeding such as SMA, Cow & Gate, Ostermilk or Milupa, which have a caloric value of 20 calories per 30 ml, are used. Infants too ill to tolerate oral feeding for a protracted period may be fed by *continuous intravenous infusion* which consists of the administration of solutions containing amino acids, vitamins, electrolytes, dextrose and fats.

TABLE 61.4   VOLUME OF FEEDINGS FOR THE NEWBORN

Age of infant	Volume per kg per day (ml)
1st day	60
2nd day	90
3rd day	120
4th day	150
5th day	150
(This is the basic fluid requirement for a term infant.)	
6th day	180
7th day	200
(This is the basic fluid requirement for a preterm infant.)	

Additives to Oral Feedings for Premature Babies

A multivitamin preparation is commenced on day 7 (DHSS vitamin drops, 10 drops per day). The vitamin supplement should be given by spoon before feeding, although it may be added to the feeding. It should never be heated.

An oral *iron preparation* is administered from the 28th day of life. The dose is 4–8 mg of sodium ironedetate daily until the infant is on a diet adequate in iron. The premature infant becomes deficient in *vitamin E* and this may result in haemolysis; to prevent this vitamin E is commenced with the first feeding.

In some institutions *folic acid*, 5 mg *weekly*, is given to premature infants beginning on the 7th day of life in order to prevent the occurrence of a deficiency anaemia.

Calcium (0.9 mmol/day) and *phosphorus* (0.8 mmol/day) supplements are commenced on day 21 of life in infants with a birth-weight of or beneath 1,500 g who are being fed with breast milk.

Commencement of Feeding

As a general rule, feeding is commenced when the infant shows signs of thirst. This is generally within 4 hours of birth. Infants who are at risk from hypoglycaemia (e.g. small for dates infants or infants of diabetic mothers) are fed earlier. On the first day of life an infant requires 30 ml per kg total feedings. This is divided by the number of feedings to be given for 24 hours and that is the volume (in rounded figures) the child is first offered. This volume simulates that which breast fed infants have been observed to obtain (see Chapter 60).

Administration of Feedings

The particular method depends upon the state of health of the infant, its maturity and the presence of congenital abnormalities that may interfere with feeding. Healthy term babies are fed via the bottle. Sick or premature babies may require tube feeding. Infants with a cleft palate require spoon feeding or feeding from a bottle with a special 'cleft palate' teat.

Bottle feeding. The temperature of the feeding is tested by allowing a little to drip onto the arm. The baby may be nursed by the mother, or if being cot-fed, the head of the cot is elevated. *At all times the bottle must be held.* The palm of the hand faces upwards and the forefinger is placed under the baby's chin to ensure an airtight junction between the teat and the mouth. Swallowed air should be brought up halfway through and at the end of the feeding. It may be necessary to do this more often. At the conclusion of the feeding, the napkin is changed if necessary, the infant turned onto either side, and the head of the cot kept elevated for an hour or so.

Intervals between Feedings

As a general rule, healthy mature babies weighing more than 2,600 g at birth are fed on demand. Those below this weight are fed more frequently, since these infants tire easily on the larger volumes required in 4-hourly regimens.

After the first day of life the fluid requirements increase daily and hence the newborn infant is offered a little more each day. Based on observations of the volumes taken by breast-fed babies, the volumes shown in table 61.4 are suggested. Feedings should be pleasurable episodes for the infant and the mother. As in breast feeding, the intervals may be dictated by the term baby. The infant can, without much difficulty, be directed into a socially acceptable schedule with respect to day and night feedings. From 6.00 pm to 6.00 am he should be allowed to choose his own feeding periods. The result is that he soon omits one night feeding and seldom awakens even once at night beyond the age of 2 or 3 months.

Length of Feedings

The best advice is that a baby is fed until satisfied, provided that no more than *30 minutes is taken for any one feeding*, including the time spent bringing up the baby's 'wind'. He may be satiated in 5 or 10 minutes, after which he is dewinded, played with and returned to bed. If he dawdles and mouths the teat without vigorous sucking, the mother should not persevere too long before returning the infant to his cot.

When the Baby Leaves Hospital

(i) Details of the recipe of the formula, method of preparation, care of bottles and teats, and addition of vitamins should be supplied on a printed leaflet.

(ii) A demonstration should be given of the preparation of the mixture, including its sterilization, either as individual feedings or the total amount required for 24 hours, according to the storage facilities in the home.

(iii) The mother should be taught how to feed the baby, and given details of the amount to be offered, the number of feedings in 24 hours, and the intervals between them.

(iv) The mother should be advised to attend a Child Health Clinic regularly. Here the baby will be weighed, progress assessed, and the mother will receive guidance on feeding matters. She must be told to report there or to her own doctor if the baby has diarrhoea, vomiting, or any other abnormal signs.

CONCLUSION

As in anatomical development, all infants follow the same basic pattern but show individual variations, and so it is with the development of the digestive functions. In feeding infants artificially, it must always be remembered that the baby is an individual with individual digestive and metabolic capabilities. *We must adapt the feeding to the baby, not endeavour to adapt the baby to the feeding.* There are many different methods of successfully feeding a baby artificially.

The feedings suggested are a little generous so the infant *does not have to finish each bottle.* If a baby is still hungry a little more of the same formula should be offered. Feedings are calculated on the basis of either 5 feedings for a schedule of 4 hours or 7 feedings for a schedule of 3 hours. If the baby is awake an extra full feeding may be offered at night. Instruct the mother to feed the baby to *appetite*, not to *capacity* in hospital and at home. At home most babies do well on a demand regimen. In hot weather, extra fluids should be offered regularly, in the form of boiled water. *The signs that feedings are satisfactory* are a contented baby who sleeps well, has good tissue turgor, and finally, the weight gain is satisfactory.

chapter sixty-two

Asphyxia and Resuscitation

OVERVIEW

Hypoxia causes 70% of perinatal deaths and hence should be prevented or its effects minimized. An important detrimental effect of hypoxia is damage to the *type 2 pneumatocyte* which worsens the severity of *hyaline membrane disease*. Hypoxia also has a strong association with *intracranial haemorrhage*.

In the *antenatal period* the effects of *intrauterine hypoxia* can often be detected by *fetoplacental function tests* (assay of plasma or urinary oestrogen, plasma HPL) or *cardiotocography* which allows the infant to be born in good condition, by selection of the appropriate time and route of delivery. *In labour*, hypoxia is detected by the clinical signs of fetal distress and is definitively assessed by cardiotocography and fetal scalp blood sampling for pH measurement — these tests indicate if it is safe to allow labour to continue or if immediate delivery (forceps or Caesarean section) is necessary. *After birth*, hypoxia is prevented or promptly treated if present by adequate and efficient *resuscitation* which usually requires only simple techniques such as *clearing of the airway* and *administration of oxygen*.

Improvements in resuscitation have resulted from the understanding that the *syndrome of shock* rather than *acidosis alone* must be treated in severely depressed infants. This is achieved by the use of *plasma volume expansion* with SPPS or blood. Although *sodium bicarbonate* is still used in larger infants, it is avoided in those with birth-weight less than 1,500 g, because of an association with *intraventricular haemorrhage* in these smaller infants.

Survival alone is not a measure of successful resuscitation. Resuscitative efforts must aim at preventing the complications due to hypoxia, in particular *hyaline membrane disease*, *intracranial haemorrhage* and *necrotizing enterocolitis*.

THE FIRST BREATH

At delivery, *the placental blood supply is abruptly arrested*, the infant assailed by a *crescendo of sensory stimuli* (chiefly tactile and thermal), the blood oxygen and pH levels fall, and the carbon dioxide tension rises. These factors stimulate chemoreceptors and cause the infant to gasp, to breathe and to establish rhythmic respirations. *Drugs* (analgesics, narcotics, tranquillizers, anaesthetics), *intrauterine hypoxia, nervous system trauma, immaturity, airway obstruction* and *congenital respiratory malformation* are influences which may inhibit the onset of respiration.

INTRAUTERINE AND NEONATAL HYPOXIA

Brain and heart are tissues especially prone to damage from hypoxia. A minor reduction in oxygen tension, with the parallel rise in carbon dioxide tension and fall in pH, has a stimulating effect on respiration. Further reduction in oxygenation is compensated by a utilization of the alternative metabolic pathway of *anaerobic glycolysis*. This, however, quickly exhausts glycogen reserves and produces a *metabolic acidosis* (see sections on intermediary metabolism and respiratory disorders of the newborn). Depressed cerebral function and even permanent injury to the brain may result, despite the infant's blood pressure being maintained. Such an infant is cyanosed and apnoeic, a clinical picture previously referred to as *asphyxia livida*. With increasing hypoxia, circulatory collapse and bradycardia supervene, and the child now clinically passes into the phase of *asphyxia pallida* (apnoea and pallor). Death is the outcome of continuing hypoxia at this stage. The causes and clinical features of fetal hypoxia have been discussed in Chapter 48.

The term 'asphyxia neonatorum' is used to describe the condition of an infant who fails to breathe within 60 seconds of delivery.

The normal neonate breathes quickly and efficiently. It is generally accepted that the infant should achieve his first breath in 20 seconds and regular respiration should be established by 90 seconds. The infant's colour 'pinks', the heart contracts strongly and regularly, muscle tone is firm and there is response in reflex fashion to stimulation. These findings form the basis of the *Apgar score*, which is widely used to estimate an infant's birth condition (table 62.1). Familiarity and accuracy are expected of the attendant midwifery staff in estimation of this score. It correlates with immediate neonatal status and also with the subsequent psychomotor development of the individual. It is an important documentation which summarizes the vital clinical findings in the immediate postnatal period. The score is recorded at 1 and 5 minutes.

An Apgar score of 10 represents optimal birth condition, and conversely a score of *3 or less* indicates a markedly asphyxiated infant. The additional 5-minute evaluation gives an assessment of the rate of recovery. The respiratory effort is the single most important feature; its volume, rate and regularity should be noted. In general, if respiration is established all will be well. The pulse, colour, tone and reflexes are dependent on this. If respiration is absent, diminished in volume or slow, the recording of the pulse becomes the most valuable assessment of the infant's progress. If the pulse rate falls, the infant's condition is deteriorating, whereas an increase in rate is encouraging. An assistant whose sole function is to indicate the heart rate is helpful. The colour can be misleading, but has been widely used as a guide to the infant's condition. The terms *asphyxia livida* and *asphyxia pallida* are now used less frequently and have been applied to the colour of nonbreathing infants, the latter state being regarded as more serious. Certainly, an infant, whether blue or pale, needs attention. A blue baby may be cold rather than hypoxic; a pale infant may be anaemic. The availability of biochemical measurement of acid-base and oxygen concentrations has made possible objective and extended assessment of the apnoeic or dyspnoeic neonate.

CAUSES OF BREATHING DIFFICULTIES

Intrauterine Hypoxia
See Chapter 48.

Respiratory Centre Depression
(i) *Maternal drug administration* — narcotics, analgesics, sedatives, anaesthetics and tranquillizers. The recording of these agents on the labour ward charts prepares those responsible for the reception of the infant for possible problems.

(ii) *Intracranial birth trauma.*

(iii) *Failure of resuscitation* will increase hypoxia and further depress the respiratory centre.

Airway Obstruction
(i) Mucus, blood, meconium and amniotic fluid may block the nasal passages, pharynx, larynx, trachea and bronchi. (ii) Stenoses and atresias (congenital malformations) are rare, but include choanal atresia, laryngeal web, and laryngeal atresia.

Parenchymal Disorders of the Lung
Intrauterine pneumonia, cystic disorders, lobar emphysema, pulmonary hypoplasia and agenesis.

Gross Cardiac Malformations

Diaphragmatic Defects
The most important malformation is diaphragmatic hernia, since prompt diagnosis allows life-saving surgery.

RESUSCITATION OF THE NEWBORN

The principles and skills of resuscitation techniques must be understood and developed by all who care for newborn infants.

Anticipation of the Infant at Risk
Specific obstetrical disorders (antepartum haemorrhage, preeclampsia, premature labour), medical diseases of the mother (diabetes mellitus), difficult or prolonged labour, operative delivery (forceps, Caesarean section) are examples where a higher incidence of resuscitative problems demands the routine attendance of a member of the paediatric staff to care for the baby.

Preparation and Availability of Resuscitation Equipment
Constant checks are made of the apparatus to ensure that it is in working order. A whole chapter could profitably be devoted to the disasters, preventable in nature, that have resulted from failure of observation of this recommendation. Oxygen catheters should be connected, suction apparatus tested, and batteries in the laryngoscope checked. The equipment available in the resuscitation boxes should be adequate for all aspects of neonatal resuscitation (figure 62.1).

Provision of Warmth
Gentle handling and provision of warmth are

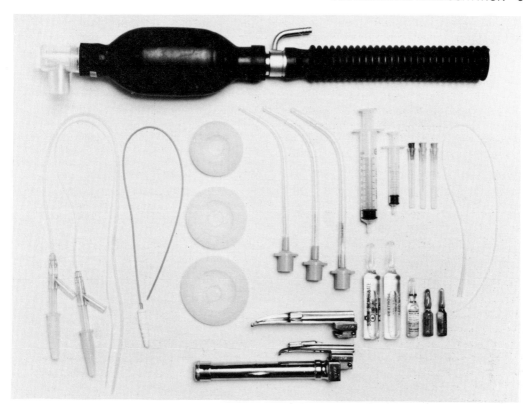

Figure 62.1 Basic equipment required for resuscitation of the newborn infant. Note bag for administration of oxygen with face-masks of various sizes (1, 2 and 3); suction catheters of different diameters (8 and 10Fr); catheter (6Fr) for administration of intranasal oxygen; endotracheal tubes of various sizes (2.5, 3 and 3.5); laryngoscope with size 1 (term infant) and size 0 (preterm infant) blades; ampoules of 4.2% sodium bicarbonate, dextrose, naloxone, adrenaline (1 in 1,000) and vitamin K_1; syringes (10 ml and 2 ml); needles (25, 23 and 18 gauges) and catheter (8Fr) for cannulation of the umbilical vein to allow administration of drugs.

Figure 62.2 Aspiration of the mouth. This is performed before aspiration of the nostrils.

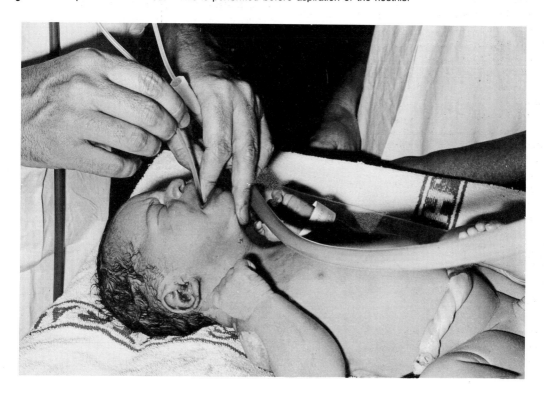

extremely important. It must be remembered that *hypothermia* significantly reduces the chance of survival and hence care must be taken to minimize this complication by (i) receiving the infant into warm wraps, (ii) drying the infant's skin quickly, (iii) keeping the infant covered as much as possible, (iv) minimizing time taken to perform procedures and (v) resuscitating in a warm and draft-free environment.

Airway Aspiration

Note that the infant breathes through the nostrils; mouth breathing develops only after the neonatal period. *Oropharyngeal suction (figure 62.2) should precede nasal aspiration* because the latter may initiate gasping and, if the pharynx is not clear of fluid material, its inhalation further impedes resuscitative measures.

Remember: (i) *Suction must be gentle*: excess suction pressure and rough catheter passage will damage the delicate mucosal lining of the infant's airway, producing haemorrhage and predisposing to infection. (ii) *Suction should be prompt*. Usually relatively small quantities of mucous fluid need removal; repeated insertions of the suction catheter are usually unnecessary and may stimulate nervous *inhibition* of respiration.

Excessively thick mucus or meconium requires careful and thorough removal. Skilled personnel may attempt tracheal aspiration of meconium after *visualization of the vocal cords* by means of a laryngoscope. Placing the baby in the head down position on the inclined plane of a resuscitation trolley facilitates gravitation of

fluid into the pharynx, as does the time-honoured grasping of the feet and holding the infant in an inverted position. *Stomach aspiration* should not be a routine procedure, but it is helpful in the following circumstances: in infants born at Caesarean section; where meconium is present at delivery (to prevent meconium gastritis); and when gastric distension with air has occurred during resuscitative attempts.

Oxygen Administration

Oxygen is usually supplied through a wall unit apparatus with metered gauges for flow measurement. However, cylinder oxygen may be the only type available. Before birth of the infant, the apparatus should be checked to ensure it is in working order, connecting tubes are attached to the outflow, and appropriate giving devices are connected. Oxygen may be administered in one of several ways.

(i) *Intranasal catheter*. This is a common method. Often the simple administration of oxygen will be sufficient to 'pink-up' the infant. The flow rate must be adjusted carefully to avoid hyperinflation of the lungs with resultant damage such as *pneumothorax*. The distance which the tube is inserted into the nostril is equal to the nostril-eye distance across the face; a flow rate of ½–2 litres per minute is used. With the intranasal catheter in situ, intermittent occlusion of the nostrils at 2-second intervals, and simultaneous closure of the mouth by an upwards extension of the chin is the simple basis for providing build-up of oxygen pressure in the air

Figure 62.3 Insertion of an oropharyngeal airway before commencement of positive pressure resuscitation using a bag and mask.

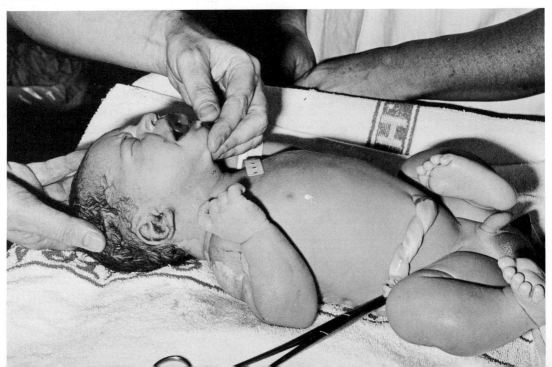

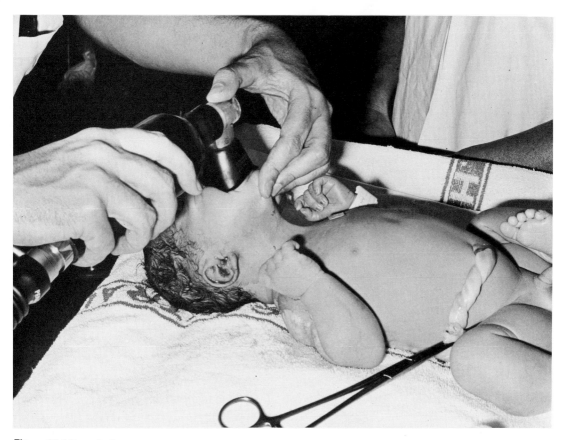

Figure 62.4 Use of a bag and mask. The lower jaw is held forward to allow easier entrance of the gases being supplied.

Figure 62.5 Endotracheal intubation. The blade of the laryngoscope is inserted down the right side of the infant's mouth gently deflecting the tongue. As it is advanced, the base of the tongue and epiglottis are visualized. The blade is then advanced into the pouch between the base of the tongue and the epiglottis, and as it is gently raised the epiglottis swings anteriorly revealing the opening of the larynx. The endotracheal tube is advanced from the right corner of the mouth and inserted into the larynx while maintaining direct visualization. The laryngoscope blade is then carefully withdrawn.

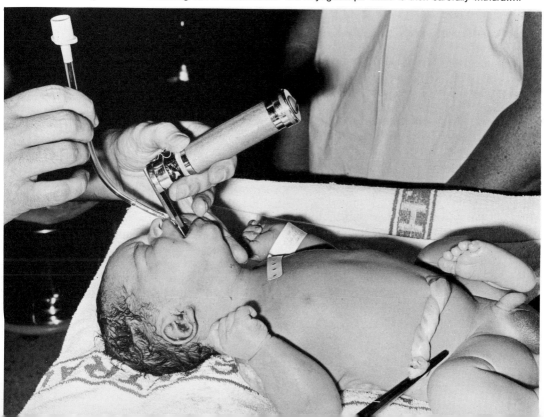

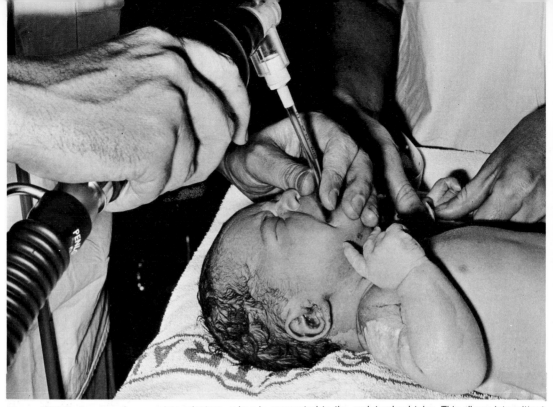

Figure 62.6 By the use of appropriate adaptors, a bag is connected to the endotracheal tube. This allows intermittent positive pressure to be applied to the lungs.

passages ('*frog breathing*'). The production of positive pressure inflates the lung and allows gaseous transfer. The flow rate of oxygen should be no more than 2 litres per minute. This effective measure of artificial ventilation should be known to all.

(ii) *Bag and mask.* An oropharyngeal airway (size according to the infant) should be inserted first (figure 62.3). The usual anaesthetic bag and mask apparatus needs experienced staff for adequate inflation. The danger of this technique is the build-up of excessive pressure (because there is no blow-off valve), with the risk of resultant pneumothorax. If this type of bag is used, a pressure manometer should be connected to the bag so that inflation pressures can be clearly monitored. *The Cardiff bag* has an inbuilt pressure valve which prevents overinflation of the lungs (figure 62.4). Bag and mask resuscitation is more efficient, quicker and safer than the intranasal catheter technique and hence is preferred.

(iii) *Endotracheal intubation.* An infant laryngoscope, blade, and endotracheal tubes of appropriate diameters should be included in the resuscitation box for use by medical staff (figure 62.5). Using this method, the principles of oxygen administration are similar to those already described, but this method ensures that maximum oxygen concentrations can be delivered directly to the lungs (figure 62.6).

(iv) *Mouth to mouth breathing.* If the equipment mentioned above is not available, cannot be connected, or does not function, this direct method should not be overlooked. Mouth to mouth breathing, at a rate of 30 breaths per minute and with the force equivalent to blowing out a match, can be lifesaving and brain-sparing. Oxygen can be added by the passing of an oxygen line into the operator's mouth.

External cardiac massage

Gentle external massage of the heart by compression between the anterior and posterior chest wall may be necessary if circulatory failure occurs.

Drugs

Generally the resuscitative value of drugs has been over-emphasized. Sometimes the painful stimulus of an injection will help to establish respiration. If there is circulatory collapse, drugs administered by intramuscular injections are poorly absorbed into the circulation. This situation will apply in the severely depressed hypoxic infant — just the circumstance where the beneficial effect of stimulant drugs is most wanted. *Naloxone (Narcan)* is an antagonist to narcotic drugs such as pethidine, morphine and omnopon. If respiratory depression in the neonate has followed administration of these substances to the mother, intravenous infusion (preferably) of 0.01–0.02 mg (0.01 mg/kg body weight) to the infant can produce dramatic improvement. Naloxone also increases ventilation in the newborn and improves sucking ability. Some obstetricians administer 0.01 mg of naloxone by intramuscular injection immediately the infant is born when the mother has received narcotic analgesia within 4 hours of delivery. Manufacturers provide neonatal ampoules containing 0.02 mg in 1 ml which should *not* be confused with the adult preparation (0.4 mg in 1 ml). Another important advantage of naloxone is that it does not have the complication of irritability, or the rarer complication of central nervous system depression shown occasionally by *nalorphine* (*Lethidrone*) which was previously the drug used to antagonize narcotics in the newborn (or the mother immediately before delivery).

Correction of acidosis

The hypoxic infant has a disordered biochemical environment, the accumulation of hydrogen ions producing an acidotic state, which may depress the respiratory centres. The provision of oxygen will restore normality, but the rapidity with which this is achieved is enhanced by neutralization of the excess acid content of the blood with an alkali such as sodium bicarbonate, 4.2% solution. *THAM* and *lactate* exert a similar action. Intravenous *alkali infusion* 5–10 ml, usually via the umbilical vein, is dramatically effective. The cyanotic infant gasps and stretches, his colour improves as the peripheral blood vessels dilate and the oxygen requirement is reduced. Recent research findings indicate that there is a relationship between sodium bicarbonate administration and *intraventricular haemorrhage* in infants with birth-weight of less than 1,500 g; since part of the reason for the acidosis is shock (from one or more causes) these infants should be treated with an infusion of plasma substitute or blood (10 ml/kg) rather than an infusion of sodium bicarbonate.

Correction of hypoglycaemia

Dextrose 10%, 20% or 50% solution may be given. Direct entry to the umbilical vein is not always possible and availability of an umbilical catheter, artery forceps and a scalpel blade will assist the doctor to cannulate the umbilical vein.

Guides to the efficacy of resuscitation include observation of chest movement, auscultatory assessment of air entry, and change in Apgar score.

POSTRESUSCITATION OBSERVATION

The asphyxiated infant is liable to many problems after resuscitation. (i) Hypothermia acquired during resuscitation. (ii) Respiratory disorders such as atelectasis, hyaline membrane disease, pneumothorax, meconium aspiration syndrome and pneumonia. (iii) Central nervous system problems of depression, failure to feed, irritability, cyanotic attacks and perhaps convulsions. (iv) Vomiting due to ingestion of meconium or blood. (v) Hypoglycaemia. (vi) Abdominal distension due to oxygen being forced into the gastrointestinal tract during resuscitation.

Hence, these infants should be transferred to a special care nursery and placed in an incubator for initial observation.

Long-term follow-up of such individuals will reveal an increased incidence of special sensory handicaps, psychomotor disability, and epilepsy. Prompt and efficient resuscitation and competent nursing care will markedly reduce the incidence and severity of both the initial complication and the above sequelae.

TABLE 62.1 APGAR SCORING CHART*

Sign	0	1	2
Heart rate	Absent	Slow (below 100)	Over 100
Respiratory effort	Absent	Weak cry, hypoventilation	Good strong cry
Muscle tone	Limp	Some flexion of extremities	Well flexed
Reflex response (i) Response to catheter in nostril (tested after oropharynx is clear) (ii) Tangential foot slap	No response No response	Grimace Grimace	Cough or sneeze Cry and withdrawal of foot
Colour	Blue, pale	Body pink. Extremities blue	Completely pink

* A score of 3 or less indicates severe asphyxia

chapter sixty-three

Respiratory Disorders

OVERVIEW

Respiratory disorders are the most important cause of neonatal mortality — they occur in approximately 3% of newborn infants and have a *mortality rate of about 1 in 5*. *Hyaline membrane disease* is the most common cause of respiratory distress and is due to a *deficiency of surfactant*, in turn the result of *prematurity* (production not commenced) or *hypoxia* (production having failed due to cellular damage). *Betamethasone* administration (6 mg IM 12-hourly × 4) to the mother enhances surfactant production by the fetus and *reduces the incidence and severity of hyaline membrane disease*, particularly in patients who deliver between 26–30 weeks' gestation; it is indicated when premature delivery before 34 weeks' gestation seems likely (premature rupture of membranes, premature labour ± polyhydramnios, multiple pregnancy, preeclampsia). *Artificial ventilation* has improved the survival rate of infants with hyaline membrane disease, but at the price of a higher incidence of pulmonary *air leaks* (interstitial emphysema, pneumothorax, pneumopericardium) and a new disorder *bronchopulmonary dysplasia*. Current trends are to develop alternative methods of ventilation rather than *intermittent positive pressure ventilation — oscillation ventilation* promises a reduction in the incidences of both air leak and bronchopulmonary dysplasia, while an *artificial placenta* (a device to permit oxygenation of tissues and removal of carbon dioxide) remains the challenge of the future for neonatologists and physiologists. *Surfactant* has recently been synthesized and produced from animals and promises to be useful in the treatment of hyaline membrane disease (instillation into the respiratory tract via an endotracheal tube).

INTRODUCTION

In most babies, breathing commences spontaneously within 1 minute of birth. Transition of respiratory function from the placenta to the lungs is the most important of all extrauterine adjustments. Unfortunately there are a number of babies who have difficulty in achieving this.

There are 2 clinical types of respiratory difficulty in newborn infants. Firstly, there is the child who is obviously depressed and has slow, shallow breathing; this depression is usually of intracranial origin and may be due to hypoxia, intracranial haemorrhage, metabolic disorders, or the effect of maternal sedation. Secondly, there is the child who is not depressed, but has rapid breathing, the rate being above the normal upper limit of 60 breaths per minute.

Respiratory distress syndrome in the newborn is a general term used to describe *any infant who develops a respiratory rate above 60 per minute, has difficulties in breathing as shown by retraction of the sternum and lower costal margin, or dilation of the anterior nares, has an expiratory grunt, and has central cyanosis. The incidence of this syndrome in a newborn population is approximately 3.3% and the mortality rate is about 1 in 5. It is the dreaded neonatal complication and claims more lives than any other cause.*

There are many causes of the respiratory distress syndrome. To give the reader perspective, the causes in a series of 1,361 consecutive cases are listed in table 63.1 according to incidence, and table 63.2 shows a simple classification of causes. The commonest cause is the *idiopathic respiratory distress syndrome, or hyaline membrane disease* (colour plates 64 and 120). The high mortality rate is related to *low birth-weight* (in turn related to *prematurity*), 70% of the deaths occurring in infants with birth-weights less than 2,000 g (table 63.4).

PRENATAL LUNG MATURATION

The glandular period. The lung originates as an outgrowth of the embryonic foregut at about 4 weeks' gestation. The lung bud divides into the right and left main bronchi and each division branches and rebranches as it grows to form the bronchial tree. This developing tree grows into a mesodermally-derived partition, formed by the

TABLE 63.1 AETIOLOGY AND MORTALITY IN A SERIES OF 1,361 CASES OF THE RESPIRATORY DISTRESS SYNDROME FROM 41,057 CONSECUTIVE LIVEBIRTHS

Aetiology	Number	Neonatal deaths	
		Number	%
Hyaline membrane disease	602	168	(27.9)
Transient tachypnoea	289	1	(0.4)
'Wet lung' syndrome	166	1	(0.6)
Aspiration pneumonitis	122	10	(8.1)
Pulmonary atelectasis	32	15	(46.8)
Pneumonia	31	13	(41.9)
Cardiac malformations	26	5	(19.2)
Spontaneous pneumothorax	25	8	(32.0)
Cerebral	17	7	(41.1)
Pulmonary haemorrhage	12	10	(83.3)
Others	39	23	(58.9)
Total	1,361	261	(19.1)

TABLE 63.2 CAUSES OF THE RESPIRATORY DISTRESS SYNDROME

1. *Airway Obstruction*
   (a) Bilateral choanal atresia
   (b) Congenital laryngeal stridor
   (c) Thyroid enlargement
   (d) Tracheo-oesophageal fistula
   (e) Pierre-Robin syndrome

2. *Pulmonary Disease*
   (a) Idiopathic respiratory distress syndrome (hyaline membrane disease)
   (b) Pneumonia
   (c) Meconium aspiration syndrome
   (d) Pulmonary haemorrhage
   (e) Pulmonary hypoplasia
   (f) Congenital emphysema

3. *Space Occupying Lesions*
   (a) Pneumothorax
   (b) Diaphragmatic hernia

TABLE 63.3 CRITERIA OF NORMAL NEONATAL BLOOD CHEMISTRY

Test		Normal arterial ranges
pH	7.35	– 7.45 units
Partial pressure of carbon dioxide	35	– 45 mm Hg (4.7–6.0 kPa)
Standard bicarbonate	22	– 26 m eq/l (mmol/l)
Base excess	– 2	– + 2 m eq/l (mmol/l)
Partial pressure of oxygen	60	– 70 mm Hg (8.0–9.3 kPa)
Percentage oxygen saturation	94	– 100

TABLE 63.4 BIRTH-WEIGHT RANGE AND MORTALITY RATE OF INFANTS WITH THE RESPIRATORY DISTRESS SYNDROME

Birth-weight (g)	Number	Neonatal deaths	
		Number	%
Below 1,500	332	156	46.9
1,500–1,999	237	52	21.9
2,000–2,499	215	21	9.7
2,500 and above	577	32	5.5
Total	1,361	261	19.1

incomplete folding of the embryo that occurs in the region of the developing thorax. This mesodermal tissue forms the mediastinum, the blood vessels of the lung, as well as the pleura, connective tissues, and lymphatics.

The canalicular period. Between 16 and 20 weeks' gestation, the originally solid bronchial tree becomes canalized. At 24 weeks' gestation, a rapid vascularization of the surrounding mesoderm occurs and a rich capillary network forms adjacent to the most peripheral areas of the bronchial tree.

The alveolar period. Beginning at 25 weeks' gestation and progressing to full term, the most distal areas of the bronchial tree produce alveoli. At this stage the developing capillary bed comes into close apposition to the developing alveoli and hence, potentially, the lung is now ready to perform its function of gaseous exchange.

The lung fluid. Initially it was taught that the lung was a collapsed organ before birth; this is now known to be incorrect. The alveoli are in fact distended, not with air, but with 'lung fluid' which is secreted by the type 1 cells of the developing alveoli.

Surfactant is a phospholipid and consists mainly of lecithin and sphingomyelin. It is produced by the type 2 cells of the developing alveoli and is essential for normal lung function. *It is not produced before 25 weeks' gestation.*

Lung structure at term. At term, the fetal lung consists of airways ending in alveoli surrounded by a dense capillary network. Due to high resistance to flow in the pulmonary capillaries, the pressure in the right side of the heart is higher than in the left and so most of the blood is shunted away from the lungs via the *foramen ovale* and *ductus arteriosus*. The alveoli are filled with lung fluid and are lined by surfactant (figure 63.1).

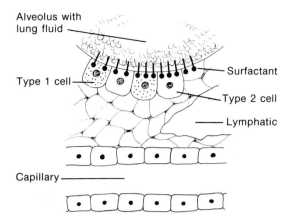

Figure 63.1 Structure of the fetal lung at term.

AERATION OF THE LUNGS

Lung fluid must be removed from the alveoli before adequate aeration of the lungs can occur. When the pregnant woman commences to labour, the infant's blood *catecholamine* levels rise; this 'turns-off' the production of lung fluid by the type 1 alveolar cell. During a vaginal delivery the thoracic cage is compressed, so squeezing the lung fluid to the pharynx. After delivery of the head, the lung fluid in the pharynx is removed by suction aspiration. Following delivery there is an immediate elastic recoil of the squeezed thorax which sucks air into the upper respiratory tract. Subsequently, the main factor contributing to aeration is the negative intrathoracic pressure created by the rhythmically-contracting diaphragm. Any excess lung fluid not removed by the squeezing mechanism is forced out of the alveoli and is removed by the lymphatics of the lung. In children born by *Caesarean section* where the mother is not in labour, lung fluid production is not 'turned-off' and the squeezing effect on the thoracic cage is minimal and hence the lung fluid has to be removed by the lymphatics. This takes 12–24 hours and is the cause of the '*wet lung*' syndrome which often occurs in infants born by Caesarean section.

As the lung inflates with air, a fall in pulmonary vascular resistance occurs. When the pulmonary pressure falls below that in the aorta, blood ceases to flow from the pulmonary artery through the ductus arteriosus, but continues along the pulmonary artery to the lung, and hence pulmonary blood flow is greatly increased. (See Chapter 58 for circulatory changes that occur after birth).

Respiration is initiated partly because of the relative hypoxia (reduced oxygen) and hypercapnia (excessive carbon dioxide) causing a fall in

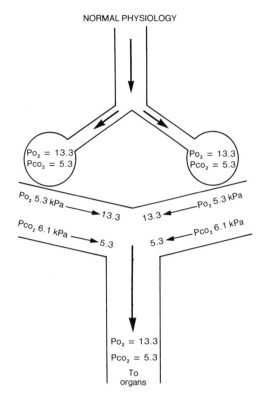

Figure 63.2 Exchange of oxygen and carbon dioxide between lung capillaries and alveoli.

blood pH which stimulates the respiratory centre in the brain and partly because of sensory stimulation from the skin (tactile and thermal).

THE PHYSIOLOGY OF RESPIRATION

The lungs are the organs of gaseous exchange. The partial pressure of oxygen is 20 kPa (150 mm Hg) in atmospheric air and 13.3 kPa (100 mm Hg) in alveolar air; the partial pressure of oxygen in the blood coming to the lungs is 40 mm Hg (5.3 kPa). Therefore, oxygen diffuses through the alveoli into the blood and is carried to all the tissues of the body by the red blood cells (figure 63.2). The partial pressures of carbon dioxide in the pulmonary capillaries and alveolar air are 6.1 and 5.3 kPa pressure (46 and 40 mm Hg) respectively, and hence carbon dioxide leaves the blood, diffuses into the alveoli and is exhaled. Carbon dioxide is more soluble than oxygen and therefore diffuses readily across the alveolar wall, although the pressure gradient is small.

It has been mentioned that *surfactant is a phospholipid* produced by the type 2 alveolar cells lining the alveolar spaces, and because of its chemical structure it alters surface tension. The lungs may be considered to be composed of many spheres (alveoli) connected by airways.

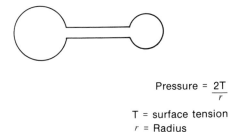

$$\text{Pressure} = \frac{2T}{r}$$

T = surface tension
r = Radius

Figure 63.3 The role of surfactant in the reduction of surface tension.

The pressure in the sphere is as shown by the formula in figure 63.3; the pressure in the smaller sphere is above that in the larger sphere because it has a smaller radius. Hence, the smaller sphere tends to collapse. It is the presence of surfactant that prevents this collapse in the human since its chemical structure is such that it causes *reduction of surface tension* as the radius of a sphere becomes smaller. Hence, alveolar pressure does not increase and small airways do not collapse and large airways do not overexpand.

Acid-base balance. The information in table 63.3 is obtained by chemical analysis of a blood sample when the acid-base balance of the body is being investigated.

THE PHYSIOLOGY OF RESPIRATORY FAILURE

The results of respiratory failure are described with reference to figure 63.4 in which, for ease of description, 50% of lung function has been removed.

There is an *increased carbon dioxide tension* in the blood. Carbon dioxide combines with water and forms carbonic acid which renders the baby *acidotic* (*respiratory acidosis*).

Reduction of the oxygen tension of the blood causes a switch to anaerobic rather than aerobic metabolism (see Chapter 35), with a decrease in stored glycogen (because the process is very inefficient), and an aggravation of the acidosis (due to the build up of lactic acid and the formation of ketoacids from the metabolism of fats after the glycogen has been used up).

The blood contains a buffering system designed to prevent serious changes in pH; 53% of the blood buffering capacity is dependent upon the bicarbonate system which is represented by the following equation:

$$CO_2 + H_2O \rightleftharpoons H_2CO_3 \rightleftharpoons H^+ + HCO_3^-$$

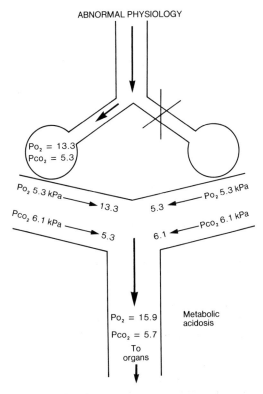

Figure 63.4 The change in blood gases in respiratory failure.

An acid is defined as a substance which donates hydrogen ions (H^+); examples are lactic acid, carbonic acid (H_2CO_3) and ketone bodies. Addition of an acid to the system depicted above pushes the equation to the left which results in reduction of the bicarbonate (HCO_3^-) concentration.

In *respiratory failure* the following *metabolic* changes occur: pH falls (acidosis), carbon dioxide tension rises (respiratory acidosis), and bicarbonate falls (buffered metabolic acidosis). Also, base excess, oxygen tension, and oxygen saturation fall. Hypoglycaemia is common because of utilization of stored glycogen.

THE RESPIRATORY DISTRESS SYNDROME

The principal causes of respiratory difficulty are summarized in table 63.2. The more important of these will be discussed in greater detail below. It should be remembered, however, that a child presenting with *tachypnoea* may have an abnormality unrelated to *primary lung disease*; 2 conditions that should be kept in mind are *cardiac abnormalities* and *methaemoglobinaemia*.

HYALINE MEMBRANE DISEASE

This is a respiratory disorder of the *premature* infant, the name being derived from the appearance of the eosinophilic (red), hyaline (glassy) membrane that lines the alveolar ducts and respiratory bronchioles (colour plate 64). It is the most common and important problem faced by premature infants. The incidence varies according to *maturity at birth*; *75% of infants born before 32 weeks' gestation will develop the condition.*

Aetiology

Hyaline membrane disease is due to a *deficiency of surfactant.* Surfactant deficiency is related to (1) *prematurity* and (2) *hypoxia*, themselves often associated with predisposing conditions such as antepartum haemorrhage, preeclampsia, maternal hypertension, multiple pregnancy, and maternal diabetes. Delivery by Caesarean section also predisposes to tachypnoea, but the respiratory distress is often transient and due to slow removal of lung fluid rather than hyaline membrane formation.

Pathophysiology. Deficiency of surfactant results in alveolar collapse and gaseous perfusion becomes inadequate. A secondary effect of the alveolar collapse is an increase in the peripheral pulmonary arterial pressure (the lungs are collapsed and solid). Hence the pressure in the right side of the heart becomes greater than the left and the foramen ovale and the ductus arteriosus reopen. Blood is then shunted away from the lungs and, not being oxygenated, further increases the hypoxia and hypercapnia.

Clinical Course

The child develops *tachypnoea and nasal flaring* within 12 hours of birth. The lungs are collapsed and because the cage formed by the ribs and sternum is pliable in premature infants, respiratory efforts cause *retraction of the xiphisternum* and *lower costal margin* (colour plate 120). Each respiration is prolonged and terminates in a *grunt*. The infant is often *oedematous* and *central cyanosis* may be present. In severe cases, the infant's condition deteriorates rapidly within the first 24 hours, cyanotic episodes develop and death occurs usually within 48 hours of birth. In those who survive, the condition remains static between 48 and 72 hours and then gradually improves.

The radiograph (figure 63.5) shows fine uniform *reticulogranular opacities* (collapsed alveoli) in the lungs and an '*air bronchogram*' which is an appearance due to collapse of alveoli around the larger divisions of the bronchial tree which remain open because their walls are rigid.

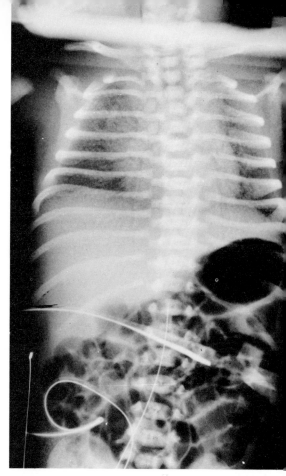

Figure 63.5 Hyaline membrane disease recognized by fine uniform reticulogranular opacities throughout the lung fields and 'air bronchograms'. The white line crossing the top of the radiograph is the edge of a plastic box surrounding the infant's head. This box is used to increase the concentration of oxygen the infant inhales. The aorta has been cannulated to allow careful monitoring of the infant's blood gas status.

Prophylaxis

The risk of hyaline membrane disease may be predicted during pregnancy by measurement of the lecithin/sphingomyelin (surfactant) ratio in a sample of amniotic fluid obtained by amniocentesis. The fetus 'coughs-up' surfactant which passes into the amniotic fluid. If the ratio is greater than 2 to 1, hyaline membrane disease is unlikely to occur. If the ratio is less than 2 to 1, hyaline membrane disease may occur. Administration of betamethasone (Betnesol) (6 mg by intramuscular injection 12-hourly × 4) to the mother for 48 hours before delivery may induce maturation of the enzyme system in the fetal lungs required for synthesis of surfactant. This may be of benefit when the need for induction of premature labour can be anticipated by 2–3 days (or premature labour inhibited for 2 days or more).

Prognosis

If the baby survives for 48 hours, death seldom occurs from hyaline membrane disease. Survivors occasionally have residual lung damage.

PNEUMONIA

Aetiology

Congenital. (i) *Transplacental.* Here a *viral* origin is most likely (rubella, cytomegalic inclusion body disease, and infections due to Coxsackie and ECHO viruses); *bacteria* such as E. coli and Listeria monocytogenes are less common causes. (ii) *Ascending infection* is much more common than transplacental infection and is likely to occur in labour when the membranes have been ruptured for 12 hours or more, particularly when there have been numerous vaginal examinations. The usual pathogens are aerobic Gram-negative bacilli (E. coli) and anaerobic streptococci. Infection with *group B, beta-haemolytic streptoccocci* causes a severe pneumonia which has a mortality rate of 50%. This organism can be cultured from the vagina in approximately 10% of pregnant women, the majority of whom are asymptomatic; 50% of infants from such pregnancies are colonized and 1% infected with the organism.

Acquired. This results from *bacteria* or *viruses* entering the upper respiratory tract (especially E. coli), or aspiration of food, infected mucus, or vomitus. A special hazard is contamination by *maternal faeces* (E. coli and other bacteria) which is most likely to occur when the patient has diarrhoea; liquid faeces are such a nuisance at delivery that *enemas should not be given as a routine to patients when they are admitted in labour.* Prompt clamping of the umbilical cord should be performed after delivery when faecal contamination is likely to occur, so that the infant can be handed (in a sterile wrap) to the safety of the mother's arms.

Clinical Features

There is likely to be a history of artificial or prolonged rupture of the membranes, multiple vaginal examinations, difficult resuscitation, or development of aspiration with a previous feeding. The onset is often gradual, the characteristic features being *tachypnoea, tachycardia, cyanosis, lethargy* and *refusal of feeding, vomiting,* and *nasal discharge.* The temperature may be elevated or depressed; the latter is usual if infection is severe and the baby is shocked. A radiograph will help establish the diagnosis.

MECONIUM ASPIRATION SYNDROME

Intrauterine hypoxia due to any cause stimulates bowel peristalsis and causes relaxation of the anal sphincter, and hence the passage of meconium. This is one of the signs of fetal distress and occurs most commonly during labour, in term and postterm pregnancies. The hypoxia also stimulates the respiratory centre in the base of the brain and respiratory movements commence. The result is aspiration of meconium, mixed with amniotic fluid, into the lungs (colour plate 63). After birth this results in a ball-valve type of obstruction, with air entering the lungs but being trapped there. The chest becomes overdistended as emphysema occurs, and pneumothorax may result as the pressure of trapped air increases. Secondarily a chemical pneumonitis occurs, followed by infection, and thus the signs of pneumonia are added to the clinical picture.

Clinical Features

The infant is born in a bath of meconium and active resuscitation is required. *Tachypnoea* and *tachycardia* occur, and the infant's *chest is over-expanded* because of emphysema as explained above. The latter finding is in contrast to hyaline membrane disease where the lungs are solid and the chest is collapsed. The radiograph shows areas of collapse, consolidation, and emphysema.

PULMONARY HAEMORRHAGE

Massive pulmonary haemorrhage has a mortality rate of about 80% and is the cause of approximately 10% of neonatal deaths. Pulmonary haemorrhage has a strong association with intrauterine growth retardation. Other associations are prematurity, asphyxia, hyaline membrane disease and erythroblastosis fetalis. Pulmonary haemorrhage is primarily due to hypoxaemia which causes damage to the myocardium, the pulmonary capillaries and the alveoli. The damage to the myocardium results in left ventricular failure with resultant increase in pressure in the pulmonary vessels which have already been weakened by hypoxaemia; the result is pulmonary haemorrhage. Infants with deficiences of *blood coagulation factors* are also prone to pulmonary haemorrhage.

Management

The disease can be anticipated and its incidence lessened by (i) *prophylactic digitalization* of infants with severe hypoxia, especially when associated with intrauterine growth retardation, and (ii) by testing growth retarded, premature and erythroblastotic infants for deficiences of blood coagulation factors; deficiences thus detected are corrected by administration of special plasma preparations.

Once a pulmonary haemorrhage has occurred, treatment is directed to minimizing further bleeding by the use of continuous positive airways pressure (CPAP), replacing the blood loss and treating the heart failure by digitalization.

PULMONARY HYPOPLASIA

This classically occurs in the condition of renal agenesis (Potter syndrome; see Chapter 21).

DIAPHRAGMATIC HERNIA AND TRACHEO-OESOPHAGEAL FISTULA (figure 63.6)

This may cause respiratory distress and require prompt diagnosis and surgical treatment (see Chapter 65).

PNEUMOTHORAX

A pneumothorax occurs when air bursts through an alveolus into the pleural cavity and the lung collapses (figure 63.7). The severity of the respiratory distress depends upon the degree of pulmonary collapse.

Aetiology

The condition usually occurs as a complication of one of the following: overenergetic resuscitation at birth, meconium aspiration syndrome, hyaline membrane disease, staphylococcal pneumonia and use of a mechanical respirator. Occasionally, the condition appears spontaneously.

Clinical Features

Pneumothorax may present either gradually or suddenly. In mild cases, the only feature may be the development of tachypnoea. In severe cases, marked respiratory distress with central cyanosis is the rule. The diagnosis should be considered in any infant with respiratory distress; it is readily confirmed by a chest radiograph (figure 63.7).

Treatment

This is by needle aspiration of the chest in an emergency (figure 63.8). To drain a pneumothorax continuously, a cannula is inserted through the chest wall (figure 63.9).

Figure 63.6 Oesophageal atresia: opaque dye shows the limit of the upper oesophagus; the excessive gas in the bowel is due to the fistula between trachea and lower oesophagus.

Figure 63.7 Bilateral pneumothoraces in a newborn infant; the lungs are collapsed and surrounded by air.

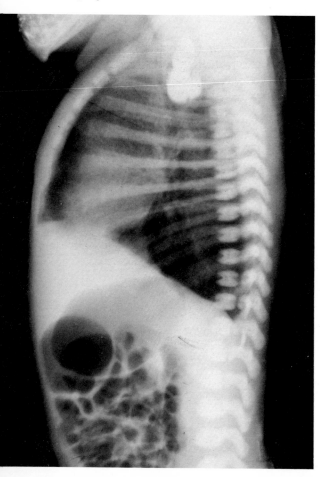

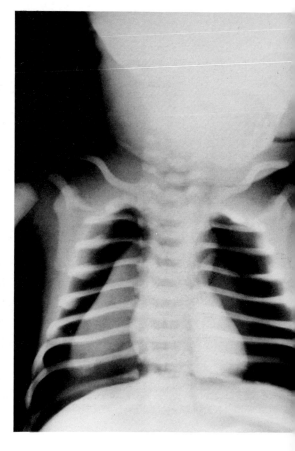

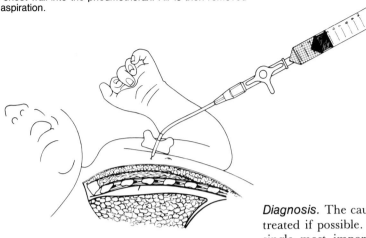

Figure 63.8 In an emergency situation a pneumothorax can be drained by the insertion of a 'scalp vein' needle through the chest wall into the pneumothorax. Air is then removed by aspiration.

TREATMENT OF RESPIRATORY DISTRESS

Dealt with here is the overall management of an infant who presents with respiratory distress. Although mechanical ventilation has become very important in the management of infants with respiratory distress, many other aspects of management must be attended to either before the ventilator is required or during its use.

Diagnosis. The cause should be determined and treated if possible. To determine the cause, the single most important investigation is a *chest radiograph.*

Minimal handling. The baby is nursed naked in an environment with controlled temperature and humidity (incubator, overhead radiant heating). This allows ease of observation with minimal disturbance.

Maintenance of body temperature. The infant is nursed in the environmental temperature at which his oxygen and calorie requirements are minimal (*neutral thermal environment* — see Chapter 64).

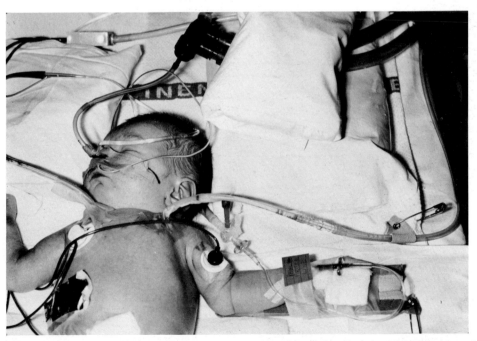

Figure 63.9 An infant with bilateral pneumothoraces receiving assisted ventilation. To drain a pneumothorax continuously, a cannula is inserted through the chest wall. Because the pneumothorax is under pressure, air bubbles along this catheter and passes through an 'underwater trap' which prevents air from being sucked back into the thoracic cavity during aspiration once the pneumothorax has been drained.

Observations. Repeated observations are made of respiratory rate, degree of chest retraction, colour of tongue, heart rate, temperature and blood pressure. To minimize handling, respiratory rate, heart rate, temperature and blood pressure can all be monitored electronically.

Maintenance of a clear airway. The infant is carefully observed in case the tongue falls back against the pharynx. Sterile suction apparatus should be on hand to remove any mucus which accumulates in the pharynx and which could obstruct the airway.

Oxygen is administered in a concentration that will maintain *arterial oxygen tension* at a satisfactory level (60–70 mmHg or 8–9 kPa). If one is unable to perform blood-gas analysis, *sufficient oxygen is given to just abolish central cyanosis.* The infant's tongue is the best area to observe for the presence of central cyanosis. Oxygen may be given *intranasally* (rarely used) at a rate of ½–1 litre per minute (an excessive rate can cause a pneumothorax), into the *canopy* of the incubator, or into a plastic *head box* which enables a 100% concentration of oxygen to surround the infant's head (figure 63.10).

If an infant requires an inspired oxygen concentration of 40% or above, arterial oxygen tension must be measured. This is performed by inserting a cannula down an umbilical artery and threading its tip into the descending aorta (figure 63.11) or percutaneously inserting a small cannula into a peripheral (radial or posterior tibial) artery. If these techniques fail, oxygen tension can be measured by a *transcutaneous oxygen electrode*, the results of which have a close correlation with arterial oxygen tension. The electrode warms the infant's skin, causes dilatation of arterial vessels which bring blood to the warm area; oxygen diffuses from the dilated arteries across the infant's thin skin to the electrode which measures its tension.

It should be remembered that *high levels of oxygen in the blood can cause retrolental fibroplasia in premature infants.* Oxygen blowing directly onto the infant is cold and chills the body. The resultant subnormal body temperature will aggravate the infant's condition; to prevent this, the oxygen is warmed and humidified by the use of a nebulizer or similar apparatus. Overheating is also dangerous and hence a nebulizer thermostatically set at *35–37°C* should be used; as an added precaution, the temperature of the humidified air is checked hourly. The advantages of humidity are that secretions in the upper respiratory tract are moistened and this facilitates aspiration, and it also helps to prevent dehydration.

Calories. *Hypoglycaemia* is common in hypoxic and ill infants due to depleted glycogen reserves (anaerobic glycolysis). To overcome this problem, the infant with respiratory distress requires glucose without delay. In mild cases of respiratory distress this may be given orally, but one must be careful to prevent aspiration of the stomach contents into the lungs; in infants with moderate or severe respiratory distress, the calories are provided as 10% glucose solution infused parenterally (peripheral vein or umbilical artery).

Figure 63.10. The plastic box surrounding the infant's head is used to increase the oxygen concentration of the inhaled gases. The oxygen is warmed and humidified before entering the plastic 'head box'.

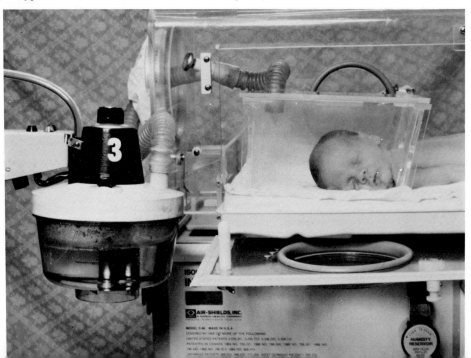

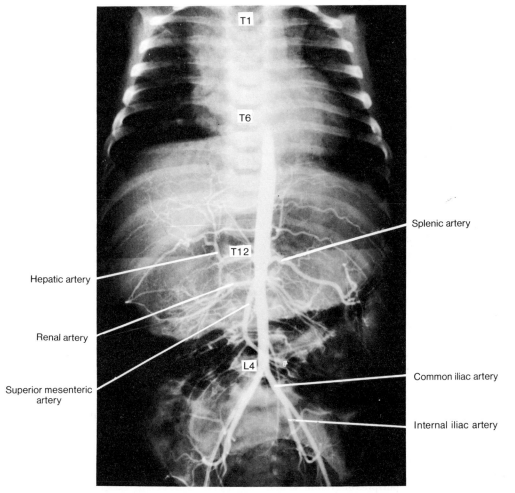

Labels on figure: T1, T6, T12, L4

Splenic artery

Hepatic artery

Renal artery

Common iliac artery

Superior mesenteric artery

Internal iliac artery

Figure 63.11 Aortogram of a newborn infant showing the main abdominal branches. The catheter is inserted via an umbilical artery and its tip should be either above or below the origin of the renal arteries (L1) to avoid the possibility of a nephrotoxic drug being injected into the renal artery.

Correction of biochemical abnormalities. Hypoxia is corrected by giving oxygen, and *metabolic acidosis* by oxygen and an intravenous infusion of sodium bicarbonate (8.7%). *Hypoglycaemia* is diagnosed by routinely performing glucose estimations on capillary blood obtained at 3-hourly intervals; treatment is by intravenous infusion of 10% glucose. *Hypercapnia*, if severe, can only be corrected by some form of mechanical respiration.

Antibiotics are used prophylactically when the infant has a condition such as hyaline membrane disease, or therapeutically when there is infection present such as in pneumonia. Because of the high mortality of infants infected with the group B, beta-haemolytic streptococcus and the fact that the disease mimics hyaline membrane disease, all infants with respiratory distress should be given penicillin (after blood has been collected for microscopy and culture) pending the diagnosis.

Mechanical Aids to Respiration

Today, in the care of babies with severe respiratory failure, assistance can be given by methods which increase the pressure of inspired oxygen delivered into the lungs.

Continuous Positive Airways Pressure (CPAP)

This is effected by supplying the gases to be inspired under pressure which forces the alveoli open, prevents collapse of alveoli in hyaline membrane disease, and forces oxygen across the alveolar membrane to the blood in the pulmonary capillaries. In this method the infant must be able to breathe spontaneously. Pressure is attained in the inspired gases by utilizing a resistance to the exhaled gases. The resistance is supplied by a screw clamp, or by flowing the gases through a water trap. Continuous positive airway pressure can be supplied by using nasal prongs, a face mask, a Gregory box or as is more common, via an *endotracheal tube.*

Intermittent Positive Pressure Ventilation (IPPV)

In this technique the lungs are repetitively expanded by increasing the pressure of the inspired gases intermittently. This intermittent pressure expands alveoli and forces oxygen across the alveolar membrane. When the pressure is withdrawn, carbon dioxide can pass from the pulmonary capillaries to the alveoli and be exhaled. If the disease process being treated is hyaline membrane disease, one must prevent the alveoli from collapsing when the pressure on the inspired gases is removed. This is done by never completely removing pressure from the inspired gases — i.e. using *positive end expiratory pressure (PEEP)*. Intermittent positive pressure ventilation (+ PEEP) is usually delivered through an endotracheal tube and administered by a mechanical ventilator (figure 63.12).

In CPAP and IPPV methods of assisted respiration it is usual to insert an endotracheal tube so that the inspired gases pass directly into the lungs. The endotracheal tube is then secured and connected to the mechanical device delivering the gases. Once a tube is in position other problems confront the nurse.

(i) *The tube must not become blocked.* This is prevented by 2–4 hourly *sterile suction* being performed via the tube. Often a 'wetting agent' such as 0.5 ml of normal saline is passed down the tube before performing the suction. A blocked tube is diagnosed by increasing central cyanosis, increasing irritability of the infant, and an obstructed breathing pattern.

(ii) *The tube must not slip out or down too far.* If it slips down too far it passes into the right main bronchus and hence the gases are only being directed to one lung.

Problems with use of IPPV are *pneumothorax* and *bronchopulmonary dysplasia (BPD)*. *Bronchopulmonary dysplasia* is a disorder where the lung is damaged by the combined effects of pressure and oxygen. In this disorder the respiratory ciliated columnar epithelium changes to that of stratified squamous epithelium. Hence secretions in the lung are removed only with difficulty, and areas of collapse, consolidation and infection occur. Once the various effects of pressure and oxygen are removed the lung heals in a majority of cases, but the healing process may take up to 2 years (figure 63.13).

Intermittent Negative Pressure Ventilation (INPV)

In this technique a negative pressure is developed around the outside of the thorax which therefore expands. This opens alveoli and aids oxygenation. When the negative pressure is withdrawn, exhalation with elimination of carbon dioxide occurs. The negative pressure is created by means of an airtight cylinder (tank) placed around the thorax. This technique has proved successful in adults, but has had only limited success in neonates because of their smaller size. Theoretically both pneumothorax and BPD would be eliminated by this technique.

Oscillation ventilation

Recently it has been discovered that if inspired gases are 'shaken', oxygenation can be improved and carbon dioxide elimination accomplished. When this is done only low inspiratory pressures are required; hence the risk of pneumothorax and BPD are minimized. This technique is still in the experimental phase.

Figure 63.12 Premature infant with respiratory distress receiving assisted ventilation. The endotracheal tube is passed through the mouth into the larynx and is held in place by the mesh bonnet.

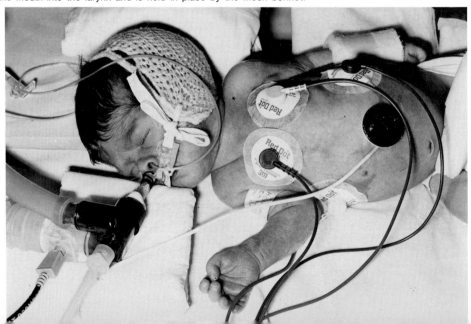

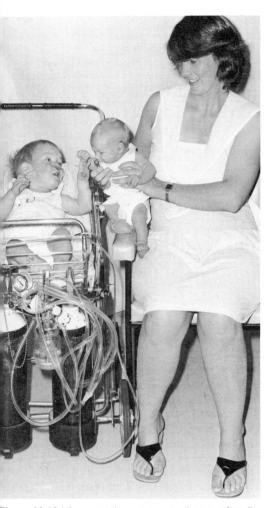

Figure 63.13 Life on continuous oxygen therapy after discharge from hospital. This infant was born at 26 weeks' gestation (birth-weight 1,300 g) when this mother suffered an antepartum haemorrhage and premature rupture of the membranes. He developed bronchopulmonary dysplasia following mechanical ventilation for hyaline membrane disease. He is shown aged 15 months, happy and apparently of high intelligence, with his loving mother and 6-week-old brother (birth-weight 3,760 g at 41 weeks' gestation). The prognosis of these infants must be guarded; in this community (population 4.5 millions) there are only 5 such children receiving oxygen therapy at home.

Statistics of Infants Requiring Assisted Ventilation

The introduction of assisted ventilation (intermittent positive pressure respiration via a mechanical ventilator, or continuous positive airways pressure via nasal prongs or endotracheal intubation) was the key to improved results of management of infants with the respiratory distress syndrome.

In one large obstetric teaching hospital, during the 7 years 1971–1977, 0.7% of all liveborn infants received assisted ventilation and the mortality rate was 45% (91 of 210); during the 3 years 1978–1980, *the proportion of infants who received assisted ventilation increased to 2.1% of all babies born alive, and the mortality rate fell to 28%* (86 of 308). Also the mean duration of assisted ventilation increased from *60 to 106* hours.

Table 63.5 shows the aetiology of the respiratory failure in the infants who required assisted ventilation — these infants *comprised 42% (308 of 732) of those with the respiratory distress syndrome. Two thirds were cases of hyaline membrane disease* and the other main indication was birth-weight below 1,500 g, this latter group of infants being electively intubated in order to minimize the effects of hypoxia — in other words the babies were ventilated as a supportive measure rather than as last minute lifesaving intervention.

TABLE 63.5   AETIOLOGY OF RESPIRATORY FAILURE, MORTALITY AND MATURITY OF 308 INFANTS REQUIRING ASSISTED VENTILATION

Diagnosis	Number (deaths)	Mean gestational age (weeks)
Hyaline membrane disease	210 (67)	32.4
Birth-weight < 1,500 g	31 (5)	28.0
Apnoeic attacks	14 (2)	32.1
Pneumonia	10 (2)	38.8
'Wet lung'	10 —	33.6
Hypoxia at birth	10 (2)	36.7
Cardiac anomaly	4 (1)	38.0
Idiopathic hydrops	2 (2)	32.5
Pulmonary haemorrhage	1 (1)	40.0
Other	16 (4)	33.6

Table 63.6 shows the *high incidence of complications* in the infants who required assisted ventilation. The combination of *pneumothorax and hyaline membrane disease accounted for 50% (43 of 86) of the neonatal deaths.* It is obvious that the prevention of air leaks is of prime importance in the management of these infants.

TABLE 63.6   COMPLICATIONS IN 308 INFANTS WHO REQUIRED ASSISTED VENTILATION*

Complications	Number	%
Pulmonary interstitial emphysema	96	31.1
Problems with the endotracheal tube	88	28.5
Pneumothorax	77	25.0
Patent ductus arteriosus	38	12.3
Retrolental fibroplasia	35**	11.3
Bronchopulmonary dysplasia	30	9.7
Pneumomediastinum	6	1.9
Pneumoperitoneum	5	1.6

* Some infants had more than 1 complication
** Retrolental fibroplasia was mild in 34 and severe in 1

chapter sixty-four

Immaturity and Disorders of Growth

OVERVIEW

A *premature infant* is defined as one born before 37 weeks of gestation. The contribution of prematurity to neonatal mortality and morbidity is monumental — the incidence of prematurity is only *8%* yet it accounts for *80% of all neonatal deaths*. The important complications of prematurity are *hyaline membrane disease* which alone accounts for 25% of all neonatal deaths, *intraventricular haemorrhage* which affects approximately 40% of infants with birth-weights below 1,500 g, *necrotizing enterocolitis*, and the complications of *oxygen toxicity* (*retrolental fibroplasia* and *bronchopulmonary dysplasia*) which are a special hazard for infants who require oxygen administration or ventilatory support because of respiratory distress.

Recent advances are: (i) the use of *ultrasonography* which when used in the first half of pregnancy provides an accurate means of assessment of fetal maturity and hence avoidance of untimely delivery, (ii) *adrenal corticosteroid* (*betamethasone*) therapy for enhancement of surfactant production and minimization of the incidence and severity of hyaline membrane disease when delivery before 34 weeks' gestation is necessary, (iii) *computerized axial tomography* or realtime ultrasonography for diagnosis of the presence and extent of intraventricular haemorrhage, (iv) the presence of a *paediatrician* at all deliveries when the birth-weight is expected to be below 1,500 g or if fetal maturity is 34 weeks or less, (v) introduction of *neonatal transport facilities* for transfer of premature infants to well-equipped centres.

The rubicon for fetal survival with regard to prematurity is a maturity of 32 weeks' gestation (figure 64.7); after this more than 96% survive.

By definition, a *low birth-weight infant* is one weighing 2,500 g or less at birth, regardless of the period of gestation. *Very low birth-weight infants* (birth-weight less than 1,500 g) *comprise 1% of births but provide 50% of perinatal deaths.* Better understanding of the physiology of the low birth-weight infant has resulted in improvements in management (adequate oxygenation, nutrition, prevention of hypoglycaemia) centred around neonatal intensive care units. Not only have survival rates increased, but the incidence of physical and/or neurological impairment in surviving infants of very low birth-weight has fallen to 6–8%. These handicaps are often due to *intraventricular haemorrhage and cerebral infarction.* In the near future, ultrasonography will enable identification of infants likely to die or to develop serious handicaps; this will allow controlled trials of treatment designed to prevent death and brain damage, and recognition of infants with severe brain damage from whom continued intensive care should be withheld.

A *growth retarded infant* is one with birth-weight below the 10th percentile for gestational age. These infants have an increased risk of *stillbirth* (× 4) and *neonatal morbidity*, especially *asphyxia* (× 2), major *congenital malformations* (× 2) and *hypoglycaemia* (× 4). However, with modern paediatric care the *neonatal mortality rate* of small for dates infants is the same as that in the overall population. Moreover, the quality of survival of these infants is satisfactory, long-term assessment having shown an incidence of major neurological handicap in only 2.2%.

INTRODUCTION

For many years, infants weighing less than 2,500 g at birth have been admitted to 'premature nurseries'. This was because of the realization that these infants were at risk and required special management. Recently, it has been appreciated that this group of infants is not a homogeneous one in terms of weight loss, complications, and length of stay in hospital. This group, once termed 'premature', is now known to consist of true premature infants, growth retarded (or small for dates) infants, and infants showing a combination of true prematurity and growth retardation.

This differentiation is important for several reasons. (i) They suffer different complications and hence require different treatment. (ii) The premature infant tends to lose weight from birth, whereas the growth retarded infant often gains weight (figure 64.1). This is relevant when estimating the child's length of stay in hospital. (iii) The premature infant is often too immature to suck, whereas a growth retarded infant of more advanced gestational age, but the same weight, can do so.

In 1961, the World Health Organization recommended that the following *definitions* be used.

An immature (or premature) infant is one born before 37 weeks' gestation, regardless of the birth-weight.

A low birth-weight infant is one weighing 2,500 g or less at birth, regardless of the period of gestation. (It should be noted that a baby can still be premature (born before 37 weeks) and behave as such, although weighing more than 2,500 g at birth, figure 64.2).

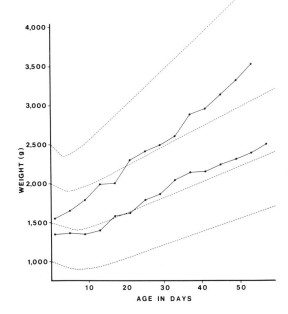

Figure 64.1 The growth charts of a small for dates and a premature infant of similar birth-weights. The small for dates infant weighed 1,550 g at 36.3 weeks' gestation and gained weight at a rate in keeping with his maturity rather than his size at birth.

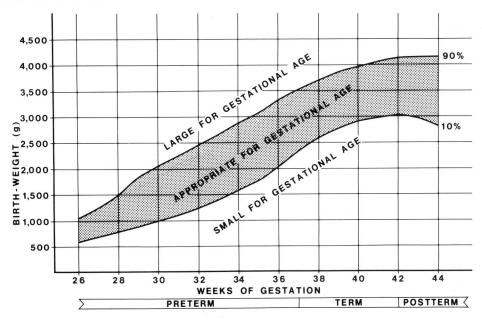

Figure 64.2 This percentile chart of birth-weight according to the period of gestation allows ready reckoning of whether an infant is small or large for dates.

A *growth retarded* (*small for dates*) *infant* is defined as one whose birth-weight is below the 10th percentile for the gestational age. Hence, in order to determine if an infant is growth retarded, 2 facts must be known — the period of gestation at birth and the birth-weight. Once gestation is determined, birth-weight is compared with that on a standard percentile chart (figure 64.2) to decide if an infant's weight is large, small, or appropriate for the gestational age.

ESTIMATION OF THE PERIOD OF GESTATION

This is one of the most difficult problems in obstetric and paediatric practice. The following are the important features on which the estimation of maturity is made.

Maternal Factors

(i) Date of the last normal menstrual period. (ii) Date when fetal movements were first noted. (iii) Size of the uterus, especially if assessed early in pregnancy.

Maternal Investigations

(i) *Ultrasonography* is the most accurate test available for assessment of fetal maturity and should be performed whenever the clinical findings are in doubt (irregular or unreliable menstrual data, uterine size not consistent with dates or time of quickening). Maturity is assessed by measurement of the size of the *gestational sac* (6–7 weeks' gestation), *crown-rump length* (8–12 weeks' gestation) or *biparietal diameter*, which is most accurate between 15–20 weeks' gestation. Ultrasonographic assessment of fetal maturity is less accurate after 26 weeks' gestation but may be of value for following fetal growth.

(ii) *X-ray.* The presence of distal femoral epiphyses indicates a fetal maturity of 36 weeks or more. Radiographic assessment of fetal maturity has been replaced by ultrasonography in most centres.

(iii) *Amniocentesis* allows prediction of *functional maturity* rather than gestational age. The amniotic fluid *lecithin/sphingomyelin ratio* or comparable index of surfactant production is estimated to predict fetal *pulmonary maturity*. Other tests of less clinical value are measurement of the *creatinine* level in amniotic fluid to assess fetal renal maturity and the percentage of '*fat cells*' which correlates with the maturity of sebaceous glands of the fetal skin.

Assessment of the Infant

Examination of the infant is the final method that is utilized, but it is not necessarily accurate. Many complicated charts have been derived for determining fetal maturity by examination, but the most useful clinical features are the following.

(i) *Head circumference.* This is the parameter least affected in growth retardation and hence is

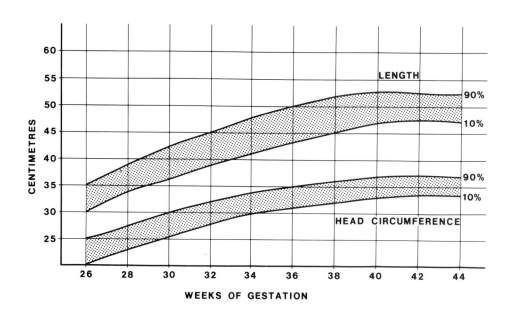

Figure 64.3 Percentile chart of length and head circumference according to gestational age.

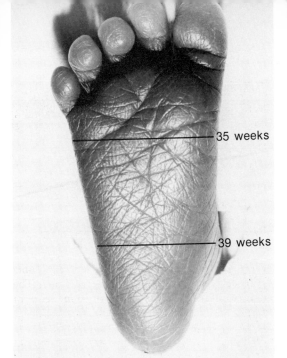

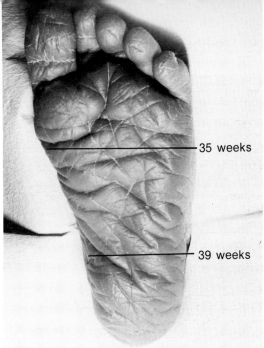

Figure 64.4 Sole of an infant born at 32 weeks' gestation; the deep creases are located only in the anterior one-third.

Figure 64.5 Sole of an infant born at full term showing deep creases over the entire surface.

the best single measurement for estimation of maturity (figure 64.3). (ii) *Breast tissue.* The diameter of the breast bud in millimetres plus 34 gives an estimate of gestational age in weeks. (iii) *Ear cartilage.* If there is none the maturity is less than 35 weeks; partial presence of cartilage indicates maturity between 35–39 weeks; complete cartilage indicates maturity of more than 39 weeks. (iv) *Testes.* If present in the inguinal canal the maturity is 35 weeks, whereas when pendulous within the scrotum the maturity is more than 37 weeks. (v) *Sole creases.* Before 35 weeks, deep skin creases are present only in the anterior third of the foot (figure 64.4); between 35 and 39 weeks, they are also present in the middle third; thereafter they are present over all of the sole (figure 64.5). (vi) *Position.* Flexion of the lower limbs is evident at about 32 weeks, and at 36 weeks all limbs are flexed (figure 64.6). (vii) *Neurological assessment.* Since the brain is the organ least affected in growth retardation assessment of brain function is a good guide to the maturity of the infant. Table 64.1 lists the most important reflexes to elicit when determining brain maturity. (viii) *General appearance.* See section below.

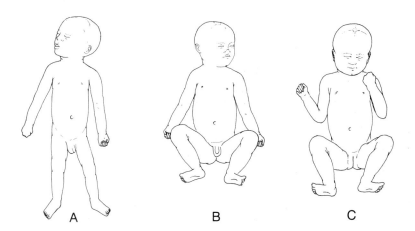

Figure 64.6 Fetal position according to maturity. **A.** At 28 weeks' maturity the infant is hypotonic. **B.** At 32 weeks the lower limbs are flexed. **C.** At 36 weeks all limbs are flexed.

TABLE 64.1   REFLEXES OF VALUE IN ASSESSING GESTATIONAL AGE

Reflex	Stimulus	Patient response	Maturity in weeks according to reflex	
			Absent	Present
Pupil reaction	Light	Contraction	< 31	29 or more
Glabella tap	Tap on glabella	Blink	< 34	32 or more
Head-turning	Light	Head-turning to light	Doubtful	32 or more
Traction	Pull up by wrists from supine	Flexion of neck on arms	< 36	33 or more
Neck-righting	Rotation of head	Trunk follows	< 37	34 or more

Adapted from R. J. Robinson

THE PREMATURE INFANT

An infant is generally considered to be viable at 28 weeks' gestation. *At this time it weighs approximately 1,000 g and is 35 cm long.* The lung development at this stage is usually just adequate to sustain life. Infants born between 23–28 weeks' gestation may also survive with modern paediatric care. The survival rates of infants born at 26 and 28 weeks' gestation are approximately 1 in 4 and 1 in 2, respectively (figure 64.7).

PHYSICAL APPEARANCE

General appearance will vary with the period of gestation. The smallest premature infants look all skin and bone since they lack subcutaneous fat and muscle tissue. The limbs look thin and spindly and there is no muscle tone. The infant's general appearance improves with gestational age.

Position (figure 64.6). At 28 weeks the infant is hypotonic; at 32 weeks flexion is present in the lower limbs, and at 36 weeks all limbs are flexed.

The *head* appears large in comparison with the body. The sutures often override and the fontanelles are wide and soft. In the smallest babies the skull seems vulnerable to palpation.

Skin. In the smallest infants the texture of the skin is very fine. The colour is often brick-red because the skin is almost transparent and shows the colour of blood in subcutaneous tissues. The skin is covered with fine downy hair called *lanugo* (figure 64.8, colour plate 119). The hair on the skull is sparse and fine and the hair line extends to the infant's brow and down past the ears as 'sideburns'. The eyelashes and eyebrows are so fine that they are almost invisible. *Vernix caseosa* is present on the skin in minimal amounts at 28 weeks, reaches its maximum at 36 weeks and thereafter is present in diminishing amounts.

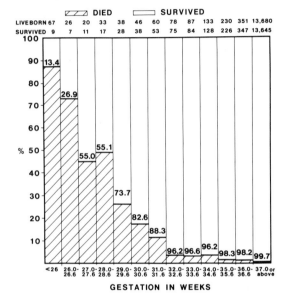

Figure 64.7 Percentage survival for each week of gestation in a series of 14,849 consecutive liveborn infants, 19784–1980. The rubicon for survival was 32 weeks' gestation after which more than 96% survived.

Breast tissue is usually not palpable before 34 weeks.

Cartilage in the ears begins to develop at 35 weeks. At 28–35 weeks' maturity the ears are thin, pliable and inelastic (figure 64.8).

The *chest* appears small and the chest wall is very yielding and tends to collapse. The *cry* is feeble and poorly sustained.

The *abdomen*, due to poor muscle tone, often appears distended.

Genitalia. (i) *Male.* The scrotum is poorly developed, has few rugae (skin folds), and the testicles may be undescended. (ii) *Female.* The labia minora and clitoris are exposed and appear large because the labia majora are poorly developed.

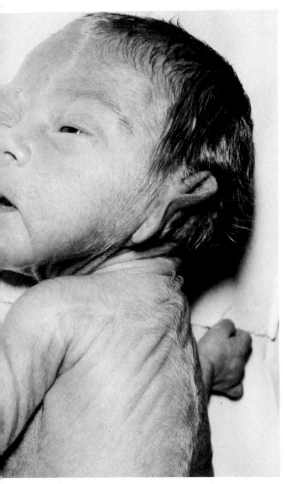

Figure 64.8 This infant was born at 29 weeks' gestation. He shows a covering of lanugo and absence of ear cartilage and subcutaneous fat; his sideburns are apparent.

PHYSIOLOGY OF THE PREMATURE INFANT

Although the premature infant has immature organs, he adapts surprisingly well to extrauterine life. The neonatal mortality rate according to birth-weight is shown in figure 64.9. The death rate falls markedly with increase in weight and levels out at 2,500 g, this being the average weight at 36 weeks' gestation (figure 64.2). *This is why the cardinal rule in obstetrics is to avoid delivery before 37 weeks' gestation whenever possible.*

Respiratory system. The *lungs* commence to develop at 4 weeks' gestation and continue to develop until full term. Alveoli (or air sacs), which are essential for transportation of gases to the blood, begin to be budded-off from the developing respiratory tree at about 26 weeks' gestation. *Surfactant,* a substance vital for normal lung function, is not produced until about 26 weeks' gestation. At 28 weeks there is a sufficient number of *capillaries* in close contact with the future air spaces to permit sufficient oxygenation of the blood for extrauterine survival, but their apposition to the developing air spaces improves with further maturity.

Periodic breathing occurs to a greater or lesser extent in 30–40% of all premature infants. Typically, the infant breathes for periods of 10–15 seconds and these alternate with apnoeic periods of 6–7 seconds. The infant does not become cyanosed during the period of apnoea. The cause is ill-understood, but is related to an immature respiratory centre in the brain.

Central nervous system. The *heat regulating centre* is immature. Therefore the infant tends to take up the temperature of the environment. Conservation of body heat is the main problem, since the premature infant has a large surface area relative to weight and also lacks subcutaneous tissue. The *sucking* and *swallowing reflexes* are poorly developed and feeding difficulties are common. The *cough reflex* is absent and thus there is the added danger of inhalation of milk.

Figure 64.9 Perinatal mortality rate according to birth-weight. These figures were derived from a series of approximately 15,000 deliveries in a teaching hospital, 1979–1981. The rate was 85% for infants under 1,000 g and was lowest (less than 1%) in the range 2,500–4,000 g.

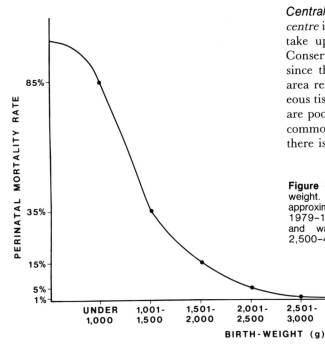

Excretory system. Kidneys. Infants have less efficient renal function, their glomerular filtration rate and tubular excretory and absorptive capacities being only 20–50% of the adult value, relative to body weight. Hence, their capacity for excretion of waste products and salts is diminished and they are unable to concentrate and acidify the urine as effectively. In premature infants renal function is even less well developed, hence they pass large amounts of dilute urine and are liable to dehydration and acidosis. The *sweat glands* are poorly developed and the infant is unable to excrete waste products via the skin or to reduce body temperature by sweating if overheated.

Digestive system. The *stomach* is of small capacity and has fewer rugae. The *cardiac sphincter* is poorly developed and immature infants readily regurgitate feedings thus increasing the risk of aspiration pneumonia. Intestinal immaturity often results in ineffective bowel peristalsis; the abdomen becomes distended and the infant requires treatment to facilitate expulsion of bowel contents. Most premature infants can digest milk readily, but they have a diminished capacity to digest fat; thus fat-soluble vitamins (A and D) given orally should be in a special water-miscible form as in DHSS vitamin drops. The *liver* is immature in several important functions: poorly developed capacity for *bilirubin* conjugation and excretion which leads to 'jaundice of prematurity'; *limited glycogen storage* which leads to hypoglycaemia; and finally, there is a *deficiency of blood clotting factors* produced in the liver (factors 2, 7, 9 and 10), so there is an increased tendency to haemorrhage.

Blood vessel fragility aggravates the tendency to bleed, leading to intracranial and pulmonary haemorrhages.

Immunity. (i) *Active immunity.* The more immature the infant the more immature is the immune system. (ii) *Passive immunity.* During pregnancy, maternal immunoglobulins pass across the placenta to the infant. After birth these play a part in the newborn infant's capacity to resist infection. The premature infant is born early and receives less maternally-derived immunoglobulins and hence is more prone to infection.

CARE BEFORE BIRTH

The mother should be delivered in a hospital with adequate facilities for premature infant care, and a paediatrician should be present at the birth. *It is much safer to transfer the mother to a suitable hospital when premature labour is expected than to transfer the baby after birth.*

In addition to the usual preparations at birth (see Chapter 59), a portable incubator (Port-O-Cot (CIG)) should be available for immediate transfer of the baby to the special care nursery.

The respiratory centre of the immature fetus is very susceptible to analgesics and anaesthetics given to the mother and these should be used as sparingly as possible during labour.

An episiotomy should be performed electively to allow delivery of the infant's soft head without moulding or undue pressure being exerted on it.

Caesarean section is advocated by many as the preferred method of delivery of premature infants due to a lower incidence of trauma. Caesarean section is not without difficulty when the fetus is small, because the lower uterine segment is often poorly formed and a vertical upper segment (classical) incision may be required.

CARE AT BIRTH

Hypoxia must be prevented or minimized at birth in premature infants since it increases the severity of hyaline membrane disease.

In addition to the usual management of the newborn, the following special measures are adopted. The mouth and pharynx are gently aspirated immediately after birth. Gastric aspiration is advisable *after* breathing has commenced.

The *umbilical cord* is clamped and cut as soon as possible after birth to ensure (i) that the infant does not receive an excessive quantity of blood that can intensify or cause jaundice, (ii) that he can be transferred quickly to the portable incubator or warmed resuscitation table with a minimum of heat loss, and (iii) that resuscitative measures can be instituted promptly if required.

The cord should be clamped 2–5 cm from the body so that the umbilical vessels are accessible for the administration of drugs, blood or fluids during the first days of life.

Vitamin K_1 (Konakion) 1mg is given by intramuscular injection as a routine to prevent haemorrhagic disease of the newborn.

Handling must be gentle and every effort is made to prevent the baby from becoming *cold* because hypothermia increases mortality sevenfold. He is transported to the special care nursery as soon as possible, with the paediatrician still in attendance. Transportation must be by a 'transport incubator' with warmth, oxygen and suction available.

CARE AFTER BIRTH (figure 64.10)

Environment. The infant should be nursed in a special care unit, preferably with facilities for

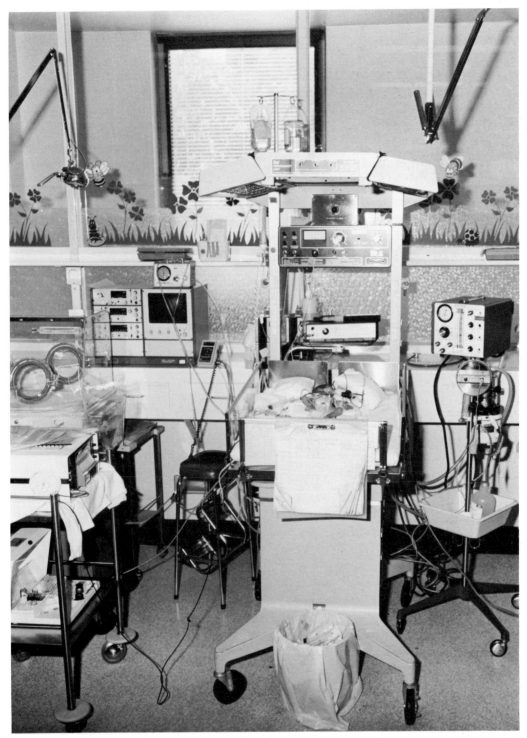

Figure 64.10 A small premature infant being cared for in an intensive care nursery. His temperature is being maintained by a servocontrolled overhead radiant heater. Vital signs are being electronically monitored. A catheter has been placed into his aorta to enable systemic blood pressure to be recorded and blood samples to be obtained painlessly for careful monitoring of his biochemical status. He is receiving a blood transfusion and the other intravenous infusion is to supply calories and electrolytes. Because of severe hyaline membrane disease his breathing is being assisted by a mechanical ventilator. To maintain his blood oxygen level within close limits, the transcutaneous oxygen level is being constantly measured.

intensive care. The unit should have temperature and humidity control (air-conditioning) to minimize the possibility of airborne infection.

Attendants. The personnel of the nursery must include staff skilled in the care of premature babies. Students should always work under the supervision of trained staff. Nursing staff should not be expected to move out of the unit and work in other ward areas. All nursing personnel must wear a clean uniform. Visitors to the unit wear a clean gown. Hand cleansing is performed by one or other of the regimens described in Chapter 67.

Parents of premature infants may be admitted to the nursery if they are free of infection, and follow the same gown and hand washing techniques as the staff members, one of whom accompanies them as they look at, and handle their infants. Mothers appear to relate emotionally better towards their infants if involved in their care and this may be important in an infant's future development (animal mothers, after even a brief separation from their offspring, may either lose interest in, kick or eat them!). There is evidence that mothers of premature infants often reject and batter their infants when they come home. It is essential for the future well-being of the family unit that the mother be sympathetically and actively encouraged to enter the nursery, to have eye to eye contact with her infant (even if in the incubator), and to handle and participate in the baby's care whenever this is possible (colour plates 99 and 100); expressing breast milk for her own infant who is too feeble to put to the breast is her unique contribution to his welfare.

Temperature. It is important to maintain the infant's body temperature; this is recorded hourly until stable, then 3-hourly. If the initial temperature of the infant is below 35°C, the true temperature is obtained by using a low reading thermometer. The temperature of the surroundings should keep the infant's skin temperature between 36.1°C and 36.6°C, in which range the infant's metabolic and oxygen requirements are minimal (*neutral thermal environment*).

Small and/or sick premature infants are nursed in a closed incubator-type cot such as the Vickers medical incubator. The smaller the infant the higher the temperature needed in the incubator. Usually an incubator temperature of 30–32°C is adequate for infants weighing more than 1,300 g; smaller babies usually require a temperature of between 32–34°C. The smallest infants are best nursed in an incubator which is equipped with a servocontrol probe (figure 64.11). The probe is taped to the infant's skin and controls the incubator temperature, thus ensuring that the

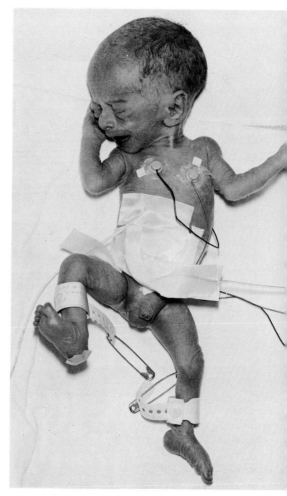

Figure 64.11 This severely small for dates infant was born at 36 weeks' gestation and weighed only 840 g. The 2 monitor leads can be seen on his chest and the servocontrol probe is strapped against his skin.

infant's temperature is constantly between 36.1–36.6°C. Babies over 2,500 g who require incubator care are best nursed in an ambient temperature between 29–31°C. *The doctor should be notified if any infant has a recorded temperature above 37°C or below 35°C.*

Pulse rate. Initially the pulse rate is recorded hourly until stable, then 3-hourly. If the infant is sick and minimal handling is desirable, the pulse rate is best recorded by a cardiac monitor. There are many types available, but the principles of use are the same. Light disposable leads are attached to the infant's chest (figure 64.11). The monitor records the heart beat audibly and in some cases visually.

There is usually an alarm system incorporated that can alert the nurse if there is bradycardia or tachycardia. If no monitor is available, it is best to record the pulse rate 3-hourly, since this avoids disturbing the baby. *If the infant is breathing his heart will be beating.* A stethoscope is used to count the apical heart beat over a full minute. *Bradycardia (below 100 beats per minute) or tachycardia (above 160 beats per minute) is reported to the doctor.*

Respiratory rate is initially recorded hourly until stable, then 3-hourly. The type of respiration should be noted as should any sternal or rib retraction or expiratory grunting (see Chapter 63). Respirations are counted over a full minute. *A rate over 60 per minute or below 20 per minute is reported to the doctor.*

In addition to observations on temperature, pulse rate and respiration, the nurse must accurately record and report the following signs: jaundice, cyanosis or pallor, excessive crying or hyperactivity, twitching or convulsive movements, excessive lethargy, suspicion of early infection ('baby does not look well'), abdominal distension, disinterest in feeding, vomiting, loose stools, no stools or voiding of urine within 30–36 hours of life.

Intravenous or intraarterial fluid. Initially, a very small or sick infant will often be given fluids by either the intraarterial (umbilical or peripheral artery) or the intravenous route (any available peripheral vein). Parenteral infusions must *never* be given to an infant without the use of a paediatric burette (e.g. Metriset (McGaw Ethicals Ltd)). A microdrip is incorporated into the set and allows accurate estimation and limitation of the amount of fluid that the infant receives. Various pumping devices are available that enable fluid to be infused at a constant rate. These include the Holter Pump (Extracorporeal Medical Specialities Inc), and the IVAC Infusion Pump (Tekmar Medical Ltd). The use of a mechanical pump does not alter the nurse's responsibility to record and adjust the rate of flow of the infusion. Any additions to the infused fluid such as sodium bicarbonate or glucose must be documented accurately. If the infusion is in the umbilical artery a notice to this effect should be displayed on the incubator. In addition to stating that the arterial infusion is in progress, the notice should list the following guides for the nursing staff. (i) All connections must be secure: loose connections are dangerous and may result in fatal haemorrhage. (ii) Tell the doctor *at once* if the infant's feet or legs become discoloured or white (this is caused by the catheter occluding arterial blood flow). (iii) Keep the flask high to counteract arterial pressure. (iv) Observe the umbilicus for bleeding.

Oxygen is given only if the baby shows *central cyanosis* (e.g. tongue looks blue). Peripheral cyanosis should be ignored, since the most common cause is cold. Oxygen is given at a rate just sufficient to relieve the central cyanosis. Babies with severe respiratory distress and little functioning lung tissue may require high concentrations of oxygen to relieve cyanosis. Remember, it is the oxygen dissolved in the arterial blood that is important, *not* the ambient (surrounding) oxygen. Blood oxygen levels (paO_2) are estimated serially if the inspired oxygen concentration exceeds 40%, and the ambient oxygen concentration is regulated so that the paO_2 is maintained between 60–80 mm Hg (7.9–10.6 kPa). To enable high concentrations of oxygen to be given to the baby, a plastic box that fits over the infant's head is sometimes used. Oxygen given via a head box should always be warmed and humidified, using individual humidifiers. Electrical humidifiers and nebulizers should *not* be used without a temperature sensor and automatic cutout to prevent accidental overheating. The ambient oxygen concentration is measured by an oxygen analyser and the rate of oxygen administration is adjusted as necessary. Administration of oxygen at a given rate (litres per minute) is not of itself a measure of the ambient oxygen concentration. Oxygen concentration should *always* be at the level ordered.

Humidity. At some institutions, the provision of humidity via the inbuilt tank in the incubator is discouraged. This area can be a reservoir for infection and it is better to give the infant individualized humidity. If the humidity tank is used, distilled water is placed in it and 2 drops of 2% silver nitrate solution are added as a bacteriostatic measure. The water is changed daily.

Position of the baby. The infant is allowed to take up a position of choice in the incubator. Initially this is usually supine (on the back) with the head turned to one side. In babies with respiratory distress, a small pad is sometimes placed under the shoulder. The head should always be in a correct position to allow free access of inspired gases. Later, the infant is nursed from side to side and prone (face downwards). Babies in cots are nursed on their sides. The cot head is tilted up after feeding to prevent regurgitation.

Handling. The time to handle and weigh the premature baby will depend on progress; a sick baby is left until recovery is under way. In general, infants nursed in incubators are left undisturbed for the first 24 hours; those in cots are left 3–6 hours, depending on temperature stability. No infant should be cleaned and weighed until the temperature has remained stable above 36°C for 3 hours. All work should be organized so as to avoid unnecessary and prolonged handling of the infant. Babies weighing less than 1,500 g should be nursed and fed in their incubator or cot to avoid unnecessary handling. Gentle firm handling is desirable. The infant who is not sick can be taken out of the incubator to be nursed by the parents for brief periods to improve parental-infant bonding.

Clothing should be easily removable and blankets *must be loose* to allow free chest movement. Infants in incubators may be nursed naked while sick to facilitate observation, and later they are clad only in a napkin.

Weighing is performed every second day. The initial weight loss depends on how soon the infant was fed and how the feedings were managed. The average weight loss is 60–90 g per kg body-weight (approximately 10% of birth-weight).

Cord care. (i) *Cot babies.* The cord clamp is left on and inspected periodically for signs of oozing. (ii) *Incubator babies.* No dressing is applied to the umbilical cord other than a cord clamp. Subsequently local toileting is performed using swabs impregnated with alcohol (Mediswab).

Prevention of infection. Since the infant is vulnerable to infection, certain measures to prevent cross-infection should be taken in the special care nursery. These are discussed in Chapter 67.

Feeding

The following physiological factors contribute to feeding difficulties in premature infants: small capacity of stomach, lax cardiac sphincter, deficient and incoordinate peristalsis, immature digestion, and finally, poor sucking and swallowing reflexes.

Time to Commence Feeding

Current paediatric practice is to feed babies as early as possible. This minimizes the dangers of hypoglycaemia and hyperbilirubinaemia. However, the everpresent dangers of vomiting, aspiration and resulting pneumonitis must be considered. Because of this danger, most infants weighing less than 1,300 g are initially fed with fluids administered parenterally. Oral feeding is then commenced about 24 hours later when the risk of vomiting is less. In an endeavour to minimize the risk of aspiration, a technique of *nasojejunal feeding* has been developed. This consists of passing a nasogastric tube into the stomach; the infant is then placed on his right side and the tube is passed through the pylorus and duodenum into the jejunum. A continuous infusion of milk is

then passed down the tube (colour plate 100). Because of the position of the tube there are 2 sphincteric mechanisms (one at the pylorus and the other at the gastrooesophageal junction) preventing aspiration, and hence, with this technique, small infants may be fed much earlier than previously. Larger premature infants are fed about 4–8 hours after birth by bottle, or intermittent tube feeding if sucking ability is weak.

Frequency of Feedings

Premature infants are usually fed 3-hourly. The smaller ones require feedings every 2 hours, and the very small ones every hour. Feeding may be performed by nasogastric tube. Infants over 2,600 g are fed 4-hourly.

Bottle Feeding

(i) The baby's napkin is changed. (ii) The mouth is checked for signs of monilial infection. (iii) The baby is kept warm but loosely wrapped. (iv) The cot is tilted head upwards and the baby turned onto his right side. (v) The teat is tested for patency and is inserted into the infant's mouth making sure that the tongue is under the teat. (vi) The infant's chin may need to be gently supported with the forefinger and occasionally the infant's cheeks may have to be held together to achieve greater suction. (vii) The infant is dewinded halfway through a feeding and at the conclusion of it; for this procedure the infant is sat upright with the spine erect and the head supported. There is no need to thump the baby on the back in order to break his wind; gentle pressure with the supporting hand is adequate. (viii) The amount of the feeding given and how it was taken is recorded on the infant's chart and then the cot is left with the head end tilted upwards. (ix) No premature infant should take more than 15–20 minutes to fully feed; if longer, the effort will be too tiring and tube feeding will be required.

Tube Feeding

Requirements. Kidney dish, 10 ml syringe, plastic nasogastric tube size 5 French gauge, 60 ml medicine glass. For babies over 2 kg requiring nasogastric feeding, a nasogastric tube size 8 French gauge may be used.

Procedure. (i) Change the infant's napkin if necessary and tilt the cot or incubator mattress head up. (ii) Take a firm hold of the infant's jaw with the forefinger and the thumb of the left hand, pinch the nasogastric tube with the right hand and pass it gently down the back of the infant's throat. (iii) In the unlikely event that the tube goes down the larynx instead of the pharynx the infant will show immediate signs of distress, cyanosis and failure to cry. If this happens remove the tube, *immediately!* (iv) Attach a 10 ml syringe barrel to the end of the nasogastric tube; aspiration can be performed at this stage if required. (v) Pour the feeding mixture from the medicine glass into the syringe barrel and allow it to run down by gravity. (vi) When the feeding is finished, pinch the end of the tube near the infant's lips and withdraw it. (vii) Wakeful infants who are becoming more vigorous sometimes swallow air while being tube fed and it is a good policy to dewind them at the end of the feeding. (viii) The infant is left lying on the right side with the head elevated, or prone with the head elevated if in an incubator. (ix) If infants are partly tube fed, they are fed by tube first and then by bottle.

If an indwelling nasogastric tube is required, a number 5 French gauge plastic tube is individually measured and attached with adhesive tape to the infant's face. The tube may be passed either through the mouth or through the nose (not recommended because of the irritation to the nasal mucosa). The tube can remain in position for 72 hours before being replaced. The method of giving the feeding via the nasogastric tube is the same. However, it is advisable to run a little normal saline down the indwelling tube to clean it, 1 ml twice per day usually being sufficient.

Type of Feeding

The initial feeding consists of sterile water. The subsequent ones may consist of expressed breast milk or simulated breast milk feedings such as SMA, Cow & Gate and Ostermilk, as previously described in Chapter 61.

Amount of Feeding

Large quantities are avoided. The amount taken will depend on the hunger and capacity of the individual baby. Generally the full caloric (120 calories per kg per day) and fluid requirements (200 ml per kg per day) are reached by the seventh day of life. The fluid requirement is determined on a weight and age basis (see Chapter 61). The total amount is divided by the number of feedings for the day.

Bowel Actions

The meconium in a tiny premature infant is often thick and sticky. Its passage might be delayed and cause the infant distress and abdominal distension. The passage of an oiled catheter or a small saline enema will usually relieve this (colour plate 60).

COMPLICATIONS OF PREMATURITY

Functional immaturity of the premature infant renders him susceptible to certain complications other than the common neonatal disorders. The following are the more important complications (not all of which are exclusive to prematurity).

1. *Birth trauma*
2. *Hypoxia*
3. *Hyaline membrane disease*
4. *Temperature instability*
5. *Feeding difficulties*
6. *Jaundice*
7. *Diminished food stores*
8. *Apnoeic episodes*
9. *Oedema*
10. *Anaemia*
11. *Rickets*
12. *Hernias — umbilical, inguinal*
13. *Oxygen toxicity*
    (i) *retrolental fibroplasia*
    (ii) *bronchopulmonary dysplasia*
14. *Intraventricular haemorrhage*
15. *Necrotizing enterocolitis*

Many of the above complications are discussed in other chapters; the remainder are described in the paragraphs which follow.

Apnoeic Episodes

These may occur at any time in the first few weeks of life. They may be due to obstruction of the airway by mucus or regurgitated feeding, hypoglycaemia, hypocalcaemia, hypomagnesaemia, cerebral conditions, metabolic acidosis, infection or an immature respiratory centre in the brain. When the infant becomes apnoeic for a period over 20 seconds, bradycardia develops and the infant becomes cyanosed. The nurse must act promptly and efficiently in such cases. (i) Aspirate the nose and pharynx quickly, gently and efficiently (remember, prolonged suction can cause laryngeal spasm). (ii) Administer oxygen into the incubator. If apnoea continues, resuscitation is provided by frog breathing or the use of a Penlon Cardiff infant inflating bag. (iii) Gentle cutaneous stimulation (e.g. flick soles of feet). (iv) Send someone to report the collapse to the doctor in charge, but not before resuscitative measures have been commenced. *Never leave the baby alone until respirations have once more become stabilized and colour has improved.* Once the episode is over, the infant is assessed to discover the cause of the apnoea so that, if possible, recurrence can be prevented. If the aetiological factor is an immature respiratory centre, further episodes may be prevented by giving a respiratory centre stimulant (eg. theophylline in a dose of 5 mg per kg per day).

Oedema

Most premature infants have some degree of generalized oedema. It is most noticeable in infants who have respiratory distress. The causes are physiological and subside spontaneously within a few days.

Anaemia

The normal haemoglobin value at birth is in the range of *14–22 g/dl*. This level progressively declines and is at its lowest at about 11 weeks of age. This is due to: (i) removal from the relative hypoxia of the intrauterine environment — this reduces release of erythropoietin which stimulates red blood cell production, (ii) the shortened life-span of the premature infant's red blood cells, and (iii) rapid body growth. During the 4th month, the condition gradually improves and a normal level is reached by 20 weeks of age. In most infants this anaemia causes no problems, but if symptoms occur (lethargy, vomiting and failure to gain weight), a blood transfusion may be needed. Oral iron therapy does *not* prevent this *early anaemia of prematurity*. Due to the small size of the premature infant at birth, his blood volume, and hence iron stores, are low. Thus, the premature infant is likely to develop iron deficiency anaemia at 6–12 months of age. This is called *late anaemia of prematurity* and is prevented by prophylactic iron therapy which is usually commenced at 40 days of age.

Rickets

Premature infants are more prone to rickets than those born at term because of deficiencies in total body calcium and phosphate ions. Calcium and phosphate are stored by the fetus in the last trimester of pregnancy. To prevent rickets, milk feedings can be supplemented with calcium and phosphate; vitamin D is also added to the infant's feeding. The mother should be aware of this need for added vitamins before the infant is discharged into her care.

Hernia

(i) *Umbilical* (figure 64.12). This is the common type and seldom needs treatment. Usually the aperture (palpable with a finger tip) closes spontaneously within 12 months of birth. The umbilicus everts when the baby cries. The mother should be reassured, but told to report if the lump becomes large or irreducible, particularly if the baby is vomiting, these signs being indicative of strangulation and the need for urgent surgery. Strapping is of no benefit.

(ii) *Inguinal*. This is not uncommon and is treated by elective surgery as strangulation is likely. The signs of this complication are distress, vomiting, disinclination to feed in a previously well baby, together with an obvious irreducible mass.

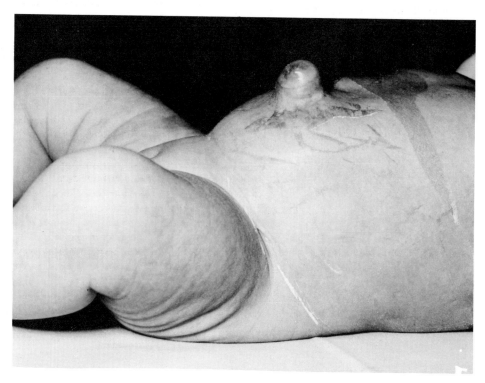

Figure 64.12 A moderate-sized umbilical hernia with bulging bowel content during crying. It was strapped to no avail. Eighty per cent of umbilical hernias spontaneously regress with no treatment.

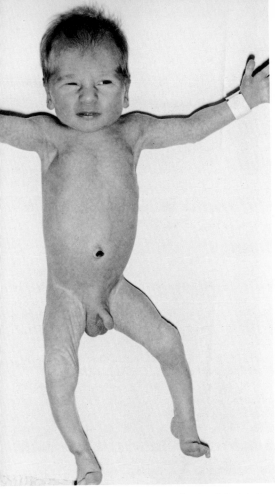

Figure 64.13 The Moro or startle reflex is elicited to test the neurological status of the infant. Its absence is indicative of extreme prematurity or cerebral damage.

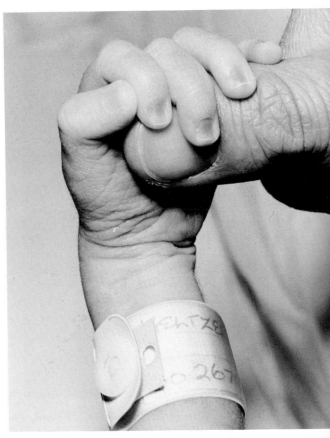

Figure 64.14 The grasp is a primitive reflex possessed by normal newborn infants.

Oxygen Toxicity

(i) *Retrolental fibroplasia* is most likely to occur in infants born before 34 weeks' gestation and weighing less than 2,000 g at birth. It is caused by excess oxygen dissolved in the blood. This leads to retinal vasospasm with consequent ischaemic injury to the retina; when oxygen administration ceases, new capillaries grow in a rapid disorganized fashion, proliferating inwards towards the lens. Later on, in severe cases, fibrous tissue develops and retinal detachment may occur. Ophthalmoscopic changes may be visible to a skilled observer as early as 10 days of age. Clinically, changes become apparent at a later date when the infant obviously has defective vision; there is nystagmus, squint, and a white mass is visible behind the lens of the eye (colour plate 121). The condition is usually bilateral.

(ii) *Bronchopulmonary dysplasia.* Prolonged oxygen administered directly to the respiratory epithelium, can damage lung tissue. The cells lining the bronchioles show the main effects and the clinical result is chronic respiratory insufficiency (colour plate 99). This condition

occurs most commonly in infants who have required mechanical pulmonary ventilation and who would have died without modern methods of intensive care (figure 63.13).

In view of the above complications, the following instructions are posted in special care nurseries for all staff members to remember. (i) High oxygen concentrations must *never* be given to small premature infants unless there is central cyanosis. (ii) Oxygen concentrations within the incubator must be constantly measured and adjusted. (iii) Oxygen should never be given for longer than is necessary to correct cyanosis. (iv) Infants receiving high oxygen concentrations (> 40%) should have arterial oxygen tensions monitored frequently, and the ambient oxygen adjusted accordingly.

Intraventricular Haemorrhage (colour plate 146)

This complication of prematurity has a high mortality rate and is second in importance only to hyaline membrane disease. The *aetiology* is multifactorial. (i) Deficiency of the mechanism

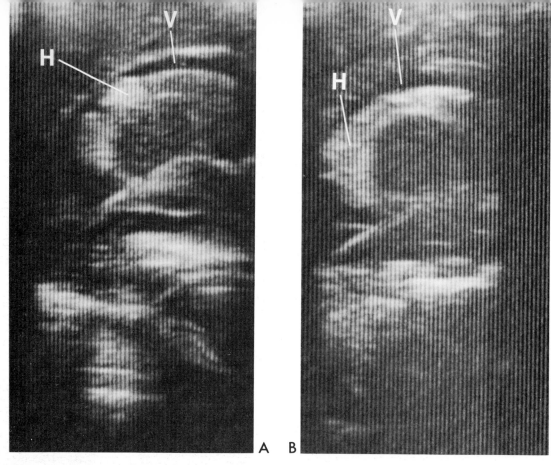

Figure 64.15 Intraventricular haemorrhages (H) demonstrated by ultrasonography. **A.** Grade 1: sagittal view showing a haemorrhage, subependymal in site which has not burst into the lateral ventricle (V). **B.** Grade 2: here the haemorrhage has extended and burst into the ventricle which however is not dilated or filled with blood. **C.** Grade 3: a larger haemorrhage has completely filled and distended the ventricle. **D.** Grade 4: coronal view showing a haemorrhage which was so extensive that it could not be contained within the ventricle and has burst into the brain substance.

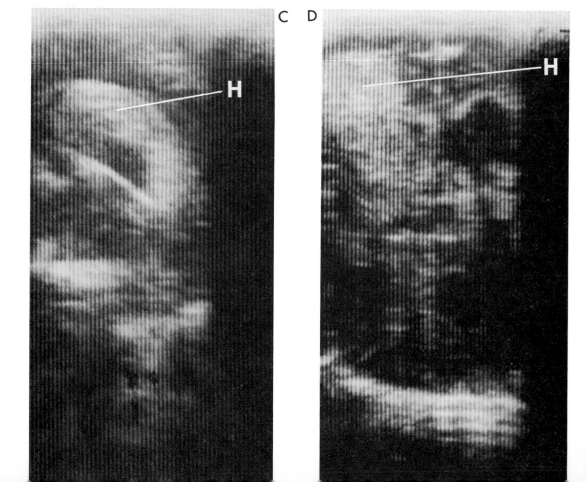

that minimizes intracranial pressure changes. In the adult, changes in systemic arterial and venous pressures are not transmitted to the intracranial vessels, but in premature infants this protective mechanism is underdeveloped and is further reduced by hypoxia. Hence, changes in systemic arterial and venous pressures are directly transmitted to the poorly-supported vessels in the germinal matrix, with the resultant risk of haemorrhage. (ii) Hypoxia. (iii) Trauma. (iv) Hyperosmolality: rapid infusion of a hyperosmolar solution (e.g. sodium bicarbonate) in very small infants causes intracellular volume changes with the resultant risk of haemorrhage. (v) Coagulopathy. (vi) Pneumothorax.

The commonest *clinical manifestations* are apnoea, paucity of normal movements and convulsions. Examination reveals a pale hypotonic infant with a tense anterior fontanelle. Diagnosis is confirmed by computerized axial tomography or ultrasonography.

The use of routine *ultrasonographic examination* of very low birth-weight infants (birth-weight < 1,500 g) has recently broadened our knowledge of intraventricular haemorrhage. The condition occurs in about 40% of such infants, but fortunately not all show the classical clinical picture described above. Many infants with lesser grades of haemorrhage have no clinical signs and long-term studies of these infants has revealed a favourable prognosis. Four grades of intraventricular haemorrhage are now recognized (figure 64.15). (i) Grade 1: subependymal, with a good long-term prognosis. (ii) Grade 2: intraventricular with no ventricular dilatation; this type also has a good long-term prognosis. (iii) Grade 3: intraventricular with ventricular dilatation; in this variety long-term prognosis is less favourable. (iv) Grade 4: intracerebral extension; here the long-term prognosis is unfavourable.

Necrotizing Enterocolitis (colour plate 147)

This disorder is not confined to premature infants, but the incidence increases with increasing immaturity. The *incidence* is 2 per 1,000 births and the *mortality rate* is about 25%. No single aetiological agent has been identified, but the following are associated factors. (i) *Hypoxia* which may be localized to the intestinal tract (thrombosis of mesenteric vessels) or is part of a generalized process (birth asphyxia). (ii) *Cow's milk feedings* (mothers should therefore be encouraged to express milk for their small premature infants). (iii) *Bowel infection.* Both Klebsiella species and the Staphylococcus aureus have been associated with this complication.

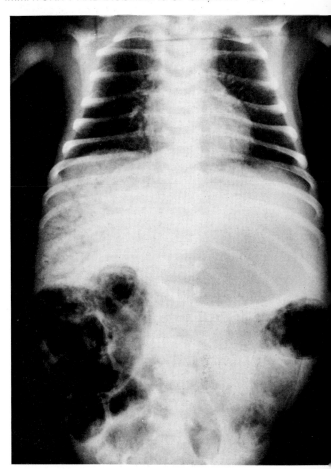

Figure 64.16 Radiographic features of necrotizing entero-colitis. There is intramural gas in the distended loops of bowel. Gas has penetrated through the intestinal wall into the portal venous system and can be seen throughout the liver; this sign indicates a poor prognosis.

(iv) *Blood hyperviscosity.* (v) *Umbilical catheterization.*

The diagnosis is suggested by abdominal distension, vomiting and bright blood in the stools. Radiographically, the characteristic features are intramural, intraperitoneal and even intrahepatic gas (figure 64.16). In about 75% of affected infants, medical measures such as the substitution of parenteral for oral feedings, antibiotic use and improvement in the perfusion of the gut, allow the bowel to recover. In the remainder, *perforation* or *massive necrosis* results in *peritonitis* and *septicaemia*; the mortality of these infants, who all require surgery, is very high.

GROWTH OF THE PREMATURE BABY

Weight. The weight loss in the first few days of life is variable as is the time taken to regain birth-weight, these depending on how soon feeding is commenced and the type of feedings given.

An infant weighing 2,500 g at birth usually regains birth-weight within 8–10 days, whereas an infant weighing 1,000 g takes up to 17 days (figure 64.1). Once birth-weight is attained, infants weighing 1,250–1,450 g gain approximately 160–200 g per week, and those weighing 1,000–1,250 g gain about 120–150 g per week.

Head circumference. The premature infant's head grows rapidly (figure 64.3). This is physiological and must not be mistaken for hydrocephaly. The average monthly increase in head circumference is 4 cm between 28–32 weeks' gestation, and 3 cm between 32–40 weeks. Thereafter the rate of growth slows; at full term the average head circumference is 35 cm and at the ages 3, 6 and 12 months the averages are 41, 44 and 47 cm, respectively.

WHEN MAY A PREMATURE INFANT BE TREATED AS ONE BORN AT TERM?

The answer to this question depends on the infant's maturity rather than on any particular weight; maturity will be judged according to ability to feed, gain weight, and maintain body temperature. Generally a baby can be treated as an 'ex-prem' after reaching 37 weeks (gestational plus neonatal age), which is equivalent to a weight of 2,600 g or above. The infant can then attempt to feed from the breast if the mother has been expressing her milk. At this stage the infant is on 4-hourly feedings, and depending on performance at sucking, home discharge is arranged when the weight is about 2,700 g.

A baby born before full term, although not premature by definition, often requires to spend the missing weeks in hospital, with the risk of infection and other complications. This emphasizes that induction of labour should never be performed without a proper medical (not social) indication.

SUBSEQUENT DEVELOPMENT

Mortality. From 1971 to 1980, inclusive, 41,057 infants were born alive in a large obstetric teaching hospital, and 563 (1.3%) died during the 28 days after birth. Although only 3,176 (7.7%) were born before the 37th completed week of gestation (i.e. premature infants), this group contributed 442 (78%) of all neonatal deaths. *These statistics are quoted because they proclaim the dangers of prematurity.*

With advances in perinatal care, the mortality rates in premature infants have fallen considerably (figures 64.7 and 64.17). However, the

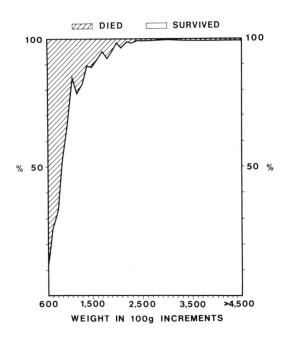

Figure 64.17 Percentage survival in a consecutive series of 13,680 liveborn infants in 100 g increments for birth-weights from 600 g to 4,500 g. The rubicon for survival was 2,500 g (the 50th percentile at 36 weeks' gestation (figure 64.2)) after which more than 98% survive.

contribution of prematurity to overall neonatal mortality remains monumental and should never be forgotten.

Many pessimistic remarks are passed regarding the long-term prognosis of surviving premature infants. However, the majority who survive develop normally. The physical and intellectual development of infants born 6 weeks or less before full term, and who had an uncomplicated course, is much the same as that of term infants. Those born between 28–34 weeks have a somewhat less favourable prognosis with a major disability rate of 6–8%. Those born before 28 weeks undeniably have an increased incidence of physical and neurological impairment, the rate being approximately 25%. It is probable that an improved quality of survival for premature infants will be reported in the future due to modern methods of intensive paediatric care.

THE GROWTH RETARDED (SMALL FOR DATES) INFANT

A growth retarded infant is defined as one whose birth-weight is below the 10th percentile for the period of gestation; such a child may therefore be born before, at, or after the due date of confinement. These infants may appear placentally insufficient or they may not.

Mortality and Morbidity

In a consecutive series of 2,566 infants with intrauterine growth retardation, the significant perinatal results in comparison with those in the overall hospital population (shown in parentheses) are shown below.

Stillbirths	5.8%	(1.2%)
Neonatal deaths	2.3%	(2.3%)
Birth asphyxia	16.5%	(8.6%)
Major malformations	7.7%	(4.0%)
Respiratory distress	9.1%	(4.9%)
Infections	14.4%	(10.9%)
Hypoglycaemia	18.0%	(3.9%)
Jaundice	15.6%	(10.0%)

Thus, fetal growth retardation is characterized by an increased risk of *stillbirth* (× 4) and *neonatal mortality*, as well as *asphyxia* (× 2), *malformations* (× 2) and *hypoglycaemia* (× 4). However, with modern paediatric care, the neonatal mortality rate of small for dates infants is similar to that in the overall population.

Cellular Characteristics

Normal cellular growth progresses through 2 phases. (1) *The phase of cellular multiplication.* The exact time when this phase is completed in the human fetus is not known, but is about the 20th week of gestation. Harmful influences operative during this stage result in fewer than normal cells in an individual, who will ultimately be small. This type of abnormality is irreversible, regardless of attempts to provide optimal nutrition at a later date. (2) *The phase of increased production of cytoplasm.* Harmful influences during this phase do not affect the *number* of cells, but the individual cells are small and hence, the individual is small. This impairment is reversible, at least to some extent, by proper nutrition after the harmful influence has been corrected.

Aetiology

(i) *Placental dysfunction* occurs typically in association with preeclampsia, maternal hypertension, chronic renal disease, diabetes, placental abruption (accidental haemorrhage) and prolonged pregnancy. (ii) *Multiple pregnancy.* (iii) *Intrauterine infections* due to toxoplasmosis, rubella, and cytomegalic inclusion disease. (iv) *Socioeconomic factors.* Low birth-weight has a strong association with addiction to nicotine, other drugs and alcohol, and poor maternal nutrition due to other causes. (v) Multiple *major malformations* including *chromosomal* abnormalities (approximately 50% of such infants are small for dates). (vi) *Genetic and racial.* Racial, socioeconomic, and nutritional factors are often difficult to separate.

Physiology

Many, but not all growth retarded infants have obtained suboptimal amounts of oxygen and nutrients throughout pregnancy. They receive enough to maintain life, but not enough to grow normally. In addition, they are deficient in body stores (e.g. liver glycogen). The suboptimal concentration of oxygen stimulates the release of *erythropoietin* from the fetal kidney which stimulates the bone marrow to produce more red cells and hence *polycythaemia* occurs. These infants are precariously placed in relation to life and death during pregnancy. The onset of labour provides a further threat to the supply of nutrients and oxygen, and signs of fetal distress frequently develop; the risk of death is appreciable at this time. The chronic deprivation of oxygen and nutrients may also affect the developing cells of the fetal brain and result in permanent damage, manifest as mental retardation.

Physical Appearance

These infants are dehydrated and have a wizened old-man appearance (figure 64.11). The syndrome is most obvious when it occurs in the large infant born weeks after the due date of confinement. The subcutaneous fat has disappeared and the skin is dry, cracked, and peeling; the latter is most pronounced on the palms and soles. The skin is often meconium-stained as a result of fetal distress due to hypoxia before or during labour. The cord is thin because Wharton's jelly has disappeared. The infant appears ruddy as a result of polycythaemia. It should be noted that the signs of placental insufficiency are evident only in a proportion (less than 50%) of infants resulting from prolonged pregnancies.

Associated Clinical Complications

(i) *Respiratory distress.* Usually this is due to *meconium aspiration pneumonitis* rather than hyaline membrane disease; *pulmonary haemorrhage* is also common.

(ii) *Haemorrhage.* Due to hypoxia and lack of substrates, the liver fails to produce adequate amounts of coagulation factors. Because of intrauterine infections, thrombocytopenia is not uncommon in growth retarded infants. These abnormalities result in a haemorrhagic diathesis.

(iii) *Hypoglycaemia.* Inadequate glycogen stores in the liver predispose to hypoglycaemia. This condition is suspected if the infant develops fine limb tremors, is 'jittery', has periods of cyanosis, is lethargic, or has a generalized convulsion. Routine blood glucose measurement using the Dextrostix (Ames) should be ordered on all small for gestational age infants after birth in order to diagnose impending hypoglycaemia. The treatment is intravenous or intraarterial administration of 10% glucose in water.

(iv) *Infection*. The possibility of rubella, cytomegalic inclusion disease or toxoplasmosis should be considered and tests carried out if facilities permit (colour plates 125–127).

(v) *Vomiting* is often a problem; swallowed meconium-contaminated liquor causes gastritis and frequently the vomitus contains blood.

(vi) The incidence of *malformations* is approximately double.

(vii) Signs of *cerebral irritation* secondary to intrauterine hypoxia are often present in the first few days of life.

(viii) *Temperature*. Due to lack of subcutaneous fat, these infants have a problem in preventing excessive heat loss.

(ix) *Polycythaemia* results in an increased tendency to jaundice, since the excessive red cell mass is removed by degradation of haemoglobin.

Nursery Care

Principles of treatment. Prevent the infant becoming *cold*. Prevent *hypoglycaemia* by commencement of feedings as soon as possible: since the blood sugar level may fall rapidly after birth it is checked 3-hourly until stable by Dextrostix analysis of capillary blood.

Subsequent Progress

A growth retarded infant has a much better prospect of survival compared with an immature infant of a similar weight. Provided hypoglycaemia is prevented or controlled, and if no major malformation is present, these infants make good intellectual progress. The incidence of all degrees of neurological abnormalities on long-term assessment is 9.5% and of major neurological handicap is 2.2%. Over the first 2 years of life 'catch-up' in growth occurs; however, the very severely affected infants tend to remain small.

LARGE FOR DATES INFANT

An infant is defined as being 'large for dates' when the birth-weight exceeds the 90th percentile for gestational age. The very large baby is typically born of a mother with diabetes mellitus, although in fact only 40% of such mothers produce large for dates infants (figures 30.7 and 30.8); *what is classical is not most common in obstetrics!* In fact the majority of large infants

are produced by mothers with normal glucose tolerance. There is far more to excessive fetal size than maternal hyperglycaemia. However, glucose *does* cross the placenta readily and high maternal blood levels would be expected to cause fetal hyperglycaemia and hyperinsulinism. It is well known that infants of diabetic mothers have signs of hyperinsulinaemia, and those who die are often found to have enlarged islets of Langerhans in the pancreas. It should be noted that diabetic mothers may produce small for dates infants, especially when the disease is long-standing and complicated by hypertension or chronic renal disease.

The Large 'Diabetic' Baby

(i) The infant is large, fat and plethoric.

(ii) The infant has a bull-neck, wrestler-like appearance and hence the shoulders tend to become impacted during birth (colour plate 53, figures 30.7 and 30.8).

(iii) The umbilical cord is thick and succulent with an abundance of Wharton's jelly.

(iv) The ear lobes and pinnae are often unusually hairy.

Clinical Problems

Before birth. (i) There is an increased risk of fetal death in late pregnancy, especially if the disease is severe or poorly controlled. (ii) The excessive fetal size can result in trauma due to mechanical difficulties at birth.

After birth. (i) *Respiratory distress* results from hyaline membrane disease. Many of these infants are born by Caesarean section at 36–38 weeks' gestation; although prematurity and excessive lung fluid partly explain the increased incidence of the respiratory distress syndrome, there is an increased incidence of hyaline membrane disease in infants of diabetic mothers born at *any* period of gestation. Thus, it is not uncommon for a large infant born at 37 weeks' gestation of a diabetic mother to develop severe hyaline membrane disease — hence the tendency to defer delivery in diabetics to at least 38 weeks' gestation unless amniocentesis has shown an L/S ratio of 2:1 or above. (ii) *Hypoglycaemia* occurs after birth since transfer of glucose from the maternal circulation ceases but hyperinsulinaemia temporarily persists. These infants require early glucose feedings and 3-hourly Dextrostix blood analyses as performed with small for dates infants. (iii) *Hyperbilirubinaemia* results from hepatic immaturity and inability to conjugate bilirubin. (iv) *Haemorrhagic disease* and *venous thrombosis* are more common, as are (v) Major *malformations* which are 2 to 3 times more common.

Nursery Care

(i) These infants are best nursed in a special care nursery because of the potential problems listed above.

(ii) They require the management usual for a premature infant.

(iii) Glucose (Dextrostix) blood analysis is carried out 1 hour after birth and then 3-hourly. Levels below 1.4 mmol/l (25 mg/dl) or signs of hypoglycaemia (twitching and sweating) are reported to the doctor.

(iv) These infants often are slow feeders and usually need to remain in hospital until the date equivalent to 40 weeks' gestation.

(v) For the first 24 hours the infant is nursed in an incubator and observed carefully. Unlike premature babies, they have a large layer of subcutaneous fat, and it is important to avoid overheating.

TRANSPORTATION OF PREMATURE OR SICK INFANTS

It has been shown in Britain, Canada and the United States that transfer of premature babies to well-equipped centres results in a 30–60% reduction in the number of deaths of babies weighing 1,000 g or more at birth and who survive for 12 hours. Infants of this size and age are candidates for transfer, particularly when there is evidence of respiratory distress and the hospital in which they were born lacks facilities for respirator care. It is considered that transport of premature and sick infants to neonatal intensive care units is the single greatest area for further improvement in neonatal survival rates. The requirements during transportation of these infants are set out in Chapter 71; it is estimated that implementation of these recommendations would prevent approximately 10% of neonatal deaths.

Recommendations when to transfer an infant

(i) *Respiratory distress.* (a) An infant with an oxygen requirement of more than 40% needs to be in a centre with facilities for monitoring blood gases. (b) An infant requiring more than 60% oxygen requires supervision in a neonatal intensive care unit (level 3 nursery). (c) An infant with respiratory distress associated with apnoea requires supervision in an intensive care nursery. (d) Respiratory distress associated with significant aspiration of meconium needs supervision in an intensive care nursery.

(ii) *Low birth-weight (< 2,500 g).* (a) Infants weighing less than 1,500 g should have an initial period of supervision in a neonatal intensive care nursery. (b) Infants weighing 1,500–2,500 g should be in a centre where specialist paediatric medical and nursing facilities are available.

It is now considered that infants of 24 weeks' gestation or above, or with birth-weight above 500 g are worthy of transfer.

(iii)   Infants with recurrent apnoeic attacks.
(iv)   Infants with convulsions.
(v)   Infants with depression following severe birth asphyxia.
(vi)   Jaundiced infants in potential or immediate need of exchange transfusion.
(vi)   Infants bleeding from any site.
(vii)   Infants of diabetic mothers.
(ix)   Infants in need of surgery.
(x)   Infants with suspected congenital heart disease.
(xi)   Infants with severe or multiple congenital anomalies.
(xii)   Unwell infants, manifested by lethargy, poor feeding, weak cry, cyanosis, jitteriness and/or vomiting.
(xiii)   Any infant in need of special diagnostic and/or therapeutic services.

chapter sixty-five

Congenital Malformations

OVERVIEW

Major congenital malformations are present in *4%* of newborn infants and account for *25% of perinatal deaths.* The survival rate of infants with malformations has increased. These facts illustrate why national congenital malformation registers are required to establish the incidence and pattern of malformations. Such monitoring is an early warning system designed to detect evidence of a new teratogen in the environment, either by the appearance of a new malformation or by an increase in the incidence of known anomalies. This information will enable research into possible causes of birth defects and approaches to prevention will emerge.

Malformations may be *inherited due to genetic factors* (40%) or *acquired due to fetal damage* during development by infections (5%), drugs (2%), irradiation or maternal metabolic disorders. A large proportion of the unexplained abnormalities (50%) are probably of genetic origin.

Chromosomal abnormalities are present in 50% of spontaneous abortions and 0.5% of liveborn infants. Thus it is Nature's law to identify and reject the imperfect. It is against this background that the philosophy of *genetic counselling* should be judged. Chromosomal abnormalities account for 10% of major abnormalities. The most important is *Down syndrome* which accounts for 30% of chromosomal abnormalities and 30% of cases of severe mental retardation. The incidence of Down syndrome is related to maternal age; 25% of cases are born to the 5% of mothers aged 35 years or more — hence the scope for *diagnostic amniocentesis* and elective abortion of affected fetuses. Screening for raised *alpha fetoprotein* levels in maternal serum, combined with *ultrasonography* also provide the possibility of diagnosis of *neural tube defects* in the second trimester and *fetoscopy* allows diagnosis of *thalassaemia*. Application of these techniques can significantly reduce the incidences of these birth defects in liveborn infants.

Screening of all newborn infants is practised to detect hypothyroidism (1 in 5,000 births), *phenylketonuria* (1 in 10,000) and *congenital dislocation of the hip* (1 in 130). The latter is the commonest of all major malformations, yet when diagnosed in the first few months of life can be cured by the use of an abduction splint for 2–3 months.

Many previously inoperable malformations can now be corrected due to recent improvements in surgical techniques and intensive care. Antenatal diagnosis of malformations, mainly by new ultrasonographic technology, has enabled operations to be carried out on the fetus for such conditions as bladder neck obstruction, hydronephrosis, hydrocephalus and diaphragmatic hernia. The scope and value of these procedures is still to be determined; furthermore, the quality of survival of infants following correction of major malformations requires assessment by long-term follow-up studies to determine cost-effectiveness (money/human misery) and thereby the proper indications for surgery.

More than 10% of infants with major abnormalities have *multiple defects*, and about 15% die within 4 weeks of birth, 50% of these due to anomalies of the heart or central nervous system.

Minor malformations occur in at least 6% of newborn infants — in addition to the relatively trivial naevus flammeus that is present in 1 in 4 infants. The apparent incidence of malformations depends upon observer interest and care with documentation. It is noteworthy that even experts detect at birth less than 50% of the malformations ultimately recognized in liveborn infants.

Minor malformations often cause significant disfigurement and parental anxiety. Minor is not synonymous with unimportant — ask the parent of the child with port-wine stain or cavernous haemangioma on the face!

The incidence of malformations can change spontaneously for no known cause, or as a result of a trend towards childbearing at an earlier age, dietary or environmental factors or antenatal screening programmes, with termination of pregnancy in appropriate cases.

Old friends can be revealed as bad enemies — *alcohol*, even in moderation, is now believed to have such teratogenic potential that total abstinence from before conception until delivery has a new band of advocates!

Rubella embryopathy is largely preventable by immunization of prepubertal girls. Immunization against *cytomegalovirus* infection is the challenge of the future — this being an important cause of severe, potentially avoidable, mental retardation.

Congenital malformations should no longer be regarded as afflictions to be accepted with resignation, but as a challenge for research and prevention.

INTRODUCTION

A major malformation is one that produces a serious loss of function or permanent interference with normal life. The incidence is about *4.0%* in the neonatal period, additional cases (e.g. congenital heart disease) being diagnosed later in childhood.

The incidences of malformations show considerable geographic and racial variation, even in the case of obvious defects that could not elude diagnosis and documentation. The best example is *anencephaly*, which has an incidence of 1 in 400 births in Northern Ireland (1974–1979) and 1 in 1,145 in Victoria (table 65.1) It should be noted that the incidence of a complication in a specialist hospital may be significantly different from that in the overall population when the abnormality is associated with one or more complications likely to result in referral for specialist care — once again the best example is anencephaly which is associated with polyhydramnios (60%), low oestrogen excretion (100%) and fetal growth retardation (50%). Comparable hospital incidences of anencephaly are 1 in 275 at the Royal Maternity Hospital, Belfast (1968–1977)

and 1 in 924 at the Mercy Maternity Hospital, Melbourne (1970–1980) (table 65.2). The incidence of a malformation can change spontaneously as a result of a trend towards childbearing at a younger age, dietary or environmental factors or antenatal screening programmes with termination of pregnancy in appropriate cases.

All of the foregoing may have contributed to the changing incidence of anencephaly (table 65.1) and other neural tube defects. Of course selective abortion does not change the real incidence of a malformation, but merely the categorization of the case as an abortion rather than a viable infant.

To give the reader perspective, the major and minor malformations recorded at or within 7 days of delivery in a series of 41,584 consecutive births at a large obstetric teaching hospital during the 10-year period 1970–1980 are shown in tables 65.2 and 65.3. In this series *the incidence of major malformations was 4.2%*; these infants had a perinatal mortality rate of 13.9% (246 of 1,769), and *more than 50% of the deaths were due to malformations of the heart or central nervous system.*

TABLE 65.1   INCIDENCE OF ANENCEPHALY IN VICTORIA — 13-YEAR REGIONAL STUDY

Year	Number of births	Cases of anencephaly	Incidence of anencephaly	
			Per number of births	Per 1,000 births
1970	73,801	68	1 in 1,085	0.92
1971	76,258	68	1 in 1,121	0.89
1972	72,649	61	1 in 1,191	0.84
1973	67,925	67	1 in 1,014	0.99
1974	66,988	76	1 in 881	1.13
1975	62,610	60	1 in 1,044	0.96
1976	61,283	53	1 in 1,156	0.86
1977	60,085	68	1 in 884	1.13
Subtotal	541,599	521	1 in 1,040	0.96
1978	59,436	51	1 in 1,165	0.86
1979	58,257	45	1 in 1,295	0.77
1980	58,653	41	1 in 1,431	0.70
1981	59,965	35	1 in 1,713	0.58
1982	60,455	39	1 in 1,550	0.65
Subtotal	296,766	211	1 in 1,406	0.71
Total	838,365	732	1 in 1,145	0.87

TABLE 65.2   INCIDENCE OF MAJOR FETAL MALFORMATIONS IN 41,584 CONSECUTIVE BIRTHS IN AN OBSTETRIC TEACHING HOSPITAL

WHO classification	Number of infants				Incidence	
	SB	NND	Survived	Total	Per number of births	Per 1,000 births
Genital organs	5	17	474	496	1 in 84	12.0
Undescended testis	1	5	284	290	1 in 143	7.0
Hypospadias	—	3	171	174	1 in 239	4.2
Epispadias	—	—	8	8		
Other (imperforate vagina 2, true hermaphrodite 1)	4	9	11	24		
Limbs	6	15	344	365	1 in 114	8.8
Dislocated hip	1	1	319	321	1 in 130	7.7
Short limb	3	6	18	27	1 in 1,540	0.7
Absent limb or digits	1	5	6	12	1 in 3,465	0.3
Other	1	3	1	5		
Heart	11	61	279	351	1 in 119	8.4
Anomalies of valves ± murmur	1	11	147	159	1 in 262	3.8
Ventricular septal defect	4	20	87	111	1 in 375	2.7
Transposition of great vessels	1	5	9	15	1 in 2,772	0.4
Pulmonary stenosis	—	2	11	13	1 in 3,199	0.3
Atrial septal defect	—	4	8	12	1 in 3,465	0.3
Other (tetralogy of Fallot 3)	5	19	17	41		
Club-foot	11	21	207	239	1 in 174	5.8
Central nervous system	60	72	54	186	1 in 224	4.5
Meningomyelocele	8	25	30	63	1 in 660	1.5
Hydrocephaly	7	24	19	50	1 in 832	1.2
Anencephaly	37	8	—	45	1 in 924	1.1
Other (microcephaly 7)	8	15	5	28		
Urinary system	11	32	84	127	1 in 327	3.1
Vesicoureteric reflux	—	—	52	52	1 in 800	1.3
Renal agenesis	5	18	—	23	1 in 1,808	0.6
Polycystic kidney	2	4	11	17	1 in 2,446	0.4
Other (ectopia vesicae 2)	4	0	21	35		
Circulatory system	—	33	134	167	1 in 249	4.0
Patent ductus arteriosus	—	19	116	135	1 in 308	3.3
Coarctation of aorta	—	6	11	17	1 in 2,446	0.4
Other	—	8	7	15		
Digestive system	10	12	154	176	1 in 236	4.2
Hernia	1	—	106	107	1 in 389	2.6
Imperforate anus/rectum	3	5	15	23	1 in 1,808	0.6
Other (exomphalos 9, duodenal atresia 5)	6	7	33	46		
Multiple Systems	12	27	64	103	1 in 404	2.5
Down syndrome	3	5	53	61	1 in 682	1.5
Other (chromosomal 9)	9	22	11	42		
Cleft palate and/or lip	6	10	48	64	1 in 650	1.5
Respiratory system	11	22	5	38	1 in 1,094	0.9
Hypoplastic lungs	9	21	2	32	1 in 1,300	0.8
Other (choanal atresia 4)	2	1	3	6		

Musculoskeletal	6	14	43	63	1 in 660	1.5
Diaphragmatic hernia	1	7	—	8	1 in 5,198	0.2
Achondroplasia	1	2	5	8	1 in 5,198	0.2
Other	4	5	38	47		
Eye	4	3	13	20	1 in 2,079	0.5
Cataract	—	1	9	10	1 in 4,158	0.2
Other (micro- phthalmos 6)	4	2	4	10		
Upper alimentary tract	—	2	16	18	1 in 2,310	0.4
Tracheo-oesophageal fistula	—	1	9	10	1 in 4,158	0.2
Other	—	1	7	8		

Other unspecified
  (epidermolysis
  bullosa 2,
  phenylketonuria 1,
  gastroschisis 1)
	11	7	9	27	1 in 1,540	0.7

Total Malformations	164	348	1,928	2,440	1 in 17	58.7
Infants	75	171	1,523	1,769	1 in 24	42.5

SB = stillbirth; NND = neonatal death.

It should be noted that *major malformations are often multiple* and occur as definite syndromes; in this series 12% of infants (213 of 1,769) had 2 or more major malformations.

The incidence of minor malformations was 7.6% (table 65.3). This figure is higher than in many series, but this was a prospective study and illustrates that the apparent incidence of malformations depends upon observer interest and care with documentation. It is salutary to note that even experts detect at birth less than 50% of the malformations present in liveborn infants.

In 1982 in a large regional survey, malformations were present in 14.5% of stillborn infants, 44.4% of infants who died in the neonatal period and 31.5% of infants who died in the first year of life. It should be remembered that malformations are second only to hypoxia as a cause of perinatal mortality and account for 25–30% of perinatal deaths (see Chapter 15).

The birth of a baby with a major malformation always causes disappointment and despair. The parents will seek information regarding the risk of recurrence in subsequent pregnancies. They may request investigation of possible causes and require expert genetic counselling. Malformations can be inherited or acquired (see Chapter 17): known genetic mechanisms can be recognized in approximately 40% of cases, teratogenic effects of intrauterine infection in 5% and a chemical teratogen in 2%; in the remaining 53% the cause is unknown.

An *inherited* abnormality means that the spermatozoon or ovum carried a flaw determined by genetic factors, and in the majority this is not demonstrable by examination of chromosomes. In this group, the embryo was abnormal from the time of conception. This group includes chromosome abnormalities, multifactorial abnormalities and Mendelian disorders. There is a variable recurrence risk in subsequent pregnancies.

An *acquired* abnormality means that the embryo was initially normal, but was damaged during its development by some injurious agent (e.g. drugs, infections, irradiation or maternal metabolic disorders). This group of abnormalities is *not* inherited and would only recur if the injurious agent was again operative.

CHROMOSOMAL DEFECTS

In screening programmes of liveborn infants the incidence of chromosomal defects ranges from 0.4–0.8% and accounts for about 10% of all major abnormalities. They are particularly important since it is possible to identify them by amniocentesis in the second trimester.

Down Syndrome (Mongolism) (figure 65.2)

This is the commonest chromosomal abnormality (about 30% of all cases) and is responsible for approximately 30% of severe mental retardation. It occurs once in every 700 births. The incidence of Down syndrome in liveborn infants depends upon the age distribution of mothers in the population concerned (table 65.4), and the proportion of those at increased risk (above 35 years of age) who have diagnostic amniocentesis performed. In the past 20 years the proportion of Down syndrome infants born to mothers aged 35 years or more in Australia has fallen from over 50% to about 25%; currently about 5% of all births occur to mothers aged 35 years or more, and about 30% of these elect to have diagnostic amniocentesis performed. The infant has 47 chromosomes instead of the usual 46; the extra chromosome is a 21 chromosome — *trisomy 21* (figure 65.3). From a genetic point of view 3 types of Down syndrome are recognizable: regular trisomy which is the most common (94%) variety, translocation of a chromosome (4%) and mosaic pattern (2%). These children all have the same clinical features. Translocations may arise de novo or be inherited. Recurrence

risks are related to the findings of chromosomal analysis. If the infant has regular trisomy, the risk for recurrence is slightly higher than the risk in the general population which increases as maternal age increases (table 65.4). If the infant has a noninherited translocation (i.e. parents have normal karyotypes) the risk of recurrence is low. If the translocation is inherited the recurrence risk varies (2%–100%) depending on the type of translocation and the sex of the parent carrying it.

TABLE 65.3   INCIDENCE OF MINOR FETAL MALFORMATIONS IN 41,584 CONSECUTIVE BIRTHS IN AN OBSTETRIC TEACHING HOSPITAL

Type of malformation	Number	Incidence	
		Per number of births	Per 1,000 births
Haemangioma/naevus	1,148	1 in 36	27.6
Skin tag	452	1 in 92	10.9
Hydrocele	298	1 in 140	7.2
Mongoloid patch	291	1 in 143	7.0
Pilonidal sinus/sacral dimple	211	1 in 197	5.1
Lacuna skull	121	1 in 344	2.9
Single umbilical artery	119	1 in 349	2.9
Webbed toes/fingers	115	1 in 362	2.8
Single palmar crease	77	1 in 540	1.9
Malformed ears	71	1 in 586	1.7
Overriding toes/fingers	48	1 in 866	1.2
Abnormally shaped digits	42	1 in 990	1.0
Nail hypoplasia	40	1 in 1,040	1.0
Supernumerary digits	37	1 in 1,124	0.9
Nasal abnormalities	33	1 in 1,260	0.8
Gastro-oesophageal reflux	33	1 in 1,260	0.8
Multiple/large fontanelles	30	1 in 1,386	0.7
Cyst under tongue/ranula	21	1 in 1,980	0.5
Teeth present at birth	15	1 in 2,772	0.4
Urinary abnormalities	14	1 in 2,970	0.3
Uterine anomalies	12	1 in 3,465	0.3
Eye/orbital anomalies	12	1 in 3,465	0.3
Penile cyst	11	1 in 3,780	0.3
Lymphangioma	10	1 in 4,158	0.24
Rib deformities	8	1 in 5,198	0.19
Pigmented lesions of the skin	8	1 in 5,198	0.19
Vaginal septum	6	1 in 6,931	0.14
Clitoral hypertrophy	6	1 in 6,931	0.14
Retinopathy/ptosis	6	1 in 6,931	0.14
Accessory nipple	4	1 in 10,396	0.10
Enlarged labia	4	1 in 10,396	0.10
Dextrocardia/situs inversus	4	1 in 10,396	0.10
Anteriorly placed anus	3	1 in 13,861	0.07
Hemihypertrophy	1	1 in 41,584	0.02
Other	33	1 in 1,260	0.8
Total Malformations	3,344	1 in 12	80.4
Infants	3,177	1 in 13	76.4

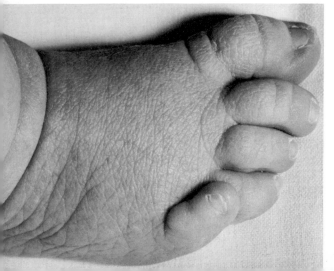

TABLE 65.4 INCIDENCE OF DOWN SYNDROME ACCORDING TO MATERNAL AGE

Maternal age (years)	Incidence	
	Per number of births	Per 1,000 births
15–19	1 in 1,850	0.5
20–24	1 in 1,600	0.6
25–29	1 in 1,350	0.7
30–34	1 in 800	1.3
35–39	1 in 260	3.9
40–44	1 in 100	10.0
45–49	1 in 20	50.0
Total	1 in 700	1.4

Figure 65.1 Full term infant with overriding toes (hammer toes).

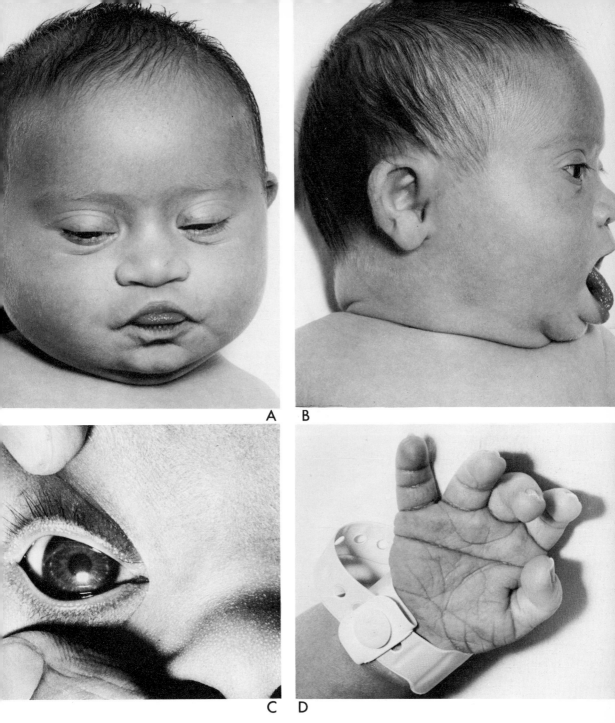

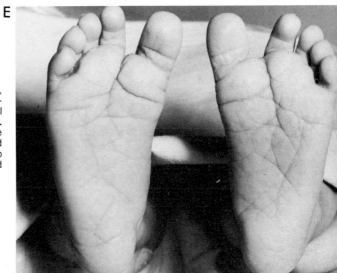

Figure 65.2 Down syndrome. **A.** The eyes slant upwards, there are epicanthic folds and the 'fish mouth' with protruding tongue is shown. **B.** Note the flattened occiput, small ears and the broad neck with the loose fold of skin. **C.** Around the margin of the iris are Brushfield spots. **D.** The hand is broad with a single transverse crease. The second phalanx of the fifth digit is small. **E.** The feet show a deep longitudinal skin crease between widely spaced first and second toes.

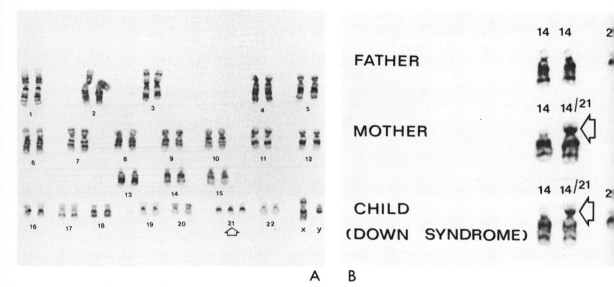

Figure 65.3 Chromosomal analysis in Down syndrome. **A.** Shows regular trisomy 21 which is the most common (94%) finding in Down syndrome. **B.** Translocation of 21 chromosome to 14 chromosome resulting in a child with Down syndrome. This translocation is inherited through the child's mother.

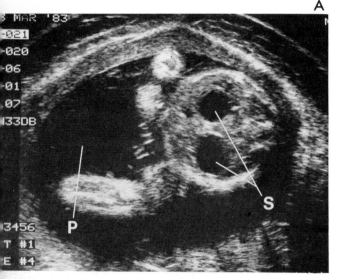

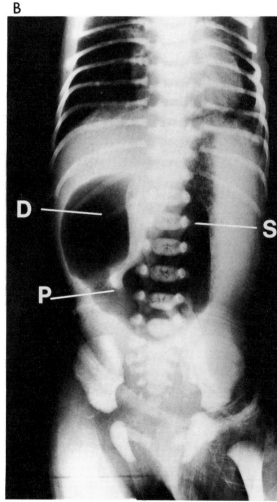

Figure 65.4 Duodenal atresia is common in Down syndrome. **A.** Transverse ultrasound scan performed at 30 weeks' gestation because of polyhydramnios (P) showing 2 sonolucent rounded areas (S) consistent with fluid containing structures in the fetal abdomen. **B.** The infant was born 8 weeks later (birth-weight 2,450 g) and this radiograph taken shortly after birth shows the classic 'double bubble' — with air distending the body and antrum of the stomach (S), the pylorus (P), and the first part of the duodenum (D) which is much more distensible than the pylorus.

Infants with Down syndrome may not show every feature classically associated with the condition, but generally they look so much alike that appearance leads to suspicion of the diagnosis. The characteristic features are as follows: small head with a flattened occiput, large anterior fontanelle with an associated middle fontanelle, and short, broad neck with a loose fold of skin at the back; eyes slanting upwards and with epicanthic folds (figures 65.2A and B); the iris of the eye speckled with white spots around its rim (Brushfield spots, figure 65.2C), protruding tongue ('adder tongue'); fingers of equal length, with the fifth curving inwards and often having a single crease; single palmar crease (simian crease, figure 65.2D); big toe widely separated from the second (simian foot, figure 65.2E); marked hypotonicity; and pot belly and umbilical hernia.

All such infants are mentally retarded with intelligence ranging from profound to borderline retardation — the majority are in the moderate range (IQ36–51). Many have other malforma-

tions such as cardiac and intestinal anomalies (e.g. duodenal atresia — figure 65.4).

The problem of management of the child with Down syndrome is one which must be faced early by parents and doctor. Everything must be done to prevent hasty rejection of the child and no effort in support and counsel should be spared in helping the parents to understand and accept the problem.

Other chromosomal abnormalities associated with physical malformations include *trisomy 13* and *trisomy 18* (figure 65.5); these lesions are usually fatal. A rare abnormality of the number 5 chromosome known as the *cri du chat syndrome* may be suspected in a dysmorphic baby with a cry like a cat mewing; such a baby is destined to be mentally retarded.

There are many other abnormalities of chromosomes that can be recognized on karyotyping and involve duplication or deletion of specific segments of chromosomes. *Children with multiple malformations or mental retardation require chromosome analysis.*

A

Figure 65.5 Trisomy 18. **A.** Note the micrognathia, prominent occiput and malformed ears. **B.** Flexion deformity of the hands. **C.** 'Rocker-bottom' feet.

B

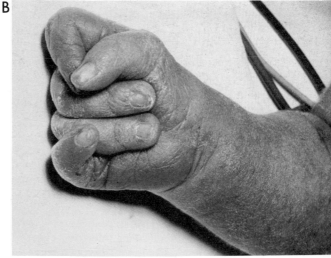

C

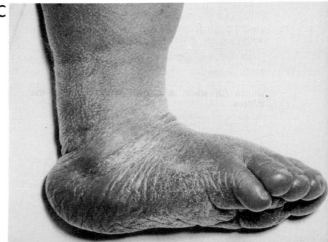

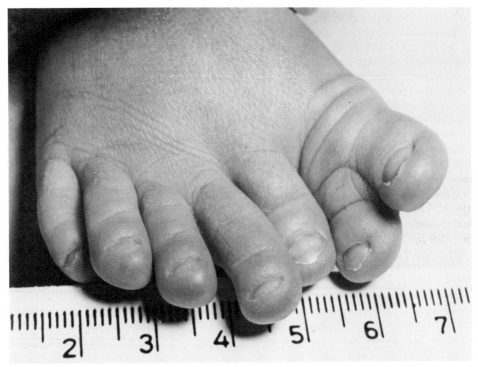

Figure 65.6 Extra digits can be due to a dominant genetic defect and therefore 'run' in families.

GENE DEFECTS

Autosomal Dominant Defects

These may be inherited from a parent or arise as a new mutation. When inherited there is a 50% chance of each subsequent child being similarly affected. Examples are skin tags, extra digits (figure 65.6), achondroplasia (figure 65.7), neurofibromatosis, tuberose sclerosis, Marfan syndrome, deafness.

Autosomal Recessive Defects

In this group, both parents carry a single 'dose' of the affected gene. The children of such a marriage have a 50% chance of being carriers (1 normal, 1 abnormal gene), a 25% chance of being affected (2 abnormal genes) and a 25% chance of being unaffected (2 normal genes). A relatively common example is *fibrocystic disease of the pancreas* which may cause meconium ileus and present in the neonatal period as a bowel obstruction (figure 65.8). The incidence is 1 in 2,500 births. *Phenylketonuria* is much less common (1 in 10,000 births) and is due to a congenital absence of the enzyme that converts the amino acid phenylalanine to tyrosine, with the result that phenylalanine and its metabolites build up in the serum and brain damage results. The *Guthrie test* is a simple and effective method of screening infants for this disorder: a heel-prick specimen of blood is dropped onto specially

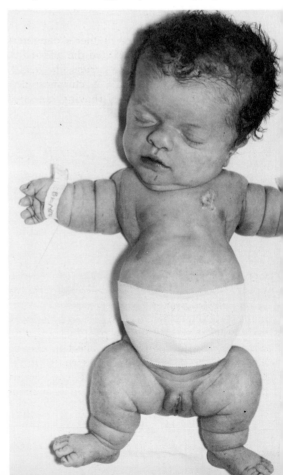

Figure 65.7 Achrondroplastic dwarf: shortening of all limbs is more marked in the proximal than in the distal portions; the head is large due to hydrocephaly (causing difficulty during breech delivery) while the trunk is of normal size.

impregnated paper to detect *hyperphenylalanin-aemia*. This test is performed on the 5th day of life in normal infants, but is postponed if the infant has been receiving parenteral fluids (no amino acid intake) or antibiotics (interference with the test). Treatment is aimed at early diagnosis and feeding with a specially prepared formula low in phenylalanine such as Lofenalac (Mead Johnson). Blood collected for the Guthrie test can also be used to screen newborn infants for *hypothyroidism* (1 in 5,000 births) and galactosaemia (1 in 50,000 births).

Polygenic Defects

This is the most common group of disorders and includes *cleft lip and palate* (figure 65.9, colour plates 111 and 112) *neural tube defects, congenital heart disease, congenital dislocated hips and pyloric stenosis*. In this group there are many genes from both parents interacting with the environment. The recurrence rate is much less.

X-linked Defects

In this group of disorders the abnormal gene is carried on the X chromosome, of which females (XX) possess 2. Because males (XY) have only one such chromosome they will develop signs of the abnormality even when the genetic defect is recessive, there being no matching normal gene on the partner chromosome to suppress the harmful influence. Examples are *Duchenne muscular dystrophy, haemophilia* and *glucose-6-phosphate dehydrogenase deficiency*. In these diseases, 50% of a carrier mother's daughters are normal (not having inherited the affected X chromosome), and 50% are carriers like herself (having inherited the affected X chromosome); 50% of her sons are affected (having inherited the affected X chromosome), and 50% are normal (not having inherited the affected X chromosome).

In some children X-linked recessive disorders arise as a result of a new mutation. Carrier detection studies can be undertaken in women at risk of having a child with Duchenne muscular dystrophy or haemophilia.

DRUGS

Certain drugs taken in the first trimester of pregnancy can result in fetal malformations, the prime example being *thalidomide* which caused many cases of phocomelia. *Progestogens* given in early pregnancy can result in *pseudohermaphroditism* in female infants. This effect is uncommon and the condition is not serious, therefore the risk does not warrant withholding progestogen therapy when indicated in patients

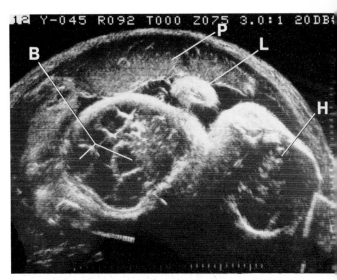

Figure 65.8 Antenatal ultrasonography (performed at 37 weeks' gestation because of polyhydramnios) showing dilated loops of fetal bowel suggestive of a bowel obstruction. The diagnosis was meconium peritonitis with obstruction and perforation secondary to meconium ileus, itself due to fibrocystic disease of the pancreas. B = loops of bowel, P = placenta, H = head, L = limb.

Figure 65.9 Severe left cleft lip and minor degree of right cleft lip with associated cleft palate.

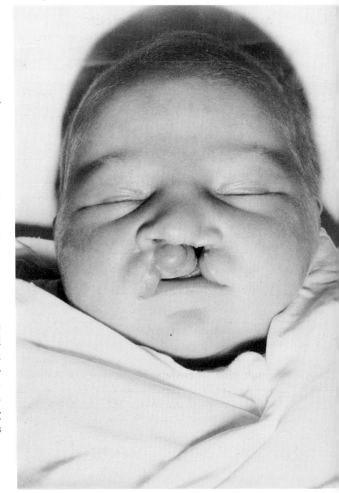

with threatened or habitual abortion. *Anti-thyroid* drugs taken to control maternal thyrotoxicosis can cause cretinism and such children may have congenital goitres large enough to cause tracheal obstruction. Enlargement of the thyroid in such cases can even result in obstructed labour. The human teratogenicity of many drugs is not known and hence the advice given to the pregnant woman is to avoid all drugs (except iron and folic acid) unless absolutely necessary.

INFECTIONS

The effects of maternal *rubella*, *cytomegalic inclusion body* virus, *toxoplasmosis*, and *syphilis* are discussed in Chapter 67 (colour plates 125–127).

CLINICALLY IMPORTANT ANOMALIES

Neonatal paediatric surgery has developed rapidly over the past 25 years. Improved anaesthesia, parenteral nutrition, and antibiotic therapy, as well as surgical skill, have accounted for this development. Hence, many babies born with developmental defects can now be saved by early surgery.

Figure 65.10 Radiograph of an infant with bowel obstruction: the loops of bowel are distended and many fluid levels are shown.

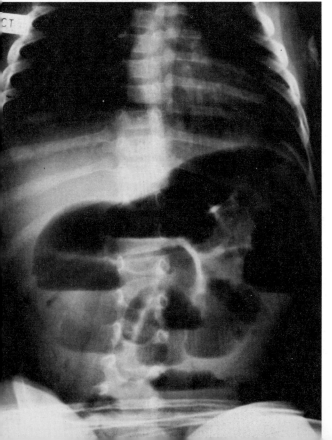

ALIMENTARY SYSTEM

Intestinal Obstruction

Clinical features. The diagnosis of intestinal obstruction is suggested by *failure to pass meconium, abdominal distension* and *vomiting*. The site of the obstruction determines the presentation: in high bowel obstruction, vomiting is an early feature, abdominal distension is not marked and the infant passes the meconium distal to the obstruction; in low bowel obstruction, vomiting is a late symptom, abdominal distension is marked and little, if any, meconium is passed. *Bile-stained vomitus is suggestive of intestinal obstruction and its occurrence should always be taken seriously.*

Causes. Intestinal obstruction may occur at any level of the alimentary tract. The lumen of the gut may be narrowed (*stenosis*) or closed (*atresia*). Abnormal rotational development of the gut can cause a *volvulus*, with obstruction. Obstruction may also be caused by pressure on the gut from abnormal external structures such as fibrous bands. Occasionally, an infant has a mucus plug at the anus too tenacious for evacuation (*meconium plug syndrome*). In the immature infant, *intestinal neuromuscular dyskinesia* may present clinically as a bowel obstruction. Both of these conditions require only conservative management (colour plate 60).

Investigations. Fluid levels in radiographs with the infant in the erect position assist in confirming the diagnosis (figure 65.10). The lesion can usually be localized and identified by more detailed study with radio-opaque dyes.

Oesophageal Atresia and Tracheo-oesophageal Fistula

In this condition development of the oesophagus is incomplete. In the most common type (90% of cases) the upper region of the oesophagus ends in a blind pouch which is usually not connected to the stomach; the stomach however, may have a fistulous connection to the trachea via a lower oesophageal rudiment. Hence, pharyngeal secretions once swallowed are unable to pass into the stomach; the blind upper pouch fills and aspiration into the trachea may occur. Classical features in the baby are therefore excess mucus and cyanotic attacks; also, since the lower gut is usually connected by the fistula to the trachea, inspired air passes to the stomach and results in abdominal distension. The infant with a tracheo-oesophageal fistula is often immature, and *polyhydramnios* (presumably from failure to swallow liquor) is such a common association that it makes exclusion of this anomaly mandatory when polyhydramnios is present. A firm 10 French gauge catheter is passed down the oesophagus; if it does not pass at least 10 cm beyond the lips the diagnosis should be suspected and confirmed radiographically by an opaque dye study. In many instances, reconstruction of the oesophagus and closure of any fistulous communication can be carried out surgically. The survival rate after operation is approximately 85%.

Diaphragmatic Hernia

This is a serious emergency in neonatal medicine. There is a defect in the diaphragm (usually the left side) through which the abdominal contents (bowel, liver, or spleen) herniate (colour plate 134). The lung on the affected side fails to develop adequately and is *hypoplastic*.

The baby presents with respiratory distress (marked cyanosis), and this worsens as swallowed air distends the gut in the chest, further displacing the mediastinum, usually to the right side, and embarrassing the good lung. The heart sounds may be heard on the right side of the chest, bowel sounds may be heard on the left side of the chest, and the abdomen appears scaphoid as it is relatively empty of contents. The condition will be confirmed by a chest radiograph (figure 65.11), and no delay should occur in organizing surgical consultation.

The resuscitation of a neonate with symptomatic diaphragmatic hernia requires endotracheal intubation to make sure inspired gases are entering the lung and not the gut as would occur with the use of a bag and mask. A nasogastric tube should be placed into the gut and an attempt made to aspirate any swallowed air to decompress the bowel.

Exomphalos (Omphalocele)

In this condition (figure 65.12), the bowel, and often a portion of the liver, herniates through the abdominal wall into the umbilical cord and is covered by a translucent membrane formed by fused layers of peritoneum and amnion. If the hernia is caused by a defect in the abdominal wall (*gastroschisis*, figure 65.13) there is no covering membrane. Surgical correction of exomphalos is preferred because there may be important coexistent abnormalities such as malrotation of the gut. Whilst awaiting surgical correction, every effort is made to prevent rupture of the sac by covering it with moist warm sterile saline packs or with thin plastic wraps. However, some are too large to manage surgically, and are treated conservatively by painting the area with 1% mercurochrome and ensuring protection from injury. The area epithelizes gradually and is usually complete in about 6–8 weeks. The infant is often operated on for further repair of the abdominal wall at about 18–24 months of age. In a gastroschisis too large for immediate surgical correction, the herniated mass is covered by a plastic wrap and gradually (several weeks) squeezed back as the abdomen enlarges until surgical correction is possible.

Care should always be taken in clamping the umbilical cord to avoid damage to skin which often extends about 1 cm along it. Any swelling at the base can be due to a small *hernia* containing intestine, and bowel obstruction or peritonitis would result if this was clamped.

Figure 65.11 Radiograph of a left diaphragmatic hernia: gas-containing loops of bowel have herniated through the defect into the left chest; the mediastinum is shifted to the right.

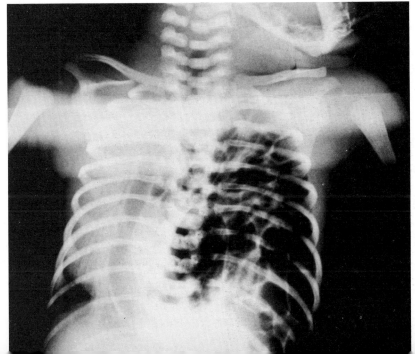

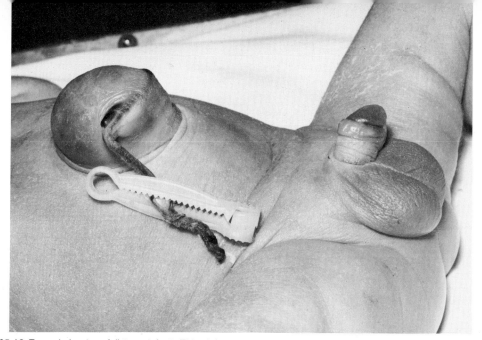

Figure 65.12 Exomphalos in a full term infant. This defect was small enough to permit surgical correction.

Hirschsprung Disease

This condition is due to absence of nerve ganglia in an area of the large bowel. This prevents peristaltic waves progressing to the rectum and thus causes obstruction. It is recognized by abdominal distension and constipation, diagnosed by rectal biopsy and treated surgically by excision of the aganglionic segment.

Imperforate Anus

This may vary from a 'web of membrane covering the rectal opening to atresia of the rectum (figure 65.14) and may be missed at birth unless the anus is inspected carefully. Attempted passage of a rectal thermometer will reveal the absence of an anal opening, but will not always exclude a higher atresia or membranous obstruction. The treatment is surgical.

CARDIOVASCULAR SYSTEM

Congenital cardiac malformations occur in 9 in 1,000 infants, and are 2-3 times more common in premature than term infants (table 65.2).

Clinical features. Cardiac lesions are suspected in the newborn infant if there is *cyanosis* which increases with crying and is not relieved with oxygen; *dyspnoea* can be present and becomes worse after handling and feeding; *tachycardia* is usual; a *heart murmur* may or may not be heard. Cardiac lesions which are *not* associated with cyanosis generally are not diagnosed until a murmur is heard on routine examination or signs of cardiac failure occur (dyspnoea, grunting, lethargy, pallor, liver enlargement, tachycardia, and peripheral oedema).

The diagnosis of a cardiac malformation may

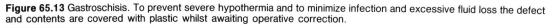

Figure 65.13 Gastroschisis. To prevent severe hypothermia and to minimize infection and excessive fluid loss the defect and contents are covered with plastic whilst awaiting operative correction.

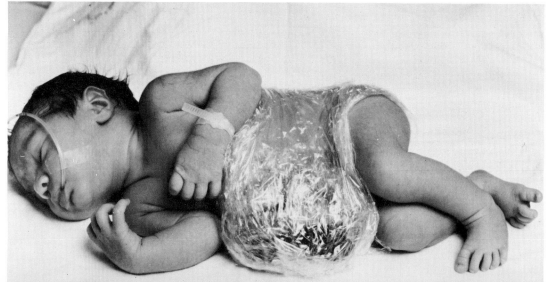

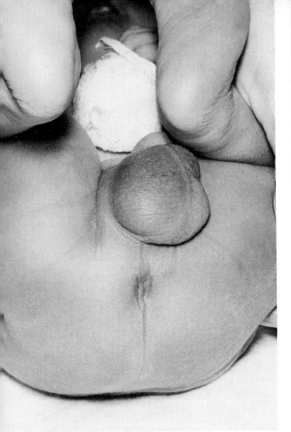 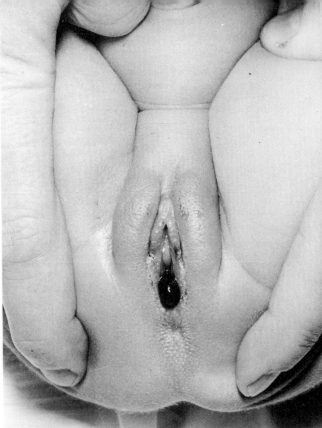

A   B

Figure 65.14 Imperforate anus. **A.** This infant had only 2 vessels in his umbilical cord. He required a colostomy which was closed after 18 months. **B.** This infant had an associated rectovaginal fistula as shown by meconium issuing from the vagina.

be established purely on clinical grounds with the help of a radiograph, echocardiograph and an electrocardiograph. Some lesions however, require angiography and pressure studies to establish the precise diagnosis.

Ventricular Septal Defect

The defect can occur anywhere in the ventricular septum, but most are found in the membranous portion. The size of the opening and hence the severity of the symptoms is variable. Symptomless infants without evidence of pulmonary hypertension are not operated on immediately. Infants who have symptoms and fail to thrive are investigated by cardiac catheterization in order to determine the volume of the shunt, the pulmonary vascular resistance, and to detect any associated anomalies, because surgery may be indicated. In uncomplicated cases with moderate-sized defects, the results of surgery are excellent. *Small defects usually close spontaneously.*

Transposition of the Great Vessels

This is an important cause of cyanotic heart disease and can be treated if recognized early. In this anomaly, the aorta originates from the right ventricle and the pulmonary artery from the left ventricle, the result being 2 separate circulations of blood. A communication is made between the 2 circulations in order to sustain life. Definitive repair of the lesion is performed at a later date.

Patent Ductus Arteriosus

This may result in heart failure, but there may be no symptoms or signs other than a heart murmur. If the ductus is patent in a premature infant, it generally closes spontaneously. A patent ductus in a term baby or one persisting in a premature infant will generally require further investigation, and medical (oral indomethacin) or surgical closure.

Coarctation of the Aorta

In this condition there is a narrowing of the lumen of the aorta nearly always at or near the attachment of the ductus arteriosus. An important sign of this condition, which should be looked for in all newborn infants, is greatly diminished or absent *pulses* in the femoral arteries. Coarctation alone seldom causes heart failure in infants. The occurrence of heart failure indicates that other major cardiac defects are likely to be present. With adequate medical management, correction of coarctation by surgery is seldom necessary before the child is aged 5 years.

SKELETAL SYSTEM

Congenital Dislocation of the Hips

Screening programmes detect instability of the hip in 2–20 per 1,000 livebirths and the incidence of congenital dislocation of the hip is about *1 in 130 births. It is the most common major malformation* (table 65.2), but when diagnosed in the first few months of life, it can be completely cured in the vast majority by the use of an abduction splint for 2–3 months. The physical signs of dislocation can be elusive and the condition is missed in about 1 in 1,000 newborn infants; therefore, continued surveillance programmes (general practitioner, health visitor) are necessary until the child is walking. Failure to diagnose the presence of a dislocated hip in the newborn infant has very serious orthopaedic consequences. The technique of hip examination is illustrated in Chapter 59 (figure 59.9). During examination, the following features may be found. (i) A fine *click* in the hip joint *not* associated with any laxity or abnormal movement between the head of the femur and the pelvis. This is very common and of no significance. However, one repeatedly examines that hip until the click has disappeared. (ii) A *laxity* in the hip joint which is not associated with any jerk on abduction of the hip. This is common in the first 2–3 days of life, especially in premature or shocked babies, and usually disappears within 7 days. It is treated with abduction of the hips (nursing the baby in 'double nappies') and regular follow-up to ensure that the hips return to normality. (iii) A *palpable, visible jerk forwards* of the upper end of the femur of about 1 cm when the flexed thigh is abducted to about 45°. The thigh can then be fully abducted. When the thigh is then adducted to 45°, the upper end of the femur jerks backwards. The head of the femur, which is 2 cm in diameter at this age, can be moved in and out of the acetabulum over the posterior rim. This is a true congenital dislocation of the hip and requires orthopaedic management which consists of holding the hips in an abducted and flexed position by means of a simple plastic and aluminium splint or one made of strapping (colour plate 136). The hips cease to be dislocated in 2–3 weeks, are stable in 4–6 weeks, and the splint is removed at about 12 weeks of age.

Talipes (figures 65.15 and 65.16)

This condition is diagnosed only when the feet cannot be manipulated easily into their normal position. If the feet can be manipulated into a normal position, the talipes is only *postural*, i.e. caused by fetal posture in utero; this form of talipes disappears without interference. The treatment of true talipes is by early manipulation

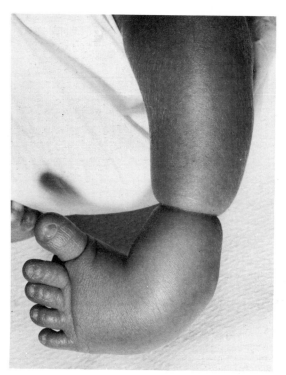

Figure 65.15 Talipes equinovarus: the constriction ring around the ankle is due to an amniotic band and is a most uncommon lesion.

and maintenance of position with Dennis Browne splints (figure 65.17).

(i) *Equinovarus deformity* is where the foot is turned inwards (inverted) throughout its length and is displaced downwards at the ankle joint. It may be bilateral in which case the soles of the feet are turned towards one another. This is the more common deformity (figures 65.15–65.17).

(ii) *Calcaneovalgus deformity* is where the feet are turned outwards (everted) and displaced upwards at the ankle joint.

Cleft Palate and Cleft Lip

These malformations are readily apparent and occur with an incidence of 1 in 500 to 1 in 1,000 births (colour plates 111 and 112). The defects (figure 65.9) can be corrected by plastic surgery during the first year of life. The lip is generally closed at about 3 months of age and the palate is left until 12 months of age to allow better surgical access. During this growing period a prosthetic device may be inserted to fill the gap in the palate or a special teat, spoon or feeding bottle is used. Mother learns to cope with the problem quite satisfactorily. Other problems include recurrent otitis media with possible deafness and difficulties in speech development which may require the assistance of a speech therapist. In the Pierre-Robin syndrome, the infant has

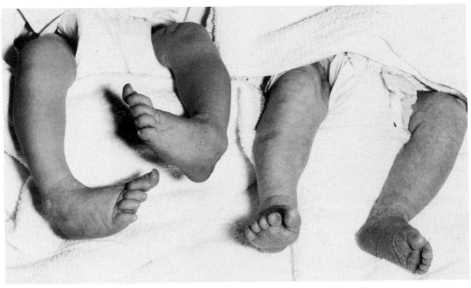

A

B

Figure 65.16 Talipes. **A.** The child on the left has postural talipes equinovarus due to compression by the uterus; there was extreme oligohydramnios and placental insufficiency. The child's feet on the right are normal. **B.** The same child with postural talipes equinovarus at 6 weeks of age. No active treatment had been instituted and the feet are now normal.

micrognathia with a wide cleft palate. The tongue tends to fall back into the palate and can obstruct the airway. These infants must be observed carefully, nursed prone, and fed very carefully to ensure that they do not asphyxiate.

Bilateral Choanal Atresia

This is a rare condition in which both posterior nares are obstructed due to bony, cartilaginous, or membranous maldevelopment. It must be remembered that the newborn infant cannot mouth-breathe unless he is awake. Hence, the child is pink when crying, but cyanosed when asleep or sucking. Emergency treatment consists of keeping the lips apart (insertion of a plastic oropharyngeal airway) whilst awaiting skilled surgical treatment.

CENTRAL NERVOUS SYSTEM

The common abnormalities of the central nervous system are *spina bifida, hydrocephaly and anencephaly*, the incidence of each being about 1 in 1,000 births (table 65.2). As noted already, neural tube defects (anencephaly and spina bifida) are at least 3 times more common in Eire and Northern Ireland than elsewhere.

Neural Tube Defects

(i) *Spina bifida occulta* is where the defect is confined to the vertebrae. This is often only seen

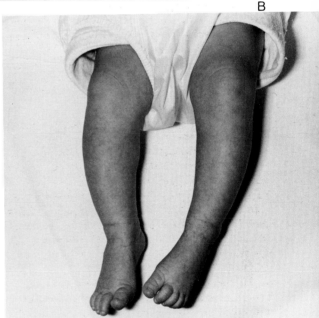

Figure 65.17 Fixed (nonpostural) talipes equinovarus requires treatment by splinting.

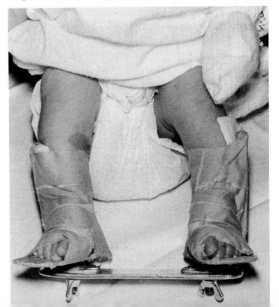

radiographically. Clinically it may present as a hairy patch or dimple on the midline of the infant's back. No treatment is needed.

(ii) *Meningocele*. In this condition, the meninges protrude and are covered by a fine membrane which may ulcerate and become infected with resulting meningitis. A meningocele is not associated with defects in the spinal cord, but can be associated with hydrocephaly. Surgery is performed as soon as possible after birth before the lesion ruptures and meningitis occurs. Treatment is to cover the lesion with warm sterile nonadherent packs whilst awaiting surgery.

(iii) *Meningomyelocele* is a malformation that not only involves the vertebrae, but also the spinal cord (colour plate 110). It is associated with severe neurological impairment or paralysis of structures below the lesion (limbs and sphincters), congenital dislocation of the hips, talipes, and hydrocephaly. A decision about operative treatment requires expert assessment. The contraindications to operation include hydrocephaly present at birth, meningitis, a high lesion (above lumbar vertebra 3) and other major malformations incompatible with life. If operation is deferred, approximately 85% of infants die within 3 months of birth. Treatment is aimed at keeping the exposed sac dry and uninfected until epithelization takes place. This is performed by daily dressings of tulle gras covered with a crepe bandage. If operation is decided upon, the aim is to protect the exposed sac with warm, sterile, nonadherent dressings until the operation is performed.

Figure 65.18 Hydrocephalus in a 7-week-old infant born at 28 weeks' gestation (birth-weight 1,220 g). Ultrasonography, performed because of rapid enlargement of the head, revealed gross dilatation of both lateral ventricles and extreme thinning of the cerebral cortex. V = lateral ventricle, F = falx cerebri, T = tentorium cerebelli. Normal size of the fourth ventricle suggested that the hydrocephalus was due to aqueduct stenosis.

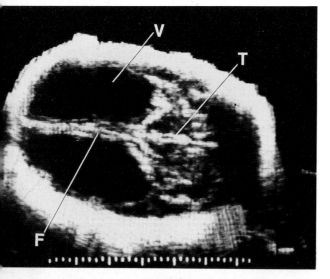

(iv) *Anencephaly*. In this malformation, the cranial vault and contents fail to develop. The death rate is 100%, most infants dying during delivery (table 65.2).

Hydrocephaly

When this condition occurs as an isolated abnormality it requires investigation. It is usually due to a blockage in the circulation of the cerebrospinal fluid, but can be due to excessive production and/or impaired absorption of the fluid. It can be diagnosed in late pregnancy, or become apparent after birth when the head enlarges rapidly. Ultrasonography confirms the diagnosis and shows the degree of thinning of the cerebral cortex (figure 65.18). The clinical features in advanced cases are a large head, thin skull bones, wide sutures, bulging fontanelles, prominent forehead, and distended scalp veins. When hydrocephaly is suspected, the head circumference is measured frequently, and if the rate of increase is abnormal, the infant is referred to a neurosurgeon. Definitive diagnosis is made either by ultrasonographic scanning or computerized tomography. Hydrocephaly in the fetus can be diagnosed by ultrasonography and the obstetrician alerted to the occurrence of possible mechanical difficulties he might have in delivering the infant. When there is a blockage in the circulation of cerebrospinal fluid, hydrocephaly can be treated by implantation of a shunt, usually from the ventricles of the brain to the peritoneal cavity or to the right atrium of the heart, in order to bypass the site of blockage.

One type of hydrocephaly seen in males is a sex-linked recessive form with aqueduct stenosis. Thus genetic counselling should be sought in this group of patients.

Microcephaly

Infants with this abnormality have small heads and severe mental retardation. X-ray of the skull shows narrow sutures. This condition occurs with intrauterine infections (rubella or cytomegalovirus) or may be inherited as an autosomal recessive disorder (colour plate 127). In many the cause is not found.

Craniostenosis (Craniosynostosis) (figure 65.19)

Affected infants have premature fusion of one or more cranial sutures, thus limiting growth of the brain. The diagnosis is confirmed by radiography and the infant is referred to a neurosurgeon. Prompt operation ensures survival without intellectual impairment. There are many different disorders with craniosynostosis and many have genetic implications.

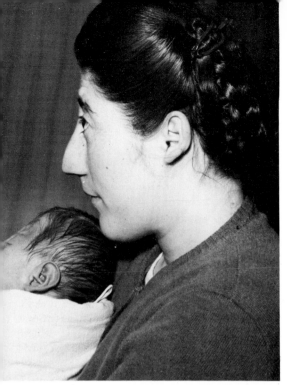

Figure 65.19 Crouzon disease shown here in mother and child is inherited as an autosomal dominant. There is premature fusion of both sides of the coronal suture (craniostenosis) causing flattening of the anteroposterior diameter of the head and deformity of the face and orbits — other features are a beak-shaped nose, maxillary hypoplasia, hypertelorism and exophthalmos.

EYES

Abnormalities of the eye include anophthalmia (absence of the eye), microphthalmia (smallness of the eye), congenital glaucoma, congenital cataracts (colour plate 98), and absence of the iris. Congenital ptosis can occur and be mistaken for facial nerve palsy.

UROGENITAL SYSTEM

Renal Agenesis (Potter syndrome)

The infant has hypoplastic lungs and absent or poorly formed kidneys. The condition is more common in males and is associated with oligohydramnios. On inspection, the baby has widely spaced eyes, sweeping epicanthic folds, turned-down tip of the nose, loose full upper lips, small jaw, and low-set misshapen-ears (figure 21.6). The infant passes no urine and dies within hours of birth from respiratory failure.

Hydronephrosis or Polycystic Kidneys

These may present at birth as abdominal masses (colour plate 56). Fetal renal masses may be diagnosed by the use of ultrasonography and the paediatrician should be alerted to the abnormality prior to birth (figure 65.21).

Ectopic Bladder (ectopia vesicae)

This is a rare, clinically obvious malformation which is treated surgically (colour plate 118).

Hypospadias

In the more common glandular form of this anomaly the urinary meatus opens just below the tip of the penis; the prepuce is incomplete and looks hooded. Penile (meatal opening on the undersurface of the penis) or scrotal (opening in the base of the scrotum) types are rare (colour plate 58). Hypospadias is often associated with urinary tract abnormality and if the infant shows symptoms of urinary tract infection, he is investigated with this in mind. Circumcision is contraindicated since the skin of the prepuce may be needed for the surgical repair. Definitive repair of the defect is undertaken when the child is about 2–3 years of age.

Clitoral Hypertrophy

The clitoris may appear to be hypertrophied in immature infants because lack of fat in the labia majora renders the organ unduly prominent. True hypertrophy is seen in infants with the adrenogenital syndrome, and in those with intersex states (figures 65.22 and 65.23).

Figure 65.20 Left inguinoperineal ectopic testis. The left scrotal sac is smaller than the right which contains a normal testis. Operation to re-site the testis is performed at 4–5 years of age.

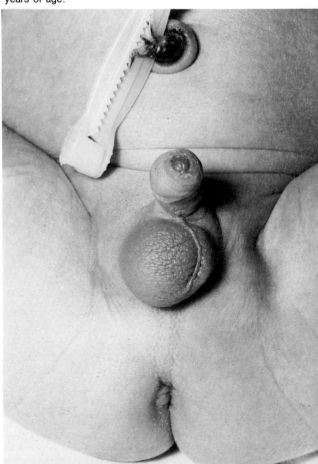

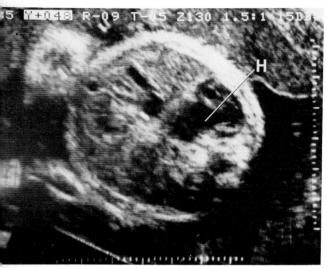

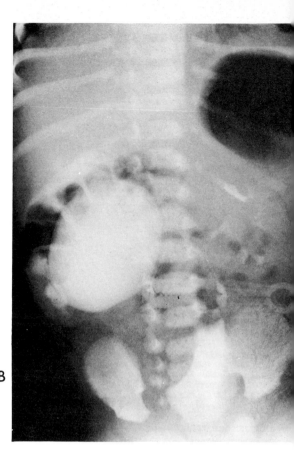

A **Figure 65.21** Unilateral hydronephrosis. **A.** Transverse ultrasound scan, performed because of uncertain maturity, showing a dilated renal pelvis (H) in a cross-section of the fetal abdomen. The infant was born 4 weeks later (birth-weight 3,730 g). **B.** Intravenous pyelogram, performed 3 days after birth, confirming the right-sided hydronephrosis. Pyeloplasty was performed 4 months later.

B

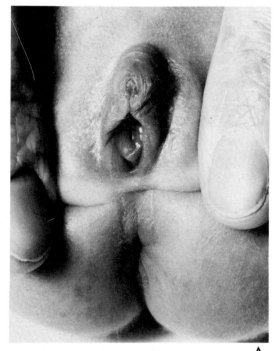

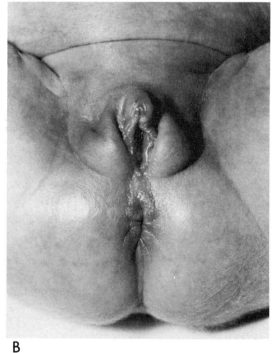

A **B**

Figure 65.22 Hypertrophy of the clitoris.

Figure 65.23 A case of intersex: the 'labia majora' were found to be a divided scrotum and contained testes.

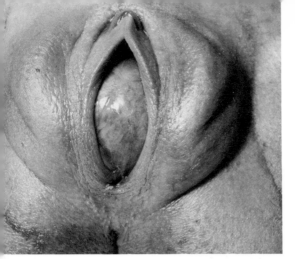

Figure 65.24 Mucocolpos causing bulging of an imperforate hymen in a 5-day-old infant. A circular disc of the occluding membrane was excised to provide drainage. If an imperforate hymen is not diagnosed until after puberty there is primary amenorrhoea and cyclical attacks of abdominal pain; retained blood balloons the vagina and sometimes the tubes which can result in inflammation, tubal occlusion and sterility.

Imperforate Hymen

This condition usually escapes recognition in the newborn unless there is a *mucocolpos* (figure 65.24) or unless vaginal patency is routinely confirmed — e.g. taking the temperature with a thermometer per vaginam.

SKIN

The commonest abnormalities seen are *naevi* (birthmarks). These are varied, can occur anywhere on the skin and may be single or multiple.

Naevi Flammei

These are the commonest of all 'birthmarks' and appear as red areas on the upper eyelids and root of the nose (colour plate 59) or on the occipital region. They are usually multiple and are present in 15–20% of newborn infants. These marks are more noticeable when the infant cries. They tend to become more marked during the first few weeks of life, and then fade away; they have usually disappeared within 12–18 months of birth.

Port Wine Naevi

These are purple or very dark and do not blanch on pressure. They occur mainly on the face and neck. These lesions are permanent.

Strawberry Naevi

These are common and may not be apparent at birth (figure 65.25). They commence as small, nonelevated red areas (colour plate 107). The naevus, soon after presentation, commences to

A   **B**

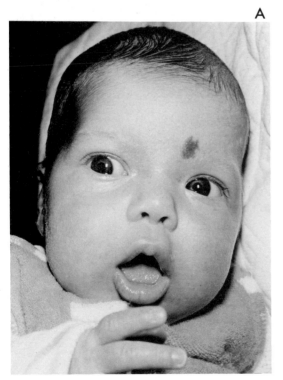
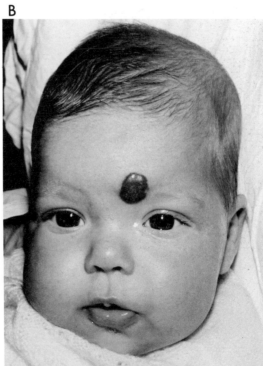

Figure 65.25 Strawberry naevus. **A.** Appearance 4 days after birth. **B.** Six weeks later the naevus has enlarged and become raised above the skin. This minor lesion can result in major psychological problems.

grow and results in a red, elevated lesion (colour plates 108 and 109). Cessation of growth and regression is the usual outcome and hence no active treatment is recommended.

Spider Naevi

These are fine 'cobwebs' of dilated blood vessels with small, bright red centres.

Pigmented Naevi

These can occur anywhere. They may be small or large, and can be covered with hair (colour plate 57). Only rarely do they become malignant.

Cystic Hygroma (figure 65.26)

These lesions form as a result of proliferation of lymphatic vessels and appear as a lump, usually in the neck; occasionally they resolve spontaneously, but usually surgical treatment is required.

HEAVY IRRADIATION OF THE FETUS

It was noted as an aftermath of the atom bombing of Hiroshima that some fetuses exposed to heavy irradiation were born with microcephaly. Therapeutic doses of irradiation for the treatment of cancer during pregnancy can also produce this effect.

Most radiographic investigations whilst best avoided during pregnancy do not give sufficient irradiation to cause problems.

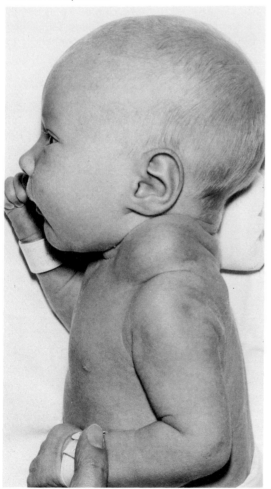

Figure 65.26 A cystic hygroma which unexpectedly disappeared spontaneously when the baby was aged 6 months and due for operation!

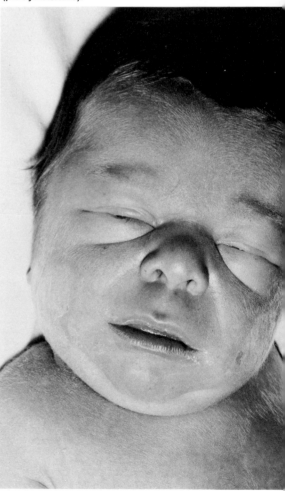

Figure 65.27 Congenital hypothyroidism (cretinism). This infant presented with hypothermia, lethargy and poor feeding. Examination revealed a depressed nasal bridge, puffy eyelids, thick, dry and cold skin, coarse hair, large tongue and abdominal distension. His cry was poor and hoarse. All infants have blood collected by heel-prick 5 days after birth to exclude hypothyroidism and hyperphenylalaninaemia (phenylketonuria).

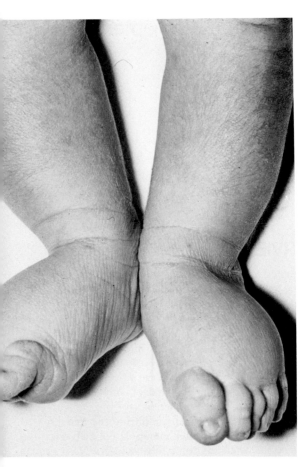

Figure 65.28 Dorsal oedema of the feet in an infant with Turner syndrome (45, XO chromosome karyotype).

MATERNAL METABOLIC DISORDERS

The incidence of congenital malformations is increased when the mother has *diabetes mellitus*. Indeed, a history of a previous malformed baby is one indication for performing a glucose tolerance test during pregnancy.

A mother who has *phenylketonuria* can produce children with microcephaly and mental retardation. This is due to the high maternal phenylalanine levels which cross the placenta and damage the developing fetus.

Only a few of the large number of abnormalities that can occur have been mentioned in this chapter. Careful early examination is mandatory in the newborn to detect the presence of such abnormalities. Genetic counselling is always warranted so that the family is aware of future risks.

Figure 65.29 Extreme hypotonia in a male infant born at 40 weeks' gestation. Muscle biopsy revealed atrophic muscle fibres with groups of giant fibres, some with central nuclei. The diagnosis was Werdnig Hoffman disease which is an inherited autosomal recessive disease with atrophy of anterior horn cells in the spinal cord and ultimately of motor nuclei in the brain stem leading to death.

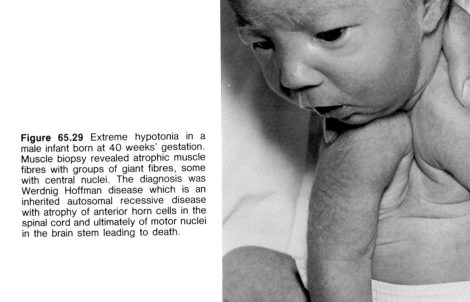

chapter sixty-six

Birth Trauma

OVERVIEW

About 5% of liveborn infants show obvious evidence of trauma at birth, mainly involving the *soft tissues of the scalp and face*. The common 'injuries' are *cephalhaematomas* (25 per 1,000 livebirths), *bruising or abrasions of the face* (12 per 1,000 livebirths) and gross *caput succedaneum* (9 per 1,000 livebirths). These lesions usually result from cephalopelvic disproportion during labour. Although these injuries are seen following spontaneous 'normal' births, the incidence is higher after manipulative deliveries (vacuum extraction, breech, forceps) (tables 66.1 and 66.2). Infants born by Caesarean section can suffer trauma from dystocia in labour or as a result of difficulty during delivery. *Fractures are uncommon* (1 per 1,000 livebirths) and like *nerve injuries* (2 per 1,000 livebirths) are usually the result of mid-forceps delivery (facial nerve palsy), impacted shoulders (fracture of clavicle/humerus, brachial plexus injury) or breech extraction (fracture of humerus, clavicle or femur). Fractures are usually felt or heard by the accoucheur during the delivery.

Caesarean section has a lower incidence of birth trauma than other manipulative deliveries, but even here there can be difficulties resulting in trauma when the fetus lies transversely, is growth retarded, of low birth-weight or has its head jammed deeply in the maternal pelvis. The fetus can also be cut with the scalpel blade when the uterus is incised!

The relatively high incidence of *intracranial haemorrhage* in infants of very low birth-weight (below 1,500 g) raises the question of whether or not Caesarean delivery can reduce this risk, especially when there is associated breech presentation or growth retardation. *Ultrasonography* and/or *computerized tomography* of all newborn infants of very low birth-weight may resolve this question, by showing whether the incidence and severity of intracranial haemorrhage is related to the mode of delivery; the technique of Caesarean section (classical or lower segment incision, epidural or general anaesthesia) also requires evaluation. The significance of the various degrees of intraventricular haemorrhage is not known — hence the need for follow-up studies to assess the incidence and severity of neurological impairment.

INTRODUCTION

Despite continuous improvement in the care of the mother during pregnancy, labour and delivery, injuries to the baby still occur. Early diagnosis is important to enable prompt treatment and adequate discussion with the parents. The incidence of birth trauma differs widely from centre to centre, depending largely on the skill of the personnel and the facilities for Caesarean section; *it occurs in about 5% of livebirths* (table 66.1).

The majority of injuries are to the region of the head (table 66.2). Table 66.1 shows that of all manipulative deliveries Caesarean section has the lowest incidence of birth injury.

TABLE 66.1 MODE OF DELIVERY AND BIRTH INJURY IN LIVEBORN INFANTS

Mode of delivery	Total livebirths	Birth injury	
		Number	%
Vacuum extraction	118	28	23.7
Breech	965	126	13.0
Forceps	10,507	1,082	10.3
Normal	24,777	702	2.8
Total vaginal	36,367	1,938	5.3
Caesarean section	4,690	151	3.2
Total	41,057	2,089	5.1

TABLE 66.2 TYPES OF BIRTH TRAUMA IN 41,057 LIVEBORN INFANTS ACCORDING TO MODE OF DELIVERY

Type of trauma	Mode of delivery				
	Normal	Forceps	Caesarean section	Breech	Vacuum extraction
Cephalhaematoma	424	542	44 (2)	5	16
Gross caput succedaneum	145 (1)	213	24	1	5
Lacerations or abrasions	40	75	18	3	2
Bruising	61	166	49	99	2
Fracture					1
clavicle	5	18	—	1	
skull	—	11	3	1	1
femur	—	1	1	3	—
Nerves					—
facial nerve palsy	9	26	4	2	
Erb	6	18	4	5	1
hemiparesis	1	—	—	—	—
cord transection	—	1 (1)	—	—	—
Intracranial haemorrhage	6 (3)	6 (2)	3 (2)	6 (5)	—
Gross periorbital oedema	1	5	1	—	—

Numbers in parentheses denote neonatal deaths

INJURIES TO THE HEAD

Head injuries are *usually associated with cephalopelvic disproportion* with compression of the head resulting in excessive moulding. This may occur during normal labour and spontaneous delivery, but is more common with prolonged labour and forceps delivery. The head may be injured either when it is the presenting part, or during breech delivery when rapid moulding is a special danger. Even when there is no bony disproportion, timely episiotomy prevents the fetal head becoming a battering ram when the mother's perineal tissues are inelastic.

EXTRACRANIAL TRAUMA

Caput Succedaneum

This is a diffuse swelling of the soft tissues of the scalp due to oedema and usually some extravasated blood (figures 2.16–2.19 and colour plate 102). It is caused by pressure of the lower uterine segment and cervix during labour and is thus present at birth; it rapidly decreases thereafter. It is boggy on palpation and may appear bruised or have overlying petechiae.

Cephalhaematoma (figure 66.1 and colour plate 142)

This lesion occurs in about 2.5% of liveborn infants (table 66.2). It could be argued that in many cases cephalhaematomas are not related to trauma, in that delivery may have been spontaneous and uneventful. However, a vessel must have been torn for the condition to develop and

the quandary may be similar to that of intracranial haemorrhage which may be due to trauma, but is predisposed to by hypoxia, with the precise relationship to the mechanism of birth being undetermined.

Figure 66.1 Cephalhaematoma overlying the right parietal bone. Milia (vernix-filled sebaceous glands) on the nose are unusually prominent.

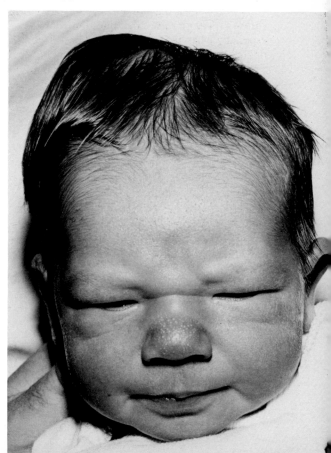

A cephalhaematoma is a fluctuant swelling due to extravasation of blood beneath the periosteum of a cranial bone (figure 2.16C). Because the periosteum is firmly attached at the margins of each bone, *the mass does not cross suture lines.* It usually presents 12-36 hours after birth, enlarges over the next few days, is not associated with bruising of the overlying skin, and there may be an underlying linear fracture of the skull. The swelling may persist for several weeks, with gradual diminution in size. *Calcification* may occur in large cephalhaematomas. The volume of blood lost into the haematoma may result in significant *anaemia* requiring blood transfusion. *Jaundice* may occur when this blood is haemolysed and absorbed into the circulation. Aspiration of the blood is unnecessary and inadvisable because of the risk of infection, and therefore treatment is conservative.

Vacuum Extractor Chignon

This resembles a caput succedaneum but is different in shape and often haemorrhagic.

CRANIAL TRAUMA

Linear fractures require no specific treatment unless associated with intracranial injury.

Depressed fractures may result in damage to the underlying brain, and hence operative elevation is undertaken as soon as possible after birth (colour plate 144).

INTRACRANIAL TRAUMA

The brain is enclosed in a bony box (the cranium) which is subdivided by strong fibrous partitions into 3 sections. The *falx cerebri* is the midline partition that divides the brain into right and left halves, and the *tentorium cerebelli* divides it into a lower posterior region and an upper region (figure 66.2). Each of these partitions is nonelastic and can easily be torn (figure 66.3). Vessels pass from the surface of the brain to the venous sinuses situated in fibrous channels attached to the inside of the skull bones. The intermediary vessels are unsupported and quite liable to be torn. Rarely the sinuses themselves or the great vein of Galen may be torn (figure 66.2). The haemorrhage is initially within the subdural space, but readily bursts into the subarachnoid space.

Causes of Intracranial Damage

The predisposing factors are chiefly prematurity (fragile vessels, lower levels of coagulation factors, and larger fontanelles predisposing to overmoulding without excessive force being

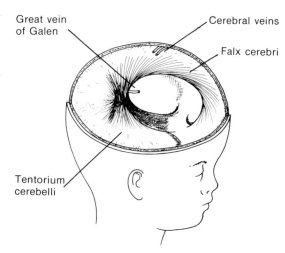

Figure 66.2 Sagittal section of the skull showing falx cerebri and tentorium cerebelli.

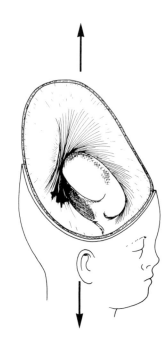

Figure 66.3 Torn tentorium cerebelli from excessive moulding as occurs in obstructed labour, especially with posterior position of the occiput.

applied), and dysmaturity (lower levels of coagulation factors, and hypoxic changes in vessels). The actual factors include precipitate labour, prolonged labour, obstructed labour, difficult forceps delivery or breech extraction, and rigid perineum, together with any other factor leading to intrauterine hypoxia.

Clinical Features

These will differ according to the extent of damage and the area of the brain involved. It may be obvious at birth or 'cerebral signs' might not be manifest for some days. There are basically 2 clinical types (i) The *agitated, irritable infant* who resents being handled, is restless, has 'tucked-in' thumbs and a shrill piercing cry. He may vomit, have head retraction, intermittent apnoeic attacks, raised tension of the anterior fontanelle, and tremors or convulsions may occur. (ii) The *somnolent, stuporous infant* who is flaccid at birth and appears pale and shocked, or extremely cyanosed, and is difficult to resuscitate. After birth he becomes a 'depressed baby' and remains flaccid. He may have tremors or convulsions, has no sucking reflex, and hence requires tube feeding.

Diagnosis

(i) The details of labour and delivery are helpful when deciding if trauma or hypoxia has occurred. (ii) The presence of injury may be revealed by clinical examination of the child which should include daily measurement of the head circumference; any increase beyond normal raises the suspicion of persistent bleeding. Transillumination of the skull is worthwhile and may show a localized haemorrhage. (iii) Two invasive diagnostic procedures may be performed: a lumbar puncture will reveal evenly blood-stained cerebrospinal fluid when there is subarachnoid haemorrhage, and a subdural tap will reveal a subdural haematoma (and also enable it to be evacuated). (iv) Ultrasonography may be helpful in localizing the lesion and demonstrating its extent. (v) Computerized tomography is the definitive method of making the diagnosis.

Treatment

The following preventive measures are important. (i) Antenatal diagnosis of conditions which may give rise to intracranial injury and the correction of these if possible. (ii) Close supervision of fetal condition during labour. (iii) Reducing the duration of the second stage of labour by forceps delivery when necessary. (iv) Elective episiotomy, especially when the infant is premature. (v) Care with forceps application and delivery, vacuum extraction, and delivery of the aftercoming head during breech delivery. (vi) Rapid resuscitation of the infant after birth. (vii) Prophylactic parenteral administration of a vitamin K preparation. (viii) Transfer of all 'at risk' babies to a special care nursery for close observation for 24 hours after birth.

The following definitive measures are employed.

(i) *Immediate.* This depends upon the general state of the infant, but resuscitation with oxygen, correction of acidosis, hypoglycaemia and shock may all be required.

(ii) *Subsequent.* Bleeding is controlled by the intramuscular injection of a vitamin K preparation and intravenous administration of blood coagulation factors. To relieve symptoms, the baby is nursed in an isolette with minimal handling; he may require sedation with a drug such as phenobarbitone, and tube or parenteral feeding may be necessary.

(iii) *Long-term.* With adequate treatment these babies often survive. Children with hypoxic cerebral injury have a much greater risk of long-term neurological sequelae than do infants who survive a traumatic intracranial haemorrhage. Periodic follow-up is essential in both groups to diagnose neurological sequelae as early as possible, and to allow early implementation of the appropriate treatment and parental advice.

INJURIES TO BONE

In general bones of newborn infants unite with surprising rapidity and good restoration of normal anatomy is the usual outcome. Hence your approach to the parents is one of optimism.

Cranial Bones

Fractures of these bones have already been discussed.

The Clavicle

This is the bone most often fractured (figure 66.4). Treatment is conservative. Within a few weeks a swelling will be noted at the fracture site: this callus formation denotes healing.

The Humerus

Fracture may occur during a breech delivery when the arms are extended, or during the treatment of impacted shoulders. The treatment is immobilization in a plaster backslab.

The Femur

Fracture may occasionally complicate a breech delivery during the management of extended legs. Treatment is with a gallows traction (figure 66.5). Within 2–3 weeks the fracture is stable and the traction is ceased. The ends of the fractured bone do not have to align accurately, but it is important that there is no overlapping since this will result in shortening of the affected limb.

Figure 66.4 This clavicle was fractured during delivery of impacted shoulders; the infant was otherwise unharmed.

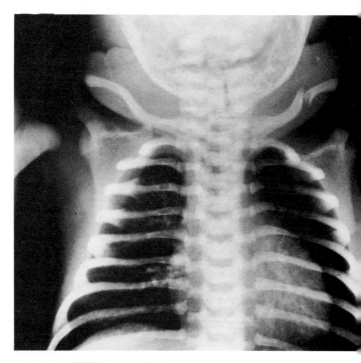

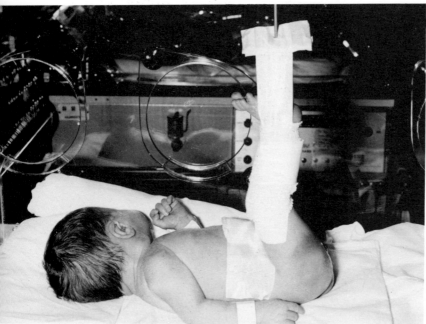

Figure 66.5 A right fractured femur treated by gallows traction. The injury occurred during a difficult extraction of extended legs in a breech presentation.

INJURIES TO NERVES

Nerve lesions occur in about 0.2% of liveborn infants. Most do *not* result in a complete anatomical separation of the nerve fibres. Hence prognosis is *good* and recovery is the rule.

Facial Nerve

Facial palsy occurs with an incidence of 0.1% livebirths. Injury to the facial nerve is usually caused by pressure of a forceps blade, but can be due to pressure from a maternal bony prominence or the fetus's own shoulder on the nerve as it branches over the face just in front of the ear. The infant is unable to close the eye on the affected side and whilst crying the unaffected side draws the angle of the mouth away from the affected side (figure 66.6). The only treatment necessary is protection of the eye from injury and instillation of eye drops. Fifty per cent show complete recovery within 24 hours of birth; ultimately, about 5% fail to recover.

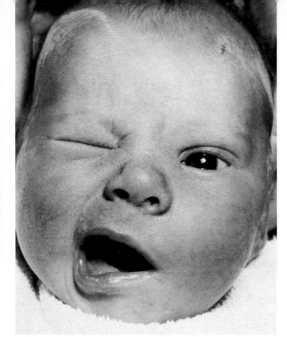

Figure 66.6 Left facial nerve paralysis; note inability to close the left eyelids. The mouth is drawn away from the affected side when the infant cries.

Brachial Plexus

Injuries to the brachial plexus occur in 0.1% of liveborn infants and account for about 50% of the nerve lesions that occur during the newborn period. The damage to the brachial plexus involves the upper nerve roots in 90%, the lower nerve roots in 4% and all the nerve roots in 6%. The brachial plexus may be damaged when traction is used in cases of delivery of impacted shoulders in a cephalic presentation or in a breech delivery when there is difficulty with the aftercoming head. Three regions of the brachial plexus may be damaged.

(i) *Upper brachial plexus damage* (C 5,6) results in an Erb paralysis in which the arm is held in the 'porter's tip' position (figure 66.7A) In 65% of cases the lesion involves the right arm. The treatment is to prevent overstretching of the paralysed muscles by tying the abducted, flexed and supinated arm to the side of the cot (figure 66.7B). With this management 93% recover fully and of those that recover, 33% do so within 24 hours of birth.

(ii) *Lower brachial plexus damage* (C 7,8, T1) results in a Klumpke paralysis in which the muscles of the hand are paralysed and hence the hand is held limply flexed at the wrist (figure 66.8). It is treated by splinting the wrist.

(iii) *Combined upper and lower brachial plexus damage* results in paralysis of the whole arm (colour plate 140). This lesion denotes severe damage to the brachial plexus and prognosis is more guarded. Physiotherapy and long-term follow-up are necessary and surgery may be required.

Sciatic Nerve

This may be damaged by injection of an irritant drug into the umbilical artery with resultant spasm of the vessels that supply the sciatic nerve. A misplaced intramuscular injection into the buttock may also damage it.

A

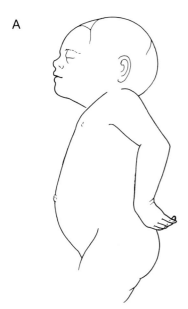

B

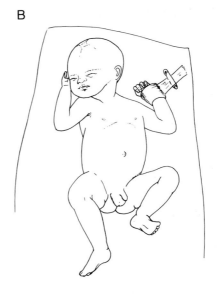

Figure 66.7 Left Erb paralysis. A. The characteristic 'porter's tip' position. B. The arm is restrained until recovery occurs to prevent overstretching of the paralysed muscles.

Spinal Cord (colour plate 145)

Fortunately, injury to the spinal cord is rare. Although it has been recorded as a complication of attempted external cephalic version, it is usually caused by traction on the head when the shoulders have impacted.

OTHER INJURIES

Muscles

A *sternomastoid tumour* may be the result of overstretching of the sternomastoid muscle. The infant lies with his head towards the affected side and palpation of the sternomastoid muscle on that side reveals a mass within the muscle substance. The condition is treated by active physiotherapy; rarely is surgical intervention necessary.

Eyes

Oedema of the eyelids is not uncommon. Red marks on the upper eyelids and forehead are not due to birth trauma, but are due to blood vessels seen beneath the skin (*naevus flammeus* — see Chapter 59). Mid-forceps delivery commonly results in *subconjunctival haemorrhages* (colour plate 139); these require no treatment other than reassurance of the mother. Rarely, severe injury can occur (colour plates 143A and B).

Skin

Pressure on subcutaneous fat beneath the skin can cause *fat necrosis* which presents as a red, firm, swollen lump. The usual cause is pressure between bones with sharp edges (mandible, tibia or radial bones) and either a maternal bony prominence or forceps. The lesion presents late in the first week and treatment is conservative with recovery being complete. The lesion must be distinguished from an area of *infection*.

Intraabdominal Viscera

Abdominal viscera may be damaged during breech delivery or during resuscitation when external cardiac massage has been used.

The liver may be torn with resultant intraabdominal haemorrhage. The usual train of events is that the liver rupture causes bleeding (initially contained by the capsule of the liver)

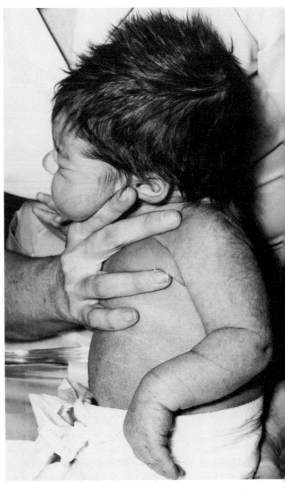

Figure 66.8 Left Klumpke paralysis in a baby born at home to a 20-year-old unmarried woman; 3 weeks later almost complete recovery had occurred.

which produces shock. Treatment then results in improvement in the infant's clinical condition. Many days later if the bleeding continues, rupture through the capsule occurs with catastrophic bleeding, shock and often death.

The spleen is at risk of injury mainly when enlarged as in erythroblastosis. The clinical presentation is one of shock and abdominal distension.

Adrenal gland. Haemorrhage may occur in the cortical zone and results in peripheral circulatory failure and shock.

chapter sixty-seven

Infection

OVERVIEW

Infections occur in approximately 14% of infants during the first 4 weeks of life and cause 4% of perinatal deaths. *Conjunctivitis, omphalitis and moniliasis* account for about 75% of infections, most of which are not life-threatening. *E.coli and other Gram-negative bacteria* continue to be responsible for most neonatal bacterial infections. However, infections due to the *group B beta-haemolytic streptococcus* have become more common (2 per 1,000 livebirths) and have a high mortality rate (50%). The limitation of hexachlorophane usage, because of the risk of neurological toxicity, may lead to resurgence of infections due to the Staphylococcus aureus.

Recent research indicates that *viruses* and *anaerobic bacteria* have previously been underestimated as causes of infection in the newborn.

It is often difficult to determine when vague ill health in a neonate is due to infection or something else (haemorrhage, metabolic disorder). Because the results of bacterial and viral cultures take 2–14 days, new techniques (use of C-reactive protein, C_3-complement activation, analysis of types and proportions of white cells in peripheral blood films) are used to provide nonspecific evidence of infection which indicates that antibiotic therapy should be commenced.

INTRODUCTION

Infection is the third most common cause of perinatal mortality after immaturity and malformations and accounts for approximately 4% of perinatal deaths. *In a consecutive series of 41,057 liveborn infants observed in an obstetric teaching hospital, 5,679 (13.8%) acquired some type of infection.* There are several reasons for the high incidence and mortality rate of infection in the first 4 weeks of life. (i) The environment in which the hospitalized neonate lives is polluted with pathogenic organisms. (ii) Infants have poorly developed natural protective mechanisms; examples are absence of the cough reflex, and thinness of the skin, especially in premature infants. (iii) A ready portal of entry is provided by such open wounds as the stump of the umbilical cord or circumcision area. (iv) The infant's immune mechanisms are incompletely developed; this is especially evident in the less mature babies. Many areas of the immune system are suboptimal in function: (a) *Opsonization* of invading organisms is inadequate leading to an inability of the granulocyte to locate the invader. (b) In the *inflammatory cycle*, polymorphonuclear cells predominate and specific immune cells are scarce; the result is poor localization of infection, allowing overwhelming septicaemia and meningitis. (c) The *serum complement sys-*

tem is poorly developed. (d) *Surface IgA* is not present at birth and is not formed until about 2 weeks later; the result is a decrease in surface (skin and gut) immunity. (e) Maternal *immunoglobulins* with large molecules (IgM) do not cross the placenta, but those with small molecules (IgG) do, and confer some protection. As the gestational age of the fetus increases, so does the amount of IgG transferred; premature infants are thus more prone to infection. Because IgM immunoglobulins do not cross the placenta they are absent from cord blood unless the fetus acquired an infection before birth and produced his own IgM. *Hence, the presence of this class of immunoglobulin in cord blood is evidence that intrauterine infection has occurred.*

TYPES OF INFECTION

Intrauterine (see also Chapter 27)

(i) *Maternal bacteraemia* (e.g. E.coli) or *viraemia* (rubella or cytomegalovirus) may result in transfer of the infecting organism across the placenta to the developing fetus. In the case of maternal syphilis, the organism reaches the fetal circulation only when a syphilitic lesion occurs in the placenta. Maternal infections can result in fetal malformation, growth retardation, infection or death.

(ii) *Maternal genital infection* can enter the

amniotic cavity and reach the fetus by *direct contact or inhalation of liquor*. This occurs when there is prolonged rupture of the membranes, especially if multiple pelvic examinations are performed.

Acquired During Birth

A fetus may become infected during passage through the birth canal if the mother has gonorrhoea, herpes cervicitis, monilial vaginitis or colonization of the vagina with the group B beta-haemolytic streptococcus.

Extrauterine

There are many types of infection that may be acquired after birth.

To gain insight into what are the common infections seen in newborn infants in a maternity hospital, a survey of the incidence and type of infection in 41,057 consecutive neonates was carried out. The results are shown in table 67.1.

It is also important to know what are the most common bacteria causing these infections, since this enables selection of an appropriate antibiotic to commence therapy before the results of bacteriological investigations (culture and sensitivities to antibiotics) are available.

Table 67.2 shows the bacteria identified in 100 consecutive positive cultures taken from infected neonates in a midwifery teaching hospital. The antibiotic sensitivities of bacteria differ from hospital to hospital but most infections in neonates are due to Gram-negative organisms.

TABLE 67.1   TYPES OF INFECTION IN 41,057 CONSECUTIVE NEWBORN INFANTS

Type of infection	Number		%
Conjunctivitis	2,400		37.7
Omphalitis	1,483	(4)	23.3
Moniliasis	868		13.6
Diarrhoea	570	(1)	8.9
Lower respiratory	261	(25)	4.1
Septicaemia	164	(20)	2.5
Urinary	147	(1)	2.3
Upper respiratory	118	(1)	1.8
Unspecified general*	83		1.3
Intrauterine	79	(32)	1.2
Meningitis	58	(9)	0.9
Skin	50		0.7
Necrotizing enterocolitis	45	(9)	0.7
Paronychia	18		0.2
Congenital syphilis	6		0.1
Total	6,350**(102)		99.3

The numbers in parentheses denote neonatal deaths
 * Type of infection not identified as cultures were not obtained
** Some infants had more than 1 infection

TABLE 67.2   BACTERIAL CAUSES OF NEONATAL INFECTIONS

Cause	
Escherichia coli	54
Klebsiella	24
Streptococcus pneumoniae	10
Pseudomonas aeruginosa	4
Staphylococcus aureus	4
Streptococcus faecalis	4
Total	100

SOURCES OF NURSERY INFECTION

(i) Staff. The staff member may be an asymptomatic carrier (e.g. excreting entero-pathogenic E.coli) or have clinical lesions such as a cold sore due to herpes simplex, or pustules due to Staph. aureus. (ii) Other babies, either carriers or with clinical infections. (iii) Feeding materials. Bottles, teats or gavage tubes may be contaminated. (iv) Ward equipment such as blankets, linen, or incubators may be contaminated. (v) The mother may be the source of infection.

TRANSMISSION OF NURSERY INFECTION

(i) *Airborne* spread by means of dust particles or droplets: epidemics of diarrhoea due to E.coli and viral rhinitis may result from this mode of spread. (ii) Direct *person to person* transmission, *particularly via the hands* of staff and mothers; this method of transmission is the most common. (iii) Via contaminated baby equipment (weighing scales, and examination and treatment benches), or communal staff equipment (auroscopes, stethoscopes and towels).

MEASURES TO PREVENT THE SPREAD OF INFECTION

(i) The neonatal nursery should ideally be situated on a floor away from infected or potentially infected patients (e.g. gynaecology patients). Babies who have gone home should be readmitted first to an isolation nursery since they may introduce organisms from outside. Only authorized persons should be allowed entry to the nursery. (ii) Staff: infected cases and carriers should be excluded from the nursery. Staff entering a special care nursery should don clean gowns. It must be emphasized that hands of personnel are of the most important carriers of infection. There are 2 alternative *regimens for hand washing*. In the first, the hands are washed for 3 minutes with an antiseptic solution before one enters the nursery; the hand washing is not repeated after examination unless the baby is known to be infected. In the second, the hands are washed with an antiseptic solution after examination of each infant. This method has the disadvantage that frequent washing with antiseptics often causes rashes and peeling of skin. (iii) Cots and incubators are cleaned daily with an antiseptic solution (e.g. 20% cetrimide hospital concentrate). When a baby is discharged, the cot or incubator is disinfected before reuse. In addition, incubators are changed weekly and disinfected, and have a monthly maintenance by hospital engineering staff. (iv) Isolation facilities should be available for infected babies. With a properly controlled and ventilated environment and strict adherence to hand washing techniques it may not be necessary to isolate all infected babies: exceptions include those suffering from gastroenteritis, gonococcal conjunctivitis, viral infections, and congenital syphilis. Rubella syndrome babies (resulting from maternal infection during pregnancy) excrete rubella virus after birth and should be isolated as a safety measure for staff members who may be in the early months of pregnancy. (v) Scales and treatment benches are potential areas of infection: scales are covered with clean paper before weighing of each infant, and are washed daily with an antiseptic solution. (vi) Overcrowding must be avoided; recommended nursery space is 10–16 m² per basinette. (vii) Individual equipment is desirable in all baby cots and incubators, and all cots must remain in the nursery area. (viii) Suction bottles are rinsed daily in antiseptic solution and again after use; suction tubing is autoclaved daily; the whole suction unit is autoclaved once a week. (ix) Oxygen tubing is autoclaved prior to reuse. (x) Feeding mixtures must be prepared carefully and terminally sterilized; alternatively, disposable feeding bottles may be used. (xi) Disposable equipment is used where possible; napkins are disposed of promptly in individual plastic napkin bags. (xii) Floors are washed with an antiseptic solution; mops used in the nursery are not used elsewhere; damp dusting is used in nurseries.

IMPORTANT BACTERIAL INFECTIONS

E.coli and other Gram-negative bacteria are responsible for most bacterial infections in the newborn. In past years, Staph. aureus (a Gram-positive bacterium) was the most important microorganism, but its incidence has declined following the widespread use of antiseptic solutions such as hexachlorophane (Phisohex). However, it appears that hexachlorophane in sufficient concentrations may be toxic to the brain. Hence, one must be selective in the choice of infants to be treated and, as a result of this, this technique has largely gone out of fashion in the United Kingdom.

E.Coli

The source is usually warm moist areas such as the interior of incubators or alternatively, staff may be intestinal carriers of the organism. The spread is by direct contact or via dust or equipment. The main portals of entry are the umbilical cord stump, eyes, and respiratory tract. Omphalitis and conjunctivits are relatively common; more serious infections include septicaemia, meningitis, peritonitis, urinary tract infection, and gastroenteritis.

Staph. Aureus

The source is usually a staff member with pustule or furuncle or an asymptomatic carrier; many people carry pathogenic staphylococci in their anterior nares, fingers, or perineal region. The spread and portals of entry are the same as for E.coli. Again, omphalitis, conjunctivitis, and rhinitis are relatively common; pneumonia, septicaemia, gastroenteritis, and osteomyelitis are less common.

Group B Beta-haemolytic Streptococcus

This organism has become more prevalent in recent years. About 10% of women carry it in the vagina at the time of delivery and about 50% of their babies become colonized during birth. Although infection occurs in only 1–5% of colonized infants (about 2 per 1,000 births) it has a *mortality rate of 50%* (see Chapter 63). The presentation is respiratory distress with a radiographic finding similar to that of hyaline membrane disease. Because of the possibility of infection with this organism, penicillin should be administered to infants with respiratory distress of unknown origin and to those in whom the diagnosis is thought to be hyaline membrane disease, after appropriate cultures are obtained.

IMPORTANT VIRAL INFECTIONS

Infection Acquired Before Birth

Rubella and cytomegalovirus are the most important viruses that cause congenital infections in the newborn. Others that can infect the fetus and cause congenital disease are mumps, chickenpox (varicella), smallpox (variola) and vaccinia. Because vaccinia virus can cross the placenta, primary smallpox vaccination during pregnancy should be avoided.

(i) *Rubella* (colour plates 125A and B). If the mother develops rubella during the first 3 months of pregnancy, the fetus can be born with microcephaly, cataracts, retinitis, deafness, congenital heart disease, pneumonitis and osteitis. These infants are usually growth retarded. Jaundice, hepatosplenomegaly and petechial haemorrhages may occur. After the first trimester, risks to the fetus are appreciably less. Babies affected with this disease may excrete the virus for up to 18 months in their urine and hence should be isolated to protect women in early pregnancy from infection.

(ii) *Cytomegalic inclusion body disease.* The affected infant can develop hepatosplenomegaly, jaundice and purpura (colour plate 126). Scattered calcification can be seen in radiographs of the skull. This classical syndrome of neonatal cytomegalic inclusion disease is in fact rare. Most congenital infections with this virus are asymptomatic, or cause minor illness at or after birth. However, a proportion of infected infants are subsequently found to be mentally retarded (colour plate 127).

Infection Acquired During Birth

Herpes simplex. The infant can become infected during delivery when the mother has *herpes genitalis.* When such maternal infection is recognized, Caesarean section is usually performed to protect the fetus from infection. A 'cold sore' (herpes labialis) may also be a source of infection *after birth* and staff with these lesions must not remain on duty in nurseries. The neonate becomes febrile and may develop diarrhoea and vomiting. Hepatomegaly, jaundice, and herpes-like sores develop. This disease has a high fatality rate.

Infection Acquired after Birth

Coxsackie virus causes myocarditis, encephalitis, gastroenteritis and respiratory infection.

Most viruses can infect the newborn infant.

OTHER INFECTIONS

Toxoplasmosis. This is a protozoal disease contracted transplacentally. It also can produce hepatosplenomegaly, petechiae, and intracranial calcification.

Congenital syphilis. The features of this infection appear weeks after birth and consist of a profuse haemorrhagic nasal discharge, generalized rash, hepatosplenomegaly, and jaundice. Treatment consists of penicillin by intramuscular injection for 14 days.

MINOR INFECTIONS IN THE NEWBORN

Conjunctivitis

The conjunctivae become reddened and the eyelids swollen. There is a sticky yellow discharge which agglutinates the eyelashes (colour plate 130). The condition may be due to irritation from meconium or chemicals and hence will respond to sterile saline instilled onto the eye with each feeding. When the standard culture is negative and the inflammation fails to improve with sterile saline instillations, a chlamydial or viral infection is the likely cause. This responds to sulphacetamide eye drops. When bacteria grow in the culture, an antibiotic to which the organism has been shown to be sensitive is instilled locally. Conjunctivitis due to gonococci is particularly severe and can result in ulceration of the cornea, or even perforation with subsequent blindness. Treatment is with penicillin administered both by intramuscular injection and by eye drops. Conjunctivitis may be associated with an inflamed tear sac (*dacrocystitis*) which presents as a swelling below the inner angle of the eye (figure 67.1). Treatment is by massage of the tear duct to overcome any blockage, and instillation of antibiotic eye drops.

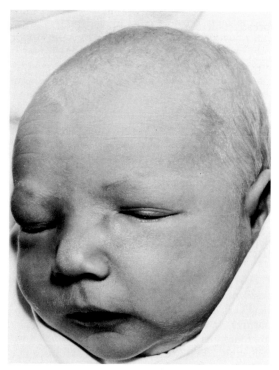

Figure 67.1 Dacrocystitis presents as a swelling below the inner angle of the eye.

Thrush

This is a common condition in neonates and is due to infection with the fungus Candida albicans. The infant may acquire the infection during birth if the mother has monilial vaginitis; another common source is contaminated feeding utensils.

The infection shows itself in the mouth as small white patches which leave raw bleeding areas if dislodged. Infection may spread down the intestinal tract and produce skin lesions on the buttocks (colour plate 131). At first these are small pink pimples each surrounded by a silvery ring. The areas may become secondarily infected and confluent, resulting in a large red excoriated surface — looking as though a potent skin irritant had flowed out of the anus.

Treatment consists of dripping 1 ml of nystatin suspension (Mycostatin 100,000 units per ml) into the mouth 4 times per day. If lesions in the mouth persist, they are painted with 0.5% gentian violet solution twice daily after feedings. Infection of the napkin area is treated with the application of an antifungal cream containing nystatin with each napkin change. If infection persists, a 1% gentian violet solution applied twice daily is usually effective.

Omphalitis

Infection of the umbilical cord stump is commonly due to E.coli, other Gram-negative bacteria, or Staph. aureus. The infection may spread to surrounding skin and subcutaneous tissues (*umbilical flare* or *cellulitis*), and can extend to the liver, or even result in septicaemia.

Initially, there is a moist, offensive, umbilical cord stump, and adjacent redness or induration indicates that the infection is spreading. When cord infection is detected, a swab is taken for bacterial culture, and local treatment is commenced with an antibiotic spray. Evidence of a spreading infection is an indication for parenteral administration of antibiotics.

Skin Infection

This may take the form of *pustules* or *cellulitis*. The entry of bacteria is facilitated by damage to skin by adhesives or abrasion by instruments (at amniotomy, forceps delivery or insertion of scalp electrodes for fetal heart rate monitoring in labour). *Paronychia* is an infection of the base of the nail and should be looked for during examination of the neonate.

Rhinitis

Infection of the upper respiratory passages may be bacterial or viral in origin. It presents as a nasal discharge ('snuffles'). It should be remembered that syphilis is a cause of persistent, watery or blood-stained nasal discharge.

MAJOR INFECTIONS IN THE NEWBORN

Babies may become sick and die of infection with little warning and therefore all staff must be vigilant for the first signs of illness. The most severe infections that occur in the neonatal period are septicaemia, meningitis, urinary tract infection, gastroenteritis, pneumonia, and some viral infections. The warning signs of these infections are similar and often special tests are required to establish the precise site of infection.

General Signs of Infection

(i) Listlessness, loss of muscle tone, anxious and drawn expression.

(ii) Fever, hypothermia, tachycardia, and tachypnoea.

(iii) Weight loss, slowness with feedings, refusal of feedings and vomiting.

(iv) Jaundice and abdominal distension.

(v) Pallor and slight cyanosis.

(vi) Coma, fitting, and hypoglycaemia.

Types of Infection

Urinary tract infection. Any infant who shows signs of infection should always have a 'bladder tap' specimen taken. When the urine is cultured the infecting organism is identified and sensitivity to a range of antibiotics is tested; the infant is then treated with the appropriate antibiotic. These infants should have radiographic investigation performed to exclude congenital malformations of the kidneys and urinary tract (vesicoureteric reflux, hydronephrosis, dysplastic kidneys), which are present in 50% of newborn infants with a urinary tract infection.

Meningitis. In the first 4 weeks of life, meningitis may be caused by Gram-negative organisms such as E. coli, Klebsiella, Proteus and Pseudomonas and less commonly by Gram-positive bacteria such as the Streptococcus. The infection can reach the meninges (membranous covering of the brain and spinal cord) from an upper respiratory tract infection, ear infection, infected meningocele, or via the blood stream (septicaemia).

Early general signs and symptoms have been listed above. The late, more specific signs are convulsions, tense fontanelle, and rigidity of the spine and neck. Lumbar puncture is performed since examination of the cerebrospinal fluid allows differentiation of meningitis from other causes of convulsions. Antibiotic therapy is commenced, although the final choice of drug will depend upon the sensitivity pattern obtained by culture of the organism from the sample of cerebrospinal fluid.

Complete recovery depends upon early diagnosis and adequate treatment. Possible sequelae are hydrocephaly, cerebral palsy, mental retardation, convulsions or deafness.

Septicaemia. The usual cause is a bacterial infection spreading from a local lesion such as an infected umbilicus. The most common infecting organisms are E.coli, pseudomonas, staphylococci and streptococci.

The onset can be insidious and the condition should be suspected in the presence of the signs listed earlier in the chapter. Antibiotic therapy is started after cultures have been taken from nose, throat, umbilicus, urine, blood and cerebrospinal fluid. It is usual for this complete range of bacteriological investigation to be undertaken when the diagnosis of septicaemia is suspected in a neonate.

Apart from chemotherapy, treatment includes the following *general measures.* (i) The infant is kept warm and has minimal handling; (ii) nutrition is maintained orally if possible and is supplemented, and if necessary wholly maintained with intravenous fluids; blood transfusion may be required if the infant is anaemic or has a haemorrhagic tendency; (iii) sedation is often needed to control restlessness and convulsions.

Pneumonia (see Chapter 63).

Gastroenteritis. Certain types of *E. coli* may cause epidemics of diarrhoea. At birth the baby's bowel becomes colonized with bacteria, including many types of E.coli and Lactobacillus acidophilus. The latter organism creates an acid environment which protects against invasion of the bowel by types of E.coli capable of causing gastroenteritis (enteropathogenic E.coli); sometimes the latter bacteria gain a foothold and epidemics of gastroenteritis may then occur in a nursery. Klebsiella, shigella, salmonella and Staph.aureus may also cause gastroenteritis, but in a large proportion of cases the infection is due to a virus.

The signs are loose or watery, offensive stools, rapid weight loss due to dehydration, abdominal distension, anorexia, and vomiting. The diagnosis is made by culture of the stools.

Treatment. (i) The infant is isolated and barrier nursed. (ii) *Milk feedings* are ceased. Fluid and electrolyte balance is maintained. Most babies will tolerate 5% glucose in boiled water orally. When the diarrhoea settles, the baby can be graded through SCM 1:8 to SCM 1:6½ and then to breast milk or weak artificial milk formulas. Some babies are unable to tolerate any lactose-containing milks after gastroenteritis due to a temporary lactose intolerance. This is diagnosed by the presence of greater than 0.75% of reducing substances found in the faeces by Clinitest tablets (Ames). These children are graded to a full strength milk which contains no lactose (e.g. Glucose Nutramigen (Mead Johnson)). (iii) Some babies require *intravenous fluids and electrolytes* for a variable period. (iv) Careful observation of the infant and the stools is necessary. (v) Antibiotics are usually not prescribed. (vi) Daily weighing is performed as a guide to the adequacy of hydration.

Necrotizing Enterocolitis (see Chapter 64).

chapter sixty-eight

Jaundice

OVERVIEW

Clinically obvious jaundice occurs in 50% of newborn infants; of these, 1 in 5 (10% of all neonates) will have a plasma bilirubin level above 150 μmol/l (9 mg/dl). *Phototherapy* will be required in 34% of such infants and *exchange transfusion* in 3%; the mortality rate is 1.5%, most deaths resulting from either the complications of *prematurity* (75%) or *erythroblastosis* (8%) (table 68.3).

The clinical problem of neonatal jaundice is to prevent *bilirubin encephalopathy* and to exclude important causes such as *erythroblastosis, infection* and *G-6-PD deficiency*. Blood group incompatibility (erythroblastosis)is responsible for *approximately 10% of cases of clinically obvious jaundice.* ABO erythroblastosis is 3 times more common than that due to the rhesus antigens but is less severe — exchange transfusion is required in 10% versus 50%; the mortality rate is 0.3% versus 3.3%.

Prevention of bilirubin encephalopathy depends upon reduction of plasma levels of toxic unconjugated bilirubin by *phototherapy* and/or *exchange transfusion* before irreversible brain damage occurs. The decision to perform an exchange transfusion has been based primarily on total bilirubin levels (conjugated plus unconjugated). Limitations of this approach are apparent, since kernicterus can occur at low plasma bilirubin concentrations in sick premature infants and minimal brain dysfunction has been reported in jaundiced term infants with plasma bilirubin concentrations considered to be 'safe'. Earlier recourse to exchange transfusion may decrease the incidence of bilirubin encephalopathy, but would also expose many infants to the risk of a procedure that carries a 1% mortality rate. It would be logical to base the decision to perform an exchange transfusion on the level of *unconjugated bilirubin* rather than the total plasma bilirubin level.

Cells and serum albumin are engaged in a continuous 'tug-of-war' for binding the miscible bilirubin pool. *Unbound bilirubin, although representing only 0.1% of the total bilirubin pool, may reflect the 'driving force' for bilirubin binding to both albumin and cells.* The concentration of unbound bilirubin is a function of 4 factors, (1) the total bilirubin concentration, (2) the concentration of albumin, (3) the affinity or tightness of the binding of albumin for bilirubin and (4) the capacity of albumin to bind bilirubin. Although it is possible to measure these 4 factors, patient management is still usually based on estimation of the total plasma bilirubin level. Further work needs to be performed to determine a test which more accurately predicts the risk of bilirubin encephalopathy.

INTRODUCTION

Jaundice is commonly seen in the first week of life, and is due to an increase in the level of bile pigments (bilirubin) in blood and tissues. Approximately 50% of infants become clinically jaundiced, but in only 20% of these (10% of all infants) does the bilirubin contained in the blood reach potentially dangerous levels. The problem with jaundice is that occasionally it may result in brain damage (figure 68.1) and hence its presence should alert one to observe the infant carefully and institute treatment when necessary.

BILIRUBIN METABOLISM

Bilirubin is produced by destruction of haem in the reticuloendothelial system of the body. Seventy-five per cent of bilirubin is produced by destruction of haemoglobin from ageing circulating red blood cells and 25% from destruction of other haem-containing compounds. The degradation of haem is through several steps to produce bilirubin, a yellow pigment which is transported in the blood attached to albumin. This form of bilirubin is insoluble in an aqueous solution, and is known as *unconjugated or indirect-*

acting bilirubin. However, it is soluble in lipid, and for this reason, when present in high concentrations, it may damage brain tissue (high lipid content) and cause *kernicterus (bilirubin encephalopathy)*. Liver cells actively 'take-up' bilirubin which is transferred to an intracellular protein used for transporting the bilirubin to the site of conjugation. The result of conjugation is

TABLE 68.1   CAUSES OF JAUNDICE IN THE NEWBORN

A. Physiological

B. Pathological
1. Prehepatic
   (a) Excessive blood destruction
       (i)   Infection
       (ii) Blood incompatibility — Rh, ABO, other incompatibilities
       (iii) Red blood cell abnormalities — hereditary spherocytosis, enzyme defects
       (iv) Enclosed haemorrhage

2. Hepatic
   (a) Deficient glucuronyl transferase
       (i)   Crigler–Najjar syndrome
       (ii) Hypothyroidism
       (iii) Breast milk jaundice
       (iv) Drugs
   (b) Hepatocellular damage
       (i)   Hepatitis
       (ii) Galactosaemia

3. Posthepatic
   Obstructive causes — biliary atresia

a water-soluble form known as *conjugated or direct-acting bilirubin* which does not affect the brain. Conjugation occurs in the presence of an enzyme *(glucuronyl transferase) and glucose* and the resultant conjugated bilirubin is actively excreted in bile into the intestine where it gives a yellow-brown colour to the stools. Some of the pigment is absorbed from the intestine, enters the blood stream and, being water-soluble, is excreted by the kidney into the urine. If an excessive amount of pigment is absorbed from the intestine, it gives the urine a mahogany colour.

When a plasma bilirubin estimation is requested, the biochemist determines the *total bilirubin* content i.e. the bilirubin bound to albumin and red cells, and that which is free in solution. It is also possible to fractionate the total bilirubin into unconjugated and conjugated varieties. *In the newborn infant over 90% of the bilirubin is the unconjugated variety* and it is only this variety that causes brain damage. *Over 99.9% of the unconjugated bilirubin is albumin-bound.* This binding to albumin prevents the unconjugated bilirubin from crossing the blood-brain-barrier. The 0.1% of the unconjugated bilirubin which is free in solution is the component of bilirubin one would like to measure since its level should correlate more closely with the risk of brain damage than would total bilirubin level. However, because free bilirubin is in such small quantities it has not been possible to measure it until recently.

TABLE 68.2   CLASSIFICATION OF JAUNDICE IN THE NEWBORN

Predominant pigment in the blood	Anatomical classification	Mechanism	Aetiology
Unconjugated bilirubin	Prehepatic	Interference with albumin: bilirubin binding	Hypoxia and drugs
		Excessive blood destruction	Rh, ABO, other blood incompatibilities Hereditary spherocytosis G-6-PD deficiency Reabsorption of extra-vasated blood Infection Drugs
	Hepatic	Deficient glucuronyl transferase	Physiological — prematurity Crigler-Najjar syndrome Hypothyroidism Drugs Breast milk jaundice
Conjugated bilirubin		Hepatocellular damage	Hepatitis Galactosaemia
		Intrahepatic obstruction	Inspissated bile syndrome
	Posthepatic	Extrahepatic obstruction	Biliary atresia

The free unconjugated bilirubin level depends on 4 factors: (i) the total bilirubin concentration, (ii) the total concentration of albumin, (iii) the capacity of albumin to bind bilirubin, and (iv) the affinity (tightness) of the binding of bilirubin with albumin. Although it is possible to measure these 4 factors, patient management is usually based on estimation of the total plasma bilirubin level.

KERNICTERUS (BILIRUBIN ENCEPHALOPATHY)

This condition is caused by high levels of unconjugated bilirubin. In each 100 ml of plasma the term infant can carry about *340* μmol (20 mg) of bilirubin and the preterm infant can carry about *300* μmol (18 mg). When these levels are exceeded the additional unconjugated bilirubin becomes *free* in solution and readily

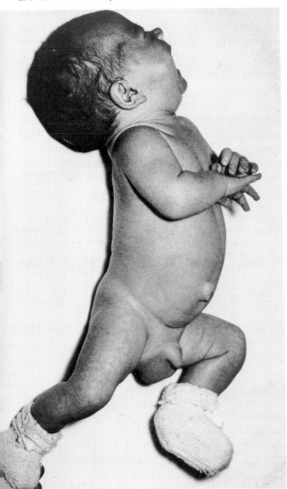

Figure 68.1 Bilirubin encephalopathy. The infant is irritable and demonstrates opisthotonic posturing.

crosses lipid membranes (such as the blood-brain barrier). Here it seriously deranges cellular metabolism by inhibiting essential enzymes, and so causes brain damage. The liberal use of *exchange transfusion* since 1950 has proved an effective method of lowering serum bilirubin levels, and hence the incidence of kernicterus has been markedly reduced. However, the problem has not been totally eradicated. There are 4 clinical stages of kernicterus.

Stage 1 is the prekernicteric stage. The jaundiced infant becomes uninterested in feedings, tends to vomit, and sucking ceases. This stage of lethargy usually lasts for 24–36 hours, and if prompt action is taken, permanent brain damage may be prevented.

Stage 2 The infant becomes febrile, and shows signs of central nervous system involvement, with restlessness and waving movements of the limbs followed by frowning, abnormal mouthing movements, and retraction of the upper eyelids, giving the 'setting sun' sign. Later, head retraction, cyanotic attacks, and increased muscle tone (figure 68.1) leading to convulsions may occur. The infant usually dies at this stage on about day 5, either from hyperpyrexia or pulmonary haemorrhage.

Stage 3 is one of apparent recovery. Jaundice abates and the child behaves in a normal manner and may do so for many months.

Stage 4 After many months of apparent normality, the infant with kernicterus begins to show signs of nervous tissue injury. He may show signs of physical damage (cerebral palsy and deafness), intellectual impairment (mental retardation), and may also develop convulsions.

Hence, it is necessary to estimate serum bilirubin levels frequently in jaundiced infants, and prophylactic measures to prevent kernicterus must be taken before dangerous levels of bilirubin are reached. *Although the plasma bilirubin level is the most important determinant of whether an infant will develop bilirubin encephalopathy, other factors increase the risk for any given bilirubin level.* These factors are immaturity, low birth-weight, age since birth, haemolysis as the cause of jaundice, general health of the infant, hypoxia, acidosis, sepsis, hypoglycaemia, hypoalbuminaemia, and the presence of certain *drugs* (sulphonamides, frusemide (Lasix), digoxin (Lanoxin)) or *free fatty acids* (produced after a few hours of starvation) which bind to albumin and displace bilirubin. *Therefore no single level of plasma bilirubin over 200 μmol/l (12 mg/dl) can be considered safe.*

CAUSES OF JAUNDICE IN THE NEWBORN

Table 68.3 was prepared to give the reader perspective with regard to jaundice in the newborn. It shows the aetiology, treatment and mortality of 4,406 jaundiced infants in a consecutive series of 41,057 livebirths in a teaching hospital. The series does not include all jaundiced infants, but only those who were shown to have a plasma bilirubin value of 150 μmol/l (9 mg/dl) or above. The following points are worthy of emphasis:

1. The incidence of infants with a bilirubin value above 150 μmol/l was 10.8%.
2. The mortality rate was 1.4%, the majority of deaths being from complications of prematurity.
3. *ABO erythroblastosis* was *more common* than that due to the rhesus group of antigens (72% versus 28%), but was *less severe* (incidence of exchange transfusion 11% versus 51%; mortality rate 0.3% versus 3.3%).
4. *Exchange transfusion* was required in 3% and *phototherapy* in 34%.
5. In approximately 1 in 3 infants no further investigation was performed and in a similar proportion the cause for the jaundice was not determined.

The terms *jaundice of prematurity* and *physiological jaundice* are often used interchangeably; however, when the plasma bilirubin level exceeds 200 μmol/l (12 mg/dl), the jaundice by definition is no longer physiological (see later). In most of these premature infants with a plasma bilirubin above 200 μmol/l, the standard investigations reveal no cause for the jaundice — approximately 60% of these infants will require *phototherapy*, but only 1–2% require an *exchange transfusion* (table 68.3).

PHYSIOLOGICAL

This is the commonest type and occurs in *both term and premature infants*, although the latter are more likely to develop it (jaundice of prematurity).

Mechanisms

(i) *Increased production of bilirubin.* The fetus has a high haemoglobin value to compensate for the relative hypoxia of the intrauterine environment. After birth, the onset of respiration provides free access to oxygen, and renders much of the haemoglobin mass redundant; thus there is a rapid breakdown of unwanted red blood cells, producing a large amount of unconjugated bilirubin. The life span of the red cell of a newborn infant (80 days) is less than that of an adult (120 days) and hence there is an increased 'turnover' of haemoglobin, again producing unconjugated bilirubin. Finally, there is a large enterohepatic circulation of bilirubin to add to the load of unconjugated bilirubin on the hepatocyte (see later).

(ii) *Hepatic immaturity.* The liver in preterm and some term infants has multiple deficiencies in function. The active uptake of unconjugated bilirubin, the intracellular transport system, conjugation and the active secretion of conjugated bilirubin all function at a level below that observed in the adult. Hence there is a build-up of uncon-

TABLE 68.3   CLINICAL DETAILS OF INFANTS WITH HYPERBILIRUBINAEMIA (> 150 μmol/l–9mg/dl) IN A CONSECUTIVE SERIES OF 41,057 LIVEBIRTHS

Aetiology	Number	Treatment		Deaths
		Phototherapy	Exchange transfusion	
Prematurity*	881	524	14	47
Erythroblastosis				
ABO	315	205	37	1
Rhesus**	120	83	67	4
Sepsis	148	75	—	3
Haematoma resorption	99	48	1	—
G-6-PD deficiency	23	15	2	—
Others	43	29	6	4
Cause unknown*	1,470	475	6	2
Not investigated*	1,307	51	—	2
Total	4,406 (10.8%)	1,505 (34.1%)	133 *(3.0%)	63 (1.4%)

* Most cases in these 3 categories had physiological jaundice
** Most infants who require exchange transfusion also receive phototherapy

jugated bilirubin in the vascular and extravascular tissues, and this gives the appearance of jaundice.

(iii) *Lack of bacteria in the gut.* Once conjugated, the bilirubin is excreted into the bowel where it is broken down by bacteria to *urobilinogen.* The bowel of the newborn, however, is sterile, and may remain so for many days. Hence, breakdown of bilirubin in the bowel does not occur. The bowel of newborn infants contains an enzyme (*beta glucuronidase*) which splits conjugated bilirubin and results in unconjugated bilirubin which is reabsorbed into the blood (*enterohepatic circulation of bilirubin*). This enzyme is important in fetal life since it permits bilirubin to reenter the circulation, cross the placenta and be excreted by the mother (conjugated bilirubin is poorly reabsorbed from the bowel). If an infant is not fed orally, the bowel contents remain sterile for longer and this tends to intensify and prolong the jaundiced state.

Diagnostic Criteria

(i) *The jaundice does not develop within the first 24 hours of life.* (ii) *The maximum plasma bilirubin level reached is 200 μmol/l (12 mg/dl).* (iii) *The jaundice disappears within 7 days of birth.* If these criteria are *not* satisfied, one must search for the cause of the infant's jaundice and not label it as physiological.

Prophylaxis

Certain measures will reduce the severity of physiological jaundice. (i) Care during delivery, including elective episiotomy to prevent hypoxia and bruising which aggravates the jaundice. (ii) Early clamping of the cord in premature infants to prevent infusion of an excessive amount of blood from the placenta which will lead to formation of more bilirubin. (iii) Care in the first week of life to prevent dehydration and infection, both of which aggravate jaundice. (iv) Avoidance of the use of large doses of vitamin K. (If the dose of such preparations (phytomenadione (Konakion)) is limited to 0.5–1.0 mg, haemolysis will not occur).

Therapy

Usually no treatment is necessary apart from adequate fluid intake, good nursing care, and careful observation.

EXCESSIVE BLOOD DESTRUCTION (HAEMOLYSIS)

Blood Group Incompatibility

Fetal red cells can enter the mother's circulation during normal pregnancy (fetomaternal haemorrhage) but are more likely to do so during delivery. A small percentage of mothers will react to this by producing antibodies against the red cells of the fetus if these cells carry antigens (inherited from the father) which are not present in the mother's blood (that is, they will be recognized as foreign). Once produced by the mother the antibodies can cross the placenta in this or a subsequent pregnancy, and enter the fetal circulation where they cause haemolysis of red cells. This haemolysis results in marked compensatory overproduction of young nucleated red cells in the fetal erythropoietic sites (liver and spleen); thus the term *erythroblastosis fetalis* was derived (see Chapter 22).

The possible blood group (antigen) systems which may cause this disease are numerous, but the vast majority of cases are due to *ABO and rhesus blood factors* (table 68.3).

Rhesus Incompatibility

The Rh antigen is carried on the red blood cells of 85% of Europeans (Rh-positive), the other 15% being Rh-negative. It is estimated that 13% of all marriages occur between Rh-negative women and Rh-positive men and that 10% of all babies born are Rh-positive babies with Rh-negative mothers. However, only 4% of these develop haemolytic disease of the newborn, which is an incidence of about 1 in 250 births. With prophylaxis by administration of anti-D gamma globulin (see Chapter 22) the incidence should fall by more than 90%. However, in major centres where rhesus isoimmunized patients are referred, the incidence remains at about 1 in 185 births — many of these patients are not severely isoimmunized and only about 50% of the infants develop jaundice sufficient to be included in table 68.3.

The likelihood of producing antibodies increases with each pregnancy. Once a mother has had an erythroblastotic child, the possibility of subsequent children being affected is determined by the Rh status of her husband. If the husband is homozygous Rh-positive (DD), then all infants will be Rh-positive, but if he is heterozygous Rh-positive (Dd), there is a 50% chance that the fetus will be Rh-negative, and therefore unaffected.

Treatment. This depends on the severity of the disease. Early exchange transfusion, which may need to be repeated, will usually prevent kernicterus in any liveborn affected infant, and result in a normal child.

Early clamping of the cord is performed at birth to prevent the infant receiving additional blood. Blood is taken from the cord into 2 tubes, one of which is heparinized. Blood group, Rh factor, direct Coombs test, haemoglobin and bilirubin levels are estimated. A positive direct Coombs test shows that the infant is affected, but does not indicate the severity of the disease.

(i) *Indications for exchange transfusion.* If the infant is born alive, and appears prehydropic (pale, oedematous, and with marked hepato-splenomegaly), transfusion is performed immediately (with Rh-negative uncross-matched blood if necessary). Otherwise, the results of the tests on the cord blood are analysed. Experience has established that one or more of the following indicate the need for an early exchange transfusion: cord blood haemoglobin value below 12 g/dl (normal 14–22 g), cord blood bilirubin level above *70 μmol/l* (4 mg/dl) (normal less than 17 μmol/l), or jaundice appearing within 12 hours of birth. A late exchange transfusion may be necessary to prevent the level of unconjugated bilirubin in the plasma from exceeding 340 μmol/l (20 mg/dl) in the term infant, and 300 μmol/l (18 mg/dl) in the preterm infant.

(ii) *Rationale of exchange transfusion.* The blood volume of the infant is approximately 90 ml per kg of body weight. During an exchange transfusion 80–90% of the baby's blood is progressively exchanged for donor blood. The aims of exchange transfusion are: (a) *replacement of vulnerable Rh-positive red cells* of the baby with nonvulnerable Rh-negative cells of the donor, (b) *removal of bilirubin*, (c) *correction of anaemia*, and (d) *removal of antibodies*. All of the bilirubin and antibodies are not free in the blood stream, a proportion having entered the extravascular tissues. After exchange transfusion has reduced the concentration of these substances, the levels in the blood will rise, as bilirubin and antibodies pass from the tissues back into the blood. Hence, further exchange transfusions may be necessary. In infants who are deeply jaundiced, 50–100 ml of the exchange transfusion may be done with salt-free serum albumin which removes more bilirubin because of its strong binding capacity for this substance.

(iii) *Technique of exchange transfusion.* Rh-negative blood of the same ABO group as the infant is used — after *cross-matching* has checked that it is compatible; the blood should be less than 48 hours old. In very anaemic infants, packed red cells are often used, the volume exchanged being reduced by half. The donor blood should be kept at 37°C to avoid a reduction of the baby's body temperature; oxygen, suction apparatus, and ampoules of 10% calcium gluconate should be available. The

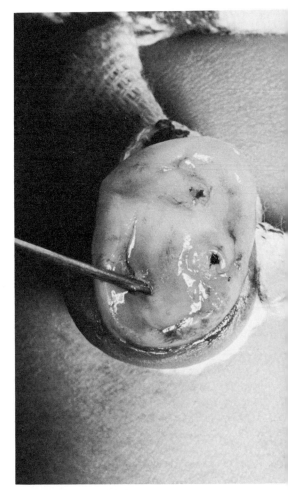

Figure 68.2 Cross-section of an umbilical cord showing the 2 thick-walled arteries and a probe in the thin-walled, patulous vein which is cannulated to perform an exchange transfusion (colour plate 124).

infant is restrained and kept warm, and cardiac function is monitored carefully during the procedure.

The exchange transfusion is carried out via the umbilical vein with strict asepsis (figure 68.2 and colour plate 124). A plastic catheter is passed into the vein, and 10 ml of blood is withdrawn, discarded, and replaced with donor blood each minute. This procedure is repeated until the desired amount has been exchanged (usually 200 ml per kg of body weight or approximately twice the total blood volume; a lesser amount is used if the infant shows he is not able to tolerate the above). Progressive totals are determined and recorded by an assistant who is supervising the baby's general condition throughout the procedure.

For some hours after an exchange transfusion the infant must be carefully observed, and when his condition is satisfactory, he may be fed. Regular haemoglobin estimations are made after exchange transfusion, since anaemia is common and many infants require a *simple blood transfusion* later. After discharge from hospital these infants should attend a follow-up clinic.

(iv) *Complications of exchange transfusion.* Death attributable to exchange transfusion is of the order of 1%. The complications are due to failure to maintain correct temperature of the donor blood, improper volume of blood exchanged, electrolyte imbalance (hyperkalaemia if donor blood is too old, hypocalcaemia if donor blood is citrated), hypoglycaemia and acidosis, air embolism, infection and necrotizing enterocolitis.

ABO Incompatibility

Erythroblastosis due to ABO incompatibility is usually mild and never causes intrauterine fetal death due to anaemia. Therefore, induction of labour before term is not indicated. The problems are those of *hyperbilirubinaemia* with the risk of kernicterus, and development of *anaemia* after the jaundice has subsided.

The mother is usually group O and the infant group A or B. Unlike erythroblastosis due to rhesus factor antibodies, that due to anti-A and anti-B antibodies can affect first born babies.

Usually the presenting sign is development of jaundice within 24–36 hours of birth. The direct Coombs test is not always positive, but the diagnosis can often be confirmed by special serological tests which show the presence of antibodies in the infant's blood. Occasionally the jaundice becomes deep and there is a risk of kernicterus, especially if the baby is premature. In these cases, exchange transfusion will be necessary (table 68.3). The blood for exchange should be group O, low in anti-A and/or anti-B, according to the baby's group.

Red Blood Cell Abnormalities

(i) *Hereditary spherocytosis.* This is an inherited, genetically dominant condition which results in abnormal red cells which are fragile and liable to haemolysis.

(ii) *Enzyme abnormalities.* The most common enzymatic abnormality is *glucose-6-phosphate dehydrogenase (G-6-PD) deficiency.* This enzyme is important in the metabolism of the red cell. Its presence results in a substance in the red cell called glutathione being kept in a reduced state. In the absence of reduced glutathione the cell envelope is damaged by contact with oxidizing agents and haemolysis occurs. Relevant

oxidizing agents are naphthalene, nitrofurantoin, sulphonamides, salicylates, antimalarials, and the fava bean. These agents can be transmitted to the infant via the placenta or breast milk or given to the child directly. The condition most commonly occurs in Mediterranean and Middle-Eastern people, and is transmitted by a sex-linked gene.

'Enclosed' Haemorrhage

Enclosed haemorrhage (such as cephalhaematoma or extensive bruising) forms a haematoma which undergoes haemolysis and the absorption and breakdown of the haemoglobin leads to the development of jaundice (colour plates 142 and 143).

HEPATIC CAUSES

Deficient Glucuronyl Transferase

(i) *Crigler-Najjar syndrome* is an inherited deficiency of glucuronyl transferase and results in extremely high levels of unconjugated bilirubin. The usual outcome is death.

(ii) *Hypothyroidism.* Cretinism results in defective glucuronyl transferase activity; it presents as *prolonged* mild jaundice.

(iii) *Drugs.* Like bilirubin, certain drugs are also conjugated by the enzyme glucuronyl transferase. These compete for the enzyme and hence may cause jaundice because removal of bilirubin is impeded. Examples are vitamin K analogue (Konakion) and the antibiotic albamycin (Novobiocin).

(iv) *Breast milk jaundice.* Occasionally prolonged jaundice, for which no cause can be found, disappears when the infant is taken off breast milk. It has been postulated that certain substances circulating in the mother's milk inhibit glucuronyl transferase activity in the baby.

Hepatocellular Damage

(i) *Neonatal hepatitis* is responsible for almost 50% of cases of persistent jaundice in the newborn. The infection may be viral (rubella and cytomegalic inclusion body disease) (colour plate 126), bacterial (E.coli), spirochaetal (syphilis), or protozoal (toxoplasmosis). The clinical features are persistent jaundice, hepatosplenomegaly, and the stigmata of the particular infecting agent.

(ii) *Galactosaemia* is a rare inherited disorder in which inability to metabolize galactose is due to deficiency of an enzyme in the liver and red blood cells. The result is that galactose accumulates in the body and damages the liver (resulting in jaundice), the eye (resulting in cataracts), and the brain. Galactose can be detected in the urine by testing for the presence of reducing substances (Clinitest (Ames) or Benedict test). The prognosis is good if a galactose-free diet is maintained.

Obstructive Causes

These are responsible for more than 50% of all cases of persistent jaundice in the newborn. *Atresia of the bile ducts* is usually congenital rather than acquired. The obstruction may be intrahepatic (which is not remediable) or extrahepatic (which is remediable in a minority of cases). It presents as persistent jaundice, but kernicterus does not develop because the bilirubin is of the conjugated variety. The stools are clay-coloured. The diagnosis is made by liver biopsy and cholangiography.

Infection

Bacterial infections may result in jaundice either by causing haemolysis, or by direct liver damage (hepatitis). This is why infection should always be looked for as a possible cause of undiagnosed jaundice, the most common sites of infection being the *umbilical cord and the urinary tract*.

OTHER THERAPY OF THE JAUNDICED INFANT

Phototherapy

This consists of the utilization of light energy *of a specific wave length (450 nm)* to convert the bilirubin molecule in the infant's skin to a form which can be excreted in the urine. In other words, the process usurps the liver's function of conjugation of bilirubin. The method consists of nursing the infant naked under fluorescent lights (figure 69.3). The eyes are covered to prevent retinal damage due to excess light and the infant is rotated at regular intervals to ensure maximum skin exposure. It is important to ensure that the infant's fluid intake is adequate during treatment. This is done by increasing fluid intake, diluting the milk and careful monitoring of weight. The method is safe and effective. *Its introduction has drastically reduced the need for exchange transfusion in controlling hyperbilirubinaemia in the neonate.* It is used when an infant's jaundice is above the ideal level but not so high as to place the infant at imminent risk of kernicterus. Charts have been prepared to help in determining how a particular jaundiced infant should be treated (figure 68.4). Complications of phototherapy consist of *overheating* of the infant, *retinal damage*, *skin rash* and the *passage of loose, green motions*.

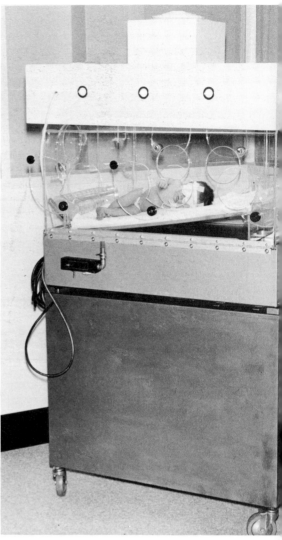

Figure 68.3 A jaundiced infant receiving phototherapy; the eyes are covered, but otherwise the child is naked, and the incubator portholes are open to prevent overheating.

Phenobarbitone

It has been shown that phenobarbitone received transplacentally by the fetus after administration to the mother induces the enzyme glucuronyl transferase to function earlier than usual. The effect occurs only after phenobarbitone has been given for some days. Therefore, phenobarbitone usage is not a form of management that can be given to the significantly jaundiced infant.

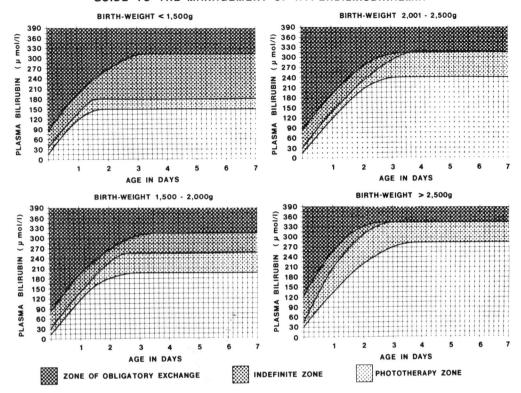

Figure 68.4 Charts prepared to aid in the management of the jaundiced newborn infant.

chapter sixty-nine

Haematology

OVERVIEW

The newborn infant has special haematological characteristics. (i) A *high haemoglobin value* (18 ± 4 g/dl). (ii) The haemoglobin is mainly of the *fetal variety* (about 70%) which was required for the relative hypoxia of the intrauterine environment i.e. it is 70–80% saturated with oxygen at the low partial pressure present in placental capillaries (25–30 mm Hg). (iii) *High red and white blood cell counts.* (iv) *Immature platelets.* (v) *Fragile vascular endothelium*, a problem which is accentuated by *hypoxia.* (vi) A tendency to a *deficiency of vitamin K* and hence *factors 2, 7, 9 and 10* which can result in *haemorrhagic disease of the newborn* — hence the rationale of routine administration of Vitamin K$_1$ (Konakion) to all newborn infants.

Major recent advances in neonatal haematology have been firstly a better understanding of the blood *coagulation mechanism*, especially in infants with very low birth-weight, and secondly, an appreciation of the significance of *hyperviscosity.*

INTRODUCTION

The blood is composed basically of 2 components: *cellular*, which includes red blood cells, white blood cells, and platelets; and *fluid or plasma*, which includes many constituents such as electrolytes, coagulation factors, and immunoglobulins.

PHYSIOLOGY

The Red Cell

Initially the fetal haemoglobin of the red blood cell is synthesized in the liver and spleen. At 20 weeks' gestation it begins to form in the medullary cavities of bones, and gradually production in these sites becomes predominant. During intrauterine life, fetal blood is oxygenated in the placenta (by transfer from maternal blood). This is a less efficient method of oxygen acquisition than via the lungs and because of this, 2 compensatory mechanisms have evolved. Firstly, *fetal haemoglobin is able to take up oxygen at a lower partial pressure* than can the adult variety because it has a different protein structure. Secondly, bone marrow stimulation (by hypoxia) results in production of more red blood cells, and hence *fetal blood has a higher haemoglobin value than adult blood.* The normal cord blood haemoglobin value is 18 ± 4 g/dl.

Expansion of the lungs after birth provides ample oxygen, and bone marrow stimulation is reduced. This, together with the shorter life span of the infant's red cells (80 versus 120 days in the adult), results in a fall of the haemoglobin value. At 8 weeks of age the level has fallen to 11 g/dl and this rises gradually to the adult level, due to recommencement of marrow activity.

White Blood Cells

These are classified into 3 groups. (i) The *myeloid* cells produced in the bone marrow; these include the *neutrophil* which is important in resistance to bacterial infection. (ii) The *lymphocyte* cells produced in the *reticuloendothelial* system (thymus, spleen, liver, lymph nodes); they are important in resistance to viral, fungal, and parasitic infections. (iii) The *monocyte* cells produced in the bone marrow; these also have a role in resistance to infections.

At birth, because of the active bone marrow, an infant has a higher total white cell count (up to 20 × 10^9/l) than an adult (5–10 × 10^9/l) and a relatively high proportion (about 70%) of these are neutrophils. During the first week of life the white cell count falls to adult levels, and only 40% of the total white cells are neutrophils.

Platelets

These are small bodies produced in the bone marrow. At birth the platelet count is similar to that of an adult (lower limit of normal 100 × 10^9/l), but they are immature in their functions and hence the process of haemostasis is less efficient than in adults.

Coagulation Factors

There are many coagulation factors, all of which do not require discussion (see Chapter 34). Briefly the first stage of coagulation results in the production of thromboplastin. In the second stage, thromboplastin in the presence of the accelerators converts prothrombin to thrombin. In the third stage, the formed thrombin acts as an enzymatic stimulus for conversion of fibrinogen to fibrin. The adequacy of the third stage is tested by performing a *thrombin clotting time* (T.C.T. — normal less than 15 seconds), the second stage by performing a *prothrombin time* (P.T. — normal less than 20 seconds) and the first stage by performing a *partial thromboplastin time* (P.T.T. — normal less than 60 seconds). Even at the moment of birth, significant alterations are present in the first and second stages of the coagulation mechanism due to deficiencies of the vitamin K-dependent clotting factors (2,7,9 and 10).

Vitamin K is required for the hepatic synthesis of factors 2,7,9 and 10. Vitamin K is initially maternally-derived. After birth it is derived from putrefactive bacteria in the gut. The gut of the newborn infant is sterile and takes some time to become colonized. Hence a deficiency of vitamin K-dependent factors occurs after birth; this is countered by the routine administration of vitamin K_1 (Konakion) to all infants after birth. In the term infant the response to vitamin K_1 administration is good, but in the preterm infant it is less predictable. The inadequate response is due to immaturity of the liver which is incapable of optimal synthesis of many of the coagulation factors.

ANAEMIA

Physiological

As mentioned previously, the haemoglobin value of the *newborn infant* falls progressively over the first 8 weeks of life. This is physiological and iron therapy *cannot* prevent it. In the premature infant this type of anaemia may be even more pronounced.

Pathological

Pathological anaemia of the newborn is due to one or more of the following: *blood loss, blood destruction*, and *failure of red cell production*.

Blood Loss

(a) *Blood loss before and during birth*. (i) *Twin to twin transfusion*. Communication of blood vessels in a twin placenta may result in one twin being born anaemic while the other is plethoric (colour plate 46). (ii) *Fetomaternal transfusion* may occasionally be large enough to cause significant fetal anaemia (colour plate 47). The diagnosis is confirmed by demonstrating the presence of fetal red cells in a smear of the mother's blood. (iii) *In vasa praevia* there is a velamentous insertion of the cord with the vessels running over the internal os. The vessels may rupture spontaneously during labour or be torn during artificial rupture of the membranes (colour plates 84 and 85). (iv) *Caesarean section*. If there is an anterior placenta praevia, the placenta may be cut or torn during the delivery and this will result in bleeding from the fetal circulation.

(b) *Blood loss after birth*. (i) *Haemorrhage from the cord*. This is nearly always due to faulty clamping and tying of the cord. Great care must be taken with this procedure. (ii) Large *cephalhaematomas* can cause anaemia. (iii) Any *haemorrhagic condition* (haemorrhagic disease of the newborn or purpura) predisposes to blood loss. (iv) Bleeding from a *circumcision* wound. (v) Spontaneous *rupture* of the *liver* or *spleen*. (vi) *Anticoagulants* given to the mother during pregnancy can cross the placenta and cause haemorrhage in the newborn; anticoagulants are also excreted in breast milk.

Blood Destruction

Haemolysis is a feature of a number of conditions. (i) *Haemolytic disease of the newborn* due to fetomaternal isoimmunization. (ii) *Congenital defects* of the red blood cell. There may be defects in the red cell membrane (e.g. hereditary spherocytosis), enzymatic defects of both the glycolytic (e.g. pyruvate kinase) or pentose phosphate (e.g. glucose-6-phosphate dehydrogenase) pathways of glucose metabolism, or defects in haemoglobin synthesis. (iii) *Acquired defects of the red cell*. An example is infantile pyknocytosis. This is a noninherited disorder related to vitamin E deficiency. It is more common in premature infants and is a transitory abnormality of the first 3 months of life. The diagnosis rests on the morphological features seen on a blood film. (iv) *Infection*, which may be either bacterial or viral.

Failure of Red Cell Production

This occurs in some congenital abnormalities (e.g. Blackfan-Diamond syndrome).

HAEMORRHAGIC CONDITIONS IN THE NEWBORN

Haemorrhage may be the result of a variety of pathological processes and a prompt and logical pathway to diagnosis is essential for effective treatment. The causes are:

(a) *Vascular abnormalities.* The blood vessels of infants are more friable than those of the adult; this is especially so in the premature infant. Hypoxia damages the endothelium of small capillaries and aggravates the bleeding tendency.

(b) *Deficiency of the coagulation mechanism.* This includes: (i) accentuation of transitory deficiences of vitamin K-dependent clotting factors — haemorrhagic disease of the newborn; (ii) transient deficiencies due to hypoxia or infection (e.g. disseminated intravascular coagulopathy); (iii) inherited permanent deficiences (e.g. haemophilia).

(c) *Quantitative or qualitative abnormalities of the platelets.*

Some of these conditions merit further consideration.

Haemorrhagic Disease of the Newborn

Previously this condition occurred in about 2 in 1,000 births, but the incidence has fallen dramatically since the introduction of prophylactic vitamin K injections at birth (maintenance of normal levels of coagulation factors 2,7,9 and 10).

Clinical features. The commonest manifestations are *haematemesis and melaena*; however, the infant can bleed from the umbilical cord, into the skin, or other parenchymal tissue, brain, and from the renal tract. Occasionally, haematemesis and melaena may be due to maternal blood swallowed at delivery (from antepartum haemorrhage or episiotomy wound), or from a cracked nipple. The *Apt test* helps to differentiate between maternal and fetal blood. The blood-stained vomitus or faeces is mixed with water to obtain a pinkish solution which is centrifuged and the resultant supernatant fluid is tested. To 5 parts of the fluid is added 1 part of 1% sodium hydroxide and the fluid is inspected after 1–2 minutes. Fetal blood is present if the fluid remains pink (fetal blood cells are alkali resistant), whereas if maternal blood is present the fluid turns a yellowish-brown colour.

Treatment. The routine use of vitamin K at delivery has been an effective prophylaxis. If bleeding occurs the steps in treatment are (i) IM injection of vitamin K_1 (Konakion) 2.5 mg, (ii) IV administration of factors 2,7,9 and 10 concentrates, and (iii) a transfusion of fresh blood if the child is anaemic.

Disseminated Intravascular Coagulopathy

This is a group of disorders in which the haemorrhagic tendency is a consequence of the acute activation of the clotting mechanism. This results in intravascular consumption of plasma clotting factors and platelets. *Activating agents include hypoxia and infection.* Upon testing the coagulation mechanism the PTT, PT and TCT are prolonged; the plasma fibrinogen is low and fibrin degradation products in the plasma are raised. The platelet count is low. The treatment is to 'turn off' the coagulation mechanism by treating the causative factor and replace the deficiencies with plasma concentrates, platelets and fresh blood infusions.

Platelet Abnormalities

A deficiency in the *number* of platelets or a *qualitative impairment of platelet function* should be suspected when small haemorrhages (purpura) occur into the superficial layers of the skin. Small (pinhead-size) extravasations are recognized as *petechiae* (colour plate 127); larger haemorrhages are called *ecchymoses* (colour plate 128).

Thrombocytopenic Purpura

Here the platelet count is reduced below $100 \times 10^9/l$. The level of platelets in the blood reflects a balance between production and destruction. Thrombocytopenia may result from *decreased production* which occurs in some rare congenital anomalies (e.g. Fanconi syndrome) or *increased destruction* which is more common. Increased destruction may be due to factors in the mother, fetus or newborn infant:

(a) *Mother.* (i) *Autoimmune maternal idiopathic thrombocytopenic purpura* is a condition where the mother has developed antibodies against her own platelets. This antibody can cross the placenta and damage fetal platelets. (ii) *Isoimmune thrombocytopenia.* Fetal platelets cross the placental barrier to the maternal circulation during pregnancy and antibodies are formed against them by the mother. These then pass back to the fetus via the placenta and damage fetal platelets in the same way as Rh antibodies cause haemolysis of fetal red blood cells. (iii) *Drugs* such as thiazides (e.g. Chlotride) taken by the mother can cause thrombocytopenia in the fetus and newborn infant.

(b) *Fetus/Newborn.* (i) *Infection*, due to either bacteria or viruses (colour plates 127 and 128). (ii) *Severe erythroblastosis* (figure 69.1). (iii) *Exchange transfusion.*

Clinical course. This is characterized by petechial haemorrhages and bruising; intracranial haemorrhage can occur.

Treatment includes specific treatment of the *underlying condition, corticosteroids*, which may prevent bleeding without correction of the platelet disorder, and finally, *platelet transfusions* may be required.

Qualitative Defects of Platelets

In qualitative defects of platelets, the platelet count is normal, but bleeding results from an impairment of platelet function. The *premature infant* has platelets which are immature in function. A variety of specific disorders of platelet function exist (e.g., Glanzmann thrombocytasthenia) and they are differentiated with the help of sophisticated tests of platelet function and electron microscopy.

PLETHORA (Polycythaemia, Hyperviscosity)

In this condition the haemoglobin value is higher than normal.

Aetiology. (i) *Late clamping of the cord*, especially with strong, ergometrine-induced

uterine contractions and positioning of the baby lower than the mother, so that little blood remains in the placenta. *The extra blood thus received by the baby is equivalent to a 1,000 ml blood transfusion in an adult.* This is especially relevant to premature babies where the placental blood volume is relatively large. (ii) *Stimulation of fetal bone marrow by chronic intrauterine hypoxia* (placental insufficiency), resulting in excessive production of red blood cells. (iii) *Bleeding from one twin to another*, either during pregnancy or at birth (colour plate 46). (iv) *Maternal diabetes.* The mechanism of the plethora is uncertain, but affected infants and their placentas are usually large for dates (colour plate 53).

Clinical course. The child appears *brick red in colour* due to the excessive number of red cells in the circulation. *Cyanosis* is not uncommon, since it takes only 5 g/dl of haemoglobin to be unsaturated with oxygen to cause this. Since the infant's haemoglobin level is very high, all of it may not be saturated with oxygen.

Since 60% of the viscosity of blood depends upon haemoglobin, *all infants with polycythaemia are hyperviscous* and hence blood flow is sluggish. The result is *cardiorespiratory difficulties* and abnormalities of the *renal* and *nervous* systems. Breakdown of the excess haemoglobin results in jaundice. At follow-up, 20–50% of infants with polycythaemia have neurological abnormalities.

Treatment. Exchange transfusion will reduce venous pressure and lower the haemoglobin level towards that of the transfused blood (colour plate 124).

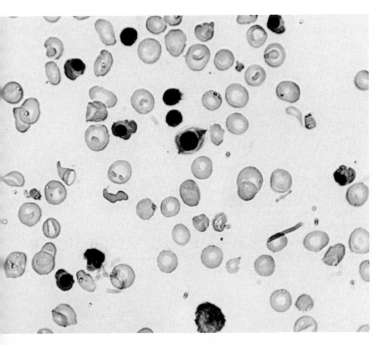

Figure 69.1 Blood smear from an infant with erythroblastosis fetalis. There is evidence of active erythroblastosis as shown by polychromasia, macrocytosis and nucleated red blood cells (erythroblasts).

chapter seventy

Convulsions and Problems in Metabolic Adaptation

OVERVIEW

Convulsions occur in approximately 0.5% of newborn infants and are associated with a mortality rate of 20% (table 70.2). In most fatal cases *cerebral hypoxia* is the underlying problem. Convulsions are frightening to the parents and tact, patience and skill are needed when counselling them.

Metabolic adaptation to life outside the uterus can go astray in a number of directions. *Hypoglycaemia* is an important example and has a 30–50% incidence of neurological sequelae if the condition produces clinical signs.

In spite of recent advances, there are many aspects of metabolic adaptation by the newborn infant where our understanding remains incomplete.

CONVULSIONS

The physiologically and morphologically immature cerebral cortex of the neonate is capable of producing seizure discharges but the clinical appearance of the seizures is noticeably *different from that seen in adults*. Classical tonic-clonic seizures are not usually seen and petit mal spells and the typical 'Jacksonian march' of motor seizures are most uncommon. Conversely, the relatively advanced maturation of the subcortical structures of the neonate's brain explains the high incidence of *apnoeic attacks, chewing, sucking* and *abnormal eye movements* as seizure manifestations.

Clinical Features

The first problem is to distinguish 'jitteriness' from convulsions. *Jitteriness* is defined as synchronous tremors or clonic movements not accompanied by other signs; it is stimulus sensitive and usually ceases when the affected limb is grasped.

Clinically, 5 types of seizures are recognized. (i) Those with *subtle manifestations*. These consist of tonic horizontal deviation of the eyes, tonic posturing of a limb, repetitive blinking of the eyelids, staring episodes, drooling and clonic movements of the chin. (ii) *Tonic seizures* which resemble decerebrate posturing seen in older patients, with stertorous breathing, eye signs, or occasional clonic movements. (iii) *Multifocal clonic seizures* which are manifested by clonic movements of one or more limbs that migrate to another part of the body in a nonorderly fashion.

(iv) *Focal seizures*. (v) *Myoclonic seizures* which are synchronous and take the form of single or multiple jerks.

Aetiology and Prognosis

The causes of convulsions are listed in table 70.1. Table 70.2 shows the aetiology and mortality rate in 235 cases occurring in a series of 41,057 livebirths. The incidence was 0.5% and the mortality rate was 20%. *The prognosis was very poor when the convulsions were due to cerebral hypoxia.*

TABLE 70.1   CAUSES OF NEONATAL CONVULSIONS

Hypoxic encephalopathy
Cerebral birth trauma
Developmental anomalies
Infection — meningitis, toxoplasmosis, cytomegalic
        inclusion disease, herpes simplex
Hypoglycaemia
Hypocalcaemia
Hypomagnesaemia
Hyponatraemia and hypernatraemia
Pyridoxine dependency
Narcotic drug withdrawal
Rare metabolic defects

In about 60% of infants in the large 'unknown' group (table 70.2) the convulsions occurred on day 4, were short-lived, and readily controlled by sedation with sodium phenobarbitone and/or phenytoin sodium. There is evidence that *zinc deficiency* is the cause of convulsions in this group.

TABLE 70.2   AETIOLOGY AND MORTALITY RATE OF NEONATAL CONVULSIONS IN 41,057 CONSECUTIVE LIVEBORN INFANTS

Aetiology	No. of infants	Neonatal death
Cerebral hypoxia	72	40
Hypoglycaemia	21	1
Meningitis	10	2
Hypo/hypernatraemia	6	—
Hypocalcaemia	6	—
Cerebral haemorrhage due to trauma	5	—
Pertussis	1	—
Cytomegalovirus infection	1	—
Battered infant	1	—
Hydrocephalus	1	1
Septicaemia	1	1
Zellweger syndrome	1	1
Unknown	109	1
Total	235	47

In many of the remaining infants in the unknown group there was some other problem such as prematurity, intrauterine growth retardation, infection or jaundice which was not the direct cause of the convulsions.

Treatment

This consists of: (i) *Resuscitation of the infant.* (ii) *Controlling the convulsions* with drugs such as phenobarbitone sodium, phenytoin sodium (Dilantin), or paraldehyde. (iii) *Further convulsions* are prevented with maintenance anticonvulsants such as phenobarbitone sodium or phenytoin sodium and (iv) *The specific cause is diagnosed and treated appropriately.*

HYPOGLYCAEMIA

The criterion for diagnosis of hypoglycaemia is a whole blood glucose value less than 1.11 mmol/l (20 mg/dl) in preterm infants, or less than 1.66 mmol/l (30 mg/dl) in term infants less than 72 hours of age. After this time, 2.22 mmol/l (40 mg/dl) is the accepted lower limit of normal.

Clinical Features

Hypoglycaemia in newborn infants can cause jitteriness or convulsions, apathy, hypotonia, refusal to suck, apnoeic attacks, cyanosis, high-pitched cry, abnormal eye movements or temperature instability.

There are various types of hypoglycaemia. (i) *Transient.* This is the most common type and occurs in *premature* and *growth retarded infants* as well as those who are *ill* or have been subjected to *hypoxia*. The pathogenesis is related to glucose supply (low body reserves of glycogen and ineffective gluconeogenesis) and demand (inordinate requirements imposed by disease and high energy needs of the low birth-weight infant). (ii) *Hyperinsulinaemia in infants of diabetic mothers.* Hypoglycaemia occurs frequently in infants of diabetic mothers soon after birth, the nadir being at 1–2 hours of age. (iii) *Hyperinsulinaemia in other syndromes.* Hypoglycaemia occurs in infants with *erythroblastosis, islet cell dysplasias* and *Beckwith syndrome.* (iv) *Other conditions.* Hypoglycaemia can occur with *hyperviscosity, galactose and fructose intolerance*, and *enzymatic disorders of glycogen storage and release.*

Incidence and Associated Conditions

Table 70.3 shows the clinical complications in 1,517 infants shown to have a blood sugar value below 1.66 mmol/l (30 mg/dl). The blood sugar value was measured by capillary blood sampling

TABLE 70.3   CONDITIONS ASSOCIATED WITH HYPOGLYCAEMIA (BLOOD SUGAR BELOW 1.66 MMOL/L (30 MG/DL) IN 41,057 CONSECUTIVE LIVEBORN INFANTS

Associated condition	No. of infants	%
Growth retardation	395	26.0
Prematurity	314	20.6
Maternal diabetes	125	8.2
Maternal low oestriol excretion	117	7.7
Hypoxia	75	4.9
Fetal distress in labour	67	4.4
Respiratory distress	55	3.6
Multiple pregnancy	46	3.0
Hypothermia	19	1.2
Erythroblastosis	19	1.2
Septicaemia	12	0.7
None	273	17.9
Total	1,517	99.4

TABLE 70.4   CLINICAL SIGNS IN INFANTS WITH HYPOGLYCAEMIA

Signs		No. of infants	%
Asymptomatic		1,261	83.1
Symptomatic*		256	16.8
Jitteriness	133		
Apnoea/cyanosis	71		
Lethargy	40		
Convulsions	21		
Collapse	1		

* Some infants showed more than 1 sign

using the Dextrostix (Ames); the test was performed only on infants considered to be at risk i.e. premature infants, infants who were ill, small for dates, born of diabetic mothers, and those with apnoea, convulsions or suffering from hypoxia.

In this series *the incidence of hypoglycaemia was 3.6%, but clinical signs were present in only 17% of the babies* (table 70.4). *The neonatal death rate was 2.4%* (37 of 1,517), but no death was directly related to hypoglycaemia.

Treatment

(i) *Prophylactic care*. The infant likely to develop hypoglycaemia is identified, has regular blood glucose estimations, and oral feedings or parenteral infusion of 10% glucose in water is commenced early. (ii) *Acute symptoms* are managed by the intravenous administration of 2 ml per kg of 50% dextrose, followed by a glucose infusion at 7–8 mg per kg per minute. (iii) *Reduction of energy needs* by treatment of sepsis, correction of acidosis and nursing in a neutral thermal environment. (iv) *Blood glucose levels* are monitored hourly until stable. (v) *Glucagon* and *steroids* are additional drugs that may be prescribed.

Prognosis

Untreated hypoglycaemia can cause damage to the central nervous system; 30–50% of survivors of 'symptomatic' hypoglycaemia have been found on follow-up to have signs of neurological impairment. There appear to be no sequelae of asymptomatic hypoglycaemia.

HYPOCALCAEMIA

Hypocalcaemia is *defined as a blood calcium level below 1.8 mmol/l* (7.0 mg/dl).

Fetal and neonatal calcium metabolism. The rate at which the fetus accumulates calcium quadruples in the last trimester of pregnancy; at birth, however, this massive calcium supply from the mother is interrupted. The following factors will affect serum calcium in the baby. (i) *Parathyroid hormone* which mobilizes calcium from bone, promotes calcium absorption from the gut and increases phosphate excretion; parathyroid activity is rarely detectable in the first 2 weeks of life. (ii) *Vitamin D* which is required for effective parathyroid hormone action on bone and gut; stores of vitamin D are adequate in the term infant, but inadequate in the preterm infant. (iii) *Calcitonin* which is secreted from the parathyroid glands and inhibits calcium mobilization from bone. High levels of the hormone are present in all newborn infants, especially those subjected to asphyxia. (iv) *Stress* or illness, which lower the level of serum calcium.

Clinical Features

Hypocalcaemia causes twitching, increased muscular tone, jitteriness, convulsions, cyanosis, vomiting and a high-pitched cry. There are several types of hypocalcaemia. (i) *Early neonatal hypocalcaemia.* This is the most common type and represents an exaggeration of the physiological fall in the serum level of calcium during the first 2 days of life. It occurs in low birth-weight infants, those subjected to stress (illness, asphyxia, trauma) and infants of diabetic mothers. (ii) *Classical neonatal tetany* which occurs towards the end of the first week of life and is associated with hyperphosphataemia due to feeding formulas containing excessive phosphorus. (iii) *Hypoparathyroidism.* This can be due to temporary suppression of the infant's parathyroid gland when the fetus has been subjected to hypercalcaemia due to maternal hyperparathyroidism. Permanent hypoparathyroidism occurs in the Di George syndrome.

Treatment

(i) *Prophylactic care* in selection of infants prone to hypocalcaemia, regular estimation of serum calcium levels and supplementation of the intake of calcium if necessary. (ii) *Treatment of acute symptoms* with intravenous administration of 1 ml per kg of 10% calcium gluconate, followed by an infusion of 50 mg calcium per kg in 24 hours or supplementation of the oral diet with calcium.

Prognosis

Unlike hypoglycaemia, there is no central nervous system damage with hypocalcaemia and thus the prognosis is excellent.

chapter seventy-one

Transport of Premature and Sick Infants

OVERVIEW

In developed countries, regionalization of perinatal services and establishment of newborn emergency transport services have lowered neonatal mortality rates. Approximately 1% of newborn infants are candidates for transport to hospitals with special care facilities (table 71.2). *The common reasons for transfer are prematurity (± respiratory distress)* and *congenital malformations requiring surgery.* However, the best transport incubator is still the uterus of the mother. To improve perinatal mortality rates further, *transportation of high risk mothers* (e.g. those with diabetes, antepartum haemorrhage, premature rupture of membranes, preeclampsia, multiple pregnancy, polyhydramnios, premature labour) to units capable of offering obstetric and paediatric intensive care facilities is essential.

Careful assessment of the mother and baby (before delivery) or of the baby (after delivery) is necessary to determine whether transport is desirable. If the latter course is adopted, it is important that the mother's and/or infant's condition be stabilized before transfer and that there is adequate supervision and facilities during transit.

INTRODUCTION

The development of neonatal intensive care units in industrialized nations has precipitated the growth of transport systems for conveying the sick newborn infant from the place of birth to specialized care centres. In the past 10 years, there have been major refinements in the construction of the transport incubator, permitting the infant to be kept warm and well-oxygenated while allowing the physician or nurse transporting the infant to render necessary care during transit.

Transport equipment has become more specialized and is usually adapted to meet local geographic and climatic conditions. Helicopters and fixed-wing aircraft supplement ground transport when appropriate. Highly sophisticated mobile intensive care vans are available to provide neonatal intensive care facilities to the infant at the referring hospital and during transit (figure 71.1). As a result of extensive educational programmes directed to staffs of peripheral hospitals, infants can receive appropriate care before the transfer team and vehicle arrive, and so are better able to withstand the journey and arrive at the special care nursery in good condition. As a result, the effectiveness of these transport systems has improved markedly with a corresponding fall in neonatal mortality rates (table 71.1).

TABLE 71.1 PERINATAL MORTALITY STATISTICS, VICTORIA (per 1,000 births)

Year	Stillbirth rate	Neonatal rate	Perinatal mortality rate
1972	11.5	10.7	22.3
1973	11.8	10.1	21.9
1974	11.7	10.7	22.5
1975*	11.3	8.7	20.1
1976	10.0	8.3	18.3
1977	9.4	7.6	17.0
1978	9.6	7.1	16.8
1979	8.4	7.2	15.6

* The commencing year of the State Newborn Emergency Transport Service (NETS)

It must be emphasized that transportation of the high-risk infant following birth is not the ideal system. Most experts in perinatal health care agree that when risk factors can be predicted, *maternal transport is far preferable to neonatal transport*; this enables delivery to be carried out in a unit equipped with neonatal intensive care facilities. There are also the problems of cost as well as concern caused by separation of mother and child. *It is far cheaper to transfer the mother before delivery; but more important is the emotional disturbance to the mother when her newborn child is taken from her and sent hundreds of kilometres away.*

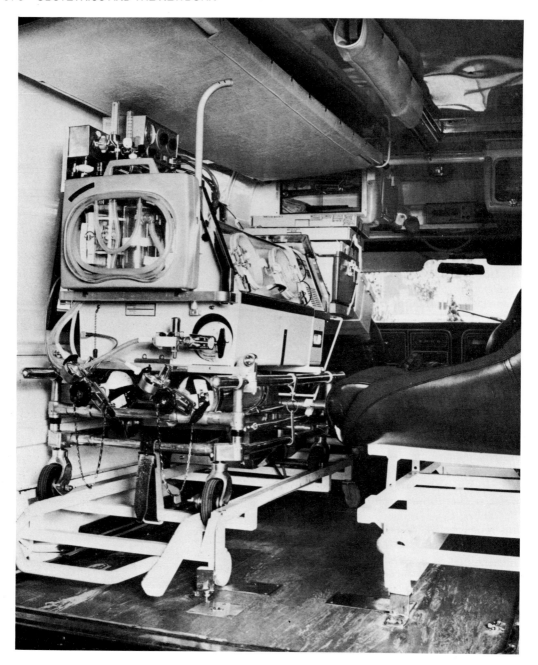

Figure 71.1 Transportation of a sick newborn infant. The ambulance must be so equipped and staffed that it becomes an extension of a neonatal intensive care nursery.

There is evidence that a policy of transfer of high risk mothers can be effected — in a 3-year regional survey, although only 25% of all births in the region occurred in the 3 maternity hospitals with perinatal intensive care facilities, 70% of all infants who weighed below 1,000 g were born in these institutions.

Approximately 1% of newborn infants are candidates for transport to hospital with special care facilities (table 71.2). The common reasons are *prematurity, respiratory complications,* and *congenital malformations* requiring surgery.

The transfer of a critically-ill newborn infant requires the provision of specially-trained personnel with special equipment. It also requires efficient coordination of communication between referring hospital staff, transport team and receiving unit and also the *stabilization of the infant's condition* by the referring hospital staff until the transport team arrives. Ideally, all suburban and rural areas should be served by a newborn emergency transport service.

TABLE 71.2 DIAGNOSIS OF INFANTS TRANSPORTED BY A NEWBORN EMERGENCY TRANSPORT SERVICE TO HOSPITALS WITH THE NECESSARY SPECIAL CARE FACILITIES

Diagnosis		Number
Respiratory distress		1,644
Prematurity		1,571
Congenital malformations		650
Heart disease	254	
Bowel obstruction	102	
Oesophageal atresia	56	
Diaphragmatic hernia	55	
Exomphalos/gastroschisis	46	
Multiple	137	
Asphyxia		423
Recurrent apnoea		142
Convulsions		131
Intrauterine growth retardation		126
Hypoglycaemia		121
Meconium aspiration		84
Necrotizing enterocolitis		57
Hypothermia		31
Hydrops		5
Others		316
Return to original hospital		229
Total		5,530*

* Many infants had more than 1 diagnosis — the total number of infants was 3,208

Indications for Transfer of a Newborn Infant

These have been listed in Chapter 64. The diagnoses in a recent survey of 3,208 transported infants are shown in table 71.2.

Principles and Practical Aspects of Transportation

The following principles should be used as a guide for the transfer of premature or sick infants to another centre.

(i) *Method of transport.* The choice of method of transfer by *road ambulance, helicopter, commercial airways flight*, or *small plane* will depend on the distance involved, the urgency of transfer, and local conditions. Rarely will a private vehicle or train be satisfactory for transport.

(ii) *Contact of referral centre.* The centre to which the infant is being transferred should be contacted and given details of the baby's condition, the type of urgent treatment that might be required, and expected time of arrival.

(iii) *Accompanying attendant.* The team should consist of a medical officer, transport nurse and ambulance attendant, all skilled in the intensive care of newborn infants. The severity of the infant's problem will dictate whether all or part of the team is required.

(iv) *Reverse contact.* The referring medical officer should be available for a reverse telephone call for further details if necessary after full admission and investigation of the infant.

(v) *Equipment and drugs.* Incubator and oxygen cylinders with fittings and power supply; laryngoscope with neonatal blade; selection of endotracheal tubes 2.5, 3.0, and 3.5 mm with adaptors; 1 breathing bag and mask of suitable size for infant; 2 or 3 oropharyngeal airways of appropriate size; selection of disposable syringes for gastric aspiration, tube feeding, injections etc; selection of needles for drawing up solutions, giving injections, and possible aspiration of intrathoracic air; 1 or 2 sterile 3-way stop cocks if aspiration of air leak is possible; No. 5 and No. 8 French feeding catheters; selection of suction catheters and means of suction (mouth or bulb type); ampoules of sterile water, saline, and sodium bicarbonate; 1 vial of heparin; 1 bottle of 50% dextrose; ampoules of phenobarbitone; 1 or 2 ampoules of adrenaline; scissors; haemostats; tape; nasal oxygen catheter and/or funnel or hood for supplying high oxygen concentration; appropriate supply of plastic or latex tubing; lancets; Dextrostix (Ames) with wash bottle; alcohol swabs; sterile disposable gloves; benzalkonium chloride (Zephiran)-impregnated towelettes; blankets and other baby linen; stethoscope; hot water bottles in case of power failure; record sheets; clinical thermometer; extra IV drip set, small vein sets and IV fluid if infant is on IV therapy; several sterile dressing towels. Ventilation equipment and equipment for continuous intravascular infusion.

(vi) *Maternal blood and operation consent.* If the mother is not being transferred with the infant, a specimen of 10 ml of clotted maternal blood and written permission for any form of treatment should accompany the infant. The blood may be required for blood group incompatibility investigation if the baby develops hyperbilirubinaemia.

(vii) *Power source.* A satisfactory source of power must be available for functioning of the incubator and for lighting. Well charged 12-volt batteries should be available in case the transporting vehicle's power supply fails. The power available in an aircraft is not always available for medical equipment and a source of supply from batteries must be available.

(viii) *Temperature control.* Adequate thermal protection during transportation must be assured. Only infants weighing more than 2,500 g and considered well should be regarded as fit for transfer clothed and in the arms of an attendant; all other infants should be transferred in a suitable incubator. Cold stress will depend on the temperature, humidity, and air flow within the incubator, as well as the surrounding temperature in the ambulance or aircraft. Overheating must be avoided also, since both cold stress and overheating can initiate a chain of biochemical effects culminating in death or permanent damage. The use of a foil blanket should be considered if a well-insulated incubator is not available (colour plate 122). In the past there have been problems due to the cots cooling during transport. The cot temperature should be approximately 33°C (91°F) for term neonates and 34°C (93°F) for premature infants (table 71.3). The infant should be adequately clothed.

TABLE 71.3 SUGGESTED INCUBATOR TEMPERATURE ON THE FIRST DAY OF LIFE

Birth-weight (g)	Temperature	
	° Celsius	° Fahrenheit
500	35.5 ± 0.5	96.0 ± 0.9
1,000	35.0 ± 0.5	95.0 ± 0.9
1,500	34.0 ± 0.5	93.5 ± 0.9
2,000	33.5 ± 0.5	92.0 ± 1.3
2,500	33.1 ± 0.9	91.5 ± 1.6
3,000	33.0 ± 1.0	91.4 ± 1.8
3,500	32.8 ± 1.2	91.0 ± 2.1
4,000	32.5 ± 1.4	90.5 ± 2.5

TABLE 71.4 WEIGHT OF INFANTS TRANSFERRED BY THE NEWBORN EMERGENCY TRANSPORT SERVICE, VICTORIA 1976–1981

Weight (g)	Number
500– 999	179
1,000–1,499	421
1,500–1,999	478
2,000–2,499	542
> 2,499	1,588
Total*	3,208*

* 0.9% of all livebirths during the period of survey

(ix) Visibility of infant. There must be adequate visibility of the infant and adequate illumination, particulary of the face and chest, during the period of transfer; hence a source of light in the vehicle is necessary.

(x) Oxygen supplies. Adequate oxygenation must be maintained during transportation; interruption of supply even for a short period must be avoided. Adequate supplies of com-

pressed oxygen must be available to cover the necessary flow for the time of the journey and also to allow for a possible delay of 1–2 hours. The oxygen cylinders in the ambulance only last 50 minutes at a flow rate of 8 l/minute. Oxygen flow rate should be sufficient to abolish central cyanosis. The oxygen concentrations achieved in an empty transport incubator (Port-O-Cot) during tests were 55% at a rate of 2 l/minute, 75% at a rate of 4 l/minute, and 85% at a rate of 8 l/minute.

(xi) Suction apparatus must be carried and it is necessary to check that this is available. Infants with respiratory distress should have pharyngeal secretions sucked out at half-hourly intervals or as required during the journey.

(xii) Fixation of crib. The crib should be fixed so that gross movement does not occur, and the surface on which the baby rests and the confining walls around him should be such that he is not injured by unexpected movement.

(xiii) Effect of motion. The effects of motion, with rapid acceleration and deceleration, noise, and vibration on the infant must always be remembered. These may lead to regurgitation in an infant who has not previously vomited and whose ability to prevent aspiration by gagging and coughing is already lowered.

(xiv) Effect of altitude. The possible expansion of air contained in body cavities, even in a pressurized plane cabin, must be remembered, in that restlessness may occur in the infant from pain originating in the middle ear, and symptoms due to pneumothorax or abdominal distension may become worse.

(xv) Risk of burning. Direct contact with a hot surface should be avoided in unconscious infants or those with shock (poor peripheral circulation) because of the increased susceptibility to burns.

(xvi) Avoidance of infection. The risk of infection during transfer should be kept to a minimum by adherence to antiseptic and aseptic techniques.

(xvii) Treatment before transfer. Because a variety of small factors during transfer can cause deterioration, an attempt should be made to correct serious disorders to the best degree possible before transfer (e.g. *convulsions* should be controlled, an attempt made to *correct severe dehydration*, an empirical dose of *bicarbonate* given in respiratory distress, IV glucose given for hypoglycaemia, *digitalization* given when the infant is in heart failure, and *assisted ventilation* commenced in infants with respiratory failure).

(xviii) *Vitamin K.* A dose of 1 mg of Konakion should be given before transfer, especially if surgery is contemplated, or there is abnormal bleeding.

(xix) *Radiographs and pathology results.* All radiographs, pathology results, or pathology specimens not yet examined should accompany the infant.

(xx) *Ambulance speed.* The ambulance driver should aim at a steady speed and must be prepared to stop when requested if motion interferes with manoeuvres such as aspiration or feeding.

(xxi) *Identification.* Adequate identification of the infant must be available. Parents' names, address, and religion should be given, as well as a statement indicating that the infant has been baptised or that this is desired. A telephone number for rapid certain contact of parents is essential.

Special Care in Particular Conditions

(i) *Severe hyperbilirubinaemia.* Avoid anoxia, cold stress, and periods of starvation.

(ii) *Apnoeic episodes.* Avoid overheating; maintain airway and have available a bag and mask for resuscitation.

(iii) *Gut obstruction.* Insert a nasogastric tube, size 8, and aspirate before and regularly during transportation.

(iv) *Meningomyelocele.* Keep covered with sterile moist gauze.

(v) *Omphalocele or gastroschisis.* Keep gut covered with sterile, moist, warm saline packs or special polythene bag.

(vi) *Respiratory obstruction.* Maintain airway with oropharyngeal or endotracheal tube or positioning.

(vii) *Pneumothorax.* (a) *Without tension*: keep in a very high oxygen atmosphere and be prepared to decompress the pneumothorax if deterioration occurs; (b) *with tension*: decompress before transfer.

(viii) *Pneumomediastinum.* Keep in a very high oxygen atmosphere and be prepared to needle and aspirate if deterioration occurs.

(ix) *Diaphragmatic hernia.* Keep in a very high oxygen atmosphere so that further intraluminal gas is absorbed. Aspirate the stomach hourly and leave the nasogastric tube open for free drainage.

(x) *Oesophageal atresia.* If a radiograph shows no gas below the diaphragm, nurse semiprone with head a little down. If no radiograph has been performed or a fistula is present, nurse with the head elevated to 45° and aspirate pharynx regularly. Keep in a high oxygen atmosphere to minimize abdominal distension.

(xi) *Suspected severe infection.* Give a large dose of a broad spectrum antibiotic which will cross the blood-brain barrier before transfer.

(xii) *Hyaline membrane disease.* Give oxygen in sufficient concentration to keep infant pink. Clear airway as indicated but avoid compulsive aspiration and handling and subsequent fall in oxygen concentration of the environment.

(xiii) *Haemorrhagic disease of the newborn.* Give 1 mg Konakion before transfer. Save all specimens of vomitus or stools obtained during the journey.

chapter seventy-two

Psychological Aspects

OVERVIEW

Modern methods of obstetric and paediatric practice have reduced perinatal mortality and improved quality of survival. These favourable results have been achieved at a price — that is, *consumer dissatisfaction with the methods of application of the new technology* and relative neglect of the psychological aspects of pregnancy and mothering by the medical and nursing professions.

It has been well documented in the animal kingdom that separation of the mother from her baby results in a failure to 'bond', with subsequent rejection of the offspring. In the human, failure to bond is a major cause of the '*battered baby syndrome*', a condition which in recent years has aroused much interest in the community. Prior to birth the intimate physical fetomaternal bond ensures optimum growth and development. After birth, in order that growth and development continue to be optimal, another type of bonding must develop. *Inflexible hospital procedures* and over-rigid attitudes to the management of the mother in the delivery suite and postnatal wards have in the past tended to impede natural bonding between mother and baby.

Lack of understanding of parents' expectations has led to pressure for a return to '*home deliveries*', regardless of the greater risks to the lives of mother and child. However, it is possible to effect a compromise between consumer demand and obstetric excellence by modifying hospital regimens so that deliveries in hospital become more relaxed and informal. Some hospitals have set up '*home childbirth centres*' within their walls; this provides parents with a less clinical atmosphere for the birth of their baby, but at the same time help is immediately available if needed in an emergency situation (obstructed labour, postpartum haemorrhage, birth of an asphyxiated infant). It would be a retrograde step to encourage home deliveries. The modification of existing regimens in our major maternity hospitals may offer the best of both worlds. It is often a simple matter to satisfy a patient's needs (colour plate 98).

INTRODUCTION

Babies cannot tell us what they feel, imagine, fear, enjoy or want; we are limited therefore in our assessment of their true needs. However, much has already been learned by careful observation of their behaviour, including interaction with their mothers. It is now accepted that the fetus, even before birth, responds to changes in its physical and chemical environment by alterations in body movements and heart rate. The newly-born infant can hear, smell and taste; though focusing of the eyes is poorly developed at birth, shapes and lights are followed from a few days of age. Primitive coordinated movements, such as stretching and yawning, and automatic walking with support are all present initially, though they disappear later. Thumb sucking and scratching of the face may be obvious within a few hours of birth. Most move-ments, however, are random and apparently purposeless and there is little control of posture. A loud noise or sudden change in position produces a startled response (Moro reflex, elicited from 28 weeks' gestation). Various other inborn reflex movements are also present (grasp reflex, tonic neck reflexes, and those concerned with feeding).

The life of the newborn baby is a constantly repeated cycle of events — much sleeping, punctuated by wakefulness, during which feeding, elimination, bodily movements and sensory experience occur. However, this description of early infant behaviour, although accurate, fails to capture the essential biological reality of the first weeks of life — that the infant exists in a reciprocal relationship with its mother (or mother substitute). Indeed, the baby is entirely *dependent* upon her for survival.

MOTHERING AND ITS VICISSITUDES

All sorts of mothers care successfully for all sorts of babies. It would be fallacious, however, to imagine that the relationship is continuously one of mutual satisfaction and enjoyment. Healthy babies are attractive, interesting, amusing and affectionate — most of the time! They may also be restless, noisy and baffling. Mothers are mostly gentle and relaxed; sometimes they are exhausted, irritable, even angry. Nevertheless, the quality we call 'motherlove' predominates, the essence of which is concern for the child's safety and physical needs, compounded with tenderness. For this to happen, a mother has to be alert to the child's needs; she has to interpret behaviour accurately and then act appropriately. It is quite common, however, for a mother to feel detached, even uninterested in her baby for some days after delivery. Very frequently she feels guilty about feelings such as these and so hides her apathy. Enormous relief and support is provided when time is taken to explain to a mother that this absence of feeling for the infant is a commonplace and temporary situation.

It must be remembered that mother and child do not exist in a separate compartment; they are part of a social group, usually a family, and this in turn is part of a community. On all sides the new mother is bombarded by example and advice, the product of tradition, culture, superstition, fashion and knowledge.

Crying by the baby becomes one of the chief ways by which the mother learns to attend to his or her needs — for instance if a baby cries long and hard, all mothers learn that the situation must be investigated. Professional advice 'to let the baby cry' is a moralistic attitude based on a fear of indulgence. Babies may be systematically deprived in this way and may become progressively more demanding — the exact opposite of what is intended. Not only does a mother quickly learn to recognize the cry of her own child, but she is quick to detect any change in the usual quality of the cry. Before speech develops, the cry may indicate hunger, fatigue, pain, cold, heat, or it may be a startle reaction. Associated signs of distress may be quick, uncoordinate movements of the body, the limbs, and the head.

Mothers also learn to recognize when the baby is at ease, relaxed, or in a state of apparent composure. Here the signs of contentment are less dramatic but quite consistent — a lessening of wild bodily movements and of loud crying, quiet 'exploratory' head-turning, gazing, and hand grasping, and soft mumbling, proceeding to drowsiness and then to sleep. Infant responses of this kind are an endorsement of the preceding maternal behaviour — talking, singing, rocking, making body and eye contact. In this way the infant educates his mother to respond to his messages and mothers learn what pleases the child. It can thus be seen that this sensitive system may go wrong if the baby fails to make his 'distress signals' clear to his mother or if the mother fails to recognize the signals or does not respond to them appropriately. When this happens, infants tend to react with disorders of crying, sleeping, feeding, and relating. They may cry incessantly or hardly at all, sleep most of the time or very little, show little interest in food, vomit frequently, or become unresponsive and apathetic. This disorder is referred to as 'colic'.

DISORDERS OF THE PARENT-INFANT RELATIONSHIP

Causes in the Baby

Some babies are unusually active and restless; they may be difficult to nurse because of backarching, and actively resist cuddling. Most mothers find ways of coping, but a few are less successful. Other infants are so undemonstrative and inactive that all initiative has to come from their mothers. Most mothers supply the extra stimuli, but some fail to do so and may become unresponsive themselves. Appreciable differences in levels of infant activity and responsiveness may reflect innate temperament, but persistent extremes of overactivity or apathy may be symptomatic of brain damage or developmental dysfunction of the nervous system.

Any *malformation* present in a newborn baby is inevitably distressing. However, it must be remembered that the mother's reaction may be quite unrelated to the clinical severity of the condition. 'Sensitization' may occur in many different ways, such as a family history of an inborn defect, a previous stillbirth, or mishap or illness during pregnancy. Sharing the consequent anxiety with an informed and sympathetic listener cannot remove maternal concern — nor should it — but ineffectual brooding and self-blame can be redirected towards a more rational acceptance and effective planning. Except where parents are very immature or unstable, rejection of such babies is comparatively rare. It is quite common, however, for a persistently overprotective attitude to develop, which often leads to emotional difficulties in the child. The time for preventive measures is when the mother and father are first told about the baby's condition, with sufficient time and continuity of contact for the exploration of the inevitable feelings of guilt, denial, rage and despair. This is a common situation where close cooperation is needed between the staff, the doctor and the distressed parents.

Causes in the Parents

Puerperal psychosis may for a time prevent the mother from coping adequately with her baby. Whether depressive or schizophrenic in type, a common leading symptom is the fear of harming the child and this must always be taken seriously. Drugs and supportive psychotherapy are rapidly effective as a rule. There is some evidence that recovery is aided by keeping the baby within sight and sound of the mother — she is, however, temporarily relieved of all caring responsibility, but can observe that her child is safe.

Parenthood may suddenly expose *personality problems* in the father and/or mother. A girl who has had a severely deprived childhood may have little capacity for mothering and tends to become clinically depressed or agitated, especially in the early months of the baby's life.

Other Causes

There are many problems in the parent/infant relationship which do not involve psychological abnormality in the parent or organic disease or disability in the child, which on listing may appear trivial, but can engender much stress and are potentially harmful. Factors to keep in mind in eliciting potential problems are whether the pregnancy was *acceptable* to both parents or whether it was *planned, wanted* or *unwanted*. The *parity* and *physical condition* of the mother and baby, *the baby's place in the birth order* and often *the sex of the baby* can influence parents' feelings as can the *emotional and mental attitudes* of all concerned — mother, father, siblings, relatives. The *socioeconomic class* of the parents is important as is the *ethnic origin* of the mother. Many mothers in immigrant families suffer from lack of social contact; their isolation can lead to depression to such a degree that caring for a baby becomes drudgery. It is important, in multicultural societies, to have some knowledge of the differing cultural beliefs associated with childbirth and child nurturing so that the regimens of management provided in a hospital can be varied when necessary.

It can thus be seen that the early days after childbirth may be a vulnerable and difficult time for some mothers. This is likely to be exaggerated if the baby is *premature or sick* and requires specialized care and is separated from the mother.

Intensive care of the neonate often involves nursing the infant in an incubator for months at a time. The equipment can appear complex and frightening and the infant is often lost in a maze of monitor leads and intravenous lines. In these circumstances, the establishment of normal bonding is very difficult and requires extra effort on behalf of nursing and medical staff to minimize psychological difficulties (colour plates 99 and 100).

It is not enough to allow parents physical access to the nursery and then sit back and assume that instant and magical bonding will occur. Parents should be prepared beforehand for what they will see. They need an appropriate explanation of the apparatus surrounding their baby. Their first sight of a premature baby may produce feelings of shock, horror, distaste and fear. These natural reactions can only be overcome gradually. Parents need time to adjust to the appearance of their premature baby; they had been expecting a rounded beautiful baby with chubby cheeks and responsive eyes; instead they are presented with a frail, almost transparent, skinny object who is nearly lost in the maze of equipment. To overcome these feelings, the parents should be encouraged to touch and stroke their baby and to visit as often as possible for as long as possible.

Once the mother is discharged from hospital, visiting can become a problem, especially if the parents live far away. Most major maternity hospitals have some type of accommodation to offer in these circumstances. This is particularly important if the mother expresses a desire to breast-feed, for she can then be accommodated when the time comes to establish the baby on the breast.

However, for a *premature baby* the situation is far from ideal. With the best intentions in the world, the baby will of necessity be deprived of normal maternal contact. Thus, it is not surprising that it is these babies in particular who are at risk of being abused and neglected. It has been estimated that of all babies neglected and battered in later life, approximately 25–30% had been separated from their mothers and had been deprived of normal maternal contact in the first few days following their birth. It can thus be seen that establishing a satisfactory maternal-infant relationship is of the utmost importance to ensure the subsequent optimal growth and development of the infant. Supportive and understanding help from caring and well-informed members of the obstetric/paediatric team can be of inestimable value in bringing about the optimum mother-infant relationship.

APPENDICES

Patient Education

Appendix I

OVERVIEW

A general introduction to the course should be given, outlining its scope, participants, hospital setting and routines, types of staff likely to be encountered and available services.

It is important that the material should be presented in a simplified manner, since few couples will have significant knowledge of the subjects to be discussed. Atlases of the anatomy and physiology of reproduction should be used freely to help the patient's understanding.

If several educators are involved, it is important that there be no conflict in the messages given.

A degree of realism is necessary in relation to the events of pregnancy, birth, and infant care. Complications are inherent in reproduction (e.g. miscarriage, 10–15%; premature birth 5–10%; fetal malformation, 5%; operative delivery (forceps, Caesarean), 15–35%; perinatal death, 1–2%); it is a disservice to the couple to gloss over these facts, since there will be a greater sense of disappointment if their expectations are not fulfilled.

Each school will develop its own syllabus and sequence of presentation. The following is a suggested framework, which can be built up to the required extent from details given in relevant sections of the text.

Anatomy

(i) *External genitalia.* Mons pubis, vulva, perineum, labia majora, labia minora, clitoris, urethral and vaginal orifices, Bartholin glands.

(ii) *Internal genitalia.* Vagina, uterus (cervix, body), Fallopian tubes, ovaries.

(iii) *Related viscera.* Bladder and rectum.

(iv) *Birth canal.* Bony and soft tissues.

(v) *Breasts.*

Physiology

(i) *Menstrual cycle, ovulation, fertilization.*

(ii) *Development of embryo and fetus.* Implantation, fetus, placenta, and liquor; fetal organs, external characteristics, sex; fetal movements, positions of the baby; fetomaternal exchange; positive and negative influences on the fetus.

(iii) *Maternal changes.* Symptoms and signs of pregnancy; diagnosis of pregnancy and duration; weight gain, changes in breasts and uterus, striae, pigmentation, prominence of veins, bladder function; psychological alterations (dependency, anxiety, mood swings); minor disorders (nausea, heartburn, constipation, haemorrhoids, varicose veins, backache, oedema, and fainting).

Antenatal Care

(i) *Objects* of care.

(ii) *Visits* (when and why).

(iii) *Routines.* History; examination of mother and fetus; clinical tests (blood, urine, ultrasonic, radiographic).

(iv) *Drugs,* X-rays and live virus vaccines in pregnancy.

(v) *Disorders specific to pregnancy.* Early pregnancy bleeding, late pregnancy bleeding, preeclampsia, multiple pregnancy, malpresentations, prematurity.

(vi) *Coexisting disease and pregnancy.* Common medical disorders (urinary tract infection, asthma, hypertension, epilepsy, diabetes).

(vii) *Well-being of the fetus.* Clinical features, laboratory tests.

(viii) *Sociology of pregnancy.* Social deprivation, the social worker, home help, maternity benefits, adoption and fostering.

(ix) *Activities.* Sport, physiotherapy, intercourse (libido changes, dangers), travelling, professional and household work, rest.

Nutrition and Hygiene of Pregnancy

(i) *Basic foodstuffs.* Proteins, fats, carbohydrates, vitamins, minerals; meats and fish, dairy produce, vegetables, fruits.

(ii) *Balanced diet.* Adequate protein, moderate carbohydrate, adequate fibre.

(iii) *Effects of food preparation.* Cooking denaturation.

(iv) *Additives.* Iron, folic acid, vitamins, calcium, fluoride.

(v) *General hygiene.* Bathing, fresh air; care of teeth; dental check-ups, changes in and care of skin and hair, care of breasts and nipples.

(vi) *Maternity clothes, baby's requirements.*

Breast Feeding

(i) *History.* Previous experience of the mother and attitudes of the couple.

(ii) *Advantages.*

(iii) *Physiology* of lactation.

(iv) *Care* of breast and nipple.

(v) *Breast expression* in late pregnancy.

Changes in Labour

(i) *Orientation.* Visit to the delivery suite; general familiarization with routines.

(ii) *The onset of labour.* Causes of labour, true and false labour, show, induction of labour.

(iii) *Stages of labour, duration.* The 3 stages — first stage (dilatation): latent phase, acceleration, deceleration; second stage (expulsion); third stage (delivery of placenta and membranes).

(iv) *Physiology.* Uterine contractions, cervical effacement and dilatation, rupture of membranes, 'mechanisms', secondary powers, positive and negative influences (parity, size and position of baby, size of pelvis, efficiency of contractions).

(v) *Pain relief.* Causes of pain, pain threshold (factors raising and lowering this), breathing patterns, effleurage, rubbing and their relation to the stages of labour, role of husband, drugs (sedatives, tranquillizers, narcotics), local analgesia (routes and time of application), inhalational analgesia (nitrous oxide, Penthrane, Trilene), anaesthesia. The patient should be aware of the rhythm of labour and work with contractions (using relaxation and breathing control ± analgesia as required) rather than denial or diversion (the hallmarks of psychoprophylaxis).

Delivery of the Baby

(i) *Normal vaginal delivery.* Bearing down, crowning, assistance at delivery of the baby and the placenta.

(ii) *Variations.* Multiple pregnancy, breech presentation, face presentation, oxytocic drugs, episiotomy and repair.

(iii) *Instrumental vaginal delivery.* Indications (delay, maternal or fetal distress), vacuum extraction or forceps.

(iv) *Abdominal delivery — Caesarean section.* Indications, anaesthesia, recovery.

(v) *Birth before arrival.* Getting to hospital in time; failing this, what to do.

The Puerperium

(i) *Returning to normal.* Uterus, afterpains, lochia, diuresis.

(ii) *Lactation.* Early congestion, milk flow, rooming-in techniques, *difficulties* (measurement of intake, breasts, nipples, baby, test feeding), suppression, artificial feeding.

(iii) *Wound care.* Perineum (icepacks, therapeutic ultrasound, bathing, heat), Caesarean section, analgesia, sutures.

(iv) *Emotional changes.* Transient depression, relation to baby, relation to husband.

(v) *Activity.* Ambulation, visitors, showering and bathing, exercises (importance of the postnatal period as a time for exercising the abdominal wall and pelvic floor), discharge home, resumption of coitus.

(vi) *Care of the baby.* Bathing (requirements, technique), bladder and bowel behaviour, napkin techniques, clothing, crying (normal and abnormal), sleeping, early development (weighing, milestones, aids to physical and mental development), special problems (twins, prematurity, intensive care).

(vii) *Family planning.* Spacing desired, methods.

(viii) *Postnatal visit.* Importance, information required concerning mother and baby.

PHYSIOTHERAPY
The Physiotherapist's Role
Better Health
Essentials of diet, rest, sleep and exercise.

Muscles and Joints
(i) Types of muscle — skeletal, smooth, cardiac; muscles of importance in reproduction. Mechanisms of control of muscle function — voluntary and involuntary; contraction and relaxation; coordination of different muscles.

(ii) Joints of importance in reproduction; effects of pregnancy, laxity, strains — flat feet, back strain.

(iii) Correct posture, lifting techniques, nursery furniture that is posturally safe, resting positions.

(iv) Exercises — control of diaphragm, abdominal, back, and pelvic muscles; special situations (e.g. postoperative).

(v) Perineal massage. Preparation of the vagina and perineum by regular antenatal stretching massage may reduce the incidence of tears and episiotomy, and facilitate the baby's birth. As with preparation of the breasts this should commence in the third trimester.

(vi) Effects of emotional tension on muscles.

Respiration

(i) *Elementary anatomy.* The upper and lower respiratory passages, the thoracic cage and diaphragm.

(ii) *Elementary physiology.* Vital capacity, tidal volume, gas exchange.

(iii) *Effect on venous blood return.* Prevention of venous thrombosis.

(iv) *Breathing techniques in labour.* Role in labour management — occupying mind during contractions; counteraction of the tendency to breathholding in the second stage; aid in the inhibition of expulsive efforts as required at delivery.

Need for proper practice and timing: early labour — slow, deep breathing; later labour — shallower and faster breathing; transition — still fast and shallow, blowing out each 4th–6th breath; second stage — deeper before pushing. The breathing pattern should be dictated by the strength of the contraction, the stage of labour and the oxygen requirements of the fetus.

(v) *Hyperventilation.* Effects and avoidance.

(vi) *Effects of smoking.* Pharmacological (nicotine, carbon monoxide); pathological (emphysema, fibrosis).

(vii) *The patient with chest pathology.* Correct aeration, adequate removal of secretions.

Contributions to Pain Relief

(i) Methods of handling pain: distraction, dissociation, denial, endurance (stoics), pharmacological.

(ii) Threshold for pain: effects of ignorance, fear, anxiety, fatigue; mental relaxation and meditation.

(iii) 'Active' muscular relaxation.

(iv) Comfortable positioning in labour.

(v) Distraction: breathing techniques, firm rubbing for back pain, effleurage = light stroking of abdomen or thighs.

(vi) Optimum use of analgesic agents, especially inhalational types.

General Advice

THE HUSBAND

Involvement in Reproductive Process
Heredity: chromosomes and genes, male has 50% responsibility, sex determination, blood groups, other heredity problems.

Overview of Relevant Anatomical, Physiological, Psychological Changes

(i) *Anatomical changes.* Early and late pregnancy, relation to symptoms.

(ii) *Physiological changes.* Nausea and vomiting, fatigue, insomnia, altered temperature appreciation due to vasodilation, need for rest.

(iii) *Psychological changes.* Lability, dependence, anxieties.

Supporting Role
Physical (greater help in the home), *psychological* (morale, understanding of pregnancy changes and upsets, help with educational and physiotherapy aspects), labour ward, the puerperium, when baby comes home, fatherhood.

Results in *consolidation of the family unit* and *closer marital ties.*

Sexual Relations
Possible changes in libido during pregnancy and after delivery; possible role in abortion and premature labour (prostaglandins, trauma); high standard of hygiene necessary; puerperium and perineal repair; family planning.

CHILDREN

If it is intended that children join the parents during labour, some prior antenatal education is desirable.

A simplified explanation is necessary of the changes during pregnancy and the process of labour. In the latter would be included some basic anatomy and physiology, examinations, labour discomfort and its alleviation, rupture of the membranes and liquor amnii, episiotomy, the birth process, including the delivery of the placenta and associated blood loss. If old enough, the child, like the father, may wish to hold the new brother or sister.

Passing the Examination

Although the details of the examination system differ from one place to another, it is necessary that all students master the techniques required in both written and oral examinations.

THE WRITTEN EXAMINATION

In each training centre, there will usually be copies of past examination papers. The student should read as many of these as are available to see the types of questions that are asked. It will quickly become obvious that the number of suitable questions is limited. In many nursing and medical schools, the *essay* type question has partly been replaced by more specific questions that have 3 or more subsections or by multiple choice questions. Because there are many parts to each question, a wide range of topics in both obstetrics and neonatal paediatrics is covered. *The candidate who has practised the art of self expression has an enormous advantage in examinations.*

It should not need emphasizing that *literacy* and *neatness* remain qualities cherished by all examiners. *Headings and important statements should be underlined.*

The Golden Rules

(i) *Read the paper carefully*. Even in postgraduate medical examinations 10% or more of candidates fail because they misread one or more questions.

(ii) Where possible, *devote equal time to each question*. When questions carry equal marks it is poor technique to spend too much time on one which you can answer in great detail. Furthermore, when the paper indicates the distribution of marks to be given for each subsection of a question, the candidate should again divide the time available in an appropriate manner.

(iii) *Interpret the examiner's intent*. 'List' or 'Enumerate' mean the same thing and an essay is *not* required. However, an answer can be too terse to be correct without qualification e.g. 'List

the causes of a high head at term'. The important causes are multiparity, incorrect menstrual data, posterior position of the occiput, placenta praevia, and cephalopelvic disproportion due to deflexion, malpresentation or pelvic contraction. In a recent examination, many candidates wrote multiple pregnancy, which is an ambiguous answer without the explanation that the mobile head belongs to the second fetus, the presenting part of the first being deep within the pelvis.

'Write notes on' indicates that the candidate should deliver as much important information as possible on the subject in the time available. Items of lesser importance can be added if time permits.

'Discuss' really means more than the above i.e. it is not just the proferring of factual material. What is required is an opinion based on such material e.g. why such an event occurs, its significance, how it can be prevented, which of several available treatments may be more applicable, and so on.

Example:
   Write notes on:
   (a) Vasa praevia   (5 marks)
   (b) Afterpains   (5 marks)
   (c) Early ambulation of the puerperal patient
                                                         (5 marks)
   (d) Vulval haematoma in the puerperal patient
                                                         (5 marks)

In (a) the candidate should define vasa praevia, stating that a *fetal vessel* runs across the *internal os* in front of the presenting part. The condition is associated with velamentous insertion of the cord, a succenturiate lobe, or a *bipartite* placenta (colour plates 84 and 85). The placenta usually encroaches upon the lower uterine segment — grade 1 or 2 *placenta praevia*. The diagnosis can be made by *amnioscopy*, during vaginal examination, or on clinical evidence if *haemorrhage* occurs when the membranes rupture, and is accompanied by fetal *bradycardia*. The fetal blood which is lost remains pink (resistant to denaturation) with 10% NaOH, in contradistinction to all other types of bleeding, which are maternal in origin. Although rare, there is a high fetal mortality rate (80%) unless prompt recognition and delivery are effected.

In (b) it should be explained that afterpains occur after delivery and are due to *uterine contractions* caused by release of *oxytocin* from the *posterior lobe of the pituitary gland* and thus occur particularly during *breast feeding* when oxytocin release is stimulated. The patient is usually a *multipara*. Treatment is by administration of mild analgesics and explanation to the patient of the cause of the pain and the value of the contractions in promotion of *involution* of the uterus.

In (c) the candidate might be aware that in former times it was not uncommon for the puerperal patient to be confined to bed for a week or more (hence the German term '*wochenbett*' or week in bed); a common legacy of this practice, fortunately now rare, was 'white leg' due to venous thrombosis — a disability often lasting for the patient's lifetime. Thus, early ambulation is important in the prophylaxis of superficial and deep *venous thrombosis* in the legs, and hence pulmonary *embolism*, which is a leading cause of *maternal death*. Predisposing factors such as maternal *age*, *obesity*, *multiparity*, *Caesarean section*, *varicose veins* and *cardiac disease* should be enumerated. It is *not* necessary to state the treatment of superficial and deep venous thrombosis or pulmonary embolism.

A vulval haematoma (d) is usually associated with an *episiotomy* or *vaginal laceration*, particularly if suturing or haemostasis is imperfect (colour plate 34). The condition can be due to tearing of a vein during insertion of a pudendal nerve block, or can occur *spontaneously* during a normal delivery, in the absence of visible trauma, probably as a result of overdistension of vessels. The lesion may result in shock due to blood loss and thus blood transfusion may be required. The haematoma causes extreme pain, may extend into the paravaginal tissues, and *acute retention* of urine may necessitate catheterization of the bladder. Treatment may be *conservative* or by *incision and evacuation* of the clot; the latter method is more likely to result in *infection* and continued haemorrhage.

A Common Failing

Some students have literal minds and tend to learn by rote, and therefore are inclined to regurgitate a prepared answer rather than the one that is wanted.

Example 1.

'Discuss the errors of techniques which may be committed during a normal vertex delivery. How would you avoid them?'

This question was found to be too difficult because the technique required for a satisfactory answer was too sophisticated for the candidates to be able to do justice to their knowledge. In fact 41 of the 43 candidates answered the question as though it was worded 'How do you conduct a normal delivery?' The examiner of course had wanted the candidates to explain the *reasons* behind the various steps in the technique of a normal delivery.

(a) Errors of positioning are avoided by helping the patient shift into the left lateral or dorsal position. The services of an assistant are also useful at this stage for supervision of inhalation analgesia.

(b) The accoucheur must don mask, gown and gloves in the approved fashion, wash down the patient's vulva, and apply drapes in the proper manner. Errors in technique may result in *infection* of the mother's genital tract.

(c) When the presenting part comes on view, vaginal and perineal *lacerations* are avoided by timely episiotomy, preceded by infiltration of the perineum with a solution of 1% lignocaine. The latter step is needed to minimize maternal pain. Lacerations are also avoided by *maintaining flexion of the head*. This allows birth of the fetus with minimal distension of the mother's genital tract, since the presenting diameters are then smaller. Deflexion in effect increases the size of the head, as the occipitofrontal diameter (12.0 cm) is 25% greater than the suboccipitobregmatic (9.5 cm).

(d) Painful postanal prodding must be avoided while waiting for the next contraction. It is impossible to 'pick-up' the chin until the scalp is well on view.

(e) Sudden *emergence of the head* is avoided by asking the mother to stop pushing, and to breathe on the mask, as soon as the accoucheur has control of the head. This prevents perineal lacerations and fetal *cerebral damage* due to explosive delivery.

(f) *Faecal contamination* of the mother's genital tract and fetal respiratory tract may occur at this stage, unless a perineal pad is used in the correct manner to push the perineum away from the baby's face.

(g) If the head is not allowed to *restitute* and *externally rotate*, then internal rotation of the shoulders may fail to occur and the shoulders may become *impacted*. The shoulders must be brought into the anteroposterior diameter of the outlet, so that the anterior shoulder may be delivered from beneath the pubic symphysis.

(h) Delivery of the *posterior shoulder* is relatively easy. A common error is to perform this step too suddenly, with the result that the perineum is torn, or the episiotomy incision unnecessarily extended.

(i) Delivery of the trunk should be in the direction of the curve of Carus. Lateral flexion of the trunk is often overdone. It is common for the baby's head to be grasped incorrectly at this stage. He should *not be throttled*, but held by the back of the neck. If the head is not *lowered* at this stage the baby, who often begins to breathe at this time, may inhale amniotic fluid or blood from the episiotomy.

(j) The commonest error of technique in a normal delivery is mismanagement of the third stage by *fiddling with the uterine fundus* after the baby is born. This results in partial separation of the placenta because the normal mechanism of placental separation by retroplacental clot formation is interfered with. The result is often *postpartum haemorrhage*. The crux of the proper management of the third stage of labour is the timely administration of an oxytocic drug immediately after the baby is born. It is proper to exclude the presence of an unsuspected second twin. It is improper to continue to palpate and knead the uterus. '*Guarding the fundus*' with the palm of the hand after completion of the second stage was a term dear to the instructors of the past. They were on the alert for the fundus enlarging due to the uterus filling with blood. With the use of oxytocics this no longer occurs. The accoucheur of course is watching the vagina; it is impossible for a patient to be bleeding heavily (in the absence of a ruptured uterus) unless there is copious visible blood loss. Another reason for guarding the fundus in the past was to identify the return of contractions so that the separated placenta could be expressed by the Dublin method of fundal pressure i.e. using the contracted uterus like a piston to expel the placenta. With the general use of oxytocic drugs and controlled cord traction as the favoured method for delivery of the placenta, this other excuse for fiddling with the fundus is no longer acceptable. *Traction* on the cord must never be performed unless the uterus is contracted because of the risk of *acute inversion of the uterus*.

(k) The patient must not be left unattended with the placenta undelivered because of the risk of *postpartum haemorrhage*.

(l) The risk of postpartum eclampsia or cerebral haemorrhage is reduced by the routine recording of the patient's *blood pressure* after delivery, and by testing the next available specimen of urine for *protein*. The signs of *preeclampsia* often occur for the first time during labour or within 2 hours of delivery, and indicate the need for the usual treatment with sedative and hypotensive drugs.

Example 2.

What is the significance of the following:
(a) Proteinuria at 32 weeks' gestation

(6 marks)
(b) Painless vaginal bleeding at 34 weeks' gestation   (6 marks)
(c) A high, mobile head in a nullipara at 40 weeks' gestation   (8 marks)

This question was answered very badly since most of the candidates were unable to explain the *significance* or *importance* of these signs i.e. what do they mean in terms of the likely causes and what influence these conditions may have on the mother and baby.

(a) However, the best answer to this part of the question was first class, and read as follows:

Protein found in the urine at 32 weeks may be significant of a *urinary tract infection*, *contamination* of the urine from vaginal discharge, *preeclampsia*, associated *chronic renal disease* such as pyelonephritis, or perhaps if the membranes have ruptured early, liquor draining into the urine will show protein. Investigations are carried out to determine the cause. In a urinary tract infection a microscopic examination and culture of the urine would give positive findings. Preeclampsia is diagnosed if the proteinuria is seen in conjunction with hypertension and oedema. The patient is hospitalized and treated depending on the cause.

The most common error was for the candidate to write a short essay on preeclampsia — for example:

'Preeclampsia is a condition when the health of the mother and fetus is in danger if not promptly controlled when first recognized'.

This type of answer was not due to deficient knowledge but to poor technique. The candidate had not grasped the point that the *significance* of a *sign* depended upon the *diagnosis*, which in turn depended upon the presence or absence of *other signs* and symptoms. For evaluation of the significance, a diagnosis must be made.

It is correct to list the possible causes of

proteinuria, and then to identify the actual one by consideration of other clinical findings, and the results of special investigations. Thus proteinuria in the third trimester is very likely to be due to preeclampsia, but not in the absence of *hypertension* and *generalized oedema* — unless treatment with hypotensives and diuretics has removed these other signs. In the absence of these other signs, proteinuria is quite likely to be due to contamination or a nonhypertensive form of renal disease. If the proteinuria was also present in a mid-stream specimen of urine, it would be reasonable to obtain a specimen for microscopy and culture by *catheterization*, particularly if speculum examination revealed that the patient did not have a vaginal discharge. Likewise, if the patient had scalding, frequency, and loin pain, the proteinuria would most likely be due to a *urinary tract infection*. The answer to this question did *not require any mention of treatment*. The objective of the question was to assess whether or not the candidate appreciated the importance of proteinuria in late pregnancy. What was the likely cause? How could this be verified by seeking the expected associated signs and symptoms?

In this examination one candidate wrote that 'the significance of proteinuria is a mother with a large family rushing around'!

Candidates often state that oedema is a sign of preeclampsia. This is *incorrect*, because *peripheral oedema*, which is the common type of oedema seen in pregnancy, is not a sign of pre-eclampsia. Oedema of the lower limbs is due to pressure of the enlarging uterus upon the pelvic veins, often in a patient who has *varicose veins*. Hence the need to inspect the fingers and face for evidence that the excessive accumulation of fluid is *generalized*.

(b) *The significance of painless vaginal bleeding at 34 weeks' gestation depends upon the cause* and *severity* of the bleeding, the state of the *fetus*, and whether or not the patient is in *labour*. Painless bleeding, particularly if recurrent, would be suggestive of *placenta praevia*, especially if a high, unstable presenting part indicated that there was a soft tissue mass preventing it from entering the pelvic brim. A diagnosis of *abruptio placentae* would be more likely if the fetal head was in the pelvis, and the uterus was *tense and tender*. It would be unusual for there to be evidence of severe abruption (fetal death, blood coagulation failure, or renal failure) in the absence of pain. Painless bleeding could be due to *incidental causes* such as vaginitis, cervical polyp or carcinoma, conditions which would be diagnosed by speculum examination 24 hours after the bleeding had settled down.

Vaginal bleeding signifies an *increased hazard to both mother and fetus*. For the mother there are the risks of shock due to blood loss and those associated with operative delivery. For the fetus there are those associated with prematurity and breech or forceps delivery. It would be relevant, in an answer to this question, to state that *ultrasonography* should be performed to see if there was a *placenta praevia*, or evidence of *retroplacental blood clot* if the placenta was normally situated.

Most of the candidates gave details of the treatment of placenta praevia or accidental haemorrhage, although this was not required. Many stated that labour could be induced by rupture of the membranes if placenta praevia was the cause of bleeding. This is quite incorrect. *Caesarean section* is always necessary when placenta praevia causes bleeding of such degree that pregnancy must be terminated in a patient who is *not in labour*.

Other peculiar answers:

(i) 'Painless vaginal bleeding at 34 weeks' gestation is an accidental haemorrhage from the placental site and usually is an indication of placenta praevia.' The candidate clearly would be unable to define the terms placenta praevia and accidental haemorrhage.

(ii) 'When bleeding is due to placenta praevia, the condition of the fetus must be observed closely as it is its blood which is being lost.'

(iii) 'The dangers of placenta praevia are mainly dangers to the fetus during labour when separation of the placenta occurs, and massive vaginal haemorrhage causes exsanguination of the fetus.'

The authors of answers (ii) and (iii) clearly did not realize that in placenta praevia, bleeding, although due to separation of the placenta, is *maternal* in origin. The normal full term fetus weighs about 3,500 g and has a total of about 350 ml of circulating blood. In placenta praevia, fetal blood loss can occur only if the placenta is damaged, as is possible at Caesarean section or if an instrument is introduced through the internal os; another possibility would be if there was tearing of an associated *vasa praevia*.

The fetus is more likely to die *in utero* when bleeding is due to placental abruption than to placenta praevia. In abruptio placentae, placental separation may be extensive, whereas with placenta praevia, bleeding is likely to be severe when only a small area of the placenta has been separated from the lower uterine segment.

The dangers faced by the fetus with placenta praevia are those of *prematurity*. In abruptio placentae there is the additional hazard of *intra-uterine hypoxia* due to placental separation.

(c) This part of the question was answered much better than the others except that most candidates only wrote a list of the causes of a high, mobile head. The complete answer would have indicated not only the *causes* but also the significance in terms of *fetal* and *maternal* prognosis. Thus a high head is likely to be due to relative or absolute cephalopelvic disproportion caused by deflexion, posterior position of the occiput, a large fetus or small pelvis. An error in the menstrual data could explain why the head had not entered the pelvis. Less common causes would be placenta praevia or tumours of uterus or ovary preventing the head from entering the pelvis. Many candidates correctly stated that an abnormally large head due to *hydrocephaly* could be the explanation, albeit quite rare. Many also stated that anencephaly could cause a high head at term, which is nonsense.

Few candidates stated that a high head indicated the need for a *trial of labour*, and that *X-ray pelvimetry* may be warranted. Other significant points would be that the patient would have an increased risk of requiring a Caesarean section or forceps delivery. The possibility of an *operative delivery* is also significant in terms of fetal morbidity and mortality.

THE ORAL EXAMINATION

The following section has been included in the book mainly to help students prepare for oral examinations. It is placed at the end of the book since it should also prove helpful for revision. The questions appear with no special order as is also the case in an examination, and in the practice of obstetrics and neonatal paediatrics. The candidate must be ready to switch onto any aspect of the subject. This chapter is fairly detailed because we believe that the learning process is assisted by exposure to such clinically orientated questions. The more difficult questions (but popular with examiners) have been collected together in a following section. The reader can move a ruler down the page and participate in an examination, and at the same time improve factual knowledge (it is useless to know the questions without the answers). The questionnaire has been designed to span the entire syllabus.

Since education is basically aimed at increasing knowledge, improving attitudes and facilitating practice, the student should try and develop a *logical framework of thinking* rather than rote memory. For example, in a discussion of the causes of fetal hypoxia, one would seek the broadest classification initially (mother, conceptus) and work to a more detailed analysis — e.g. *mother*: conditions in the heart, lungs, blood, uterus; *baby*: placenta, umbilical cord, fetus itself.

Examination Questions and Answers

Most of these questions highlight an important clinical problem. Do not read them merely to learn the answer but, after reading the question, see if you have understood the problem and its management, by reading the answer after you have decided on a course of action. These are the common questions asked in clinical examinations or in the short answer written papers which have replaced multiple choice questions in many centres. In many cases the answers are deliberately not exhaustive — it is the headlines that are important!

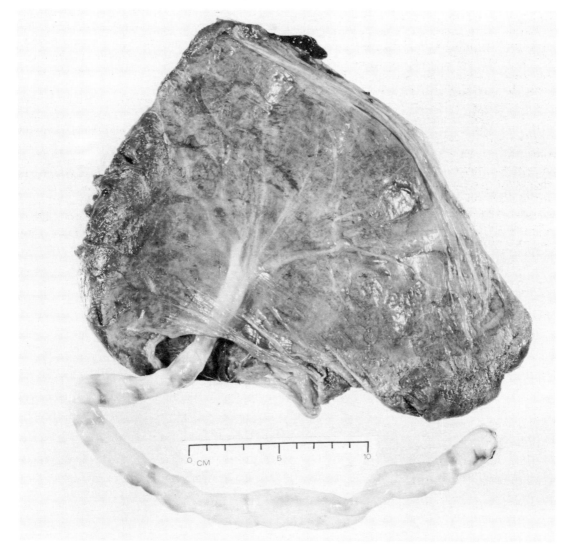

Figure IIIA.1 This placenta was delivered with difficulty after failed controlled cord traction (Brandt-Andrews method) and catheterization of the bladder, by pressure on the contracted uterine fundus (i.e. the Dublin method — see figure 43.4 and Question 88, Appendix IIIA). The patient was a 29-year-old para 2 in whom labour was induced at 37 weeks' gestation because her previous pregnancy had resulted in intrauterine death at 40.3 weeks' gestation. The placental edge was not palpated at amniotomy; 4 hours later the patient had a normal delivery of a healthy female infant, birthweight 3,100 g. Note that the hole of fetal exit in the membranes abuts upon the edge of the placenta (weight 740 g) — which is indicative of a marginal (grade 1) placenta praevia. This patient had neither antepartum, intrapartum nor postpartum haemorrhage — about 10% of cases of placenta praevia are diagnosed in such patients (no antepartum haemorrhage) by inspection of the secundines after vaginal delivery (see Question 66, Appendix IIIA and Chapter 19).

1. Q. **How would you estimate the expected date of confinement?**
    A. By adding 9 months and 7 days to the first day of the last menstrual period.

2. Q. **If the patient has irregular cycles, or has not menstruated since the birth of her last baby, how would you estimate the maturity of her pregnancy?**
    A. In early pregnancy, by the size of the uterus on bimanual examination and by noting the date on which *quickening* occurred. Special tests (compound ultrasound scanning) could also be used. In later pregnancy, information from the fundal height can be assisted by further tests (ultrasonography, radiography; lecithin/sphingomyelin (L:S) ratio for functional maturity).

3. Q. **How may the contraceptive pill 'cause' prolonged pregnancy?**
    A. When the pill is discontinued there is a hormone withdrawal menstruation, and ovulation may be delayed 2 to 8 weeks. The patient then conceives, but her pregnancy is less mature than the duration of amenorrhoea would indicate.

4. Q. **What are the signs of preeclampsia?**
    A. Hypertension, generalized oedema and proteinuria which is not explained by urinary contamination or infection. Note that oedema must be generalized, and that excessive weight gain is *not* one of the 3 signs, although it is a frequent precursor.

5. Q. **What uses have fetal fontanelles?**
    A. They allow *moulding* in labour and *growth* of the enclosed brain after birth. They are also useful in the diagnosis of *position* of the head in labour and the state of intracranial tension after birth.

6. Q. **What are the commonest causes of acute variation in intracranial tension in the neonatal period?**
    A. Respiration, crying and defaecation. You can see the anterior fontanelle bounce up and down at these times.

7. Q. **When does the anterior fontanelle close? (i.e. when is the phase of rapid growth of the infant's brain completed?).**
    A. At about 18 months of age.

8. Q. **What would lead you to suspect the diagnosis of oesophageal atresia after birth?**
    A. If there was polyhydramnios and no visible explanation such as anencephaly, hydrocephaly or hydrops fetalis. A firm 10-gauge catheter would be passed immediately to see if the oesophagus was patent (if diagnosis is delayed, feeding would cause cyanotic attacks due to inhalation of the feeding).

9. Q. **What are Braxton Hicks contractions? (figure 38.3).**
    A. Painless uterine contractions which occur throughout pregnancy, but are more obvious in the later months. They are not accompanied by dilatation of the internal os.

10. Q. **What is the cause of the show of blood at the start of labour?**
    A. It is due to commencement of cervical dilatation and taking up of the cervix. The operculum (mucus plug) is shed (colour plate 83), and there is a little bleeding as the membranes are stripped away from the cervix.

11. Q. **What do you tell a patient when she asks: When do I come into hospital to have the baby?**
    A. The patient should come in when she has either regular painful contractions, bleeding, or leakage of amniotic fluid. It is best to err on the side of coming in too soon. She can always go home and most husbands fear the possibility of having to deliver their wife at home.

12. Q. **What would make you suspect that a patient had twins at 30 weeks' gestation?**
    A. (a) Excessive weight gain and development of anaemia.
    (b) *Undue uterine enlargement*, palpation of many limbs or more than 2 fetal poles, or feeling a small engaged head when the fetal mass above seemed disproportionately large.

(c)   The diagnosis would also be considered if a multipara developed preeclampsia when she had never done so in previous pregnancies.

13.   Q.   **What antenatal complications are more common in multiple pregnancy?**
A.   Preeclampsia, anaemia (iron and folic acid deficiency), pressure symptoms, premature labour, and malpresentations.

14.   Q.   **What are the contraindications to external cephalic version?**
A.   (a)   Antepartum haemorrhage.
(b)   Multiple pregnancy.
(c)   Fetal malformations easier to deliver as a breech (anencephaly and hydrocephaly).
(d)   Ruptured membranes — cord prolapse could occur.
(e)   Maturity less than 32 weeks — there is the risk of premature labour and in any case the fetus may turn spontaneously.
(f)   Planned Caesarean section — (see Question 56 Appendix IIIB).
(g)   Severe hypertension or preeclampsia.

15.   Q.   **What are the complications of attempted external cephalic version?**
A.   (a)   Premature labour or rupture of the membranes.
(b)   Placental abruption or uterine rupture due to the use of excessive force are most likely to occur when general anaesthesia is used, and the patient's abdominal and uterine walls are relaxed.
(c)   Fetomaternal haemorrhage (see Question 167 Appendix IIIA).
(d)   Fetal hypoxia due to cord entanglement.

16.   Q.   **How would you recognize that labour has become obstructed?**
A.   (a)   *Failure of progress* of cervical dilatation and descent of the presenting part in spite of good contractions. This applies particularly to multiparas, since obstruction is likely to result in uterine exhaustion (inertia) in nulliparas.
(b)   The presence of a retraction ring, visible and palpable at about the level of the umbilicus, above the distended lower segment and bladder (figure 52.4).
(c)   Signs of fetal and maternal distress are likely to be present due to prolonged labour.
(d)   Vaginal examination would show marked *caput and moulding* and possibly a malpresentation or posterior position of the occiput. There may be an oedematous anterior lip of cervix.
(e)   The head is probably palpable abdominally and *not engaged*.

17.   Q.   **What causes the increase of physiological vaginal discharge during pregnancy?**
A.   Hypertrophy of the cervical glands and increased vascularity of the lower genital tract.

18.   Q.   **What are the 2 common causes of vaginal infection during pregnancy — both often causing irritation?**
A.   Trichomonas and monilia.

19.   Q.   **What symptoms would cause you to suspect that the patient had a vaginal infection?**
A.   A yellow or white discharge, especially if associated with pruritus vulvae.

20.   Q.   **What is the typical appearance of monilial vaginitis as seen during speculum examination?**
A.   The vaginal epithelium is oedematous and has *white patches* like curds, which when dislodged leave reddened areas (figure 27.2). The appearance is similar to thrush in a baby's mouth and the same fungus is the cause of both conditions.

21.   Q.   **What is the treatment of monilial vaginitis?**
A.   Application with a cotton wool swab of *gentian violet* 1% aqueous solution, after cleansing with 1% solution of acetic acid. The other effective method is the use of *nystatin* or similar pessaries, one of which is inserted each night, for 2 weeks.

22.   Q.   **What is the typical appearance of trichomonas vaginitis as seen during speculum examination?**
A.   There is a frothy, greenish-yellow, offensive discharge which tends to collect in the posterior fornix. The vagina has many small, red 'strawberry' spots (figure 27.3).

23. **Q. What is the treatment of trichomonas vaginitis?**
    A. Metronidazole 200 mg tablets by mouth, 1 three times daily for one week, or tinidazole 2 g orally (4 × 500 mg tablets) as a single dose.

24. **Q. Why do vaginal infections recur after treatment?**
    A. Reinfection from the husband who should be treated at the same time as his wife if infection recurs, or if he has symptoms. Another possibility in monilial infections is that the patient may have a predisposing cause such as *diabetes mellitus*, which is excluded by performing a glucose tolerance test. Systemic (oral) treatment of the patient may be necessary.

25. **Q. What symptoms may the husband have when his wife has trichomonas or monilial vaginitis?**
    A. Penile and scrotal rash with intolerable itching. He is prescribed metronidazole, nystatin cream or gentian violet solution according to the cause of his symptoms.

26. **Q. What are condylomata?**
    A. They are warts which differ in size and are usually multiple; they are found usually in the vagina and on the vulva and perineum.

27. **Q. What are the causes of condylomata?**
    A. The common variety are *condylomata acuminata* (figure 6.2) which are due to a papilloma virus infection, but occur in association with vaginitis due to trichomonas or monila. *Condylomata lata* are due to *syphilis* which should always be excluded in patients with genital warts. Pregnancy predisposes to the rapid growth of condylomata acuminata.

28. **Q. What is the significance of vaginal bleeding during the first trimester?**
    A. By definition the patient has a *threatened abortion* (even if speculum examination reveals a cervical erosion as the possible site of haemorrhage). If there are no associated painful uterine contractions and the cervix is closed the risk of spontaneous abortion is at least *20%*. If bleeding is heavier and associated with *pain*, the risk of abortion is at least *80%*, even if the cervix is closed.

29. **Q. What are the causes of spontaneous first trimester abortion?**
    A. (a) Usually there is death or developmental failure of the fetus. The cause of this is usually not known although *chromosomal abnormalities* are present in about 40% of cases. This may be Nature's method for rejection of the imperfect. Usually no *fetus* is present in first trimester abortions.
       (b) Infection of the fetus (rubella) or pyrexia due to maternal infection (influenza, hepatitis or pyelonephritis).
       (c) Defective corpus luteum.
       (d) Uterine malformation.
       (e) Physical or emotional trauma.

30. **Q. What are the causes of second trimester abortion?**
    A. The important cause is an *incompetent cervix* which may be treated by cervical ligation (colour plate 35). Other causes are uterine abnormalities and intrauterine fetal death due to maternal pyrexia, cord entanglements or erythroblastosis (colour plate 89). Retroplacental haemorrhage and placenta praevia are other causes.

31. **Q. What are the signs of maternal distress in labour?**
    A. Tachycardia, oliguria and ketonuria. These are the signs of dehydration and starvation and are often associated with signs of obstructed labour. Hypertension is not a sign of distress, but of preeclampsia.

32. **Q. What are the causes of maternal collapse in labour in the absence of visible blood loss?**
    A. Accidental haemorrhage, postural hypotension, uterine rupture, cardiac failure, pulmonary venous or amniotic fluid embolism and septicaemia. Also the patient may have had a convulsion (eclamptic or epileptic) or a cerebral (usually subarachnoid) haemorrhage.

33. **Q. What is the explanation of postural hypotension in late pregnancy or labour?**
    A. When the patient lies on her back the enlarged uterus compresses the inferior vena cava

and reduces venous return to the heart (figure 48.1). There is a fall in cardiac output and blood pressure, then bradycardia occurs and the patient faints.

34. Q. **What is the treatment of the postural hypotensive syndrome?**
    A. Turn the patient onto her side until she has recovered. Instruct her to avoid lying on her back for any length of time. Administration of oxygen may also be helpful.

35. Q. **What are the clinical signs of fetal distress in labour?**
    A. Fetal heart rate above 160 or below 120 beats per minute, the passage of meconium, or both. Convulsive fetal movements are usually quoted as a sign of fetal distress, but have little clinical importance since it is unlikely that there would be time to act.

36. Q. **What are the causes of fetal bradycardia?**
    A. (a) *Pressure* on the base of the brain causes reflex slowing of the heart (mediated by the vagus nerve). Because of the fontanelles and suture lines, pressure is transmitted to the fetal brain during a uterine contraction or abdominal palpation (Pawlik grip).
    (b) *Hypoxia* is the important cause of fetal bradycardia and causes slowing towards the end or after a uterine contraction, rather than during the height of the contraction.

37. Q. **How may the fetal condition be investigated when signs of distress are present in labour?**
    A. The *fetal blood pH* can be measured and the heart rate monitored accurately in relationship to the timing of contractions, with special electronic equipment. This enables the clinician to decide if labour may safely be allowed to continue, or if immediate delivery is necessary.

38. Q. **What is the usual cause of delay in the second stage of labour?**
    A. Tense pelvic floor musculature ('tight perineum') in a nullipara.

39. Q. **What is the treatment of delay in the second stage of labour which results from a tight perineum?**
    A. Episiotomy, after infiltration of the perineum with 1% lignocaine, followed by spontaneous or forceps delivery. If maternal exhaustion has occurred, contractions will be weak and infrequent and forceps are required to prevent further delay.

40. Q. **What are the fetal risks when delivery is delayed in the second stage of labour?**
    A. Brain damage or death due to hypoxia. Continued retraction of muscle fibres in the upper uterine segment impairs placental transfer and there is compression of the head in the lower birth canal. Another possibility is acute hypoxia due to *placental separation* or tightening of a knot in the cord or a cord tangled around the baby.

41. Q. **What would you do if called to a patient delivered 4 days ago who has a temperature of 39°C?**
    A. (a) Ask if there were symptoms of infection of the respiratory or genitourinary tracts, or of the breasts.
    (b) Inspect the vulva for signs of an infected *episiotomy wound* or vaginal laceration, and ask if there was an excessive or offensive vaginal discharge. Palpate the uterus for tenderness suggestive of severe endometritis.
    (c) Look for evidence of venous thrombosis in the legs, and engorgement or infection of the breasts.

42. Q. **What investigations are performed when a patient has puerperal pyrexia?**
    A. (a) A smear and culture (aerobic and anaerobic) of a high vaginal swab.
    (b) Microscopy and culture of a mid-stream or less commonly a catheter specimen of urine.
    (c) Culture of the milk.
    (d) Blood culture if the cause of the infection remains elusive or the patient is seriously ill.
    (e) Blood examination to exclude anaemia.

43. Q. **What conditions are associated with the occurrence of striae in the skin?**
    A. Pregnancy, rapid weight gain in adolescence, adrenal steroid therapy, and Cushing syndrome.

44. Q. **In what areas do striae gravidarum occur most commonly?**
    A. The abdominal wall below the level of the umbilicus, upper and outer aspects of the thighs, and the lower quadrants of the breasts (colour plates 65–74).

45. Q. **What are the advantages of an episiotomy?**
    A. (a) The risks of trauma to the fetal head and fetal hypoxia are reduced by hastening the birth of the baby.
       (b) Overdistension of maternal tissues is avoided thus minimizing the risks of genital prolapse.
       (c) Perineal and vaginal lacerations are prevented; these are often more painful than an episiotomy, and are more difficult to suture.

46. Q. **What are the disadvantages of an episiotomy?**
    A. The patient has a sore perineum for 5 days, and often experiences *dyspareunia* for 2 or 3 months after coitus is resumed. Also the average *blood loss* is increased by 150 ml, and there are the possibilities of *infection* and *haematoma* formation (colour plate 34).

47. Q. **Does continued lactation delay the return of the menses after childbirth?**
    A. Yes, usually by 2–4 months or more, and therefore lactation has some value in 'family planning' in that the return of ovulation is also delayed.

48. Q. **Can a patient conceive while still lactating, if no menstruation has occurred since her baby was born?**
    A. Yes. The first menstruation after childbirth is usually (80%) preceded by ovulation. Some women can identify the 'at risk of conception' time by noting changes in the nature of the *cervical mucus*. Apart from this, the 'safe period' method of birth control cannot be used during lactational amenorrhoea.

49. Q. **In breech delivery what is the position of the sacrum when the breech emerges from the vagina?**
    A. It is *lateral* because the buttocks are born by *lateral flexion of the trunk*, through the 90° curve of Carus (figure 50.7). If the sacrum was anterior the breech would not be able to negotiate the curve of the birth canal.

50. Q. **What treatment is indicated when a patient is found to have acetone or ketones in the urine during labour?**
    A. The mother's condition should be improved by *hydration* and caloric replacement (intra-venous infusion of 5% dextrose) and *sedation*; the labour may need to be terminated (forceps or Caesarean section) if the maternal distress persists. Diabetic ketosis may also be a rare cause.

51. Q. **What are the indications for intravenous fluid therapy in labour?**
    A. Apart from the conditions requiring or likely to require blood transfusion (e.g. multiple pregnancy), intravenous therapy is required before epidural analgesia is commenced and when there is maternal or fetal distress, prolonged labour, or if general anaesthesia is likely to be required at delivery. An intravenous oxytocin infusion may be used to initiate or accelerate labour, usually when amniotomy has failed to do so, and also to accelerate labour if uterine action is ineffective.

52. Q. **What conditions predispose to hyperemesis gravidarum?**
    A. Multiple pregnancy, hydatidiform mole and infection, especially of the urinary tract. It is usual to exclude these in all patients admitted to hospital with this diagnosis.

53. Q. **What are the warning signs and symptoms that suggest that a patient with nausea and vomiting should be admitted to hospital?**
    A. Evidence of dehydration and starvation (oliguria, loss of weight and tissue turgor, and ketonuria), jaundice, proteinuria, or peripheral neuritis.

54. Q. **What are the principles in the treatment of hyperemesis gravidarum in a patient who requires admission to hospital?**
    A. Parenteral antiemetic and sedative drugs; replacement of fluids, electrolytes, vitamins and calories; and isolation (from in-laws and perhaps the husband!).

55. Q. **At what stage of pregnancy do patients usually complain of heartburn?**
    A. In late pregnancy when pressure of the enlarging uterus causes reflux of stomach contents into the oesophagus. The symptom is worst at night when the patient lies down.

56. Q. **What is the treatment of heartburn?**
    A. Antacid preparations and advice to sleep propped up with several pillows and/or raising of the head end of the bed.

57. Q. **Why are all babies given a vitamin K preparation (Konakion 1 mg) by intramuscular injection soon after birth?**
    A. To reduce the incidence of *haemorrhagic disease* of the newborn, since *vitamin K* is required for production of blood coagulation factors by the liver. (Vitamin K is normally produced in the gut by bacteria which colonize it only some days after birth).

58. Q. **What is a cephalhaematoma?**
    A. A collection of blood *beneath* the periosteum of a cranial bone (usually the parietal), and therefore the mass does not cross a suture line (colour plate 142).

59. Q. **What is the treatment of a large cephalhaematoma?**
    A. Haemoglobin estimation to exclude anaemia of such severity as to warrant blood transfusion. Occasionally haemolysis of the blood may result in jaundice requiring phototherapy or exchange transfusion; otherwise treatment is conservative and the mother is assured that the blood will be reabsorbed.

60. Q. **Why is it important for a patient to be admitted to hospital when the membranes rupture, even though she is not having contractions?**
    A. So that vaginal examination can be performed to exclude prolapse of the umbilical cord, and an oxytocin infusion given if uterine contractions do not occur spontaneously. If the patient is less than 36–37 weeks' pregnant, speculum rather than digital examination is performed and the patient is treated conservatively (rest in bed in hospital) until the baby is more mature.

61. Q. **How is progress in labour assessed?**
    A. (a) By observing the frequency, duration and strength of *uterine contractions*.
       (b) By abdominal, vaginal, and postanal palpation to note *descent and rotation of the presenting part*.
       (c) By vaginal examination to assess progressive *dilatation of the cervix*.

62. Q. **How do you recognize the onset of the second stage of labour?**
    A. (a) Positively if vaginal examination shows the cervix to be fully dilated.
       (b) When the patient involuntarily wants to bear-down. There is often a bright show of blood as the cervix tears, and the membranes typically rupture at this time.
       (c) When the presenting part can be felt by postanal palpation, its greatest diameter is at the level of the ischial spines, and it may be inferred that the cervix is fully dilated.

63. Q. **What are the indications for a glucose tolerance test during pregnancy?**
    A. (a) Strong family history of diabetes.
       (b) Maternal obesity or *age over 35 years*.
       (c) Unexplained intrauterine fetal death.
       (d) Persistent or heavy glycosuria.
       (e) Polyhydramnios.
       (f) History of large (above 4,000 g) or malformed infants.

64. Q. **What conditions are associated with excessive placental size?**
    A. (a) Severe erythroblastosis fetalis.
       (b) Maternal diabetes mellitus (colour plates 92E and F).
       (c) Large fetus — multiple pregnancy also belongs in this category if the placentas are joined.
       (d) Maternal anaemia.
       (e) Syphilis and other infections (e.g. cytomegalovirus).
       (f) Nonimmunological hydrops fetalis (colour plate 11).

65.   Q. **When and why should vaginal examination be performed in labour?**
      A. (a) When signs of *fetal distress* are first recognized to exclude cord prolapse, and to
             ascertain whether conditions are suitable for vaginal delivery.
          (b) When the *membranes rupture* if the presenting part is high, or if there is polyhydram-
             nios or a malpresentation, to exclude cord prolapse.
          (c) Before a second dose of *narcotic* analgesic or *epidural block* for pain relief is ordered.
          (d) When *labour is prolonged* or the mother distressed, in order to *assess progress*, and
             decide whether Caesarean section is required.
          (e) Before any *manipulative* procedure such as forceps delivery, internal version, or
             manual removal of the placenta is undertaken.

66.   Q. **How can you make a positive diagnosis of placenta praevia by inspection of the
         secundines after a normal delivery?**
      A. The hole in the membranes will be close to the placental edge if the placenta has
         encroached onto the lower uterine segment (Appendix IIIA, figure 1).

67.   Q. **What are the causes of impacted shoulders?**
      A. (a) Big shoulders or a small pelvis.
          (b) Failure of the mechanism of internal rotation of the shoulders. This may be due to
             the accoucheur 'externally rotating' the head in the wrong direction, thus preventing
             the shoulders turning into the anteroposterior diameter of the pelvis.

68.   Q. **How do you diagnose impacted shoulders?**
      A. When the head is born the neck fails to appear — the *chin burrows* into the mother's
         buttocks and the usual degree of traction on the head fails to cause further descent.

69.   Q. **How would you manage a case of impacted shoulders?**
      A. Make more *room* (episiotomy), get *help* from above if available (fundal pressure by an
         assistant), allow *restitution* of the head, and then apply *traction* to it to bring the shoulders
         into the anteroposterior diameter of the pelvis. Traction is directed backwards and down-
         wards to get the *anterior shoulder* past the symphysis pubis (this is easier in the left lateral
         or lithotomy positions).

70.   Q. **How do you distinguish true from spurious labour?**
      A. In spurious labour cervical dilatation and effacement do not occur, although the patient
         may be distressed by the contractions.

71.   Q. **What is the treatment of spurious labour?**
      A. Administer a potent analgesic drug such as morphine (15 mg) or pethidine 100 mg by
         intramuscular injection. The patient is then sent home after a good rest if the contractions
         cease, after excluding fetoplacental dysfunction (which may indicate delivery) by
         cardiotocography.

72.   Q. **How do you determine if the head is engaged? (figures 6.7 and 6.8).**
      A. (a) Pawlik grip reveals less than 3 cm of head palpable abdominally when the greatest
             diameter has entered the pelvic brim, and the occiput is no longer palpable.
          (b) Vaginal examination or postanal palpation may show that the head is below the level
             of the ischial spines.

73.   Q. **What does the term perinatal mortality mean?**
      A. The number of stillbirths plus neonatal deaths in the first week of life.

74.   Q. **What is the perinatal mortality rate?**
      A. About 10–15 per 1,000 total births in developed countries.

75.   Q. **What are the positive clinical signs of pregnancy?**
      A. Palpable fetal movements, palpable fetal parts and auscultation of fetal heart sounds.

76.   Q. **What important conditions are associated with polyhydramnios?**
      A. (a) Malformations in which the ability of the fetus to swallow amniotic fluid is impaired
             e.g. *anencephaly*.
          (b) Maternal diabetes mellitus.
          (c) Multiple pregnancy. *Acute* polyhydramnios occurs only with uniovular twins during

the second trimester (figure 25.12).

   (d) Severe erythroblastosis.

77. Q. **What are the indications for forceps delivery?**
A. (a) Delay in the second stage of labour.
   (b) Fetal or maternal distress.
   (c) Constitutional maternal disorder such as cardiac disease.

78. Q. **What conditions are necessary for forceps application and delivery?**
A. (a) The presentation and position must be favourable. In a vertex presentation, forceps
   or manual rotation is performed if the occiput is not already in the anterior position.
   (b) The cervix must be fully dilated, else there is a grave risk of trauma to mother and
   fetus.
   (c) The head must be engaged.
   (d) The membranes should be ruptured, the bladder empty, and analgesia adequate.

79. Q. **Why is regional analgesia (pudendal nerve block or epidural) preferred for forceps delivery?**
A. To avoid the risk of inhalation of gastric contents during induction of general anaesthesia.

80. Q. **Why should exercises in the knee-elbow position be avoided by patients during the puerperium?**
A. When the patient stands up, contraction of perineal muscles raises pressure within the
vagina and fatal uterine venous *air embolism* can occur.

81. Q. **What are the principles in the treatment of a patient with an incomplete abortion?**
A. (a) Stop the bleeding by administration of ergometrine 0.5 mg by intravenous or intramuscular injection.
   (b) *Resuscitation* with intravenous fluid or blood if the patient is shocked.
   (c) With the patient in the left lateral or dorsal position a speculum is passed and clotted
   blood and placental tissues are removal from the vagina and cervix with sponge-
   holding forceps.
   (d) Antibiotic therapy is commenced (after taking a cervical swab for bacteriological
   examination) if there is evidence of infection.
   (e) *Curettage* is performed to remove remaining placental tissue.

82. Q. **What is the strength of a 'physiological' solution of oxytocin used to induce labour?**
A. Two units per litre.

83. Q. **What is the commonest cause of neonatal death?**
A. Idiopathic respiratory distress syndrome (hyaline membrane disease) which is almost
always due to *prematurity*.

84. Q. **What are the causes of death associated with breech delivery?**
A. (a) Hypoxia due to delay in delivery, cord compression, or placental separation.
   (b) Intracranial trauma.

85. Q. **What is achieved by exchange transfusion in an infant with severe erythroblastosis?**
A. (a) Correction of anaemia and congestive cardiac failure.
   (b) Removal of harmful maternal antibodies.
   (c) Removal of bilirubin and the risk of kernicterus.
   (d) Provision of blood which will not be haemolysed by antibodies remaining in the
   infant's circulation (e.g. in rhesus erythroblastosis, rhesus negative blood of the
   appropriate ABO blood group).

86. Q. **What is the force which drives fetal blood from the placenta back to the fetal heart?**
A. The blood pressure due to the fetal heart beat. Uterine contractions do *not* influence blood
flow in the fetus, which, being surrounded by fluid, is incompressible. There is a high
capillary pressure in the placental blood vessels.

87. Q. **What is the differential diagnosis of an eclamptic fit?**
A. (a) Epilepsy, meningitis, or intracranial tumour.
   (b) Cerebral haemorrhage due to a ruptured aneurysm.

    (c) Hypertensive encephalopathy or haemorrhage as may occasionally be caused by ergometrine.

    (d) Convulsions due to intravenous injection of local analgesic solution during an epidural or pudendal nerve block.

88. **Q. What would you do if a patient had a sudden postpartum haemorrhage of 800 ml immediately after the baby was born?**

  A. (a) *Rub* up the uterine fundus, administer 0.5 mg *ergometrine* by intravenous injection, pass a *catheter*, then deliver the *placenta* by controlled cord traction or by pressure on the contracted uterine fundus (the Dublin method).

    (b) If bleeding continued although the placenta was delivered, and the uterus well contracted, then the perineum, vagina and cervix would be inspected for *lacerations*.

    (c) Blood *coagulation failure* would be excluded by a clot observation test.

    (d) *Blood transfusion* and *manual exploration* of the uterus (for rupture or retained placental fragments) would be required if bleeding continued (colour plate 33).

    (e) Firm *bimanual compression* of the uterus allows time for the above to be organized, and may itself solve the problem.

89. **Q. When would you cut an episiotomy?**

  A. During a *contraction* when the perineum is stretched and thinned out.

90. **Q. What are the indications for an episiotomy?**

  A. Many obstetricians perform episiotomy almost routinely but the procedure is mandatory if a laceration appears inevitable, or when an inelastic perineum causes delay in the second stage of labour. Episiotomy is required to provide extra room when delivery is likely to be difficult, as in breech or forceps delivery, or when there is a persistent occipitoposterior position. It is performed to prevent pressure on the head during delivery, and is necessary for premature as well as term infants.

91. **Q. Why is a 'footling' the least favourable type of breech presentation?**

  A. There is a high (about 10%) incidence of cord prolapse, and the body is often delivered before the cervix is fully dilated. *Never* pull on a footling breech as the head may extend and be caught in an incompletely dilated cervix.

92. **Q. What are the 5 leading causes of maternal mortality?**

  A. (a) Haemorrhage.

    (b) Pulmonary embolism.

    (c) Preeclampsia and eclampsia.

    (d) Ectopic pregnancy.

    (e) Caesarean section complications (a,b,d above, plus anaesthetic problems).

93. **Q. How would you distinguish between abruptio placentae and placenta praevia by abdominal examination in a patient who has had an antepartum haemorrhage?**

  A. In abruption the uterus is likely to be hard and tender, the presenting part entering or in the pelvis, and the fetal heart inaudible or difficult to hear. In placenta praevia the uterus will not be tender, and the presenting part is likely to be high, and the lie unstable.

94. **Q. What factors may precipitate heart failure during pregnancy in a patient with rheumatic heart disease?**

  A. (a) The increased blood volume and cardiac output characteristic of pregnancy.

    (b) Respiratory tract infection.

    (c) Hypertension or preeclampsia.

    (d) Subacute bacterial endocarditis.

    (e) Anaemia.

    (f) Expulsive maternal effort during the second stage of labour.

    (g) Engorgement of the right side of the heart due to acceleration of venous return during the third stage of labour.

95. **Q. What symptoms may cause the patient with a hydatidiform mole to present?**

  A. (a) Vaginal bleeding or passage of vesicles.

    (b) Nausea and vomiting.

    (c) Headaches and visual disturbance due to severe preeclampsia.

    (d) Dyspnoea due to cardiac failure or pulmonary metastases.

96. Q. **What are the clinical signs of placental insufficiency?**
   A. (a) Failure of maternal weight gain, or weight loss although the patient is not dieting or on diuretic drugs.
   (b) Failure of normal fundal height increase. Often the uterus is irritable, there is oligo-hydramnios and the fetus is small for dates.
   (c) Minimal fetal movements.

97. Q. **What tests may be of value in assessment of fetal well-being before the onset of labour?**
   A. (a) Plasma or urinary oestriol assay (figure 23.2B).
   (b) Rate of growth can be assayed by serial ultrasonography.
   (c) Cardiotocography (figures 13.12–13.18).
   (d) Amnioscopy or amniocentesis.

98. Q. **What are the causes of subinvolution of the uterus?**
   A. Retained fragments of placenta or membranes, with associated infection. The patient is likely to develop *secondary postpartum haemorrhage*. Submucous fibroids are an uncommon cause of subinvolution. Subinvolution is more likely to occur if lactation is not established.

99. Q. **What is a missed abortion?**
   A. The fetus has died but the cervix remains closed. The conceptus may be entirely absorbed or shed piecemeal when spontaneous abortion eventually occurs. Missed abortion is usually preceded by an episode of bleeding (threatened abortion).

100. Q. **What are the routine blood tests performed during pregnancy, and why are they necessary? (table 6.1).**
   A. (a) Rhesus and blood group determination is necessary in case blood transfusion is required urgently.
   (b) Indirect Coombs test to exclude rhesus isoimmunization.
   (c) Full blood examination (including red cell indices) to exclude anaemia and haemoglobinopathies.
   (d) Serological test to exclude syphilis which may harm the unborn child.
   (e) In some centres all patients have a glucose tolerance test performed to exclude diabetes mellitus.
   (f) Rubella antibodies may be estimated to determine the level of immunity and to indicate if a rubella contact or rash is of significance.
   (g) In some centres hepatitis B antigen is tested for to select the fetus at risk of postnatal infection so that immunization can be given.

101. Q. **When do the membranes usually rupture?**
   A. At the end of the first stage of labour, but it is common for rupture to occur during the first stage. Early rupture, especially before the onset of contractions, suggests the possibility of cephalopelvic disproportion, with a poor fit of the presenting part in the pelvic brim. Prolapse of the umbilical cord must be excluded.

102. Q. **What does the term 'lightening' mean?**
   A. It means that the patient finds it easier to breathe — engagement of the head into the pelvis has 'lightened' the pressure of the uterine fundus on her diaphragm.

103. Q. **What structures may be damaged if an episiotomy incision begins in the labium majus rather than at the fourchette of the perineum?**
   A. Bartholin gland and duct.

104. Q. **How do you distinguish between the anterior and posterior fontanelles on vaginal examination?**
   A. The anterior fontanelle is diamond-shaped and much larger than the triangular-shaped posterior fontanelle (figure 2.15).

105. Q. **What symptoms indicate the onset of generalized oedema as occurs in preeclampsia?**
   A. *Puffiness under the eyes* in the morning when the patient gets out of bed, and rapid onset of *swelling of the fingers* (*rings tight* and/or have to be removed).

106. Q. **How may puerperal psychosis be prevented?**
   A. (a) Childbirth preparation and parenting classes.
   (b) By avoiding infection and prolonged labour (pain and fatigue).
   (c) By preventing sleeplessness and anxiety by adequate sedation at night and reassurance. The puerperium is a difficult time for the primipara and she requires emotional support from nursing and medical staff as well as from the husband.

107. Q. **How would you diagnose a posterior position of the fetus on abdominal examination at term?**
   A. (a) The sinciput is felt nearer to the surface of the abdomen than the occiput.
   (b) The head is often deflexed, and not engaged before the onset of labour.
   (c) The anterior shoulder is out in the mother's flank; this causes *subumbilical flattening* (figure 52.4).
   (d) The fetal heart sounds are best heard 5–8 cm from the midline.
   (e) In the occipitosacral position the small, hard, irregular sinciput may feel like the sacrum, and result in misdiagnosis as a breech with extended legs.

108. Q. **Why may ballottement of the fetal head be impossible in a breech presentation?**
   A. (a) Because the head is splinted by *extended legs*.
   (b) The head may be out of reach under the costal margin if the uterus or abdominal muscles are tense, as in many nulliparas.
   (c) *Tenderness* over the head, a common sign in breech presentation, may preclude accurate palpation.
   (d) The head may be impalpable due to maternal obesity, an anterior placenta or malformation (anencephaly).
   (e) Movement of the head may be restricted by lodgement in a malformed uterus (bicornuate horn, unicornuate) especially when there is *oligohydramnios*.

109. Q. **What conditions predispose to primary postpartum haemorrhage?**
   A. (a) Prolonged labour, or when there is uterine exhaustion. Uterine atony is commoner when labour is induced with an oxytocin infusion (thus always run the infusion for 1–2 hours after completion of the third stage).
   (b) Full bladder — pass a catheter!
   (c) Overdistension of the uterus due to a large baby, multiple pregnancy or polyhydramnios.
   (d) General anaesthesia with the uterus relaxed.
   (e) Operative vaginal delivery.
   (f) Conditions causing hypofibrinogenaemia (colour plate 91).

110. Q. **What conditions predispose to fetal growth retardation (intrauterine malnutrition or infant small for dates)?**
   A. (a) Preeclampsia.
   (b) Hypertension and chronic renal disease.
   (c) Diabetes mellitus with maternal vascular disease.
   (d) Malnutrition due to socioeconomic factors, heavy smoking, other drugs of habit.
   (e) Retroplacental haemorrhage which may be chronic and subclinical.
   (f) Major fetal malformations and infections.
   (g) In many cases the patient has had an apparently normal pregnancy.

111. Q. **Are the infants of mothers with diabetes mellitus always large for dates?**
   A. No, only in 40% of cases. *What is classical is not most common*, and this statement is true in many other situations in obstetrics.

112. Q. **What complications may result from mismanagement of the third stage of labour?**
   A. (a) *Postpartum haemorrhage* when fundal fiddling causes partial separation of the placenta and breakdown of the retroplacental clot.
   (b) *Retained placenta* due either to premature attempts at delivery or bad timing in the administration of ergometrine.
   (c) Maternal *shock* due to rough handling of the uterine fundus to promote placental separation.

(d) *Inversion of the uterus* by pulling on the cord when the uterus is not contracted and held safely by the abdominal hand.

113. Q. **If a breech presentation was suspected on abdominal palpation how would the diagnosis be confirmed?**
     A. (a) Vaginal examination.
     (b) X-ray or ultrasonic examination of the fetus.

114. Q. **What are the dangers to the mother if anaemia is not diagnosed and treated?**
     A. (a) Mainly that she is less able to withstand acute blood loss before, during, or after delivery.
     (b) Severe anaemia can precipitate heart failure in any patient; lesser degrees can do so when the patient has cardiac disease or severe preeclampsia.

115. Q. **What would you do when the signs of fetal distress occurred in labour?**
     A. (a) Give the mother *oxygen* by mask and lie her on her side, especially if there was evidence of postural hypotension.
     (b) Arrange for *vaginal examination* to be performed to exclude cord prolapse and to ascertain if conditions were favourable for immediate vaginal delivery.

116. Q. **What are the indications for catheterization in obstetric practice?**
     A. (a) Acute retention of urine. Rarely this is due to incarceration of a retroverted uterus which occurs at about 14 weeks' gestation. Retention also occurs in labour, especially when there is cephalopelvic disproportion. In the puerperium, retention is due to a painful perineum or Caesarean section wound (i.e. reflex in origin).
     (b) Retained placenta, especially when accompanied by postpartum haemorrhage.
     (c) To distinguish between proteinuria due to preeclampsia and that due to urinary infection or contamination.
     (d) Before Caesarean section and vaginal manipulations such as forceps delivery, breech extraction, and manual removal of the placenta.

117. Q. **What abnormalities may be detected by abdominal examination of the pregnant woman in late pregnancy?**
     A. (a) Abnormal uterine shape or size indicative of polyhydramnios, multiple pregnancy, fibromyomas, or a bicornuate uterus (colour plates 70–72).
     (b) Breech presentation, transverse or oblique lie.
     (c) Mobile presenting part suggestive of cephalopelvic disproportion or placenta praevia.
     (d) Oligohydramnios and a uterus small for dates indicating placental insufficiency.
     (e) Posterior position of the occiput.

118. Q. **What are the indications for oestriol assay (plasma or urine) during pregnancy?**
     A. Fetoplacental function ideally should be assessed biochemically in all pregnancies. It is mandatory when there are complications known to be associated with an increased risk of intrauterine death: important amongst these are hypertension and chronic renal disease, preeclampsia, postterm pregnancy (testing should begin at 41 weeks), clinical evidence of fetal growth retardation, diabetes mellitus, rhesus isoimmunization, bad obstetric history, antepartum haemorrhage.

119. Q. **What is the average head circumference of a normal infant at *full* term?**
     A. 35 cm.

120. Q. **What is the average birth-weight of a normal infant at full term?**
     A. 3,500 g.

121. Q. **What is the definition of a premature infant?**
     A. One born before *37 weeks'* gestation.

122. Q. **What are the clinical features of prematurity? (figure 64.8).**
     A. (a) The *head* appears large in comparison with the rest of the body, the *chest* appears small, and the *abdomen* appears distended.
     (b) The *cartilage* of the ears is poorly developed.
     (c) The *skin* is red, thin and delicate and is covered by fine, downy hair called lanugo.
     (d) The *hair-line* tends to be low over the forehead and extends down the temples.

    (e) *Breast* tissue is poorly developed.
    (f) The labia majora are thin and poorly developed, and therefore the *labia minora* appear unduly prominent.
    (g) The limbs are thin and spindly.
    (h) Lack of skin creases on the soles of the feet (figure 64.4)
    (i) Undescended *testes.*
    (j) The cry is feeble and poorly sustained.

123. Q. **What complications are premature infants likely to encounter?**
    A. (a) *Hyaline membrane disease* (idiopathic respiratory distress syndrome).
    (b) Imperfect *temperature* control — they tend to take on the temperature of their surroundings.
    (c) *Feeding problems* due to vomiting, inability to suck, and immature digestion.
    (d) Increased risk of *infection.*
    (e) Hepatic enzymatic immaturity leading to the development of *jaundice.*
    (f) Lack of development of blood vessels and deficiency of blood coagulation factors increasing the risk of *haemorrhage.*
    (g) Inadequate *food stores* resulting in iron deficiency anaemia and rickets.

124. Q. **What is a 'dysmature infant'?**
    A. One who has suffered retarded intrauterine growth and as a result is '*small for dates*' (i.e. one whose birth-weight is below the 10th percentile for the gestational age) (figures 20.1, 21.4 and 64.11).

125. Q. **What complications may occur in the dysmature infant after birth?**
    A. (a) Intrapartum *hypoxia* resulting in *cerebral irritation* and the passage of *meconium* with subsequent *inhalation* into the lungs causing the *meconium aspiration syndrome.*
    (b) Chronic intrauterine hypoxia leading to *polycythaemia* and hence an increased incidence of jaundice.
    (c) An increased *haemorrhagic* tendency due to deficiency of blood coagulation factors.
    (d) An increased incidence of *hypoglycaemia* due to diminished glycogen stores in the liver.
    (e) Poor heat conservation due to lack of subcutaneous fat.
    (f) An increased incidence of *congenital malformations.*

126. Q. **What are the causes of redness on the anterior abdominal wall of the baby above the umbilicus?**
    A. Local pressure from the cord clamp or an 'umbilical flare'.

127. Q. **What is the significance of an 'umbilical flare'?**
    A. It indicates spread of *infection* from the umbilicus along the umbilical vein and suggests the possibility of septicaemia.

128. Q. **What is the management of a 'sticky cord'?**
    A. A swab is taken for bacterial culture, the area is cleansed at each change of napkin, and an antibiotic preparation (e.g. neomycin sulphate — Neotracin) is applied locally.

129. Q. **What is the management of an infant after circumcision?**
    A. The area is inspected frequently for evidence of haemorrhage. The infant is sponged rather than bathed for 4 days when the dressing is soaked in a bath and removed. Vaseline may be applied at each napkin change until healing has occurred.

130. Q. **What is phototherapy?**
    A. A means of isomerization of excess unconjugated bilirubin pigment in the infant's skin by energy derived from light resulting in a product which can be directly excreted.

131. Q. **How can high levels of oxygen administration cause harm to any infant?**
    A. (a) By causing *retrolental fibroplasia* which can result in *blindness* in premature infants.
    (b) By causing damage to lung tissue (*bronchopulmonary dysplasia*).

132. Q. **The dextrostix is commonly used in neonatology. What is it?**
    A. A glucose oxidase impregnated paper strip used for the estimation of the level of *blood glucose.* It is used especially in infants liable to develop hypoglycaemia.

133. Q. **What infant is liable to develop hypoglycaemia?**
   A. (a) A dysmature infant.
   (b) The infant of a diabetic mother.
   (c) Any very sick infant (e.g. one with respiratory failure).
   (d) An infant with an infection.
   (e) An infant with rhesus erythroblastosis (colour plate 123).

134. Q. **How would you manage a baby with idiopathic respiratory distress syndrome (hyaline membrane disease)?**
   A. (a) Nurse in an *incubator*.
   (b) Minimal and gentle *handling*.
   (c) Regular *observations* of oxygen concentration, respiratory and heart rates, temperature, and the presence of central cyanosis.
   (d) Administration of the minimal amount of *oxygen* required to prevent central cyanosis.
   (e) Maintenance of a clear *airway*.
   (f) Oral or intravenous *feedings* depending on the severity of the condition.
   (g) Correction of the metabolic acidosis with *bicarbonate*.
   (h) *Antibiotics*.

135. Q. **Why are all premature infants given iron therapy?**
   A. Because they are prone to iron deficiency anaemia due to diminished stores of iron and the rapid demands for iron in postnatal life; neither breast nor cow's milk is adequate in such infants.

136. Q. **What is physiological jaundice?**
   A. Jaundice that is *not* present on the first day of life and disappears within 7 days of birth, the maximum plasma bilirubin not exceeding 150 μmol/l (9 mg/dl) in term infants, and 200 μmol/l (12 mg/dl) in preterm infants. The jaundice is due to poor development of the glucuronyl transferase enzyme system in the infant's liver, which normally handles bilirubin, a breakdown product of the haemoglobin in the red blood cell.

137. Q. **What are the common causes of neonatal jaundice?**
   A. (a) Physiological.
   (b) Excessive breakdown of red blood cells such as when the infant has erythroblastosis due to ABO blood group or rhesus incompatibility.
   (c) Absorption of extravasated blood (cephalhaematoma or bruises due to birth trauma).
   (d) Infection (general sepsis, syphilis, toxoplasmosis).
   (e) Liver malfunction due to hepatitis or metabolic disturbance (galactosaemia — a hereditary disorder).
   (f) Obstruction to the biliary tree.

138. Q. **What is the management of a 'sticky' eye? (colour plate 130).**
   A. After a swab is taken for bacterial culture, an appropriate antibiotic is administered locally to the eyes (ointment or drops) at the time of each feeding.

139. Q. **What are the advantages of breast feeding?**
   A. (a) Human milk has a composition appropriate for the infant's digestive capacity.
   (b) There is no expense and less preparation is required.
   (c) Mother and child enjoy mutual psychological satisfaction.
   (d) Human milk contains *antibodies* which protect the baby from infection.
   (e) Involution of the *uterus* is aided by pituitary hormone release initiated by stimulation of the nipples during suckling.

140. Q. **What are the contraindications to breast feeding?**
   A. (a) When the baby requires special care (e.g. the premature baby), or when there is a cleft lip and palate.
   (b) The mother does not wish to breast-feed or the baby is being adopted.
   (c) Breast abnormalities such as inverted, cracked or hypersensitive nipples which are unresponsive to treatment.
   (d) Open maternal tuberculosis or poorly controlled epilepsy.
   (e) Puerperal *psychosis*; the mother may harm the child.
   (f) Previous breast abscess requiring surgery.

(g) Drugs transmitted in milk which may be harmful to the baby (antithyroid drugs, tetracyclines or anticoagulants).

141. Q. **What is the correct method of storing multivitamin preparations?**
A. Away from direct sunlight and heat which may destroy the vitamins.

142. Q. **What facilities does incubator care provide?**
A. (a) Maintenance of body *temperature*.
(b) Ease of observation and hence minimal handling of the infant.
(c) Isolation from cross-infection.
(d) Control of humidity and oxygen concentration.

143. Q. **What is the major complication of life in an incubator?**
A. *Infection*. The sterilization of an incubator is difficult and the humidity favours infection, although the baby is isolated from other infants.

144. Q. **What is thrush and how may it present in the newborn infant?**
A. (a) It is an infection due to the fungus *Monilia albicans*.
(b) It presents as *white patches* on the buccal mucosa which leave a raw bleeding surface if removed. The infection may pass down the intestinal tract and produce an eruption on the buttocks.

145. Q. **What is the treatment of thrush?**
A. (a) Lesions in the mouth are treated with 1 ml of nystatin (100,000 units per ml) dropped into the mouth 4 times per day; if the infection persists, the lesions are painted with 0.5% gentian violet solution twice daily after feedings.
(b) Infection of the napkin area is treated by application of an antifungal cream containing nystatin at each napkin change; if infection persists, application of 1% gentian violet solution twice daily is commenced (colour plate 131).

146. Q. **What is the Guthrie test?**
A. A test performed on blood obtained by a heel-prick, to detect excessive amounts of phenylalanine which occurs in the disease *phenylketonuria* (PKU).

147. Q. **What is the Apgar score?**
A. A numerical assessment of the infant's condition after birth based on *heart rate, respiratory effort, muscle tone, reflex response,* and *colour*.

148. Q. **What are the signs of placental insufficiency in the newborn infant?**
A. Those due to *malnutrition* before birth, and *distress* (passage of meconium) during birth. The baby has wrinkled or peeling skin, absence of subcutaneous fat, and birth-weight below the 10th percentile for the period of gestation. The cord is thin and the infant has polycythaemia. Meconium may have stained the cord and skin, and irritated the stomach (*gastritis* with coffee-ground vomitus) and eyes (*conjunctivitis*) (colour plate 20, figures 20.1, 21.4 and 64.11).

149. Q. **What are the signs of intracranial trauma in a newborn infant?**
A. Raised tension of the anterior fontanelle together with one of the following 2 patterns:
(a) The *agitated, irritable* infant who resists handling, is restless, has 'tucked-in' thumbs and a shrill piercing cry. He may vomit, have head retraction, intermittent apnoeic attacks, and tremors or convulsions may occur.
(b) The *somnolent, stuporous* infant who is flaccid at birth and appears pale and shocked, or extremely cyanosed, and is difficult to resuscitate. He remains flaccid and becomes a 'depressed baby'. He may have tremors or convulsions, has no sucking reflex, and hence requires tube feeding.

150. Q. **Why is cord blood collected at birth when the mother is rhesus negative?**
A. To determine the infant's blood group and whether the direct Coombs test is positive. The cord blood haemoglobin and bilirubin values are measured if the infant is Coombs positive, to see if immediate *exchange transfusion* is indicated.

151. Q. **What is kernicterus?**
A. Brain damage and yellow staining due to excessive levels of *unconjugated bilirubin*.

152. Q. **Are there any indications for circumcision in the newborn infant?**
      A. Only social factors ('all his brothers have been done') and religious considerations.

153. Q. **What are the complications of circumcision?**
      A. *Haemorrhage, infection* and rare surgical catastrophes such as damage to the glans penis.

154. Q. **What is tube feeding?**
      A. Feeding through a tube placed into the stomach or jejunum when an infant cannot suck, usually as a result of prematurity (colour plate 100).

155. Q. **What is the main complication of tube feeding?**
      A. Aspiration pneumonia.

156. Q. **What would cause you to suspect that a nasogastric tube was in the trachea and not in the oesophagus?**
      A. Continued *coughing* and *cyanosis* of the baby. The aspirate, not being acidic, would *not* turn blue litmus paper red.

157. Q. **What are the common causes of an apparently healthy baby continuing to cry after feeding?**
      A. The baby may still be *hungry*, have *colic*, a *dirty* napkin, be *emotionally unsatisfied*, or full of *wind*.

158. Q. **What is the hazard of being born in a caul?**
      A. Death from asphyxia or '*drowning*'. The fetus is born with the membranes intact, and has no access to air unless the amnion is removed (figure 42.10).

159. Q. **If caput and moulding obscure the fetal fontanelles during the second stage of labour, how can a deep transverse arrest be diagnosed by vaginal examination?**
      A. By feeling for the *ear* beneath the pubic symphysis. The direction of the auricle indicates whether the occiput is to the left or right.

160. Q. **What are the signs of infection in a newborn infant?**
      A. (a) Signs of *major infection* are hypothermia, pyrexia, dyspnoea, collapse.
         (b) Signs of *minor infection* are sticky eye or umbilicus, white plaques in the mouth, nappy rash, diarrhoea, umbilical flare.

161. Q. **Why is vaginal examination performed at the first antenatal attendance?**
      A. To confirm the diagnosis of pregnancy and the period of gestation by assessment of the size and consistency of the uterus; to assess pelvic dimensions and exclude pelvic pathology (ovarian cyst, fibromyomas, uterine or vaginal abnormality); to exclude vaginal infections, cervical incompetence and carcinoma (macroscopic appearance and cytological examination).

162. Q. **What are advantages of routine vaginal examination when the patient is admitted to hospital in labour?**
      A. Baseline observation of cervical dilatation and effacement, diagnosis of a previously unrecognized malpresentation (breech, face, brow, shoulder, umbilical cord) or vasa praevia.

163. Q. **What are the causes of secondary postpartum haemorrhage?**
      A. Retained placental tissue or membranes with or without infection.

164. Q. **What is the treatment of secondary postpartum haemorrhage?**
      A. Resuscitation if required, antibiotic therapy and curettage if haemorrhage is heavy or persistent.

165. Q. **What are the risks of curettage for secondary postpartum haemorrhage?**
      A. Perforation, and infertility due to denudation of the uterine lining causing adhesions and perhaps obliteration of the cavity (*Asherman syndrome*).

166. Q. **What problems may be associated with a poorly-fitting presenting part in labour?**
      A. Premature rupture of the membranes, prolapse of the umbilical cord, cephalopelvic disproportion (big or deflexed head, malposition, malpresentation, abnormal pelvic shape or size), prolonged labour, incoordinate uterine action, fetal and maternal distress, infection

(mother and child) and the risk of operative delivery.

167. Q. **What are the indications for administration of anti-D gamma globulin in obstetric practice?**
A. (a) Antenatally in Rh-negative patients when fetomaternal haemorrhage is likely to occur — threatened, incomplete or therapeutic abortion, ectopic pregnancy, antepartum haemorrhage, amniocentesis, external cephalic version.
(b) To all nonimmunized Rh negative mothers within 72 hours of delivery of an Rh positive infant.
(c) In some centres anti-D is given antenatally to all Rh negative mothers in the third trimester (unless the father of the child is known to be Rhesus negative).

168. Q. **What is the treatment of prolapse of the umbilical cord in a multipara in labour at term?**
A. (a) If the patient is in the second stage urge her to push and deliver spontaneously, otherwise perform forceps delivery (if the head is engaged) or breech extraction.
(b) If the patient is not deliverable vaginally, push the presenting part off the cord and take her to theatre for Caesarean section, if the fetus is alive and not known to be seriously malformed.

169. Q. **Why may external cephalic version fail?**
A. (a) Tight abdominal muscles and/or tense uterus (usually in a nullipara).
(b) Bicornuate or unicornuate uterus (colour plate 72).
(c) Oligohydramnios.
(d) Very large baby or very obese mother.
(e) Breech with extended legs, especially when the buttocks are deeply engaged in the pelvis.
When these conditions are present it is often prudent not to attempt external cephalic version.

170. Q. **Why is it preferable to deliver the baby's head between contractions rather than during a contraction?**
A. To avoid a perineal tear or extension of an episiotomy incision — it is better for the patient to have a relaxed pelvic floor, because when she bears down the vagina is taut and readily torn.

171. Q. **When is it safe to allow vaginal delivery when there is a placenta praevia?**
A. When a patient is in established labour (preferably a multipara), with *minimal bleeding*, ruptured membranes, and the degree of praevia is minor (types 1–2).

172. Q. **What are the causes of premature rupture of the membranes?**
A. Cervical incompetence, poorly-fitting presenting part (transverse lie, footling breech, cephalopelvic disproportion), increased intrauterine tension (multiple pregnancy, polyhydramnios), membranes weakened by infection.

173. Q. **What is the differential diagnosis of premature rupture of the membranes?**
A. Urinary *stress incontinence* (this often occurs for the first time late in pregnancy and the patient may be uncertain of the origin of the fluid), discharge caused by physiological *leucorrhoea* or by irritation of the cervix by bulging membranes (incompetent cervix) or discharge due to *vaginitis*.

174. Q **What are the causes of acute urinary retention in obstetric practice?**
A. (a) Perineal or abdominal pain postpartum (episiotomy or Caesarean section).
(b) *Occlusion of the urethra* by pressure of the fetal head in labour, a pack inserted after delivery to control bleeding from vaginal lacerations, a large paravaginal haematoma or pressure from an incarcerated uterus (figure 37.2).

175. Q **How would you investigate a patient with polyhydramnios at 30 weeks' gestation?**
A. (a) Ultrasonography ± radiography for fetal malformations, multiple pregnancy and hydrops fetalis (figure 21.2).
(b) Glucose tolerance and indirect Coombs tests to exclude diabetes and rhesus isoimmunization.
(c) Perhaps amniocentesis (amniography, fetography, culture of amniotic fluid for

cytomegalovirus) (colour plate 126 and figure 25.7).

176. **Q. How do you exclude contamination as a cause of proteinuria?**
A. Obtain a mid-stream or catheter specimen of urine or even perform a suprapubic bladder puncture. Also pass a speculum to examine the vagina for discharge or vaginitis.

177. **Q. How do you ensure flexion of the aftercoming head in a breech delivery so that minimal diameters present?**
A. Allow the baby to hang free (Burns-Marshall manoeuvre — figure 50.4).

178. **Q. At what times during pregnancy are the signs of preeclampsia most likely to occur or intensify?**
A. In labour when the uterine contractions force the unknown aetiological agent from the placenta into the maternal circulation; and within 1–2 hours of delivery while the agent remains active.

179. **Q. When should an oxytocin infusion be turned off?**
A. The onset of fetal distress; when contractions are strong, less than 2 minutes apart and of more than 1 minute in duration; uterine tenderness not associated with a contraction (?impending uterine rupture), and 1–2 hours after delivery of the placenta when the risk of atonic postpartum haemorrhage becomes minimal.

180. **Q. What are the indications for delivery in a patient with an antepartum haemorrhage?**
A. Heavy continuing haemorrhage, onset of labour, critical fetal reserve on cardiotocography, a dead fetus or fetal maturity at or beyond 37 weeks' gestation if the cause is placenta praevia.

181. **Q. Why is 37 weeks' gestation the rubicon for elective delivery when pregnancy is complicated by antepartum haemorrhage, preeclampsia, hypertension, diabetes etc?**
A. The risk of neonatal death from hyaline membrane disease becomes markedly reduced.

182. **Q. When should the obstetrician be called to a patient in labour?**
A. The onset of fetal distress, rupture of the membranes, failure of progress, or when it is time for delivery (see Question 24, Appendix IIIB).

183. **Q. Why does vaginal haemorrhage occur when the patient has a placenta praevia?**
A. As the lower segment takes up in late pregnancy or in labour it is almost inevitable that the placenta separates and haemorrhage occurs.

184. **Q. What are the major indications for ultrasonography in obstetric practice?**
A. (a) Assessment of gestational age, multiple pregnancy, placental localization, diagnosis of hydatidiform mole, polyhydramnios, fetal anomalies, growth and viability (threatened abortion, suspected intrauterine death).
(b) For detection of fetoplacental function and to guide intrauterine manipulative procedures (chorion biopsy, amniocentesis, intrauterine fetal transfusion — figure 13.7).

185. **Q. What anaesthetic agents relax the uterus?**
A. Halothane and ether — curare-like voluntary muscle relaxants do not!

186. **Q. How would you conduct the delivery of the second twin?**
A. (a) Check the lie, presentation and station by abdominal and vaginal examination. Note whether the membranes are intact and exclude cord prolapse.
(b) Listen to the fetal heart rate.
(c) Most patients will continue to labour and deliver spontaneously cephalically or by assisted breech delivery.
(d) Persistent transverse lie, cord prolapse, haemorrhage etc will require immediate delivery (see Question 55, Appendix IIIB).
(e) If contractions are weak or absent, in the absence of the above complications, there is the choice of *amniotomy* when conditions are favourable (see Question 73, Appendix IIIB), or *waiting* — if the latter course is adopted oxytocin should be added to the intravenous infusion.
(f) After the second twin is born, careful management of the third stage is essential to avoid *postpartum haemorrhage*.

Advanced Questions and Answers

1. Q. **What conditions are more likely to be associated with preeclampsia?**
   A. (a) Parity — the patient is usually a nullipara.
   (b) Hypertension or chronic renal disease.
   (c) Multiple pregnancy.
   (d) Erythroblastosis.
   (e) Diabetes mellitus.
   (f) Hydatidiform mole.
   (g) Change of marital partner (i.e. for multiparas).

2. Q. **What tests would be performed on the mother to investigate the cause of recurrent intrauterine death in late pregnancy?**
   A. (a) Serological testing of the blood to exclude syphilis.
   (b) An indirect Coombs test to exclude rhesus isoimmunization.
   (c) A glucose tolerance test to exclude subclinical diabetes mellitus.

3. Q. **What methods are available for improvement of fetoplacental function in normal and abnormal pregnancies?**
   A. (a) *Rest*, especially in the left *lateral position* (figure 48.1).
   (b) Adequate *nutrition* — vitamins, minerals and calories (especially from foods high in protein). Intravenous infusion of dextrose to the mother is of particular value when the fetus has severe placental insufficiency, or when there is fetal distress in labour.
   (c) Correction of maternal anaemia by administration of iron or folic acid or by blood transfusion.
   (d) Correction of *fetal anaemia* due to erythroblastosis by intrauterine blood transfusion.
   (e) Improvement of placental blood flow by control of hypertension.
   (f) Administration of oxygen to the mother when there is fetal distress in labour.
   (g) Anticoagulant therapy in patients with recurrent intervillous thrombosis.

4. Q. **Does lactation usually occur after spontaneous abortion?**
   A. No, because most abortions occur in the first trimester, and in these patients lactation does not occur, presumably because there has been inadequate hormone preparation of the breasts. Lactation usually does occur after second trimester abortions.

5. Q. **What would you suspect to be the cause if lactation occurred during late pregnancy?**
   A. Fetal and placental death from any cause.

6. Q. **How is the diagnosis of fetal death established?**
   A. The diagnosis is suspected if fetal movements or fundal growth cease. The fetal heart cannot be heard even with the sensitive Doppler instrument, heart motion cannot be seen on ultrasonography, X-ray signs may be positive (figure 23.4), and the urinary oestriol excretion falls below 3.5 μmol (1 mg)/24 hours.

7. Q. **Why is the prognosis of the second twin said to be worse?**
   A. (a) Reduction in uterine size causes placental separation or diminution of uterine blood flow resulting in *hypoxia*.
   (b) Also there is a higher incidence of malpresentations and hence greater risks of *trauma* due to manipulative delivery, especially internal version followed by breech extraction (tables 53.1–53.4).

8. Q. **How may the number of fetal deaths due to prematurity be reduced?**
    A. (a) By ligation of the *incompetent cervix*.
       (b) By adequate treatment of essential hypertension.
       (c) By early diagnosis of *multiple pregnancy*, and resting the patient in hospital.
       (d) By treatment of *premature labour* with rest and sedation, and drugs which relax the uterus.
       (e) By prevention and early treatment of *preeclampsia*, minimizing its incidence and severity, and thus lessening the need for premature induction of labour.
       (f) By avoidance of social (elective) inductions of labour where it is always possible that the dates are wrong.
       (g) By performing an amniotic fluid *L:S ratio* when the indication for induction of labour is not absolute and when fetal maturity is in doubt — the same applies to the timing of delivery by repeat elective Caesarean section, especially in diabetics.
       (h) Adequate maternal diet, avoidance of smoking and prevention of anaemia.
       (i) *Betamethasone* therapy if premature delivery is imminent (premature rupture of membranes, premature labour) or there is a need for delivery when the L:S ratio is less than 2:1.
       (j) Rest in hospital when the patient has gross *polyhydramnios* — often the uterine tension subsides and the liquor volume decreases.
       (k) Use of ultrasonography to confirm fetal maturity in early pregnancy when premature delivery is likely to be required and/or if menstrual data is uncertain.
       (l) Extended use of Caesarean section when delivery is more hazardous (breech ± fetal growth retardation and/or distress).
       (m) Special care of the neonate with respiratory distress, and transfer to a special care nursery (see Question 72, Appendix IIIB).

9. Q. **How may oesophageal atresia and exomphalos be diagnosed before the fetus is born?**
    A. Fetal anomalies should be suspected when polyhydramnios is present. If X-ray shows no skeletal abnormality, soft tissue defects can be sought by amniocentesis and introduction of both water- and fat-soluble radio-opaque materials into the amniotic fluid. The fat-soluble dye will adhere to vernix and show the outline of an exomphalos. Oesophageal atresia is suspected when the water-soluble dye does not appear within and outline the fetal gut 24 hours later. Structural defects such as exomphalos may also be diagnosed by *ultrasound scanning* — this allows early surgery before distension with air makes surgical reduction more difficult.

10. Q. **Why is the baby of a diabetic mother likely to develop signs of hypoglycaemia after birth?**
    A. The mother being hyperglycaemic during pregnancy transfers extra glucose across the placenta, and so the fetus also has hyperglycaemia. Because of this the fetal pancreas secretes extra insulin to reduce the blood glucose level. After birth this increased output of insulin causes *hypoglycaemia* because the baby is no longer receiving an excessive amount of glucose from the maternal circulation.

11.a Q. **Why is glycosuria more common in pregnancy?**
     A. The renal threshold is lower in pregnancy.
11.b Q. **What is the physiological explanation for the above change.**
     A. In pregnancy there is a 30–50% increase in cardiac output, renal blood flow, and a similar increase in glomerular filtration rate. Therefore, more glucose reaches the renal tubules and the maximum ability of the tubules to reabsorb it is more likely to be exceeded with the result that glucose appears in the urine. Damage to the tubules (chronic pyelonephritis) aggravates this tendency.

12. Q. **Why does a patient not menstruate at the time of the first missed period and abort the recently implanted embryo?**
    A. Because the trophoblastic cells have produced sufficient *chorionic gonadotrophic hormone* to maintain the corpus luteum in the mother's ovary. The corpus luteum therefore continues to produce oestrogen and progesterone which sustain the endometrium. Normally, menstruation occurs because the corpus luteum regresses towards the end of the cycle.

13.   Q. **What is the classical history from which the diagnosis of an incompetent cervix may be made?**
      A. The patient has a history of cervical trauma such as dilatation for termination of pregnancy (colour plate 35). She has had second trimester abortions which were preceded by a copious serosanguineous or mucoid discharge. Then the patient felt the membranes bulge into the vagina and burst, and the fetus was aborted. The main feature was that the abortion was *not preceded by episodes of bleeding or pain.*

14.   Q. **What are the indications for X-ray pelvimetry?**
      A. (a) A high mobile head at term in a nullipara.
      (b) Short stature (below 150 cm) or history of injury or disease of the pelvis (figure 49.3).
      (c) Breech presentation when external cephalic version has failed, particularly in a nullipara.
      (d) Clinical evidence of pelvic contraction.
      (e) History of previous difficult deliveries or unexplained stillbirths.
      (f) Previous Caesarean section when it is planned to allow the patient to attempt vaginal delivery.

15.   Q. **What is the significance, from the fetal point of view, of supine hypotension syndrome in the mother?**
      A. The transfer of *oxygen* and *nutriments* from the maternal blood is likely to be impaired. All patients with high risk pregnancies should lie in the left lateral position when resting (figure 48.1).

16.   Q. **Before the introduction of forceps how was vaginal delivery effected when labour was prolonged?**
      A. By destructive operations or internal version and breech extraction. The latter procedure provided a part of the fetus which the accoucheur could pull upon. Fundal pressure 'sitting on the patient' was also used.

17.   Q. **What is a bipolar version?**
      A. When a foot of the fetus is grasped through the partially dilated cervix. The manoeuvre was described by Braxton Hicks as a means of controlling bleeding from *placenta praevia*, in the days before safe Caesarean delivery. Pressure of the thigh compressed the placental edge and stopped bleeding from blood vessels in the uterine wall (figure 50.11).

18.   Q. **Can placental abruption be shown to be the cause of fetal death immediately before birth?**
      A. Probably not, because the retroplacental clot is not old and looks the same as the fresh clot which is usually seen. Also it would be difficult to distinguish between the pain of uterine contractions, and that due to placental abruption.

19.   Q. **What are the indications for amniocentesis?**
      A. (a) To obtain amniotic fluid for genetic counselling (e.g. Down syndrome, neural tube defect), assessment of the severity of *erythroblastosis*, or the degree of *fetal maturity*.
      (b) To administer drugs to treat a sick fetus or to evacuate an unwanted one.
      (c) To relieve acute polyhydramnios.
      (d) To inject water- and fat-soluble radio-opaque dyes prior to an X-ray when fetal malformations are suspected (figures 21.9 and 25.7).
      (e) To insert a catheter to monitor intrauterine pressure.
      (f) To diagnose intrauterine infection in labour.

20.   Q. **What factors provoke an increase in the incidence of monilial vaginitis?**
      A. (a) Pregnancy or oral contraceptives.
      (b) Broad-spectrum antibiotics.
      (c) Diabetes mellitus.
      (d) Corticosteroids.

21.   Q. **Is hypoplasia of the uterus a cause of spontaneous abortion?**
      A. Possibly. Many women give a history of late heavy periods, preceded by nausea and breast tenderness, before their first baby is conceived.

22. Q. **Why is there no mechanism of delivery in a face presentation when the chin is posterior?**
    A. To negotiate the curve of Carus further extension of the head would be required and this is not possible because extension is already complete (figure 51.7).

23. Q. **What conditions predispose to prolapse of the umbilical cord?**
    A. (a) A mobile presenting part at the time when the membranes rupture.
    (b) A poorly-fitting presenting part (footling breech presentation or transverse lie).
    (c) Multiple pregnancy.
    (d) Polyhydramnios.
    (e) Early rupture of the membranes.
    (f) Obstetrical manipulations.
    (g) Low cord implantation (e.g. battledore insertion in a low-lying placenta).

24. Q. **How does the charge sister know when to call the accoucheur for the delivery?**
    A. (a) In the case of a *nullipara*, when the head can be felt by postanal palpation, or is visible after parting the labia.
    (b) In the case of a *multipara*, as soon as the patient begins to *push*.

25. Q. **What is the best time during pregnancy to perform a glucose tolerance test to diagnose gestational diabetes?**
    A. At about 30–32 weeks — the diabetogenic effect of pregnancy has had time to operate, and there is still time to terminate the pregnancy at the optimum time of 37–38 weeks' gestation, after stabilization of the disorder. When there are strong clinical indications (Question 63, Appendix IIIA) the test should be performed earlier (before 20 weeks' gestation).

26. Q. **Abnormal glucose tolerance usually reverts to normal after delivery. What is the explanation?**
    A. Patients destined to develop *diabetes* in middle-age may become temporarily diabetic during pregnancy due to the effect of *placental hormones* and increased activity of the *adrenal glands*. Pregnancy is nature's 'cortisone stress' test. (Likewise women destined to suffer from *essential hypertension* tend to develop high blood pressure during their first pregnancy).

27. Q. **What are the clinical signs characteristic of Clostridium welchii infection in a patient with a septic abortion?**
    A. (a) Jaundice and 'port-wine' urine due to intravascular haemolysis; oliguria is common.
    (b) Extreme uterine tenderness or crepitus.

28. Q. **What are the causes of failed forceps?**
    A. (a) Cervix not fully dilated.
    (b) Head not engaged.
    (c) Unrecognized occipitolateral or occipitoposterior position, or cephalopelvic disproportion.

29. Q. **What are the dangers of grand multiparity?**
    A. (a) Those of a lax abdomen and strongly contracting uterus — malpresentations and uterine rupture.
    (b) Cephalopelvic disproportion due to excessive fetal size.
    (c) The diseases that are commoner with advancing years — hypertension, thromboembolism, chronic renal disease, and diabetes mellitus.

30. Q. **What conditions are associated with blood coagulation failure in obstetrics?**
    A. (a) Major *placental abruption* (accidental haemorrhage).
    (b) Prolonged retention of a dead fetus.
    (c) Amniotic fluid embolism (colour plate 62).
    (d) Septicaemia particularly when due to Cl. welchii or E. coli (both cause haemolysis of red blood cells and thus release thromboplastin into the circulation).
    (e) Incompatible blood transfusion, tissue trauma, and other causes of shock.

31. Q. **What are the indications for internal version and breech extraction?**
    A. (a) Delivery of the second twin.
    (b) Cord prolapse or transverse lie if the cervix is fully dilated and the pelvis is adequate.

32. Q. **When would internal version and breech extraction be indicated for delivery of the second twin?**

A. When immediate delivery is indicated because of haemorrhage or fetal distress, and the presentation is unsuitable for forceps delivery or breech extraction; in other words when the lie is transverse, or when the head is not engaged in a vertex presentation (see also Question 55, Appendix IIIB).

33. Q. **During breech delivery what is the cause of delay in delivery of the head and intracranial trauma?**

A. (a) Cephalopelvic disproportion due to pelvic contraction, or a large or deflexed head.

(b) Obstruction due to an incompletely dilated cervix: here the baby is usually premature and the relatively small buttocks slip through the cervix before full dilatation; this is especially common in footling presentations.

34. Q. **What is the mechanism of hydrops fetalis in severe erythroblastosis?**

A. Heart failure due to profound anaemia together with low levels of plasma proteins.

35. Q. **What factors are considered in deciding when to induce labour in a patient who is rhesus isoimmunized?**

A. (a) The past obstetric history.

(b) The husband's genotype.

(c) The indirect Coombs antibody titres.

(d) The level of bilirubin in the liquor.

(e) The presence of clinical complications such as preeclampsia and polyhydramnios.

(f) Fetal function tests (ultrasonography, cardiotocography).

36. Q. **What are the situations in which classical Caesarean section may be required?**

A. (a) Transverse lie.

(b) Poorly developed lower uterine segment (e.g. prematurity especially with breech presentation).

(c) Adhesions due to previous lower segment Caesarean section.

(d) Constriction ring.

(e) Fibromyomas or large veins in the lower uterine segment (e.g. due to placenta praevia especially when anterior — figure 13.11).

(f) If hysterectomy is to be performed see Question 68, Appendix IIIB).

(g) Postmortem.

37. Q. **How may complications of preeclampsia result in fetal or maternal death?**

A. (a) Fetal death may result from placental insufficiency or abruption (accidental haemorrhage).

(b) Maternal death may be due to cardiac failure, or cerebral, renal, or hepatic complications (usually ischaemic necrosis and haemorrhage).

38. Q. **What are recurring indications for Caesarean section?**

A. (a) Pelvic contraction.

(b) Diabetes mellitus.

(c) Previous classical operation.

39. Q. **What are nonrecurring indications for Caesarean section?**

A. (a) Placenta praevia.

(b) Brow presentation or transverse lie.

(c) Incoordinate uterine action.

(d) Fetal distress or placental insufficiency.

40. Q. **What tests are used to assess maturity of the fetus?**

A. (a) Ultrasonic measurement of biparietal and other diameters and fetal volume — assessment of fetal maturity is by far the most common indication for ultrasonography (table 13.1).

(b) Estimation of lecithin and sphingomyelin levels in amniotic fluid (pulmonary maturity).

(c) X-ray. The indices are the size and degree of calcification of the skeleton, and the presence or absence of epiphyses around the knee joint (figure 49.6).

41. Q. **What is an incarcerated uterus, and how may it present?**
A. Incarceration occurs when the gravid uterus is retroverted and becomes jammed in the pelvic cavity. At about 14 weeks' gestation it fills the pelvis and compresses the urethra, causing acute retention of urine (figure 37.2). Spontaneous abortion or sacculation of the uterine wall may occur.

42. Q. **What conditions may reduce the supply of oxygen to the fetus before birth?**
A. (a) Maternal cardiovascular or respiratory disease.
(b) *Maternal* anaemia or hypotension due to any cause.
(c) Tonic or prolonged *uterine* contractions, especially due to misuse of oxytocic drugs.
(d) *Placental* dysfunction or separation (abruptio placentae — figure 23.1).
(e) Knotting, compression, or prolapse of the *umbilical cord* (figure 48.2).
(f) Fetal anaemia due to erythroblastosis, fetomaternal haemorrhage, or bleeding from a vasa praevia (colour plates 47, 84, 85 and 123).

43. Q. **What are the dangers of induction of labour?**
A. (a) The morbidity and mortality of unsuspected *prematurity*.
(b) *Prolapse of the umbilical cord* (table 44.3).
(c) *Infection* of mother and fetus if the membranes have been ruptured, especially when there is delay in delivery.
(d) Sensitivity to or overdosage of oxytocin may result in generalized tonic contraction or rupture of the uterus.
(e) The risks of any intravenous infusion — infection, air embolism, thrombophlebitis, and overhydration.

44. Q. **What fetal malformations are most likely to be diagnosed before the mother comes into labour?**
A. (a) Anencephaly and other neural tube defects: polyhydramnios or very low oestriol values are the usual clues.
(b) Hydrocephaly: in severe cases abdominal palpation indicates that the fetal head is abnormally enlarged (figure 49.4 A)
(c) Conditions recognized by amniocentesis (e.g. Down syndrome) and/or ultrasonography.

45. Q. **What would cause you to suspect that uterine rupture has occurred during labour?**
A. The onset of severe abdominal pain and tenderness at the height of a strong contraction. Usually there is vaginal haemorrhage. The patient will probably collapse, contractions will cease, and the fetal heart will become inaudible (colour plate 23).

46. Q. **What are the causes of cyanosis in the newborn infant?**
A. (a) *Cold* — due to peripheral vasoconstriction.
(b) Inadequate respiration due to *intracranial haemorrhage*, or the effect of *hypoxia* or *drugs* given to the mother on the infant's brain.
(c) *Hyaline membrane* disease, meconium aspiration and pneumonia by impeding oxygen exchange, and *pulmonary hypoplasia* and *diaphragmatic hernia* by preventing expansion of the lungs.
(d) Severe *cardiac abnormalities* such as transposition of the great vessels.
(e) *Methaemoglobinaemia*.

47. Q. **What are the common causes of excoriation of the buttocks in newborn infants?**
A. (a) Frequent loose stools.
(b) Poor hygiene with continual dampness.
(c) Contact dermatitis due to reactions to soaps.
(d) Ammoniacal dermatitis.
(e) Moniliasis (colour plate 131).
(f) Seborrhoeic dermatitis of the napkin area.

48. Q. **What are the signs of hypoglycaemia in the newborn infant?**
A. Sweating, undue restlessness, twitching, convulsions or attacks of apnoea.

49. Q. **What are the contraindications to circumcision?**
    A. (a) *Hypospadias*. The prepuce is required for repair.
    (b) *Jaundice*. Haemorrhage may be excessive.
    (c) *Prematurity*. The baby has enough to contend with.
    (d) If the mother is taking *anticoagulant* drugs and the baby is breast-fed or the baby has a bleeding diathesis.
    (e) An infant too *ill* to tolerate the procedure.
    (f) Local *infection*.

50. Q. **What is the advantage of Kielland forceps?**
    A. There is only a *small pelvic curve* and rotation with forceps (for which the instrument was designed) is therefore less likely to cause vaginal lacerations (figure 46.2).

51. Q. **How can the diagnosis of constriction ring be made?**
    A. (a) The ring may be palpable in the lower uterus at the time of vaginal examination.
    (b) It may be seen at Caesarean section performed for fetal or maternal distress if the anaesthetic agent has not relaxed the uterus.
    (c) The diagnosis would be suspected if the head receded (lost station) during a contraction, or if attempted forceps delivery failed when there was no evidence of cephalopelvic disproportion.

52. Q. **What is the significance of continued pulsation of the arteries in the umbilical cord after birth?**
    A. It means that *respiration* has not commenced. The physiological stimulus causing closure of umbilical arteries (and ductus arteriosus) is an increase in *oxygen saturation* of the blood which occurs when the lungs expand with air.

53. Q. **Why may the ductus arteriosus remain patent or reopen when the baby has the respiratory distress syndrome?**
    A. Because the lungs are poorly expanded, there is inadequate gaseous exchange, blood oxygenation is impaired, and thus the stimulus causing contraction of the muscle in the wall of the ductus is abolished.

54. Q. **Explain the mechanism of closure of the foramen ovale after birth.**
    A. The onset of respiration lowers resistance to pulmonary blood flow and the pressure in the right side of the heart falls sharply. The increase in return of blood from the lungs to the left atrium (the ductus has closed so the shunt from pulmonary trunk to aorta has ceased) increases pressure in this chamber and so the septum primum is pushed against the foramen ovale (figure 58.1).

55. Q. **What are the indications for immediate delivery of the second twin?**
    A. (a) Patient anaesthetized for forceps, breech extraction or Caesarean delivery of the first twin.
    (b) Fetal distress (cord prolapse, meconium, fetal heart rate abnormality).
    (c) Transverse lie which cannot be corrected.
    (d) Haemorrhage from uterus (placental separation) or episiotomy performed for delivery of the first twin.
    (e) Uniovular monoamniotic twins (risk of knotted cords) (figure 53.2).

56. Q. **When is breech presentation favourable for delivery?**
    A. At Caesarean section or vaginal delivery when the fetus is hydrocephalic, anencephalic or dead.

57. Q. **When is a repeat Caesarean section performed if the period of gestation is uncertain and the patient presents too late for accurate ultrasonographic estimation of fetal maturity?**
    A. When she comes into labour or if tests show fetoplacental compromise (e.g. cardiotocography).

58. Q. **What are the disadvantages of delaying a repeat Caesarean section until the patient comes into labour?**
    A. Scar dehiscence is more likely to occur, and there is the inconvenience and hazards of an emergency procedure (colour plate 87).

59. Q. **What factors occurring at Caesarean section can influence the condition of the infant at birth?**
    A. The interval from induction of anaesthesia until delivery (type of abdominal and uterine incision, skill of surgeon — see Questions 60 and 68 Appendix IIIB), effect of *drugs* (premedication, thiopentone, halothane, epidural rather than general anaesthesia), intermittent positive pressure ventilation (maternal hyperventilation or hypoventilation causing acid-base changes in the fetus), *posture* (aortocaval compression causing maternal hypotension and fetal hypoxia from poor placental perfusion), and *trauma* due to difficulty in delivery of the head.

60. Q. **What are the advantages and disadvantages of the Pfannenstiel incision for Caesarean section?**
    A. (a) Advantages are cosmetic (a bikini covers the scar), a lower incidence of wound dehiscence, and less postoperative pain.
    (b) Disadvantages are a longer induction-delivery interval (especially at repeat sections), delivery of the baby is more difficult, poor access to the upper segment if a classical (upper segment) incision or hysterectomy is required, and a higher incidence of wound haematoma ± infection.

61. Q. **What factors determine the timing of delivery in patients with placenta praevia?**
    A. Severe or continuing haemorrhage, the onset of labour, fetal condition (cardiotocography, ultrasonography) and maturity.

62. Q. **What are the advantages of the left lateral position for delivery?**
    A. Patient more comfortable and less exposed than in the lithotomy or dorsal positions, less risk of aortocaval compression, easier to pick up the chin and maintain flexion of the head since the perineum is accessible, easier to deliver the anterior shoulder, and safer if the mother has cardiac disease, sciatica or vomits (less risk of inhalation).

63. Q. **What is the explanation when a fetal head which is on view in the occipitoanterior position at the height of a contraction, recedes to the midpelvis and rotates to the occipitolateral position after the contraction (and the mother's voluntary expulsive efforts) cease?**
    A. *Occipitoposterior position* where the shoulders have failed to rotate when the occiput rotated 135° to the anterior position — i.e. the twist of the neck on the shoulders due to internal rotation is undone 90° when the force of the contraction fades — beware of impacted shoulders in such patients when the head is delivered (by episiotomy ± forceps) — it is usual for the head to recede to a lesser degree after a contraction when the perineal floor recoils with cessation of the expulsive efforts.

64. Q. **Why is the umbilical cord sometimes avulsed with minimal force during attempted delivery of the placenta by controlled cord traction?**
    A. Weak attachment due to velamentous insertion, or friable cord due to prematurity, intrauterine infection or fetal death.

65. Q. **If the cord pulls off how do you proceed to deliver the placenta?**
    A. By the Dublin method of pressure on the contracted uterine fundus ± catheterization of the bladder. If this fails manual removal will be required.

66. Q. **Why does a baby with Potter syndrome die?**
    A. From hypoxia due to pulmonary hypoplasia — death occurs before renal agenesis can cause problems!

67. Q. **What complications are unique to uniovular twin pregnancies?**
    A. Conjoined twins, fetofetal transfusion syndrome, and acute polyhydramnios (colour plates 12, 45, 46 and 50).

68. Q. **What are the indications for Caesarean hysterectomy?**
    A. (a) Uterine rupture.
    (b) Placenta accreta/increta/percreta (figure 13.11).
    (c) Uncontrollable postpartum haemorrhage not due to blood coagulation failure.
    (d) Invasive cervical carcinoma.

(e) Multiple fibromyomas.

(f) Elective as a means of sterilization is not favoured because of increased morbidity.

69. Q. **What conditions predispose to placenta accreta?**

A. (a) Scarring of the uterine wall (poor decidua formation) due to previous damage at curettage, manual removal or Caesarean section.

(b) Placenta praevia because the lower segment tends to lack decidua — beware of the patient who has an anterior placenta praevia and a lower segment Caesarean section scar (figure 13.11).

70. Q. **What are the indications for delivery of the second twin by Caesarean section?**

A. (a) Caesarean delivery of the first twin!

(b) Obstructed labour with conditions unsuitable for forceps delivery.

(c) As an alternative to internal version and breech extraction.

71. Q. **How may neonatal deaths and disabilities due to congenital malformations be lessened?**

A. (a) Optimal diet, avoidance of drugs, and stabilization of blood sugar levels in diabetics from before conception until delivery.

(b) Prepregnancy immunization against rubella.

(c) Genetic counselling:

(i) Avoid marriages between carriers of identifiable inheritable diseases (e.g. thalassaemia, sickle cell anaemia).

(ii) Contraception/sterilization of high risk patients.

(iii) Selective abortion of fetuses with severe abnormalities (e.g. Down syndrome, neural tube defects, homozygous haemoglobinopathies).

72. Q. **What are the conditions for which consultation and transfer to a neonatal intensive care unit should be considered, because of increased mortality and morbidity rates?**

A. (a) Birth-weight less than 2,000 g or maturity less than 35 weeks.

(b) Requirement of oxygen at 30% concentration or higher for longer than 3 hours.

(c) Suspicion of infection.

(d) Severe asphyxia (Apgar score of 3 or less).

(e) Significant congenital anomalies.

(f) Seizures or serious birth trauma (colour plates 140, 143 and 144).

(g) Hypoglycaemia, hypocalcaemia, significant jaundice.

73. Q. **When is it safe to rupture the membranes to hasten delivery of the second twin?**

A. When the head is engaged, the breech presents, or the patient already has a general anaesthetic and thus conditions are favourable for internal version and breech extraction if required.

74. Q. **What are the complications of severe placental abruption?**

A. (a) Fetal death from hypoxia due to separation of the placenta by retroplacental blood clot.

(b) Maternal shock from blood loss (concealed ± revealed).

(c) Entry of thromboplastin from the retroplacental clot into the maternal circulation can cause *disseminated intravascular coagulopathy* resulting in renal cortical/tubular necrosis, pituitary necrosis, eclampsia and (d)

(d) Blood coagulation failure and *postpartum haemorrhage* if delivery occurs before this is corrected by transfusion of blood and plasma concentrates (colour plate 91).

75. Q. **When is placenta praevia likely to be complicated by blood coagulation failure?**

A. When the praevia is accreta and haemorrhage occurs — the blood is retained and simulates the clinical features of placental abruption (pain, tenderness, rigid and enlarging uterus).

76. Q. **Why does vaginal bleeding occur in ectopic pregnancy?**

A. Death of the placenta as a result of tubal bleeding causes hormone withdrawal haemorrhage (like menstruation) from the uterus when the decidua separates.

77. Q. **How is the correct amount of anti-D gamma globulin calculated for administration to a patient who has had a fetomaternal haemorrhage?**

A. By the Kleihauer test on maternal blood to assess the relative number of fetal red cells (these remain stable at an acid pH — figure 22.1).

78. Q. **How can you determine that a patient has been given sufficient anti-D gamma globulin to prevent rhesus isoimmunization?**
A. Perform a papain enzyme test (more sensitive than the indirect Coombs test) on the patient's blood to show that her circulation contains anti-D globulin i.e. it was not all used to inactivate the fetal blood.

79. Q. **What is appropriate advice regarding contraception when the patient is breast feeding?**
A. She is 'safe' for 10 weeks after delivery if the infant is fully breast-fed; then she may rely on the use of a *condom* until the first menstruation occurs, or have an *intrauterine* device inserted. When menstruation occurs an *oral contraceptive pill* (progesterone-only if still breast feeding) is commenced. If use of a condom is not favoured, the contraceptive pill should be commenced 6 weeks after delivery. The *Billings mucus observation method* is also suitable for some patients (figure 56.4A).

80. Q. **When may it be necessary to perform a Caesarean section when the fetus is dead?**
A. A major degree of placenta praevia, ruptured uterus, conjoined twins, neglected transverse lie with generalized tonic uterine contraction (figure 49.5).

81. Q. **How is the risk of the acid aspiration (Mendelson) syndrome lessened in obstetric practice?**
A. (a) Administration of *magnesium trisilicate*, 15 ml orally, 2-hourly to all patients in labour and 30 ml before going to theatre for delivery under general anaesthesia.
(b) Use of *epidural analgesia* rather than general anaesthesia for manipulative procedures (forceps, manual removal, Caesarean section).
(c) Avoidance of food when the patient is in established labour.
(d) Use of cricoid cartilage pressure to close the oesophagus during induction of general anaesthesia.

82. Q. **What observations are necessary after insertion of an epidural nerve block for pain relief in labour?**
A. (a) Pulse and respiratory rate, blood pressure,and ability to move the limbs (exclude total spinal block, or hypotension due to paralysis of sympathetic nerve fibres).
(b) Fetal heart rate.
(c) Degree of pain relief.
(d) Bladder distension — often catheterization is required.
(e) Signs of obstructed labour and of the onset of the second stage of labour — often there is loss of the bearing-down reflex.
(f) The intravenous infusion ± oxytocin.

83. Q. **What are the routine observations after a normal delivery and why are they performed?**
A. (a) Check that the uterine fundus is contracted and central in position — not atonic, filling with blood or displaced by a broad ligament haematoma.
(b) Observe between the patient's thighs and inspect her perineum — to exclude *primary postpartum haemorrhage* and haematoma of the vulva (colour plate 34).
(c) Record the blood pressure — to exclude *hypotension* due to blood loss, uterine inversion etc, and hypertension due to preeclampsia or ergometrine.
(d) Test urine for *protein* — the signs of severe preeclampsia or eclampsia may first appear after delivery.
(e) The *placenta* is inspected for completeness, abnormalities and weighed.
(f) The *infant* receives the usual care after birth and a rapid initial inspection for significant anomalies (see Chapter 59).

84. Q. **What is the incidence and significance of a low lying placenta identified by ultrasonography in early pregnancy?**
A. In 20–30% of patients the placenta encroaches upon the lower uterine segment at 15–25 weeks' gestation, but in 95% it moves upward as the lower segment develops (figure 19.7) — at term the incidence of placenta praevia is about 1%. Note that a central placenta praevia (one entirely within the lower part of the uterus reaching both anterior and posterior walls) *never* migrates upwards (figure 13.11).

85. Q. **What are the functions of amniotic fluid?**
     A. (a) Buffer zone between fetus and uterine wall allowing equal growth and *protection* from all but severe localized *trauma* (figure 23.1).
        (b) Allows *swallowing*, limb movement, *urination* and *respiration* (pulmonary hypoplasia occurs when there is extreme oligohydramnios — Potter syndrome, longstanding premature rupture of membranes).
        (c) Barrier to ascending infection; also the fluid has bactericidal qualities.
        (d) Source of calories — especially protein (the term fetus swallows about 500 ml of liquor/day).
        (e) Flushes out the vagina with a sterile fluid before the fetus is born!

86. Q. **What is the cardiotocographic evidence of fetal hypoxia?**
     A. (a) Loss of spontaneous accelerations and short-term variability (beat to beat variation) (figures 13.14–13.16).
        (b) Heart rate decelerations related to Braxton Hicks contractions — the ominous type (type 2) is when the deceleration persists after the contraction has ceased (figures 13.16–13.18).
        (c) Combination of (a) and (b) is the most critical pattern indicating severe fetal hypoxia (figures 13.15 and 13.16).

87. Q. **How may a vasa praevia be diagnosed before delivery? (see legends of colour plates 84 and 85)**
     A. (a) The occurrence of a small, bright antepartum haemorrhage (usually when the membranes rupture) associated with the onset of fetal bradycardia is suggestive — immediate delivery is mandatory.
        (b) When the Apt test shows vaginal blood (passed spontaneously or after a pelvic examination) to be fetal in origin (resistant to alkali desaturation — see Chapter 19).
        (c) Rarely a fetal vessel is seen at amnioscopy or palpated when vaginal examination is performed preparatory to amniotomy, or in labour to assess progress.

Midwifery Notes

1. THE MIDWIFE AND THE NATIONAL HEALTH SERVICE

While early legislation for midwives in the Midwives Acts of 1918 and 1926 provided improvements in training and conditions, so, in a broader context, were social conditions for the working classes very gradually improving as trade unions were developed and state insurance schemes were introduced. Midwifery training and practice were put on a much better basis with the passing of the 1936 Midwives Act, which not only increased the duration of training but also required local authorities to employ sufficient staff of adequately paid domiciliary midwives, a real social need at a time when two-thirds of births took place in the home.

These important changes in the pattern of midwifery were barely launched when the Second World War began, and before long the need for major post-war reconstruction came to be appreciated. It was in 1942 that the committee under the chairmanship of Sir William Beveridge, reviewing social insurance and certain allied subjects, published what is now well known as the Beveridge Report. This report, a lengthy and historically important social document, is perhaps best remembered for recommending 'the provision of a comprehensive health service'. It was on this basis that the present National Health Service was built, its architect being Aneurin Bevan, Minister of Health in the post-war government.

The National Health Service

The National Health Service Act, was passed in 1946 and implemented in 1948. Its structure, three divisions under the then Ministry of Health, now the Department of Health and Social Security,

is outlined in figure 1. The hospital and specialist services were provided by the regional hospital boards, their hospital management committees and the boards of governors of the teaching hospitals; the general medical services by executive councils; and the remainder of the community services by the local health authorities, namely the county councils and the county borough councils. These services, all provided without charge, were supported by massive legislation giving insurance cover and allowances.

This welfare state pattern developed rapidly, with enormous improvements in standards of health and impressive advances in both curative and preventive medicine. The midwife, whether in hospital or in domiciliary practice, was now a member of a well-established team of specialists, all concerned, either immediately or indirectly, with the welfare of mother and child.

In hospital, the team included the obstetrician, paediatrician, anaesthetist and physiotherapist, on the one hand, and the domestic orderly, porter

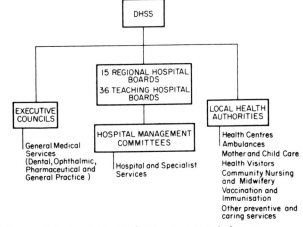

Figure 1 National Health Service structure before re-organisation in 1974.

and kitchen staff on the other. In the community, the family doctor, health visitor, ambulance driver and home help are all team members, with the consultant obstetrician and emergency obstetric unit ('flying squad') to be called upon in emergency.

If, as has often been stated, the standard of a nation's health can be judged by its perinatal mortality figures, these and the other vital statistics in the 1950s and 1960s speak for themselves. The Beveridge concept had come to realize tremendous dividends in terms of health.

But the tripartite structure of the National Health Service shown in figure 1 was in question from the outset. The hospital, local health authority and general practitioner services were separately financed and administered, and misgivings that liaison might be impeded and artificial barriers to good health care created were soon seen to be valid. The financial and administrative constraints were often frustrating, sometimes absurd and usually difficult to overcome. To give one simple example, a patient's antenatal appointments could take her to the doctor's surgery, to the local authority clinic and to the hospital antenatal clinic. An anxious woman could have her antenatal examinations triplicated—a time-wasting exercise, during which conflicting statements could only aggravate her anxiety; a more casual patient could default repeatedly, her absences ascribed to attendances elsewhere and her health deteriorating, sometimes disastrously.

In 1959 the Cranbrook Committee, reviewing possible unification of the maternity services, recommended the continuation of the three-part structure, but with better collaboration and liaison at all levels—a decision which evoked considerable adverse criticism.

1974 Reorganization of the National Health Service

By the late 1960s the case for unification of the entire service was much clearer. After elaborate high-level discussion and prolonged and detailed preparation, full integration was started in April 1974.

This event coincided with the implementation of the recommendations of a Royal Commission set up under Lord Redcliff-Maud to review the structure of local government outside Greater London. This commission recommended a massive streamlining of the local authorities. The large conurbations were to become metropolitan counties, each being subdivided into a number of metropolitan districts. The remainder of the country—cities, towns and surrounding rural areas—would be administrative counties, some having boundaries corresponding with the erstwhile county, some incorporating two smaller counties and some having a simpler boundary than previously. Parishes retained their traditional councils, though in an advisory but no longer executive capacity—a gesture to many thousands of villages, a good number having a history predating the Domesday Book.

These local authorities did not have health service responsibilities, but they retained administration of the social services departments set up after the Seebohm Committee's recommendations were legislated for in the Local Authority Social Services Act of 1970.

The service had a three-tier statutory structure; the Department of Health and Social Security, 14 regional health authorities and 90 area health authorities (figure 2). For operational purposes

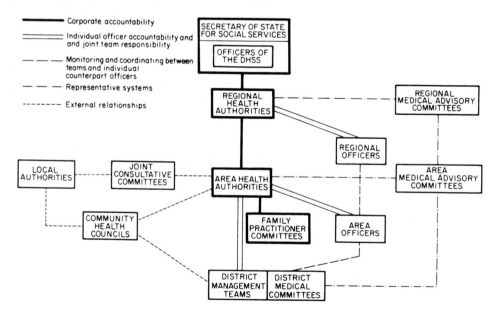

Figure 2 Framework of the National Health Service 1974–1982 organizational structure in England.

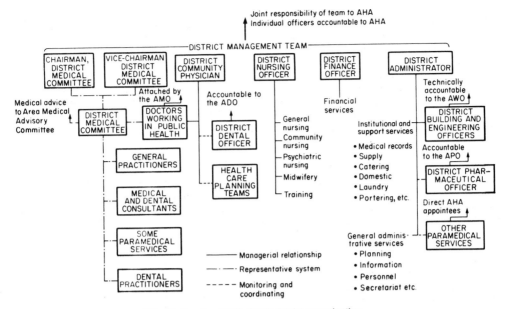

Figure 3 Framework of the National Health Service 1974–1982 district organization.

most of the areas were divided into districts.

The regional health authorities oversaw geographical areas corresponding with those of the Regional Hospital Boards but having local government boundaries. Each was directly responsible to the Secretary of State, and supervised the work of a number of area health authorities (varying between three and eleven). The regional health authority was responsible for allocating resources within its areas, reviewing area plans, coordinating certain research facilities, providing blood transfusion and certain specialist services, managing major building schemes, deciding terms of employment of senior professional staff and other top-level administration.

The area health authorities, several to each region, had the revised local government boundaries, with one area to each county or metropolitan district. Within the areas were the operational districts, each district having a population of 250 000–300 000. Thus some areas (those having a relatively small population) were single-district areas, while the more populous were multi-district areas.

Each area health authority had a chairman appointed by the Secretary of State and members appointed by the regional health authority, the local authority and one or more university nominees. These members gave part-time service and were clearly distinguished from the professional team employed by the area health authority. This team comprised the area medical officer, the area nursing officer, the area treasurer and the area administrator. The members were responsible for policies, plans and allocation of resources within the area, the appointment of senior officers, the assessment of the services and the maintenance of the best possible standard of service.

It was at district level that the reorganized service operated. A district in this context, comprised a group having a population of 250 000–300 000 served by the community health services together with the specialist services of a district general hospital.

The district services were planned and coordinated by a district management team, responsible to the area health authority and comprising a district community physician, a district nursing officer, a district finance officer and a district administrator with two representatives of the district medical committee (figure 3). As well as local policy-making and planning, this team was responsible for implementing the plans that the area health authority had approved. The district medical committee, representative of all local medical staff, took responsibility for coordinating the various medical aspects of health care. Health care planning teams were groups of experts appointed to determine the needs of special groups of patients, to review the services in general and to recommend any necessary modifications.

These important health care planning teams included consultants and general practitioners, hospital and community nurses, health visitors, social services representatives and various paramedical staff, supported by the district community physician and an administrator.

The framework of a district organization up to 1982 is shown in figure 3. The detail of its structure varied from one district to another.

Royal Commission of the NHS 1979

This recommended certain changes in the 1974 structure, to simplify lines of communication and responsibility at local level. This was accepted by the government who published a consultative paper—*Patients First*.

Patients First (December 1979)

In this document suggestions were made for rearrangement of the administrative structure which appeared top-heavy.

1. Abolishment of area health authorities (AHAs).
2. Setting up district health authorities (DHAs) to combine the functions of AHAs and district management teams (DMTs).

Structure from 1 April 1982 (figure 4)

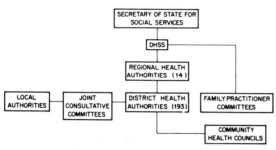

Figure 4 National Health Service structure from 1 April 1982.

District Health Authorities (DHAs)

These number 193 in England, and they are the basic units for management and planning in the NHS.

Composition:

The chairman is chosen by the Secretary of State and receives a 'part time' salary.

The members are unpaid, and number between 16 and 19. They should include:

Two medical practitioners—one a consultant and one a general practitioner, both of whom are employed by the DHA.
A nurse, midwife or health visitor, who may not be employed by the DHA.
A nominee of the university medical school in the region.
A trade unionist.
Four to six appointees of the local authorities.

District Management Team (DMT)

Composition

District administrator ⎫
District nursing officer ⎬ Appointed
District community physician ⎪ officers
District finance officer ⎭

General practitioner ⎫ Elected by
Consultant ⎬ district colleagues

Department of Health and Social Security (DHSS)

The Department has national responsibility for:

1. Social security.
2. Personal social services.
3. The National Health Service.

The *political head* is the Secretary of State for Social Services. He or she is both a member of Parliament and the Cabinet, is appointed and dismissed by the Prime Minister, and is accountable to Parliament for the work of the DHSS. He or she is supported by a number of junior ministers, including a Minister of State for Health and civil servants. The 7000 civil servants include the Permanent Secretary, who is an administrator, and a doctor, who is the Chief Medical Officer.

The DHSS functions in relation to the NHS are:

1. Policy making and the issue of advice.
2. Allocation of resources to regions, in line with the recommendations of the Resource Allocation Working Party (RAWP), published in 1976. This is to try to share out money in a fairer way. Health circulars and policy documents such as *Care in Action 1981* inform the RHAs of the way the money should be spent.

Social Service Committee. This is a select committee set up in 1979 to investigate various aspects of the work of the DHSS. It has produced a number of reports, including the Short Report on perinatal mortality.

Regional Health Authorities

Composition. There are approximately 20 members, appointed by the Secretary of State after consultation with interested organizations. Only the chairman is paid. Each authority is served by paid officials led by the regional team of officers (RTO). The full team and their responsibilities can be seen in figure 5.

Apart from a few services such as blood transfusion, their main responsibilities are:

1. Allocation of resources to DHAs.
2. Planning development of health services.
3. Designing major capital projects.
4. Employing senior medical staff in non-teaching hospitals.
5. Setting up and reviewing community health councils (CHCs).

In 1981, when the latest reorganization was taking place, the government stated its intention to allow each DHA flexibility for the framework of the structure. However, the financial constraints militated against satisfactory district management and administration. This has proved to be especially so for small midwifery units. Many have been combined with a varied selection of other specialities.

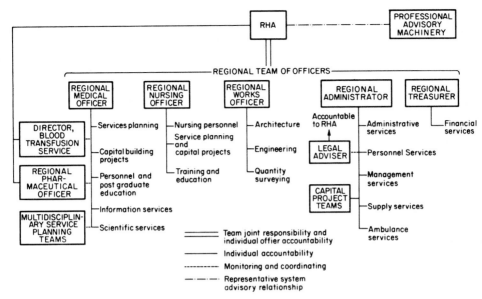

Figure 5 Framework of the National Health Service 1974–1985 regional organization.

Both the regional team of officers (RTOs) and the district management teams (DMTs) reached decision by consensus, with each member having equal status and the right to veto. This system of management practice was subject to an inquiry in February 1983 led by Roy Griffiths, Managing Director of Sainsbury's.

The *Griffiths' Report* was published on 25 October 1983. This was subsequently accepted by the Government, as a lack of real evaluation of performance of the NHS was observed, as well as a lack of general management function which was leading to extreme difficulties in achieving change. The devolution of responsibility was also very slow.

Recommendations of the Griffiths' Report

These are being carried out at three levels:

1. DHSS as set up

   (a) *Health Services Supervisory Board*

   Composition:
   Secretary of State
   Minister of State for Health
   Permanent Secretary
   Chief Medical Officer (CMO)
   Chief Nursing Officer (CNO)
   NHS Management Board Chairman
   Two or three non-executive members

   (b) *NHS Management Board.* This is under the direction of, and accountable to, the Supervisory Board.

   Composition:
   National General Manager (Chairman)
   Small multi-professional group

2. (a) *Regional Health Authority level.* Each RHA has appointed a general manager. These are either administrators, doctors or nurses, but so far the latter are in the minority.

   (b) *District Health Authority level.* Each DHA has appointed a general manager.

   The RHA and DHA managers are appointed for a fixed number of years only. Their remit is to:

   (i) Initiate major cost improvement programmes.
   (ii) Devolve decision making and responsibility down to unit level where patient needs are met directly.
   (iii) Review and reduce need for functional management structures.
   (iv) To organize a management structure best suited to local needs.

3. *Unit Management level.* Managers are being appointed in each unit where all day-to-day decisions are to be taken and where clinicians are more closely involved in the management process and budgets. It is likely that the Boards of Directors will not include professional managers. The effects of this new reorganization is intended to deliver improved services to patients and clients and better managerial support to staff in direct patient contact.

2. THE REGULATION OF TRAINING AND PRACTICE OF THE MIDWIFE

The title of midwife is an ancient one; we may read about midwives, and even learn their names, as early as the beginning of the Old Testament.

Through the centuries the midwife sometimes received a little instruction in her work, but more often none. The profession thus has a chequered history, in which the midwife is sometimes clearly an honoured and respected member of the community, while at others she emerges as a drunken, disreputable and thoroughly undesirable character.

In Great Britain, during the seventeenth and eighteenth centuries, there were a few attempts—mostly unsuccessful—to train midwives and to obtain for them some kind of state recognition, but it was not until the latter part of the nineteenth century that any real progress was made. The 30 years from 1872 saw the London Obstetrical Society's training and examination in midwifery, the General Medical Council's efforts to gain state recognition for the profession and the formation in 1881 of the Midwives Institute, now the Royal College of Midwives.

At this time various public-spirited people obtained the introduction of a number of Bills to Parliament. Eight were unsuccessful; the ninth, passed in 1902, brought about the formation of the Central Midwives Board and only then was midwifery organized on a national basis with state certification. The midwife in those days was a lone worker in the health field, attending her patients in labour and in the lying-in period—antenatal care was to come later—and calling a doctor only when serious complications arose.

Nurses, Midwives and Health Visitors Act 1979

This Act resulted from the Report of the Committee on Nursing, published in 1972. This report suggested that the establishment of one unified structure would make for more effective patterns of training, after examining the interrelationship between basic and specialist training. The Act brought into being the United Kingdom Central Council for Nursing, Midwifery and Health Visiting (UKCC), composed of 33 members, and four National Boards having 20 members each. The 1979 Act provided for an overlap of two to three years with the existing bodies, which included the Central Midwives Boards, General Nursing Councils, the Council for Education and Training of Health Visitors and the Joint Board of Clinical Nursing Studies. After this period these bodies were dissolved.

UKCC Main Responsibilities

These are:

1. To establish and improve standards of training and professional conduct for nurses, midwives and health visitors.
2. To establish the rules for registration.
3. To maintain a single professional register.
4. To issue a code of conduct to maintain standards of professional conduct.
5. To protect the public from unsafe practitioners by means of the professional conduct or health committees.

Midwifery Training

Midwifery training came under statutory control in 1902, consequent upon the passing of the first Midwives Act. At its inception the training lasted only three months: over the years it has expanded steadily, being increased in 1926 to six months and in 1936 to 12 months for state registered nurses. Non-nurses received a longer training. In 1936 the training was divided into two parts: a first period of six months for those nurses who required some knowledge of the subject, but who did not wish to become midwives: and a second period of six months for those who wished to qualify and practise. For women who were not nurses the first period lasted 18 months and for state enrolled nurses a 12-month first period was devised.

In 1961 obstetric nurse training was introduced to provide a short period of midwifery experience for student nurses, in accordance with a plan jointly agreed by the General Nursing Council and the Central Midwives Board, the training being implemented by the Central Midwives Board. This has now been superseded by maternity care experience, which is a European Economic Community (EEC) Nurses Directive requirement. It was foreseen that in due course the first-period midwifery training would become unnecessary, and in 1968 a single-period training was introduced. This single-period training was introduced extensively while the separate first- and second-period training were phased out.

The single-period training for state registered nurses and registered sick children's nurses was completed within a year, which included five weeks' holiday and the qualifying examination. For state enrolled nurses and for women who were not nurses, the single-period training lasted 18 months and two years respectively.

As time passed, it became apparent to most tutors and their students that a longer training time was essential. The subject matter had increased and, as technology grew, there was a need for a greater depth of understanding and application of behavioural sciences.

Eighteen-Month Training

For some 10 years the Central Midwives Board had pressed for an extension of training of state registered nurses from one year to 18 months. The EEC Midwives Directives brought about the lengthening with effect from September 1981, and it is now mandatory for general nurses. Registered sick children's nurses, registered mental nurses/registered nurses for mental defectives, state-enrolled nurses and orthopaedic nurses are no longer eligible for this shortened training.

The training falls into three sections—(1) initial, (2) community and (3) final periods:

Initial period. This is fundamentally concerned with the physiology and psychology of normal childbirth. It consists of 18–24 weeks' clinical experience in conventional as well as modern techniques.

Community period. The aim is to consolidate knowledge of normal childbirth in the family and social setting. The student midwife should be attached to a teaching midwife for antenatal, labour and postnatal care, which includes the preparation of the home for confinement and conducting parentcraft sessions. This period must be not less than 12 weeks up to a maximum of 18 weeks. It can be divided into two sections, provided that the first is at least eight weeks.

Final period. During this time of 26.5–38.5 weeks, the student should be introduced to her/his role as a practising midwife. Complications and their psychological effects should be included. A two-week study period is included and six weeks' experience in a special care baby unit as well as six weeks in an antenatal clinic or ward, labour ward and postnatal ward.

Documentation of clinical experience has greatly increased to meet the requirements of the European Community, who define the minimum range of activities.

European Economic Community (EEC)

The official journal of the European Communities published on 11 February 1980, L33, volume 23, contains the Midwives Directives (signed in January 1980) which were implemented by 23 January 1983. The purpose of these is to aid freedom of movement of midwives between EEC member states. In order to achieve mutual recognition of formal qualifications, certain changes had to be made and, even with the UK 18-month programme for general nurses, a midwife requires a certificate of one year's satisfactory professional practice after qualification. She will then—provided she is a national of a member state, and has a document showing good character—be recognized.

Those who are not general trained nurses, must take a three-year full-time course for recognition. If they do not possess educational qualifications equivalent to university admission, they will, in addition to their qualification, need a certificate on completion of two years satisfactory professional practice.

The activities the midwife may undertake are laid down in Article 4 of the EEC Midwives Directives.

3. COMMUNITY MIDWIFERY AND OTHER COMMUNITY SERVICES

Historical Background

The term 'midwife' means 'with woman', and therefore any who chose to help a woman through the trials of labour and delivery of the baby could set herself up to be the local midwife. Her knowledge was largely gained by practice, until, on the formation of the Midwives Institute in 1881, it became possible to acquire some form of training on a voluntary basis.

The first Midwives Act (of 1902) required all midwives to be trained, but some were able to be certified then due to skills already acquired and in practice. Anyone wishing to practise after that date had first to undergo the training and examination as laid down by the newly formed Central Midwives Board. Once qualified, midwives were free to practise independently or through one of the voluntary agencies which were usually associated with the church.

In 1936 the local authorities, in their capacity as local health authorities, were required to provide an adequate number of midwives to care for mothers and babies in their own homes, in accordance with the rules of the Central Midwives Board. This they did, either by employing them direct or by making arrangements with the established agencies.

Domiciliary midwives, as they were then known, worked from their own homes, although accommodation was often provided, and indeed it was sometimes specially built for them. When the midwife left home, she pinned to her door a list of addresses to be visited. Anyone requiring her services, went from house to house until they located her. While the midwife went to the labouring mother, the husband was often dispatched to her house to collect the necessary equipment. The local authorities provided this equipment, which meant it varied considerably according to the resources of the councils.

Nearly all babies were born at home, and midwives generally had their own 'area'. They were expected to be available at all times except for their weekly day off, when their colleague in the next door area took the calls. The local health authority was also the supervising authority responsible for the statutory supervision of midwives in their area. There was usually a medical supervisor (medical officer) and a non-medical supervisor (a midwife) of midwives. The services of the midwife were free but medical services had to be paid for if the midwife had to summon medical aid.

The implementation of the National Health Services Act 1946 in 1948 left domiciliary midwifery with the local authority. As far as the mothers were concerned, the major change came in being entitled to free medical coverage. The trend towards hospital confinement had already begun and this continued, accelerated by the Cranbrook Report (1959) which recommended the provision of sufficient maternity beds for 70 per cent of the confinements. By 1967, hospital confinements had in fact risen to 75 per cent and, with a steadily rising birth rate, the maternity units were overburdened. This situation was resolved by shortening the stay and passing the care of the mother and baby over to the domiciliary midwife. Initially this was done haphazardly, but it was not long before the confusion necessitated a more formal arrangement. It appeared that many mothers and babies could return to their own homes within ten days with no ill-effects to either, and to many women this became an attractive idea, combining the safety of hospital with the freedom to return to their family more quickly.

The decline in home confinements and the reduced stay in hospital meant that domiciliary midwives were largely providing postnatal care only, and by the 1960s they felt their traditional role had been eroded and they were merely maternity nurses. Not only did this create job dissatisfaction, but, more significant, the domiciliary midwives were in danger of losing their traditional skills and missing out on advances in midwifery and obstetrics.

Far-sighted managers realized that the needs of mothers and midwives could best be met by domiciliary midwives conducting deliveries in hospitals and then providing continuity of care for the mother and baby once they were transferred home. In order for this to be accomplished, domiciliary midwives had to be given honorary appointments to hospitals, and many had to spend periods working in the unit to familiarize themselves with current practices. These ideas were the forerunner of an integrated midwifery service, which had been seen to be desirable many years before.

Present-day Community Midwifery

In 1974, as a result of the 1973 National Health Service Act, all community health services became part of the National Health Service. The newly formed regional health authority was designated the local supervising authority, and the domiciliary midwifery service was taken over by the District, the head of service being the district nursing officer. According to local situations, domiciliary midwives came into either the community or the midwifery division. The embryo schemes for midwives to conduct deliveries in the unit flourished, and today there are many such schemes. It became accepted practice to call domiciliary midwives 'community midwives', reflecting more accurately their role. In some areas midwives are attached to GP practices; in others they have retained their geographic area. They are expected to work in close liaison with health visitors, and should be considered members of the primary health care team.

The changes in management structures brought about in 1982, with the abolition of the Area Health Authorities and the introduction of District Health Authorities, had little effect on community midwifery, except that community midwives found themselves part of a larger structure at local level. Community midwifery was incorporated into the most appropriate Unit.

PATTERNS OF MATERNITY CARE INVOLVING COMMUNITY MIDWIVES

Home Confinement

A woman wishing to have a home confinement should discuss the idea with her general practitioner; if he is agreeable, either she or the doctor informs the community midwifery service. As soon as possible the midwife will visit the woman in her own home and 'book' her. All antenatal care will be by the general practitioner (provided he is on the obstetric roll) and the midwife. Should the general practitioner not undertake maternity care, the woman has the right to engage a general practitioner obstetrician (GPO) for maternity services only.

Use can be made of specialist hospital facilities as necessary (e.g. ultrasonography). The woman is provided with a home confinement box, and is given a list of things she should have in readiness. During the last month of the pregnancy the midwife visits the house, and together they discuss the most suitable preparation of the room in which the confinement is going to take place.

In the interests of safety, the midwife should ensure that a third person is present at the delivery. The midwife should remain in the house until she is satisfied with the condition of the mother and baby, and for at least 1 hour after delivery. She is expected to return within 2 hours to ensure that neither has deteriorated. The remainder of the care during the postnatal period is carried out according to the recommendation of the UKCC Midwife's Code of Practice.

General Practitioner Booking

In many parts of the United Kingdom there are small maternity units where obstetric care is provided by general practitioner obstetricians. In others, part of the hospital unit is set aside for use by the general practitioners, or they may use the main delivery suite. Antenatal care is provided by the GP and the community midwife, and the delivery is conducted either by the community midwife or a midwife working in the unit—whichever is going to provide more continuity. It is the GP who examines the mother and baby as being fit to return home for the postnatal care to be carried on there by the community midwife.

Domino Booking

The term was coined originally to describe the situation where the community midwife brings the mother in when labour is established and then returns home with her any time from 6 to 48 hours after delivery (domiciliary midwife in and out). This scheme was intended to encourage women who were unsuitable for home confinement on obstetric grounds to accept a hospital bed. It also enabled the community midwife to practise her full range of skills and keep up with modern day obstetrics. Once the woman is booked at the hospital the community midwife visits her at home and discusses the Domino scheme. Together they plan her antenatal care, which is often shared between the GP, hospital obstetrician and the community midwife. When labour commences, the community midwife either visits the woman at home to confirm that labour has commenced or meets her in the hospital delivery ward. The community midwife conducts the delivery but any obstetric care is provided by the hospital obstetrician, who also has the responsibility of examining the mother and baby prior to allowing them to return home. (The examination of the baby may be carried out by the paediatrician.) The actual length of stay is determined to some extent by the time of day at which the woman is delivered. Care during the postnatal period is provided by the community midwife both in the unit and when the mother returns home. The midwife must visit until the 10th postnatal day and may continue until the 28th day.

Planned Early Transfer

The trend towards postnatal care in the community has continued. In many units mothers and babies are transferred home as soon as both are fit for the community midwife to complete their care. Ideally the midwife visits the woman during pregnancy to discuss what help is available and to offer advice.

Following confinement, the midwife is informed of the impending transfer home of mother and baby, enabling her to fulfil her responsibilities.

Community midwives now have contact with some 80% of maternity patients, which increases their role as health educators.

Equipment provided for Community Midwifery (examples)

Antenatal bag

Sphygmomanometer
Adult stethoscope
Fetal stethoscope
Urine-testing equipment
Syringes, needles
Specimen bottles
Stationery (case sheets, etc.—see below)

Delivery bag

Many of these may be replaced by the use of a ready-sterilized CSSD pack.

Artery forceps, 2 pairs
Dissecting forceps, 1 pair
Episiotomy scissors, 1 pair
Cord scissors, 1 pair
Thermometers (1 adult, 1 low-reading)
Lotion thermometer
Selection of gallipots, dishes and a measuring jug
Urinary catheters
Mucus extractors
Masks
Gloves (sterile)
Medicine glass
Nail brush, soap and towel
Razor
Antiseptic (usually cetrimide)
Antiseptic cream (obstetric)
Surgical spirit
Chloral hydrate tablets
Ergometrine tablets
Ergometrine preparation for injection
Drugs approved by the particular authority for resuscitation of the baby e.g. Naloxone
Plastic apron
Disposable enema or equipment for simple enema
Syringes, needles and assorted sample bottles

Infant resuscitation

1. Oxygen
   Preset flow meter
   Rubber tubing
   Connecting piece and face mask
2. Neonatal resuscitator e.g. Laerdal or Penlon Bag
3. Infant airway

Stationery

Register of cases to record (a) all professional visits made or attempted, and (b) all personal deliveries.

Case notes
Drug record book
Statistical return forms
Information (assorted) for distribution to mothers
Assorted forms relevant to the employer

Nursing bag

Artery forceps, 1 pair
Dissecting forceps, 1 pair
Stitch scissors, 1 pair
Thermometers, 2 (1 adult, 1 low-reading)
Selection of gallipots
Urinary catheters
Mucus extractors
Masks
Gloves
Antiseptic (usually cetrimide)
Surgical spirit
Ergometrine tablets
Ergometrine preparation for injection
Aperients
Syringes and sample bottles (assorted)
Cord powder
Cord ligatures
Guthrie cards, lancets and plasters

Inhalation analgesia

Entonox machine
Entonox cylinders, 2.

The midwife practising in the community should be aware of other community services available to her patients. Some are part of the NHS and others the local authority.

COMMUNITY SERVICES WITHIN THE NHS

Health Visiting

This comes within the community nursing unit. A health visitor is a state registered nurse with 10 weeks' approved obstetric experience, who has undergone a further year's training and obtained the Certificate for Health Visiting.

Her role is preventive, and can be described under four broad headings:

1. The prevention of mental, physical and emotional ill-health and all their consequences.
2. The early detection of ill-health and surveillance of high-risk groups.
3. The recognition of need and mobilization of resources.
4. Health education.

The health visitor works either attached to a group practice or in a geographic area. She has a special responsibility towards families where there are young children, and she takes over the care of the new baby from the midwife. Around the 10th day after birth the health visitor will make her first visit to the home. The mother will be advised of the child health clinic facilities, and any feeding problems will be discussed. In some areas the hand-over from midwife to health visitor is done at this time. It is customary to obtain consent for the child to participate in the immunization programme, and the health visitor may examine the baby. Unless further home visits are indicated, the child is seen subsequently at the child health clinic.

At the other end of the scale, her work includes regular visits to the elderly and the housebound. She also has a supportive role towards the mentally or physically handicapped, and to those families with special problems.

District Nursing

District nurses are either state registered or state enrolled nurses who have undertaken an extra, mandatory course leading to the District Nursing Certificate. They provide nursing services to people in their own homes and are part of the community nursing unit. They either work in a geographical area or are attached to a group practice.

Much of their work is concerned with the elderly, but they also provide a valuable follow-up for surgical patients, often enabling them to return home earlier. In midwifery the district nurse occasionally takes over where there is some infection, the midwife retaining her statutory responsibility.

General Practitioner Services

General practitioners are responsible for the provision of a 24-hour service for the treatment of illness. Their contract with the Family Practitioner Committee requires them to provide: 'all necessary and appropriate personal medical services of the type usually provided by general medical practitioners . . . to their patients'.

Some general practitioners work alone, others work in group practices and the rest work from health centres. In the last there may be as many as 12 doctors engaged in practice. Many general practitioners use some form of deputizing service to cover the night hours.

To register with a general practitioner the person takes their medical card to the chosen surgery, and, provided there is room on the list, he will be accepted. Should there be any difficulty in registering with a doctor, an application is made to the Family Practitioner Committee. They will allocate the person to a practice with a vacancy.

With the increase in group practice there is a trend towards the various members of the partnership specializing in that branch of general practice which particularly interests them, e.g. maternity, paediatrics, geriatrics.

In order to be classified as a general practitioner obstetrician (GPO), additional experience or qualification in obstetrics is required. A GPO is entitled to provide maternity services to anyone who applies to him, and he is prefixed 'M' in the family practitioner list.

COMMUNITY SERVICES PROVIDED BY THE LOCAL AUTHORITY

Social Services

The Local Authority Social Services Act of 1970 required local authorities to establish a social services committee (department). This department provides for:

1. The elderly.
2. The mentally and physically handicapped.
3. Children in need of care and protection.
4. Children for adoption.
5. Anyone or any family in temporary or long-term social need.

Social services departments were set up in 1971. The head in each such department is the director of social services. He is supported by assistants, and below that the fieldworkers are qualified and trainee social workers.

In addition, he is responsible for the home help service, residential care, day care and meals on wheels.

The department is able to provide adaptations to the home to enable the elderly and/or handicapped to live as normal and independent a life as possible, and they can make special payments in cases of acute need. Social workers can help people obtain benefits and grants which might be due to them through the Department of Health and Social Security.

Referral is generally through the health visitor or general practitioner, or sometimes the community midwife, although an individual may also apply direct.

Environmental Health Department

The purpose of this department is to ensure that the environment in which we all live is suitable for us to remain free from disease. To this end environmental health officers supervise commercial food preparation and working conditions. They inspect and report on premises which may be considered unfit for human habitation, and monitor the levels of noise and pollution in the atmosphere. Wherever there is an infestation of rats, mice, lice, etc., they can be called in.

Occasionally they will have to investigate the outbreak of an infectious disease.

Housing Department

Community midwives will visit many mothers and babies in local authority housing. Housing is allocated to people in order of priority, and in almost all areas the supply of houses is inadequate for the need. Under the Homeless Persons Act (1977) the local authority has a responsibility to house anyone made homeless through no fault of their own.

THE USE OF PETHIDINE BY COMMUNITY MIDWIVES

Since 1951, practising midwives have been allowed to use pethidine on their own responsibility, provided they abide by the UKCC Handbook of Midwives Rules relating to the use of drugs in general, and by anything laid down by Acts of Parliament.

The Misuse of Drugs Act 1971 classifies drugs into schedules and the one into which pethidine comes is Schedule 2.

The Misuse of Drugs Regulations 1973 (with amendments in 1974 to allow for the terms used in the reorganized health service) specify the authorization given to midwives.

Paragrah 11: (1) A midwife who has notified her intention to the local supervising authority may:

(a) so far as necessary for the practice of her profession or employment as a midwife, have pethidine in her possession;
(b) so far as necessary as aforesaid, administer pethidine;
(c) surrender to the appropriate medical officer any stocks of pethidine in her possession which are no longer required by her.

(2) Nothing in paragraph (1) authorizes a midwife to have in her possession pethidine which has been obtained otherwise than on a midwife's supply order signed by the appropriate medical officer.

For the purposes of paragraph (2), the medical officer includes the midwife appointed by the local supervising authority to exercise supervision over midwives.

Paragraph 21: (3) A midwife authorized to have pethidine in her possession shall:

(a) on each occasion on which she obtains a supply of pethidine enter in a book kept by her and used solely for the purposes of this paragraph the date, the name and address of the person from whom the drug was obtained, the amount obtained and the form in which it was obtained; and
(b) on administering pethidine to a patient, enter in the said book as soon as practicable the name and address of the patient, the amount administered and the form in which it was administered.

The safe-keeping of pethidine is spelt out in the Misuse of Drugs (Safe Custody) Regulations 1973. Paragraph 5 relates to safe-keeping where the regulations for storage on a large scale are not in force.

'... any person ... having possession of the drug shall ensure that, so far as circumstances permit, it is kept in a locked receptacle which can be opened only by him or by a person authorised by him.'

Interpretation of the Act in Relation to Community Midwifery

When a midwife requires a supply of pethidine, she applies to her supervisor of midwives. Together they check the entries in the midwife's personal register and drug book. Provided they tally, the remaining stock is checked, and all being in order the supervisor issues a supply order form, signed by her. It is normal practice to issue the smallest practicable amount, often two ampoules The midwife takes the drug book and order form to the agreed chemist or hospital pharmacist, who issues the new stock. Both he and the midwife make the appropriate entries. The midwife should have been introduced to the pharmacist, and he should have a sample of the supervisor's signature.

A midwife who wishes to return drugs should first check these with the supervisor and then approach an authorized person, i.e. a police officer, an inspector of the Home Office Drugs Branch, an inspector of the Pharmaceutical Society, a regional pharmaceutical officer, or a senior administrative officer of a National Health Service hospital.

HEALTH BENEFITS

The DHSS provides a range of financial and other benefits designed to help the expectant mother and the family maintain a satisfactory level of health.

Maternity Benefits

Maternity grant. A lump sum of £25 is payable to the expectant mother whose pregnancy continues to the 27th week, provided she has been resident in the United Kingdom for a minimum of 6 months. The grant can be claimed from the 27th week of pregnancy up until 3 months after the birth of the baby. A certificate signed by a doctor or midwife is required, to be sent with the claim form. The woman who is delivered of a live baby before the 27th week of pregnancy is also entitled to the maternity grant.

Maternity allowance. A weekly sum is payable to the expectant mother on her own class 1 or class 2 National Insurance contributions for 18 weeks, commencing 11 weeks before the expected date of confinement. Further benefit may be allowed for dependants. The maternity allowance is only paid for weeks in which the woman does not work.

Welfare Milk, Vitamins, Dental Treatment and Prescriptions

Any expectant mother receiving supplementary benefit, or in the low income group, is entitled to free milk and vitamins. The allowance is for 1 pint of milk daily and vitamin tablets as required.

All expectant mothers are entitled to free prescriptions and free dental care throughout their pregnancy and up until 1 year afterwards. A form signed by a doctor, health visitor or midwife is forwarded to the Family Practitioner Committee.

Family Benefits

Child benefit. A weekly sum is payable for each child under 16 years, or for longer if the child continues with studies full time up until the age of 18 years. Additional amounts may be available for single-parent families.

Supplementary benefit. A means-tested weekly amount is payable to anyone not working who has insufficient money on which to live according to a national scale.

Family income supplement. A weekly sum is payable to a family where there is at least one child, and where the parent is in work (for a couple the man must work at least 30 hours) but whose total income falls below a level set by the DHSS.

Attendance allowance. Where one or other parent is required to provide a continual level of supervision (e.g. for a severely handicapped child), a claim may be lodged once the child is 22 months old. A decision is based on the results of a medical examination; where the claim is accepted, a weekly payment is made.

Hospital fares. For anyone needing to attend hospital and who is unable to afford the fares, it is possible to claim from the Department of Health and Social Security. (Those receiving supplementary benefit or family income supplement are automatically entitled to fares.)

Miscellaneous Benefits

All women may attend antenatal and postnatal clinics and take their children to child health clinics without payment. The services of the midwife, health visitor and general practitioner are free. Home helps are available for maternity patients, payment being according to means. Expectant mothers are entitled to free ambulance service and a hospital bed for confinement.

4. THE UNSUPPORTED MOTHER AND HER CHILD

The midwife is often consulted about the care of babies and children deprived of a normal home environment, and she should have some knowledge of the legislation and services which exist to help and protect the mother and her child.

The unsupported mother may be single. She may, on the other hand, be married and without the support of her husband. The number of single-parent families is a growing problem. The child of an unsupported parent may sometimes be 'at risk'. Poor housing, lack of emotional stimulation and social isolation contribute to this problem. The midwife should put the mother in contact with a social worker either from the local social services or from a voluntary organization (e.g. Welcare organized by the Church of England).

This mother may, whether insured or uninsured, claim the State maternity grant. The mother who is fully insured may also claim the State maternity allowance. If she is only entitled to the maternity grant, she may apply for supplementary benefit if she is in a low income bracket or unemployed.

She can continue her work if she places the child in a day nursery run by the local authority, and where her request will be given priority; day nurseries are very popular and women are glad to take advantage of them.

If there is a crèche at her place of work, the problem is settled. Many factories, hospitals and stores have, in recent years, helped to solve their labour problems by opening and staffing a crèche.

She can also leave the child with a child-minder or a foster mother, again continuing to work.

A schoolgirl may receive home tutoring in order that her studies may not be interrupted.

Child-minders and Foster Parents

Child-minders are persons undertaking for reward, the care of children other than their own offspring, whereas Foster parents receive payment that does not allow a profit to be made. Both categories are required to notify the local authority of their undertaking, giving full details, and they must allow the local authority social services department to see their homes and the children for whom they are caring.

Affiliation

The responsibility for maintaining an illegitimate child rests with its mother. She may, however, apply, by way of summons, to a Court of Summary Jurisdiction for an affiliation order on the putative father of the child. If the court grants such an order, the father, is thereby compelled to contribute a weekly sum towards the cost of the child's maintenance, continuing until the child is 16 or, if he is still receiving full-time education, 21 years old. Paternity must be admitted, or some corroborative evidence (e.g. an admission by the putative father to a third person) is necessary. Failure to comply with an affiliation order is a punishable offence though it is not always possible either to oblige the defaulter to pay or to enforce the punishment. If a mother claims supplementary benefit, the Department of Health and Social Security, through their liable relative clause, will take out their own summons.

Adoption

As an alternative to all these possibilities, whereby she keeps her baby, the mother may place the child for adoption, thus relinquishing all claim upon him.

Third party and private adoptions have become illegal since 1 February 1982. Midwives, in the past, were occasionally asked to arrange such adoptions.

An adoption order, made usually by a county court or a court of summary jurisdiction, puts the adopted child into the position of a legitimate child of the adopter or adopters. The mother now has no claim whatsoever over the child.

The Adoption Acts of 1958 and 1960 are designed to protect in every possible way the child's interests.

The Adoption Act 1958 does not allow an adoption order to be made unless the applicant:

1. is the mother or father of the infant;
2. is a relative of the infant, and has attained the age of 21 years;
3. has attained the age of 25 years.

A married couple may be granted an adoption order:

1. if either of the applicants is the mother or father of the infant;
2. if one applicant satisfies the requirements of criteria 1 or 2, above, and other has attained the age of 21 years.

Only in exceptional circumstances may a man adopt a female child.

The infant must have been continuously in the care of the applicant for at least 3 months before the order is made, not counting the first 6 weeks of life.

The applicant, at least 3 months before the date of the order, must have given written notice to the local authority in whose area he was then living, of his intention to apply for an adoption order in respect of the infant.

More recently, the Children Act 1975 was introduced to put the welfare of the child first. Decisions must take into consideration the child's long-term interest. It is now mandatory for local authorities to run an adoption service. The Act also makes it easier for children to be adopted who have been in long-term care. The number of children currently being put up for adoption is small. The Abortion Act 1965, and the current trend for single parents to keep their families, have contributed to this. When an adopted person reaches the age of 18, he has the right of access to his own birth records. A counselling service is provided by the Registrar General. The social workers who are employed for this purpose have a heavy responsibility, as they can add further details to complete the family background. They also have to take into consideration the effect on the natural and the adoptive parents.

Foster Parents

New rights have been granted to foster parents under the Children Act. Where a child has been fostered for 6 months, the natural parents must give 28 days' notice before removing him from care. This has alleviated the 'tug of love' situation where, in the past, the child could be removed without any warning at all. Under the Children Act 1975, from 1 December 1985 those who have cared for a child for 3 years will be able to apply for a custodianship order with or without the consent of either parent or the local authority. This will give the foster parents the rights and duties of a natural parent and the ability to make decisions about a child's day-to-day care and upbringing in the same way as a parent.

The three groups who will be able to apply for custodianship orders are:

1. Relatives e.g. grandmothers.
2. Stepmothers, who will then be able to share with their partners the responsibilities of a parent.
3. Foster parents.

With the recent streamlining and vast increase in scope of the social services departments, any unsupported mother, whatever her means, nationality or social background, should be able to approach a social worker who will give her expert advice and put her in touch with the particular authority from which she may claim monetary or other assistance.

5. DRUGS USED IN MIDWIFERY AND NEONATAL PAEDIATRICS

Drugs of any description should be avoided in pregnancy if possible because of the risk of their harmful effect on the fetus. This is especially relevant during the first trimester, when the fetus is undergoing development. There are times, however, when the benefits of a drug outweigh the risks—for example, in epilepsy where there is little choice but to continue the anticonvulsant therapy.

Following the thalidomide tragedy, a Committee on the Safety of Drugs was set up in 1962 to ensure that every new drug is tested for toxicity on pregnant animals in a laboratory before it is considered safe to be prescribed to the pregnant woman.

The need for drugs in midwifery and paediatrics can be divided into five categories:

1. To relieve pain in labour—an effective analgesic which does not adversely affect the mother, the contractions or the fetus.
2. To induce labour.
3. To prevent/treat haemorrhage.
4. To resuscitate the neonate.
5. To treat medical conditions.

Legislation
1. Medicines Act 1968 regulates use of all medicinal products.
2. Misuse of Drugs Act 1971 is concerned with abuse of controlled drugs (formerly classified as 'dangerous drugs').

3. Misuse of Drugs Regulations 1973 lays down conditions whereby controlled drugs may be used by medical practitioners and certain others (e.g. certified midwife is authorized to be in possession of pethidine).
4. Misuse of Drugs (Amendment) Regulations 1974 outline safe custody of controlled drugs and the procedure whereby midwives must surrender unwanted stock.
5. Medicines Prescription Only Order 1977 prescribed only by a doctor but midwives are authorized to obtain certain ones (e.g. ergometrine maleate, oxytocin, naloxone, pentazocine, promazine, chloral hydrate, dichloralphenazone, lignocaine).

Controlled drugs are stored in a locked compartment within a locked cupboard, the keys of which are held by the midwife in charge to prevent unauthorized access to them.

Midwives and Pethidine

A certified midwife may possess and administer pethidine as far as necessary for the practice of her profession. Supplies may only be made to her on the authority of a midwife's supply order signed by:

1. The appropriate medical officer who is authorized in writing by the local supervising authority.
2. Her supervisor of midwives.

The order must specify the midwife's name, the purpose for which the pethidine is required and the quantity obtained. The midwife is required to keep a record of supplies received and administered. She must surrender any surplus stock to the 'appropriate medical officer'.

The foregoing applies to midwives working in the community; midwives in hospital are governed by the 'standing orders' for that particular unit.

Further information regarding the legislation on the use of drugs by a midwife can be found in the UKCC Handbook of Midwives Rules and Midwife's Code of Practice.

'Topping-up' Epidurals

Midwives were permitted by the UKCC to top up epidurals provided that:

1. The midwife had been fully instructed in the technique.
2. There were written instructions regarding the dose to be given.

3. The drug and the dose were checked by one other person.
4. She had been instructed by the anaesthetist as to the patient's position, blood pressure recordings and steps to take if there were side effects.
5. The ultimate responsibility rested with the anaesthetist concerned.

Drugs Commonly Used

The drugs mentioned in the following table are those which are commonly used in midwifery and paediatrics, and the doses given are those most frequently employed. These may vary according to the purpose for which a drug is administered.

The categories of drugs are listed in alphabetical order.

Drug	Proprietary name	Dose	Mode of administration	Uses/remarks
Anaesthetics, general				
Halothane		0.5–3%	Inhalation	Postpartum haemorrhage may result due to relaxation of the uterus
Methohexitone sodium	Brietal Sodium	1 mg/kg body weight	IV	—
Thiopentone sodium	Intraval Sodium	4 mg/kg body weight	IV	2.5% solution only must be used
Anaesthetics, local				
Bupivacaine hydrochloride	Marcain Plain	0.25%, 0.5% 0.75%	Epidural Intrathecal	Greater duration than lignocaine, so useful where prolonged analgesia is required. Used for Caesarean section.
Lignocaine hydrochloride	Xylocaine	0.5%, 1% 2%	Infiltration Epidural	10 ml 0.5% solution or 5 ml 1% solution may be used by midwives for infiltration prior to episiotomy and prior to perineal repair
Prilocaine hydrochloride	Citanest	0.5%, 1%	Infiltration	For nerve blocks
Analgesia, inhalational				
Methoxyflurane	Penthrane	0.35% in air	Cardiff inhaler	Pain relief in labour. Oliguric renal dysfunction is associated with excessive total dosage of methoxyflurane
Nitrous oxide + oxygen	Entonox	50% of each gas (in a cylinder)	Entonox apparatus	Safe and effective. Excreted via the lungs.
Analgesics				
Dihydrocodeine tartrate		30 mg qds 50 mg	Oral IM	Side effects: headache, nausea, vertigo. Avoid in asthmatics, as it causes histamine release
Fentanyl citrate	Sublimaze	0.05–0.1 mg	IV	For intra- and postoperative pain

Drug	Proprietary name	Dose	Mode of administration	Uses/remarks
Analgesics cont.				
Mefenamic acid	Ponstan	2 capsules tds	Oral	Anti-inflammatory as well as analgesic
Methadone hydrochloride	Physeptone	5–10 mg	IM	May be prescribed to drug addicts in pregnancy as a maintenance drug
Papaveretum	Omnopon	10–20 mg	IM/IV	For postoperative pain
Paracetamol	Panadol	2 tablets qds	Oral	Mild. Antipyretic as well as analgesic
Pentazocine hydrochloride Pentazocine lactate		50–100 mg qds 30–60 mg qds	Oral IM/IV	Relief of moderate to severe pain. Relief is variable
Pethidine hydrochloride		25–150 mg 25–50 mg	IM IV	Short-acting but effective. May cause depression of respiratory centre of baby
Anticoagulants				
Heparin		Prophylaxis: 10 000 units bd Treatment: up to 40 000 units daily	SC IV infusion	Heparin assay: not above 0.4 units/ml Protamin sulphate neutralization test: 0.5–1.5 units/ml. Useful in pregnancy, does not cross placenta
Warfarin		Maintenance: 2–15 mg daily (dose depends on prothrombin time)	Oral	In general: contraindicated in pregnancy and labour but may be given at 16–36 weeks' gestation if heparin not available. Dose should control prothrombin time to 2.5–3.5 times above normal
Anticonvulsants				
Chlormethiazole edisylate	Heminevrin	0.8% solution, 60 drops per minute until patient drowsy, then maintenance at 15 drops per minute	IV infusion	Hypnotic as well as anticonvulsant. Useful in eclampsia and status epilepticus
Phenobarbitone sodium		60–300 mg daily	Oral	Avoid in early pregnancy
Phenytoin sodium		100 mg bd/tds (max. 600 mg daily)	Oral	Avoid in early pregnancy if possible unless potential benefits outweigh risk of congenital abnormality

NB. The use of barbiturates should be avoided, except when required as anticonvulsants, because dependence and tolerance occur readily.

Drug	Proprietary name	Dose	Mode of administration	Uses/remarks
Antiemetics				
Perphenazine	Fentazin	4 mg tds 5–10 mg	Oral IM	Avoid in 1st trimester
Promazine hydrochloride	Sparine	25–100 mg qds	Oral	May be given in conjunction with pethidine in labour
Promethazine hydrochloride	Phenergan	25–50 mg	IM/IV	May be given in conjunction with pethidine in labour
Antihistamines				
Ranitidine	Zantac	50 mg	IM	Histamine blocker (H$_2$), used to reduce gastric pH in labour

Drug	Proprietary name	Dose	Mode of administration	Uses/remarks
Antihypertensives				
Hydralazine hydrochloride	Apresoline	20–40 mg	IV (physiological saline)	Contraindicated in early pregnancy and in women with tachycardia
Methyldopa	Aldomet	250 mg tds (max. 3 g daily)	Oral	Crosses placenta but no evidence that it affects fetus

NB. Beta blockers (e.g. propranolol) have been used successfully in pregnancy to lower the blood pressure. They are, however, associated with side effects such as acute fetal distress, neonatal hypoglycaemia and intrauterine growth retardation.

Drug	Proprietary name	Dose	Mode of administration	Uses/remarks
Antimicrobials				
Amoxycillin trihydrate	Amoxil	250 mg qds	Oral	Same action as ampicillin but better absorption
Ampicillin trihydrate	Penbritin	250–500 mg qds 0.5–1 g	Oral IM/IV	Broad-spectrum antibiotic
Cefuroxime sodium	Zinacef	750 mg tds	IM/IV	Active against both gram-positive and gram-negative bacteria
Cephradine	Velosef	500 mg qds 2–4 g daily	Oral IM/IV	Active against both gram-positive and gram-negative bacteria
Chloramphenicol	Chloromycetin ophthalmic	2 drops to affected eye every 3 hours	Topically	For bacterial conjunctivitis
Clotrimazole	Canesten	200 mg daily × 3 500 mg daily × 1	PV	Antifungal. Antitrichonomas (not as effective as metronidazole)
Erythromycin stearate	Erythrocin	1–2 g daily (divided doses) 100 mg qds (max. 5–8 mg/kg per 24 hours)	Oral Deep IM	Highly effective in the treatment of a wide variety of clinical infections
Flucloxacillin sodium	Floxapen	250 mg qds	Oral IV/IM	Active against most staphylococci and streptococci, including majority of penicillinase-producing staphylococci
Metronidazole	Flagyl	400 mg tds	Oral	For anaerobic infections and *Trichonomas vaginalis*
Miconazole nitrate	Gyno-Daktarin	200 mg nightly	PV	For vulvovaginal candidiasis
Nystatin	Nystan	1–2 pessaries	PV	For *Candida albicans*
Spectinomycin dihydropentahydrate	Trobicin	4 g (females) 2 g (males)	Deep IM	For gonorrhoea

NB. The sulphonamides have not been included because—due to the large selection of relatively safe and effective antibiotics, and the many contraindications and side effects of the sulphonamides—they are rarely used in midwifery.

Drug	Proprietary name	Dose	Mode of administration	Uses/remarks
Antiseptics				
Benzalkonium chloride	Roccal	0.05% antiseptic 1% disinfectant		Skin antiseptic and general disinfectant. Not effective against viruses, fungi, spores
Cetrimide	Cetavlon Savlon	1% solution 1:100 solution 1:30 solution		Skin antiseptic Swabbing Disinfection of wounds
Chlorhexidine hydrochloride/gluconate	Hibitane	1:2000 solution 1% obstetric cream 1% solution in spirit		Potent antibacterial Vaginal examinations Cleansing umbilical cord
Glutaraldehyde	Glutarol	10% solution		For viral warts

Drug	Proprietary name	Dose	Mode of administration	Uses/remarks
Antithyroid				
Carbimazole	Neo-Mercazole	5–60 mg daily	Oral	For thyrotoxicosis. May cause fetal hypothyroidism
Antituberculous				
Ethambutol hydrochloride	Myambutol	15 mg/kg per day	Oral	
Isoniazid	Rimifon	200–300 mg daily	IM/IV Intrathecal Intrapleural	All three drugs given together
Rifampicin	Rifadin	450–600 mg daily	Oral	Teratogenic
Contraceptives				
Medroxyprogesterone	Depo-Provera	150 mg	IM	Effective for 12 weeks. A useful single-dose contraceptive to be given following rubella vaccination or to the woman whose husband has had vasectomy performed
Progesterone-only pill		1 tablet daily	Oral	Not as reliable as combined pill but can be prescribed to postnatal mothers even if breast-feeding
Combined progesterone/ oestrogen pill		1 tablet daily for 21 days starting on 5th day of menstrual cycle	Oral	Can be commenced 7–12 days postpartum. Contraindicated if breast-feeding
Corticosteroids				
Betamethasone sodium phosphate	Betnesol	24 mg in divided doses	IM	Thought to stimulate the production of surfactant in the immature fetal lungs
Diabetic				
		Determined by patient's requirements	SC	Requirements rise in 2nd and 3rd trimesters

NB. Oral hypoglycaemic agents are contraindicated in pregnancy.

Drug	Proprietary name	Dose	Mode of administration	Uses/remarks
Diuretics				
Frusemide	Lasix	20–40 mg	IM/IV	May inhibit lactation. Should be reserved for pulmonary oedema and selected oliguric patients
Hypnotics/sedatives				
Dichloralphenazone	Welldorm	1300 mg	Oral	For insomnia; early stages of labour
Temazepam		10–30 mg	Oral	Should not be given in 1st trimester. Otherwise, effective hypnotic with no side effects
Iron				
Ferrous fumarate 100 mg + folic acid 0.35 mg	Pregaday	1 tablet daily	Oral	
Ferrous sulphate 150 mg + folic acid 0.5 mg	Fefol	1 spansule daily	Oral	Prophylaxis against iron deficiency and megaloblastic anaemia in pregnancy
Ferrous sulphate 325 mg + folic acid 0.35 mg	Ferrograd Folic	1 tablet daily	Oral	

Drug	Proprietary name	Dose	Mode of administration	Uses/remarks
Iron cont.				
Iron dextran	Imferon	According to body weight and Hb level	IV infusion	Test dose must be given first at rate of not more than 5 drops per minute for 10 minutes under supervision
Laxatives				
Danthron	Dorbanex	5–10 ml	Oral	Restoring bowel habit in puerperium; for painful defecation associated with haemorrhoids
Ispaghula	Fybogel	1 sachet bd	Oral	Increases faecal mass
Senna	Senokot	2–4 tablets	Oral	
Glycerine	—	1–2 suppositories	PR	Gentle bowel evacuation
Myometrial relaxants				
Isoxsuprine hydrochloride	Duvadilan	100 mg in 500 ml saline	IV infusion	Start at 0.5 ml per minute; increase every 10 minutes until labour arrested
Ritodrine hydrochloride	Yutopar	0.05 mg per minute	IV infusion	Increase by 0.05 mg every 10 minutes. Effective dose: 0.15–0.35 mg
Salbutamol sulphate	Ventolin	4 mg qds 5 ml/500 ml sodium chloride/dextrose	Oral IV infusion	Contraindicated in preeclampsia and antepartum haemorrhage
Myometrial stimulants				
Dinoprostone	Prostin E2	1 mg/ml 10 mg/ml	IV infusion IV infusion/ extraamniotic	Induction of labour Termination of pregnancy
		1 mg hourly until labour is established 2.5 mg pessary	Oral PV	In use only where they can be produced by the pharmacist. Not available commercially, as they must be kept at a temperature of + 4°C until use
Ergometrine maleate		0.5 mg	IV IM	Acts in 45 seconds, so is useful in prevention/treatment of postpartum haemorrhage Acts in 7 minutes and gives sustained contraction of uterus
Oxytocin	Syntocinon	1 i.u. in 1 litre solution at 15 drops per minute = 1 milliunit per minute	IV infusion	Induction of labour— stimulates contraction of uterine muscle
Syntometrine		1 ml	IM	Consists of oxytocin 5 units + ergometrine maleata 0.5 mg, and so has rapid and sustained action. Active management of 3rd stage of labour
Thyroid				
Thyroxine sodium	Eltroxin	50–300 μg, adjusted monthly until normal metabolism is maintained	Oral	For hypothyroidism

Drug	Proprietary name	Dose	Mode of administration	Uses/remarks
Neonatal medicines (premature neonates and term neonates less than 7 days old) (dose per kilogram of body weight)				
Amikacin sulphate	Amikin	7.5 mg bd	IV/IM	For serious gram-negative infections resistant to gentamicin
Ampicillin trihydrate	Penbritin	62.5 mg qds 30 mg qds	Oral IM/IV	For some gram-positive and gram-negative organisms. It is mostly used for the treatment of urinary tract infections, otitis media, chronic bronchitis, invasive salmonellosis, and gonorrhoea
Cefuroxime sodium	Zinacef	25 mg bd	IM	For infections due to sensitive gram-positive and gram-negative bacteria, particularly *Hemophilus influenzae* and *Neisseria gonorrhoeae.*
Ceftazidime	Fortum	25 mg 12-hourly	IM/IV	For greater activity against gram-negative bacilli
Chloramphenicol	Chloromycetin	1st injection 25 mg; then 12.5 mg bd	IV	For meningitis
Chloramphenicol eye drops	Chloromycetin eye drops	2 drops to affected eye every 3 hours	Topical	For bacterial conjunctivitis
Diazepam	Valium	0.25 mg/kg 8-hourly	IM/IV slowly	Not to be used in jaundiced babies, as it competes for albumin-binding sites, and so increases hyperbilirubinaemia
Dexamethasone sodium phosphate	Decadron	1 mg 6-hourly	IV	Suppression of inflammatory and allergic disorders; cerebral oedema
Digoxin	Lanoxin	Digitalizing dose: 20 μg/kg $\times$ 1; then 10 μg/kg $\times$ 2 *or* 15 μg/kg $\times$ 1; then 8 μg/kg $\times$ 2 Maintenance dose: 5 μg/kg 12-hourly 4 μg/kg 12-hourly	 Oral Oral IM IM Oral IM	For heart failure
Frusemide	Lasix	1 mg/kg/day	IM/IV	Inhibits resorption
Gentamicin sulphate	Genticin	4.5 mg 18-hourly	IM/IV	For urinary tract infection, respiratory tract infections, septicaemia, neonatal sepsis, meningitis, biliary tract infection, acute pyelonephritis or endocarditis. Blood levels need careful monitoring in neonatal use
Naloxone hydrochloride	Narcan	0.01 mg/kg	IV/IM	To counteract respiratory depression in neonate, resulting from pethidine given to mother in labour
Neomycin sulphate	Nivemycin	1/2 drops to eyes 3–4 times daily	Topical	For 'sticky' eyes due to *pseudomonas aeruginosa*
Nystatin	Nystan	100 000 units qds	Oral	For *Candida albicans*

Drug	Proprietary name	Dose	Mode of administration	Uses/remarks
Neonatal medicines cont.				
Paraldehyde		0.1 ml/kg	IM deep/IV/PR	To abort prolonged or recurrent fits
Benzylpenicillin sodium penicillin G	Crystapen	100 000 units qds	IM/IV	For streptococcal, pneumococcal, gonococcal and meningococcal infections
Phenobarbitone	Gardenal	Stat dose 10 mg/kg; then 5 mg/kg/24 h	IM/IV	To control fits; accumulation may occur, need to check serum level regularly
Phenobarbitone elixir (5 mg/ml)		1.25 mg/kg qds	Oral	Anticonvulsant
Phytomenadione	Konakion	0.5–1 mg	IV/IM/oral	Prevention and treatment of haemorrhage due to vitamin K deficiency
Alprostadil (prostaglandin E_1)	Prostin VR	0.02–0.03 µg/kg/min	IV infusion	To maintain patency of the ductus arteriosus in neonates with congenital heart defects, prior to corrective surgery
Sodium bicarbonate		Amount based on the severity of the degree of acidosis	IV infusion	For metabolic acidosis
Choline theophyllinate	Choledyl	Stat dose 6.2 mg/kg; maintenance dose 1.5 mg/kg 6-hourly	Oral Oral	Bronchodilator, for reversible airways obstruction. Useful in weaning infants off ventilatory support
Tolazoline hydrochloride	Priscoline	Stat dose 1–2 mg/kg; then 1 mg/kg/h	IV infusion	For pulmonary hypertension. It reduces pulmonary artery pressure and total peripheral resistance, and increases cardiac output, leading to a decrease in thoracic gas volume and an increase in arterial oxygen tension
Vitamin E		2–10 mg daily	Oral	Recent studies suggested vitamin E can aid recovery in bronchopulmonary dysplasia. Need to monitor serum level weekly

6. IMMUNIZATION SCHEDULE

Immunization cannot be commenced until a baby is 3 months old, as the production of the specific antibodies will not occur effectively until this age. Infectious diseases which can be avoided by immunization are listed below.

Smallpox

World-wide vaccination has been so successful that the disease has virtually been eradicated, so it is no longer given as a routine.

Whooping Cough (Pertussis)

In about 1974 anxiety grew about the danger associated with immunization. A nationwide inquiry since then has revealed that there is a risk of 1 in 110,000 children developing serious neurological damage. These rare cases were given so much prominence in the media that many parents have not had their children immunized. An epidemic of whooping cough has resulted. The illness may last as long as 8 weeks, and most children recover without apparent long-term ill-effects, but fatalities occur in babies under 6 months of age. Health authorities are being exhorted by the Department of Health and Social Security to run local campaigns to improve the uptake of immunization. It is given as a triple antigen with diphtheria and tetanus toxoids.

Triple Antigen

This contains dead organisms of whooping cough (*Bordetella pertussis*) together with the toxoids of diphtheria and tetanus. The dose is 0.5 ml on three occasions.

Contraindications. The triple vaccine should not be given if there is a family history of epilepsy, disease of the central nervous system, fits or other abnormality of the baby's own central nervous system. Any severe reaction from the first injection such as dyspnoea, fits or encephalopathy, indicates that the programme should continue with *only* diphtheria and tetanus toxoids.

Storage. The triple vaccine should not be frozen, but refrigerated between 2° and 10°C.

Rubella

In 1970 the Joint Committee on vaccination and Immunization (JCVI) recommended the routine use of rubella vaccine for girls between 11 and 14 years of age. The proportion vaccinated by 14 is now 83 per cent, and in an effort to improve this figure, from 1 September 1981, the younger age of 10 is now DHSS policy. Screening is now carried out in many family planning and antenatal clinics in order to detect those at risk.

Poliomyelitis

This is given as a syrup on a lump of sugar, usually at the same time as the triple antigen initially, but needs a booster dose on leaving school (as does tetanus).

Typical Scheme of Immunization

Age	Avoidable disease
4–6 months (1st)	Diphtheria, tetanus, pertussis and poliomyelitis
6–8 months (2nd)	As above
10–14 months (3rd)	As above
1–2 years	Measles
5 years (school entry)	Diphtheria, tetanus and polio boosters
10–13 years	Tuberculosis
	BCG (if immunity tests are negative)
10–14 years (girls only)	Rubella (German measles)
15–19 (school-leaving age)	Tetanus, poliomyelitis

7. USEFUL ADDRESSES

United Kingdom Central Council for Nursing, Midwifery and Health Visiting, 23 Portland Place, London W1N 3AF
    Tel. 01-637 7181
English National Board for Nursing, Midwifery and Health Visiting, Victory House, 170 Tottenham Court Road, London W1P 0HA
    Tel. 01-388 3131
National Board for Nursing, Midwifery and Health Visiting for Scotland, Trinity Park House, South Trinity Road, Edinburgh EH5 3SF
    Tel. 031-552 6255
Welsh National Board for Nursing, Midwifery and Health Visiting, 13th floor, Pearl Assurance House, Greyfriars Road, Cardiff CF1 3AG
    Tel. 0222-395 535
National Board for Nursing, Midwifery and Health Visiting for Northern Ireland, 123/137 York Street, Belfast BT15 1JB
    Tel. 0232-246333 and 247861
British Medical Association, BMA House, Tavistock Square, London WC1
    Tel. 01-387 4499

Various Midwifery and Nursing Organizations

ACCEPT—The Alcoholism Community for Education, Prevention and Treatment, Western Hospital, Seagrave Road, London SW6
    Tel. 01-381 3155
    (Offers complete counselling services and treatment centre.)
Association of Breast Feeding Mothers, 131 Mayrow Road, London SE26
    Tel. 01-778 4769
Association of British Adoption and Fostering Agencies, 4 Southampton Row, London WC1B 4AA
    Tel. 01-242 8951
Association for Improvements in the Maternity Services, 67 Lennard Road, London SE20 7LY
    Tel. 01-778 0175
Association of Nurse Administrators, 13 Grosvenor Place, London SW1X 7EN
    Tel. 01-235 5258
Association for Postnatal Illness, Queen Charlotte's Hospital, Goldhawk Road, London W6 0XG
    Tel. 01-741 5019
Association of Radical Midwives, c/o Haringey Women's Centre, 40 Turnpike Lane, London N8
    Tel. 01-889 3912
    (This is a support and skill-sharing group—not a private midwifery service.)
Association for Spina Bifida and Hydrocephalus, 2nd floor, Tavistock House North, Tavistock Square, London WC1 9HJ
    Tel. 01-388 1382
Birth Centre, 101 Tufnell Park Road, London N7
    Tel. 01-609 7466
    (Gives information on home and hospital birth for those seeking an alternative to the increasing policy of intervention.)
British Council for the Rehabilitation of the Disabled, 25 Mortimer Street, London W1
    Tel. 01-637 5400
British Diabetic Association, 10 Queen Anne Street, London W1
    Tel. 01-323 1531

British Guild for Sudden Infant Death Study, Pathology Department, Royal Infirmary, Cardiff CF2 1SZ
    Tel. 0222-492233
    (The Guild acts as a source of information and support for parents and children lost through the sudden infant death syndrome and campaigns for improvements in the administrative and legal handling of such deaths.)
British Postgraduate Medical Federation, 33 Millman Street, London WC1
    Tel. 01-831 6222
British Pregnancy Advisory Service, Austry Manor, Wootton Wawen, Solihull, West Midlands B95 6BX
    Tel. 056 42-3225
British Red Cross Society, 9 Grosvenor Crescent, London SW1X YEJ
    Tel. 01-235 5454
Brook Advisory Centre, 233 Tottenham Court Road, London W1P 9AE
    Tel. 01-580 2911 and 01-323 1522
DHSS, Alexander Fleming House, Elephant and Castle, London SE1 6BY
    Tel. 01-407 5522
Down's Children's Association, 4 Oxford Street, London W1
    Tel. 01-580 0511
Emergency Bed Service, 28 London Bridge Street, London SE1
    Tel. 01-407 7181
Family Planning Association, Margaret Pyke House, 27-35 Mortimer Street, London W1N 7RJ
    Tel. 01-636 7866
Family Welfare Association, 501-505 Kingsland Road, Dalston, London E8 4AU
    Tel. 01-254 6251-4
Foundation for the Study of Infant Deaths, 5th Floor, 4 Grosvenor Place, London SW1X 7HD
    Tel. 01-235 1721 or 01-245 9421
Gingerbread, Minerva Chambers, 35 Wellington Street, London WC2E 7BN
    Tel. 01-240 0953
    (One parent families)
Her Majesty's Prisons and Borstal Institutions Nursing Service, Her Majesty's Prison, Holloway, London N5 1PL
    Tel. 01-607 4251
Her Majesty's Stationery Office, 49 High Holborn, London WC1
    Tel. 01-211 5656
International Confederation of Midwives, 57 Lower Belgrave Street, London SW1W 0LR
    Tel. 01-730 6137/8
Invalid Children's Aid Association, 126 Buckingham Palace Road, London SW1W 9SB
    Tel. 01-730 9891
King Edward's Hospital Fund for London, 2 Palace Court, London W2 4HT
    Tel. 01-727 0581
King's Fund Centre, 126 Albert Street, London NW1 7NF
    Tel. 01-267 6111
Let Live Association, 56a Kyverdale Road, London N16
    Tel. 01-806 1984
    (Counselling and practical help on the alternative to abortion as a way out of a problem pregnancy.)
Margaret Pyke Centre, 27-35 Mortimer Street, London W1A 4QW
    Tel. 01-580 3077
Marie Stopes Clinic, Well Woman Centre, 108 Whitfield Street, London W1P 6BE
    Tel. 01-388 0662 and 2585

Midwife Teachers Training College, High Coombe, Warren Road, Kingston Hill, Surrey
Tel. 01-942 1446

Midwives Information and Resource Service (MIDIRS), National Temperance Hospital, 112 Hampstead Road, London NW1 2LT
Tel. 01-387 3755

National Association for Maternal and Child Welfare, 1 South Audley Street, London W1Y 6JS
Tel. 01-491 2772 and 1315

National Association of State Enrolled Nurses, 1 Vere Street, London W1
Tel. 01-629 0870

National Blood Transfusion Service, Moor House, London Wall, London EC2
Tel. 01-628 4590

National Childbirth Trust, 9 Queensborough Terrace, London W2 3TB
Tel. 01-221 3833

National Council for One Parent Families, 255 Kentish Town Road, London NW5 2LX
Tel. 01-267 1361

New Life Foundation Trust, The Red House, Kelham, Newark NG23 5QP
Tel. 0636 2807 and 3029
(Counselling and rehabilitation of addicts)

NSPCC, 1 Riding House Street, London W1
Tel. 01-580 8812

Nuffield Foundation, Nuffield Lodge, Regent's Park, London NW1
Tel. 01-722 8871/9

Nursing Education Research Unit, Chelsea College Road, London SW3 6LX
Tel. 01-351 2488

Nursing and Hospital Careers Information Centre, 121 Edgware Road, London W2 2HX
Tel. 01-402 5296/7

Nursing Practice Research Unit, Northwick Park Hospital, Watford Road, Harrow, Middlesex HA1 3UJ
Tel. 01-864 5311

Office of Population Censuses and Surveys, St. Catherine's House, 10 Kingsway, London WC2B 6TP
Tel. 01-242 0262

Open University, Milton Keynes MK7 6AA
Tel. Milton Keynes 74066

Poisons Unit, New Cross Hospital, Avonley Road, London SE14
Tel. 01-639 4380

Pregnancy Advisory Service, 40 Margaret Street, London W1N 7FB
Tel. 01-409 0281

Royal College of General Practitioners, 14 Prince's Gate, London SW7
Tel. 01-581 3232

Royal College of Midwives, 15 Mansfield Street, London W1M 0BE
Tel. 01-580 6523/4/5

Royal College of Nursing and National Council of Nurses of the United Kingdom (Rcn) (Secretary), 1 Henrietta Place, Cavendish Square, London W1M 0AB
Tel. 01-409 3333

Royal College of Nursing and National Council of Nurses of the United Kingdom (Rcn) Scotland, 44 Heriot Row, Edinburgh EH3 6EY
Tel. 031-225 7231

Royal College of Nursing and National Council of Nurses of the United Kingdom (Rcn) Welsh Board, Ty Maeth, King George V Drive East, Cardiff CF4 4XZ
Tel. 0222-751374/5

Royal College of Obstetricians and Gynaecologists, 27 Sussex Place, London NW1
Tel. 01-262 5425

Royal College of Pathologists, 2 Carlton House Terrace, London SW1
Tel. 01-930 5861

Royal College of Physicians, 11 St Andrew's Place, London NW1
Tel. 01-935 1174

Royal College of Surgeons, 35 Lincoln's Inn Fields, London WC2
Tel. 01-405 3474

Royal National Institute for the Blind, 224 Great Portland Street, London W1N 6AA
Tel. 01-388 1266

Royal National Institute for the Deaf, 105 Gower Street, London WC1E 6AH
Tel. 01-387 8033

Royal Society of Medicine, 1 Wimpole Street, London W1
Tel. 01-580 2070

Society for Registered Male Nurses, 38 Marland Avenue, Oldham, Lancs
Tel. Main 2799

Stillbirth and Perinatal Death Association, 37 Christchurch Hill, London NW3
Tel. 01-794 4601

Student Nurses Association, Royal College of Nursing, 1 Henrietta Place, Cavendish Square, London W1M 0AB
Tel. 01-409 3333

Womens Royal Voluntary Service, 17 Old Park Lane, London W1Y 4AJ
Tel. 01-499 6040

Nursing Organizations Abroad

Canadian Nurses' Association, 50 The Driveway, Ottawa K2P 1EA, Canada

Frontier Nursing Service, Wendover, Kentucky, USA

International Council of Nurses, 37 Rue Vermont, 1202 Geneva, Switzerland, Postal Address: PO Box 42, 1211 Geneva 20
Tel. Geneva 33 64 00

New Zealand Nurses' Association, GPO Box 2128, 504/505, Brandon House, Featherston Street, Wellington, New Zealand

Royal Australian Nursing Federation, 132–6 Albert Road, South Melbourne, Victoria 3205, Australia

South African Nursing Association, Private Bag X105, Pretoria, South Africa

Trained Nurses' Association of India, L-16 Green Park, New Delhi 100 16, India

Trained Nurses' Association of Pakistan, Midwifery Tutor, c/o The College of Nursing, Jinnah Postgraduate Medical School, Karachi 35, Pakistan

United States Information Service, 24 Grosvenor Square, London W1
Tel. 01-499 9000

Navy, Army and Air Force Nursing Services

Princess Mary's Royal Air Force Nursing Service, Ministry of Defence, First Avenue House, High Holborn, London WC1V 6HE
Tel. 01-430 5639

Queen Alexandra's Royal Army Nursing Corps, Ministry of Defence, First Avenue House, High Holborn, London WC1V 6HD
Tel. 01-430 5555

Queen Alexandra's Royal Naval Nursing Service, Ministry of Defence, First Avenue House, High Holborn, London WC1V 6HD
    Tel. 01-430 5555

Insurance Societies and Benevolent Organizations

Federated Superannuation Scheme for Nurses and Hospital Officers (Contributory) (Secretary), Rosehill, Park Road, Banstead, Surrey
    Tel. 25-57272

Health Services Superannuation Division, Hesketh House, 200–220 Broadway, Fleetwood, Lancs FL7 8LG
Hospital Savings Association, 30 Lancaster Gate, London W2 3LT
    Tel. 01-723 7601
National Fund for Nurses, 1 Henrietta Place, Cavendish Square, London W1M 0AB
    Tel. 01-580 3965
Royal National Pension Fund for Nurses, Burdett House, 15 Buckingham Street, Strand, London WC2N 6ED
    Tel. 01-839 6785

8. PUBLICATIONS OF CURRENT INTEREST

Of the many publications of particular topical interest to the midwife, a few are listed below.

Report on Confidential Enquiries into Maternal Deaths in England and Wales (HMSO). Each edition of this report covers three years, the most recent, the ninth, dealing with 1976, 1977 and 1978, having been published in 1982. Every maternal death in each three-year period is studied confidentially, individually and impartially by an expert committee, all the circumstances being closely reviewed, in an attempt to assess possible avoidable factors. These widely read reports are greatly respected and the adoption of their various recommendations has undoubtedly led to a steady decrease in the maternal mortality rate.

On the State of the Public Health (HMSO). This is the annual report of the Chief Medical Officer of the Department of Health and Social Security, a sizeable document which can usually be borrowed from a hospital library. Every aspect of public and community health is reviewed, including vital statistics, sexually transmitted diseases, all aspects of maternal and child health, and many other, wider, health issues.

Health and Personal Social Services Statistics for England (HMSO). This is an annual publication presenting health statistics and related social services data. As well as vital statistics, finance, manpower and administration, a range of services are included with hospital and community maternity services, and other data of interest to a midwife.

Drugs in Pregnancy: Their Possible Effect on the Fetus. R. S. Illingworth, London: Royal College of Midwives. Much has been learnt, especially in the last few years, about the adverse effects on the fetus of drugs taken by the mother during pregnancy and labour. This short reprint summarizes all the latest valid information in a long list of drugs and their effects which makes alarming but salutary reading.

The Common Market and the Common Man. European Community: The Facts. London: European Communities Press. These two small booklets set out, in outline only, a great deal of factual information about the European Economic Community, which midwives (and others) could learn with advantage.

Official Journal of the European Communities, L33, volume 23, 1980 (HMSO). This publication contains the midwifery directives, which concern freedom of movement in the Community and the training programme. (The requirements for the latter are included in the changes made in the United Kingdom 18-month training which came into effect in September 1981.)

Domiciliary Midwifery and Maternity Bed Needs (HMSO). Better known as the Peel Report, after its chairman, Sir John Peel, this report of the Subcommittee of the Standing Maternity and Midwifery Advisory Committee of the Central Health Services Council was published in 1970 and is well known to many midwives. The title is self-explanatory and, although the committee's recommendations were widely publicised some time ago, they remain the subject of much discussion.

Report of the Expert Group on Special Care for Babies (HMSO). This expert committee reviewed the history and the facilities at present available for the nursing of special care babies and considered in detail how the needs of the future might best be met. Their important recommendations are of interest to midwives whether or not they are wanting to work in special care baby units.

Report of the Committee on Senior Nursing Staff Structure (HMSO). This, the well-known Salmon Report of 1966, has now acquired the quality of a historical document. Through it has been created not only a completely new pattern of hospital management, but a whole new hospital language. It is still remarkably readable, partly on account of its exceptional attention to detail, with its glossary of precise definitions of the terms used; and partly because, for the young midwife who knows only Salmon structure, it will put the whole process of development into perspective with commendable clarity.
    Anyone reading the Salmon report for the first time (and, of course, those to whom 'Salmon' is familiar) should also study the booklet below.

Progress on Salmon (DHSS Welsh Office). This booklet, published in 1972, is indeed a commentary on progress, giving a succinct but comprehensive review of the implementation of the Salmon structure, the pilot scheme experience and how Salmon was then working. Here the reviewers note many favourable factors and some adverse features. It is of interest to note that the latter relate very largely to lack of understanding of the original Salmon intention.

Report on the Committee on Nursing (HMSO). In October 1972 this committee, under the chairmanship of Professor Asa Briggs, published a lengthy but very readable report, which makes a number of recommendations which are creating radical changes in the careers of nurses and midwives. While much of the report had a very favourable reception, there remain a number of controversial issues. The report might well be borrowed from a hospital or public library.

Local Government Reform, Short Version of the Report of the Royal Commission on Local Government in England (HMSO). Lord Redcliffe-Maud and his committee published in 1969 a ponderous volume, an admirable précis of which is presented in this 22-page booklet. It should be read with frequent reference to its accompanying map. It is of immediate interest, not only to nurses and midwives but to all English citizens.

Law Notes for Nurses, S. R. SPELLER. *Supplement for Scotland*, R. A. BENNETT. London: Royal College of Nursing. This little book is well set out, lucidly presented and concise. In view of the litigation problems of the present day, its importance to nurses and midwives cannot be gainsaid.

Industrial Relations, a Guide to the Industrial Relations Act (DE). *Code of Practice* (HMSO). While not necessarily essential reading for all midwives, these booklets will certainly help to clarify the complexities of this controversial piece of legislation, both for those who are interested and for those who, as employers, are more directly involved.

Present-day Practice in Infant Feeding (HMSO). A short report submitted by a panel of experts on child nutrition set up by the DHSS Committee on Medical Aspects of Food Policy. This report gives unequivocal support to the value of breast-feeding, supplies much succinct information about problems related to artificial feeding and obesity, and underlines the need for improved education, both of mothers and of all professional personnel. Since its publication in 1974, breast-feeding has greatly increased in popularity.

Journal of the Office of Population Censuses and Surveys [OPCS]. *Population Trends*. This is published quarterly and regularly contains tables of statistics as well as articles of medical interest. The OPCS library produces many other publications, and details are obtainable from St Catherine's House, 10 Kingsway, London WC2B 6TP.

The Family in Society—preparation for parenthood, October 1972–February 1973 (HMSO). An account of consultations with professional, voluntary and other organizations on whether a policy of 'improved preparation for parenthood' could break the 'cycle of deprivation'. Many suggestions and ideas were put forward to deal with this very serious and complex issue.

Report of the Committee on Child Health Service (HMSO). This report was produced by an eminent committee of professionals concerned with children, under the chairmanship of Emeritus Professor S.D.M. Court. Regrettably there was no midwife representative, although evidence was taken from the Royal College of Midwives. It examined issues concerning children and their families, their state of health and the quality of services provided for them, in the context of those offered in other industrialized countries. The range of maternity services was assessed, and areas of concern were highlighted. The inadequacy of preparation for parenthood, deprivation of choice in some areas of institutionalized maternity care were particularly noted. Early contact between the mother and her baby was advocated, as was the provision of regional neonatal intensive care centres to reduce the sequelae of neonatal illness. Many major recommendations were made, a number of which have yet to receive attention. These are contained in volume 1, volume 2 being the statistical appendix.

A Service for Patients—Royal Commission on the National Health Service, 1979 (HMSO). Written and oral evidence was taken on many issues, including services to patients, manpower and relationships with other services and institutions. This booklet, containing Chapter 22, gives the conclusion and recommendations made by the Commission.

Patients First—a consultative paper on the structure of the National Health Service in England and Wales, December 1979 (HMSO). This is a booklet produced after the Royal Commission on the National Health Service made certain criticisms of the health service: too many tiers, too many administrators, slow decision-making and money wasted. This consultative document formed the basis of the 1981 reorganization outlined in Appendix 1.

Second Report from the Social Services Committee, Session 1979–80, Perinatal and Neonatal Mortality, volume 1 (HMSO). An enquiry resulting from public concern over the differences in the mortality rates between different socio-economic groups and different areas in England and Wales. Other developed countries' rates were falling more quickly, and a large number of conclusions were reached by the Committee, under the chairmanship of Renee Short. Recommendations were made for improving antenatal clinics, redrafting the criteria for admission to the Obstetric List of General Practitioners, and making better use of the skills of the midwife.

Current Awareness Service (Royal College of Midwives). This is a bimonthly publication which contains a very full list of recent literature on midwifery and allied subjects.

See How They Grow, D. MORLEY and M. WOODLAND. Macmillan: London. Published in 1979, this very useful book was written for health and community workers in tropical and subtropical developing countries. There is much practical and well illustrated advice on monitoring child growth in regions where there is a high rate of neonatal and infant mortality, and the book has much to offer a midwife intending to work in such an area.

Child Abuse. Edited by C. LEE. Open University Press: Milton Keynes. This is a reader and source book compiled to form part of a course on child abuse. The aim is to assist professional workers, including midwives, who can play a part in the prevention or detection of child abuse.

Maternity Care in Action (HMSO). A series of three handbooks on policies and priorities for the health and personal social services in England. Part 1 (Antenatal Care) was published in 1982, Part 2 (Care During Childbirth) in 1984, and Part 3 (Care of the Mother and Baby) in 1985. These handbooks provide guidance to the chairman and members of district health authorities from the Secretary of State for Social Services. They set out government policies and priorities to be met within the limits of resources available.

Social and Statistical Facts for Student Midwives. MEMBERS OF THE EDUCATION ADVISORY GROUP OF THE SCOTTISH BOARD OF THE ROYAL COLLEGE OF MIDWIVES (1982). London: Pitman Medical. This useful little book contains both statistics and information about social services and state benefits throughout the United Kingdom.

The Warnock Report. A report by the Committee of Enquiry Into Human Fertilisation and Embryology, 1984 (HMSO). This report examines the social, ethical and legal implications of recent and potential developments, including research experimentation on human embryos, and makes recommendations to Parliament.

Griffiths Report. A report commissioned by Mr Norman Fowler, Secretary of State for Social Services to enquire into management and cost effectiveness within the National Health Service. The main proposal was that business style management be applied, with managers being responsible for implementation of policies within a prescribed budget. This is currently being implemented.

The Judge Report. RCN Report on the Education of Nurses, 1985 (RCN). This report looks at problems inherent in the training and education of nurses. It recommends fundamental reforms of the curriculum, the educator and student status.

English National Board (ENB) Strategy Document. A consultative paper on professional and educational training. The following are but a few of its proposals: (a) A common core training programme which is theory centred; (b) that there be a single category of teacher; (c) Formation of collaborative links, between professions and institutes of higher and advanced further education; and (d) that students be supernumerary for a large part of their training.

Project 2000. A review set up by the United Kingdom Central Council in 1985 to look into the future of education and professional practice for nursing, midwifery and health visiting, with a view to making recommendations to meet the needs of society in the 1990s and into the next century.

9. ABBREVIATIONS

Much controversy still exists over the use of abbreviations. In years gone by it was accepted that in oral and written reports, in examinations and in similar fairly formal statements, abbreviations were entirely inappropriate. Though this time is long past, the tradition remains. But, in the quickened tempo of life today and with an increasing multiplicity of committees and councils, of titles and designations and, indeed, of drugs, equipment and procedures, many having long and complex names, it is small wonder that conversation and reports appear often to be reduced to lists of initial letters.

In a hospital which has evolved its own code, describing its own particular treatments and procedures, the message is perfectly clear; elsewhere it is incomprehensible. In other words, though some abbreviations are nationally or even internationally recognized, others most certainly are not.

The midwife, trying to negotiate this maze of initial letters and short words, less obvious than NATO and UNO, for example, which evolved from those initials, may wonder when an abbreviation is or is not acceptable. There is no absolute answer, but a few guidelines may help her:

1. The more formal the occasion, the more abbreviations should be avoided. Those which may pass in casual conversation may well be unsuitable for a written statement.
2. Nationally recognized abbreviations are often acceptable where those coined locally are undesirable.
3. Above all, the communication must be clear to the recipient, who may be British or foreign, intelligent or slow-witted. If the abbreviated message is not clear or if there is any doubt as to its clarity, then it should be presented in full. Failure to observe this fundamental fact has led to many serious errors in communication.

There follows a list, necessarily incomplete, of some of the abbreviations in common use in the health service in the United Kingdom.

Titles, Diplomas and Organizations

ABPN	Association of British Paediatric Nurses
ADM	Advanced Diploma in Midwifery
ADMS	Assistant Director of Medical Services
AIDS	Advice and Information for the Deaf
AIDS	Acquired immune deficiency syndrome
AIMS	Association for the Improvement of the Maternity Services
AMS	Army Medical Service
ANA	Association of Nurse Administrators
ARRC	Associate of the Royal Red Cross
ARSH	Associate of the Royal Society of Health
ASH	Action on Smoking and Health
BA	Bachelor of Arts
BAO	Bachelor of the Art of Obstetrics
BAON	British Association of Orthopaedic Nurses
BC, BCh	Bachelor of Surgery
BChD	Bachelor of Dental Surgery
BDA	British Dental Association
BDS	Bachelor of Dental Surgery
BDSc	Bachelor of Dental Science
BHyg	Bachelor of Hygiene
BM	Bachelor of Medicine
BMA	British Medical Association
BP	British Pharmacopoeia
BPC	British Pharmaceutical Codex
BPharm	Bachelor of Pharmacy
BRC	British Red Cross
BRCS	British Red Cross Society
BS	Bachelor of Surgery
BSc	Bachelor of Science
BSI	British Standards Institute

BTA	British Thoracic Association
BVP	British Volunteer Programme
CAMO	Chief Administrative Medical Officer
CCHE	Central Council for Health Education
CCNS	Committee for Clinical Nursing Studies
CETHV	Council for the Education and Training of Health Visitors
ChB	Bachelor of Surgery
CHC	Community Health Council
ChD	Doctor of Surgery
ChM	Master of Surgery
CHSC	Central Health Services Council
CM	Master of Surgery
CMB	Central Midwives Board
CNF	Commonwealth Nurses Federation
CNN	Certified Nursery Nurse
CNO	Chief Nursing Officer
CSP	Chartered Society of Physiotherapy
CStJ	Commander of the Order of St John of Jerusalem
DA	Diploma in Anaesthetics
DA	District Administrator
DCh	Doctor of Surgery
DCH	Diploma in Child Health
DCP	Diploma in Clinical Pathology
DCP	District Community Physician
DFO	District Finance Officer
DGH	District General Hospital
DGO	Diploma in Gynaecology and Obstetrics
DHA	District Health Authority
DHSS	Department of Health and Social Security
DMC	District Medical Committee
DMT	District Management Team
DN	Diploma in Nursing
DNO	District Nursing Officer
DNS	Director of Nursing Services
DObst	Diploma in Obstetrics
DPH	Diploma in Public Health
DPM	Diploma in Psychological Medicine
DPT	District Planning Team
DRCOG	Diploma of the Royal College of Obstetricians and Gynaecologists
DT	District Treasurer
EEC	European Economic Community
ENB	English National Board for Nursing, Midwifery and Health Visiting
ENT	Ear, nose and throat
FFA	Fellow of the Faculty of Anaesthetists
FICS	Fellow of the International College of Surgeons
FIGO	International Federation of Gynaecology and Obstetrics
FPA	Family Planning Association
FPC	Family Practitioner Committee
FRCOG	Fellow of the Royal College of Obstetricians and Gynaecologists
FRCP	Fellow of the Royal College of Physicians
FRCPath	Fellow of the Royal College of Pathologists
FRCS	Fellow of the Royal College of Surgeons
FRS	Fellow of the Royal Society
GMC	General Medical Council
GNC	General Nursing Council
GP	General Practitioner
HAS	Health Advisory Service

HASAW	Health and Safety at Work Act
HCPT	Health Care Planning Team
HMSO	Her Majesty's Stationery Office
HSA	Hospital Savings Association
HSC	Health and Safety Commission
HSE	Health and Safety Executive
HV	Health Visitor
HVA	Health Visitor's Association
HVCert	Health Visitor Certificate
ICM	International Confederation of Midwives
ICN	International Council of Nurses
ICRC	International Committee of the Red Cross
INR	Index of Nursing Research
ISD	Information Services Division
ITU	Intensive therapy unit
IVS	International Voluntary Service
JBCNS	Joint Board of Clinical Nursing Studies
JCC	Joint Consultative Committee
JCPT	Joint Care Planning Team
JLC	Joint Liaison Committee
KFC	King's Fund Centre
KFC	King's Fund College
LA	Local authority
LSA	Local supervising authority
MA	Master of Arts
MAO	Master of the Art of Obstetrics
MB	Bachelor of Medicine
MC, MCh	Master of Surgery
MD	Doctor of Medicine
MIDIRS	Midwives' Information and Resource Service
MO	Medical Officer
MRC	Medical Research Council
MRCOG	Member of the Royal College of Obstetricians and Gynaecologists
MRCS	Member of the Royal College of Surgeons
MS	Master of Surgery
MTD	Midwife Teacher's Diploma
NAHA	National Association of Health Authorities
NAMCW	National Association for Maternal and Child Welfare
NB	National Board
NCT	National Childbirth Trust
NCW	National Council of Women
NCUMC	National Council for the Unmarried Mother and her Child
NERU	Nursing Education Research Unit
NHS	National Health Service
NO	Nursing Officer
NSC	National Staff Committee (Nurses and Midwives)
OHNC	Occupational Health Nursing Certificate
ONC	Orthopaedic Nursing Certificate
OPCS	Office of Population Censuses and Surveys
OStJ	Officer of the Order of St John of Jerusalem
PGCEA	Postgraduate Certificate in the Education of Adults
PHI	Public Health Inspector

PMRAFNS	Princess Mary's Royal Air Force Nursing Service		BBA	Born before arrival
PNO	Principal Nursing Officer		b.d.	*bis in die* (twice a day)
PSW	Psychiatric Social Worker		BF	Breast-fed
QARANC	Queen Alexandra's Royal Army Nursing Corps		BMR	Basal metabolic rate
			BPD	Biparietal diameter
QARNNS	Queen Alexandra's Royal Naval Nursing Service		C	Celsius
QIDN	Queen's Institute of District Nursing		CAT	Computerized axial tomography
QNI	Queens' Nursing Institute		CCT	Controlled cord traction
			CDH	Congenital dislocation of the hip
RA	Regional Administrator		CIP	Continuous inflating pressure
RAWP	Resource Allocation Working Party		CNP	Continuous negative pressure
RCGP	Royal College of General Practitioners		CPAP	Continuous positive airways pressure
RCM	Royal College of Midwives		CPD	Cephalopelvic disproportion
Rcn	Royal College of Nursing and National Council of Nurses of the United Kingdom		CRL	Crown–rump length
			CS	Caesarean section
RCT	Registered Clinical Teacher		CSU	Catheter specimen of urine
RGN	Registered General Nurse		CTG	Cardiotocograph
RHA	Regional Health Authority		Cx	Cervix
RHB	Regional Hospital Board			
RM	Registered Midwife		D & C	Dilatation and curettage
RMN	Registered Mental Nurse		D & V	Diarrhoea and vomiting
RMO	Regional Medical Officer		DIC	Disseminated intravascular coagulation
RMO	Resident Medical Officer		DTA	Deep transverse arrest
RNMS	Registered Nurse for the Mentally Subnormal		DVT	Deep vein thrombosis
RNO	Regional Nursing Officer		E_1	Oestrone
RNT	Registered Nurse Tutor		E_2	Oestradiol 17ß
RoSPA	Royal Society for the Prevention of Accidents		E_3	Oestriol
			EBM	Expressed breast milk
RSCN	Registered Sick Children's Nurse		ECV	External cephalic version
RT	Regional Treasurer		EDC	Expected date of confinement
RTO	Regional Team of Officers		EDD	Expected date of delivery
RWO	Regional Works Officer		ERPC	Evacuation of retained products of conception
			EUA	Examination under anaesthesia
SCBU	Special care baby unit			
SCM	State Certified Midwife		F	Fahrenheit
SEN	State Enrolled Nurse		FACH	Forceps to the after-coming head
SHHD	Scottish Home and Health Department		FBS	Fetal blood sample
SHO	Senior House Officer		FD	Forceps delivery
SNO	Senior Nursing Officer		FH(H)	Fetal heart (heard)
SRN	State Registered Nurse		FHR	Fetal heart rate
			FHS	Fetal heart sounds
UKCC	United Kingdom Central Council (for Nursing, Midwifery and Health Visiting)		FSH	Follicle-stimulating hormone
UN	United Nations		GTT	Glucose tolerance test
UNDP	United Nations Development Programme		Hb	Haemoglobin
UNICEF	United Nations International Children's Emergency Fund		HCG	Human chorionic gonadotrophin
			HPL	Human placental lactogen
			HVS	High vaginal swab
WHO	World Health Organization		ICD	International classification of disease
WRVS	Women's Royal Voluntary Service		IMV	Intermittent mandatory ventilation

Medical, Midwifery and Nursing Terms

ACH	After-coming head (in breech presentation)		INAH	Isonicotinic acid hydrazide
			IPPV	Intermittent positive pressure ventilation
ACTH	Adrenocorticotrophic hormone		IPVH	Intraperiventricular haemorrhage
AF	Artificially fed		IUCD	Intrauterine contraceptive device
AFP	Alpha-fetoprotein		IUD	Intrauterine death
AID	Artificial insemination (donor)		IUGR	Intrauterine growth retardation
AIH	Artificial insemination (husband)		IUT	Intrauterine transfusion
AN	Antenatal		IVF	In vitro fertilization
ANC	Antenatal care; antenatal clinic		IVP	Intravenous pyelogram
AP	Anteroposterior			
APH	Antepartum haemorrhage		LBW	Low birth weight
ARM	Artificial rupture of membranes		LFD	Light-for-dates
ASD	Atrial septal defect		LFT	Liver function test
AV, A/V	Anteverted		LH	Luteinizing hormone
			LMA	Left mentoanterior

LML	Left mentolateral	RDS	Respiratory distress syndrome
LMP	Left mentoposterior	Rh	Rhesus
LMP	Last menstrual period	RMA	Right mentoanterior
LOA	Left occipitoanterior	RML	Right mentolateral
LOL	Left occipitolateral	RMP	Right mentoposterior
LOP	Left occipitoposterior	ROA	Right occipitoanterior
L/S ratio	Lecithin/sphingomyelin ratio	ROL	Right occipitolateral
LSA	Left sacroanterior	ROP	Right occipitoposterior
LSCS	Lower segment caesarean section	RSA	Right sacroanterior
LSL	Left sacrolateral	RSL	Right sacrolateral
LSP	Left sacroposterior	RSP	Right sacroposterior
		RV, R/V	Retroverted
MSU	Midstream specimen of urine		
		SB	Stillborn
NAD	No abnormality detected	SB	Serum bilirubin
ND	Normal delivery	SCBU	Special care baby unit
NND	Neonatal death	SID	Sudden infant death syndrome
NNU	Neonatal unit	s.o.s.	si opus sit (if necessary)
NTD	Neural tube defect	stat.	statim (immediately)
		SVD	Spontaneous vaginal delivery
OA	Occipitoanterior		
OCT	Oxytocin challenge test	t.d.s.	ter die sumendus (three times a day)
OP	Occipitoposterior	TENS	Transcutaneous electrical nerve
OPD	Outpatient department		stimulation
OT	Occipitotransverse		
		URTI	Upper respiratory tract infection
PA	Per abdomen	US	Ultrasound, ultrasonic
P_{CO_2}	Partial pressure of carbon dioxide	USS	Ultrasound scan
PE	Pre-eclampsia	UTI	Urinary tract infection
PGE_2	Prostaglandin E_2 pessary		
PKU	Phenylketonuria	VD	Venereal disease
PM	Post mortem	VE	Vaginal examination
PMR	Perinatal mortality rate		
PNC	Postnatal clinic	△	Diagnosis
PND	Perinatal death	♂	Male (symbol of Mars)
P_{O_2}	Partial pressure of oxygen	♀	Female (symbol of Venus)
POP	Persistent occipitoposterior	<	less than
PPH	Postpartum haemorrhage	>	more than
PR	Per rectum	+ve	positive
p.r.n.	pro re nata (when necessary)	−ve	negative
PUO	Pyrexia of unknown origin		
PV	Per vaginam		
PVH	Periventricular haemorrhage		

ACKNOWLEDGEMENTS

The *Midwifery Notes* are derived from *Baillière's Midwives' Dictionary*, 7th edition (1983) by Margaret Adams. The material used has been revised and updated by Margaret Adams SRN, SCM, MTD, DN(London) (Sections 1 and 6), Marguerite Burfitt SRN, SCM, MTD (Section 3), Esther Davidson SRN, SCM, ADM, PGCEA, MTD, FETC (Sections 2 and 4), Karissa Man-Ying Jowaheer SRN, SCM, FETC, Janet Weston SRN, SCM, ADM, PGCEA, MTD and Ann Wraight RGN, SCM, MTD (Section 5), Valerie Anne Smith ARCM, SRN, SCM, MTD (Sections 7 and 9), and Rita McDonald SRN, SCM, ADM, PGCEA, MTD (Section 8).

INDEX

All figures in upright type refer to page numbers. All figures in bold type refer to numbers of illustrations and tables (the colour plates are gathered in 3 sections, and the prefix identifies the chapter number of monochromes and tables). Q denotes the question number in italics with the page number following in parenthesis.